Clinical Nutrition and Dietetics

Clinical Nutrition and Dietetics

SECOND EDITION

Frances J. Zeman, Ph.D., R.D.
Professor of Nutrition
University of California, Davis

With contributions by Robert J. Hansen, Ph.D., Denise M. Ney, Ph.D., R.D.,
Robert B. Rucker, Ph.D., and Bruce M. Wolfe, M.D.

MACMILLAN PUBLISHING COMPANY
NEW YORK

COLLIER MACMILLAN
TORONTO

MAXWELL MACMILLAN INTERNATIONAL PUBLISHING GROUP
NEW YORK   OXFORD   SINGAPORE   SYDNEY

Every effort has been made to ensure that drug-dosage schedules and indications are correct at time of publication. Since ongoing medical research can change standards of usage, and also because of human and typographical error, it is recommended that readers check the *PDR* or package insert before prescription or administration of the drugs mentioned in this book.

Editor in Chief: Linda Jones
Production Supervisor: Betsy Keefer
Cover Designer: Patrice Fodero

This book was set in Palatino by Progressive Typographers, printed and bound by Halliday.
The cover was printed by Phoenix Color Corporation.

Macmillan Publishing Company
866 Third Avenue, New York, New York 10022

Collier Macmillan Canada, Inc.
1200 Eglinton Avenue East
Suite 200
Don Mills, Ontario M3C 3N1

Library of Congress Cataloging-in-Publication Data
Zeman, Frances J.
  Clinical nutrition and dietetics / Frances J. Zeman with contributions by Robert J. Hansen . . . [et al.]. — 2nd ed.
    p. cm.
  Includes bibliographical references.
  ISBN 0-02-431510-9
  1. Diet therapy. 2. Diet in disease. 3. Dietetics. I. Title.
  [DNLM: 1. Dietetics. 2. Nutrition. WB 400 Z526c]
RM216.Z47 1991
616.3'9 — dc20
DNLM/DLC
for Library of Congress   90-5444
                  CIP

Printing: 1 2 3 4 5 6 7   Year: 1 2 3 4 5 6 7

Contributors

Robert J. Hansen, Ph.D.
Professor of Physiological Sciences
School of Veterinary Medicine
University of California, Davis

Denise M. Ney, Ph.D., R.D.
Assistant Professor of Nutrition
University of Wisconsin, Madison

Robert B. Rucker, Ph.D.
Professor of Nutrition
University of California, Davis

Bruce M. Wolfe, M.D.
Professor of Surgery
School of Medicine
University of California, Davis
and
Attending Surgeon
University of California, Davis, Medical
  Center
Sacramento

Contents

Preface and Acknowledgments *xix*

Section I: General Principles of Nutritional Care 1

CHAPTER 1. INTRODUCTION TO PATHOLOGY 3
Normal Tissues and Tissue Changes 3
Normal Morphology and Function 4
Physiologic Changes in Cells 5
General Principles of Pathology 6
Types of Abnormalities 6
Manifestations of Disease 6
Diagnosis 6
Cellular Responses to Injury 6
Healing 13
References 15
Bibliography 15

CHAPTER 2. FLUID, ELECTROLYTE, AND ACID-BASE BALANCE 16
Water 17
Content and Distribution 17
Requirements 17
Intake 19
Fluid Transfer 19
Fluid Shifts 22
Excretion 22
Volume Disturbances 23
Electrolytes 23
Sodium 24
Potassium 28
Chloride 29
Other Electrolytes 29
Acid-Base Balance 29
Sources of Hydrogen Ion 30
Determination of pH 30
Control of Hydrogen Ion Concentration 30
Clinical Disturbances of Acid-Base Balance 31
Blood Gas Analysis 33
Procedures for Prevention of Fluid and Electrolyte Imbalances 33
Procedures for Correction of Fluid and Electrolyte Imbalances 34
Volume Disturbances 34
Concentration Disturbances 35
Composition Disturbances 36
Other Nutritional Concerns in Fluid and Electrolyte Imbalances 38
Solutions Used in Therapy 38

Energy Supply 39
Study Questions 42
References 42
Bibliography 42

CHAPTER 3. NUTRITIONAL ASSESSMENT 44
Documentation of Nutritional Care 45
Problem-Oriented Medical Record 45
Source-Oriented Medical Record 48
Nutritional Assessment 48
Assessment Procedures 49
Evaluation of Nutritional Status 77
Identification of Other Problems 81
Case Study: Nutritional Assessment 82
References 82
Bibliography 84
Sources of Current Information 85

CHAPTER 4. DRUGS AND NUTRITIONAL CARE 86
General Principles of Pharmacology 87
Mechanisms of Drug Action 87
Factors Influencing Rate and Magnitude of Drug Effects 87
Drug Metabolism and Excretion 91
Drug Safety and Effectiveness in Individuals 93
Classification and Terminology 94
Nutrition-Drug Interrelationships 94
Effects of Drugs on Nutrition 95
Effects of Food and Nutrients on Drugs 101
Study Questions 113
References 115
Bibliography 116

CHAPTER 5. METHODS OF NUTRITIONAL SUPPORT 117
Planning Nutritional Care 118
Implementation of the Nutritional Care Plan 118
Conventional Feeding 119
Tube Feeding 123
Parenteral Feeding 132
Transitional Feeding 144
Study Questions 144
References 145
Bibliography 146

Section II: Nutritional Care in Specific Clinical Disorders 147

CHAPTER 6. NUTRITION IN DISEASES OF THE IMMUNE SYSTEM 149
The Normal Immune System 149
Components of the Immune System 150
The Immune Response 153

Disorders of the Immune System   160
  Immunoproliferative Disease   160
  Immunologic Deficiency   161
  Hypersensitivity   163
Summary   181
Case Study: Allergy   181
References   182
Bibliography   185
Sources of Current Information   185

CHAPTER 7. THE ORAL CAVITY, ESOPHAGUS, AND STOMACH   186
  Components of the Alimentary Tract   186
  The Oral Cavity   187
    Normal Anatomy and Physiology   187
    Abnormalities of the Oral Cavity   190
    Effect of Aging on the Oral Cavity   196
  The Esophagus   197
    Normal Anatomy and Physiology   197
    Esophageal Disease   197
  The Stomach   201
    Normal Anatomy and Physiology   201
    Nausea and Vomiting   203
    Peptic Ulcer Disease   205
  Case Study: Lower Esophageal Sphincter Incompetence   214
  Case Study: Dumping Syndrome   215
  References   215
  Bibliography   215

CHAPTER 8. THE INTESTINAL TRACT AND ACCESSORY
            ORGANS   218
  Normal Anatomy and Physiology   219
    The Small Intestine   219
    The Biliary Tract   227
    The Pancreas   228
    The Large Intestine   230
  Conditions Common to Many Gastrointestinal Disorders   230
    Malabsorption Syndromes   230
    Intestinal Antigen Absorption   238
    Diarrhea   239
    Protein-Losing Enteropathies   242
    Intestinal Lymphangiectasia   242
    Intestinal Fistulas   243
  Diseases Affecting Primarily the Small Intestine   244
    Gluten-Induced Enteropathy   244
    Tropical Sprue   245
    Inflammatory Bowel Disease   245
    Short Bowel Syndrome   248
    Carbohydrate Intolerance   252
    Abetalipoproteinemia   255

Endocrine-Secreting Tumors of the Gastrointestinal Tract   855
Acquired Immune Deficiency Syndrome (AIDS)   256
Diseases of the Gallbladder and Bile Ducts   258
Diseases of the Pancreas   259
  Diagnosis   259
  Acute Pancreatitis   260
  Chronic Pancreatitis   260
  Cystic Fibrosis of the Pancreas   261
Diseases of the Large Intestine   265
  Fiber and Related Substances   265
  Intestinal Gas   267
  Constipation   268
  Diverticular Disease   270
  Colon Surgery   271
  Rectal Surgery   274
Case Study: Malabsorption   275
Case Study: Gluten Intolerance   276
References   276
Bibliography   279
Sources of Current Information   279

CHAPTER 9. THE URINARY SYSTEM   280
The Normal Kidney   281
  Renal Anatomy   281
  Renal Physiology   283
Renal Disease   287
  Diagnostic Tests   287
  Renal Failure   289
  Glomerulopathy   327
  Diabetic Renal Disease   332
Case Study: Renal Failure   334
References   334
Bibliography   338
Sources of Current Information   338

CHAPTER 10. THE CARDIOVASCULAR SYSTEM   339
          DENISE M. NEY, PH.D., R.D.
The Normal Circulatory System   340
  Heart   340
  Vascular System   342
  Blood Pressure   346
Hypertension   354
  Classification   354
  Consequences of Uncontrolled Hypertension   357
  Management   358
Hyperlipidemia   363
  Cholesterol   363
  Lipoproteins   364
  Effects of Diet on Plasma Lipids   371
  Classification and Treatment   375

Atherosclerosis   382
  Etiology   382
  The Lesion   383
  Pathogenesis   383
Coronary Heart Disease   385
  Angina Pectoris   385
  Myocardial Infarction   386
Congestive Heart Failure   387
  Pathogenesis   388
  Salt and Water Retention   388
  Clinical Manifestations   389
  Management   389
Cerebrovascular Disease   389
Peripheral Vascular Atherosclerotic Occlusive Disease   390
Cardiac Cachexia   390
  Clinical Manifestations and Pathogenesis   390
  Treatment   391
Rheumatic Heart Disease   391
Congenital Heart Disease   392
  Clinical Manifestations and Pathogenesis   392
  Nutritional Management   392
Heart Disease and Alcoholism   393
Case Study: Acute Myocardial Infarction   393
References   394
Bibliography   396
Sources of Current Information   397

CHAPTER 11. DIABETES MELLITUS, HYPOGLYCEMIA, AND OTHER
         ENDOCRINE DISORDERS   398
         FRANCES J. ZEMAN, PH.D., R.D. AND ROBERT J. HANSEN, PH.D.
Diabetes Mellitus   399
  Classification   400
  Etiology   402
  Pathology   403
  Diagnosis   417
  Nutritional Assessment and Monitoring of Control   420
  Management   422
  Self-Management   449
  The Diabetic Child   452
  Diabetes and Reproduction   452
  The Diabetic Patient in Surgery   457
  Diabetes and Nutritional Support   457
Hypoglycemia   458
  Clinical Manifestations   458
  Classification   458
  Diagnosis   459
  Nutritional Care   459
The Adrenal Cortex   461
  Adrenocortical Insufficiency   461

Adrenocortical Hyperfunction 462
Adrenocorticotropic Hormone or Glucocorticoid Therapy 462
Thyroid Dysfunction 462
Hyperthyroidism 463
Hypothyroidism 463
Other Nutrition-Endocrine Interrelationships 463
Case Study: Insulin-Dependent Diabetes Mellitus 463
Case Study: Diabetes Mellitus in the Elderly 464
References 465
Bibliography 469
Sources of Current Information 469

CHAPTER 12. DISORDERS OF ENERGY BALANCE AND BODY
          WEIGHT 470
Adipose Tissue 471
Some Definitions of Terms 473
Control of Energy Balance 473
Control of Food Intake 474
Control of Energy Expenditure 477
Obesity 479
Diagnosis 479
Classification of the Obesities 482
Hazards of Obesity 486
Metabolic Alterations in Obesity 486
Treatment 487
Psychological Factors in Obesity 503
Aspects of Nutritional Assessment and Monitoring 504
Prevention of Obesity 504
Effects of Repeated Cycles of Weight Loss and Gain 504
Underweight 504
Underweight in General 505
Anorexia Nervosa 505
Bulimia Nervosa 509
Case Study: Obesity 510
Case Study: Anorexia Nervosa 510
References 511
Bibliography 516
Sources of Current Information 516

CHAPTER 13. LIVER DISEASE AND ALCOHOLISM 517
Normal Anatomy and Physiology of the Liver 518
Normal Liver Structure 518
Functions of the Liver 520
Diagnosis of Liver Disease 522
Hepatitis 524
Clinical Manifestations 524
Treatment 525
Nutritional Care 525
Complications 525

Jaundice   526
Alcoholism and Alcoholic Liver Disease   526
  Alcohol Intake   526
  Absorption and Distribution   527
  Metabolism and Excretion   527
  Mechanism of Injury   529
  Nutritional Status of the Alcoholic   530
  Acute Adverse Effects of Alcohol Intoxication   531
  Alcoholic Liver Disease   531
  Nutritional Care of Alcoholics   532
  Fetal Alcohol Syndrome   532
Cirrhosis   533
  Classification   533
  Clinical Manifestations   533
  Care of the Cirrhotic Patient   540
  Specific Forms of Cirrhosis   545
Nutrition Support in Hepatic Failure   547
Nutritional Assessment   548
Liver Transplant   549
Case Study: Alcoholic Cirrhosis   549
References   550
Bibliography   552
Sources of Current Information   553

CHAPTER 14. NUTRITION IN HYPERMETABOLIC CONDITIONS   554
        Bruce M. Wolfe, M.D.
The Hypermetabolic Response   554
  Metabolic Effects of Starvation   554
  Metabolic Effects of Injury or Sepsis   557
Nutritional Requirements in Hypermetabolic Illness   559
  Energy   559
  Protein   561
  Protein-Energy Ratio   561
  Micronutrients   561
Sepsis   562
  Agents That Produce Infection or Inflammation   562
  Specific Infectious Diseases   563
The Patient Undergoing Major Surgery   563
  Preoperative Nutrition   564
  Postoperative Nutrition   564
The Burn Patient   564
  Estimation of the Extent of Injury   564
  Pathophysiology of Burn Injury   565
  Management of the Burn Patient   567
References   568
Bibliography   570
Sources of Current Information   570

CHAPTER 15. NUTRITION AND CANCER   571
  Reproduction of the Normal Cell   571
  Classification of Neoplasms   572
  Natural History of Neoplastic Growth   574
  Pathogenesis of Cancer   574
  Etiology of Cancer   575
    Nutrition and Diet   575
    Hormone-Nutrient Interactions   576
    Stress   576
    Radiation   577
    Inflammation and Infections   577
  Host Effects on Carcinogenesis   577
  Metabolic and Nutritional Alterations in Malignancy   577
    Systemic Effects   577
    Effects on Specific Organ Systems   580
    Nutritional Consequences of Cancer Therapy   581
  Cause of Death from Cancer   585
  Nutritional Management of the Cancer Patient   585
    Nutritional Assessment   588
    Nutritional Care   588
  Special Considerations in Leukemia   590
  Case Study: Leukemia and Chemotherapy   594
  References   595
  Bibliography   597
  Sources of Current Information   598

CHAPTER 16. NUTRITION IN PULMONARY DISEASES   599
  Anatomy of the Respiratory System   599
    Structure of the Airways   599
    Lungs   600
    The Pump   600
  Physiology of the Respiratory System   601
    Respiration   601
    Ventilation   602
    Other Functions   603
  Diagnosis of Pulmonary Disease   603
  Effect of Malnutrition on Respiration   605
  Chronic Obstructive Pulmonary Disease   605
    Etiology and Pathogenesis   606
    Nutritional Assessment   606
    Management of COPD   607
  Respiratory Failure   608
    Nutritional Assessment   608
    Nutritional Care   609
    Monitoring Response to Therapy   610
  Bronchopulmonary Dysplasia   611
    Pathology   611
    Prevention   611

Nutritional Assessment 612
Nutritional Care 612
Case Study: Respiratory Failure 612
References 613
Bibliography 614

CHAPTER 17. INBORN ERRORS OF METABOLISM 615
Fundamentals of Genetics 616
  Transmission of the Genetic Code 616
  Expression of the Genetic Code 618
Introduction to Inborn Errors of Metabolism 621
  Pathophysiology 621
  Clinical Manifestations 623
  Diagnosis 623
  Management 624
Disorders of Amino Acid Metabolism 625
  The Hyperphenylalaninemias 625
  Disorders of Tyrosine Metabolism 640
  Branched-Chain Ketoaciduria 644
  Isovaleric Acidemia 650
  The Homocystinurias 650
  Urea Cycle Disorders 656
  Other Disorders of Amino Acid Metabolism 659
Disorders of Carbohydrate Metabolism 659
  Disorders of Galactose Metabolism 663
  Disorders of Fructose Metabolism 666
  Glycogen Storage Diseases 668
Disorders of Lipid Transport 671
  Refsum's Disease 671
Disorders of Purine and Pyrimidine Metabolism 672
  Gout 673
  Hereditary Xanthinuria 674
Vitamin Dependency Disorders 674
  Folate Dependency 674
  Vitamin B_{12} Dependency 674
  Pyridoxine Dependency 675
  Vitamin D–Dependent Rickets 675
  Familial Vitamin D–Resistant Rickets 675
Disorders of Mineral Metabolism 676
  Wilson's Disease 676
  Acrodermatitis Enteropathica 676
Case Study: Phenylketonuria 677
References 677
Bibliography 682
Sources of Current Information 682

CHAPTER 18. NUTRITIONAL ANEMIAS 683
        ROBERT B. RUCKER, PH.D.
Erythropoiesis and Hemoglobin Synthesis 683

Sites and Developmental Stages of Red Blood Cell Formation 683
Red Blood Cell Maturation 684
Hemoglobin Synthesis and Degradation 687
Important Nutrients Involved in Erythropoiesis 687
The Anemias 691
Normocytic Anemias 691
Megaloblastic Anemias 693
Sickle Cell Anemia and Other Hemoglobinopathies 696
Hemolytic Anemia 697
Concluding Comments 699
Anemia and Athletic Performance 699
References 700

CHAPTER 19. NUTRITIONAL CARE IN NEUROLOGICAL,
                   MUSCULAR, AND SKELETAL DISORDERS 701
Cleft Lip and Palate 702
Prenatal Development 702
Nutritional Care of the Affected Infant 702
Nutritional Care and Surgical Repair 703
Neuromuscular and Nervous System Disorders 703
Developmental Disabilities 704
*Neurological and Neuromuscular Problems in the Older Child or
Adult* 719
Psychosis 734
Schizophrenia 735
Mood Disorders 736
Drug Addiction 736
Diseases of the Musculoskeletal System 737
Osteoarthritis 737
Rheumatoid Arthritis 737
Juvenile Rheumatoid Arthritis 738
Comment 738
References 739
Bibliography 741
Sources of Current Information 741

Section III: Appendixes 743

A. RECOMMENDED NUTRIENT INTAKES 746
   Table A-1. Recommended Dietary Allowances, Revised 1989 746
   Table A-2. Median Heights and Weights and Recommended Energy
          Intake 748
   Table A-3. Estimated Safe and Adequate Daily Dietary Intakes of
          Selected Vitamins and Minerals 749
   Table A-4. Estimated Sodium, Chloride, and Potassium Minimum
          Requirements of Healthy Persons 749
   Table A-5. Recommended Nutrient Intakes for Canadians 750

B. VOCABULARY AND ABBREVIATIONS 751
   Table B-1. Vocabulary 751

Table B-2. Abbreviations Used in Medical Records   753
Table B-3. Quantitative Symbols   759

C. NORMAL LABORATORY VALUES   760
    Table C-1. Whole Blood, Serum, and Plasma   760
    Table C-2. Urine   763
    Table C-3. Hematology   764
    Table C-4. Typical Test Panels   765

D. CONVERSION FACTORS   767

E. OSMOLALITY AND SPECIFIC GRAVITY   768

F. CAFFEINE   769

G. FORMULA-FEEDING PRODUCTS   771
    Table G-1. Oral Supplementary Feedings   771
    Table G-2. Sources of Single Nutrients   774
    Table G-3. Complete Liquid Formula Diets   779

H. REVISED DAILY FOOD GUIDE FOOD GROUPS   786

I. AGE-SPECIFIC LIPID VALUES   790

J. EXCHANGE LISTS FOR PROTEIN-, SODIUM-, AND POTASSIUM-
    RESTRICTED DIETS   792
    Table J-1.   Average Nutrient Values Summarized for Quick
                 Calculations   792
    Table J-2.   High-Sodium Meat List   792
    Table J-3.   Low-Sodium Meat List   793
    Table J-4.   Dairy List   793
    Table J-5.   Regular Bread, Cereal, and Starch List   794
    Table J-6.   Low-Sodium Bread, Cereal, and Starch List   795
    Table J-7.   Vegetable List 1   795
    Table J-8.   Vegetable List 2   796
    Table J-9.   Vegetable List 3   796
    Table J-10. Vegetable List 4   797
    Table J-11. Fruit List 1   797
    Table J-12. Fruit List 2   798
    Table J-13. Fruit List 3   799
    Table J-14. "Protein-Free" List   800
    Table J-15. Miscellaneous List   800
    Table J-16. Low-Sodium Specialty Items   802
    Table J-17. High-Salt Items   803

K. APPROPRIATE SERVING SIZES OF USUAL FOODS FOR INFANTS
    AND CHILDREN   805
    Table K-1. Guidelines for Evaluation of Infant Diets   805
    Table K-2. Guidelines for Evaluation of Diets in Childhood   806

L. GROWTH AND DEVELOPMENT CHARTS FOR INFANTS AND
CHILDREN 807

INDEX 815

Preface and Acknowledgments

This second edition of *Clinical Nutrition and Dietetics* has been updated and expanded to include new developments in clinical nutrition. The basic purpose of the text remains the same, to integrate the theoretical basis for nutritional care with the biological sciences, biochemistry, physiology, pharmacology, immunology, and genetics. Since usual university programs in dietetics do not require course work in pharmacology, immunology, and genetics, some basic background information in these areas is provided.

The content has been divided into two major parts with some new chapters in each section. Part I — General Principles of Nutritional Care — provides background on principles and procedures of nutritional care necessary for understanding of the chapters that follow. To strengthen this background, a new chapter reviewing fluid, electrolyte, and acid-base balance has been included. General principles of nutritional assessment and nutrition support have been divided into separate chapters, allowing consideration in greater detail. Tube feeding and parenteral feeding are introduced in an early chapter to which chapters in Part II refer.

Part II — Nutritional Care in Specific Clinical Disorders — considers nutritional care as an important component of treatment in specific diseases, largely organized on the basis of organ systems such as digestive, urinary, cardiovascular, and pulmonary. Material that does not lend itself to this type of organization is based on similarities of pathological processes, such as the chapters on hypermetabolic conditions and cancer. The chapter on immune disorders has been placed first in this section because it is useful in understanding the disease processes described in some subsequent chapters.

A new chapter that considers nutrition in pulmonary disease has been added, and a chapter on neurological, muscular, and skeletal disorders has been greatly expanded. In general, it is intended that the chapters in Part I will be studied first, largely in the order as written. The chapters in Part II may be taken in variable sequence. They assume a knowledge of the material in Part I and provide further information applicable specifically to the disorders under consideration.

This book attempts to provide background that will assist the student in future learning. It provides less emphasis on details of procedure. Therefore, with few exceptions, it does not include specific diets. The instructor may wish to include a laboratory manual, a diet manual, or both for course series intended to be comprehensive in both theory and practice.

The book also contains, at the ends of chapters, lists of useful journals and additional references for the reader seeking further information. Some case studies and review questions are included for the instructor who chooses to use them. The appendix material was judged to be of value for increased understanding by the student, but it is not intended to be a comprehensive reference.

While intended primarily as a text for students in dietetics, this book may be useful as a desk reference for dietitians and public health nutritionists and for pharmacists and medical students or practitioners with an interest in nutrition. As a consequence, the term **nutritional care specialist** has been used as a generic term to include all members of this heterogeneous group.

Thanks are extended to the reviewers of the new and revised chapters and to those graduate students in nutrition at the University of California at Davis who provided information and insight based on their own experiences in dietetics. In particular, I should like to mention Lesley Fels Tinker, M.S., R.D., and Francene Myers Steinberg, M.S., R.D., for their thoughtful comments.

F.J.Z.

Davis, California
March 1990

Clinical Nutrition and Dietetics

I. General Principles of Nutritional Care

1. Introduction to Pathology

I. Normal Tissues and Tissue
   Changes
   A. Normal morphology
      and function
      1. Epithelium
      2. Muscle tissue
      3. Nervous tissue
      4. Connective tissue
         a. intercellular
            material
         b. cells of the
            connective tissue
         c. cartilage and bone
         d. blood cells
   B. Physiologic changes in
      cells
II. General Principles of
    Pathology
    A. Types of abnormalities
    B. Manifestations of
       disease
    C. Diagnosis
    D. Cellular responses to
       injury
       1. Growth disturbances
       2. Developmental
          disorders

3. Inflammation
   a. vascular response
   b. cellular response
   c. systemic manifes-
      tations
   d. factors modifying
      the inflammatory
      response
4. Necrosis
   a. anoxia
   b. protein precipita-
      tion
   c. osmotic injury
   d. accumulation of
      certain metabolic
      products
5. Degeneration
   a. degeneration
      involving water
   b. degeneration
      involving
      carbohydrate
      (1) glycogen
          deposits
      (2) mucin
          degenerations

   c. degeneration
      involving lipids
      (1) obesity and
          adiposity
      (2) fatty meta-
          morphosis
      (3) atherosclero-
          sis
   d. degeneration
      involving protein
   e. degeneration
      involving calcium
      (1) dystrophic
          calcification
      (2) metastatic
          calcification
E. Healing
   1. Healing processes
      a. resolution
      b. sloughing
      c. repair
         (1) regeneration
         (2) organization

   2. Factors that affect
      healing

A knowledge of the effect of disease on body tissue and its reaction to injury is fundamental to an understanding of the basis for nutritional care of patients. Therefore, this text will begin with a brief review of the fundamentals of pathology. By definition, **pathology** is a study of "the nature of disease, especially of the structural and functional changes in tissues and organs of the body which cause or are caused by disease."[1]

NORMAL TISSUES AND TISSUE CHANGES

The body develops from the union of the ovum and the sperm. A single new cell is produced which has the properties of other single cells. As the fertilized ovum divides, the cells diversify and acquire individual characteristics. This process is known as **differentiation**. As cells differentiate, they undergo morphological changes—that is, they change in form and structure.

During the early development of the embryo, there is a stage during which the embryo consists of three "germ layers." One of these is the **ectoderm** (outer layer), which differentiates to form the nervous system, including the eye and ear, and the epidermis (skin) and related structures such as hair, nails, and the glands of the skin. Another layer is the **endoderm** or **entoderm** (inner layer), which forms the lining of the gut, respiratory system, and urinary tract. The

mesoderm (middle layer) lies between the other two germ layers and gives rise to muscle, connective tissue, cartilage, bone, blood cells, adipose cells, lymphoid tissue, and the linings of the major body cavities, joint cavities, and blood vessels.

Normal Morphology and Function

There are four primary tissues in the body, and these are, of course, derived from the three germ layers. They are epithelium, muscle, nervous tissue, and connective tissue. The body also contains intercellular substances, which are formed by the cells and body fluids.

Epithelium

Epithelial cells are closely apposed and have very little cementing substance between them. Many are arranged as sheets of tissue called **membrane**, which cover or line surfaces. The mucous membrane in the mouth and the peritoneal membrane lining the abdominal cavity are examples. The word *membrane*, in this context, has a meaning that is very different from its meaning when referring to a cell membrane.

The epithelial membranes lie on a **basal lamina** or **basement membrane**, which separates the epithelium from the underlying connective tissue. There are no blood or lymph vessels in epithelial membranes, so nutrients must be obtained by diffusion through the basal lamina from the underlying connective tissue. This concept is important in some diseases, such as diabetes mellitus (Chapter 11).

Endothelium, originating from the mesoderm, is a special subclassification of epithelium. Endothelial cells line the cavities of the heart, blood vessels, and lymph vessels. The **mesothelium** is a thin flat layer of cells, also derived from mesoderm, that covers the surface of the peritoneum (lining of the abdominal and pelvic cavities and covering their contained organs), the pericardium (sac en-

closing the heart), and the pleura (lining of the thoracic cavity and covering for the lungs). Endothelium and mesothelium are capable of some functions different from those of simple squamous epithelium, which they resemble. They are less differentiated and can form **fibroblasts**, a primitive type of connective tissue cell. They are also phagocytic.

Some epithelial cells are specialized further and have a secretory function. These are **exocrine** glands, or if they lose their connection with the epithelial surface of their origin and have no duct system, they are the **endocrine** glands.

The main functions of epithelial tissue are protection, absorption, and secretion. Further details of the structure and function of epithelial cells are included in later chapters related to individual organ systems.

Muscle Tissue

There are three types of muscle. **Smooth** muscles (also known as **involuntary** or **non-striated** muscles) are found in areas of involuntary movement such as in the digestive system, arteries, and veins. **Skeletal** muscles (also known as **voluntary** or **striated** muscles) have a striped or striated appearance under the microscope. They also have rich blood vessel and nerve supplies supported by connective tissue. **Cardiac** (heart) muscle is striated but involuntary. It has less connective tissue, its own intrinsic contractility, and a unique blood supply, in that all arteries are end arteries with no overlap into adjacent areas. This anatomical structure is important in cardiac disease such as myocardial infarction (see Chapter 10).

Nervous Tissue

The major functioning cell of the nervous system is the **neuron**. In addition to neurons, other types of cells are included in the nervous system. Many nerve fibers are surrounded by a layer of **Schwann** cells, the plasma membranes of which are known as **myelin** and which cover peripheral nerves. In the central nervous system (CNS), there are a variety of connective tissue cells called **glial cells**. They form the myelin of the central nervous system, provide valuable metabolic and nutritive functions, act as supporting structures, and are phagocytic.

Connective Tissue

The mesoderm layer is the source of a meshwork of embryonic connective tissue known as **mesenchyme**. Mesenchymal cells can differentiate along various lines and can produce many different kinds of cells; therefore, they are **pluripotential** cells. They serve as the source of connective tissue proper and certain specialized cells: blood cells, bone, cartilage, and adipose tissue.

Intercellular Material. Connective tissue cells produce abundant amounts of intercellular material so that the cells themselves are widely separated. The intercellular material or **matrix** includes fibers and an amorphous ground substance. These are nonliving materials that form the structure in which the body's cells live. They also act as a medium through which tissue fluid diffuses from blood to cells.

The fibrous or formed intercellular materials are proteins in long chains of three types. **Collagen** is secreted by fibroblasts and forms the meshwork of fibrillar material present in the stroma (structure) of all organs. In more concentrated form, it makes up tendons and fascia (bands or sheets connecting muscles). **Reticular fibers**, formed by primitive reticular cells similar to mesenchymal cells, create a fine supporting network around other cells. **Elastin** is an elastic material that, in fibrillar form, is associated with collagen in connective tissue. It also forms sheetlike layers in the walls of blood vessels.

The amorphous intercellular material exists in the form of a stiff gel. It provides support and strength and is a medium through which nutrients and waste products must diffuse. It is synthesized by connective tissue cells and contains collagen and other proteins, mucopolysaccharides, carbohydrates, lipids, water, and other materials.

Cells of the Connective Tissue. There are a number of different types of cells that make up the connective tissue. Fibroblasts are very numerous. They are believed to secrete the various connective tissue fibers, and most or all of the amorphous ground substance. They retain, throughout their lives, a capacity for growth and regeneration and also are capable of some movement. **Adipose cells** (fat cells) occur singly or in clumps. If present in large numbers, they form adipose tissue, the formation and metabolism of which are discussed in Chapter 12.

Cartilage and Bone. Cartilage and bone consist of cells, fibers, and ground substance, as do other body tissues, but their matrix (intercellular substance) is much more rigid.

Blood Cells. The blood cells, or formed elements of the blood, also are differentiated forms of connective tissue. The formation and function of **erythrocytes** (red blood cells) are described in Chapter 18. **Leukocytes** (white blood cells) are discussed in Chapter 6.

Physiologic Changes in Cells

Differentiated cells vary in their ability to reproduce. In some tissues, there is a constant turnover of cells. These cells are very **labile**—that is, they proliferate continuously throughout life. For example, simple squamous epithelial cells on surfaces are shed and replaced from cells in deeper layers, red and white blood cells die and are replenished from undifferentiated stem cells, and cells lining the lumen of the intestinal tract are sloughed and replaced continuously. In many other tissues, cells can be replaced by division of adjacent cells. These cells are **stable** and proliferate very little in adult life unless stimulated by tissue injury. There is great variability within the category of stable cells. Liver cells, for example, have an extensive replacement capability and will replace a whole lobe of liver. In contrast, renal glomerular cells will proliferate to some extent but will not do so sufficiently to develop new glomeruli. **Permanent cells** are highly specialized cells such as neurons and cells in the heart and some glands, which do not replicate in postnatal life.

Some cells are capable of increases in size or activity when appropriately stimulated. The increase in muscle size with increased activity is an example, as is the increase in adrenal function in stress.

GENERAL PRINCIPLES OF PATHOLOGY

Diseases are abnormalities of the structure or function of the body or any of its parts. The study of the causes of disease in general is known as **etiology**, but when a specific disease-producing agent is referred to, it is said to be a **cause** rather than an etiology; for example, the tubercle bacillus is the **cause** of tuberculosis. The causes of many diseases are unknown but are generally one of three types. **Biologic** causes include microorganisms and antibodies. Among **physical** causes are heat, cold, and radiation. **Chemical** causes include materials such as acids, alkalies, and poisons. The **pathogenesis** of a disease is the response of the body to injury, since it is these reactions, rather than the injury, that produce the manifestations of disease. In the response to injury, no new biochemical or physiologic mechanisms are created. Instead, cellular reactions to injury occur by increasing or decreasing the rate of existing reactions.

Types of Abnormalities

An abnormality may occur in a cell, a tissue, or an entire **organ**. The abnormality may be **structural** (a broken leg, for example) or **functional** (such as the inability to produce enough insulin). Structural abnormalities are called **lesions** and may be anatomic, such as a missing hand, or **morphological**, a large number of dead cells in the liver, for example.

Manifestations of Disease

The detectable indications of the presence of disease are its **manifestations**. They include both structural and functional abnormalities and may be classified into one of three categories:

1. **Symptoms** are manifestations verbalized by the patient (e.g., "I have a pain in my chest").
2. **Signs** are observations by a qualified examiner (e.g., the physician hears an irregular heart beat).
3. **Laboratory abnormalities** are abnormal results of tests of composition or function (e.g., high blood urea levels).

Diagnosis

Under ideal circumstances, the diagnosis will indicate the cause of the abnormal condition and define the reactions that are producing the manifestations of the disease. If a single manifestation is specific for a certain disease and if a positive accurate diagnosis can be made on the basis of the existence of that manifestation, then that manifestation is said to be **pathognomonic** for that disease. However, most diseases have nonspecific manifestations. Pain, fever, swelling, or rash, for example, occur in association with many diseases.

Cellular Responses to Injury

Although there are many specific agents that can injure the body, there are only a limited number of possible cellular responses. These are (1) growth disturbances, (2) abnormal development, (3) inflammation and repair, (4) cell degeneration, and (5) cell death.

Growth Disturbances

The process by which an organ completely fails to develop is known as **aplasia** or **agenesis**. Given a differentiated tissue or organ, disturbances of growth can be controlled or uncontrolled. In controlled changes, a stimulus can cause an increase in cell number (**hyperplasia**) or cell size (**hypertrophy**). In some circumstances, the absence of normal stimuli may result in **hypoplasia** (the failure to achieve normal development or size), whereas removal of the stimuli causes a decrease in the size of a tissue or organ (**atrophy**). Atrophy may result from a decrease in cell number or size or both.

In uncontrolled growth (**neoplasia**), cell replication does not cease when the original stimulus is removed. It involves an increase in the number of cells. This increase differs from normal physiologic growth in that it involves a change in the heredity of the cells, producing cells that are less subject to the normal regulatory mechanisms. Nutritional care of patients with neoplastic diseases is described in Chapter 15.

Developmental Disorders

A developmental abnormality is a structural or functional abnormality that results from the prenatal action of an injurious agent. Injuries occurring during birth are not included. The injury can become apparent before, during, or after birth. Thus some developmental abnormalities are not observed until years after birth.

Developmental abnormalities can be classified four ways, including the following:

By cause of the abnormalities: A chemical, physical, or biologic agent may be the injurious factor. These may affect the genes or chromosomes or may injure the developing embryo or fetus directly. However, most causes are unknown.

By age at onset: A **congenital** condition is one that is present at birth. Developmental disorders that become evident later in life are **noncongenital**.

By pathogenic mechanism: Developmental abnormalities may be caused by intrauterine injury or by alterations in genes or chromosomes. Chromosomal diseases may be related to autosomes or to sex chromosomes. Autosomal changes involve gross structural abnormalities evident at birth, whereas sex chromosome changes may produce abnormalities that become evident during later sexual maturation. Other conditions, such as maternal infections during pregnancy, can cause congenital or noncongenital abnormalities that are not genetic or chromosomal.

By type of structural or functional abnormalities: Structural and functional abnormalities can be subclassified as (1) **gross body deformities**, evident on physical examination; (2) **gross organ deformities** having obvious structural defects that are evident if the organ can be examined directly; (3) either **diffuse** or **focal tissue reactions**, which can be seen with a microscope; and (4) physiologic or biochemical defects detectable with physiologic or biochemical tests. Biochemical defects in which nutritional care is important are discussed in Chapter 17.

Inflammation

Inflammation is a vascular and cellular response produced when cells are injured or destroyed by biologic, chemical, or physical agents (Table 1-1). It can occur anywhere in the body. Signs and symptoms are pain, heat, redness, and swelling. It is distinct from infection, in which there is invasion of the body by pathogenic microorganisms. The reactions to infection may include inflammation, but degeneration or necrosis, described later in this chapter, also may occur.

Vascular Response. When cells are injured or killed, chemical mediators and acids are released. The chemical mediators cause the dilation of the nearby capillaries and increase their permeability (see Table 1-1). **Histamine**, released from mast cells and basophils, initiates the vascular response, but is short-acting. Long-acting responses are mediated by the blood-clotting mechanism and plasma **kinins**, released from the plasma protein **alpha-2-globulin**. The capillary dilation increases the blood in the area and causes heat and redness. Increased capillary permeability allows fluids, protein, and blood cells to exude into the surrounding tissue and causes swelling. The material escaping from the capillaries under these conditions is an **exudate**. An exudate must be distinguished from a **transudate**, which is fluid that is forced out of the capillaries as a result of increased pressure.

An exudate can cause further cell damage. It also causes pain by irritation of the local nerve endings through fluid pressure and the presence of kinins and acids released from dead cells.

Cellular Response. As fluid exudes from the capillaries, the flow of blood slows and certain white blood cells (neutrophils and monocytes) emigrate into the damaged area (see Table 1-1). They attack and ingest or digest the offending agents and remove the killed cells in preparation for repair. Digestion makes the debris soluble so that it can be carried away by plasma.

Other cells important in the inflammatory response occur in the tissues. Macrophages, similar to and derived from the monocytes in the blood, also are phagocytic. They multiply rapidly when tissues are injured. Giant cells form from the fusion of macrophages or by amitotic division to ingest large pieces of debris. Lymphocytes and plasma cells also

participate in the body's defenses. Their actions are described in Chapter 6.

Systemic Manifestations. Some inflammations are localized and others are diffuse. When they are diffuse, they cause a number of systemic manifestations. Chemical agents called **pyrogens**, some of which are released from certain types of cells, including bacteria, affect the thermoregulatory center in the brain and produce a fever. Fever also occurs in infections, tissue necrosis, hemorrhage, some neoplasms, and other conditions. It increases the metabolic rate and often is accompanied by loss of appetite. As a result, there may be depletion of body tissue, with muscle wasting and loss of body fat. Fluid losses may lead to dehydration. The nutritional consequences of fever are described in Chapter 14.

Fluid and protein that escape from the capillaries are taken up by the lymphatics and carried to the lymph nodes. These become enlarged and painful, a condition known as **lymphadenitis**.

Factors Modifying the Inflammatory Response. Inflammations vary in duration, location, degree of localization, and type of exudate. These are influenced by the amount of the damaging agent, the duration of exposure, and the **pathogenicity** of the agent (its inherent ability to cause disease and its ability to invade the tissue).

Several factors in the host also modify the inflammatory response. One of these is the overall health of the host. It is generally accepted that advanced age, poor nutrition, and the presence of preexisting disease are negative influences. In addition, the immunity of the host modifies the inflammatory response.

The vascularity of the injured tissue and its location also have an effect. The spread of disease is reduced in dense compact tissue such as bone, and the defensive response is poor when blood supply is poor.

Table 1-1. Summary of the Inflammatory Response

Response	Mediator or Mechanism					
	Neurogenic	Vasoactive Amines[a]	Plasma Proteases[b]	Arachidonic Metabolites[c]	Leukocyte Products[d]	Miscellaneous
Vasodilation	X	X	X	X	X	
Altered vascular permeability	X	X	X	X	X	Increased hydrostatic pressure; oxygen-derived free radicals; platelet-activating factor
Margination			X	X		
Chemotaxis			X	X	X (Lymphokines)	Bacterial products
Phagocytosis			X		X (Lymphokines; opsonins)	
Fever	X			X	X (Interleukin 1)	
Pain			X	X (Prostaglandin E2)		
Depressed appetite					X	
Muscle catabolism					X	

[a] Histamine, serotonin
[b] Kinins, complement, coagulation-fibrinolytic system
[c] Prostaglandins, leukotrienes
[d] Lysosomal enzymes, lymphokines

The duration of inflammation is classified as **acute** (hours to weeks), **subacute** (weeks to a month), or **chronic** (months to years). The term *acute* sometimes is used to suggest great severity instead of duration.

Inflammations persist only as long as damaging agents are present. Chronic inflammations must be caused, then, by agents that persist. These agents must be (1) resistant to phagocytosis or digestion, (2) continually produced in the body, or (3) present in the environment and therefore make exposure constant. The inflammation also tends to persist when host defenses are poor such as in impaired immune function or decreased blood supply. In chronic inflammation, the inflammatory response is less pronounced than is the case in acute conditions. Fibroblasts proliferate and may cause scarring, adhesions, or obstructions. Some injurious agents induce a response called **chronic granulomatous inflammation**, in which some microorganisms or foreign materials that are resistant to phagocytosis or digestion become surrounded by macrophages, thus causing small nodules or granulomas to develop, walling off the injurious agent. Some inflammatory disorders are described in Chapters 8, 9, and 14.

Necrosis

Cell death is the irreversible permanent cessation of the vital functions such as respiration, maintenance of homeostasis, and protein synthesis. Two types of irreversible changes indicative of cell death are **rupture of the cell membrane** and **nuclear changes**. These can be seen with a microscope.

The death of the patient is **somatic death**, whereas **necrobiosis** or **physiologic cell death** occurs as part of normal turnover. **Necrosis**, on the other hand, refers to the abnormal death of cells within a living body. It does *not* include either the gradual death of some cells in the aging process or cell death that occurs after the patient has died.

When a portion of the body becomes necrotic, the surrounding area becomes congested and inflamed. Under these circumstances, necrosis and inflammation coexist.

There are four general modes of action by which necrosis is produced. These may occur singly or in combination.

Anoxia. **Anoxia** (lack of oxygen) is the most common cause. It is produced by interference at any step in the process of supplying oxygen and therefore may be local, regional, or systemic. In some circumstances, the alteration is metabolic. In others, there is a localized functional or mechanical interference with the blood supply known as **ischemia**. When ischemia results in the death of all cells in an area, the lesion is called an **infarct**. An example is a myocardial infarct, described in Chapter 10. **Gangrene** can result from tissue anoxia in diabetes mellitus, as will be seen in Chapter 11.

Some organs have components that are more susceptible to injury than others. When anoxia is systemic or regional rather than localized, these susceptible portions are more likely to be injured, even if the anoxia is not sufficiently severe to kill all the cells. The result is called **selective necrosis**. These same cells often are also easily injured by toxic compounds. In the kidney, for example, the resulting condition is called **acute tubular necrosis** (see Chapter 9). In mild, prolonged regional ischemia, there is a reduction in organ size (**ischemic atrophy**).

Protein Precipitation. Some toxic substances cause necrosis by precipitating proteins in cells with which they come in contact. An example is ingestion of caustic chemicals.

Osmotic Injury. Three mechanisms can disrupt the maintenance of osmotic homeostasis by the cell membrane: (1) physical trauma that disrupts the cell membrane; (2) exposure to hypertonic or hypotonic solutions in excess of the cell's ability to adjust, resulting in cell shrinkage or bursting; and (3) antigen-antibody reactions on cell surfaces with possible complement activation leading to lysis of the membrane (see Chapter 6).

Accumulation of Certain Metabolic Products. Excess production of some metabolic products or reduced ability to remove metabolic wastes can result in cell death by interfering with the normal metabolism of the cell.

Degeneration

Degeneration, in contrast to necrotic changes, refers to detrimental cellular alterations that are potentially reversible. Often, however, degenerative changes precede cell death, and there is a continuous progression from reversible degeneration to irreversible loss of function to irreversible changes to death.

Acute degenerations generally are caused by milder forms of the same factors that cause necrosis, anoxia being the most common. In **chronic degeneration**, a variety of substances accumulate within the cell or extracellularly. Deposited materials may be protein, fat, carbohydrate, or minerals. The materials deposited usually are inert; otherwise, they would cause necrosis. They may be intracellular or interstitial deposits or consist of alterations of existing interstitial materials. As extracellular deposits accumulate, normal cells often atrophy.

Some degenerations are processes in which the accumulated materials are produced locally and are referred to as **accumulation** or **storage**. In others, the material is brought to the tissue and is referred to as a **deposit** or **infiltration**.

Degeneration Involving Water. Acute degenerations due to increased cellular water content with increased cell size is called **cloudy swelling** if mild or **hydropic degeneration** if more severe. In cloudy swelling,

organ weight increases; the organ increases in opacity or cloudiness and may be pale. There is tension on organs with nonelastic capsules such as the kidney. Cloudy swelling occurs in most tissues following mild injury.

Chronic degeneration with intracellular water accumulation is unknown. Water that accumulates between cells (**edema**) is classified as a hemodynamic disorder, not a form of degeneration.

Degeneration Involving Carbohydrate. There are two types of carbohydrate involved in degenerations. **Glycogen** accumulates in cells in some inherited metabolic disorders. For example, in some of the glycogen storage diseases, enzymes involved in glycogen breakdown are deficient and glucose mobilization is poor. As a result, glycogen accumulates in the tissue.

In a different form of carbohydrate degeneration, the materials that accumulate are **carbohydrate-protein complexes**. These materials are found in extracellular ground substance and in mucus-secreting epithelial cells. Their accumulation is not considered to be a degeneration in the narrow sense of the term. Rather, the term **mucin degenerations** is loosely used to include the following:

1. Plugged excretory ducts from which mucin cannot be removed. (This condition occurs in cystic fibrosis of the pancreas, which is discussed in Chapter 8.)
2. Mucin-producing cancers, which spill mucin into connective tissue. (Nutritional care of cancer patients is discussed in Chapter 13.)
3. Myxomas, connective tissue tumors that produce ground substance.
4. Atrophy of connective tissue with a *relative* increase in ground substance.

Degeneration Involving Lipids. Lipids involved in degenerations may occur as liquid droplets, protein-bound complexes, or cholesterol crystals. They are found within the cell except for the cholesterol crystals and accidentally inhaled oils. The extracellular lipids are removed by macrophages, if possible. Otherwise, the area is walled off by fibrous tissue. If adipose tissue is accidentally injured, the triglyceride escaping from ruptured adipose cells is removed by macrophages.

Degenerations involving triglyceride accumulation may occur in adipose tissue cells or in **hepatocytes** (functional cells of the liver). Accumulation of triglyceride (**adiposity**), which takes the form of a general and severe increase in lipid content of adipose tissue cells, is called **obesity**.

Another form of adiposity is the replacement of **parenchymal tissue** (functional cells) by normal-appearing adipose tissue. Some adiposity occurs in the heart muscle and pancreas with aging but is not considered to be important clinically. Adipose tissue cells are not found in the parenchyma of the brain, lung, liver, kidney, or spleen.

Fatty metamorphosis of the liver is seen in many patients who come to the attention of the nutritional care specialist. This condition consists of the accumulation of globules of neutral lipid within the hepatocytes which then resemble adipose tissue cells. Thus the response of the liver to fat accumulation is fatty metamorphosis, not adiposity. Factors promoting fatty metamorphosis in the liver are (1) increased lipid input, (2) decreased utilization of lipid for energy, and (3) inability to export it due to defective lipoprotein synthesis.

Mild to moderate fatty metamorphosis usually is not accompanied by detectable changes in liver function. Severe fatty metamorphosis, however, is likely to be prolonged and associated with liver enlargement, changes in function, and sometimes jaundice (high bilirubin levels in the blood, skin, and mucous membrane with a yellow appearance in the patient). It tends to be chronic in alcoholism (Chapter 13), prolonged protein deficiency, and diabetes (Chapter 11).

Atherosclerosis is characterized by lipid deposits in the walls of large and medium-sized arteries. The lesions are called **atheromas**. In early formation, they consist largely of foam cells containing much cholesterol. These cells later break down, and cholesterol crystals are formed. This condition and its extensive consequences are described in Chapter 10.

Degeneration Involving Protein. Accumulations of protein or proteinlike materials may be extracellular or intracellular. **Hyaline** is an adjective used to describe protein deposits that are homogeneous and translucent in appearance under the microscope. The material deposited is called **hyalin**. Most hyaline deposits are composed of collagen, fibrin, **amyloid** (a homogeneous, translucent glycoprotein), edema fluid with a high protein content, some foreign bodies, and compacted platelets. Fibrin masses are associated with inflammatory lesions where fibrin has time to accumulate. The presence of collagen is considered a degeneration only when dense masses of old acellular scar tissue accumulate.

Amyloid is associated with inflammations and some malignant tumors. It occurs in the walls of small blood vessels, between muscle fibers of all three types of muscle, and between cells of such organs as liver, spleen, kidney, and adrenal glands. The condition is called **amyloidosis**, a term that refers to a group of rare, slowly progressing conditions in which a material composed of alpha and gamma globulins and glycoproteins is deposited. It may be **primary** (no previous cause known) or **secondary** to other diseases. Primary amyloidosis commonly affects cardiac muscle, smooth muscle of the small blood vessels and gastrointestinal tract, and skeletal muscle of the tongue. Secondary amyloidosis occurs in patients who have long-standing inflammations such as rheumatoid arthritis, but the amyloid deposits occur in organs remote from the site of the inflammations, commonly in the liver, kidneys, spleen, or adrenal glands.

Degeneration Involving Calcium. Degeneration may involve deposits of calcium, phosphorus, iron, or unidentified crystals. The most common of these is calcification. In **dystrophic calcification**, the deposits occur at sites of tissue necrosis or degeneration, but the metabolism of calcium itself is normal. In **metastatic calcification**, calcium metabolism has been affected by a disease process, and serum calcium levels are elevated. Calcium then precipitates at sites such as the kidney, gastrointestinal tract, or lung, and can cause disease in these organs.

Healing

Healing is the process by which normal structure and function are restored after an injury. Complete restoration is not always possible, but the attempt to do so is a form of healing.

Healing Processes

The processes involved in healing include the following:

1. *Resolution:* The resorption of exudates and liquefied debris.
2. *Sloughing:* The separation of dead tissue or exudate from an internal or external surface.
3. *Repair:* The replacement of dead or injured tissue by new parenchymal (functional) or stromal (structural) cells.

Resolution occurs as part of the cellular response to inflammation. Resolution and sloughing may precede or accompany repair.

Parenchymal cells are much more susceptible to injury than are stromal cells. When parenchymal cells are killed, there may be permanent loss of function following resolution, even if the stroma is intact.

The kind of repair that occurs is determined primarily by the proliferative capacity of the cells involved. **Regeneration** is replacement of lost cells by proliferation of the remaining parenchymal cells. The lost cells must, then, be labile or stable cells. Regeneration is not possible if the lost cells are permanent cells, such as neurons in the brain. The types of cells in each category are listed in Table 1-2. In contrast to regeneration, connective tissue repair or **organization** consists of replacement of the lost cells by proliferation of the connective tissue (stroma) of the organ. Typically, there is growth of capillaries and fibroblasts. Later, fibrous tissue forms. This process can occur in any organ to provide strength when it is permanently injured. When exudates are organized, there is an unnecessary loss of normal structure and function. In scarring, the replacement is with collagenous tissue in its entirety, with no significant parenchymal replacement.

As a general rule, parenchyma of glandular organs such as renal tubules, secretory glands of the digestive tract, and endocrine organs, and most mesenchymal tissues, such as stroma, bone, cartilage, adipose tissue,

Table 1-2. Regenerative Capacities of Tissues and Organs

Labile cells
Epithelium of skin, gastrointestinal and genitourinary tracts, renal tubule, exocrine gland ducts
Red blood cells, white blood cells, platelets in bone marrow
Liver parenchyma
Lymphoid tissues
Endothelium
Bone
Peripheral nerves

Stable cells
Skeletal and smooth muscle
Lung parenchyma
Renal glomeruli
Endocrine glands
Gonadal parenchyma

Permanent cells
Cardiac muscle
Neurons of central nervous system
Retinal tissue and other special sense organs
Permanent teeth

and glia, contain stable cells. Muscle tissue varies in its regenerative capacity. Smooth muscle is capable of some regeneration, whereas cardiac muscle is not. In striated muscle and in nerves, if the **sarcolemma** (sheath covering the muscle fiber) or **neurilemma** (sheath covering myelinated nerves) is intact, and if the nucleus is intact, the cell can regenerate the injured portion.

Regeneration can be **orderly** and thus restore normal structure and function, but it is **disorderly** in some circumstances — that is, the regeneration is a combination of parenchymal regeneration and connective tissue repair resulting in disorganized structure and loss of function. A fibrotic liver (Chapter 13) is an example of disorderly regeneration.

The invading reparative tissue produced early in organization is called **granulation tissue**. It consists primarily of fibroblasts and endothelial cells and results in formation of a scar. Granulation tissue has many cells and a rich blood supply. In time, collagen is laid down and rearranged; the wound is contracted and, thus, smaller; and the blood vessels are pinched off. Cellularity and vascularity thereby are reduced. Scar formation is familiar on the skin, but it also can occur in internal organs with consequent permanent loss of function.

The type and severity of injury are important in determining the type of regeneration that will occur, if any. First, there must be some remaining parenchymal tissue to regenerate. Second, if the stroma is intact, orderly regeneration is more likely to occur. If the stroma also is damaged, disorderly regeneration will ensue. In summary, for orderly regeneration to occur, there must be labile or stable cells, some living parenchyma, and an intact stroma. The reparative response is summarized in Figure 1-1.

Factors That Affect Healing

Three factors are necessary for rapid wound healing: good apposition of the margins of the wound, a minimum of necrotic tissue,

Figure 1-1. Pathways of reparative response. (Reprinted with permission from Robbins, S.L., Angell, M., and Kumar, V., Basic Pathology, 3rd ed. Philadelphia: W.B. Saunders, 1981, p. 57.)

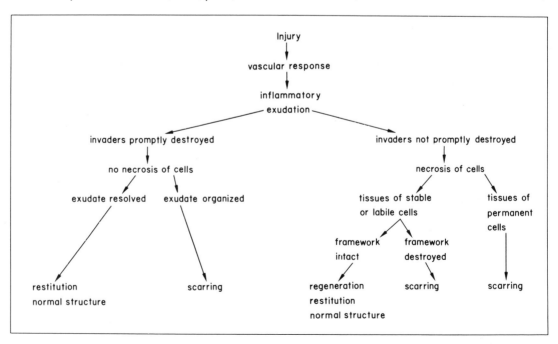

and minimum infection. If these conditions are not met, the early healing may break down and then heal more slowly with a larger scar. The repair rate is influenced by the blood supply and temperature of the damaged tissue; tissues with a poor blood supply heal slowly. Deficiencies of nutrients (especially protein and vitamin C), old age, corticosteroid medications, and the presence of debilitating illness also interfere with healing.

References

1. *Dorland's Illustrated Medical Dictionary* (26th ed.). Philadelphia: W.B. Saunders, 1981.

Bibliography

Bloom, W., and Fawcett, D.W. *A Textbook of Histology*, 11th ed. Philadelphia: W.B. Saunders, 1986.

Braunstein, H., Ed. *Outlines of Pathology*. St. Louis: Mosby, 1982.

Frohlich, E.D., Ed. *Pathophysiology: Altered Regulatory Mechanisms in Disease*, 3rd ed. Philadelphia: J.B. Lippincott, 1984.

Ham, A.W. *Histology*, 8th ed. Philadelphia: J.B. Lippincott, 1979.

Hill, R.B., Jr., and LaVia, M.F., Eds. *Principles of Pathobiology*, 3rd ed. New York: Oxford University Press, 1980.

Junqueira, L.C., Carneiro, J., and Contopoulos, A.N. *Basic Histology*, 4th ed. Los Altos, CA: Lange Medical, 1983.

Ramsey, J.M. *Basic Pathophysiology*. Menlo Park, CA: Addison-Wesley, 1982.

Robbins, S.L., Angell, M., and Kumar V. *Basic Pathology*, 3rd ed. Philadelphia: W.B. Saunders, 1981.

Snell, R.S. *Clinical and Functional Histology for Medical Students*. Boston: Little, Brown, 1984.

Sodeman, W.A., and Sodeman, T.M. *Pathologic Physiology: Mechanisms of Disease*, 7th ed. Philadelphia: W.B. Saunders, 1985.

Weiss, L., and Greep, R.O. *Histology*, 5th ed. New York: McGraw-Hill, 1983.

Woodburne, R.T. *Essentials of Human Anatomy*, 7th ed. New York: Oxford University Press, 1983.

Woolf, N. *Cell Tissue and Disease: The Basis of Pathology*, 2nd ed. London: Baillière Tindall, 1986.

2. Fluid, Electrolyte, and Acid-Base Balance

I. Water
   A. Content and distribution
   B. Requirements
   C. Intake
   D. Fluid transfer
   E. Fluid shifts
   F. Excretion
   G. Volume disturbances
      1. Water deficit
      2. Water excess
II. Electrolytes
   A. Sodium
      1. Content and distribution
      2. Requirements
      3. Intake
      4. Function
      5. Homeostasis
      6. Excretion
      7. Concentration disturbances
   B. Potassium
      1. Content and distribution
      2. Intake and requirements
      3. Function
      4. Homeostasis

      5. Alterations in serum potassium
   C. Chloride
   D. Other electrolytes
III. Acid-Base Balance
   A. Sources of hydrogen ion
   B. Determination of pH
   C. Control of hydrogen ion concentration
      1. Blood buffers
         a. buffering of acid
         b. buffering of base
      2. Respiratory system
      3. Renal system
   D. Clinical disturbances of acid-base balance
      1. Respiratory acidosis
      2. Respiratory alkalosis
      3. Metabolic acidosis
      4. Metabolic alkalosis
   E. Blood gas analysis
IV. Procedures for Prevention of Normal Fluid and Electrolyte Imbalances
V. Procedures for Correction of Fluid and Electrolyte Imbalances
   A. Volume disturbances

      1. Hypovolemia
      2. Hypervolemia
   B. Concentration disturbances
   C. Composition disturbances
      1. Hypokalemia
      2. Hyperkalemia
      3. Hypocalcemia
      4. Hypercalcemia
      5. Hypomagnesemia
      6. Hypermagnesemia
      7. Hypochloremia
      8. Hyperchloremia
      9. Hydrogen and bicarbonate ion imbalances
         a. metabolic acidosis
         b. metabolic alkalosis
   D. Other nutritional concerns in fluid and electrolyte imbalances
   E. Solutions used in therapy
      1. Categories of intravenous fluids
   F. Energy supply

Water and electrolyte imbalances occur in a large number of disorders including renal, liver, and gastrointestinal disease, burns, surgical trauma, fever, thyroid disease, congestive heart failure, respiratory disorders, and some drug therapies. The imbalances discussed in this chapter are relevant to an understanding of many of the conditions to be discussed in later chapters.

The imbalances may be divided into three types:

1. *Volume imbalances.* The patient has a deficit or excess of body fluid, but the electrolyte concentration and composition are normal.

2. *Concentration imbalance* is a disturbance of **sodium** concentration. Sodium receives this emphasis since it comprises 90% of cations in the ECF and largely controls the movement of water in the body.

3. *Composition imbalance.* The amount of fluid and concentration (of sodium) is normal, but the relative amounts of electrolytes are changed.

Although these types of imbalances are defined separately above, it must be recognized that they commonly occur together. In the interests of clarity, the various components will first be discussed separately.

WATER

Water in the body serves as a carrier of materials in solution (including nutrients and waste products), serves as a medium for chemical reactions, acts as a lubricant, provides form to cells, and participates in the maintenance of body temperature. It also is one of the building materials in growth. Water is important in maintaining the constancy of the internal environment; thus the appropriate amounts of water must be present in the proper compartments.

Content and Distribution

In an average normal adult, water makes up about 60% of the total body weight in the male and 50% in the female. Between sexes and also within each sex, body water is lower with decreased muscle mass and increased body fat. Thus most women have a lower proportion of body water than men. Therefore, a person who is obese contains less water than if he or she were of normal weight. Water content also varies with age. A newborn infant is 70–75% water, an amount which decreases progressively with age. If an adult maintains a constant weight of 70 kg, body water will decrease about 1 kg per decade.[1]

The water in the body is divided into several compartments:

1. **Intracellular fluid**, or ICF, exists within the cells and makes up about 40% of body weight or about two-thirds of total body water.
2. **Extracellular fluid**, or ECF, exists outside the cells and makes up about 20% of body weight or one-third of total body water.

The ECF is further divided into 3–5% of **intravascular fluid** within the blood vessels, 12–15% **interstitial fluid** (ISF) in the intercellular space, and 1–5% **transitional** or **transcellular fluid**. Transitional fluid consists of water in the excretory portion of the kidney, secretions of the gastrointestinal tract, the cerebrospinal fluid, aqueous humor of the eye, secretion of glands, and water in bones and potential spaces. A summary of normal body fluid compartments is given in Table 2-1. Examples of body composition are shown in Figure 2-1.

The body does not contain open, unoccupied spaces, since organs normally lie immediately adjacent to each other. However, there are some areas, such as the pericardial, thoracic, and peritoneal cavities and in the joints and bursae, where the adjacent tissues are not continuous and can be forced apart by accumulated water. These areas where fluid can accumulate are the potential spaces, or "third spaces." In a patient with liver failure, for example, a large amount of fluid can accumulate in the peritoneal cavity. "Third spacing" also occurs in some gastrointestinal, renal, and cardiovascular diseases.

Requirements

Water balance in the body is normally maintained by the interactions among the kidneys, brain, gastrointestinal tract, and the posterior pituitary gland's antidiuretic hormone (ADH). For clinical purposes, the

Table 2-1. Typical Water Distribution in the Adult Body

Water Compartment	Adult Male (% total body weight)	Volume in 70-kg Man (liters)	Adult Female (% total body weight)	Volume in 54-kg Woman (liters)
Extracellular	20–23	14	16–17	9
Intravascular	3–5	3.0	2.5–5.0	2.0
Interstitial	12–15	10.0	9–13	6.3
Transcellular	1–5	1.0	1–4	0.7
Intracellular	35–40	28	24–34	18
Total	55–60	42	45–50	27

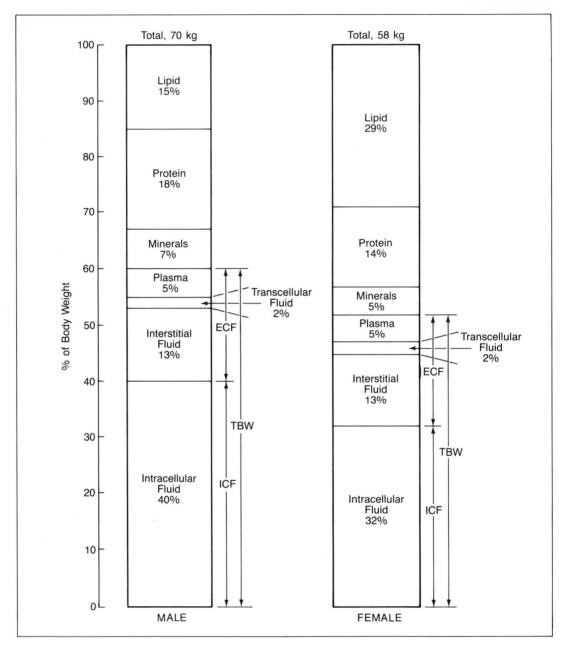

Figure 2-1. Approximate body composition of young adult males and females.

water requirement has been estimated by one of the following methods:

1. Based on body surface area: 1,500 ml/m². Body surface may be obtained from a nomogram for adults[2] or children.[3] Alternatively, it may be estimated from one of the

following equations based on the work of Dubois:[4]

$$S = W^{0.425} \times H^{0.725} \times 71.84 \qquad \text{(2-1)}$$

or

$$\log S = (\log W \times 0.425)\,(\log H \times 0.725) + 1.8564 \qquad \text{(2-2)}$$

where S = cm² body surface area, W = kg body weight, and H = cm height.

Alternative equations require simpler arithmetic for clinical situations:[5]

$$S\ (m^2) = \frac{\text{height (in.)} \times \text{weight (lbs.)}}{3,131} \quad (2\text{-}3)$$

or

$$S\ (m^2) = \frac{\text{height (cm)} \times \text{weight (kg)}}{3,600} \quad (2\text{-}4)$$

These simplified equations vary from the Dubois equation (2-1) by about 2% only.

2. Based on energy intake: 1 ml/kcal.
3. Based on body weight:

Adolescents	40–60 ml/kg
Young active adults, 16–30 years	35–40 ml/kg
Average adult	30–35 ml/kg
Adult, 55–65 years	30 ml/kg
Adult, >65 years	25 ml/kg
Child, 1–10 kg	100–150 ml/kg
11–20 kg	add 50 ml/ each kg > 10
21 kg or more	add 25 ml/ each kg > 20

4. Based on nitrogen plus energy intake: 1 ml/kcal + 100 ml/g nitrogen intake. This formula is especially useful with high-protein feedings.

Intake

There are three sources of water to the body:

1. *Liquid food and drink.* The water content may vary from about 50% in some alcoholic beverages to almost 100% in fruit juices. Water as a beverage is also included in this category.
2. *Solid foods.* Most solid foods contain some water, and some may be largely water (see Table 2-2).
3. *Metabolism of protein, fat, and carbohydrate.* In the metabolism of foods, 100 g protein will produce 41 g water, 100 g carbohydrate produces 55 g water, and

Table 2-2. Water Content of Food Groups

Food Item	Water Content (%)
Meat, fish, poultry, cooked fresh	40–65
Legumes and cereals, cooked	64–87
Fruits and vegetables, fresh	73–95
Moist bakery products, fresh	24–37
Milk, juices, coffee, tea, soft drinks	87–100

100 g fat produces 107 g water. The total is about 200–300 ml/day for the average diet or 10–14 g/100 kcal.

Water is sometimes produced from body protein if the patient is catabolizing protein. Since the extent of protein catabolism is not easily measured, this amount is often not included in clinical estimates of water balance. It is estimated that 100 g of nonfatty tissue will give rise to 15 ml of water of oxidation and will release about 73 ml of intracellular water for every 100 g of tissue. On the other hand, 100 g of fat will again give rise to 107 ml of water of oxidation but contains almost no preformed fluid. A patient who loses 1 kg of body tissue, half fatty and half nonfatty, will give rise to about 975 ml of water [(15 + 73 + 107) × 5]. Metabolic water may have to be considered in patients with impaired water excretory ability.

Water intake is normally controlled by sensations of thirst. These sensations are controlled by receptors in the hypothalamus, heart, and large blood vessels. However, difficulties arise when patients are unable to sense or respond to thirst, such as infants or patients who are comatose or senile.

Fluid Transfer

The methods by which substances cross cell membranes are diagramed in Figure 2-2. Water and some solutes may be transferred from one fluid compartment to another by **diffusion** or **osmosis**. In diffusion, a solute, solvent, or both move within a fluid compartment or across a permeable membrane to another compartment. The process does not require energy expenditure. The rate of

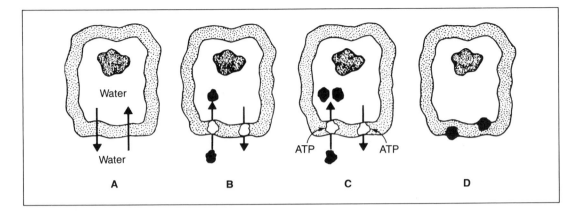

Figure 2-2. Methods of transfer across cell membranes. **A**. *In* **diffusion**, *the material, such as water, crosses the cell membrane freely, moving to equalize the concentrations of the material inside and outside the cell.* **B**. *In* **facilitated diffusion** *(or passive transport) a specific carrier is required. The carrier may shuttle a material across a membrane or affect membrane permeability. The net result is to achieve equal concentrations on the two sides of the membrane.* **C**. **Active transport** *is required to achieve a higher concentration of a substance within than outside the cell. The process requires energy obtained from ATP.* **D**. *In* **pinocytosis**, *the membrane engulfs the particle, which is then surrounded by membrane.*

movement is greater from areas of higher to lower concentration than movement in the opposite direction. Smaller molecules diffuse more rapidly than larger molecules. Diffusion rate also increases with increasing temperature. The cell controls water transport by controlling sodium concentration by **active transport**, and water follows passively.

Water and some solutes, but not all, will pass through body membranes freely. These membranes are thus **semipermeable**. Osmosis is the movement of the solvent (water) molecules from an area of low concentration to an area of high concentration of solutes *that do not cross the membrane*. In body fluids, there is always solute, since body water does not occur in pure form. As the water moves, the compartment with the low concentration of solute becomes more concentrated, and

the other becomes more dilute, until the solute concentrations in the two compartments are equivalent.

Osmotic pressure is the force that "pulls" water through a semipermeable membrane toward the more concentrated solution. It is defined as the amount of pressure necessary to stop the solvent flow across the membrane and is directly proportional to the *number* of particles in solution, regardless of their charge, and inversely proportional to the **molecular weight** of the solute. Osmotic pressure is measured in milliosmols (mOsm). If a solute does not dissociate in solution, one millimole will have an osmotic pressure of one milliosmol. If a solute dissociates (ionizes) into more than one particle, it will exert a proportionately greater osmotic pressure. NaCl, for example, will dissociate into two particles, Na^+ and Cl^-, and one millimole will exert a pressure of 2 milliosmols.

Osmotic pressure is expressed as **osmolarity**, the milliosmols of solute per liter of total **solution** (solute plus solvent), or **osmolality**, defined as milliosmols of solute per kg of **solvent**. Tissue fluids are very dilute, and there is little difference between these two expressions, but osmolality is usually used. In more concentrated solutions, such as those used for tube feedings described in a later chapter, osmolarity is used, and it may be as low as 80% of osmolality.

The normal osmolality of serum is 285–295 mOsm/kg of water, but a range of 280–320 mOsm/kg is usually considered acceptable and not requiring treatment. Serum osmolality can be estimated in serum using the equation

$$mOsm = 2(Na + K) + \frac{glucose}{18} + \frac{BUN}{2.8}$$

$$(2-5)$$

where Na and K are given in mEq/L, and glucose and blood urea nitrogen (BUN) are given in mg/dl. The values for sodium and potassium are doubled in Equation 2-5 because each is accompanied by another ion, mostly chloride, to achieve electroneutrality. Therefore, serum osmolality is provided largely by its content of small particles of sodium, potassium, and chloride. Using representative normal values, Equation 2-5 might show:

$$mOsm = 2(140 + 4) + \frac{90}{18} + \frac{5.6}{2.8}$$

$$mOsm = 288 + 5 + 2 = 295$$

Glucose and BUN contribute little, as demonstrated by this calculation. Nondiffusable particles, such as protein, have a small influence known as **colloid osmotic pressure**.

Figure 2-3. Diagram of pressure contributing to fluid exchange across a capillary membrane.

Solutions used in treatment that have an osmolality within normal physiologic range are **isotonic**. A 5% glucose solution and 0.85% sodium chloride solution are each isotonic. A **hypertonic** solution will have a higher concentration of solute than the corresponding isotonic solution, and a **hypotonic** solution will be less concentrated.

Sodium and its anion provide 90–95% of the osmotic pressure in the ECF. In the ICF, the major ions are potassium and phosphate. The osmotic pressures of the ECF and ICF are assumed to be approximately equivalent in the steady state. It is not possible to measure osmolality of the ICF; therefore, osmolality of ECF is taken to indicate either.

Another force that affects movement of body fluids is **hydrostatic pressure**. When the hydrostatic pressures on two sides of a membrane are different, water and diffusable solutes move across the membrane from the side with higher pressure. This movement is called **filtration**. As an example, at the arterial end of capillaries, hydrostatic pressure is higher than is the pressure in the extravascular space, and it is also higher than the osmotic pressure within the capillary (see Figure 2-3). Therefore, fluid and diffusable solids move out of the capillary. At the venous end, the flow is in the opposite direction, since hydrostatic pressure in the capillary is lower and osmotic (colloid osmotic or

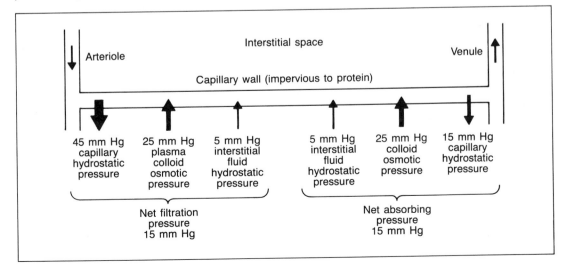

oncotic) pressure is higher. The interstitial fluid also has hydrostatic and colloid osmotic pressures in the opposite direction from that in the plasma. The net effect is slightly in favor of fluid movement into interstitial space. These processes function not only in maintenance of an appropriate amount of body water, but also in influencing its location.

Fluid Shifts

The nutritional care specialist must understand the imbalances that occur when fluid shifts from the plasma to interstitial fluid and when the shift is in the opposite direction. Abnormal fluid shift **from plasma to interstitial space** results in edema, ascites, or anasarca. These can occur in gastrointestinal bleeding or obstruction, blood vessel occlusion, infections including peritonitis, surgery, trauma, such as burns or crushing injury, and any condition that increases capillary permeability. As fluid moves from the blood, reducing blood volume, the patient presents with hypovolemia, shock, pallor, weakness, tachycardia (rapid heart rate), and oliguria (small urine output).

Treatment consists of restoration of blood volume. Often, this is accomplished by administration of intravenous fluids, whose composition resembles that in ECF. Improvement of the patient's condition is indicated by normalization of body weight, blood pressure, heart rate, hematocrit, hemoglobin, serum plasma, and urine output.

On the other hand, the shift of fluid **from interstitial fluid to plasma** may result in circulatory congestion, especially if renal and cardiac functions are impaired. The patient presents with engorged peripheral veins, cardiac dilation, a bounding pulse, and decreased hemoglobin, hematocrit, and red blood cell count. Treatment may consist of the reduction of fluid intake and use of diuretics to promote urinary excretion.

This condition may occur as the patient rebounds from a plasma to ICF fluid shift. In patients recovering from burns, surgery, and crushing injuries, water balance may be monitored by observing body weight. A weight change of 1 kg represents a change of 1 L of fluid in the same direction.

Excretion

Water may be eliminated from the body via the lungs and skin. These are the **insensible** (invisible) losses. Water is also lost via the feces and urine, and these are the **sensible**, visible, or measurable losses. Daily water losses average 250 ml in feces, 800–1,500 ml in urine, and 600–900 ml in insensible losses, of which 75% is via the skin and 25% from the lungs. Normally, total water intake and water loss are equivalent in the adult. A representative fluid balance is given in Table 2-3.

Urinary water excretion is divided into two types, referred to as obligatory and facultative. **Obligatory** water excretion is the minimum amount necessary to remove the waste materials to be excreted in the urine. The materials that must be excreted in large amounts are sodium, potassium, and chloride, as well as urea and other products of protein metabolism. In total, these materials are called the **renal solute load** (RSL).

Each gram of dietary protein contributes 5.7 mOsm to the RSL in adults. When a person is synthesizing protein, such as in growing children, each gram of protein contributes only 4.0 mOsm, and the remaining protein is used to form tissue. Each milliequivalent of sodium, potassium, or chloride excreted contributes 1 mOsm to the RSL.[6]

Table 2-3. Representative Fluid Balance

Water Intake	(ml)	Water Loss	(ml)
Sensible		*Sensible*	
Oral fluids	1,500	Urine	1,500
Solid foods	700	Intestinal	250
Insensible		*Insensible*	
Metabolic water	250	Lungs and skin	700
Total	2,450		2,450

The total RSL for an adult therefore may be calculated from the equation[7]

$$RSL\ (mOsm) = (g\ protein \times 5.7) + mEq \\ (Na + K + Cl) \qquad (2\text{-}6)$$

where all values are given as the amount per day.

The RSL determines the volume of water needed for excretion. The adult kidney has a concentrating ability that is limited to 1,200–1,400 mOsm/liter, while the kidneys of infants and some diseased kidneys have a lower concentrating ability. Once the maximum possible concentration is reached, more water must be provided to excrete any additional solute. If this water is not provided from external sources, it is extracted from body water, and the patient becomes dehydrated or hypernatremic. Thus the excess electrolyte and protein content of the diet normally determines the volume of obligatory fluid excretion.

If the patient is not fed, catabolic processes continue. The minimum renal solute load in such an adult patient is about 600–700 mOsm. With a renal concentrating ability of 1,200–1,400 mOsm/L, the obligatory fluid excretion is thus about 500 ml or 20 ml/hr.

If a person takes in more water than is needed for obligatory excretion and for growth, the excess must be excreted. This amount is known as **facultative** excretion. It can vary greatly in amount depending upon the intake.

Volume Disturbances

Fluid may be deficient or in excess. Here we will discuss the effect of changes in the amount of water, ignoring changes in sodium for clarity at the moment.

Water Deficit

Excessive fluid losses leading to **water deficit**, or **hypovolemia**, may occur by a variety of routes. Fluid is lost from the lungs in diseases involving fever or increased respira-tory rate. Fluid is also lost from the skin when burned. Other abnormal routes of losses include drainage tubes, ostomies, and fistulas described in Chapters 7 and 8. Nausea, vomiting, and hemorrhage also cause fluid loss. Selected kidney diseases and endocrine disorders such as diabetes mellitus and diabetes insipidus are additional causes of extensive fluid loss. Large amounts of solutes act as osmotic diuretics, causing obligatory water loss.

Clinical manifestations are listed in Table 2-4. Some simple rules to estimate loss are as follows:

1. If a patient is thirsty and clinical signs are minimal, deficit is about 2% of body weight. A 70-kg man would thus need 1,400 ml of replacement fluid plus current needs.
2. If the patient has not had water for 3–4 days and has a dry mouth and oliguria, the deficit may be about 6% of body weight. The 70-kg man now needs a 4,200-ml replacement.
3. If the patient has marked weakness and mental changes, the deficit may be 7–14%, or 5–10 liters. Death usually occurs from respiratory failure when water losses are 15–25% of body weight.

Water Excess

Also known as **water intoxication, overhydration, dilution syndrome**, or **hypervolemia**, **water excess** occurs when the patient gets more water than the kidneys can excrete. It can occur in patients with excess secretion of antidiuretic hormones, some central nervous system diseases, some endocrine disorders, renal diseases, and responses to selected drugs. Clinical manifestations are listed in Table 2-4.

ELECTROLYTES

Water does not exist in pure form in the body. The materials in solution are classified in two groups. If the molecule remains intact, it is a nonelectrolyte. Compounds such as

Table 2-4. Clinical Manifestations of Fluid and Electrolyte Imbalances

Fluid or Electrolyte	Clinical Manifestations of Deficit	Clinical Manifestations of Excess
Extracellular fluid volume	Increased pulse rate; decreased body temperature; increased respiration rate; anorexia; nausea and vomiting; weight loss (500 ml of fluid = 1 lb.); urine flow < 20–40 ml/hr; systolic blood pressure 10 mm Hg less when standing than when supine; dry skin; dry mucous membrane; fatigue, apathy; longitudinal wrinkles in skin; depressed fontanel in infant; shock and coma if very severe deficit	Puffy eyelids; peripheral edema; ascites; pleural effusion; pulmonary edema; acute weight gain; increased central venous pressure; dyspnea; tachycardia (symptoms vary with cause)
Sodium	Abdominal cramps; anorexia; diarrhea; lethargy; apprehension; confusion; convulsions; coma	Firm rubbery tissue turgor; dry sticky mucous membranes; oliguria; agitation, convulsions
Potassium	Muscle weakness (skeletal, intestinal, heart, respiratory); cardiac arrhythmias; electrocardiographic abnormalities; apnea and respiratory arrest; nephropathy; nausea; paralytic ileus	May be none. Symptoms similar to hypokalemia. Muscle weakness; intestinal colic; diarrhea; oliguria, anuria; electrocardiographic changes
Calcium	Muscle cramps; tingling of fingers; tetany; convulsions	Nausea and vomiting; relaxed muscles; kidney stones; pathologic fractures; bone pain; cardiac arrest; stupor, coma
Magnesium	Hyperactivity; neuromuscular irritability; tremor; disorientation; convulsions	Anorexia, weight loss; loss of muscle tone; depression
Bicarbonate	Metabolic acidosis: weakness; deep, rapid breathing; shortness of breath; disorientation, coma	Metabolic alkalosis: depressed respiration; hypertonic muscles; tetany
Carbonic acid	Respiratory alkalosis: deep, rapid breathing; tetany; unconsciousness	Respiratory acidosis: decreased respiration; disorientation

glucose, urea, and creatinine are in this category. If the material ionizes in solution, it is an electrolyte. Electrolytes of major importance are Na^+, K^+, Cl^-, and HCO_3^-.

Electrolytes function in four basic physiologic processes:

1. Maintenance of body fluid osmolarity.
2. Distribution of body fluids among fluid compartments.
3. Regulation of acid-base balance.
4. Promotion of neuromuscular irritability.

Normally, the total number of cations (positive ions) in body fluids is 155 mEq/L, and total anions (negative ions) also total 155 mEq/L. If electrolytes are lost, there may be less than 155 mEq/L of anions and cations, or there may be more if water is lost, but the number of anions and cations are equivalent, and electroneutrality is always maintained.

As shown in Figure 2-4, the major electrolyte in ECF is sodium ion (Na^+), and potassium ion (K^+) is the major electrolyte in the intracellular fluid.

Sodium

Sodium is very important in nutritional care of a number of diseases. Cardiovascular, renal, and liver diseases are particularly likely to present problems of sodium balance.

Content and Distribution

The average adult body contains 52–60 mEq/kg of sodium in males and 48–55 mEq/kg in females. Each milliequivalent

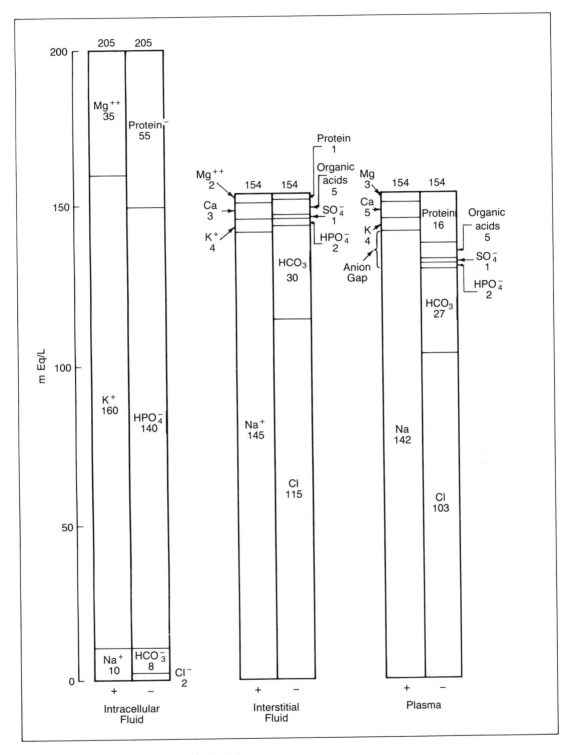

Figure 2-4. Electrolyte contents of body fluid compartments.

Table 2-5. Electrolyte Composition of Gastrointestinal Secretions and Other Body Fluids

Fluid	Electrolytes (mEq/L)			
	Sodium	Potassium	Chloride	Bicarbonate
Saliva	20–46	16–23	24–44	12–18
Gastric juice	31–90	3.6–5.5	100–105	24.6–28.8
Bile	134–156	3.9–6.3	83–110	38
Pancreatic juice	113–153	2.6–7.4	54–95	110
Small intestine (by suction)	72–120	3.5–6.8	69–127	30
Ileal fluid	90–140	6–30	82–125	25–30
Feces	<10	<10	<15	<15
Sweat	18–97	1–15	18–97	0
Cerebrospinal fluid	135–147	2.5–3.4	116–132	21–25

Modified from Lockwood, J.S., and Randall, H.T., The place of electrolyte studies in surgical patients. *Bull. N.Y. Acad. Med.* 25:228, 1949; Randall, H.T., Water and electrolyte balance in surgery. *Surg. Clin. North Am.* 32(3):445, 1952; and Maxwell, M.H., and Kleeman, C.R., Eds., *Clinical Disorders of Fluid and Electrolyte Metabolism*, 2nd ed. New York: McGraw-Hill, 1972.

equals 23 mg (see Appendix D). Sodium is the major cation in the ECF. In addition to comprising 90% of all ECF cations, it is also contained in gastrointestinal secretions (see Table 2-5). About 35–40% of total body sodium is in the skeleton, but this is not freely exchangeable with serum sodium.

Requirements

The daily requirement for sodium is unknown, but 1,100–3,300 mg has been suggested as a safe and adequate intake. The true minimum requirement is believed to be very much less.

Intake

The intake of sodium varies greatly. It has been estimated that intake in the United States is between 6 and 18 g/day for most of the population, but may be as high as 40 g/day. Sodium occurs naturally in food, but the largest amount is obtained from salt (sodium chloride) added to food in manufacturing or at the table. Sodium may also be obtained in some drugs and in the water in some areas. In some conditions, sodium intake from the diet must be restricted (see Chapters 9, 10, and 13).

Function

Sodium is important in regulating action potentials and is necessary for transmitting impulses in nerve and muscle. Therefore, in sodium deficit, there is muscle weakness. Also, sodium is the most osmotically active solute in the ICF and ISF and is thus a major factor in determining ECF volume.

Homeostasis

The level of sodium in the plasma is controlled initially by thirst, diffusion of sodium across capillary membranes, and fluid shifts across cell membranes. Hormonal controls occur more slowly but are of major importance.

Antidiuretic hormone (ADH), or **vasopressin**, secreted by the posterior pituitary, functions to maintain the osmolality of the extracellular fluid (ECF). It is secreted in increased quantities if (1) ECF osmolality is increased, or (2) ECF volume is decreased. As the name indicates, it reduces fluid excretion by the kidney. The retained fluid increases ECF volume and lowers its osmolality.

Conversely, decreased ECF osmolality or increased ECF volume will result in decreased ADH secretion. The resulting increase in fluid excretion will increase ECF osmolality and decrease ECF volume.

Aldosterone, from the adrenal cortex, influences sodium more directly. It acts on the renal tubules to increase sodium absorption.

Excretion

Since the intake is usually in excess of need, sodium balance is maintained largely by the control of its excretion. Most sodium is excreted in the urine under the control of aldosterone and natriuretic hormone. Excretion may be compromised in kidney, liver, and cardiovascular disease.

Concentration Disturbances

Fluid balance and sodium balance must clearly be considered at the same time. It is a rare situation for a water deficit or water excess to occur without concurrent electrolyte changes. Situations in which sodium and water balances are changed, separately or together, are listed in Table 2-6.

The amount of water and its movement across cell membranes are strongly affected by the concentration of sodium ions. Thus the changes are known as **concentration disturbances**. At normal serum sodium concentration (132–145 mEq/L), retention of

Table 2-6. Causes of Alterations in Sodium and Water Balance

Hypernatremia	
Pure water depletion	Inadequate water intake (e.g., improperly fed infants, comatose patients, difficulty in swallowing, impaired sense of thirst)
	Increased loss via skin or mucous membranes (e.g., burns)
	Renal loss:
	Normal kidneys (e.g., diabetes insipidus, alcoholism, excess water intake due to solute excess as in tube-fed patients or with bleeding ulcers; infections)
	Impaired kidneys (e.g., with decreased concentrating ability in pyelonephritis, polycystic kidneys, diuretic phase of acute renal failure, primary aldosteronism, amyloidosis, multiple myeloma, certain drug and chemical toxicities)
	Losses via lungs (e.g., in hyperventilation consequent to cerebral injury, fever, or heat exposure)
Hypotonic fluid loss	Vomiting
	Diarrhea
	Excessive sweating
	Renal loss from osmotic diuresis (glucose or urea)
Salt gain	IV bicarbonate or hypertonic saline
	Excess salt ingestion
	Excess mineralocorticoid
Hyponatremia	
With plasma hypertonicity	Hyperglycemia
With plasma hypotonicity	Vomiting
	Diarrhea
	Burns
	Diuretic therapy
	Salt-losing nephritis
	Addison's disease
Acute water overload	Stress, hemorrhage, burns, some drugs, hypothyroid, cortisol deficiency, renal insufficiency
Chronic water overload	Some drugs, chronic renal failure, hypothyroid, glucocorticoid deficiency
Edematous conditions	Congestive heart failure
	Nephrosis
	Cirrhosis of the liver
Isotonic dehydration	
Via skin	Burns, excessive sweat
Via digestive tract	Vomiting, diarrhea, fistula
Via kidney	Diuretic therapy, osmotic diuresis, salt-losing nephritis
Third-spacing	Ileus, peritonitis, pancreatitis, crush injury, ascites

1 g of sodium causes the accumulation of 310 ml of water.

Normally the kidney and hormonal mechanisms maintain plasma sodium concentration within normal range, and alterations in diet have little effect on total body sodium. However, there are a number of abnormal conditions that cause variations in body sodium and water content. Water and sodium deficits and excesses tend to occur together so that, although the total amount changes, the serum sodium concentration does not change markedly. Fluid and sodium deficit, occurring together, are known as **isotonic dehydration**. There are circumstances in which the changes are not proportional. There may be an increase in sodium concentration (**hypernatremia**) resulting from fluid loss in excess of sodium loss or sodium increase in excess of fluid. Conversely, **hyponatremia** (decreased serum sodium) can occur with sodium loss in excess of fluid. Situations causing these alterations are listed in Table 2-6. Clinical manifestations are also given in Table 2-4.

Potassium

Potassium balance is also important in a great number of conditions, including renal failure and congestive heart failure. Alterations in potassium levels relative to other electrolytes are examples of **composition disturbances**.

Content and Distribution

The mean body content of potassium is 31 – 57 mm/kg or about 70 mmol/kg of lean body mass. Of this amount, less than 2% is in the ECF. Although potassium is the major cation in the intracellular fluid, it cannot be measured in that location. Therefore, the concentration in the extracellular fluid is used to indicate intracellular concentration. Normal serum potassium is 3.5 – 5.0 mEq/L. Potassium is important in maintaining the fluid content of the cells, in transmitting impulses along nerve and muscle cell membranes, and in controlling hydrogen ion concentration.

Intake and Requirements

A dietary deficiency of potassium is not likely. However, a deficit can result from the dehydration or acidosis that accompanies many disorders. The average diet in the United States contains 2,000 – 6,000 mg, while a safe and adequate intake is estimated to be 1,875 – 5,625 mg. Rich sources of potassium are fruits and vegetables, including bananas, oranges, fruit juices, potatoes, and tomatoes.

Function

Potassium is the principal intracellular positive ion. It has important functions in muscle contraction and nerve impulse transmission. Therefore, an early sign of potassium deficit is muscle weakness. A more severe deficit can cause death from failure of the heart muscle. Other signs of potassium deficit are given in Table 2-4.

Homeostasis

Potassium distribution and maintenance of plasma K^+ levels are controlled via control of the gradient between ECF and ICF and control of renal potassium excretion. The distribution of potassium between the intracellular and extracellular fluids is maintained by a sodium-potassium pump. This is an active transport process which involves Na/K ATPase. Alterations in acid-base balance, that is, alterations in hydrogen ion concentration (H^+), also affect the distribution. When H^+ concentration is increased (acidosis), one hydrogen ion and two sodium ions enter the cell, and three potassium ions leave to maintain electroneutrality. In alkalosis, potassium enters the cells. Insulin and epinephrine promote cellular uptake of potassium.

Urinary excretion of potassium is influenced by aldosterone, renal tubular flow, and acid-base balance. These are discussed further in Chapter 9.

Alterations in Serum Potassium

High or low serum potassium values (hyperkalemia or hypokalemia) are life-threatening conditions that must be treated promptly. Because of the need for speed, treatment is not dietary.

The serious consequences of potassium imbalances make prevention important. Dietary manipulation is a possible approach to prevention. Potassium values should be monitored carefully in patients whose condition places them at risk. Some conditions that may result in altered serum potassium levels are listed in Table 2-7, and clinical manifestations are summarized in Table 2-4.

Chloride

Chloride is the major anion in the extracellular fluid. It is also found inside the cells, associated with potassium, and in the hydrochloric acid in the gastric juice. It is present in the diet primarily as salt (NaCl) and is excreted largely in the urine. Its intake and output are thus closely related to sodium, and it is also related to bicarbonate. In general, chloride concentrations vary directly with changes in sodium concentrations and inversely with bicarbonate levels. There are, however, some exceptions to this generalization. Safe and adequate intake is estimated to be 1,700–5,100 mg/day.

Other Electrolytes

Clinical manifestations of alterations in calcium and magnesium balance are given in Table 2-4. The mechanisms by which these conditions are produced will be discussed in later chapters.

ACID-BASE BALANCE

Acid-base balance refers to the control of hydrogen ion concentration, at a normal pH of 7.35–7.45. **Acidosis** is defined by a pH of 6.8–7.35, indicating an increase in hydrogen ions. **Alkalosis** is defined by a pH of 7.45–

Table 2-7. Causes of Altered Serum Potassium Levels

Hyperkalemia (>5.5 mEq/L)	Hypokalemia (<3.5 mEq/L)
Diabetes mellitus	Prolonged vomiting
Renal failure with urine output < 400–500 ml/day	Diarrhea
K$^+$-sparing diuretics	Gastric suction
Excessive parenteral K$^+$ administration	Intestinal fistulas
Adrenal cortical insufficiency	Renal tubular acidosis
Acidosis	Potassium-losing nephritis
Blood transfusion	Excessive treatment with some diuretics
K$^+$-containing drugs	Insulin therapy
Tissue damage (burns, trauma)	Alkalosis
Drugs (digitalis, succinyl choline, arginine HCl, indomethacin)	Familial periodic paralysis
Hyperkalemic periodic paralysis	Drugs (catecholamines, vitamin B$_{12}$, carbenecillin, amphotericin B, gentamycin)
Hypoaldosteronism (e.g., Addison's disease, congenital adrenal hyperplasia, K$^+$ transport defects)	Villous adenoma of colon
	Excessive sweat
	Burns
	Mineralocorticoid excess (e.g., primary hyperaldosteronism, ectopic ACTH, excess renin)
	Acute leukemia
	Magnesium deficit

7.9, indicating a decrease in hydrogen ions. If the normal limits are not maintained, the resulting fluctuation in hydrogen ion concentrations has marked effects on cellular enzymes. The rates of glycolysis and of PFK enzyme increase as H^+ concentration is reduced (pH rises). Blood pH lower than 6.8 or higher than 7.8 is thus not compatible with life.

Sources of Hydrogen Ion

Body cell metabolism normally produces acids that must be buffered. These acids may be classified into two types, nonvolatile and volatile.

Nonvolatile, or "fixed," acids are produced largely from metabolism of methionine and cystine to form H_2SO_4, organic phosphorus compounds to form phosphates and nucleoproteins to form uric acid. Other sources may be organic acids resulting from incomplete metabolism of carbohydrates and fats. Each of these then can release hydrogen ions when it ionizes in solution. The total amount is estimated to be 1 mEq hydrogen ion per kg body weight per day in the adult and 1.5–2.0 mEq/kg in the infant. Thus the total lies between 50 and 100 mEq hydrogen ion per day for most normal adults.

In the production of **volatile** acids, the carbon dioxide in metabolism of protein, fat, and carbohydrate in the cells becomes a source of hydrogen ion by reacting with water:

$$CO_2 + H_2O \longrightarrow H_2CO_3 \longrightarrow H^+ + HCO_3^-$$
$$\text{(2-7)}$$

The total amount of CO_2 produced per day is estimated to be 15,000 mmol.

Determination of pH

Blood is drawn without exposure to air into a heparinized syringe to prevent loss of CO_2. The hydrogen ion and carbon dioxide of the blood sample are measured in the laboratory. Bicarbonate may be measured directly

Table 2-8. Normal Arterial Values Related to Blood pH

Indicator	Mean	Range
pH	7.4	7.35–7.45
H^+, nEq/L	37–43	
pCO_2, mm Hg	40	35–45
HCO_3^-, mEq/L	24	22–26
pO_2, mm Hg	90	80–100

or calculated with the Henderson-Hasselbalch equation, which may be found in any elementary biochemistry text. The normal ranges of these values in arterial blood are given in Table 2-8.

Control of Hydrogen Ion Concentration

In order to control acid-base balance, the body has three lines of defense, the buffer system (the fastest), the respiratory system, and the kidneys (the slowest).

Blood Buffers

There are several pairs of substances in the buffer system: bicarbonate-carbonic acid, phosphates, hemoglobin-oxyhemoglobin, and blood proteins. Of these, the bicarbonate system in the ECF is very important and can be used as a model.

The body is able to control separately the plasma bicarbonate concentration and the partial pressure of carbon dioxide in the blood. Therefore, the carbonic acid–bicarbonate system is the principal buffer in the ECF. When the pH is normal, the ECF contains a ratio of 1 part carbonic acid to 20 parts bicarbonate.

Buffering of Acid. The following equation is an example of the buffering of an acid by bicarbonate:

$$2H^+ + SO_4^{2-} + 2Na^+ + 2HCO_3^- \longrightarrow Na_2SO_4 + Na_2CO_3 \quad \text{(2-8)}$$

This process decreases the bicarbonate and increases carbonic acid, altering the normal

$1:20$ ratio. The H_2CO_3 produced is converted to water and carbon dioxide by the reaction $H_2CO_3 \rightarrow H_2O + CO_2$. The carbon dioxide is excreted by the lungs. The kidney acidifies the urine, synthesizes bicarbonate ion, and excretes the sulfate. As a consequence, the buffer ratio returns toward normal.

Buffering of Base. A base may be buffered by the carbonic acid fraction, as shown by this example:

$$NaOH + H_2CO_3 \longrightarrow H_2O + NaHCO_3 \tag{2-9}$$

In this case, the acid fraction decreases and bicarbonate increases. The $NaHCO_3$ is converted to a salt such as NaCl, which, along with bicarbonate, is excreted in the urine. The kidney also decreases its synthesis of bicarbonate. Thus the $1:20$ ratio returns toward normal.

The Respiratory System

The respiratory system is also useful for the control of the pH. As rate and depth of respiration increase, more CO_2 is exhaled, and there is less to combine with water to form carbonic acid. In consequence, increased respiration serves to compensate for high hydrogen ion concentration. It will return pH from 7.0 to $7.2 - 7.3$ in about a minute.

The Renal System

The kidneys also contribute to maintenance of acid-base balance. Either hydrogen or bicarbonate ions can be excreted into the urine. The ion exchanges by which H^+ is excreted in the urine are diagramed in Figure 2-5. The kidneys, however, excrete acid more slowly than do the buffers and respiratory system.

Clinical Disturbances of Acid-Base Balance

There are four basic forms of acid-base imbalance:

1. Respiratory acidosis.
2. Respiratory alkalosis.
3. Metabolic acidosis.
4. Metabolic alkalosis.

In addition, there are mixed forms that are beyond the scope of this text.

Respiratory Acidosis

Respiratory acidosis results from an inadequate gas exchange in the lungs with carbon dioxide retention. As a consequence, there is increased carbonic acid, producing increased H^+. Some of the conditions leading to respiratory acidosis include foreign objects in the airway, emphysema, pneumonia, or depression of respiration by disease or drugs.

Signs of this condition include weakness, respiratory distress, anxiety and confusion, unconsciousness, and ventricular fibrillation. The direction of change, if the condition is uncompensated, is shown in Table 2-9.

Even though the respiratory system is compromised, as buffers and kidneys compensate for acidosis, the pH will return to normal. The kidneys excrete H^+ ions and conserve bicarbonate. The main treatment is restoration of a patent airway and normal respiration to promote adequate CO_2 exhalation.

Respiratory Alkalosis

Respiratory alkalosis results from hyperventilation, leading to a deficit of bicarbonate ion. It is an uncommon condition, often following severe exercise or an anxiety reaction.

Table 2-9. *Laboratory Findings in Acid-Base Disturbances*

Acid-Base Disturbances	pH	pCO$_2$	HCO$_3^-$	Urine pH
Respiratory acidosis	↓	↑	Nl or ↑	↓
Respiratory alkalosis	↑	↓	Nl or ↓	↑
Metabolic acidosis	↓	Nl or ↓	↓	↓
Metabolic alkalosis	↑	↑	↑	↑

Nl = normal

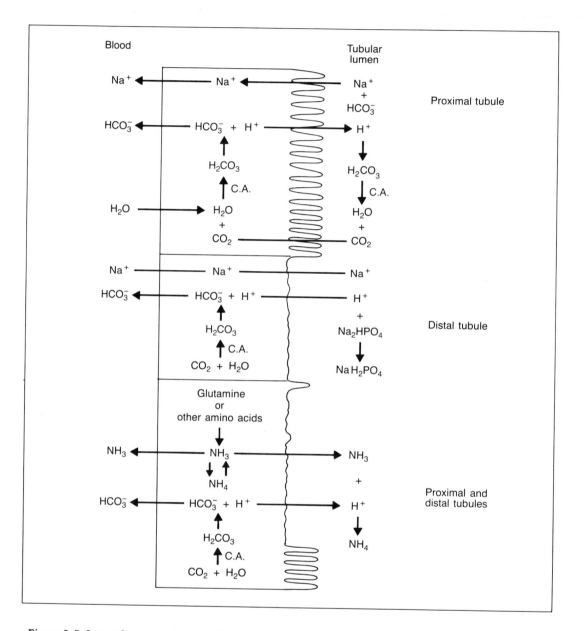

Figure 2-5. Ion exchanges to acidify urine for excretion of hydrogen ion (C.A. = carbonic anhydrase).

Signs and symptoms include tingling of fingers and toes (early), palpitation, perspiration, tetany, and arrhythmias of the heart. Laboratory values include elevated blood pH and depressed pCO_2.

In compensation, the kidneys retain hydrogen ion and excrete bicarbonate.

Metabolic Acidosis

Metabolic acidosis results from a decrease in the bicarbonate (alkali reserve) or a marked increase in hydrogen ion production. It may result from bicarbonate loss from the gastrointestinal tract or kidneys or from excessive production of acid, such as may occur in uncontrolled diabetes (see Chapter 11).

In order to distinguish between these two types of causes, the anion gap (AG) may be calculated from serum electrolyte concentrations in mEq/L:

$$AG = (Na^+ + K^+) - (Cl^- + HCO_3^-) \quad (2\text{-}10)$$

As an example, assume a patient has the following serum values: sodium, 138 mEq/L; potassium, 4 mEq/L; chloride, 103 mEq/L; and bicarbonate, 20 mEq/L. The anion gap calculation in Equation 2-11 would then be

$$AG = (138 + 4) - (103 + 20)$$
$$= 142 - 123 = 19.$$

Normal anion gap is 12–16 mEq/L. If the anion gap is greater, as it is in the example, the decrease in bicarbonate is balanced by added, but unmeasured, H^+. This condition is **normochloremic acidosis** or **anion gap acidosis**. If the patient's loss of bicarbonate is balanced by an increase in chloride, anion gap will be 12–16 mEq/L. This condition is **hyperchloremic acidosis** or **non–anion gap acidosis**.

There may be no symptoms of metabolic acidosis at first with progression to general malaise, weakness, headache, nausea, vomiting, abdominal pain, confusion, and unconsciousness. As the low pH stimulates the respiratory center, the patient has deep, gasping respirations.

As compensation occurs, pH rises toward normal, pCO_2 falls, and the kidneys may conserve HCO_3^- if kidney disease does not interfere.

Metabolic Alkalosis

Metabolic alkalosis occurs when there is excessive basic bicarbonate. It can occur when hydrochloric acid is lost from the gastrointestinal tract or if excess bicarbonate is administered.

Signs and symptoms include sensations of numbness and prickling, restlessness, confusion, and tetany. Blood pH is increased, and bicarbonate and CO_2 are above normal.

Blood Gas Analysis

Acid-base status is determined in clinical situations by measuring arterial blood gases (ABG). Blood is obtained from an artery to assay for partial pressures of carbon dioxide (pCO_2) oxygen (pO_2) and pH. Blood bicarbonate is measured at the same time. The pCO_2 represents the acid, and the bicarbonate represents the base in acid-base calculations. Means and ranges of normal values are given in Table 2-8, and effects of acid-base disturbances are shown in Table 2-9. The value for pO_2 is an indicator of oxygenation.

For interpretation of acid-base status, one must first examine the pH. As a reminder, since pH represents a negative logarithm of the hydrogen ion concentration, a *lower* pH represents a *higher* H^+ concentration (acidosis). Conversely, a higher pH indicates alkalosis.

The ABG values may also be used to determine the type of acidosis or alkalosis. The pCO_2 value indicates the respiratory effect on pH. If respiration is depressed, CO_2 will be retained and pCO_2 will rise, contributing to acidosis. A drop in pCO_2 indicates hyperventilation and contributes to alkalosis.

As an example, let us assume ABG values for a patient as follows:

pH, 7.32; pCO_2, 50; HCO_3; 24

The pH is depressed from normal. Therefore, the values indicate acidosis. The pCO_2 is elevated, indicating *respiratory* acidosis.

The bicarbonate value represents the metabolic or nonrespiratory effect on the pH. A low value indicates acidosis, and a high value, alkalosis.

PROCEDURES FOR PREVENTION OF FLUID AND ELECTROLYTE IMBALANCES

Some patients are temporarily unable to take food or fluids by mouth but do not have abnormal fluid or electrolyte losses, abnormal renal function, or preexisting imbalances. The need of these patients is for provision of normal requirements.

The daily water needs of these patients are equal to the total loss of water each day. All sources of water and all routes of loss must be considered. At least 500 ml of urine must be produced each day to excrete a usual renal solute load. Adding the insensible losses of 600 to 900 ml, the patient must then be given 1.25 to 1.50 liters of water per day. Since insensible losses may be higher in the hospital environment, a common practice is to provide 35 ml/kg of body weight per day. Thus, a 70-kg man would need 2,450 ml.

If the patient has abnormal losses, the volume of that fluid must also be included in the calculation of fluid need, to prevent development of a deficit. Some of these losses include the following:

1. There may be increased evaporation from the skin as a result of fever, high room temperature with low humidity, or hyperventilation. These and sweat losses are difficult to estimate. Approximately 500 ml/day may be lost if the body temperature is elevated to 38°C, and losses may be approximately 500 ml/day if the room temperature is higher than 32°C. Evaporative losses may be replaced with 5% glucose in water, and losses in sweat, by hypotonic saline.
2. Gastrointestinal losses are incurred if the patient is vomiting or has diarrhea, a draining fistula, or similar losses of gastrointestinal fluids. The composition of gastrointestinal secretion is given in Table 2-5, which also indicates electrolyte replacement needs.
3. Internal shifts may cause fluid to be sequestered in some compartments, creating a deficit in others, even if the amount of total body water is not altered. Replacement needs may be greatly increased in patients with infectious diseases such as peritonitis, in those with pancreatitis, extensive burns, nephrotic syndrome, enteritis, ileus, or portal vein thrombosis,

and in surgical patients in the postoperative period.
4. Urinary losses of fluid, sodium, or potassium may be excessive in a variety of renal diseases, in patients receiving corticosteroid medication, and in hyperaldosteronism.

In hypermetabolic conditions, **sodium** normally is well preserved by the kidney, but losses continue in the feces and sweat. Approximately 70 mEq of sodium ion or 4 g of sodium chloride per day usually will provide replacement and prevent a deficit.

Potassium excretion in the urine, normally 20 to 60 mEq/L, continues at the rate of 30 to 40 mEq/day even if the patient has been on a potassium-free diet for as long as a week. In addition, approximately 10 mEq are excreted in stools and sweat. These amounts can be replaced by at least 40 mEq of potassium. Commonly, 60 mEq or more are given if renal function is normal.

PROCEDURES FOR CORRECTION OF FLUID AND ELECTROLYTE IMBALANCES

In order to clarify this material, a sample case will be given.

Volume Disturbances

Hypovolemia

Extracellular fluid volume deficit or **hypovolemia** can develop in patients in the circumstances previously described and may be accompanied by increased, decreased, or normal electrolyte levels. Signs of volume depletion are given in Table 2-4. Laboratory values show increased blood urea nitrogen (BUN), serum creatinine, and hematocrit. Urine chloride is less than 10 mEq/L, and urine specific gravity is high.

Let us assume a patient (described in Table 2-10) as an example in estimating replacement need. A common procedure to calculate fluid deficit is to assume that Mrs. M.G.

Table 2-10. Case Report: Mrs. M.G., Prolonged Vomiting

Sex	Female			
Age	29 years			
Normal weight	121 lb. (55 kg)			
Present weight	105 lb. (49 kg)			
Blood pressure	95/65			
Arterial blood gases	Current	Normal		
pH	7.5	7.34–7.45		
pO$_2$	85 mm Hg	80–100 mm Hg		
pCO$_2$	45 mm Hg	35–45 mm Hg		
Bicarbonate ion	33 mEq/L	24–31 mEq/L		
	Serum		Urine	
	Current	Normal	Current	Normal
Sodium	115 mEq/L	136–145 mEq/L	26 mEq/L	40–90 mEq/L
Potassium	1.9 mEq/L	3.5–5.0 mEq/L	65 mEq/L	20–60 mEq/L
Chloride	75 mEq/L	100–106 mEq/L	8 mEq/L	40–120 mEq/L
Urea nitrogen	43 mg/dl	8–25 mg/dl		
Creatinine	1.7 mg/dl	0.7–1.5 mg/dl		
Specific gravity			1.03	1.003–1.030

pO$_2$ = arterial oxygen tension; pCO$_2$ = arterial carbon dioxide tension.

is approximately 50 percent water, since she is a young adult woman. She has lost 6 kg. The deficit of total body water can be determined by the following calculations:

Normal body weight × 50% = 55 kg
    × 0.5 = 27.5 liters total body water

Present body weight × 50% = 49 kg
    × 0.5 = 24.5 liters total body water

Fluid deficit = 27.5 − 24.5 = 3.0 liters

In the ensuing 24 hours, the patient will also need replacement of daily sensible and insensible losses. If we calculate maintenance need on the basis of normal body weight, Mrs. M.G.'s total need is 3 liters plus 2,375 ml, or slightly more than 5 liters. Generally, at least half of this should be replaced within 24 hours. More severe deficits are replaced intravenously.

Hypervolemia

The opposite condition, **volume excess** or **hypervolemia**, occurs in cardiac or renal insufficiency. It can occur when water and electrolytes shift from interstitial space to the plasma. It usually is treated with fluid and sodium restrictions and diuretics. It may be iatrogenic. The exact procedure for treatment depends on the cause.

Concentration Disturbances

It is important to recall that sodium moves water, so that a sodium deficit in the ECF (actually in the plasma, since that is the only place it can be measured) will cause fluid to move into the ICF to stabilize the osmotic pressure. Sodium excess in the plasma will draw water from the ICF. Thus concentration disturbances are disorders of sodium concentration.

Hyponatremia (sodium deficit, low-sodium syndrome, or **hypotonic dehydration)** is defined by a serum sodium level of less than 130 mEq/L. Identifiable signs of hyponatremia (see Table 2-4) can occur only when the condition is severe.

In Mrs. M.G. (see Table 2-10), the total sodium deficit can be calculated first by determining her deficit in sodium concentration (normal sodium concentration [142] minus measured serum sodium [115]), and then multiplying the result by her present fluid volume of 24.5 liters:

$$(142 - 115 \text{ mEq/L}) \times 24.5 \text{ liters} = 661.5 \text{ mEq}$$

In addition to this 661.5 mEq, the sodium in her fluid loss of 3 kg must be provided, as well as the 90 mEq that will be lost in the next 24 hours: 3 liters × 142 mEq = 426 mEq for a total of 661.5 + 426 + 90 mEq or 1,177.5 mEq. Other losses associated with her illness must be added to this amount.

Hypernatremia (pure water deficit or hypertonic dehydration), with serum sodium less than 160 mEq/L, may be treated with water, but in more marked hypernatremia, sodium-free intravenous fluid, such as 5% dextrose in water, may be used.

The volume of water necessary to correct hypernatremia may be calculated:

$$\frac{\text{normal serum sodium} \times \text{normal TBW}}{\text{measured serum sodium}} = \text{current TBW}$$

where TBW = total body water.   (2-11)

In a patient weighing 70 kg, assuming that person is 60% water, total body water equals 42 liters. If the patient's serum sodium is 162 mEq/L, current TBW is calculated using this equation:

$$\frac{142 \text{ mEq} \times 42 \text{ liters}}{162 \text{ mEq}} = 36.8 \text{ liters}$$

The deficit thus is 42 − 36.8 or 5.2 liters.

Composition Disturbances

Changes in concentration of ions other than sodium can occur without significantly altering the osmotic pressure; therefore, they are classified as changes in composition rather than concentration. A number of disorders are included in this category. Their clinical manifestations are given in Table 2-4.

Hypokalemia

Clinical manifestations of hypokalemia rarely develop until serum potassium levels have fallen below 3.0 mEq/L. Potassium depletion cannot be estimated on the basis of serum potassium alone, since that value varies with the acid-base balance. Moderate deficits may be replaced orally, usually with 10% potassium chloride mixed with fruit juice and given after meals to reduce gastric irritation. When the deficit is severe or if oral intake is not possible, intravenous therapy may be necessary.

In either case, since ECF levels of potassium are less than 2% of the total body potassium, the deficit is estimated on the basis of total body weight. A woman's total body potassium is approximately 35 mEq/kg of body weight. Therefore, Mrs. M.G.'s total potassium (see Table 2-10) may be calculated:

$$35 \text{ mEq} \times 55 \text{ kg} = 1,925 \text{ mEq}$$

Since she has a weight deficit of 6 kg, or 11% of her normal body weight (6/55 ≅ 0.11), an additional amount of potassium must be added, as follows:

$$1,925 \text{ mEq} \times 0.11 \cong 212 \text{ mEq}$$

The amount of potassium lost daily as a further consequence of her illness must be added, also. If her losses were 50 mEq, for example, her replacement need would be 1,925 + 212 + 50 or 2,187 mEq. Because of the effect of potassium on the heart and other muscles, the deficit must be made up slowly, over a period of two to three days or as much as a week. During this time, the daily losses of 40 to 60 mEq must be added to the amount being replaced.

Hyperkalemia

In hyperkalemic patients, the underlying cause is treated, and potassium administration, including dietary sources, are stopped. To avoid the effects of hyperkalemia (see

Table 2-4), insulin often is given to increase cellular uptake of glucose and potassium. An intravenous solution of sodium lactate, calcium gluconate, and dextrose in water is used less often. Calcium gluconate antagonizes the effects on the heart. Lactate is metabolized into bicarbonate, thereby raising the blood pH. This shift, combined with the glucose, helps to move potassium back into the cells.

Treatment may involve removing potassium from the body, forcing potassium into the cells, or antagonizing potassium's effects. The use of **cation exchange resins** removes potassium ion slowly. In extreme circumstances, hemodialysis may be used. Sodium bicarbonate, sometimes provided as sodium lactate, causes movement of potassium ion into the cells very rapidly, as do glucose infusions. Calcium, which antagonizes the cardiac and neuromuscular effects of hyperkalemia, may be injected as 10% calcium gluconate. This is a temporary measure, however, and should be followed by the other forms of therapy.

Hypocalcemia

Hypocalcemia is defined as a serum calcium level of less than 8 mg/dl. It is seen in malabsorption syndromes, acute pancreatitis, infections, intestinal fistulas, and hypoparathyroidism. Intravenous 10% calcium gluconate or 10% calcium chloride is used in treatment. Losses from gastrointestinal drainage may be particularly high; these patients may require 400 to 500 mg/day. Coexisting hypomagnesemia must be corrected simultaneously to reverse hypocalcemia.

Hypercalcemia

Hypercalcemia is seen most often in hyperparathyroidism and cancer of the bone. Calcium levels are lowered by dilution when other ECF deficits are treated.

Hypomagnesemia

Hypomagnesemia occurs in malabsorption syndromes, gastrointestinal losses, and deficient magnesium intake. Replacement of magnesium is provided with 10 to 40 mEq of the sulfate salt per 24 hr.

Hypermagnesemia

Hypermagnesemia can accompany renal insufficiency or excessive use of magnesium-containing drugs such as some laxatives and antacids. The condition may be treated with a slow calcium infusion to counteract the neuromuscular effects plus isotonic saline to stimulate urine flow and magnesium excretion.

Hypochloremia

Hypochloremia can be produced in severe vomiting with loss of hydrogen and chloride ions. Needs can be replaced when intravenous sodium chloride is administered. Bicarbonate serves as the replacement anion in metabolism when chloride is deficient.

Hyperchloremia

Hyperchloremia, an excess of chloride in the blood, results from fluid deficit when the kidney compensates for the dehydration by reabsorbing large amounts of water. The chloride dissolved in the water is absorbed at the same time.

Chloride retention tends to occur in:

1. renal bicarbonate loss (e.g., in renal tubular acidosis, use of carbonic anhydrase inhibitors).
2. gastrointestinal loss of bicarbonate (e.g., in diarrhea, fistulas of small intestine or pancreas, obstruction of ileum, use of anion exchange resins).
3. brain stem injury.
4. diabetes insipidus.
5. excess loading (e.g., in total parenteral nutrition, HCl with drugs, excess admin-

istration of ammonium chloride or sodium chloride).

Symptoms resemble those seen in metabolic acidosis (see Chapter 11). The acute condition is treated with sodium bicarbonate.

Hydrogen and Bicarbonate Ion Imbalances

Metabolic Acidosis. In metabolic acidosis, serum bicarbonate is less than 24 mEq/L, plasma pH is less than 7.35, and the patient retains fixed acid or loses base. Hyperventilation, which is a compensatory mechanism, causes a fall in pCO_2.

In calculating the bicarbonate deficit, the ECF space is used. The normal serum bicarbonate level is 26 mEq/L. If a 65-kg man has a plasma bicarbonate level of 16 mEq/L, we can calculate his deficit as $26 - 16$, or 10 mEq/L. The ECF constitutes approximately 20% of his total body weight or 13 liters. Theoretically, then, his bicarbonate deficit equals 10 mEq/L $\times$ liters or 130 mEq. One liter of $\frac{1}{6}$ molar sodium lactate provides 166 mEq. Sometimes, the physician elects to use bicarbonate directly. It can be added to dextrose and water from ampules containing 45 mEq/50 ml.

Metabolic Alkalosis. Metabolic alkalosis usually is defined as a plasma bicarbonate level in excess of 29 mEq/L, plasma pH higher than 7.45, and a potassium level of less than 4 mEq/L. Comparison of these values with those of Mrs. M.G. (see Table 2-10) indicates that she has metabolic alkalosis. The body attempts to compensate for this condition by retaining CO_2 via shallow breathing, and pCO_2 rises to 44 to 48 mm Hg.

Treatment is influenced by the cause and accompanying imbalances. When the patient has prolonged vomiting, saline and potassium chloride infusions are used. The sodium reduces hydrogen ion excretion in the kidneys, and the chloride frees bicarbonate

for renal excretion. The vomiting patient will also have lost potassium, which is replaced along with the chloride.

Other Nutritional Concerns in Fluid and Electrolyte Imbalances

The nutritional care specialist should be aware that these fluid and electrolyte alterations affect the desire for food and water. Anorexia is seen in potassium or protein deficit and in hypercalcemia. Thirst is seen in sodium excess, hypercalcemia, and in blood volume deficit whether it is due to hemorrhage or heart failure. Absence of thirst occurs in sodium deficit.

Solutions Used in Therapy

Isotonic solutions of low concentration for short-term supplementation or substitution for oral intake may be given into a peripheral vein. These solutions are used primarily to maintain fluid and electrolyte balance but also provide a limited supply of energy substrates. Sometimes, low concentrations of amino acids are included.

Categories of Intravenous Fluids

For maintenance or correction of fluid and electrolyte balance, there are four categories of intravenous fluids that are most often used in supplemental peripheral venous alimentation. Each of these is described briefly, so that the nutritional care specialist becomes familiar with the purpose for which the physician orders their use and the nutrients provided.

Dextrose in water solutions (Table 2-11) provide calories and water. The dextrose is hydrated (glucose monohydrate) and yields only 3.4 kcal/g. As a consequence, each liter of 5% dextrose in water (D5W) provides only 170 kcal $(1,000 \times 0.05 \times 3.4)$. To supply more energy, a higher concentration of dextrose would be needed but would cause irritation in the vein. When D5W is infused, the dextrose is metabolized rapidly, leaving water to reduce plasma osmotic pressure. Water then moves from the plasma into the cells. The use of D5W, then, is primarily for replacement of volume deficits, not as an energy source.

Saline solutions (see Table 2-11) are available in several concentrations. A concentration of 0.9% sodium chloride often is referred to as **isotonic saline, normal saline,** or **physiologic saline**. It has the tonicity of plasma (308 mOsm/L), but its sodium ions and chloride ion contents are higher in concentration than in plasma. This high concentration is necessary because other plasma ions are lacking. Isotonic saline is used to replace ECF deficits, to treat sodium depletion, and to treat metabolic alkalosis. **Hypotonic saline** (0.45% sodium chloride) supplies normal salt and water requirements, whereas **hypertonic saline** (3% or 5% sodium chloride) is used in small amounts to treat water overload and severe sodium depletion.

Dextrose in saline solutions (see Table 2-11) contain both dextrose and sodium chloride in the same solution. A mixture of 5% dextrose in 0.45% saline is used to replace fluid losses and to assess the adequacy of renal function. Mixtures of 5% or 10% dextrose in normal saline provide replacement of sodium ion and chloride ion and some kilocalories to reduce catabolism.

Multiple electrolyte solutions (see Table 2-11) are used for maintenance or replacement. Maintenance solutions contain approximately normal needs, whereas replacement solutions contain some electrolytes in excess of normal needs. Almost all contain potassium and either lactate, citrate, or acetate, which are metabolized to bicarbonate. These solutions are used in cases of gastrointestinal losses, burns, acidosis, dehydration, or sodium depletion.

Other available solutions sometimes used contain alcohol, artificial plasma extenders, ammonium chloride, and calcium gluconate.

All intravenous solutions can be classified as hypertonic, isotonic, or hypotonic in the same manner as described for the saline solutions. Hypertonic solutions contain electrolytes in excess of the concentrations in plasma and are used to provide replacement. Hypertonic solutions are 5% dextrose in normal saline, 5% dextrose in Ringer's lactated injection, and 10% or 20% dextrose in water. Isotonic solutions are used to expand ECF volume. Normal saline, D5W, and Ringer's lactated solution are isotonic. Hypotonic solutions are useful to shift fluid from plasma to the interstitial fluid. The primary example is half-normal (0.45%) saline.

Energy Supply

The energy supply available from the solutions used for supplemental peripheral venous feeding is limited for two reasons. First, the total amount of solution that can be administered per day is limited by the danger of fluid overload. Second, the osmolality of the solution must be low, since highly concentrated solutions cause inflammation and sclerosis in the vein at the site of the administration. Consequently, 5% to 10% glucose solutions are used for administration into peripheral veins. Since each liter of intravenous solution of 5% glucose provides 170 kcal, 9 liters of solution would be required to meet a minimal maintenance requirement of 1,500 kcal/day. This amount of solution is unlikely to be tolerated. Hence, as a source of energy, supplemental peripheral venous feeding is useful only for patients who need limited support for a short period.

As an alternative, Blackburn et al.[8] have suggested the use of a glucose-free amino acid solution to reduce the stimulation for insulin release. The procedure is known as **protein-sparing therapy**. Assuming that the patient has adequate fat reserves, the reduced insulin levels would result in increased fat mobilization for energy, reduce the mobilization of amino acids for energy, and make the administered amino acids available for protein synthesis. The method has not been generally accepted as standard

Table 2-11. *Characteristics of Intravenous Fluids*

Type of Fluid	Cations			Anions		Kilocalories per Liter	pH (approximate)	Osmolarity (mOsm/L)	Notes
	Sodium (mEq/L)	Potassium (mEq/L)	Calcium (mEq/L)	Chloride (mEq/L)	Bicarbonate (mEq/L)[a]				
Dextrose in water solutions									
5% dextrose in water						170	4.8	252	5%: No replacement of electrolytes or correction of fluid deficits
10% dextrose in water						340	4.7	505	10%, 20%, 50%: Hypertonic solutions act as osmotic diuretics, increasing body fluid loss
20% dextrose in water						680	4.8	1,010	
50% dextrose in water						1,700	4.6	2,525	All: Dextrose provides calories
Dextrose in saline solutions									
5% dextrose and 0.2% sodium chloride	34			34		170	4.6	320	All: Provides calories, water, sodium, and chloride. Dextrose provides calories.
5% dextrose and 0.45% sodium chloride	77			77		170	4.6	406	5%, 0.45%: Used to treat hypovolemia and to promote diuresis in dehydrated patients
5% dextrose and 0.9% sodium chloride	154			154		170	4.4	559	
10% dextrose and 0.9% sodium chloride	154			154		340	4.8	812	

Saline solutions									
0.45% sodium chloride	77			77		0	5.9	154	0.45%: Supplies maintenance salt and water requirements
0.9% sodium chloride	154			154		0	6.0	154	0.9%: Widely used as a routine electrolyte replacement solution or to correct mild metabolic acidosis
3% sodium chloride	513			513		0	4.5–7.0	1,026	3%, 5%: Used for correction of severe salt depletion only
5% sodium chloride	855			855		0	4.5–7.0		
Multiple electrolyte solutions									
Ringer's solution	147	4	5	155		0	4.0–7.5	309	Replaces potassium, calcium, sodium, and chloride; chloride is in excess of normal plasma level
Lactated Ringer's solution (Hartmann's)	130	4	3	109	28	9	6.5	273	Closely resembles ECF
5% dextrose in lactated Ringer's solution	130	4	3	109	28	179	5.1	524	Replaces ECF deficits; replaces losses from vomiting or gastric suction
10% dextrose in lactated Ringer's solution	130	4	3	109	28	349	4.9	776	Dextrose provides calories
1.9% Darrow's solution	122	35		104	53				Useful in treatment of acidosis and potassium deficiency; useful in diarrhea and diabetic coma

ECF = extracellular fluid.

a Or its equivalent in lactate, acetate, or citrate.

procedure. In the opinion of many clinicians, the high cost of amino acids compared to glucose is not justified by the limited advantage gained.

For patients whose needs are greater than those described here, other methods of support are required. The need for such support may be established using methods described in the next chapter. Methods of such support are discussed in Chapter 5.

Study Questions

1. List the sources of water to the body and routes of water loss.
2. If a patient has a diet containing 90 g protein, 80 g fat, and 250 g carbohydrate, how much water would be obtained if all were metabolized?
3. Laboratory values for a patient are as follows:

   108 mg/dl glucose

   11.2 mg/dl blood urea nitrogen

   142 mg/dl sodium

   4 mg/dl potassium

   Calculate the serum osmolality. How does your result compare to normal?
4. An adult patient has daily intakes of 90 g protein, 4,600 mg sodium, 4,000 mg potassium, and 4,900 mg chloride.
   a. What is the renal solute load?
   b. Describe the consequences if the patient's *total* fluid intake (including metabolic water) were as follows, and explain your reasoning:
      (1) 2,000 ml.
      (2) 4,000 ml.
5. A patient has arterial blood gases and serum electrolytes as follows:

pH	7.21
pCO_2, mm Hg	26
Sodium mEq/L	132
Potassium, mEq/L	5.2
bicarbonate, mEq/L	11.1
Chloride mEq/L	35

   BUN is 37.
   Evaluate the patient's acid-base status and hydration state.
6. Describe how the kidneys and lungs maintain acid-base balance.

References

1. Moore, F.D., Oleson, K.H., McMurrey, J.D., et al. *Body Cell Mass and Its Supporting Environment: Body Composition in Health and Disease.* Philadelphia: W.B. Saunders, 1963.
2. Wilmore, D.W. *Metabolic Management of the Critically Ill.* New York: Plenum, 1977.
3. Behrman, R.E., and Vaughn, V.C., III, Eds. *Nelson Textbook of Pediatrics,* 13th ed. Philadelphia: W.B. Saunders, 1987. p. 1521.
4. DuBois, D., and DuBois, E.F. A formula to estimate the approximate surface area if height and weight be known. *Arch. Int. Med.* 17:863, 1916.
5. Mosteller, R.D. Simplified calculation of body-surface area. *New Engl. J. Med.* 317:1098, 1987.
6. Bergman, K.E., Ziegler, E.E., and Fomon, S.J. Water and renal solute load. In *Infant Nutrition,* 2nd ed., S.J. Fomon, Ed. Philadelphia: W.B. Saunders, 1974.
7. Ziegler, E.E., and Fomon, S.J. Fluid intake, renal solute load and water balance in infancy. *J. Pediatr.* 78:561, 1971.
8. Blackburn, G.L., Flatt, J.P., Clowes, G.H.A., and O'Donnell, T.E. Peripheral intravenous feeding with isotonic amino acid solutions. *Am. J. Surg.* 125:447, 1973.

Bibliography

Arieff, A.I., and DeFronzo, R.A. *Fluid, Electrolyte and Acid-Base Disorders.* New York: Churchill Livingstone, 1985.

Christensen, H.N. *Body Fluids and Acid-Base Balance.* Philadelphia: W.B. Saunders, 1964.

Goldberger, E. *A Primer of Water, Electrolyte and Acid-Base Syndromes,* 6th ed. Philadelphia: Lea & Febiger, 1980.

Kokko, J.P., and Tannen, R.L. *Fluids and Electrolytes.* Philadelphia: W.B. Saunders, 1986.

Pestano, C. *Fluids and Electrolytes in the Surgical Patient,* 2nd ed. Baltimore: Williams & Wilkins, 1981.

Richards, P., and Truniger, B. *Understanding*

Water, Electrolyte and Acid-Base Balance. London: Heinemann, 1983.

Shapiro, B.A., Harrison, R.A., Cane, R.D. and Templin, R. *Clinical Applications of Blood Gases,* 4th ed. Chicago: Year Book Medical, 1989.

Scribner, B.H., Ed. *Teaching Syllabus for the Course on Fluid and Electrolyte Balance.* Seattle: University of Washington, 1953.

Talbot, N.B., Crawford, J.D., and Butler, A.M. Homeostatic limits to safe parenteral fluid therapy. *New Engl. J. Med.* 248:1100, 1953.

Talbot, N.B., Kerrigan, G.A., Crawford, J.D., Cochran, W., and Terry, M. Application of homeostatic principles to the practice of parenteral fluid therapy. *New Engl. J. Med.* 252:898, 1955.

Walmsley, R.N., and Guerin, M.D. *Disorders of Fluid and Electrolyte Balance.* Bristol: Wright, 1984.

3. Nutritional Assessment

I. Documentation of
   Nutritional Care
   A. Problem-oriented
      medical record
      1. Data base
      2. Problem list
      3. Initial care plans
      4. Progress notes
      5. Other pertinent
         information
   B. Source-oriented
      medical record

II. Nutritional Assessment
   A. Assessment procedures
      1. Weight in relation
         to height
         a. height
         b. weight
         c. interpretation
      2. Estimation of
         energy stores
      3. Estimates of
         somatic protein
         a. circumference
            of midarm muscle
         b. midarm muscle
            area
         c. creatinine-
            height index
      4. Measurement of
         visceral protein
      5. Nitrogen balance
      6. Cell-mediated
         immune function
      7. Hematological
         assessment
      8. Vitamin assays
      9. Evaluation of
         hydration status
      10. Functional tests
      11. Clinical observa-
         tions
      12. Dietary assessment
         a. methods to
            obtain data
            (1) twenty-
               four-hour
               recall
            (2) food fre-
               quency lists
            (3) food records
            (4) nutrition
               history
            (5) observa-
               tions of
               food intake
         b. evaluation of
            the diet
   B. Evaluation of nutri-
      tional status
      1. Diagnosis of
         protein-calorie
         malnutrition
      2. Evaluation of
         requirements
         a. energy balance
         b. nitrogen balance
      3. Estimate of clinical
         risk

III. Identification of Other
   Problems

IV. Case Study

The most important function of the nutritional care specialist is to assure that all patients, regardless of specific diagnosis, are adequately nourished, either by the actual provision of nutrients or by counseling patients in their own food choices. Not only must the normal nutritional requirements of healthy persons be considered, but also the increased or decreased needs mandated by the nature of the patient's illness must be met. In addition, the individual characteristics and preferences of patients cannot be disregarded. In providing for patients' needs, nutritional care specialists must integrate their own activities with those of other members of the health care team.

In practice, an initial evaluation, applied to all patients, identifies those who require nutritional care. Nutritional care, then, consists of four basic steps:

1. **Assessment** to identify the patient's specific nutritional problems.
2. **Planning** for care.
3. **Implementation** of the plans for care.
4. **Evaluation** of the results of care.

Evaluation involves reassessment, making nutritional care a cyclic process.

All steps in nutritional care should be documented in the medical record; therefore, it is important that the nutritional care specialist be familiar with the recording procedures used.

The chapters in this part will provide an overview of the nutritional care process, without regard to specific diagnosis, and a discussion of the means of documenting that care. This chapter will discuss nutritional assessment and its documentation. The succeeding chapters will discuss the major components of planning and implementing steps, that is, methods of nutritional support and patient education.

DOCUMENTATION OF NUTRITIONAL CARE

Information on the patient's medical care is recorded in the **medical record** or medical **chart**. The medical record must be accurate because it is considered to be a legal document. It serves a number of purposes:

1. Documenting all aspects of medical care.
2. Facilitating communication and promoting coordination of the activities of the members of the health care team. This team consists, at a minimum, of a physician, nurse, nutritional care specialist, and, usually, a pharmacist. For a given patient it might also include a social worker, physical and occupational therapists, clinical psychologist, speech therapist, and a variety of other allied health professionals.
3. Promoting education of members of the health care team by documenting the reasoning processes leading to care decisions.
4. Serving as a basis for the evaluation of health care delivery, including hospital accreditation and peer review.[1]
5. Providing data for financial management.

In the present atmosphere of attempting to control health care costs, documentation of nutritional care is essential. Medicare and Medicaid, programs of the U.S. government, provide major support of health care. In order to reduce cost, the Medicare Prospec-

tive Payment System was established. Under this program, conditions treated are classified into diagnosis-related groups (DRGs), and payment, based on severity of the condition and typical length of hospital stay, is made according to the diagnostic classification. Some examples are as follows:[2]

Condition	Severity Factor	Length of Stay (days)
Tonsillectomy	0.3100	1.5
Liver transplant	4.1790	20.8
Underweight	0.7923	6.0

Malnutrition has been shown to cause longer lengths of stay, higher costs, and increased mortality rate. If malnutrition is listed among the diagnoses as a complication or a co-morbidity factor, it may be possible to increase the reimbursement for the care of that patient.

Under the prospective payment system, there is strong incentive to reduce costs, and the effectiveness of nutritional services must be demonstrated in order to justify their existence. Evidence of effectiveness might include decreased average length of hospital stay, decreased hospital admissions or clinic visits, and decreased mortality rate. The necessary supporting data are obtained from the medical record. Therefore, the nutritional care specialist must be accurate and dependable in documenting nutritional care services.

Two formats of medical records are in common use, the **problem-oriented medical record** (POMR) and the **source-oriented medical record** (SOMR). The problem-oriented record is the newer system and is thought by many to be superior.[3,4]

Problem-Oriented Medical Record

The POMR is particularly useful in assuring recognition of all the patient's problems and promoting coordination of the activities of all members of the health care team. It consists of four major parts: the data base, a problem list, the initial care plan, and progress notes.[5] In addition, the record will include flow sheets and a discharge summary.

Data Base

The data base is established at the time that care is initiated. It is the basis for the diagnosis and treatment plan. It includes a **patient profile**—that is, a description of the patient along with relevant environmental, social, and family factors—the patient's perception of his purpose in seeking care (the chief complaint), previous medical history, and family medical history. It also contains the review of systems, a series of focused screening questions arranged by organ systems. In addition, the results of physical examination, the results of laboratory tests and other diagnostic procedures, and the nutrition history are included. The original nutritional assessment is included in the data base. A list of commonly used abbreviations is given in Appendix B.

Problem List

Based on these data, a master problem list is established by the physician. A problem is anything that requires diagnostic procedures or management. Problems may be symptoms, an abnormal physiologic or laboratory test result, a diagnosis, or social, nutritional, or psychiatric factors. **Current problems** are those for which an initial plan will be written, whereas **inactive problems** are those that require no further management. New problems are added to the current list as they become known, and those that are resolved are moved to the inactive list.

Allergies, sensitivities, and intolerances to foods and drugs, such as gluten intolerance, milk allergy, or penicillin allergy, should be included in the problem list. Problems related to previously prescribed diets or drugs also are listed. These might include the diabetic patient who does not follow a given diet, for instance.

The problem list is usually kept at the front of the chart and acts as a table of contents, with each problem bearing its own number. In most institutions, only the physician adds items to or removes an item from the problem list, while in other institutions, other professionals may add to the list.

Initial Care Plans

Plans for dealing with each problem are written by the physician in a standardized format containing the following elements, known by the acronym SOAP:

Subjective data: Any information obtained from the patient or the patient's family that is pertinent to the listed problem is recorded, including the patient's perception of how he or she feels and his or her description of symptoms and other concerns (e.g., "I get diarrhea every time I drink milk").

Objective data: Data obtained from tests, analyses, or observations made by members of the health care team that can be confirmed by others are listed (e.g., blood or urine analyses, roentgenograms, diet analysis, measures of intake or output, observations of behavior).

Assessment: The physician gives the interpretation (diagnosis), if known, or his or her impression of the significance of the problem.

Plan: Specific plans are stated for dealing with each problem.

For each problem, plans may be of several types. If the diagnosis is unknown, plans are made to obtain further information leading to diagnosis. These plans are listed under the subheading **Dx**. Specific treatment plans under the subheading **Rx**, including nutritional care such as a modified diet, may be instituted. Referral to the nutritional care specialist may be made at this time. Patient education, including nutritional counseling of the patient or significant other, is included under the subheading **Pt. Ed. (Significant**

other is a sociologist's term referring to important persons in the individual's social system. In nutrition, this usually means those with whom the patient lives and shares meals or other close family members.)

Progress Notes

Once the initial problem list is established, the continuing care of the patient is documented chronologically in the POMR by those involved in that care. Progress notes, marked with the number of the problem to which they are related, are contributed by the physician, nursing staff, nutritional care specialist, physical therapist, occupational therapist, social worker, or any other professional involved in the care of that patient. The type of note (for example, nutrition note, nutrition consult, or dietitian's note) is stated also.

Progress notes are also written in SOAP format. In this fashion, all members of the health care team are aware of the functions, contributions, and activities of all the others. Coordination and cooperation are thus fostered. It should be obvious that, since thought processes must be documented, the POMR also is an educational tool for the health professionals who read these notes.

Table 3-1 suggests items which are appropriate for inclusion in progress notes. The nutritional care specialist must include only those items which are relevant to a problem in the problem list.

Table 3-1. Suggested Items for a Nutritional Care Progress Note

Subjective and Objective Data	Assessment	Plan

Significant history:
  Eating habits
  Life style
	Pertinent prior intake and relationship to current problem	*Dx:*
		Recommend consultation or evaluation by others
		Recommendation for more comprehensive nutritional assessment

Pertinent laboratory values	Eating habits	
Adequacy of prior intake	Life-style influences	
Current intake	Current dietary intake	

Previous experience with modified diet	Current nutritional status:
	  Anthropometric data
	  Weight (change)
		Rx:
		Diet recommended
		Provision of special equipment

Patient comments about prescribed diet	Interpretation of significant laboratory values	Recommendation of feeding route Volume and frequency of nutrient delivery

Contraindicated foods:
  Allergies
  Drug interactions
	Patient's ability to accept and understand diet counseling	Referrals for public aid or other social services

Ethnic food preferences	Factors that limit food intake	*Pt. Ed.:* Nutrition education Referral for follow-up
Anthropometric data (weight, height, and ideal weight are always given)		

Psychosocial problems:
  Alcoholism
  Drug addiction
  Advanced age
  Poverty
  Psychosis		

Accidents or unusual events		
Error in diet control		
Error in feeding schedule		

Factors limiting food intake:
  Impaired ability to feed self
  Impaired ability to eat		

Prepared from information in Zeman, F.J., and Ney, D.M., *Applications in Clinical Nutrition.* Englewood Cliffs, N.J.: Prentice Hall, 1988.

Using the example of a particular male patient, selected items appropriate to narrative notes might be:

S: A statement from the patient or significant other, pertinent to the problem, that reflects changes in his symptoms, concerns, and feelings. *Example:* "I felt very hungry and light-headed yesterday afternoon."

O: Data that indicate the patient's response to treatment and education. *Example:* Blood glucose level in midafternoon measured 40 mg/dl.

A: Interpretation of subjective and objective data that reveals the patient's progress and the causes of new problems. *Example:* The subjective and objective data suggest hypoglycemia in the midafternoon.

P: Suggestions for formulation of new or revised plans based on the new assessment. Plans may be directed toward obtaining more information (Dx), treatment (Rx), or education (Pt. Ed.). *Examples:* Rx: Redistribute the carbohydrate in the diet to provide a midafternoon snack that will prevent hypoglycemia. Pt. Ed.: Instruct the patient on the change in his diet.

Development of skill in writing appropriate SOAP notes requires opportunity for practice.[6]

Other Pertinent Information

Two other items of interest to the nutritional care specialist are also contained in the medical record. **Flow sheets** are records of data that are obtained periodically. Some examples of this type of data are temperature, pulse, respiration, medications, and nutrient intake. These may accompany or follow the progress notes. The **discharge summary** includes a note in SOAP format on each problem and summarizes the level of resolution of that problem at the time the patient is discharged. This is written by a physician.

Source-Oriented Medical Record

The SOMR is organized so that similar types of information from similar sources are filed together. There may or may not be a problem list. The components of the SOMR are patient identification data, admission notes, physician's orders, laboratory reports, medication records, consents, consultations, operating room records, progress notes, and flow sheets. The patient identification data and admission notes contain the same information as the data base of the POMR.

NUTRITIONAL ASSESSMENT

The first step in the nutritional care process is the assessment of the patient's current status. A great deal of evidence in recent years has shown that protein-calorie malnutrition is distressingly prevalent in hospital patients[7-10] and that patients often deteriorate during hospitalization.[8] The evidence also indicates that aggressive nutritional care with promotion and maintenance of good nutritional status results in more rapid wound healing and decreased incidence of infections and other complications, with a decreased mortality rate.

It is possible, but rare, for vitamin and mineral deficiencies to exist in hospitalized patients in the absence of coexisting protein or calorie deficits.[11] In addition, vitamin and mineral deficiencies can be more rapidly treated than can protein-calorie malnutrition. As a result, assessment of protein and calorie nutritional status is given highest priority. An important function of nutritional assessment, therefore, is to identify patients who are protein-calorie malnourished or who have exceptionally high needs and are likely to become protein-calorie malnourished (Table 3-2). Once identified, these patients can be provided with special nutritional support. It is obvious from Table 3-2 that many patients are potential candidates for special attention.

Conditions resulting from protein and calorie malnutrition were once thought to be confined to underdeveloped countries, but marasmus (or cachexia) or a kwashiorkor-like syndrome, or a combination of these two syndromes, has been found in hospitalized

Table 3-2. Conditions Suggesting Nutritional Risk

Inadequate nutrient intake (quantity or quality)	*Increased nutrient losses*
Alcoholism	Abnormal metabolism (selected hepatic, renal, and endocrine disorders)
Drug addiction	
Avoidance of specified food groups (meat, eggs, milk; fruits and vegetables; grains)	Alcoholism
	Blood loss
Constipation, hemorrhoids, diverticulosis	Ascitic and pleural taps (centesis)
Poor dentition	Diarrhea
Food idiosyncrasies	Draining abscesses, fistulas, and wounds
Poverty; isolation	Diabetes (uncontrolled)
Anorexia (from disease process, drugs, emotional problems)	Peritoneal dialysis or hemodialysis
	Recurrent vomiting
Recent weight loss or gain	Exudative enteropathy
Allergies	*Increased nutrient requirements*
Inappropriate food choices from lack of information	Fever
Following head or neck trauma, gastrointestinal surgery	Hyperthyroidism
	Athetosis
Loss of senses of taste or smell	Surgery, trauma, burns, infections, pulmonary diseases with dyspnea
Ill-fitting dentures	
	Tissue hypoxia
Inadequate nutrient absorption	Normal physiologic stresses (infancy, childhood, adolescence, pregnancy, lactation)
Related to drug use (antacids, anticonvulsants, laxatives, neomycin, cholestyramine)	
	Multiple birth
Malabsorption (diarrhea, steatorrhea)	Frequent conceptions
Intestinal parasites	Previous stillbirth, prematures
Gastrointestinal surgery (gastrectomy, intestinal resection)	Malignancy
	Other
Pernicious anemia	Radiation treatment
Pancreatic disease	Aging
	Conditions related to overnutrition (excessive vitamin intake; obesity)
Decreased nutrient utilization	
Inborn errors of metabolism	Failure to thrive
Alcoholism	Mental illness
Related to drug use (anticonvulsants, antimetabolites, oral contraceptives, isoniazid)	Hypertension; Hyperlipemia

patients.[12] The detection and differentiation of these conditions have been shown to be important in the further treatment of the patient.

These findings have led to a more general appreciation of the importance of good nutrition in the care of patients and greater participation by nutritional care specialists in that care. At the same time, financial limitations require that nutritional support be directed to those patients whose need for such support is greatest.

Assessment Procedures

There is no good single test that provides a measure of nutritional status. Instead, a variety of somewhat nonspecific indicators are used to provide the basis for evaluation.[13] Those in current use will be described. Further study should provide more precise procedures in the future.

The assessment process consists of data gathering followed by an interpretation of the data for the identification of the problems. The methods used to gather the data necessary to assess nutritional status are classified as anthropometric, biochemical, clinical, and dietary. These sometimes are referred to as the ABCDs of nutritional assessment.

Some parameters of value include body weight in relation to height, an estimate of fat stores, an estimate of body proteins, and a nutritional history. For convenience in assessment of protein-calorie status, the body proteins are considered to exist in two compartments—the **somatic proteins** (in skeletal muscle) and the **visceral proteins**, consisting of all others. A measure of **cell-mediated immunity**, a subdivision of the visceral protein compartment, has been found to be especially important in indicating the potential for infection (see Chapter 6). These data currently are used in nutritional assessment in many institutions. Their limitations as well as their functions will be discussed.

Weight in Relation to Height

Height. The patient's height may be obtained with a vertical measuring rod or length may be measured on the bedfast patient. It is sometimes difficult to accurately measure height of patients who have large fat deposits on the back or deformities caused by vertebral collapse, arthritis, kyphosis, osteoporosis, or pulmonary disease. There is also a shortening of stature with advancing age. These conditions alter trunk length primarily but have little effect on limb length. For all such patients, true stature may be estimated from limb length. In one method, stature is obtained by doubling the distance from the patient's sternal notch to the fingertips.

An alternative method uses **knee height**, the distance from the bottom of the heel to the top of the knee when the knee is bent 90°. Total stature is calculated using these equations:

For men: height = 64.19 − (0.04 × age)
  + (2.02 × knee height)   (3-1)

For women: height = 84.88 − (0.24 × age)
  + (1.83 × knee height)   (3-2)

where knee height and total height are in centimeters and age is rounded to the nearest whole year.

If measurements are not available, it may be necessary to ask the patient or a family member for this information. Accurate height data are necessary for evaluation of body weight and in the calculation of creatinine-height index, body mass index, and basal energy expenditure, described in the following sections. The use of height is essential in evaluation of growth in children.

Weight. Body weight is obtained with the patient standing on a scale, or by use of a bed scale for bedridden patients. The patient's body weight may be evaluated in several ways.

1. Compared to a standard weight for height. The most commonly used table has been published by the Metropolitan Life Insurance Company, reproduced in Table 3-3. The tables give weight ranges at ages 25–59 years based on lowest mortality and subdivided into three frame-size categories, small, medium, and large. The table also assumes the person is wearing shoes with 1-inch heels. Women are assumed to be wearing 3 pounds of clothing, and men, 5 pounds of clothing.

   Body frame size may be estimated by measuring elbow breadth, the distance between the two prominent bones on either side of the elbow. Table 3-4 gives elbow breadth for medium frame. Lower values indicate a smaller frame, and higher values, a large frame. Alternatively, the wrist circumference is measured just distal (toward the hand) to the styloid process at the wrist crease of the right hand. The ratio (r) of body frame size to wrist circumference is calculated with the formula

$$r = \frac{H}{C} \qquad (3\text{-}3)$$

where H = height in centimeters and C = wrist circumference in centimeters. Frame size is determined from the following:

	r Value	
Frame Size	Men	Women
Small	>10.4	>10.9
Medium	10.4–9.6	10.9–9.9
Large	<9.6	<9.9

An alternative set of standards is based on

Table 3-3. 1983 Metropolitan Height and Weight Tables

Men					Women				
Height		Small Frame	Medium Frame	Large Frame	Height		Small Frame	Medium Frame	Large Frame
Feet	Inches				Feet	Inches			
5	2	128–134	131–141	138–150	4	10	102–111	109–121	118–131
5	3	130–136	133–143	140–153	4	11	103–113	111–123	120–134
5	4	132–138	135–145	142–156	5	0	104–115	113–126	122–137
5	5	134–140	137–148	144–160	5	1	106–118	115–129	125–140
5	6	136–142	139–151	146–164	5	2	108–121	118–132	128–143
5	7	138–145	142–154	149–168	5	3	111–124	121–135	131–147
5	8	140–148	145–157	152–172	5	4	114–127	124–138	134–151
5	9	142–151	148–160	155–176	5	5	117–130	127–141	137–155
5	10	144–154	151–163	158–180	5	6	120–133	130–144	140–159
5	11	146–157	154–166	161–184	5	7	123–136	133–147	143–163
6	0	149–160	157–170	164–188	5	8	126–139	136–150	146–167
6	1	152–164	160–174	168–192	5	9	129–142	139–153	149–170
6	2	155–168	164–178	172–197	5	10	132–145	142–156	152–173
6	3	158–172	167–182	176–202	5	11	135–148	145–159	155–176
6	4	162–176	171–187	181–207	6	0	138–151	148–162	158–179

Source of basic data: 1979 Build Study, Society of Actuaries and Association of Life Insurance Medical Directors of America, 1980. Reproduced with permission from Metropolitan Life Insurance Company.

Weights at ages 25–59 based on lowest mortality. Weight in pounds according to frame (in indoor clothing weighing 5 lb. for men and 3 lb. for women; shoes with 1″ heels).

population surveys.[14] The standards are given for individuals aged 18–24 and for 10-year intervals to age 75. Various percentile values are also given to aid in interpretation. For children, a number of "growth charts" are available. They relate height (length) and weight to age, weight to height, and head circumference to length and weight (see Appendix L). Spe-

Table 3-4. An Approximation of Frame Size

Height in 1″ heels	Elbow Breadth
Men	
5′2″–5′3″	2½″–2⅞″
5′4″–5′7″	2⅝″–2⅞″
5′8″–5′11″	2¾″–3″
6′0″–6′3″	2¾″–3⅛″
6′4″	2⅞″–3¼″
Women	
4′10″–4′11″	2¼″–2½″
5′0″–5′3″	2¼″–2½″
5′4″–5′7″	2⅜″–2⅝″
5′8″–5′11″	2⅜″–2⅝″
6′0″	2½″–2¾″

Reproduced with permission from Metropolitan Life Insurance Company.

cial growth charts are used to evaluate growth of premature infants.[15]

2. If tables are not available, a standard that will be called here the optimum body weight (OBW) may be quickly estimated using one of the following equations:

For men: OBW = 106 lb. + 6 lb. for each inch over 60 (+10% over age 50) **(3-4)**

For women: OBW = 100 lb. + 5 lb. for each inch over 60 (+10% over age 50) **(3-5)**

The results of these equations differ from values given in Table 3-3. Values for body weights similar to those in the table may be obtained from the equations:

For men: OBW = 135 lb. + 3 lb. for each inch over 63 **(3-6)**

For women: OBW = 119 lb. + 3 lb. for each inch over 60 **(3-7)**

A range of ±10% is allowed for frame size.

A factor must be added to the measured weight if the patient has an amputation. Estimated weights of body parts are as follows:

Entire leg	18.6% of total body weight
Above-knee amputation	11.0%
Below-knee amputation	7.0%
Foot	1.7%
Entire arm	6.2%
Forearm and hand	2.6%
Hand	0.3%

The total body weight (TBW) would be calculated with the equation:

$$TBW = \frac{\text{measured weight}}{100 - \text{\% weight of amputation}} \times 100 \quad \textbf{(3-8)}$$

For example: A man has a below-the-knee amputation. His measured body weight is 170 lb. His total weight without amputation would be

$$TBW = \frac{170 \times 100}{100 - 7} = 182.8 \text{ lb.}$$

Interpretation. The patient's body weight as a proportion of the standard is calculated with the equation:

$$\% \ OBW = \frac{\text{current weight}}{OBW} \times 100 \quad \textbf{(3-9)}$$

Many patients are obese at the onset of their illness. Significant weight loss may not be noted in these patients if they are still at or above OBW. Height-weight relationships are also invalid if the patient is retaining fluid and has edema or is dehydrated. Therefore, weight **change** and **direction** of change, rather than absolute weight, are often more useful. The percentage of change from usual to present body weight can be calculated

using the equation

$$\% \text{ weight change} = \frac{\text{usual weight} - \text{present weight}}{\text{usual weight}} \times 100$$

$$\textbf{(3-10)}$$

One basis for interpretation of the change in weight is given in Table 3-5. If 20% of a patient's body weight is lost, that patient's risk of mortality increases.[16,17]

In another approach to interpretation, Tables 3-6 and 3-7 provide weight-for-height data at various ages. Values at the 50th, 15th, and 5th percentiles are given. Weights above the 15th percentile have been interpreted to be within normal range; weights between the 5th and 15th percentiles indicate that the patient is at risk of malnutrition. Patients below the 5th percentile in weight for height are considered malnourished.

In some cases, it is necessary to evaluate the degree of the patient's obesity. Procedures used, including the body mass index (Equation 12-3), are discussed in Chapter 12.

Estimation of Energy Stores

For patients who require further assessment, the thickness of skinfolds gives an indication of subcutaneous fat and is considered an index of stored energy.[18-23] Conversely, the results may suggest the severity and duration of inadequate energy intake.

Table 3-5. Evaluation of Weight Change

Time	Significant Weight Loss (% of change)	Severe Weight Loss (% of change)
1 week	1–2	>2
1 month	5	>5
3 months	7.5	>7.5
6 months	10	>10

Reprinted with permission from Blackburn, G.L., Bistrian, B.R., Maini, B.S., et al., Nutritional and metabolic assessment of the hospitalized patient. *JPEN* 1:15, 1977. © 1977, American Society of Parenteral and Enteral Nutrition.

Table 3-6. Weight (pounds) for Height (inches), Males

Height in Inches	Percentile	Age Group in Years					
		18−24	25−34	35−44	45−54	55−64	65−74
62	50	130	141	143	147	143	143
	15	102	109	115	118	113	116
	5	85	91	98	100	96	100
63	50	135	145	148	152	147	147
	15	107	113	120	123	117	120
	5	90	95	103	105	100	104
64	50	140	150	153	156	153	151
	15	112	118	125	127	123	124
	5	95	100	108	109	106	108
65	50	145	156	158	160	158	156
	15	117	124	130	131	128	129
	5	100	106	113	113	111	113
66	50	150	160	163	164	163	160
	15	122	128	135	135	133	133
	5	105	110	118	117	116	117
67	50	154	165	169	169	168	164
	15	126	133	141	140	138	137
	5	109	115	124	122	121	121
68	50	159	170	174	173	173	169
	15	131	138	146	144	143	142
	5	114	120	129	126	126	126
69	50	164	174	179	177	178	173
	15	136	142	151	148	148	146
	5	119	124	134	130	131	130
70	50	168	179	184	182	183	177
	15	140	147	156	153	153	150
	5	123	129	139	135	136	134
71	50	173	184	190	187	189	182
	15	145	152	162	158	159	155
	5	128	134	145	140	142	139
72	50	178	189	194	191	193	186
	15	150	157	166	162	163	159
	5	133	139	149	144	146	143
73	50	183	194	200	196	197	190
	15	155	162	172	167	167	163
	5	138	144	155	149	150	147
74	50	188	199	205	200	203	194
	15	160	167	177	171	173	167
	5	143	149	160	153	156	151

Reprinted with permission from Ross Laboratories, Columbus, OH 43216. From *Nutritional Assessment Summary Sheet*, © 1982 Ross Laboratories.

The skinfolds over the triceps muscle, biceps muscle, superiliac crest, or the subscapular are sometimes measured to provide greater reliability. However, for practical purposes, it is more common to use the triceps skinfold (TSF) only. Changes in the patient's state of hydration, edema, and variations in technique serve as sources of error. Therefore, it is suggested that the same person take repeated measurements to reduce variation and determine the direction of change with treatment. Although it often is recommended that these measurements be made with the patient standing,[18,24] measurements made on supine patients have also been found to be acceptable.[25] The TSF

Table 3-7. Weight (pounds) for Height (inches), Females

Height in Inches	Percentile	Age Group in Years					
		18–24	25–34	35–44	45–54	55–64	65–74
57	50	114	118	125	129	132	130
	15	85	85	89	94	97	100
	5	68	65	67	73	77	82
58	50	117	121	129	133	136	134
	15	88	88	93	98	101	104
	5	71	68	71	77	81	86
59	50	120	125	133	136	140	137
	15	91	92	97	101	105	107
	5	74	72	75	80	85	89
60	50	123	128	137	140	143	140
	15	94	95	101	105	108	110
	5	77	75	79	84	88	92
61	50	126	132	141	143	147	144
	15	97	99	105	108	112	114
	5	80	79	83	87	92	96
62	50	129	136	144	147	150	147
	15	100	103	108	112	115	117
	5	83	83	86	91	95	99
63	50	132	139	148	150	153	151
	15	103	106	112	115	118	121
	5	86	86	90	94	98	103
64	50	135	142	152	154	157	154
	15	106	109	116	119	122	124
	5	89	89	94	98	102	106
65	50	138	146	156	158	160	158
	15	109	113	120	123	125	128
	5	92	93	98	102	105	110
66	50	141	150	159	161	164	161
	15	112	117	123	126	129	131
	5	95	97	101	105	109	113
67	50	144	153	163	165	167	165
	15	115	120	127	130	132	135
	5	98	100	105	109	112	117
68	50	147	157	167	168	171	169
	15	118	124	131	133	136	139
	5	101	104	109	112	116	121

is measured with calipers, usually on the nondominant arm, halfway between the olecranon and acromial processes (Figure 3-1).[17,26,27]

There is more than one approach to interpretation of TSF, and also of other anthropometric measurements. One approach is to compare the measurements with the reference values (Table 3-8) using the following equation:

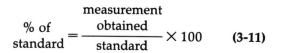

$$\% \text{ of standard} = \frac{\text{measurement obtained}}{\text{standard}} \times 100 \qquad \textbf{(3-11)}$$

However, it must be kept in mind that the "standards" used are not true standards. They were adopted from Jelliffe's data,[28] which were designed for use in developing

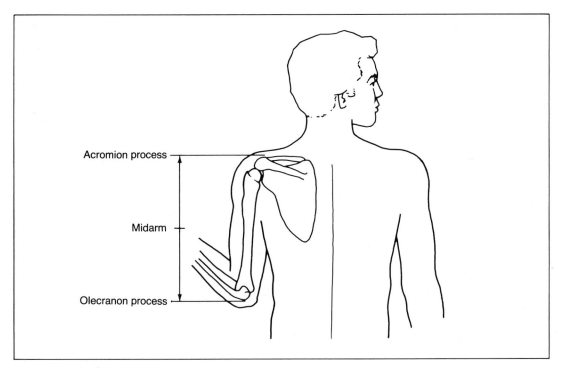

Figure 3-1. Finding the midarm point.

countries. Sometimes the terms **reference data** or **reference values** are considered preferable.

One approach to interpretation of the

Table 3-8. Standards for Anthropometric Measurements

Sex	Triceps Skinfold (mm)	Midarm Circum-ference (cm)	Midarm Muscle Circum-ference (cm)
Standard			
Men	12.5	29.3	25.3
Women	16.5	28.5	23.2
80% of standard			
Men	10.0	23.4	20.2
Women	13.2	22.8	18.6
60% of standard			
Men	7.5	17.6	15.2
Women	9.9	17.1	13.2

values obtained is given in Table 3-9. Mild, moderate, and severe malnutrition are not well defined, and the numerical definitions given in Table 3-9 have not been rigidly validated. As a consequence, percentile values, obtained from a large population in the United States,[29] have been suggested[29,30] to serve as better standards. They also provide for adjustments for age. The percentile values are given in Tables 3-10 and 3-11. Malnourished subjects may be considered to have TSF at the 5th percentile or below, and to be at risk if between the 5th and 15th percentiles.[28] An alternative interpretation provides the following guidelines:[31]

Mild deficiency	35th–40th percentile
Moderate deficiency	25th–35th percentile
Severe deficiency	<25th percentile

A variation of the use of TSF to indicate energy reserve is the use of midarm fat area (MAFA). This method requires the measure, first, of midarm circumference (MAC) with a tape measure (Figure 3-2). The TSF measure

Table 3-9. Interpretation of Nutritional Assessment Values

Observation[a]	Deficit			
	None	Mild	Moderate	Severe
TSF (% of standard)	>90	90–51	50–30	<30
AMC (% of standard)	>90	90–81	80–70	<70
CHI (% of standard)	>90	90–81	80–71	70–60
Serum albumin (g/dl)	>3.5	<3.5–3.2	<3.2–2.8	<2.8
Transferrin (mg/dl)	>200	<200–180	<180–160	<160
TIBC (µg/dl)	>214	<214–182	<182–152	<152
Total lymphocytes (per mm³)	>1,500	1,500–1,201	1,200–800	<800

Values compiled from Blackburn, G.L., Bistrian, B.R., Maini, B.S., et al., Nutritional and metabolic assessment of the hospitalized patient. *JPEN* 1:11–22, 1977; and Blackburn, G.L., Nutritional assessment: An overview. *Clin. Consult. Nutr. Support* 1:10, 1981.

[a] TSF = thickness of triceps skinfold; AMC = arm muscle circumference; CHI = creatinine-height index; TIBC = total iron-binding capacity.

is also used to calculate the MAFA with the equation

$$MAFA \ (cm^2) = \left[\frac{MAC \times TSF}{2} \right]$$
$$- \frac{3.14 \times (TSF)^2}{4} \qquad (3\text{-}12)$$

Percentile values for arm circumference are given in Table 3-12, and MAFA, in Table 3-13. It has been suggested that MAFA is more useful than the TSF.[32]

None of the criteria described have been rigidly validated. Under these circumstances, the TSF measurements must be combined with other assessment procedures and seasoned well with good clinical judgment.

Estimates of Somatic Protein

There are several methods for estimating skeletal muscle mass.

Circumference of Midarm Muscle. Midarm muscle circumference (MAMC) may be calculated using the triceps skinfold and midarm circumference (see Figures 3-2 and 3-3) to indicate muscle mass or somatic protein[18] using the equation

$$MAMC = MAC - (0.314 \times TSF) \qquad (3\text{-}13)$$

where MAMC and MAC are in cm and TSF in mm.

Standards for MAMC are given in Table 3-8 with suggested interpretations in Table 3-9. Percentile values are given in Table 3-12.

Midarm Muscle Area. The midarm muscle area (MAMA) can also be calculated from data described previously, with the equation

$$MAMA = \frac{(MAC - 3.14 \ TSF)^2}{4 \times 3.14} \qquad (3\text{-}14)$$

where MAMA is in mm² and MAC and TSF in mm. Percentile standards of comparison are given in Table 3-13. Muscle area has also been suggested to be more useful than MAC.[32]

Creatinine-Height Index. An additional test of somatic protein requires the collection of a 24-hour urine sample, a procedure that must be ordered by the attending physician. From this sample, the amount of creatinine excreted is determined by chemical analysis. Creatinine normally is formed in an amount proportionate to muscle mass, and its urinary excretion is related to the amount of skeletal muscle. In patients of ideal body

Table 3-10. Percentiles for Triceps Skinfold (mm)[a]

Age Group	Males								Females							
	n	5	10	25	50	75	90	95	n	5	10	25	50	75	90	95
1–1.9	228	6	7	8	10	12	14	16	204	6	7	8	10	12	14	16
2–2.9	223	6	7	8	10	12	14	15	208	6	8	9	10	12	15	16
3–3.9	220	6	7	8	10	11	14	15	208	7	8	9	11	12	14	15
4–4.9	230	6	6	8	9	11	12	14	208	7	8	8	10	12	14	16
5–5.9	214	6	6	8	9	11	14	15	219	6	7	8	10	12	15	18
6–6.9	117	5	6	7	8	10	13	16	118	6	6	8	10	12	14	16
7–7.9	122	5	6	7	9	12	15	17	126	6	7	9	11	13	16	18
8–8.9	117	5	6	7	8	10	13	16	118	6	8	9	12	15	18	24
9–9.9	121	6	6	7	10	13	17	18	125	8	8	10	13	16	20	22
10–10.9	146	6	6	8	10	14	18	21	152	7	8	10	12	17	23	27
11–11.9	122	6	6	8	11	16	20	24	117	7	8	10	13	18	24	28
12–12.9	153	6	6	8	11	14	22	28	129	8	9	11	14	18	23	27
13–13.9	134	5	5	7	10	14	22	26	151	8	8	12	15	21	26	30
14–14.9	131	4	5	7	9	14	21	24	141	9	10	13	16	21	26	28
15–15.9	128	4	5	6	8	11	18	24	117	8	10	12	17	21	25	32
16–16.9	131	4	5	6	8	12	16	22	142	10	12	15	18	22	26	31
17–17.9	133	5	5	6	8	12	16	19	114	10	12	13	19	24	30	37
18–18.9	91	4	5	6	9	13	20	24	109	10	12	15	18	22	26	30
19–24.9	531	4	5	7	10	15	20	22	1,060	10	11	14	18	24	30	34
25–34.9	971	5	6	8	12	16	20	24	1,987	10	12	16	21	27	34	37
35–44.9	806	5	6	8	12	16	20	23	1,614	12	14	18	23	29	35	38
45–54.9	898	6	6	8	12	15	20	25	1,047	12	16	20	25	30	36	40
55–64.9	734	5	6	8	11	14	19	22	809	12	16	20	25	31	36	38
65–74.9	1,503	4	6	8	11	15	19	22	1,670	12	14	18	24	29	34	36

Reproduced from Frisancho, A.R., New norms of upper limb fat and muscle areas for assessment of nutritional status. *Am. J. Clin. Nutr.* 34:2541, 1981, © *Am. J. Clin. Nutr.*, American Society for Clinical Nutrition.

[a] Data collected from whites in the United States Health and Nutrition Examination Survey I (1971–1974).

Table 3-11. Thickness of Triceps and Subscapular Skinfolds at 1 to 36 Months of Age

Age (months)	Percentiles	Triceps (mm)		Subscapular (mm)	
		Males	Females	Males	Females
1	2.5	2.9	3.5	3.1	3.8
	10	4.0	4.5	4.2	4.9
	25	4.7	5.2	4.8	5.4
	50	5.3	5.8	5.6	6.2
	75	6.2	6.7	6.5	7.0
	90	7.0	7.6	7.5	7.9
	97.5	8.1	8.3	8.3	9.0
3	2.5	4.5	5.0	3.5	4.7
	10	6.0	6.2	4.9	5.9
	25	6.8	7.2	5.8	6.9
	50	8.1	8.2	6.9	8.0
	75	9.2	9.2	8.1	8.6
	90	10.3	10.5	9.0	9.4
	97.5	11.7	11.8	10.7	11.1
6	2.5	6.3	6.7	3.8	4.0
	10	7.8	8.2	5.5	5.9
	25	8.6	9.0	6.2	6.9
	50	9.7	10.4	7.1	8.1
	75	11.1	11.3	8.4	8.9
	90	11.8	12.7	10.1	10.3
	97.5	13.5	13.9	11.0	12.4
9	2.5	6.0	6.7	3.4	4.7
	10	7.5	7.9	5.3	6.0
	25	8.7	8.8	6.0	6.7
	50	9.9	10.1	7.1	7.6
	75	11.2	11.3	8.5	8.8
	90	12.5	12.5	9.7	10.1
	97.5	14.0	13.5	11.4	11.1
12	2.5	6.2	6.4	3.8	4.5
	10	7.8	7.6	5.3	6.0
	25	8.6	8.7	6.0	6.5
	50	9.8	9.8	7.2	7.5
	75	11.1	11.2	8.6	8.7
	90	12.2	12.2	9.6	9.8
	97.5	13.8	13.6	11.0	10.9
18	2.5	6.4	6.8	3.9	4.2
	10	7.7	7.9	5.3	5.7
	25	8.6	8.9	6.0	6.2
	50	9.9	10.3	6.8	7.1
	75	11.4	11.3	7.9	8.0
	90	12.2	12.3	9.3	9.0
	97.5	13.6	13.6	10.3	10.2
24	2.5	5.8	6.5	3.0	3.9
	10	7.4	8.3	4.6	5.3
	25	8.5	8.9	5.4	5.6
	50	9.8	10.1	6.5	6.5
	75	11.6	11.6	7.4	7.3
	90	13.1	12.8	8.3	8.4
	97.5	14.2	14.1	10.2	9.5
36	2.5	6.6	6.4	2.9	2.6
	10	7.8	8.2	4.5	4.7
	25	9.0	9.4	5.0	5.2
	50	9.8	10.3	5.5	6.1
	75	11.0	11.5	6.4	7.2
	90	12.2	12.5	7.1	8.6
	97.5	13.4	14.4	8.9	10.6

Adapted from Karlberg, P., et al., The development of children in a Swedish urban community: A prospective longitudinal study. III. Physical growth during the first three years of life. *Acta. Pediatr. Scand.* 187:48, 1968; in Palmer, S. and S. Ervall, Eds., *Pediatric Nutrition in Developmental Disorders*, 1978. Courtesy of Charles C Thomas, Publisher, Springfield, IL.

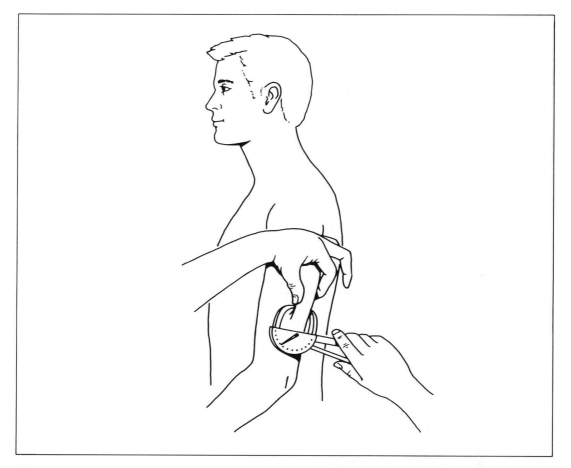

Figure 3-2. Measuring the triceps skinfold.

weight, the creatinine coefficient is 23 mg/kg ideal body weight for men and 18 mg/kg ideal body weight for women. These values have been used to make a table of ideal creatinine excretions for patients whose weights and body compositions are ideal for their heights (Tables 3-6 and 3-7). Comparison of the actual urinary creatinine excretion per 24 hours and the expected excretion of a person of the same height and sex provides a **creatinine-height index** (CHI). This calculation provides a sensitive measurement of somatic protein:

$$\text{CHI} = \frac{\substack{\text{actual} \\ \text{urinary creatinine}}}{\substack{\text{ideal urinary} \\ \text{creatinine for height}}} \times 100 \qquad \textbf{(3-15)}$$

The CHI gives an estimate of lean body mass compared to ideal body mass. Values for interpretation are provided in Table 3-9, and ideal urinary-creatinine-for-height values are given in Table 3-14. These standards are based on a small number of patients and apply only to patients with normal renal function.[29] Since the test correlates well with MAMC, it may be unnecessary duplication of information.[29] Also, since 24-hour urine samples are difficult to obtain, this test is rarely done.

Measurement of Visceral Protein

Visceral protein is often measured by biochemical assays on serum. The most commonly used values are those which are usually available.

Table 3-12. Percentiles of Upper Arm Circumference and Estimated Upper Arm Muscle Circumference[a]

Age Group	Midarm Circumference (mm)							Midarm Muscle Circumference (mm)						
	5	10	25	50	75	90	95	5	10	25	50	75	90	95
Males														
1–1.9	142	146	150	159	170	176	183	110	113	119	127	135	144	147
2–2.9	141	145	153	162	170	178	185	111	114	122	130	140	146	150
3–3.9	150	153	160	167	175	184	190	117	123	131	137	143	148	153
4–4.9	149	154	162	171	180	186	192	123	126	133	141	148	156	159
5–5.9	153	160	167	175	185	195	204	128	133	140	147	154	162	169
6–6.9	155	159	167	179	188	209	228	131	135	142	151	161	170	177
7–7.9	162	167	177	187	201	223	230	137	139	151	160	168	177	190
8–8.9	162	170	177	190	202	220	245	140	145	154	162	170	182	187
9–9.9	175	178	187	200	217	249	257	151	154	161	170	183	196	202
10–10.9	181	184	196	210	231	262	274	156	160	166	180	191	209	221
11–11.9	186	190	202	223	244	261	280	159	165	173	183	195	205	230
12–12.9	193	200	214	232	254	282	303	167	171	182	195	210	223	241
13–13.9	194	211	228	247	263	286	301	172	179	196	211	226	238	245
14–14.9	220	226	237	253	283	303	322	189	199	212	223	240	260	264
15–15.9	222	229	244	264	284	311	320	199	204	218	237	254	266	272
16–16.9	244	248	262	278	303	324	343	213	225	234	249	269	287	296
17–17.9	246	253	267	285	308	336	347	224	231	245	258	273	294	312
18–18.9	245	260	276	297	321	353	379	226	237	252	264	283	298	324
19–24.9	262	272	288	308	331	355	372	238	245	257	273	289	309	321
25–34.9	271	282	300	319	342	362	375	243	250	264	279	298	314	326
35–44.9	278	287	305	326	345	363	374	247	255	269	286	302	318	327
45–54.9	267	281	301	322	342	362	376	239	249	265	281	300	315	326
55–64.9	258	273	296	317	336	355	369	236	245	260	278	295	310	320
65–74.9	248	263	285	307	325	344	355	223	235	251	268	284	298	306

Females

Age	5	10	25	50	75	90	95	5	10	25	50	75	90	95
1–1.9	138	142	148	156	164	172	177	105	111	117	124	132	139	143
2–2.9	142	145	152	160	167	176	184	111	114	119	126	133	142	147
3–3.9	143	150	158	167	175	183	189	113	119	124	132	140	146	152
4–4.9	149	154	160	169	177	184	191	115	121	128	136	144	152	157
5–5.9	153	157	165	175	185	203	211	125	128	134	142	151	159	165
6–6.9	156	162	170	176	187	204	211	130	133	138	145	154	166	171
7–7.9	164	167	174	183	199	216	231	129	135	142	151	160	171	176
8–8.9	168	172	183	195	214	247	261	138	140	151	160	171	183	194
9–9.9	178	182	194	211	224	251	260	147	150	158	167	180	194	198
10–10.9	174	182	193	210	228	251	265	148	150	159	170	180	190	197
11–11.9	185	194	208	224	248	276	303	150	158	171	181	196	217	223
12–12.9	194	203	216	237	256	282	294	162	166	180	191	201	214	220
13–13.9	202	211	223	243	271	301	338	169	175	183	198	211	226	240
14–14.9	214	223	237	252	272	304	322	174	179	190	201	216	232	247
15–15.9	208	221	239	254	279	300	322	175	178	189	202	215	228	244
16–16.9	218	224	241	258	283	318	334	170	180	190	202	216	234	249
17–17.9	220	227	241	264	295	324	350	175	183	194	205	221	239	257
18–18.9	222	227	241	258	281	312	325	174	179	191	202	215	237	245
19–24.9	221	230	247	265	290	319	345	179	185	195	207	221	236	249
25–34.9	233	240	256	277	304	342	368	183	188	199	212	228	246	264
35–44.9	241	251	267	290	317	356	378	186	192	205	218	236	257	272
45–54.9	242	256	274	299	328	362	384	187	193	206	220	238	260	274
55–64.9	243	257	280	303	335	367	385	187	196	209	225	244	266	280
65–74.9	240	252	274	299	326	356	373	185	195	208	225	244	264	279

a Data collected from whites in the United States Health and Nutrition Examination Survey I (1971–1974).

Table 3-13. Percentiles for Estimates of Upper Arm Fat Area and Upper Arm Muscle Area[a]

Age Group	Arm Muscle Area Percentiles (mm²)							Arm Fat Area Percentiles (mm²)						
	5	10	25	50	75	90	95	5	10	25	50	75	90	95
Males														
1–1.9	956	1,014	1,133	1,278	1,447	1,644	1,720	452	486	590	741	895	1,036	1,176
2–2.9	973	1,040	1,190	1,345	1,557	1,690	1,787	434	504	578	737	871	1,044	1,148
3–3.9	1,095	1,201	1,357	1,484	1,618	1,750	1,853	464	519	590	736	868	1,071	1,151
4–4.9	1,207	1,264	1,408	1,579	1,747	1,926	2,008	428	494	598	722	859	989	1,085
5–5.9	1,298	1,411	1,550	1,720	1,884	2,089	2,285	446	488	582	713	914	1,176	1,299
6–6.9	1,360	1,447	1,605	1,815	2,056	2,297	2,493	371	446	539	678	896	1,115	1,519
7–7.9	1,497	1,548	1,808	2,027	2,246	2,494	2,886	423	473	574	758	1,011	1,393	1,511
8–8.9	1,550	1,664	1,895	2,089	2,296	2,628	2,788	410	460	588	725	1,003	1,248	1,558
9–9.9	1,811	1,884	2,067	2,288	2,657	3,053	3,257	485	527	635	859	1,252	1,864	2,081
10–10.9	1,930	2,027	2,182	2,575	2,903	3,486	3,882	523	543	738	982	1,376	1,906	2,609
11–11.9	2,016	2,156	2,382	2,670	3,022	3,359	4,226	536	595	754	1,148	1,710	2,348	2,574
12–12.9	2,216	2,339	2,649	3,022	3,496	3,968	4,640	554	650	874	1,172	1,558	2,536	3,580
13–13.9	2,363	2,546	3,044	3,553	4,081	4,502	4,794	475	570	812	1,096	1,702	2,744	3,322
14–14.9	2,830	3,147	3,586	3,963	4,575	5,368	5,530	453	563	786	1,082	1,608	2,746	3,508
15–15.9	3,138	3,317	3,788	4,481	5,134	5,631	5,900	521	595	690	931	1,423	2,434	3,100
16–16.9	3,625	4,044	4,352	4,951	5,753	6,576	6,980	542	593	844	1,078	1,746	2,280	3,041
17–17.9	3,998	4,252	4,777	5,286	5,950	6,886	7,726	598	698	827	1,096	1,636	2,407	2,888
18–18.9	4,070	4,481	5,066	5,552	6,374	7,067	8,355	560	665	860	1,264	1,947	3,302	3,928
19–24.9	4,508	4,777	5,274	5,913	6,660	7,606	8,200	594	743	963	1,406	2,231	3,098	3,652
25–34.9	4,694	4,963	5,541	6,214	7,067	7,847	8,436	675	831	1,174	1,752	2,459	3,246	3,786
35–44.9	4,844	5,181	5,740	6,490	7,265	8,034	8,488	703	851	1,310	1,792	2,463	3,098	3,624
45–54.9	4,546	4,946	5,589	6,297	7,142	7,918	8,458	749	922	1,254	1,741	2,359	3,245	3,928
55–64.9	4,422	4,783	5,381	6,144	6,919	7,670	8,149	658	839	1,166	1,645	2,236	2,976	3,466
65–74.9	3,973	4,411	5,031	5,716	6,432	7,074	7,453	573	753	1,122	1,621	2,199	2,876	3,327

Females														
1–1.9	885	973	1,084	1,221	1,378	1,535	1,621	401	466	578	706	847	1,022	1,140
2–2.9	973	1,029	1,119	1,269	1,405	1,595	1,727	469	526	642	747	894	1,061	1,173
3–3.9	1,014	1,133	1,227	1,396	1,563	1,690	1,846	473	529	656	822	967	1,106	1,158
4–4.9	1,058	1,171	1,313	1,475	1,644	1,832	1,958	490	541	654	766	907	1,109	1,236
5–5.9	1,238	1,301	1,423	1,598	1,825	2,012	2,159	470	529	647	812	991	1,330	1,536
6–6.9	1,354	1,414	1,513	1,683	1,877	2,182	2,323	464	508	638	827	1,009	1,263	1,436
7–7.9	1,330	1,441	1,602	1,815	2,045	2,332	2,469	491	560	706	920	1,135	1,407	1,644
8–8.9	1,513	1,566	1,808	2,034	2,327	2,657	2,996	527	634	769	1,042	1,383	1,872	2,482
9–9.9	1,723	1,788	1,976	2,227	2,571	2,987	3,112	642	690	933	1,219	1,584	2,171	2,524
10–10.9	1,740	1,784	2,019	2,296	2,583	2,873	3,093	616	702	842	1,141	1,608	2,500	3,005
11–11.9	1,784	1,987	2,316	2,612	3,071	3,739	3,953	707	802	1,015	1,301	1,942	2,730	3,690
12–12.9	2,092	2,182	2,579	2,904	3,225	3,655	3,847	782	854	1,090	1,511	2,056	2,666	3,369
13–13.9	2,269	2,426	2,657	3,130	3,529	4,081	4,568	726	838	1,219	1,625	2,374	3,272	4,150
14–14.9	2,418	2,562	2,874	3,220	3,704	4,294	4,850	981	1,043	1,423	1,818	2,403	3,250	3,765
15–15.9	2,426	2,518	2,847	3,248	3,689	4,123	4,756	839	1,126	1,396	1,886	2,544	3,093	4,195
16–16.9	2,308	2,567	2,865	3,248	3,718	4,353	4,946	1,126	1,351	1,663	2,006	2,598	3,374	4,236
17–17.9	2,442	2,674	2,996	3,336	3,883	4,552	5,251	1,042	1,267	1,463	2,104	2,977	3,864	5,159
18–18.9	2,398	2,538	2,917	3,243	3,694	4,461	4,767	1,003	1,230	1,616	2,104	2,617	3,508	3,733
19–24.9	2,538	2,728	3,026	3,406	3,877	4,439	4,940	1,046	1,198	1,596	2,166	2,959	4,050	4,896
25–34.9	2,661	2,826	3,148	3,573	4,138	4,806	5,541	1,173	1,399	1,841	2,548	3,512	4,690	5,560
35–44.9	2,750	2,948	3,359	3,783	4,428	5,240	5,877	1,336	1,619	2,158	2,898	3,932	5,093	5,847
45–54.9	2,784	2,956	3,378	3,858	4,520	5,375	5,974	1,459	1,803	2,447	3,244	4,229	5,416	6,140
55–64.9	2,784	3,063	3,477	4,045	4,750	5,632	6,247	1,345	1,879	2,520	3,369	4,360	5,276	6,152
65–74.9	2,737	3,018	3,444	4,019	4,739	5,566	6,214	1,363	1,681	2,266	3,063	3,943	4,914	5,530

Reproduced from Frisancho, A.R., New norms of upper limb fat and muscle areas for assessment of nutritional status. *Am. J. Clin. Nutr.* 34:2543, 1981, © *Am. J. Clin. Nutr.*, American Society for Clinical Nutrition.

[a] Data collected from whites in the United States Health and Nutrition Examination Survey I (1971–1974).

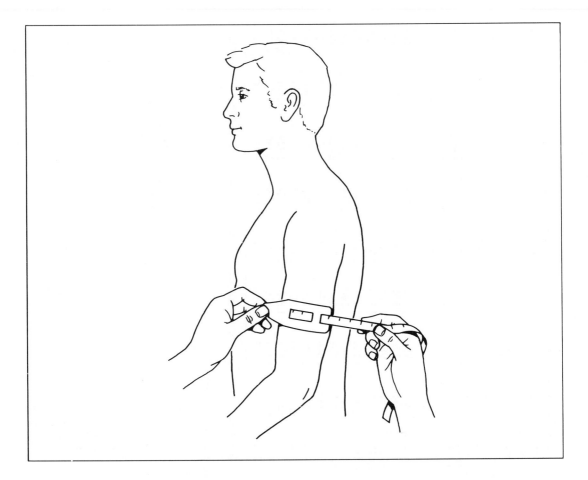

Figure 3-3. Measuring the midarm circumference.

A number of automated test panels are used, often for diagnosis or to obtain baseline data when the patient is admitted to the hospital. One of these, as an example, is the SMA 6, which provides values for bicarbonate (CO_2), sodium, potassium, chloride, blood urea nitrogen, and blood glucose. In addition, serum albumin and a complete blood count (CBC) are usually ordered when a patient is admitted. The CBC provides red cell and white cell counts, hematocrit, red cell morphology, and a differential count that gives proportions of different white cells. As a result, these values are easily available from the patient's medical record. Other tests may be available, depending on the patient's disease, or may be ordered by the physician. In particular, the serum albumin and CBC are useful in nutrition screening.

Serum albumin concentration, measured in grams per deciliter, is used in preliminary screening as an indication of visceral protein, that is, all protein other than structural protein. Normal concentration is 3.5 to 5.5 g/dl. Synthesis requires an adequate supply of amino acids and adequate hepatic function. Since albumin has a half-life of 20 days,[33] a deficit is considered an indication of impairment in protein synthesis in the liver due to a deficiency in quantity or quality of substrate, provided the patient does not have diagnosed liver disease, renal disease, congestive heart failure, or inflammation.[33,34] This value, obtained from a test ordered by the physician, is routinely available to nutritional care specialists from the patient's medical record. The severity of any deficit may be measured by comparison of the actual value and the values in Table 3-9. Total serum protein is not an adequate sub-

Table 3-14. Normal 24-Hour Urinary Creatinine Excretion Relative to Height

Children (0–9 years)		Men[a]		Women[b]	
Height (cm)	Creatinine (mg)	Height (cm)	Creatinine (mg)	Height (cm)	Creatinine (mg)
50.0	36	157.5	1,288	147.3	830
53.5	45	160.0	1,325	149.9	851
56.9	55	162.6	1,359	152.4	875
60.4	66	165.1	1,386	154.9	900
64.4	79	167.6	1,426	157.5	925
66.4	85	170.2	1,467	160.0	949
69.6	96	172.7	1,513	162.6	977
73.8	113	175.3	1,555	165.1	1,006
76.3	124	177.8	1,596	167.6	1,044
80.7	143	180.3	1,642	170.2	1,076
84.7	165	182.9	1,691	172.7	1,109
88.5	189	185.4	1,739	175.3	1,141
94.1	231	188.0	1,785	177.8	1,174
98.0	264	190.5	1,831	180.3	1,206
102.2	290	193.0	1,891	182.9	1,240
105.6	308				
108.7	337				
113.2	385				
117.2	408				
121.5	478				
124.5	528				
126.0	557				
129.0	617				

Compiled from Blackburn, G.L., Bistrian, B.R., Maini, B.S., et al., Nutritional and metabolic assessment of the hospitalized patient. *JPEN* 1:15, 1977; Viteri, F.E., and Alvarado, J., The creatinine height index. Its use in the estimation of the degree of protein depletion and repletion in protein calorie malnourished children. *Pediatrics* 46:696–706, 1970; and Graystone, J.E., Creatinine excretion during growth. In D.B. Cheek, *Human Growth, Body Composition, Cell Growth, Energy and Intelligence.* Philadelphia: Lea & Febiger, 1968, pp. 182–197.

[a] Creatinine coefficient = 23 mg/kg of ideal body weight.
[b] Creatinine coefficient = 18 mg/kg of ideal body weight.

stitute, since variation in serum globulin levels, which make up part of total protein, may introduce a large error.

Serum transferrin may be a useful alternative to serum albumin. Transferrin is synthesized in the liver and has a half-life of 8 to 10 days.[33] Normal concentration is 170 to 250 mg/dl. The measurement of plasma **total iron-binding capacity** (TIBC), a less expensive laboratory assay, sometimes is used. Serum transferrin can be calculated from TIBC, but, since the values vary proportionately, the calculation probably is not necessary. Direct measurement of transferrin is not often done. It is assayed by radioimmunodiffusion, a method not commonly available.

Normal concentration of TIBC is 250 to 410 µg/dl. A deficit in transferrin is believed to be a more sensitive indicator of visceral protein than is serum albumin because of its shorter half-life.[35-37] However, transferrin levels are affected by hepatic and renal disease, congestive heart failure, and inflammation, as is serum albumin, limiting the usefulness of either measure in these conditions. In addition, transferrin concentration is influenced by iron status. The use of prealbumin with a 2-day half-life,[38] retinol-binding protein with a 12-hour half-life,[39] fibronectin with a half-life of 12–24 hours, or somatomedin C with a half-life of 1–3 hours as an alternative to serum albumin has been suggested, but the short half-lives cause the serum values to vary with recent intake instead of longer-term protein nutrition. Values are also affected by dehydration and liver dysfunction.

The amino acid 3-methylhistidine (3-MH) is found primarily in myofibrils of the muscle. During muscle breakdown, 3-MH is released and excreted in the urine. This amino acid is not recycled. Thus the 3-MH in a 24-hour urine sample may indicate muscle turnover. The 24-hour urine collection presents a problem, and the sample also contains sarcoplasmic protein breakdown products. Excretion of 3-MH is also affected by sex, age, diet, starvation, and infection. As a consequence, this method is not used to a great extent.

Nitrogen Balance

The measurement of urea in the collected urine sample, when combined with protein intake data, can be used to give a rough estimate of **nitrogen balance**, the difference between nitrogen intake and output. When patients have high rates of protein catabolism, the increased losses of nitrogen are reflected in increased urinary excretion of urea,[40] which therefore is considered a good indicator of nitrogen excretion.[41] An additional 4 g/day is added to account for nonurea nitrogen in the urine (2 g) and the nitrogen losses in the feces (1 g) and through the integument (0.2 g). This value is relatively stable except in patients with diarrhea. Thus the equation for estimation of nitrogen balance is

$$\text{nitrogen balance} = \frac{\text{24-hour protein intake}}{6.25} - (\text{UUN} + 4)$$

(3-16)

in which grams of protein, which is 16% nitrogen, are converted to grams of nitrogen by dividing by 6.25, and UUN is urinary urea nitrogen in grams per 24 hours. This equation estimates the degree of catabolism in relation to the patient's protein intake. It is useful for planning nutritional care and evaluating the adequacy of that care by estimating nitrogen retention or loss. It has, however, a limitation in that, like the CHI, it requires collection of a 24-hour urine sample from patients being fed orally or receiving intermittent or cyclic infusions. A 12-hour urine sample is sufficient for a patient being fed continuously (see Chapter 5). The result is doubled to represent values for 24 hours.

Cell-Mediated Immune Function

The **total lymphocyte count** is used in a preliminary screening to provide an estimate of immune function (see Chapter 6). A **complete blood cell count** (CBC), which is ordered routinely on admission of most patients, provides the total number of white blood cells (leukocytes) per cubic millimeter of blood. It also provides a **differential count**, which states the percentages of the different types of white blood cells that make up the total. For assessment purposes, total lymphocyte count is obtained by the following calculation:

$$\text{total lymphocyte} = \frac{\text{\% lymphocytes} \times \text{total WBC/mm}^3}{100}$$

(3-17)

A lymphocyte count of more than 1,500/mm^3 is considered adequate. Values may be interpreted in comparison to those in Table 3-9, but consideration should be given to the fact that conditions other than nutrition, such as viral infections, may have an effect.

For those patients requiring further assessment, **recall antigen skin testing** or **delayed cutaneous hypersensitivity** (DCH) for cell-mediated response to various injected substances sometimes is used.[42] This procedure usually is done by a nurse but occasionally may be the responsibility of the nutritional care specialist. Typically, several antigens are injected intradermally in the forearm, and the amount of **induration** (hardening due to inflammation) in millimeters is measured in 48 hours. Three to five antigens may be used for testing. Useful antigens are streptokinase-streptodornase (SK-SD), *Candida* sp., *Trichophyton* sp., mumps, and tuberculin. A positive skin test consists of a raised and hardened area, **induration**, or **wheal** of at least 5 mm or more in diameter in 24 and 48 hours. This is surrounded by a reddened area of the skin (**erythema** or **flare**) which usually is not considered in evaluating the response.

The results are not yet standardized for interpretation. In one system, two positive responses of five tests are interpreted as a normal immune reactivity. One positive response only is considered to be "relative anergy," a suboptimal response. The absence of induration is **anergy**. If only three antigens are used in testing, patients are classified as reactive or anergic. In another system, the following classification may be used:[43]

4+	>20 mm induration
3+	11–20 mm induration
2+	7–10 mm induration
1+	1–5 mm induration (or >10 mm erythema)

The physiologic basis for this procedure is explained in Chapter 6.

Undernutrition is not the only cause of decreased DCH. It also is affected by surgery and anesthesia, drugs, gastrointestinal hemorrhage, infection, liver disease, shock, trauma, extensive burns, malignancy, myocardial infarction, renal failure, and age.[44] Nevertheless, patients who remain anergic have been shown to have increased morbidity and mortality rates. Antibody-producing capacity also is affected in protein-calorie malnutrition, but less severely. Ongoing research may find a more accurate and sensitive indicator of immune competence.

Hematological Assessment

Certain tests of the morphology and physiology of blood cells may be useful in nutritional assessment, although these tests are also influenced by a variety of other factors. Iron deficiency, for example, can result from impaired absorption, increased loss, and increased requirements, as well as insufficient intake. From a nutritional perspective, the purposes of hematologic assessment are

(1) to detect the presence of anemia and indicate its type, (2) to detect associated nutritional deficiencies, (3) to indicate the appropriate nutritional support, and (4) in selected patients, to screen for alcoholism and for hypoxia in the obese.

In the CBC, the **hematocrit** (Hct) or **packed cell volume** (PCV) is the proportion of the total volume of blood that is blood cells. The assay for hemoglobin gives the amount in grams per deciliter. The number of erythrocytes, or red blood cells (RBC), is counted and reported in numbers per cubic millimeter. In addition, the blood cells may be examined under the microscope and classified in the following ways:

Size: small (microcytic), normal (normocytic), or large (macrocytic).
Color: pale (hypochromic) or normal (normochromic).
Shape: normal (normocytosis) or irregular (poikilocytosis).

Some additional calculations may be reported based on the numerical indices.

1. The size of the RBC is indicated by mean corpuscular volume (MCV) recorded in cubic microliters (μ^3) or femtoliters (F):

$$MCV\ (\mu^3) = \frac{Hct \times 10}{RBC\ (millions/mm^3)}$$

(3-18)

   MCV is decreased in microcytic anemia and increased in megaloblastic anemia.
2. The hemoglobin content per cell is indicated by the mean corpuscular hemoglobin (MCH) given in picograms (pg):

$$MCH\ (pg) = \frac{Hb\ (g/dl \times 10)}{RBC\ (millions/mm^3)}$$

(3-19)

MCH is decreased in the small cells of iron deficiency and generally in hypochromic cells. It is high in the large cells of megaloblastic anemia.

Table 3-15. Laboratory Tests in the Differential Diagnosis of Anemia

Type of Anemia	Hb	Hct	MCV	Serum Iron	TIBC	Transferrin Saturation	Ferritin	Marrow Hemosiderin	Sideroblasts	RBC	Retic	Other
Iron deficiency	D	D	D	D	I	D	D	D	D	N	D	Hypochromic, microcytic, or normocytic
Vitamin B$_{12}$	D	D	I	I	D or N	I, D, or N	N	I	I	D	D or N	Macrocytic, megaloblastic, hypersegmented neutrophils, low-serum B$_{12}$, thrombocytopenia, leukopenia
Folic acid	D	D	I	I	D or N	I, D, or N	D	I	I	D	D or N	Macrocytic, megaloblastic, normal or slightly low B$_{12}$, decreased red cell folate
Vitamin E	D	D	I or N	I	D	N	N	I	I	D	I	Hemolytic anemia, low serum vitamin E, increased RBC, hemolysis, normochromic, normocytic
Anemia of chronic disease	D	D	N	D	D	D	N	N or I	D	D	D	Usually normocytic, normochromic, may be hypochromic, microcytic
Anemia of chronic infection	D	D	N or D	D	D	D or N	I or N	I, N, or D	D	D	D	Normochromic and normocytic, may be hypochromic and microcytic

Reproduced with permission from Walker, W.A., and Hendricks, K.M., *Manual of Pediatric Nutrition.* Philadelphia: W.B. Saunders, 1985.
D: decreased; N: normal; I: increased.

3. The hemoglobin content per volume of red blood cells is indicated by the mean corpuscular hemoglobin concentration (MCHC) given in percent:

$$\text{MCHC (\%)} = \frac{\text{Hb (g/dl)} \times 100}{\text{Hct}} \quad \text{(3-20)}$$

A low value is seen when hemoglobin is decreased more than hematocrit.

A summary of the results of these tests as they may be used to differentiate among the anemias is given in Table 3-15 with more quantitative values in Table 3-16. When the patient is iron deficient, MCV, MCH, and MCHC are low. If folate or vitamin B_{12} is deficient, producing a macrocytemia, these values may be high or normal. The patient may have several deficiencies, such as iron

Table 3-16. Current Guidelines for Laboratory Evaluation of Hematologic Data

Nutrient and Units	Age of Subject (years)	Criteria of Status		
		Deficient	Marginal	Acceptable
Hemoglobin (g/dl)[a]	1 week			13–20
	1 month			≥14
	6–23 months	<9.0	9.0–9.9	10.0+
	2–5	<10.0	10.0–10.9	11.0+
	6–12	<10.0	10.0–11.4	11.5+
	13–16 M	<12.0	12.0–12.9	13.0+
	13–16 F	<10.0	10.0–11.4	11.5+
	16+ M	<12.0	12.0–13.9	14.0+
	16+ F	<10.0	10.0–11.9	12.0+
	Pregnant			
	2nd trimester	<9.5	9.5–10.9	11.0+
	3rd trimester	<9.0	9.0–10.5	10.5+
Hematocrit (packed cell volume in %)[a]	1 week			43–66
	1 month			>50
	3 months			>35
	6 months–5 years			>38
	6–12	<30	30–35	36+
	13–16 M	<37	37–39	40+
	13–16 F	<31	31–35	36+
	16+ M	<37	37–43	44+
	16+ F	<31	31–37	33+
	Pregnant	<30	30–32	33+
Mean corpuscular volume (μm^3)	All ages			80–94
Mean corpuscular hemoglobin (μg)	All ages			27–35
Mean corpuscular hemoglobin concentration (%)	All ages			32–36
Serum iron ($\mu g/dl$)[a]	<2	<30		30+
	2–5	<40		40+
	6–12	<50		50+
	12+ M	<60		60+
	12+ F or pregnant	<40	40	40+
Transferrin saturation (%)[a]	<2	<15.0		15.0+
	2–12	<20.0		20.0+
	12+ M	<20.0		20.0+
	12+ F or pregnant	<15.0	15	15.0+
Serum folic acid (ng/ml)[b]	All ages; pregnant	<2.0	2.1–5.9	6.0+
Serum vitamin B_{12} (pg/ml)[b]	All ages; pregnant	<100	100	100+

Compiled from King, J.W., and Faukner, W.R., Eds., *Critical Resources in Clinical Laboratory Sciences*. Cleveland: CRC Press, 1973, p. 116; and Ney, D., Nutritional assessment. In D.G. Kelts, and E.G. Jones, Eds., *Manual of Pediatric Nutrition*. Boston: Little, Brown, 1984.
[a] Adapted from the Ten-State Nutritional Survey.
[b] Criteria may vary with different methodology.

Table 3-17. Current Guidelines for Laboratory Evaluation of Vitamin Status

Nutrient and Units	Age of Subject (years)	Criteria of Status		
		Deficient	Marginal	Acceptable
Serum ascorbic acid (mg/dl)[a]	All ages	<0.1	0.1–0.19	0.2+
Plasma vitamin A (μg/dl)[a]	All ages	<10	10–19	20+
Plasma carotene (μ/dl)[a]	All ages	<20	20–39	40+
	Pregnant		40–79	80+
Serum folic acid (ng/ml)[b]	All ages; pregnant	<2.0	2.1–5.9	6.0+
Serum vitamin B$_{12}$ (pg/ml)[b]	All ages; pregnant	<100	100	100+
Thiamine in urine (μg/g of creatinine)[a]	1–3	<120	120–175	175+
	4–5	<85	85–120	120+
	6–9	<70	70–180	180+
	10–15	<55	55–150	150+
	16+	<27	27–65	65+
	Pregnant	<21	21–49	50+
Riboflavin in urine (μg/g of creatinine)[a]	1–3	<150	150–499	500+
	4–5	<100	100–299	300+
	6–9	<85	85–269	270+
	10–16	<80	70–199	200+
	16+	<27	27–79	80+
	Pregnant	<30	30–89	90+
RBC transketolase-TPP effect (ratio)[b]	All ages	25+	15–25	<15
RBC glutathione reductase-FAD effect (ratio)[b]	All ages	1.2+		<1.2
Tryptophan load (mg xanthurenic acid excreted)[b]	Adults (Dose: 100 mg/kg body weight)	6 hr 25+		<25
		24 hr 75+		<75
Urinary pyridoxine (μg/g of creatinine)[b]	1–3	<90		90+
	4–6	<80		80+
	7–9	<60		60+
	10–12	<40		40+
	13–15	<30		30+
	16+	<20		20+
Urinary N'methyl nicotinamide (mg/g of creatinine)[a]	All ages	<0.2	0.2–5.59	0.6+
	Pregnant	<0.8	0.8–2.49	2.5+
Urinary pantothenic acid (μg)[b]	All ages	<200		200+
Vitamin E (serum tocopherol) (mg/dl)	Birth			0.22
	2 mo.			0.33
	2–12 yr.			0.72
	Adults			0.85
Transaminase index (ratio)[b]				
EGOT	Adult	2.0+		<2.0
EGPT	Adult	1.25+		<1.25

Compiled from J.W. King and W.R. Faukner, Eds., *Critical Resources in Clinical Laboratory Sciences.* Cleveland: CRC Press, 1973, p. 116; and Ney, D., Nutritional assessment. In *Manual of Pediatric Nutrition.* ed. D.G. Kelts and E.G. Jones. Boston: Little, Brown, 1984, p. 119.

M = male subjects; F = female subjects; RBC = red blood cells; TPP = thiamine pyrophosphate; FAD = flavin adenine dinucleotide; EGOT = erythrocyte glutamic oxaloacetic transaminase; EGPT = erythrocyte glutamic pyruvic transaminase.

[a] Adapted from the Ten-State Nutritional Survey.
[b] Criteria may vary with methodology.

and folate, which tend to cancel out each other's effects on these indices.

In the assessment of nutritional anemias, serum iron, folate, vitamin B_{12}, ferritin, and transferrin saturation values are sometimes available. Some guidelines for interpretation of these values in relation to nutritional status, deficient, marginal or acceptable, are given in Table 3-16. Further discussion of anemias is in Chapter 18.

Vitamin Assays

A number of biochemical tests are available to evaluate vitamin status. These are not routinely done, but are sometimes useful. They may be informative, for example, when the patient is taking a medication that interferes with vitamin nutrition. Table 3-17 gives values for interpretation.

Evaluation of Hydration Status

In conditions that affect fluid and electrolyte balance, such as cardiac, renal, and hepatic diseases, it may be necessary to evaluate the patient's hydration status. **Serum osmolality**, calculated from laboratory values, is one method for this purpose. It may be estimated from the values found in the patient's chart for serum sodium, blood glucose, and blood urea nitrogen (BUN). The equation for calculation is given in Chapter 2 (see Equation 2-5).

Abnormal values are the result of changes in concentration of serum sodium, the significance of which will be discussed in later chapters. Other laboratory indicators of dehydration include low urine output and elevated hemoglobin, hematocrit, and serum albumin, indicating hemoconcentration. High serum albumin values always suggest hemoconcentration, but normal or even low values do not exclude the possibility of dehydration. Clinical features of mild (4% deficit) dehydration include thirst, dryness of mucous membranes, and low urine output with high osmolality. Severe dehydration (8–10% deficit) is indicated by loss of skin turgor, sunken eyeballs, hypotension, increased pulse rate and a urine output less than 20 ml/hr. A deficit of 5–8%, or 4–6 liters in a 70-kg man, is a moderate dehydration.

Functional Tests

A number of tests of physiological function may reflect nutritional status, but they are not in common use. In many cases, they are expensive and insufficiently specific.

One function test which may be useful is the determination of skeletal muscle function. A hand-grip dynamometer measures grip strength and endurance, but the test is not useful for patients with diseases affecting neuromuscular or connective tissue such as myasthenia gravis, systemic lupus erythematosus, or multiple scleroderma. Hand-grip standards are 35 kg or more for adult males and 23 kg or more for adult females. Hand-grip dynamometry below 85% of standard has been associated with increased risk of morbidity and mortality.[45]

Clinical Observations

Many clinical signs of malnutrition are nonspecific (Table 3-18). They may result from deficiencies of more than one nutrient or from causes unrelated to nutrition. Nevertheless, they may be useful to indicate which patients need further evaluation. Many of these signs will be noted on the patient's chart by the physician. When interviewing patients, as well as when reviewing the medical record, the nutritional care specialist should be alert to their presence. When nutrient deficiencies are suspected to be severe, based on other data, the patient may be observed for specific clinical signs.

Dietary Assessment

A dietary evaluation is an important part of the nutritional assessment, as is observation of the current intakes of the hospitalized patient. The process most often involves inter-

Table 3-18. Clinical Evaluation of Nutritional Status

Tissue	Clinical Findings	Deficiency	Differential Diagnosis
Skull	In infants; bossing of the skull over ossification centers, delayed closure of anterior fontanelle	Vitamin D, calcium	Syphilis, sickle-cell disease, positional deformity, hydrocephalus
	Decreased head circumference	Protein-calorie	
Hair	Dry, wirelike, easily pluckable, brittle, depigmented, sparse	Protein-calorie	
	Impaired keratinization (hair is "steely")	Copper	
	Hair loss	Zinc, biotin, protein, essential fatty acids	
Skin	Malar pigmentation (darkened pigment over malar eminences)	Calories, B complex, especially niacin	Melasma in pregnancy or from oral contraceptives, Addison's disease
	Nasolabial seborrhea	Niacin, riboflavin, B_6	
	Ecchymosis ⎫ Perifollicular petechiae ⎭	⎧ Vitamin C ⎨ ⎩ Vitamin K	Hematologic disorders (thrombocytopenia), trauma, liver disease, anticoagulant overdose, orthostatic purpura, Fabry's disease, emboli, stasis, clotting factor deficiency
	Follicular hyperkeratosis (skin is rough, surrounding skin is dry)	Vitamin A	Fungus infection, perifolliculitis or scurvy, keratosis pilaris, Darier's disease
	Xerosis (skin is dry, with fine flaking)	Vitamin A, essential fatty acids	Aging, environmental drying, hypothyroidism, uremia, poor hygiene, ichthyosis
	Hyperpigmentation (seen more frequently on hands and face)	Niacin, folic acid, B_{12}	Addison's disease, environmental factors, trauma
	Scrotal dermatitis	Riboflavin, zinc	Fungus infection
	Pellagrous dermatitis (lesions are symmetric and in areas exposed to the sun)	Niacin	Chemical injury, sunburn, thermal burn
	Thickened skin at pressure points (predominantly in belt area)		
	Delayed wound healing	Zinc, vitamin C, protein	
Eyes	Circumcorneal injection (bilateral)	Riboflavin	
	Xerophthalmia (conjunctiva is dull, lusterless, exhibits a striated or rough surface)	Vitamin A	
	Bitot's spots (small circumscribed, dull, dry lesions usually seen on the lateral aspect of the bulbar conjunctiva)	Vitamin A	Pterygium
	Keratomalacia	Vitamin A	
	Night blindness	Vitamin A	
	Xanthomatosis, hyperlipidemia, and hypercholesterolemia leading to localized deposits of lipids	Excess intake of fat with elevated serum lipoproteins	
Lips	Cheilosis (lips may be swollen)	Niacin, riboflavin	Herpes simplex, arid or arctic environmental exposure
	Angular fissures (corners of mouth broken or macerated)	Niacin, riboflavin, iron, B_6	Herpes, syphilis

(continued)

Table 3-18. (continued)

Tissue	Clinical Findings	Deficiency	Differential Diagnosis
Gums	Bleeding gums (spongy)	Vitamin C	Dilantin toxicity, periodontal disease
Teeth	Dental caries	Fluoride	Poor oral hygiene
	Mottled enamel	Excess fluoride	Staining from tetracyclines
Tongue	Glossitis (red, painful tongue—may be fissured)	Folic acid, niacin, riboflavin, B_{12}, B_6, iron	Uremia, antibiotics, malignancy, aphthous stomatitis, monilial infection
	Atrophy of filiform papillae (low or absent)	Niacin, folic acid, B_{12}, iron	Nonnutritional anemias
	Hypertrophy of fungiform papillae	General malnutrition	Dietary irritants
	Pale, atrophic tongue	Iron, folic acid, B_{12}, niacin, riboflavin, B_6	Nonnutritional anemias
Exocrine	Parotid enlargement	Protein (?)	Mumps
Endocrine	Goiter	Iodine	Thyroglossal duct cyst, bronchial cleft cysts and tumors, hyperthyroidism, thyroiditis, thyroid carcinoma
Oral	Dysgeusia (disordered taste) Hypogeusia (loss of taste acuity)	Zinc	Cancer therapy
Nails	Koilonychia (spoon nails; nails are thin, concave)	Iron	Cardiac or pulmonary disease
Cardiac	Cardiac enlargement, tachycardia	Thiamine, iron	
Abdominal	Hepatomegaly	Chronic malnutrition	Liver disease
Skeletal	Rickets (bowed legs, deformities may also be seen in pelvic bones)	Calcium, phosphates, vitamin D	Renal rickets, malabsorption, congenital deformity
	Costochondral beading (?)	Calcium, vitamin D	
	Scorbutic rosary (costochondral junctions may have sharp edges caused by epiphyseal separation)	Vitamin C	
	Epiphyseal swelling secondary to epiphyseal hyperplasia (in rickets, secondary to tenderness and swelling caused by hemorrhage)	Vitamin D, calcium, vitamin C	Renal disease, malabsorption, congenital deformity
Neurologic	Absence of tendon reflexes (bilateral) Absence of vibratory sense (bilateral)	Thiamine, B_{12}	Peripheral neuropathy from other causes
	Calf tenderness	Thiamine	
	Pseudoparalysis (movement restricted because of pain)	Vitamin C	Hypokalemia
Extremities	Calf tenderness	Thiamine	Muscle strain, trauma, other causes of peripheral neuropathy, deep venous thrombosis
	Bilateral edema of lower extremities	Protein (occurs late in deficiency)	Congestive heart failure, renal failure, protein-losing enteropathy
Growth	Nutritional dwarfism, subcutaneous fat loss	Calories, protein	
	Dwarfism, hypogonadism	Zinc	

From Palmer, S., and Ekvall, S., *Pediatric Nutrition in Developmental Disorders,* 1978. Courtesy of Charles C Thomas, Publisher, Springfield, IL.

viewing the patient. Skilled interviewing is important in many steps of patient care but is beyond the scope of this text. Excellent information on interviewing techniques is available elsewhere.[46-50]

Methods to Obtain Data. The procedure chosen to obtain the data varies with the circumstances. It is important to use a method that provides as much (*but not more*) detailed information as is required to achieve the purpose.[46] Commonly used procedures include the following:

Twenty-four-hour recall. The patient is asked to describe the food eaten in the previous 24 hours or on a "typical day." In some illnesses, however, the recent diet may be atypical, and it is important to be aware of this. A frequently used technique is to ask the patient about activities in a typical day and explore the content of meals and snacks in the context of a day's usual activities. Questioning may begin with, "What time do you usually get up in the morning?" Later questions include, "When do you eat first?" and, "What kinds of food do you usually eat then?" Information on the amount, preparation, form, and other details are obtained for each food. Sometimes, pictures or food models are helpful to the patient in describing the size of portions. It is important to elicit information on consumption of alcoholic beverages, coffee, candy, soft drinks, chewing gum, other snack foods, and vitamin and mineral medications. A sample form that might be used in recording this information is shown in Figure 3-4.

Food frequency lists. The patient is asked how often he or she eats foods in each of a number of groups on a standardized list (see Figure 3-5). For example, "How many times in a day (or week) do you drink milk?" The results can be used as a cross-check on the information obtained in the 24-hour recall; therefore, these two methods often are used together.

Food records. Occasionally, a patient may be asked to keep a record of his or her food intake for a special period, usually three or seven days. This technique is often used in nutritional consultation with ambulatory patients. It is important to recognize, when evaluating the diet, that the process of keeping the record may cause an alteration in the intake. Patients may be stimulated to change their diets when required to give more thought to their meals. Others may alter the record to avoid embarrassment.

Nutrition history. A nutrition history is a more complete assessment. It usually includes a 24-hour recall plus the food frequency list. In addition, it includes information about other factors that influence food intake, nutritional needs, and nutritional adequacy. Some of these factors are the patient's financial resources, occupation, physical activity, allergies, appetite, chronic diseases, medications, dental health, handicaps, home life and living conditions, cultural background, and other socioeconomic factors. Obtaining a useful and accurate nutrition history requires a great deal of skill in interviewing.

Observations of food intake. When a patient is hospitalized, his or her current intake may be determined by direct observation. It is important, in addition, to inquire about consumption of foods brought to the patient by visitors or given to the patient by a roommate. The nursing staff is helpful in providing such information. Nursing records provide information on fluid intake and output.

A request may appear in the patient's medical record for a **calorie count** or a **calorie-protein count**. For this purpose, the nutritional care specialist or a technician observes or weighs the content of the tray as it is served and as it is returned. The difference presumably represents the patient's intake. The energy and protein content of food eaten is then calculated and entered into the medical record.

When greater precision is needed, foods may be weighed before being put on the tray, and foods not eaten may then be weighed when the tray is returned. Again, the degree of precision varies with the purpose. A graduated cylinder and spring balance are suffi-

Patient's name _____ Date _____

Activity level: Very active _____ Active _____ Moderate _____

Inactive _____ Ambulatory bed rest _____

Person responsible for shopping? _____ Food preparation? _____

Dentition (circle one):

Normal; Dentures, partial or complete; Edentulous

List of food eaten yesterday:

Wake-up time? _____ Is this usual? _____

Name foods eaten in order for 24 hours.

Time	Where eaten	Food	Description	Amount

Figure 3-4. Twenty-four-hour recall.

(continued)

Was this day typical? _____

If not, why not? _____

Do you eat differently on weekends? _____

If so, describe _____

How much salt do you add to your food at the table? _____

Do you take vitamins? _____

What kind and how much? _____

Are there foods you do not eat because of religious beliefs or other reasons? _____

Figure 3-4. (Continued)

ciently accurate for most purposes. Some patients, however, are subjects for research projects and are housed in a research unit. Their nutrient intake is measured with precision if the research protocol so requires.

Other methods, such as determination of "household consumption," used in population surveys, generally are not useful for application to individuals.

Evaluation of the Diet. Any of these data-gathering methods can provide valuable information if the nutritional care specialist is skillful, but the information still requires interpretation. An estimate of the nutrient content of the foods eaten may be obtained and compared to the patient's requirements.

As a practical matter in clinical practice, the translation from food intake to nutrient content is not often done in great detail for several reasons. First, the diet information obtained usually is approximate. The patient may not recall eating some items,[51-53] his or her estimates of quantities frequently are inaccurate, and the content of many mixtures is unknown. Second, our knowledge of the nutrient content of foods is very approximate. Last, knowledge of the individual's nutrient requirements also is approximate. Under these circumstances, precision in evaluation is not possible. In addition, other demands on the time of the nutritional care specialist usually do not permit detailed calculations. The most common types of quantitative data obtained are the intake of so-dium, the amount and type of carbohydrate, and the intake of saturated fat when they are related to the specific disease state. The number and timing of meals is recorded for obese patients or patients with diabetes mellitus.

A common practice in diet evaluation is to compare the diet with guidelines such as the Daily Food Guide,[54] familiar to all nutritionists as the "basic four," but the limitations of this guide must be recognized. A recent study demonstrated that the basic four provides only 60% or less of the National Research Council's (NRC) Recommended Dietary Allowances for energy, vitamins E and B_6, magnesium, zinc, and iron.[55] A modification is suggested that can be used in evaluation of diets. It includes the following:

Two servings of milk and milk products.
Four servings of protein foods (two animal protein and two legumes or nuts).
Four servings of fruits and vegetables, including one serving rich in vitamin C and one serving dark green.
Four servings of whole grain cereal products.
One serving of fat or oil.

When more detail is required, the protein, fat, and carbohydrate content of the diet may be calculated using "exchange lists." The procedure is described in Chapter 11.

Even greater detail can be provided by using extended tables of food values. These contain information on a broad spectrum of nutrients.[56-60] Other tables contain data on single nutrients.[61-64] Commercial manufacturers often provide data on nutritive values of their products, and many research papers give information on individual items. However, these tables of food values also are limited in accuracy. They represent average values obtained from laboratory determinations sometimes performed with varying methods and in different places. The foods analyzed can differ in variety, geographic source, season of the year, and subsequent processing and storage, all of which can affect their nutritive content. The nutritional value of the foods the individual patient eats also is influenced by the preparation methods in the home and the recipes used.

Given the many sources of error in the data and the time constraints placed on the nutritional care specialist in practice, only limited use is made of calculations in the detail provided in this type of table, unless the patient is the subject of research. Recently, however, nutrient information has been housed in some computer data banks. If the nutritional care specialist has access to such a system, more detailed diet analyses are possible.

Once the nutrient content of the diet is determined, it must then be compared to the patient's needs. In this process, the NRC table of Recommended Dietary Allowances[65] (Appendix A, Table 1) or the Dietary Standard for Canada[66] (Appendix A, Table 5) often is used as a starting point, even though neither was designed to be applied to individuals. Except for energy, U.S. recommended allowances are deliberately set high to include most of the population. They do not represent the average or minimal requirement. When the amount of a nutrient consumed by an individual falls below the amounts given in either of these tables, it cannot be assumed that the individual is deficient.[65,66] The effect of the patient's disease and of any medications or other treatment must also be considered. These matters require knowledge and experience and will be discussed in the remaining chapters of this text.

Evaluation of Nutritional Status

In practice, a stepwise procedure of nutritional assessment is used to ensure the most efficient use of resources. A routine screening process, consisting of some of the simpler methods, is applied to all patients to identify those in need of further study. In addition, the routine screening establishes baseline values for use in later evaluation. Candidates for complete assessment include those with conditions that place them "at nutritional risk" (see Table 3-2) and those whose preliminary assessment show the following:

Serum albumin less than 3.2 g/dl.
Total lymphocytes less than 1,500/mm³.
Nonvoluntary weight loss.
A history of nutritional deficiency.
A statement from the patient of change in
    appetite.

Even if not malnourished on original assessment, patients who are hospitalized for lengthy periods should be reevaluated at intervals.

With the collective data obtained from the previously outlined procedures, the patient's nutritional status is evaluated. The more severe forms of protein-calorie malnutrition often are considered to be analogous to primary protein and energy deficiencies in childhood. Thus the terms **marasmus** and **kwashiorkor** commonly are used, but it is important to remember that many patients, even if depleted, will be less severely affected than the use of these terms implies.

Diagnosis of Protein-Calorie Malnutrition

Marasmus or **cachexia** results from a calorie deficit that often has extended over months or years. The patient experiences severe wasting of fat and muscle. Arm muscle circumference and skinfold thickness are diminished, indicating loss of muscle tissue and of fat stores. The patient also has reduced immune function. Serum proteins

Name _____   Date _____

How often do you eat the following foods?

Food	Servings per Day	Servings per Week	Seldom	Never
Meat, poultry, rice				
Beef, hamburger				
Pork, ham				
Bacon				
Liver				
Lamb				
Veal				
Lunch meat				
Poultry				
Fish				
Shellfish				

Food	Servings per Day	Servings per Week	Seldom	Never
Potatoes				
Dried beans, peas				
Fruit or juice				
Citrus				
Other				
Tomatoes				
Dried fruit				
Fats & oils				
Margarine				
Butter				
Cooking fat/oil				

Dairy products _____
  Cheese (type) _____
  Milk (type) _____
  Yogurt _____
  Ice cream _____
  Ice milk _____

Breads & cereals _____
  Bread (type) _____
  Cereal (type) _____
  Pasta (type) _____
  Baked goods (type) _____

Vegetables _____
  Dark green _____
  Dark yellow _____
  Other _____

Salad dressing _____
Salt pork _____
Cream (type) _____
Fried foods _____
Other _____
  Nuts _____
  Seeds _____
  Sprouts _____
  Snack foods _____
  Soft drinks _____
Coffee (decaf?) _____
Tea _____
Alcohol (type) _____

Are there other foods not listed that you eat regularly?

_____

_____

_____

Do you drink water? _____   How often? _____   How much? _____
Do you add salt to your food? _____   How much? _____

Figure 3-5. Food frequency checklist.

Table 3-19. Indicators of Protein and Energy Malnutrition

Condition	Deficit	Indicators				
		Body Weight	Body Fat	Somatic Protein	Visceral Protein	Immune Function
Marasmus	Energy	↓	↓	↓	Slightly ↓ or WNL	↓
Kwashiorkor	Protein	↓	WNL	WNL	↓	↓
Marasmic kwashiorkor	Protein and energy	↓	↓	↓	↓	↓

↓ = decreased; WNL = within normal limits.

may be moderately reduced or normal. The prognosis is good if the patient is provided with adequate oral nutritional support, but with additional stress, the patient can develop marasmic kwashiorkor very rapidly.

A **kwashiorkor-like syndrome** develops much more rapidly than does marasmus, sometimes within weeks, as a consequence of a protein deficit concurrent with severe stress, such as those described in Chapter 14. In these patients, fat reserves and muscle mass tend to be normal and may even be above normal; however, laboratory tests will indicate severely depressed serum albumin and transferrin and depressed immune function. The patient may be edematous and have delayed wound healing. Aggressive nutritional support is needed, sometimes by means other than simply supplying the patient with a tray of food. Prognosis is poor compared to the patient with marasmus.

Marasmic kwashiorkor is the combined form of protein-calorie malnutrition that occurs when a stress is superimposed on a chronically starved patient. The prognosis is very poor. The mortality rate increases as a result of increased infections and poor wound healing. The relationship of these conditions and results of nutritional assessment procedures is summarized in Table 3-19.

Evaluation of the patient's diet can be used to confirm a diagnosis obtained from anthropometric and biochemical parameters. Dietary data also provide information basic to planning for nutritional intervention.

Evaluation of Requirements

Nutritional assessment data also provide information for calculations of present and potential future needs. Thus these data improve planning for nutritional support.

Energy Balance. An estimate of basal energy expenditure (BEE) may be calculated from anthropometric data. BEE is slightly higher than basal metabolic rate (BMR), which is not used since basal conditions are difficult to achieve. Basal energy expenditure is obtained by use of one of the following formulas:

$$\text{For men: BEE} = 66 + (13.7 \times W) + (5 \times H) - (6.8 \times A) \qquad (3\text{-}21)$$

$$\text{For women: BEE} = 665 + (9.6 \times W) + (1.8 \times H) - (4.7 \times A) \qquad (3\text{-}22)$$

where W = kg body weight, H = height in centimeters, and A = age in years.

In order to estimate the total energy expenditure, a factor must be included for activity. To allow for activity, the BEE is multiplied by the following activity factors (AF):

Bed rest	1.2
Ambulatory	1.3
Normal activity	1.5–1.75
Extremely active	2.0

The result will give an approximation of the energy requirement for maintenance.

If the patient is depleted and anabolism is

desired, the "injury factors" (IF) in the following list should be applied. These factors should be used as soon as the stress is applied, if possible.

Minor surgery	1.2
Skeletal trauma	1.33
Elective surgery	1.44
Major sepsis	1.6 – 1.9
Trauma plus steroids	1.88
Severe thermal burns	2.1 – 2.5

Thus the total daily energy expenditure (TDE) is obtained from the equation

$$TDE = (BEE)\,(AF)\,(IF) \tag{3-23}$$

It is very important to keep clearly in mind that the equation for BEE and the applied factors that are described here are estimates and should not be taken as absolute accurate values.

Nitrogen Balance. Nitrogen balance, calculated as previously described (see Equation 3-16), may be used as a basis for estimation of protein requirements. An existing negative nitrogen balance indicates the need for an increase in protein intake. As a preliminary estimate, protein need for nitrogen balance $\times 1.5$ will provide for anabolism.

An alternative method of estimation of protein need is based on total energy need. For maintenance, 1 g nitrogen (6.25 g protein) is provided for 200 kcal. For anabolism, 1 g nitrogen is provided for 150 kcal.

Estimate of Clinical Risk

A **prognostic nutritional index** (PNI) has been developed that provides a quantitative estimate of risk of anergy, sepsis, and death.[17] It is expressed as a percentage and is calculated from the following formula:

$$PNI = 158\% - [(16.6 \times ALB) + (0.78 \times TSF) + (0.2 \times TFN) + (5.8 \times DCH)] \tag{3-24}$$

where ALB = serum albumin concentration

(in g/dl), TSF = triceps skinfold (in mm), TFN = transferrin (in g/dl), and DCH (delayed cutaneous hypersensitivity) = grade of reactivity to any of three antigens (mumps, *Candida*, or SK/SD). Reactivity is graded as **nonreactive** if induration equals 0, 1 if induration is less than 5 mm, and 2 if induration is greater than or equal to 5 mm.

The following comparative values of a well-nourished and a malnourished patient are exemplary:

Well-Nourished Patient

ALB	4.7 g/dl × 16.6 =	78.0
TSF	15.0 mm × 0.78 =	11.7
TFN	245 g/dl × 0.2 =	49.0
DCH	2 × 5.8 =	11.6
Total		150.3
PNI	158 − 150.3 =	7.7%

Malnourished Patient

ALB	2.8 g/dl × 16.6 =	46.5
TSF	10.2 mm × 0.78 =	8.0
TFN	160 g/dl × 0.2 =	32.0
DCH	1 × 5.8 =	5.8
Total		92.3
PNI	158 − 92.3 =	65.7%

According to this method, the malnourished patient has eight and one-half (65.7 ÷ 7.7) times the risk of complications as does the well-nourished patient.

IDENTIFICATION OF OTHER PROBLEMS

In addition to the data base for identification of nutritional problems—which includes a nutritional assessment with anthropometric, biochemical, clinical, and dietary data—psychological, social, economic, and educational factors must be carefully evaluated to assure that all the needs of the patient will be met. This evaluation requires skillful integration of the biological and social science knowledge of the nutritional care specialist plus practice and experience in application.

An estimation of the patient's immediate

nutritional needs and comparison with intake are required. The patient's nutrient needs are affected by (1) current nutritional status, (2) current or projected stress factors, and (3) the method of feeding. There is no condition in which malnutrition is a desirable goal of treatment.

In addition, problems related to the patient's food choices, education, and financial problems, together with any other factor influencing the patient's nutritional state, must be identified. The influence of these factors is unpredictable, and the nutritional care specialist must judge their relevance in each case. The chronic use of certain drugs that place the patient at nutritional risk must also be included in the assessment. Information on drug-nutrient interactions is the subject of the next chapter.

In summary, nutritional assessment is used to

1. Identify malnourished patients.
2. Identify patients at risk of becoming malnourished.
3. Provide data to serve as a basis for planning nutritional support to correct or prevent malnutrition.
4. Provide information for evaluation of the effectiveness of nutritional support.

Case Study: Nutritional Assessment

Mr. K. is a 47-year-old man who was admitted to the hospital after an automobile accident. His injuries included a broken arm, a broken nose, and multiple bruises.

The medical record states that Mr. K. is unemployed and has no health insurance. When you talk to him, you learn that he is a widower who lives in one room. He cooks his meals on a one-burner gas plate in his room. He has dentures that do not fit well. He denies any allergies and states he has no food dislikes. He admits he has lost 15 pounds since the death of his wife six months ago.

The medical record gives the following data:

Height, in.	68
Weight, lb.	135
Serum albumin, g/dl	3.0
Lymphocytes, %	25
Hemoglobin, g/dl	12.0
Hematocrit, %	39
Red blood cells, $\times 10^6/mm^3$	4.2
White blood cells/mm^3	4,800

You obtain the following measurements:

Elbow breadth, in.	2.75
Triceps skinfold, mm	7.5
Midarm circumference, cm	17.6

Exercises

1. List the factors that place this patient at risk of malnutrition.
2. Calculate the patient's midarm fat area, midarm muscle circumference, and midarm muscle area.
3. Calculate the patient's total lymphocyte count.
4. What procedures would you use to gather data for a dietary assessment for this patient? Why?
5. Calculate the patient's mean corpuscular volume, mean corpuscular hemoglobin, and mean corpuscular hemoglobin concentration. Evaluate the patient's hematological status.
6. Calculate the BEE for this patient. Assume he is ambulatory.
7. What is your assessment of this patient's nutritional status?
8. You write a SOAP note in the patient's medical record. What items would you give as subjective data? As objective data? Assume you were unable to interview the patient concerning his previous diet. What would you write in your assessment of his diet?

References

1. Schiller, R., and Behm, V. Auditing dietetic services. *Hospitals* 53:122, 1979.
2. Escott-Stump, S. *Nutrition and Diagnosis-Related Care.* Philadelphia: Lea & Febiger, 1985.
3. Atwood, J., Mitchell, P.H., and Yarnall, S.R. The POR. A system for communication. *Nurs. Clin. North Am.* 9:229, 1974.
4. Fowler, D.R., and Longabaugh, R. The problem-oriented record. Problem definition. *Arch. Gen. Psychiatry* 32:831, 1975.
5. Weed, L.L. *Medical Records, Medical Education and Patient Care.* Chicago: Year Book Medical Publishers, 1969.

6. Zeman, F.J., and Ney, D.M. *Applications of Clinical Nutrition.* Englewood Cliffs, N.J.: Prentice-Hall, 1988.
7. Bistrian, B.R., Blackburn, G.L., Hallowell, E.H., and Heddle, R. Protein status of general surgical patients. *J.A.M.A.* 230:858, 1974.
8. Bistrian, B.R., Blackburn, G.L., Vitale, J., et al. Prevalance of malnutrition in general medical patients. *J.A.M.A.* 235:1567, 1976.
9. Weinsier, R.L., Hunker, E.M., Krumdieck, C.L., and Butterworth, C.E., Jr. Hospital nutrition. A prospective evaluation of general medical patients during the course of hospitalization. *Am. J. Clin. Nutr.* 32:418, 1979.
10. Bollet, A.J., and Owens, S.D. Evaluation of nutritional status of selected hospitalized patients. *Am. J. Clin. Nutr.* 26:931, 1973.
11. Blackburn, G.L., and Bistrian, B.R. Nutritional care of the injured and/or septic patient. *Surg. Clin. North Am.* 56:1195, 1976.
12. Weinsier, R.L., and Butterworth, C.E., Jr. *Handbook of Clinical Nutrition.* St. Louis: C.V. Mosby, 1981.
13. Blackburn, G.L., Bistrian, B.R., Maini, B.S., et al. Nutritional and metabolic assessment of the hospitalized patient. *JPEN* 1:11, 1977.
14. Bishop, C.W., Bowen, P.E., and Ritchey, S.J. Norms for nutritional assessment of American adults by upper arm anthropometry. *Am. J. Clin. Nutr.* 34:2530, 1981.
15. Dacis, J., and O'Connell, J.R. A grid for recording the weight of premature infants. *J. Pediatr.* 33:570, 1948.
16. Studley, A.O. Percentage of surgical risk in patients with chronic peptic ulcer. *J.A.M.A.* 106:458, 1936.
17. Mullen, J.L., Buzby, G.P., Waldman, M.T., et al. Prediction of operative morbidity and mortality by preoperative nutritional assessment. *Surg. Forum* 30:80, 1979.
18. Jelliffe, D.B. *The Assessment of the Nutritional Status of the Community.* Geneva: World Health Organization, 1966.
19. Fomon, S.J. *Nutritional Disorders of Children: Prevention, Screening and Follow-up.* D.H.E.W. Publication No. (HSA) 78–5104. Washington, D.C.: U.S. Government Printing Office, 1978.
20. Brozek, J. Physique and nutritional status of adult men. *Hum. Biol.* 28:124, 1956.
21. Tanner, J.M. The measurement of body fat in man. *Proc. Nutr. Soc.* 18:148, 1959.
22. Ward, G.M. Krzywicki, H.J., Rahman, D.P., et al. Relationship of anthropometric measurements to body fat as determined by densitometry, potassium-40 and body water. *Am. J. Clin. Nutr.* 28:162, 1975.
23. Cahill, G.F. Starvation in man. *N. Engl. J. Med.* 282:668, 1970.
24. Ruiz, L., Colley, J.R.T., and Hamilton, P.J.S. Measurement of triceps skinfold thickness — and investigation of sources of variation. *Br. J. Prev. Soc. Med.* 25:165, 1971.
25. Jenson, T., Dudrick, S., and Johnston, D. A comparison of triceps skinfold and arm circumference values measured in standard and supine positions. *JPEN* 3:513, 1979.
26. Standard, K.L., Wills, V.G., and Waterlow, J.C. Indirect indicators of muscle mass in malnourished infants. *Am. J. Clin. Nutr.* 7:271, 1959.
27. Reindorp, S., and Whitehead, R.G. Changes in serum creatinine kinase and other biological measurements associated with musculature in children recovering from kwashiorkor. *Br. J. Nutr.* 25:273, 1971.
28. Jelliffe, D.B. *The Assessment of the Nutritional Status of the Community: With Special Reference to Field Surveys in Developing Regions of the World.* WHO Monograph 53. Geneva: World Health Organization, 1966.
29. Stoudt, H.W., Damon, A., McFarland, R.A., and Roberts, J. *Skin Folds, Body Girths, Biacromial Diameters, and Selected Anthropometric Indices of Adults: United States, 1960–1962.* Vital and Health Statistics Series II, National Health Survey No. 35. Washington, D.C.: U.S. Public Health Service, 1970.
30. Gray, G.E., and Gray, L.K. Anthropometric measurements and their interpretation. Principles, practices, and problems. *J. Am. Diet. Assoc.* 77:534, 1980.
31. Bernard, M.A., Jacobs, D.O., and Rombeau, J.L. *Nutritional and Metabolic Support of Hospitalized Patients.* Philadelphia: W.B. Saunders, 1986.
32. Frisancho, A.R. New norms of upper limb fat and muscle for assessment of nutritional status. *Am. J. Clin. Nutr.* 34:2540, 1981.
33. Guyton, A.C. *Basic Human Physiology: Normal Function and Mechanism of Disease,* 2nd ed. Philadelphia: W.B. Saunders, 1977.
34. Wallach, J.B. *Interpretation of Diagnostic Tests: A Handbook Synopsis of Laboratory Medicine,* 3rd ed. Boston: Little, Brown, 1978.
35. Reeds, P.J., and Laditan, A.A.O. Serum albumin and transferrin in protein energy malnutrition. *Br. J. Nutr.* 36:255, 1976.
36. Kaminski, M.V., Fitzgerald, M.J., Murphy, R.J., et al. Correlation of mortality with serum transferrin and anergy. *JPEN* 1:27A, 1977.
37. Mullen, J.L., Gertner, M.H., Buzby, G.P., et al. Implications of malnutrition in the surgical patient. *Arch. Surg.* 114:121, 1979.
38. Ingenbleek, Y., DeVisscher, M., and DeNayer, P. Measurement of prealbumin as index of protein-calorie malnutrition. *Lancet* 2:106, 1972.

39. Ingenbleek, Y., Van Den Schrieck, H.G., DeNayer, P., and DeVisscher, M. The role of retinol-binding protein in protein-calorie malnutrition. *Metabolism* 24:633, 1975.
40. Cuthbertson, D.P. The disturbance of metabolism produced by bony and non-bony injury with notes on certain abnormal conditions of bone. *Biochem. J.* 24:1244, 1930.
41. Kaminski, M.K., Jr. Enteral hyperalimentation. *Surg. Gynecol. Obstet.* 143:12, 1976.
42. Meakins, J.L., Pietsch, J.B., Bubenick, O., et al. Delayed hypersensitivity. Indicator of acquired failure of host defenses in sepsis and trauma. *Ann. Surg.* 186:241, 1977.
43. Bates, S.E., Sven, J.Y., and Tranum, B. L. Immunological skin testing and interpretations. A plea for uniformity. *Cancer* 43:2306, 1979.
44. Blackburn, G.L., and Thornton, P.A. Nutritional assessment of the hospitalized patient. *Med. Clin. North Am.* 63:1103, 1979.
45. Klidjian, A.M., Archer, T.J., Foster, K.J., et al. Detection of dangerous malnutrition. *JPEN* 6:119, 1982.
46. Derelian, D. Interviewing the patient. In F.J. Zeman and D.M. Ney, *Applications of Clinical Nutrition.* Englewood Cliffs, N.J.: Prentice-Hall, 1988.
47. Mason, M., Wenberg, B.G., and Welsch, P.K. *The Dynamics of Clinical Dietetics,* 2nd ed. New York: Wiley, 1982.
48. Froelich, R.E., and Bishop, F.M. *Medical Interviewing.* St. Louis: C.V. Mosby, 1969.
49. Bernstein, L., and Bernstein, R. *Interviewing and the Health Professions,* 4th ed. New York: Appleton-Century-Crofts, 1985.
50. Bird, B. *Talking with Patients,* 2nd ed. Philadelphia: J.B. Lippincott, 1973.
51. Campbell, V.A., and Dodds, M.L. Collecting dietary information from groups of older people. Limitations of the 24-hour recall. *J. Am. Diet. Assoc.* 51:29, 1967.
52. Madden, J.P., Goodman, S.J., and Guthrie, H.A. Validity of the 24-hr recall. Analysis of data obtained from elderly subjects. *J. Am. Diet. Assoc.* 68:143, 1976.
53. Beal, V.A. The nutritional history in longitudinal research. *J. Am. Diet. Assoc.* 51:426, 1967.
54. Food and Nutrition Service, Agriculture Research Service. *A Daily Food Guide.* FNS–13. Rev. July 1975. Washington, D.C.: U.S. Department of Agriculture, 1975.
55. King, J.C., Cohenour, S.H., Corruccini, C.G., and Schneeman, P. Evaluation and modification of the basic four food guide. *J. Nutr. Educ.* 10:27, 1978.
56. Watt, B.K., and Merrill, A.L. *Composition of Foods—Raw, Processed, Prepared.* Rev.

57. U.S.D.A. Handbook No. 8. Washington, D.C.: U.S. Department of Agriculture, 1976.
57. Consumer and Food Economics Research Division, Agriculture Research Service. *Nutritive Value of Foods.* S1, rev. U.S.D.A. Home and Garden Bull. No. 72. Washington, D.C.: U.S. Department of Agriculture, 1971.
58. Pennington, J., and Church, H.N., Eds. *Food Values of Portions Commonly Used,* 13th ed. New York: Harper and Row, 1980.
59. Adams, C.F. *Nutritive Value of American Foods in Common Units.* U.S.D.A. Handbook No. 456. Washington, D.C.: U.S. Department of Agriculture, 1976.
60. Leveille, G.A., Zabik, M.E., and Morgan, K.J. *Nutrients in Foods.* Cambridge, Mass.: Nutrition Guild, 1983.
61. Food and Agriculture Organization of the United Nations, Food Policy and Food Science Service. *Amino Acid Content of Foods and Biological Data on Proteins.* Rome: Food and Agriculture Organization, 1970.
62. Orr, M.L., and Watt, B.K. *Amino Acid Content of Foods.* U.S.D.A. Home Economics Research Report No. 4. Washington, D.C.: U.S. Department of Agriculture, 1957.
63. Orr, M.L. *Pantothenic Acid, Vitamin B_6 and Vitamin B_{12} in Food.* U.S.D.A. Home Economics Research Report No. 36. Washington, D.C.: U.S. Department of Agriculture, 1969.
64. Teopfer, E.W., Zook, E.G., Orr, M.L., and Richardson, L.R. *Folic Acid Content of Foods.* U.S.D.A. Handbook No. 29. Washington, D.C.: U.S. Department of Agriculture, 1951.
65. Food and Nutrition Board, National Research Council. *Recommended Dietary Allowances,* 10th rev. ed. Washington, D.C.: National Academy of Sciences, 1989.
66. Committee for Revision of the Canadian Dietary Standard, Bureau of Nutritional Sciences, Department of National Health and Welfare Canada. *Recommended Nutrient Intakes for Canadians.* Ottawa: Information Canada, 1983.

Bibliography

Gibson, R.S. *Principles of Nutritional Assessment.* New York: Oxford University Press, 1990.
Grant, A. *Nutritional Assessment Guidelines,* 2nd ed. Seattle: Anne Grant, 1979.
Grant, J.P., Custer, P.B., and Thurlow, J. Current techniques of nutritional assessment. *Surg. Clin. North Am.* 61:437, 1981.
Jensen, T.G., Englert, D.M., and Dudrick, S.J. *Nutritional Assessment. A Manual for Practitioners.* Norwalk, Conn.: Appleton-Century-Crofts, 1983.

Krey, S.H., and Murray, R.L., Eds. *Dynamics of Nutrition Support, Assessment, Implementation, Evaluation.* New York: Appleton-Century-Crofts, 1986.

Silberman, H., and Eisenberg, D. *Parenteral and Enteral Nutrition for the Hospitalized Patient.* New York: Appleton-Century-Crofts, 1982.

Simko, M.D., Cowell, C., and Gilbride, J.A. *Nutrition Assessment.* Rockville, Md.: Aspen, 1984.

Wright, R.A., and Heymsfield, S., Eds. *Nutritional Assessment.* Boston: Blackwell, 1984.

Sources of Current Information

American Journal of Clinical Nutrition
Annals of Internal Medicine
Annual Review of Nutrition
Archives of Internal Medicine
Clinical Nutrition
Human Nutrition: Applied Nutrition
Human Nutrition: Clinical Nutrition
Journal of the American Dietetic Association
Journal of the American Medical Association
Journal of the Canadian Dietetic Association
Journal of Human Nutrition
Journal of Nutrition
Journal of Nutrition Education
JPEN. Journal of Parenteral and Enteral Nutrition
Medical Clinics of North America
New England Journal of Medicine
Nursing Clinics of North America
Nutrition Abstracts and Reviews
Nutrition International
Nutrition and Metabolism
Nutrition in Clinical Practice
Nutrition Research
Nutrition Reviews
Nutrition Today
Pediatric Nutrition and Gastroenterology
Postgraduate Medicine
Topics in Clinical Nutrition
World Review of Nutrition and Dietetics

4. Drugs and Nutritional Care

I. General Principles of Pharmacology
   A. Mechanisms of drug action
   B. Factors influencing rate and magnitude of drug effects
      1. Size and frequency of drug dosage
      2. Methods of administration
      3. Absorption
         a. solubility
         b. concentration
         c. properties of the drug molecule
            (1) size of molecules
            (2) lipid solubility
            (3) ionization
         d. effect of gastric emptying
         e. blood supply at injection site
      4. Distribution
         a. volume of distribution
         b. blood supply to target organ
         c. plasma protein binding
         d. concentration in adipose and other tissues
         e. blood-brain barrier
         f. placental barrier
         g. inflammation
   C. Drug metabolism and excretion

      1. Excretion
      2. Drug biotransformations
         a. nonsynthetic reactions
         b. synthetic reactions
         c. factors influencing rate of metabolism
   D. Drug safety and effectiveness in individuals
      1. Factors modifying drug effects in individuals
      2. Individual variations in drug response
      3. Drug interactions
   E. Classification and terminology

II. Nutrition-Drug Interrelationships
   A. Effects of drugs on nutrition
      1. Drug effects on taste, appetite, and food intake
         a. anatomy of taste and odor
         b. effect of disease on taste and odor perception
         c. drug effects on taste and odor perception
         d. drug effects on appetite and food intake

      e. nutritional care of patients with altered taste and depressed appetite
      2. Drug effects on nutrient absorption
      3. Drug effects on nutrient metabolism
         a. protein
         b. lipids
         c. carbohydrates
         d. vitamins and minerals
      4. Nutritional care

   B. Effects of food and nutrients on drugs
      1. Effects of food on drug absorption
         a. food in the digestive tract
         b. specific nutrients
      2. Effects of nutritional status on drug metabolism and excretion
         a. protein
         b. lipids
         c. minerals
         d. vitamins
      3. Detrimental systemic food-drug interactions
         a. vasoactive compounds and monoamine oxidase inhibitors
         b. alcohol-drug interactions

The existence of interrelationships between nutrition and drugs has become increasingly clear in recent years. At the same time, the need has grown for practitioners in the health professions to have a knowledge of these interrelationships. In order to provide appropriate nutritional care to patients receiving drugs, to work as a member of a health care team, and to understand advances in this important field of knowledge, an appreciation of some basic principles of pharmacology and a command of current knowledge of drug-nutrient interrelationships is required. This chapter provides an introduction to the fundamentals of pharmacology, followed by a discussion of drug-nutrient interrelations. In later chapters, the effects of drugs on nutrition in specific disease states will be reviewed.

GENERAL PRINCIPLES OF PHARMACOLOGY

Pharmacology is the study of the activity and effects of chemicals in living matter. One of its branches is **pharmacy**, the preparation and dispensing of these chemicals for therapy. As used in medicine, a **drug** is any chemical used in the prevention, diagnosis, or treatment of disease.

Mechanisms of Drug Action

Drugs do not create new metabolic processes. Instead, they act by increasing or decreasing a naturally occurring process. They may inhibit an enzyme, facilitate enzyme action by acting as a coenzyme, activate an inactive part of the DNA molecule to stimulate synthesis of a protein, alter membrane permeability, or act as a chelator.

The pharmacologic effect of a drug is often correlated with its concentration in the blood. Blood, serum or plasma levels may be monitored, even though the drug's effect is on a tissue other than blood.

The usual mode of drug action requires the formation of a drug-receptor complex, which then produces one or more reactions. The amount of the response depends on the number of drug-receptor reactions which, in turn, depends on the concentration of the drug near the receptor. A few drugs do not form a drug-receptor complex. An example is sodium bicarbonate, which neutralizes gastric acidity by direct reaction with the gastric hydrochloric acid. Another example is a chelating compound such as penicillamine, which chelates copper and is useful in the treatment of Wilson's disease.

Usually a drug can bind to more than one type of receptor and thereby produce more than one effect. Any effects other than those the drug was intended to produce are its **side effects**. These vary in nature and degree of severity. As a general rule, serious side effects are acceptable only when there is no equally effective alternative drug and the disease being treated also is serious. For example, more severe side effects are acceptable in the drug treatment of cancer than in the treatment of a less serious disease. Side effects are frequently a major concern in nutritional care, since they very often include nausea, vomiting, diarrhea, and other symptoms that influence nutritional status.

Factors Influencing Rate and Magnitude of Drug Effects

Size and Frequency of Drug Dosage

The rate and magnitude of drug effect is influenced by the dosage of the drug. The drug dose varies in amount and frequency and is influenced by the maximum effect of which the drug is capable.

A basic tool for determining the amount of a drug necessary to produce a given effect is the **logarithmic dose-response curve** (Figure 4-1). In that part of the curve marked *A*, there is a small increase in dose and a small increase in response. The dose at which a response is first measured is the **threshold dose**. In part *B* of the dose-response curve, there is a large increase in response in proportion to the increase in dose. It is in this part of the curve that the minimum dose necessary to produce a maximum response is found. In part *C*, there is no further response regardless of the amount of increase in dose. At this dose level, receptor sites are saturated and no further response is possible. It usually is in part *C* that toxic side effects occur. In some drugs, such as anticancer drugs, toxic side effects may occur in part *B* of the curve.

The duration of action of the drug must be considered in determining the frequency of dose administration. A few drugs may be

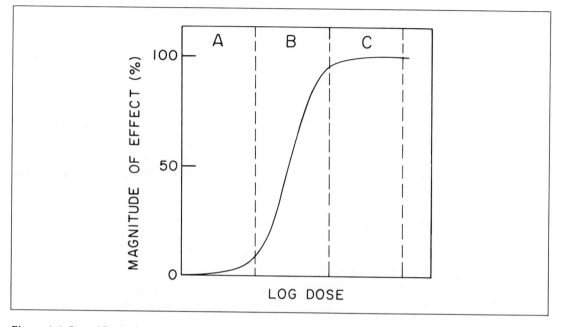

Figure 4-1. Logarithmic dose-response curve.

given only once. Prolonged action of some drugs is needed, and so they must be given repeatedly. The size and frequency of the dose is established at a level to maintain concentration of the drug above its threshold but below its toxic level. The frequency of administration is affected by the rate at which the drug is excreted or inactivated; rapidly excreted drugs must be given more frequently.

Methods of Administration

The route by which a drug is administered affects the rate at which it is transferred to the vicinity of its receptor sites. Some drugs, such as ointments, liniments, powders, paints, eye drops, and nose drops, are used for a local effect on the skin or mucous membranes. This is called **topical** administration. However, most drugs have more general or **systemic** effects or an effect at a site other than the site of administration.

Systemic administration of drugs has been divided into two categories. One of these is **enteral** administration, that is, via the gastrointestinal tract. More specifically, this can include giving medication by mouth (p.o.), sublingually by allowing it to dissolve under the tongue, or by a tube into the stomach or intestines. Drugs may also be given rectally in the form of suppositories. It is estimated that approximately 80 percent of all drugs are taken by mouth. The other major category of systemic administration is **parenteral** (outside of the gastrointestinal tract). This includes injecting medication (1) **subcutaneously** (s.c.) or under the epidermis, (2) **intradermally,** or into the dermis just below the epidermis, (3) **intramuscularly,** or into a muscle (i.m.), (4) **intrathecally,** or into the spinal fluid, and (5) **intravenously** (i.v.), or into a vein. In addition, a few drugs can be administered by **inhalation.** Probably the most familiar example of drugs that are inhaled are certain anesthetics.

Regardless of the means of administration, the drugs must then be absorbed and transported to their site of action. Those given enterally or by inhalation must cross the epithelial cells of the gastrointestinal tract or lungs. They also must cross the endothelial cells of the capillaries to reach the bloodstream, as must drugs given subcutaneously, intradermally, or intramuscularly. After they reach the bloodstream, most drugs, including those given intravenously, must again cross endothelial cells of the capillaries to reach the target cells. When a drug is given intravenously, it can be expected to cause a more rapid response than if it is given intramuscularly or subcutaneously, because the latter must be absorbed into the bloodstream first. The absorption is slowed down even further if the site of administration has a poor blood supply.

Absorption

The rate and magnitude of a drug effect also is influenced by factors affecting its absorption. We shall use the term **absorption** to include the processes by which a drug is transferred from the lumen of the gastrointestinal tract, the muscles, dermis, or similar site to the blood or lymph. These processes, defined and described in elementary biochemistry and physiology texts, are **passive transfer** by simple diffusion or filtration, **specialized transport** by facilitated diffusion or active transport, and **pinocytosis**. They apply to transfer to and from the capillaries, into and out of target cells, and into excretory pathways (such as into the urine), as well as to absorption from the gastrointestinal tract. Many properties of drugs affect their absorption.

Solubility. Drugs may be administered in the form of solutions, suspensions, capsules, or tablets. If a drug is not in solution, it must be dissolved before it can be absorbed. This process will affect the rate at which it will be absorbed. The structure of the drug can often be manipulated to affect the speed of solubility. For example, protamine sulfate is added to insulin to form a suspension and decrease its rate of absorption. Food in the stomach or taken concurrently affects the solubility of some drugs taken orally.

Concentration. Absorption of most drugs from the gastrointestinal tract is by diffusion, and the rate is proportionate to the concentration. Thus larger more frequent doses will result in higher concentrations and more rapid absorption. On the other hand, the concentration of drugs taken by mouth may be decreased by dilution with gastric contents if the drug is taken with or immediately following meals.

Properties of the Drug Molecule. Several properties of drugs affect the rate at which they are transported across membranes and thereby affect their absorption.
Size of molecules. Smaller molecules generally are absorbed more rapidly than large molecules. The rate of absorption of a drug can therefore be slowed if it is bound to some material that increases the size of the molecules.
Lipid solubility. Lipid-soluble compounds cross cell membranes easily and therefore are absorbed more rapidly than are water-soluble drugs.
Ionization. Ionized drugs are absorbed more slowly than those that are not ionized. For example, many drugs are weak acids or weak bases and are absorbed in the stomach or small intestine. Drugs that are either strongly acidic or basic are more ionized and cross lipid membranes poorly. Thus they are poorly absorbed.

Effect of Gastric Emptying. Drugs that retard gastric emptying, such as chloroquine (an amebicide), will have decreased rates of absorption from the intestine.

Blood Supply at Injection Site. The rate of absorption from an injection site will vary with the blood supply at that site. Absorption from muscle is more rapid than absorption from subcutaneous fat.

Distribution

The term **distribution** includes the processes by which a drug, given for its systemic effect, is distributed in the body from the site at which it enters the circulatory system. The distribution of a drug influences its concentration and thus the rate and magnitude of its effects. When the drug is absorbed from the gastrointestinal tract or another site, it is distributed by the bloodstream or lymph. When it reaches the area of its target cell, the drug again must cross membranes to make contact with its receptor. These membranes usually are capillary cells but sometimes include the membranes of the target cells themselves. Those factors, previously listed, that affect absorption by their effect on the ability of the drug to cross cell membranes also influence the distribution of drugs by their effect on the drug's ability to cross membranes at the target cell.

There are additional factors that must be considered in drug distribution.

Volume of Distribution.

When a specified dose of a drug is given and absorbed into the circulatory system, it becomes diluted by the blood, and its concentration decreases. If a drug could not be transferred out of the circulatory system, it would be diluted by the fluid of the blood plasma, approximately 3 liters in an average adult. This 3 liters is its volume of distribution. If the drug diffuses throughout the extracellular fluid, its volume of distribution could be approximately 12 liters in the same adult. If the drug can diffuse across all membranes and is evenly distributed within the cells as well, its volume of distribution might be approximately 40 liters, and its concentration in that fluid would be correspondingly reduced if the dose were the same.

Blood Supply to Target Organ.

Many drugs are used for their effect on a specific organ. If the target organ has a large blood supply, such as the liver or kidneys, it will receive a larger proportion of the drug. In the liver and kidneys, endothelial linings of the liver sinusoids and renal glomerular capillaries permit faster transport of drugs; therefore, the liver and kidneys are associated with faster drug distribution than are other organs.

Plasma Protein Binding.

Drugs bind to plasma protein and protein other than their specific receptors. The binding to plasma albumin is quantitatively the most important of these, although some binding to globulin does occur. When a drug is bound to such a protein, it does not cross membranes and may not reach its active site. Alternatively, some drugs have an affinity for a cellular constituent, such as certain nucleoproteins in cells that are not necessarily target cells. The net effect of protein binding is to reduce the concentration of free, or active, drug produced by a given dose. However, the bound and free drug forms are in equilibrium. As the free drug is absorbed from the circulatory system, the drug–plasma protein complex dissociates to restore the equilibrium and provide free drug. Therefore, protein binding tends to prolong the action of a drug. There are, however, limits to the capacity for protein binding. Once the system becomes saturated, additional drug may reach toxic levels quickly. A patient with decreased levels of plasma proteins—as a result of malnutrition, for example—may require smaller doses of drugs, since smaller amounts will be bound. Toxic levels will also be more easily reached in these patients.

Concentration in Adipose and Other Tissues.

Lipid-soluble drugs may concentrate in adipose tissue but will be in equilibrium with the drug concentration in the plasma. This may increase the length of time a drug is active, a factor that may be important in patients who are severely under or over normal weight.

Some drugs, such as quinacrine hydrochloride, localize in the liver and are protected against degradation. Thus their half-lives are prolonged. A drug that precipitates in the gastrointestinal tract is distributed more slowly, and so its action may be prolonged.

Blood-Brain Barrier. The capillaries in the brain are more tightly bound to each other and are surrounded by a thicker basement membrane than are the capillaries in other organs. They are enveloped by **glial cells**, which act as a barrier to many water-soluble compounds. These factors are referred to collectively as the **blood-brain barrier**. They form a barrier to absorption by passive diffusion of water-soluble or ionized drugs. The blood-brain barrier interferes with drug transfer to the central nervous system, cerebrospinal fluid, and the aqueous humor of the eye.

Placental Barrier. The placenta serves as a barrier to some drugs. In general, the placenta presents a greater barrier to large molecules and a lesser barrier to drugs composed of small molecules. This can be an important consideration when drugs are prescribed for pregnant women.

Inflammation. The permeability of some membranes to drugs changes in the presence of inflammation. Penicillin, for example, will penetrate into the cerebrospinal fluid of a patient with meningitis more easily than in a person without infection.

Drug Metabolism and Excretion

The discussion thus far has been based on an idealized model in which termination of drug activity, which begins almost immediately following its administration, has not been considered. A drug must be either excreted or inactivated to stop its activity. A common unit of measure for a drug's activity is **half-life**, the time in which the concentration of a drug in the plasma is reduced to half its original concentration.

Excretion

Most drugs or their metabolites are in solution and are excreted in the urine. Some are excreted into the bile and thence into the intestine to be excreted in the feces; however, many of these are reabsorbed from the intestine and recycled so that urinary excretion remains the primary excretory pathway. Some other, usually minor, excretory pathways include the lungs for volatile compounds, and other body fluids such as sweat, tears, saliva, and milk. Excretion in milk may be an important consideration for the infants of nursing mothers but is not usually a major excretory pathway for the mother herself.

Various methods may be used to alter the rate of excretion of a drug, including changing the pH of the urine and decreasing renal tubular secretion of the drug. These methods may be used to decrease the excretion rate and prolong drug action or to increase the excretion rate to eliminate toxic materials.

Drug Biotransformations

Many drugs undergo one or more molecular changes while they are in the body. These changes are referred to as **biotransformations** or **metabolism** and often involve specific nutrients (Table 4-1). Some of these reactions are therefore influenced by nutritional status. The effects of some drugs are produced before or during such transformations. Other drugs undergo a biotransformation to produce a metabolic product which is the active compound. Many drugs undergo a biotransformation for purposes of **detoxification** — that is, altering the drug so as to stop its action. Many of these reactions also convert lipid-soluble drugs into more polar and more water-soluble drugs that can be excreted in the urine. Otherwise, lipid-soluble drugs might remain in the body almost indefinitely.

The reactions that occur in biotransformations commonly are classified into two categories, **nonsynthetic** and **synthetic** reactions.

Nonsynthetic Reactions. Nonsynthetic reactions, including oxidation, reduction, and hydrolysis, may make the drug more active or less active or may increase its toxicity. The

Table 4-1. Nutrients Used in Drug Oxidation and Conjugation

Nutrient	Oxidation	Conjugation
Carbohydrate		Glucose
Lipid	Lecithin	Acetyl (also from protein and carbohy-drate)
Amino acids and derivatives	Glycine Protein	Glycine Glutamic acid, glutamine Cysteine, cystine Methionine Serine Arginine Alanine Some peptides
Minerals	Iron, copper, calcium, zinc, magne-sium	
Vitamins	Pantothenate Niacin Riboflavin Ascorbic acid(?)	Pantothenate Niacin Folate Vitamin B_{12}

reactions are catalyzed by specific enzymes, such as esterases, or by nonspecific enzymes. The latter are the microsomal enzymes, found mostly in the liver in the smooth endoplasmic reticulum of the hepatocytes.

Most oxidations are accomplished by the

Figure 4-2. Mixed-function oxidizing (MFO) system. RH = a substrate; C = an unidentified electron acceptor; ROH = the oxidized RH substrate. (Adapted with permission from Williams, R.T., Nutrients in drug detoxication reactions. In J.N. Hathcock and J. Coon, Eds., Nutrition and Drug Interrelationships. New York: Academic Press, 1978. p. 306.)

mixed-function oxidizing (MFO) **system** (Figure 4-2), which requires (1) cytochrome P-450, (2) NADPH-cytochrome c reductase (a flavoprotein), (3) lecithin, (4) NADPH, and (5) oxygen. Some reduction reactions occur in the microsomal fraction of cells and others in the cytosol. Hydrolysis reactions occur in the blood plasma and in the soluble fraction of cells. The nutrients needed for oxidation reactions are shown in Table 4-1; those required for reduction or hydrolysis are less well understood but seem to be similar.

Synthetic Reactions. Synthetic reactions, including acetylation, sulfation, methylation, or combination with glycine, glutamine, or glucuronic acid, are called **conjugations** and consist of the combination of two materials in the body to form a new compound. In drug metabolism, one of the components involved in a conjugation reaction is the drug or a metabolite produced by one of the nonsynthetic reactions. The other component, the **conjugating agent**, is provided by the body.

One of the most important of the conjugating agents is glucuronic acid, which is derived from carbohydrate. Protein provides glycine, glutamine, cysteine, glutathione, and methionine as sources of conjugating agents and also serves as a source of sulfate. Acetyl groups can be derived from protein, fat, or carbohydrates. Other nutrients necessary for some of the common conjugations are shown in Table 4-1.

Factors Influencing Rate of Metabolism. Drugs usually are metabolized at rates de-

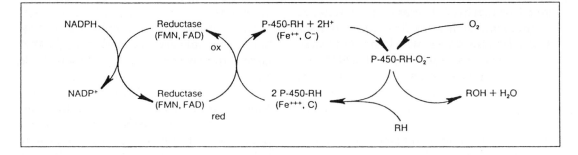

pendent on their concentration, but there are several factors that influence and alter this generalization. First, decreased concentration of the circulating free drug, such as that resulting from protein binding or concentration in adipose tissue, will reduce the rate of drug biotransformation. Second, the metabolism of drugs is dependent on the nutrient supply, and so clinical conditions that compromise the supply of these nutrients may affect the biotransformations of drugs. Third, depressed levels of drug-metabolizing enzymes resulting, for example, from liver disease, or occurring in a newborn infant will lower the rate of drug metabolism. Finally, one drug may alter the metabolism of another. Drug interactions with nutrients will be discussed in more detail in the next section.

Drug Safety and Effectiveness in Individuals

Factors Modifying Drug Effects in Individuals

A number of factors modify the effect of drugs in individuals. Some of these apply to all persons, and some only to selected individuals.

Body weight: In individuals of normal weight, a larger person will require a larger dose of a given drug than will the smaller person to maintain an equal concentration of the drug.

Body composition: If a person is seriously overweight or underweight, efficacy of drugs may be altered because of the differences in proportions of body fat and body water.

Age: In addition to its obvious effect on body size, in the early years age has a significant effect on drug metabolism. Some enzyme systems for drug metabolism are underdeveloped in infants, resulting in increased and prolonged drug action. The elderly may also have altered absorption or metabolism of drugs.

Gender: Women normally have more fat and less water than do men of equal weight and usually will require less drug. In addition, if the woman is pregnant or lactating, the effect of the drug on the fetus or on the nursing infant is an important consideration.

General physical condition: Severe renal or liver disease decreases the ability to excrete many drugs and thus will prolong their effect. Diseases that reduce the hydration of the body may affect drug action as a result of the change in the volume of distribution. For example, as the water content of the body is decreased, the volume of distribution also decreases, with a consequent increase in drug concentration. Conversely, if the patient is edematous, the volume of distribution may be expanded.

Individual Variations in Drug Response

Some patients may develop an allergy to a drug. The allergic reaction is an unusual response of the immune system, the mechanism of which is described in Chapter 6. The magnitude of the response is not related to the size of the dose, but, in order for an allergic response to occur, the patient must have had a previous exposure to the drug or a molecule of similar structure.

Some individuals react to a drug in a manner that is different from the usual but is not an allergy. This is called an **idiosyncrasy** and is believed to be the result of a mutation. It differs from a **toxicity** in that a toxicity will occur in all persons. In both an idiosyncrasy and a toxicity, unlike allergy, the magnitude of the response is related to the size of the dose, and the first dose can elicit the abnormal response.

After repeated exposure to some drugs, a patient may develop a drug **tolerance**; that is, an increasing amount is needed to cause the same response. This occurs especially with those drugs acting on the central nervous system. The mechanisms by which drug tolerances develop are not understood completely. It has been suggested that there may be a decrease in the rate of absorption, in the rate of transfer to the active site, or in the response of the receptor cells, resulting in diminished or slower reaction, or a drug may induce the enzymes of the MFO system. The phenomenon of drug tolerance is relevant to the abuse of "hard" drugs.

Drug Interactions

Patients frequently receive more than one drug at a time. There are several types of drug interactions that may be important. **Summation** occurs when two or more drugs elicit the same response, and the combined response is the sum of the effect of each. If each of these drugs elicits the response by acting via the same mechanism, the effect is **additive**. An additive response is, therefore, a form of summation.

Sometimes, two or more drugs that elicit the same response, such as raising blood glucose, have a greater effect together than the sum of each separately. This is called **synergism**. If, on the other hand, the effect of two or more drugs is less than the sum of each separately, the effect is referred to as an **antagonism**. Antagonistic reactions may be (1) pharmacologic (the drugs compete for the same receptor); (2) physiologic (the drugs have opposing actions at different receptors); or (3) chemical (the drugs react with each other to produce an inactive substance).

Classification and Terminology

Drugs may be classified in several ways. One of the simplest systems is a grouping into three categories:

1. *Drugs that fight infection:* These are the only drugs that actually cure a disease. They are toxic to the infecting organism, with little or no toxicity to the host.
2. *Drugs that replace inadequate materials:* Hormones, for example, sometimes are administered in amounts to replace inadequate levels in the body. When a drug is given at a dose level to provide replacement only, the amount is called a **physio-**

logic dose. A much larger **pharmacologic dose** is used for some purposes, but side effects will be more severe.
3. *Drugs that affect regulation:* Most drugs fall into this category. Examples include drugs that control blood pressure and those that control water and electrolyte balance.

Drugs may also be classified on the basis of the organ or tissue affected or on the basis of their type of action. The latter includes categories such as anti-infectives, anticonvulsants, hypotensive drugs, and anesthetics.

The naming of specific drugs within these categories has presented some problems. Drugs, as chemical compounds, have names that indicate their structure, but these names often are long and too difficult to pronounce or remember for common use. Therefore, when a drug is accepted for therapeutic use, it is assigned a name that is shorter and usually more pronounceable but still gives some indication of its chemical structure. This **generic** name is available for use in referring to the drug regardless of the manufacturer. In addition, manufacturers give their particular products names which only that manufacturer can use. Usually these names, the **proprietary** (or brand or trade) names, are the easiest to pronounce. In this book, the generic names of drugs are used, and an indication of the type of action of the drug is provided whenever possible. The professional in nutritional care may need to know the proprietary names that are equivalent to the various generic drug names. This information is contained in recent issues of one or more of various pharmaceutical indexes, some of which are listed in the Bibliography of this chapter.

NUTRITION-DRUG INTERRELATIONSHIPS

The interrelationships between nutrition and drugs may be examined broadly from two perspectives. One of these is the effects of drugs on the nutrition of the patient. The other is the influence of nutrition on drug action. Either or both of these may be important in a given patient.

In the material that follows, the tables contain extensive detail on drug-nutrient interactions. For the practicing nutritional care specialist, these may serve as general references. Those practicing with patients in specific categories (e.g., renal or oncology) will become familiar with the nutritional effects of drugs used frequently by those patients. In general, the most commonly used drugs in the United States are, in order, (1) prescription drugs acting on the central nervous system, (2) nonprescription cough and cold "remedies," (3) nonprescription internal analgesics, (4) anti-infectives, (5) prescription neoplasm and endocrine drugs, (6) prescription digestive and genitourinary drugs, and (7) prescription cardiovascular drugs.

Effects of Drugs on Nutrition

The specialist in nutritional care must be alert to medications that may contribute, either directly or indirectly, to malnutrition. This is true, of course, primarily when the drug is given over a long period of time. Drugs may affect nutritional status by changing nutrient intake, absorption, transport, metabolism, catabolism, or excretion. Some drugs interfere with protein, enzyme, or coenzyme synthesis and compete with nutrients for binding sites.

Drug Effects on Taste, Appetite, and Food Intake

Some drugs, described in Chapter 12, are used specifically for the purpose of increasing or decreasing the food intake of the patient. Other drugs, used for purposes unrelated to food intake regulation, affect food intake as a side effect of their primary function. It is these drugs that will be discussed in this chapter.

Anatomy of Taste and Odor. The **flavor** of food is a sensation that is thought to combine the effects of stimulation of sensory receptors in the tongue, palate, and pharynx, pro-

viding a sense of taste (**gustation**), stimulation of receptors for **odor** in the nose, providing the sense of smell (**olfaction**), and also temperature, texture, and color. The relative importance of the perception of taste and odor are not understood completely.

The sensory structures of the tongue and their innervation are depicted in Figure 4-3. Taste perception results from combinations of varying amounts of the sensations traditionally called *sweet, salty, sour,* and *bitter* and probably others. The ability to detect and recognize the "traditional" tastes are measured using pure chemicals — sugar, sodium chloride, citric acid, or caffeine — in solution, for convenience and to make comparisons possible. However, chemosensory scientists generally believe there are other tastes but have not agreed on terminology.

Taste buds located in the back of the tongue innervated by the ninth cranial (glossopharyngeal) nerve are more sensitive to bitter compounds and generally less sensitive to those classified as sweet, salty, or sour, in comparison to taste buds located on the anterior portion of the tongue. These anteriorly located taste buds are innervated by the **chorda tympani** (a branch of the facial or seventh cranial nerve). Within the individual taste buds, there are approximately sixty individual taste bud cells. Most of these respond to many stimuli but to varying degrees. The final taste perceived is the result of a complicated pattern of individual nerve fiber responses to stimuli.

Basic odors are much less precisely defined. It has been suggested that some of these may be **putrid, ethereal, musky,** and **camphoric.**[1] Detection and recognition of these odors are tested using butylmercaptan, diethyl ether, butylbenzene, or camphor in an odorless solvent. In addition, modern researchers classify odors on the basis of the molecular structure of the compounds and on the basis of portions of the molecule. Receptors are located in the mucosa high in the nose and are innervated by the olfactory nerve. Oral and nasal cavities are richly innervated also with free nerve endings (pain receptors), which respond to noxious stimuli

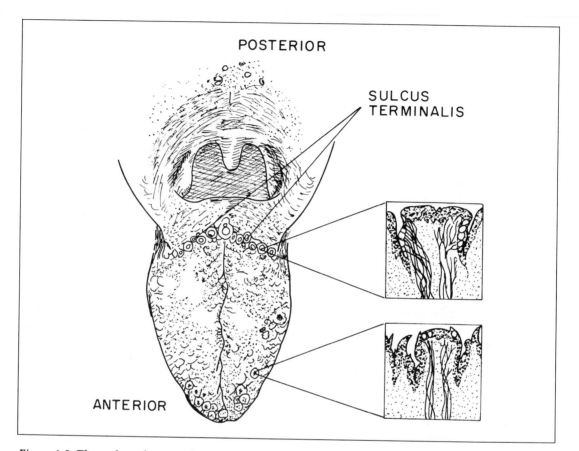

POSTERIOR

SULCUS
TERMINALIS

ANTERIOR

Figure 4-3. The surface of a normal tongue and palate. Filiform papillae may be seen covering the entire lingual surface. Fungiform papillae, somewhat larger and raised, may be seen covering the anterior two-thirds of the surface; they terminate at a V-shaped groove, the sulcus terminalis. Circumvallate papillae are seen over the posterior one-third of the lingual surface. Papillae may also be seen covering the area of the palate near the junction of the hard and soft palates. **Lower insert:** *Light microscopic appearance of a fungiform papilla. The taste buds, innervated by the chorda tympani branch of the facial nerve, are located at the top of the papilla only; free nerve endings may also be seen.* **Upper insert:** *Light microscopic appearance of a circumvallate papilla. The number of taste buds, innervated by a branch of the glossopharyngeal nerve, is much greater than in a fungiform papilla. These taste buds usually are located along the sides of the papilla. Free nerve endings may also be seen and are greater in number than in a fungiform papilla. (Adapted from Henkin, R.I., The role of taste in disease and nutrition. Borden's Rev. Nutr. Res. 28:71, 1967, pp. 72–73.)*

from materials such as pepper, chili, and ammonia.

Effect of Disease on Taste and Odor Perception. Even before a diagnosis is made and before any drugs are prescribed, the disease process itself may affect the patient's sensitivity to taste. If the membrane characteristics of the taste bud cells or olfactory receptors are altered or if electrical activity of the nerve cells involved in sensations of taste or smell is distorted, the message may be misinterpreted by the brain. "Salty" may be interpreted as "bitter," for example. If the electrical activity is blocked, reduced, or increased in intensity, the perception of the taste or odor would be absent, decreased, or increased accordingly. The descriptive terms used to define alterations in these senses, also known as **chemical senses**, are listed in Table 4-2.

Table 4-3 lists various conditions that may

Table 4-2. Alterations in Senses of Taste and Smell

Term		
Taste	Odor	Definition
Ageusia	Anosmia	Total loss of the perception
Hypogeusia	Hyposmia	Decreased ability to detect or identify a taste or odor
Hypergeusia	Hyperosmia	Increased sensitivity in detecting or recognizing a taste or odor
Dysgeusia	Dysosmia	Distortion (usually unpleasant) in the perception
Cacogeusia	Cacosmia	Obnoxious sensation most commonly elicited by egg, meat, poultry, fish, garlic, onions, tomatoes, coffee, chocolate, fried foods
Prantogeusia	Prantosmia	Sensation perceived without external stimuli
Heterogeusia	Heterosmia	Inappropriate but consistent sensation, e.g., all foods taste salty

cause alterations in taste or odor sensitivity. It is important to recognize that the symptoms may or may not be seen in an individual patient. In addition, these data are obtained from studies of responses to threshold levels of the stimulant. In a practical situation, stimuli are well above threshold concentrations, and so data on threshold responses may not be meaningful.

Drug Effects on Taste and Odor Perception.

In addition to patients with the conditions listed in Table 4-3, patients who are receiving any of a wide variety of drugs may suffer from alterations in taste or odor perceptions. Table 4-4 lists a number of these drugs.

Some drugs, such as potassium iodide and those containing bromides, are secreted into the saliva and thereby produce an unpleasant taste in the mouth. Others produce an unpleasant aftertaste or are themselves simply unpleasant tasting. These include penicillin, clofibrate, chloral hydrate, paraldehyde, and B-complex vitamins.

Drug Effects on Appetite and Food Intake.

Some drugs tend to decrease appetite as a side effect. Included among these are the drugs previously listed that have an unpleasant taste in the mouth. Additionally, drugs and other compounds can be borne to the taste receptors intravascularly via the capillaries supplying the receptors. As a consequence, there may be a lingering sensation after the stimulation from the inhaled or ingested substance is over. Other drugs depress food intake because they cause nausea, and some produce **anorexia** (abnormal absence of the desire for food) by mechanisms that are not understood. March[2] notes that an extensive number of drugs can cause nausea, vomiting, and anorexia. Table 4-5 lists those in which the action is frequent or more severe. Many antineoplastic agents cause severe nausea and vomiting as well as other symptoms that tend to decrease nutrient intake. They are discussed in greater detail in Chapter 15.

Some drugs tend to increase appetite as a side effect, but there are no safe and effective drugs whose primary function in humans is to increase food intake.[3] Those that have some appetite-stimulating side effects are listed in Table 4-6.

Nutritional Care of Patients with Altered Taste and Depressed Appetite.

Improved food intake can sometimes be achieved by altering meal schedules and catering to patients' likes and dislikes. Specific techniques are discussed further in Chapter 15, since cancer patients are often seriously affected. Patients receiving drugs that alter taste and appetite are candidates for repeated monitoring of nutritional status.

Drug Effects on Nutrient Absorption

Some drugs adversely affect the absorption of nutrients and thereby influence the nutri-

Table 4-3. Conditions That Might Alter Taste or Odor Sensitivities

Increased detection threshold[a]
Advanced age
Burns
Congenital defect
Copper deficiency
Zinc deficiency
Familial dysautonomia
Facial paralysis
Head injuries
Trauma (head injuries, gunshots, burns)
Sjögren's syndrome
Hypothyroidism
Mental depression
Chronic renal insufficiency
Cystic fibrosis of the pancreas (↓ odor; normal taste?)
Decreased detection threshold
Adrenocortical insufficiency
Panhypopituitarism
Congenital adrenal hyperplasia
Cystic fibrosis of the pancreas (↑ odor and taste?)
Congenital defect
Epileptic syndromes
Specific alterations in sensitivity
Turner's syndrome (↓ sour, ↓ bitter)
Gonadal dysgenesis
Pseudohypoparathyroidism (↓ sour, ↓ bitter)
Congenital cretinism
Congenital taste blindness
Drug-induced
Lesions of tongue or palate (tumor, infection, trauma, granuloma, irradiation, postsurgery) (↓ salt, ↓ sweet)
Maxillary dentures (↓ sour, ↓ bitter)
Menses
Pregnancy
Diabetes mellitus (↓ sweet if ↑ blood sugar)
Cancer (↓ sweet, ↓ salt, altered bitter)
Renal failure (↓ sweet, ↓ salt, ↓ sour)
Sjögren's syndrome (↓ bitter, ↓ sour, ↓ salt)
Schizophrenia

Compiled from Campanella, G., Filla, A., and DeMichele, G., Smell and taste acuity in epileptic syndromes. Eur. Neurol. 17:136, 1978; Henkin, R.I., The role of taste in disease and nutrition. Borden's Rev. Nutr. Res. 28:71, 1967; Henkin, R.I., and Christiansen, R.L., Taste thresholds in patients with dentures. J. Am. Diet. Assoc. 75:118, 1967; and Hertz, J., Cain, W.S., Bartoshuk, L.M., and Dolan, T.F., Jr., Olfactory and taste sensitivity in children with cystic fibrosis. Physiol. Behav. 14:89, 1975.

[a] Detection threshold is the lowest concentration of a substance that a person can discriminate as being different from water. Increased threshold indicates decreased sensitivity.

tional status of the patient. The resulting malabsorption defects have been classified as **primary** or **secondary**.[4]

Primary malabsorption is caused by action in the lumen or on the intestinal mucosa. The most severe primary malabsorption results from actions of drugs that damage the absorptive cells of the small intestine. Other mechanisms of action include (1) altering transit time, (2) binding bile acids and decreasing micelle formation, (3) acting as a physical barrier, and (4) altering the pH in the lumen of the gastrointestinal tract. Table 4-7 contains a list of drugs that cause malabsorption of various nutrients.

Secondary malabsorption of a nutrient is due to the interference of a drug with the absorption or metabolism of another nutrient. The primary example involves the interrelationship of drugs and vitamin D metabolism, which results in calcium malabsorption.[5]

Some drugs cause gastrointestinal upsets and diarrhea by causing changes in the intestinal flora.

Drug Effects on Nutrient Metabolism

The desirable effects of some drugs are based on their action of interfering with the activity of a nutrient. Some anticoagulant drugs, for example, are antagonists to vitamin K action. Other drugs affect nutrient metabolism as a side effect.

Alcohol, in particular, has a wide range of effects on nutrient metabolism. However, in view of its wide use as a social beverage and its association with liver disease, the nutritional effects of chronic alcoholism will be discussed in Chapter 13.

Protein. A number of drugs affect the metabolism of proteins and amino acids (Table 4-8). A few stimulate protein synthesis, but the majority have the opposite effect. The mode of action of many of these drugs is unknown. For patients receiving long-term therapy, it is important that their protein status be monitored frequently.

Lipids. Drugs that influence lipid metabolism may be divided roughly into those that raise plasma triglyceride or cholesterol levels and those that lower them. Some drugs are used for the primary purpose of lowering

Table 4-4. Drugs That May Alter Taste Sensations

Drug Category	Drug	Decreased Taste Acuity	Specific Alterations
Amino acid	Histidine		Induces bad taste
Anesthetic	Amydricaine	x	↓ bitter, ↓ salt
	Benzocaine		↑ sour
	Chloral hydrate		Bad taste
	Cocaine	x	↓ bitter, ↓ sweet
	Eucaine	x	↓ bitter, ↓ sweet
	Lidocaine	x	↓ sweet, ↓ salt
	Lincomycin · HCl		↓ sweet
	Procaine · HCl	x	↑ sweet
	Tetracaine · HCl	x	↓ bitter, ↑ sweet
Anorexic	Amphetamines		↓ sweet, ↑ bitter
Antiarrhythmic	Quinidine		Induces bad taste
Antiarthritic, anti-inflammatory	Phenylbutazone	x	
	Gold compounds		Induces bad taste
Antibiotic	Clindamycin		
	Lincomycin · HCl	x	
	Penicillin		Induces bad taste
	Streptomycin sulfate		
	Sulfasalazine	x	
Anticoagulant	Phenindione	x	
Anticonvulsant	Carbamazepine	x	
	Phenytoin	x	
Antidepressant	Nortriptyline · HCl		Unspecified bad taste
Antifungal	Griseofulvin	x	
Antigout	Allopurinol		Induces bad taste
Anti-infective	Metronidazole	x	Induces metallic, sharp taste
Antineoplastic	Fluorouracil		Altered bitter and sour, ↓ sweet
Antiparkinsonism	Bromocriptine mesylate		Induces bad taste
	Captopril		Induces bad taste, sweet tastes salty
	Levodopa	x	
Antithyroid	Methimazole	x	
	Methylthiouracil	x	
Antitubercular	Ethambutol · HCl		Induces bad taste
	Ethionamide		Induces metallic taste
	Rifampin	x	
Chelating agent	Penicillamine	x	↓ sweet, ↓ salt
Cholinergic-blocking	Anisotropine methyl-bromide	x	
	Oxyphencyclimine	x	
Diuretic	Furosemide		↓ sweet
Hormone	Insulin		↓ salt, ↓ sweet with prolonged use
Hypolipemic	Cholestyramine	x	
	Clofibrate		Unpleasant aftertaste
Immunosuppressant	Azathioprine	x	
Skeletal muscle relaxant	Baclofen	x	
Sedative	Triclofos sodium		↑ bitter
Tranquilizers/antipsychotics	Chlorpromazine		Induces bad taste, metallic taste
	Lithium carbonate		Unpleasant metallic taste; dairy products taste spoiled
	Thioridazine		Induces bad taste

Table 4-5. Drugs That May Cause Nausea, Vomiting, or Anorexia as a Side Effect

Adrenergic blocking agents	*Antifungal*	Busulfan	*Chelating agent*
Isoproterenol	Griseofulvin	Chlorambucil	Penicillamine
Metaproterenol	*Antihistamines*	Cis-Platinum	*Cholinergic blocking agents*
Analgesics	Brompheniramine	Cyclophosphamide	Anisotropine
Mefenamic acid	Chlorpheniramine	Cytarabine	Glycopyrrolate
Morphine sulfate	Cyproheptadine · HCl	Dactinomycin	Oxyphencyclimine
Oxycodone · HCl	Diphenhydramine · HCl	Daunorubicin	Procyclidine
Oxymorphone · HCl	Tripelennamine	5-fluorouracil	*Diuretic*
Pentazocine · HCl	*Anti-infective*	Hydroxyurea	Furosemide
Propoxyphene	Cephalexin	Lomustine	Spironolactone
Salicylates	Cephalothin	Mechlorethamine	*Hormones*
Anorexic	Cephalosporin	Melphalan	Estrogen
Amphetamine	Clindamycin	Methotrexate	*Hypnotic*
Phendimetrazine tartrate	Erythromycin	Mithramycin	Glutethimide
Antiarrhythmic	Kanamycin	Nitrogen mustard	*Hypocholesterolemic*
Amiodarone (Cordarone)	Lincomycin	Pipobroman	Cholestyramine
Digitalis	Metronidazole	Procarbazine	Nicotinic acid
Mexiletine (Mexitil)	Nitrofurantoin	Vinblastine	*Hypoglycemic*
Procainamide	Nystatin	Vincristine	Acetoheximide
Propranolol	Pyrvinium	*Antiparkinsonism*	*Hypolipemic*
Anticonvulsants	Sulfasalazine	Amantadine · HCl	B-sitosterol
Carbamazepine	Tetracyclines	Benztropine mesylate	Clofibrate
Ethosuximide	Penicillins:	Diphenhydramine	Probucol
Ethotoin	Ampicillin	Levodopa	*Hypotensive*
Methsuximide	Carbenicillin	Trihexyphenidyl	Captopril
Phenacemide	Methicillin	*Antispasmodic*	Deserpidine
Phenobarbital	Oxacillin	Diclomine · HCl	Guanethidine
Phensuximide	*Anti-inflammatory*	Methocarbamol	Hydralazine
Primidone	Benemid (for gout)	*Antitubercular*	Methyldopa
Trimethadione	Ibuprofen	Ethambutol	Propranolol
Antidepressants	Indomethacin	Ethionamide	Reserpine
Amitriptyline	Noprofen	Isoniazid	*Tranquilizers*
Desipramine	Oxyphenbutazone	P-aminosalicylic acid	Chlordiazepoxide
Doxepin · HCl	Phenylbutazone	Pyrimethamine	Lithium carbonate
Imapramine	Zomeperac	Rifampin	Loxapine · HCl
Isocarboxazide	*Antineoplastic*	*Bronchodilators*	Meprobamate
Nortriptyline	Actinomycin D	Brompheniramine	Thioridazine · HCl
Phenelzine · SO₄	Azathioprine	Dyphylline	*Vasodilators*
Antiemetic	BCNU (Carmustine)	Metaproterenol	Dipyridamole
Diphenhydramine	Bleomycin	Theophylline	

blood lipid levels. These will be discussed in Chapter 10. Others affect lipid metabolism as a side effect. These are listed in Table 4-9 and are categorized according to the direction of their effects.

Carbohydrates. Drugs that affect carbohydrate metabolism may be divided into those that increase blood glucose levels and those that lower them. Some affect blood glucose levels as side effects of their intended actions (Table 4-10), whereas it is the primary purpose of others, such as insulin and the oral hypoglycemic agents, to lower blood glucose levels.

Vitamins and Minerals. Some drugs are useful primarily as a result of their relationship to minerals or vitamins in the body. As previously mentioned, penicillamine is a chelating agent used in the treatment of Wilson's disease to remove excess copper. There are diuretics that function primarily because of their effects on sodium excretion.

However, drugs may have important side effects as a result of their actions on mineral

Table 4-6. Drugs That Tend to Increase Appetite

Drug	Function	Suggested Mechanism
Alcohol	Social beverage	Stimulate sense of taste; increase flow of secretions in digestive system; promote relaxation
Androgens	Hormone	
Benzodiazepines	Antidepressant; tranquilizer	Promote relaxation
Corticosteroids	Hormone	
Cyproheptadine hydrochloride	Antihistamine	Direct effect on hypothalamus or hypoglycemic effect
Insulin	Hormone	Hypoglycemic effect
Phenothiazines	Antipsychotic; tranquilizer	Promote relaxation; antiemetic
Sulfonylureas (e.g., tolbutamide, chlorpropamide)	Hypoglycemic agents	Stimulate insulin release

or vitamin metabolism. When these alterations result in increased nutrient requirements, the possibility of deficiency results, particularly in patients who have had marginal diets over extended periods or in those whose nutritional status has been damaged by the disease process. The nutritional care specialist should be alert to the increased needs of such patients, particularly when treatments involve long-term, high dosages of the drugs listed in Table 4-11.

Nutritional Care

Patients receiving drugs that affect nutrient absorption or metabolism for a long period should be monitored for changes in nutritional status. Many interactions of drugs and nutrients cause only changes in serum levels of nutrients but no clinical signs or symptoms. If deficiencies of vitamins and minerals cause specific signs or symptoms, the attending physician may order supplements.

Effects of Food and Nutrients on Drugs

Food or specific nutrients sometimes affect the action of drugs.

Effects of Food on Drug Absorption

Most drugs are taken on an empty stomach one hour before or two hours after a meal. However, drugs that cause unpleasant side effects in the stomach are sometimes exceptions to the rule.

Food in the Digestive Tract. Many drugs acts as gastric irritants when taken orally (Table 4-12). It is recommended that these drugs be taken with food.[6] The presence of food may alter the pH, osmolality, amount of various secretions, or motility of the gastrointestinal tract. Any of these changes, as well as differences in volume, temperature, and viscosity of stomach contents, can, in turn, alter the absorption of drugs by causing alterations in their ionization, stability, solubility, or transit time. There is no constant effect of food on drug absorption. It may be decreased, delayed, or increased (Table 4-13), depending on the drug involved. As Table 4-13 suggests, the more frequent effect is a reduction in the amount or rate of drug absorption. Such changes reduce the blood level of the drug, thus reducing its effectiveness. When the rate of absorption is reduced, the action of the drug is prolonged. Conversely, when absorption is increased, the blood level may be increased, perhaps to toxic levels. These effects are of clinical importance when fast action of the drug is needed. Concomitant use of food and drugs can also delay drug absorption, resulting in a later peak concentration. This may or may not be accompanied by a reduction in the total amount of drug absorbed.

Table 4-7. Intestinal Absorption Defects Induced by Drugs

Drug	Nutrients Lost	Mechanism	Notes on Nutritional Care
Antacids (containing magnesium)	Riboflavin	Increases pH	Monitor serum riboflavin
Anticonvulsant (Phenytoin, primidone, phenobarbital)	Folate, vitamin B_{12}, Ca	Accelerates vitamin D metabolism in liver; mechanism in folate absorption unclear	Monitor nutrient levels; supplement as necessary
Antihypertensive (Methyldopa)	Folate, vitamin B_{12}, Fe	Autoimmune	
Anti-infectives			
Neomycin, Cycloserine, Erythromycin, Kanamycin	Nitrogen, fat, Ca, Na, K, Mg, Fe, vitamins A, B_{12}, folate	Structural defect; bile acid sequestration	Monitor nutrient levels; supplement as necessary
Sulfasalazine	Folate	Mucosal block	Monitor for anemia (uncommon)
Tetracyclines		Forms chelates with di- and trivalent cations (effect on Fe absorption not clinically significant)	Take medication 1 hour a.c. or 2 hours p.c.
Anti-inflammatory (gout) (Colchicine)	Fat, carotene, Na, K, vitamin B_{12}	Mitotic arrest; structural defect; enzyme damage	Monitor vitamins A and B_{12} and electrolyte status; supplement as necessary
Antineoplastic (Methotrexate)	Folate, vitamin B_{12}, Ca	Mucosal damage	Monitor folate and B_{12} status
Antitubercular (Paraaminosalicylic acid)	Fat, Ca, Mg, Fe, folate, vitamin B_{12}	Mucosal block in B_{12} uptake; can cause megaloblastic anemia; mechanism in fat absorption unclear	Monitor nutrient levels; supplement as necessary
Contraceptive (Estrogen containing)	Vitamin C		
Glucocorticoid (Dexamethasone)	Folate		Megaloblastic anemia
Hypocholesterolemic Cholestyramine	Fat, fat-soluble vitamins, carotene, vitamin B_{12}, Fe	Binding of bile acids, salts and nutrients	Monitor B_{12}, A and Fe status; supplement as necessary
Clofibrate	Vitamins A, D, E, B_{12}	Unknown action on liver	Monitor nutrients; supplement as necessary
Colestipol	Fat, fat-soluble vitamins	Binds and promotes excretion of bile acids	Monitor nutrient levels
Laxatives			
Castor oil	Ca, K		Ca and K supplements
Milk of magnesia	Ca, K		Ca and K supplements
Mineral oil	Carotene, vitamins A, D, K	Physical barrier; nutrients dissolve in oil and are lost	Avoid use near meal times
Phenolphthalein	Vitamin D, Ca	Intestinal "hurry," K depletion; structural changes	Monitor serum K and Ca; supplement K and Ca
Potassium repletion (KCl)	Vitamin B_{12}	Change in ileal pH to inhibit B_{12} absorption	Monitor B_{12} status
Sedative (Glutethimide)	Ca		Acute folacin deficiency

Compiled from Roe, D.A., *Drug-Induced Nutritional Deficiencies.* Westport, Conn.: AVI, 1976; Utah Dietetic Association, *Handbook of Clinical Dietetics,* 1977; Bernard, M.A., Jacobs, D.O. and Rombeau, J.L., *Nutritional and Metabolic Support of Hospitalized Patients.* Philadelphia: W.B. Saunders, 1986; Holtzapple, P.G., and Schwartz, S.E., Drug-induced maldigestion and malabsorption. In D.A. Roe and T.C. Campbell, Eds., *Drugs and Nutrients. The Interactive Effects.* New York: Dekker, 1984; Grant, A., *Nutritional Assessment Guidelines,* 2nd ed. Seattle: Anna Grant, 1979; and Moore, A.O., and Powers, D.E., *Food-Medication Interactions,* 3rd ed. Tempe, Ariz.: Food-Medication Interactions, 1981.

Table 4-8. Drugs That Affect Protein Metabolism

Drug	Action
Analgesic	
Salicylates	Produces aminoaciduria
Antibiotic	
Tetracyclines	Inhibits protein synthesis
Antifungal	
Amphotericin B	Accelerates catabolism
Chloramphenicol	
Antineoplastic	
Azaribine	Inhibits protein synthesis
Bleomycin	Inhibits DNA and RNA synthesis
Cis-platin, mitomycin	Cross-links DNA helix
Cytarabine	Inhibits DNA polymerase
Dactinomycin; daunorubicin; doxorubicin	Prevents DNA template activity; inhibits RNA synthesis
5-fluorouracil	Inhibits pyrimidine synthesis
L-asparaginase	Deaminates asparagine
6-mercaptopurine, thioguanine	Inhibits purine ring synthesis; inhibits nucleotide interconversion reactions
Methotrexate	Inhibits purine ring synthesis
Vinblastine, vincristine	Inhibits microtubular function
Hormone	
Anabolic steroids, insulin	Stimulate synthesis
Corticosteroids	Increases gluconeogenesis; increases urinary nitrogen
Thyroid	Increases urinary nitrogen

Specific Nutrients. Individual nutrients also affect the absorption of some drugs. The interactions of certain nutrients with tetracycline, griseofulvin, or tetrachloroethylene may be of particular clinical importance.

The antibiotics tetracycline and oxytetracycline form insoluble complexes with calcium, magnesium, iron, or aluminum, which inhibit absorption of the drug; therefore, it usually is recommended that tetracycline or its derivatives be taken without milk or milk products. Tetracycline can cause serious

Table 4-9. Drugs with Side Effects Altering Serum Lipid Levels

Drug	Increased Serum Level	Decreased Serum Level
Analgesic		Ampicillin
		Oxacillin
		Penicillin
Antibiotic		Chlortetracycline · HCl
Anticoagulant		Phenindione
Anticonvulsant		Carbamazepine
Anti-inflammatory		Colchicine
		Nonsteroidal
		Steroids
Antiobesity		Fenfluramine · HCl
Antitubercular		P-aminosalicylic acid
		Rifampin
Hormone	Corticosteroids	Glucagon
	Growth hormone	
	Vitamin D	
Hormone antagonist	Thiouracil	
Tranquilizer	Chlorpromazine	
Uricosuric		Sulfinpyrazone

Table 4-10. Drugs Altering Blood Glucose as a Side Effect

Drug	Hyperglycemic	Hypoglycemic
Analgesic	Morphine	Aspirin, phenacetin, acetaminophen
Anticoagulant	Coumarin derivatives	
Anticonvulsant	Phenytoin	
Antidepressants/antihypotensive		Monoamine oxidase inhibitors
Anti-infective		Sulfonamides
Anti-inflammatory		Phenylbutazone
Antiobesity		Fenfluramine
Antiparkinsonism	Levodopa	
B-adrenergic blocker		Propranolol · HCl
Diuretic	Thiazides	
Hormones	Corticosteroids, estrogen	Anabolic steroids
Hypotensive	Diazoxide, clonidine	
Sedatives		Barbiturates
Tranquilizers	Phenothiazines	
Uricosuric	Probenecid	

nausea and vomiting, and sodium bicarbonate, which some patients may take for their gastrointestinal symptoms, seems to reduce tetracycline absorption. Possibly, the mechanism of action involves the change in pH of the gastric contents. In any case, there is danger that the drug will be rendered ineffective, with potentially serious consequences. Newer tetracycline derivatives such as doxycycline and monocycline are less affected by food, but serum levels may be reduced by concomitant use of antacids and iron preparations.

Griseofulvin (an antifungal agent) and tetrachloroethylene (an anthelmintic) are absorbed more rapidly if taken with a high-fat meal.

Effects of Nutritional Status on Drug Metabolism and Excretion

The malnutrition that often can occur in hospitalized patients may have a detrimental effect on the metabolism of many drugs.[7–9] Many nutrients can be involved.

Protein. Protein deprivation can affect drug binding in two ways. First, it reduces the amount of plasma albumin available for binding. Since the unbound, or free, drug is the active component, a decrease in plasma albumin results in an increase in the amount of drug available to react with binding sites, to be metabolized, and to be excreted. The net effect is an increase in drug potency in a shorter time. Second, other substances such as nonpolar amino acids and free fatty acids carried by albumin may affect drug binding.[10] The clinical significance of altered levels of these substances is unknown.

In addition to the effects on drug binding, protein deficiency depresses both the cytochrome P-450 content and P-450 reductase activity in the MFO system.[11] The consequences of these actions vary. If the MFO system detoxifies a drug, the protein deficiency would have the effect of making the drug more toxic. If, however, the MFO system metabolizes a drug to a more toxic compound, protein deficiency would decrease the toxicity of the drug. These statements, however, assume a simple one-step metabolic pathway. The effects of protein deficiency in more complex systems need additional study.

Lipids. Lipids have been reported to be essential for normal functioning of the MFO system,[12] although their precise function is not understood entirely.[13] A fat-free diet has

Table 4-11. *Vitamin and Mineral Interactions in Chronic Drug Use*

Drug	Nutrient	Mechanism	Possible Signs and Symptoms	Notes on Nutritional Care
Analgesics Aspirin, APC, indomethacin	Vitamin D, Ca	↓ D absorption; 2° low serum Ca	Decreased serum D	Do not use in K deficiency
	Vitamin K		Can induce hypoprothrombin-emia	C supplement if needed Avoid alcohol; take with meals, milk, or antacids
	Vitamin C Fe	1–3 g/day may produce GI bleeding	Decreased C in platelets Fe deficiency	Folate supplement if needed
	Folate	Alters transport by competing for binding sites	Folate deficiency	
Antacids Aluminum hydroxide	Thiamine	Destruction; decreased absorption	Thiamine deficiency	Thiamine supplement if needed
	Phosphate	Deplete phosphorus; ↑ Ca absorption	Hypercalciuria, osteomalacia, and stones	Increase phosphate intake except in renal failure
Antiarrhythmic (Digoxin and Quinidine)	All vitamins	Diarrhea	Deficiency	Maintain high potassium diet for patient taking digoxin/digitoxin to avoid K depletion toxicity
Anticoagulants (Coumarin and derivatives)	Vitamin K		Hemorrhage	Avoid excess vitamin K in excess clotting disorders (thrombosis, embolism); avoid cabbage, kale, leafy vegetables, cauliflower, liver, cheese, fish, egg yolks, soybean oil; check multivitamin preparations for K content; monitor vegetarian diets; do not take with alcohol
Anticonvulsants	Folate	↓ absorption?; competitive inhibition of coenzymes; enzyme induction	Megaloblastic anemia	Vitamin supplements if needed
Phenytoin Primidone Phenobarbital	Vitamin C Vitamin D Vitamin K Vitamin B$_{12}$	Increased excretion Enzyme induction Enzyme induction	Deficiency Rickets, osteomalacia Neonatal hemorrhage	Supplement folate, vitamin B$_{12}$, vitamin D if needed

(continued)

Table 4-11. (Continued)

Drug	Nutrient	Mechanism	Possible Signs and Symptoms	Notes on Nutritional Care
Anti-infective				
Chloramphenicol	Folate	↓ utilization	Rb and B₁₂ deficiency	
	Vitamin B₆	Inactivate		
	Vitamin K and protein	↓ synthesis		
Neomycin	Vitamin B₁₂	Mucosal damage; inhibition of intrinsic factor	Malabsorption	
	Vitamin A	Mucosal damage; inhibition pancreatic lipase; binding bile salts	Malabsorption	
Penicillins	Vitamin K	↓ synthesis		
	Folate	↓ utilization		
	Vitamin B₆	Inactivate		
Sulfonamides	Vitamin K	↓ bacterial synthesis	Hypoprothrombinemia	
Tetracyclines	Vitamin C	↑ excretion		
	Folate	Malabsorption	Anemia	
	Vitamin K	↓ bacterial synthesis	Hypoprothrombinemia	
Trimethoprim	Folate	Inhibition of dihydrofolate reductase	Megaloblastic anemia	
Anti-inflammatory				
Colchicine (for gout)	Vitamin B₁₂, carotene	Absorptive enzyme damage; mucosal damage	B₁₂ deficiency; ↓ serum carotene	B₁₂ supplements if needed; low purine diet?
Phenylbutazone	Folate	Malabsorption	Megaloblastic anemia	
Antimalarial (Pyrimethamine)	Folate	Inhibition of dihydrofolate reductase	Megaloblastic anemia	Treat anemia with folate > 25 mg/week or supplement with folinic acid which bypasses the metabolic blocks if needed
Antineoplastic				
Methotrexate	Folate	Inhibition of dihydrofolate reductase	Megaloblastic anemia	See Chapter 15 for further information
Cis-platin and other heavy metal	Mg, Zn, K		Mineral depletion	Foods high in Fe; Fe supplement if needed
Antiparkinsonism (Levodopa)	Vitamin B₆	↑ vitamin-drug complex excretion	Peripheral neuropathy	B₆ may limit drug effectiveness; may need to limit foods rich in vitamin B₆; avocado, beans, beef liver, dry skim milk, malted milk, oatmeal, pork, tuna, yams, cheese, wine, yeast, wheat germ

Drug category	Vitamin/Mineral	Mechanism	Effect
Antitubercular (Isoniazid, Cycloserine, ethionamide, pyrazinamide)	Vitamin B_6	↑ Vitamin-drug complex excretion; interferes with pyridoxal kinase to cause decreased pyridoxal phosphate synthesis	Peripheral neuropathy; anemia; generalized convulsions (infants)
	Niacin	Competitive inhibition of vitamin coenzymes 2° to B_6 deficiency	Pellagra
Chelating agent (Penicillamine)	Vitamin K	↓ bacterial synthesis	Peripheral neuropathy
	Vitamin B_6	↑ vitamin-drug complex excretion	
	Zn, Cu		Mineral depletion
Contraceptive (Estrogen-containing)	Folate	Inhibition of absorptive enzymes; ↑ synthesis of folate-binding macroglobulin; enzyme induction	Megaloblastic anemia
	Vitamin B_{12}	Alters tissue distribution	
	Vitamin B_6	Tryptophan oxygenase induction; competition for apoenzyme binding sites	Depression
	Vitamin C	↑ serum ceruloplasmin, altered tissue distribution	
Diuretics Furosemide	K, Mg, Zn, Ca		Mineral depletion
Thiazides	K, Mg, Zn		Mineral depletion
Triamterene	Folate	Inhibition of dihydrofolate reductase	Megaloblastic anemia
Hypnotic (Glutethimide)	Vitamin D	Enzyme induction	Osteomalacia
Hypolipemic (Cholestyramine)	Folate	Complexation	
	Vitamin B_{12}	Inhibition of intrinsic factor	
	Vitamins A,D,K, electrolytes, Fe	Binding bile salts	Malabsorption
Hypotensives Hydralazine	Vitamin B_6	↑ excretion of vitamin-drug complex	Peripheral neuropathy; anemia
Reserpine	All vitamins	Diarrhea	Deficiencies
Laxatives Bisacodyl, cascara, castor oil, mineral oil	Vitamins A, D, E, K	Complexation; increased peristalsis; mucosal damage	Osteomalacia, rickets
Senna, phenolphthalein	All vitamins K, Ca	Diarrhea	Deficiencies Mineral depletion

Compiled from Avesen, L., Drugs and vitamin deficiency. *Drugs* 18:293, 1979; Bernard, M.A., Jacobs, D.O., and Rombeau, J.L., *Nutritional and Metabolic Support of Hospitalized Patients*. Philadelphia: W.B. Saunders, 1986; Decker, E.L., Effect of food on serum drug levels. *RD* 2:2–3, 1982; Grant, A., *Nutritional Assessment Guidelines*, 2nd ed. Seattle: Anne Grant, 1979; Moore, A.O., and Powers, D.E., *Food-Medication Interactions*, 3rd ed. Tempe, Ariz.: Food-Medication Interactions, 1981; and Weiner, B., Effects of drugs on vitamin/micronutrient absorption. *RD* 3:2–4, 1983.

Table 4-12. Drugs That May Be Gastric Irritants

Analgesic
Aspirin
Aspirin-phenacetin-caffeine (APC)
Percodan
Anorexic
Amphetamines
Anticoagulants
Coumarin
Antifungal
Metronidazole
Antihistamine
Trimeprazine tartrate
Antihypertensive
Reserpine
Anti-infective (urinary tract)
Nalidixic acid
Anti-inflammatory
Steroidal:
   Hydrocortisone
   Prednisolone
   Prednisone
Nonsteroidal:
   Indomethacin
   Phenylbutazone
Antiparkinsonism
Procyclidine · HCl
Trihexyphenidyl
Antitubercular
Isoniazid
P-aminosalicylic acid
Diuretic
Hydrochlorothiazide
Spironolactone
Triamterene
Hypoglycemic
Chlorpropamide
Tolazamide
Tolbutamide
Iron replacement
Ferrous fumarate, gluconate, lactate or sulfate
Potassium replacement
Potassium bicarbonate, chloride, gluconate, etc.
Tranquilizers
Chlorpromazine
Uricosuric
Sulfinpyrazone

been shown to decrease the activity of the drug-metabolizing enzyme system in the rat, and drug-metabolizing enzymes are induced in rats fed diets with added polyunsaturated fatty acids.[14-16]

Minerals. There is a paucity of information concerning the effects of mineral nutrition on drug metabolism in humans. Experiments with animals have indicated that dietary deficiencies of calcium, magnesium, and zinc alter the rate of metabolism of a variety of drugs, and iron deficiency stimulates hepatic drug metabolism.[17] Hypokalemia alters the plasma half-life of some drugs. The significance of these changes in human patients is unknown, and the effects of multiple deficiencies also need investigation.

Vitamins. There is evidence that several vitamins affect the drug-metabolizing enzyme system. These include ascorbic acid (vitamin C), riboflavin, and alpha-tocopherol (vitamin E).[18] Niacin deficiency may also be included, possibly in relation to NADPH levels. Further investigation is needed on (1) the function of these vitamins in the drug-metabolizing enzyme system, (2) the possible involvement of other vitamins, and (3) the effects of multivitamin deficiencies and of combined mineral-vitamin deficiencies.

Two more specific reactions of clinical importance may be used as examples. Pyridoxine blocks the effects of the drug levodopa, used in the treatment of Parkinson's disease. Foods do not contain enough pyridoxine to inhibit levodopa, but supplementation with 1.0 mg or more of pyridoxine should be avoided. Vitamin K interacts with and decreases the effect of warfarin sodium (an anticoagulant). Vitamin K supplementation or excessive intake should be avoided.

Detrimental Systemic Food-Drug Interactions

Some interactions between drugs and certain foods or alcohol result in systemic reactions that may be unpleasant or even life-threatening. Four types of these reactions are listed in Table 4-14.

Vasoactive Compounds and Monoamine Oxidase Inhibitors. There are a number of compounds found naturally in food that can cause a marked increase in blood pressure if they appear in the circulation. They include

Table 4-13. *Effects of Food on Drug Absorption*

Drug Category	Reduces Absorption	Delays Absorption	Increases or Speeds Absorption	Notes on Specific Foods
Analgesic	Aspirin	Acetaminophen Aspirin	Propoxyphene	
Antiarrhythmic	Digoxin/digitoxin	Digoxin/digitoxin		Quinidine potentiated when combined with antacids or alkaline ash diet; may recommend acid ash diet Take digitalis-related drugs with meals to reduce drug toxicity
Anticoagulant			Dicoumarol	
Anticonvulsant			Carbamazepine	
Antifungal		Metronidazole	Griseofulvin	Water intoxication occurs
Antihypertensive			Hydralazine Metoprolol Propranolol	
Anti-infective	Amoxicillin Ampicillin Cephalexin Demeclocycline Demethylchlortetracycline Doxycycline Erythromycin Methacycline · HCl Oxytetracycline Penicillin G Penicillin V Phenethicillin Pivampicillin · HCl Sulfadiazine Tetracycline	Amoxicillin Cephalexin Cephradine Dicloxacillin Lincomycin Oxacillin Sulfadiazine Sulfadimethicone Sulfanilamide Sulfasoxazole Sulfasymazine Toleandromycin	Erythromycin	Penicillins, erythromycin, lincomycin chemically destroyed if taken with low pH foods (e.g., fruit juice); avoid citrus fruits, antacids Chloramphenicol has antabuse reaction with alcohol
Antiparkinsonism	Levodopa			
Antitubercular	Isoniazid Rifampin			
Bronchodilator	Theophylline			
Diuretic		Furosemide	Chlorothiazide Spironolactone	
Peptic ulcer treatment	Propantheline bromide			
Potassium replacement		Potassium ion		
Tranquilizer			Diazepam	
Urinary germicide			Nitrofurantoin	
Vasodilator	Dipyridamole			

Table 4-14. *Drug-Food and Drug-Alcohol Incompatibilities*

Reaction Classification	Reactants		Effect
	1	2	
Tyramine reactions	Monoamine oxidase inhibitors, antidepressants (e.g., phenelzine sulfate), procarbazine hydrochloride, isoniazid (INH)	Foods rich in tyramine or dopamine: Cheese, red wines, chicken liver, broad beans, yeast extracts	Flushing, hypertension, cerebrovascular accidents
Disulfiram reactions	Aldehyde dehydrogenase inhibitors: Disulfiram (Antabuse), calcium cyanamide, metronidazole, nitrofurantoin, *Coprinus atramentarius* (inky cap mushroom), sulfonylureas, furazolidone, quinacrine hydrochloride, chloramphenicol	Alcohol: Beer, wine, liquor, foods containing alcohol	Flushing, headache, nausea, vomiting, chest and abdominal pain
Hypoglycemic reactions	Insulin releasers: Oral hypoglycemic agents, sugar (as in sweet mixes)	Alcohol	Weakness, mental confusion, irrational behavior, loss of consciousness
Flush reactions (see disulfiram reactions)	Miscellaneous: Chlorpropamide (diabetes), griseofulvin, tetrachlorethylene	Alcohol	Flush, dyspnea, headache

Adapted from Roe, D.A., Interactions between drugs and nutrients. *Med. Clin. North Am.* 63:988, 1979.

the psychoactive drugs, dopamine and norepinephrine, and, in addition, the vasoactive amines tyramine, histamine, serotonin (5-HT), isoamylamine, and phenylethylamine (see Figure 4-4). These amines can be synthesized by some plants and also appear in animal products in which there is some fermentation or microbial contamination. Of these compounds, tyramine has been found to be the most clinically significant. As a result of sympathetic overstimulation, tyramine produces a marked elevation in blood pressure along with occipital headache, nausea, and vomiting. If severe, the effects cause a hypertensive crisis which can be life-threatening.

Monoamine oxidase (MAO) is found in the liver, gastrointestinal tract, and adrenergic nerve endings where it metabolizes norepinephrine, tyramine, and other pressor amines. Normally, MAO metabolizes the tyramine in food before it reaches the systemic

circulation. The action of MAO is inhibited by a number of drugs known as **monoamine oxidase inhibitors** (MAOIs). This category of drugs includes the antidepressants isocarboxazid, nialamide, phenelzine sulfate, and tranylcypromine sulfate; the anti-infective drug furazolidone; an anticancer drug, procarbazine; and an antihypertensive, pargyline. If a patient is taking any of these drugs and eats food containing tyramine, the tyramine is not metabolized, reaches the systemic circulation, and causes the symptoms described previously.

Because of the hazards of the reaction, the patient should avoid foods that contain tyramine and other foods with which MAOIs are thought to react, such as raisins. Similar reactions have been reported in patients who have eaten broad beans (*Vicia fava*), presumably due to the presence in the beans of dopa, which is metabolized to dopamine. As a result, it also is recommended that these be avoided. Table 4-15 lists foods that contain tyramine or dopamine and that should be avoided by patients taking MAOIs. Blood

Figure 4-4. Vasoactive amines in food.

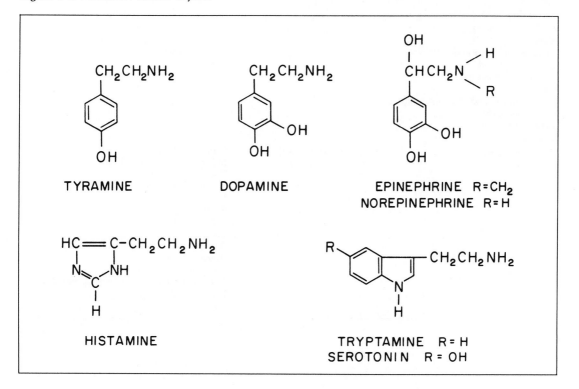

Table 4-15. Foods Reported to Contain Tyramine or Dopamine

Foods to Be Avoided	Foods to Use in Limited Amounts	Other[a]
Cheeses		
Cheddar		Brie
Camembert		Cottage
Emmenthaler		Cream
Swiss		
Stilton blue		
Processed		
Gruyere		
Gouda		
Brick, natural		
Mozzarella		
Bleu		
Roquefort		
Boursault		
Parmesan		
Romano		
Provolone		
Beer and ale		
Wines		
Chianti	Red wines	
	White wines	
	Port	
	Sherry	
Vermouth		
Marmite yeast and yeast extract		Products made with large amounts of yeast (e.g., homemade bread)
		Cookies
Fish		
Salted dried cod, herring		
Pickled herring		
Meat		
Meat extracts, bouillon		Canned meat
Beef liver (stored)		Egg, boiled
Chicken liver (stored)		
Aged game		
Salami, fermented (hard) sausage, bologna, summer sausage		
Pepperoni		
Vegetables		
Italian broad beans	Avocado	Chinese pea pods
Sauerkraut	Legumes	Mixed Chinese vegetables
		Tomato
		Green bean pods
		Eggplant
		Mushroom
		Sweet corn
		Beets
Fruit	Raspberries	Banana
		Pineapple, fresh
		Red plums
		Orange (limit to 1 small orange per day)
		Figs (overripe or canned)
		Raisins

(continued)

Table 4-15. (Continued)

Foods to Be Avoided	Foods to Use in Limited Amounts	Other[a]

Miscellaneous	Chocolate
	Yogurt (from
	  unpasteurized
	  milk)
	Soya and soy
	  sauce
	Peanuts
	Unpasteurized
	  cream
		Cola drinks
		Coffee
		Curry powder
		Worcestershire sauce
		Salad dressings
		Junket

Compiled from Lovenberg, W., Some vasoactive and psychoactive substances in food. Amines, stimulants, depressants and hallucinogens. In *Toxicants Occurring Naturally in Foods.* Washington, D.C.: National Academy of Sciences, 1973, pp. 172–174; Horwitz, O., Lovenberg, W., Engelman, K., and Sjöerdsma, A., Monoamine oxidase inhibitors, tyramine and cheese. *J.A.M.A.* 188:1108, 1964; and McCabe, B.J., Dietary tyramine and other pressor amines in MAOI regimens. A review. *J. Am. Diet. Assoc.* 86:1059, 1986.

[a] These foods have been reported to contain tyramine but evidence for restriction is weak.

pressure can be increased by 6 mg tyramine, and 25 mg produces severe hypertension.[19]

There is uncertainty concerning some other food items. Studies on rats indicate that methylxanthines found in coffee, tea, cocoa, and cola drinks react with MAOIs. The patient's physician may decide that it is necessary to eliminate these beverages from the diet.

The inhibition of monoamine oxidase by MAOIs is irreversible. The enzyme is synthesized slowly. Hypertensive reactions have been known to occur three weeks after the drug is withdrawn. Therefore, it is recommended that the diet continue for four weeks following drug withdrawal.[20]

Little is known about the metabolism of other amines, such as histamine, serotonin, and norepinephrine. It may become necessary to restrict other foods as the interactions between these substances and drugs become known. If a drug acted as a histaminase inhibitor, for example, a diet restricted in histamine might be necessary. The diet would require the elimination of fermented foods such as chocolate and sauerkraut.

Alcohol-Drug Interactions. Although alcohol has been considered both a drug and a nutrient, it will be considered here as a beverage that can interact with various drugs (Table 4-16). It has been shown to decrease the absorption of many nutrients and to alter the metabolism of drugs. Some of the types of reactions are described in Table 4-14. The reactions with alcohol of disulfiram and of hypoglycemic drugs are particularly important. Patients taking these drugs may need to be counseled concerning alcohol intake.

In addition to beverages, many over-the-counter (OTC) drugs contain large amounts of alcohol. In counseling patients taking drugs that interact with alcohol, patients should be questioned concerning their use of such nonprescription medications. Alcohol content can be obtained from the label or from the literature.[21]

Study Questions

1. Describe and explain the significance of the drug-receptor complex.
2. List the general methods of drug administration and explain their relationships to speed of action.
3. How do the following affect drug action:
   a. Plasma protein binding?
   b. Blood-brain barrier?
   c. Placental barrier?
4. Define and differentiate among a drug idiosyncrasy, allergy, and toxicity.
5. Describe the mechanism of production of side effects of monoamine oxidase inhibitors.

Table 4-16. Drugs Reported to Interact with Alcohol

Drug	Possible Reactions
Analgesics Glycodone Meperidine Narcotic drugs Propoxyphene Salicylates	Excess sedation, stomach irritation, gastrointestinal bleeding, risk of hemorrhage, liver damage
Anorexic Amphetamines Fenfluramine · HCl	Excess high blood pressure Excess CNS stimulation
Anticoagulants Coumarin	Increased drug effect
Anticonvulsants Carbamazepine Phenytoin Primidone Valproic acid	Excess sedation Decreased drug effect
Antidepressants Amitriptyline · HCl Imepramine · HCl Isocarboxazide Nortriptyline Tranylcypromine	Drug increases alcohol effects
Antifungal Griseofulvin	Flushing, tachycardia
Antihistamines Chlorpheniramine Dramamine	Increases sedation
Anti-infectives Chloramphenicol Chloromycetin Furazolidone Metronidazole Nalidixic acid	Flushing, headache, hypertension, nausea and vomiting, confusion Drug increases alcohol effects
Anti-inflammatory Butazolidone Dexamethasone Hydrocortisone Ibuprofen Indomethacin Oxyphenbutazone Phenylbutazone	As with anti-infective drugs Stomach irritation/bleeding Stomach irritation/bleeding Stomach irritation/bleeding Stomach irritation/bleeding
Antineoplastic Methotrexate Procarbazine · HCl	Increased liver toxicity, excess sedation
Antispasmodic Chlorzoxazone Propantheline bromide	Excess sedation
Antitubercular Ethionamide Isoniazid	Decreased drug effect, increased incidence of hepatitis
Cardiovascular agents Nitroglycerin Digoxin Digitoxin	Increased absorption, possible hypotension, cardiac arrhythmias
Bronchodilators Brompheniramine maleate	

(continued)

Table 4-16. (Continued)

Drug	Possible Reactions
Diuretics	Excess orthostatic hypotension
Ethycrinic acid	
Spironolactone	
Thiazide diuretics	
Hypnotic	
Glutethimide	
Pentobarbitol	Excess sedation
Hypoglycemics	
Chlorpropamide	Increased drug effect
Tolbutamide	Increased drug effect
Hypolipemics	
Clofibrate	
Hypotensives	Increased drug effects, hypotension
Conidine	
Guanethidine	
Hydralazine	
Pargyline	Excess orthostatic hypotension
Other	
Allopurinol	
Tranquilizers and antidepressants	Excess sedation, incoordination
Chlorpromazine	Intoxication inhibits drug
Chlorprothixene	
Diazepam	Intoxication inhibits drug
Haloperidol	
Lorazepam	
Meprobamate	
Phenothiazines	
Reserpine	
Thiothixene	
Trifluoperazine · HCl	
Vasoconstrictor	
Ergotamine	Reduced drug effect
Vasodilator	
Tolazoline	

References

1. Maller, O., and Cardello, A. The sick senses. Functions of taste and smell. *The Professional Nutritionist* 10:1, 1978.
2. Roe, D.A. *Handbook: Interactions of Selected Drugs and Nutrients in Patients*, 3rd ed. Chicago: American Dietetic Association, 1982.
3. Pawan, G.L.S. Drugs and appetite. *Proc. Nutr. Soc.* 33:239, 1974.
4. Roe, D.A. Effects of drugs on nutrition. *Med. Clin. North Am.* 63:985, 1979.
5. Roe, D.A. Effects of drugs on nutrition. *Life Sci.* 15:1219, 1974.
6. Visconti, J.A. Drug-food interaction. In *Nutrition in Disease*. Columbus, Ohio: Ross Laboratories, 1977.
7. Bistrian, B.R., Blackburn, G.L., Hallowell, E., and Heddle, R. Protein status of general surgical patients. *J.A.M.A.* 230:858, 1974.
8. Bistrian, B.R., Blackburn, G.L., Vitale, J., et al. Nutritional status of general medical patients. *Clin. Res.* 22:692A, 1974.
9. Bistrian, B.R., Blackburn, G.L., and Sherman, M. Therapeutic index of nutritional depletion in surgical patients. *Surg. Gynecol. Obstet.* 141:512, 1975.
10. Spector, A.A., and Fletcher, J.E. Nutritional effects on drug-protein binding. In J.N. Hathcock and J. Coon, Eds., *Nutrition and Drug Interrelations*. New York: Academic Press, 1978.
11. Campbell, T.C. Effect of dietary protein on drug metabolism. In J.N. Hathcock and J. Coon, Eds., *Nutrition and Drug Interrelations*. New York: Academic Press, 1978.
12. Wade, A.E., and Norred, W.P. Effect of dietary lipid on drug-metabolizing enzymes. *Fed. Proc.* 35:2475, 1976.
13. Wade, A.E., Norred, W.P., and Evans, J.S.

Lipids in drug detoxication. In J.N. Hathcock and J. Coon, Eds., *Nutrition and Drug Interrelations.* New York: Academic Press, 1978. p. 476.

14. Norred, W.P., and Wade, A.E. Dietary fatty acid-induced alterations of hepatic microsomal drug-metabolizing enzymes. *Biochem. Pharmacol.* 21:2887, 1972.

15. Century, B., and Horwitt, M.K. A role of dietary lipid in the ability of phenobarbital to stimulate hexobarbital and aminopyrine metabolism. *Fed. Proc.* 27:349, 1968.

16. Marshall, W.J., and McLean, A.E.M. A requirement for dietary lipids for induction of cytochrome P-450 by phenobarbitone in rat liver microsomal fraction. *Biochem. J.* 122:569, 1971.

17. Becking, G.C. Hepatic drug metabolism in iron-, magnesium-, and potassium-deficient rats. *Fed. Proc.* 35:2480, 1974.

18. Zannoni, V.G., and Sato, P.H. The effect of certain vitamin deficiencies on hepatic drug metabolism. *Fed. Proc.* 35:2464, 1974.

19. Blackwell, B. Hypertensive interactions between monoamine oxidase inhibitors and foodstuffs. *Br. J. Psychiatry* 113:349, 1967.

20. McCabe, B.J. Dietary tyramine and other pressor amines in MAOI regimens. A review. *J. Am. Diet. Assoc.* 86:1059, 1986.

21. Dukes, G.E., Kuhn, J.E., and Evans, R.P. Alcohol in pharmaceutical products. *American Family Physician* 16:97, Sept., 1977.

Bibliography

AMA Department of Drugs. *AMA Drug Evaluations,* 5th ed. Chicago: American Medical Association, 1983.

Avery, G.S. *Drug Treatment,* 2nd ed. Sydney: Adis Press, 1980.

Csaky, T.Z. *Introduction to General Pharmacology,* 2nd ed. New York: Appleton-Century-Crofts, 1979.

Dukes, M.N.G. *Meyler's Side Effects of Drugs Annual,* 10th ed. Amsterdam: Excerpta Medica, 1984.

Food and Nutrition Board. *Toxicants Occurring Naturally in Foods,* 2nd ed. Washington, D.C.: National Academy of Sciences, 1973.

Gilman, A.G., Goodman, L.S., Rall, T.W., and Murad, F. *Goodman and Gilman's Pharmacological Basis of Therapeutics,* 7th ed. New York: Macmillan, 1985.

Goth, A. *Medical Pharmacology,* 11th ed. St. Louis: C.V. Mosby, 1984.

Hartshorn, E.A. Food and drug interactions. *J. Am. Diet. Assoc.* 70:15, 1977.

Hathcock, J.N., and Coon, J., Eds. *Nutrition and Drug Interrelations.* New York: Academic Press, 1978.

Levine, R.R. *Pharmacology: Drug Actions and Reactions,* 3rd ed. Boston: Little, Brown, 1983.

Long, J.W. *The Essential Guide to Prescription Drugs,* 4th ed. New York: Harper and Row, 1985.

5. Methods of Nutritional Support

I. Planning Nutritional Care
II. Implementation of the
   Nutritional Care Plan
   A. Conventional feeding
      1. Adaptations for
         disease
         a. purposes of
            modified diets
         b. types of diets
            (1) routine diets
            (2) modified diets
            (3) test diets
            (4) quantitative
                and qualita-
                tive diets
         c. increasing
            nutrient intake
         d. adaptations for
            individual
            characteristics
            (1) vegetarianism
            (2) cultural
                factors
   B. Tube feeding
      1. Physical properties
         of tube feeding
         formulas
         a. osmolality
         b. renal solute load
         c. residue
         d. viscosity
      2. Ingredient and
         nutrient content
         a. caloric density
         b. carbohydrate
         c. fat
         d. protein
         e. specific amino
            acids
         f. vitamins and
            minerals
      3. Products available
      4. Evaluation of tube
         feeds
      5. Techniques of
         administration
         a. routes
         b. delivery systems
         c. types of tubes
         d. rate, frequency,
            and concentration
            of feeding
      6. Contraindications to
         tube feeding
      7. Complications
      8. Patient monitoring
   C. Parenteral feeding
      1. Central venous
         alimentation
         a. placement of the
            catheter
         b. preparation and
            administration of
            the solutions
         c. composition of
            solutions
            (1) amino acids
            (2) carbohydrate
            (3) lipids
            (4) vitamins and
                minerals
         d. osmolarity of the
            infusate
         e. estimating
            nutritional
            needs
         f. complications
      2. Peripheral venous
         alimentation
      3. Cyclic parenteral
         nutrition
      4. Monitoring the TPN
         patient
   D. Transitional feeding

When the initial nutritional assessment is complete, the data to provide the subjective, objective, and assessment portions of the SOAP note are at hand. The next step is to plan the nutritional care process, to be followed by implementation of these plans. This circular process may thus be diagramed as shown in Figure 5-1. The process ends when care is terminated. This event is recorded by the attending physician in a discharge note.

The first step in planning is to establish goals and objectives for dealing with each problem identified in the assessment. A **goal** states the general purpose of the effort, whereas an **objective** states a specific measurable and verifiable step toward achieving the goal. In order that procedures for implementation and evaluation follow logically from the goals and objectives, it is necessary that the objectives be patient-centered. They should be stated in terms of what the patient will achieve if the objective is met, and they should be stated in quantitative terms whenever possible. Here is an example:

Problem No. 1: Patient lacks knowledge of the principles of a gluten-free diet.
Goal: Understanding of and ability to apply the principles of the gluten-free diet.
Objective: Patient will demonstrate understanding of and ability to apply the princi-

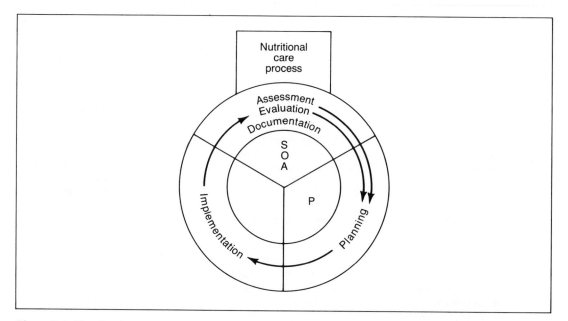

Figure 5-1. The circular nature of the nutritional care process.

ples of his gluten-free diet by selecting proper foods from the hospital menu on Tuesday, Wednesday, and Thursday of this week.

There may be more than one goal per problem and more than one objective necessary to reach each goal.

PLANNING NUTRITIONAL CARE

When the objectives related to each problem have been determined, the procedure to be used to help the patient to reach these objectives must be established. The general types of activity or interventions that are used in nutritional care are (1) gathering further information (recorded under "P-Dx" in the SOAP note), (2) methods of nutrition support such as prescription of a modified diet or other methods of providing nutrients, and referrals for public aid, nutrition follow-up, or other social services (recorded under "P-Rx" in the SOAP note), and (3) provision for patient education ("P-Pt. Ed."). Each intervention should be related to one of the established objectives and should be stated in specific terms.

IMPLEMENTATION OF THE NUTRITIONAL CARE PLAN

A person's **diet** is defined as that person's intake of food and drink. The term does not necessarily imply that the patient's usual food intake has been altered in any way. For many patients a normal unrestricted intake is an adequate diet, but for others, an important aspect of nutritional intervention is an alteration in their usual diets or in the method by which nutrients are provided.

The patient may eat and drink in normal fashion, by mouth, referred to as "conventional feeding." Some patients are unwilling or unable to take sufficient food by mouth, but have a functioning gastrointestinal tract. These may be fed through a tube into the gastrointestinal tract. Those patients in whom digestion and absorption are not possible may be fed directly into the circulation, a process known as parenteral feeding. These procedures will be discussed in turn, without reference to a specific diagnosis.

Conventional Feeding

In planning for the diet of patients, it is important to use the normal unrestricted diet as the starting point whenever possible. Only those alterations are made that are required to achieve the objectives. This procedure has several advantages. It makes for easier planning for nutritional adequacy; shows to the patients as clearly as possible the relationship to a normal diet and reduces a sense of alienation, of being "different"; clarifies and simplifies the procedures for providing meals either in an institution or in the home; and reduces the number and variety of special items that must be prepared.

Adaptations for Disease

Purposes of Modified Diets. The patient's diet may be modified for one or more of the following reasons:

1. To maintain or restore good nutritional status. This should be an objective in feeding all patients.
2. To rest or relieve an affected organ (e.g., a soft or liquid diet in gastritis).
3. To adjust to the body's ability to digest, absorb, metabolize, or excrete (e.g., a low-fat diet for fat malabsorption).
4. To adjust to tolerance of food intake by mouth (e.g., a liquid diet for sore throat).
5. To adjust to mechanical difficulties (e.g., a soft diet for the patient without teeth).
6. To increase or decrease body weight (e.g., a 1,200-calorie diet for obesity).

It is important to realize that modification of the diet does not cure any disease except in nutrient deficiency disease and perhaps in simple obesity. The diet may reduce symptoms, make the patient more comfortable and, in some circumstances, prolong life. A diabetic diet, for example, does not cure diabetes, but it may be instrumental in prolonging the patient's life and improving the quality of that life.

Types of Diets. The diets served in institutions commonly are classified as standard, modified, or test diets. These categories are established for convenience and efficiency of service and are explained in detail in the diet manual of each institution.

Routine diets. The **standard, routine,** or **progressive diets** are used in all acute care hospitals and usually are served to relatively large numbers of patients. The foods included in these diets are fairly consistent from one institution to another, but the terminology varies. Some of the alternative terms are indicated here. All of these diets are based on the normal adequate diet, but they differ in consistency.

The **clear liquid diet** is the most limited of the routine diets. It is used to relieve thirst, to provide some fluid for the prevention of dehydration, to minimize stimulation of the gastrointestinal tract, and to serve as the initial feeding when a patient is returned to oral feeding following surgery or a period of intravenous feeding. Foods commonly included are listed in Table 5-1. The diet may contain 600–900 kcal/day, primarily from carbohydrate. A small amount of incomplete protein is obtained from gelatin. Since the diet is nutritionally inadequate, it seldom is used for more than one or two days. For patients requiring a residue-free liquid diet for longer periods, a commercial low-residue feeding may be added (see Appendix G).

The **full liquid diet** (see Table 5-1) is the next in the progression to the unrestricted diet. It provides food for the patient who is unable to chew, swallow, or digest more solid foods. It is given to postoperative patients, those with gastrointestinal inflammations and those with pathologic conditions of the head and neck. It is composed of those foods allowed on the clear liquid diet plus others that are liquid at body temperature (37°C) or at any lower temperature, and it includes a large amount of milk and milk products. The caloric density (kilocalories per milliliter) is low, and feedings between meals often are included to increase the nutrient content. As usually served, the diet is

Table 5-1. Summary of Routine Hospital Diets

Food Group	Clear Liquid	Full Liquid	Pureed	Soft	House
Soup	Broth, bouillon (fat-free)	Broth, bouillon (fat-free), strained cream soups	Broth, bouillon (fat-free), strained cream soups	Broth, bouillon (fat-free), strained cream soups	All
Cereal		Refined or strained in gruels	Refined or strained	Refined cooked, cornflakes, rice, pasta products	All
Bread			White bread	White breads, rolls, crackers	All
Meat and substitutes		Pasteurized eggs in milk drinks, eggs in custards; strained meat or poultry in soup	Eggs, ground meats, or poultry, white fish (not fried); no pork	Eggs, milk, cheese, tender beef, lamb, veal, bacon, poultry (not fried)	All
Milk		Milk, milk drinks, cream, plain yogurt	Milk, milk drinks, cream, plain yogurt	Milk, milk drinks, cream, plain yogurt	All
Vegetables		In strained cream soups only; vegetable juices	Potatoes (not fried); strained or pureed bland cooked vegetables	Potatoes (not fried); whole tender or chopped bland cooked vegetables	All
Fruits	Bland clear juices; fruit ades	All juice	All juice; pureed bland cooked fruit	All juice; whole bland cooked fruit; raw banana; oranges and grapefruit sections (no membrane)	All
Desserts	Plain gelatin desserts; fruit ices; Popsicles	Foods from preceding column, plus plain ice cream, sherbet, custard, pudding	Foods from preceding columns, plus plain cake	Foods from preceding columns, plus plain cookies	All
Miscellaneous	Soft drinks; decaffeinated coffee, tea; cereal beverage; sugar, honey; hard candy; salt; low-residue defined formula (on prescription only in some institutions)	Foods from preceding column; butter, margarine, oil in cream soups; honey, syrup; cocoa, chocolate syrup	Foods from preceding columns, plus salt, pepper, jelly	Foods from preceding columns, mayonnaise or similar dressing	All

adequate in protein and energy for maintenance. It can be modified for an increase in calories and protein, to reduce the sodium content, and to fit into a diabetic diet. Cholesterol level is high; iron is low. The diet is also fiber-free.

In some institutions, the full liquid diet is modified further into **medical liquid diet**,

surgical liquid diet, or other variations. The details of these diets, designed to meet the needs of patients in a particular institution, are found in the diet manuals of those institutions.

The **soft diet**, more solid than the liquid diet, is made up of foods reputed to be easily digested, without strong seasoning and containing a limited amount of fiber. The soft diet may be subdivided into two subcategories. In one, allowed meats, fruits, and vegetables are served whole. In the other, the meat is ground and vegetables and fruits are pureed (see Table 5-1). In this form, the diet sometimes is called the **pureed diet** or **strained soft diet**. The soft diet is used for patients with difficulties in chewing and swallowing, acute infections, or some gastrointestinal disturbances, and as a transitional step from the liquid to an unrestricted diet in postoperative patients. The diet is nutritionally adequate.

The **house diet** (see Table 5-1) is also known as the **general**, **regular**, or **full diet**. It is an adequate normal diet, used for patients whose food intake can be unrestricted in kind or amount and who do not need additional nutritional support. As served in most institutions, it provides 2,000 to 2,500 kcal with 60 to 80 g protein, 80 to 100 g fat, and 200 to 300 g carbohydrate for adults. Some institutions use instead the "prudent diet" recommended by the American Heart Association (see Chapter 10). Most institutions allow patients to select their meals from a **menu**. Those that have a pediatrics unit have a series of diets adjusted for the ages of the children (see Appendix K).

Modified diets. The **modified diets** are available for patients needing diets that differ from the routine diets. There is a wide variety of alterations that can be made. In general, each modified diet is used for a much smaller number of patients and often requires more individualized planning. For convenience, they have been classified according to the types of alterations:

1. Kilocalories (e.g., high calorie or low calorie).
2. Consistency (e.g., low fiber, high fiber, soft, or liquid).
3. Single constituents or balance among nutrients (e.g., low fat, sodium restricted, low fiber, diabetic, low protein).
4. Method of preparation (e.g., soft).
5. Specific food restriction (e.g., milk-free).

6. Number, size, and frequency of meals (e.g., six small meals per day).

As is apparent from this list, some diets fit into more than one of these categories. It also is seen that the routine diets can be included in this classification, particularly in the category of changes in consistency.

Test diets. **Test diets** are single meals or diets lasting only one or a few days that are given to patients in connection with certain laboratory tests. They are used when the results of a test are affected by variations in food intake. For example, for the fecal fat excretion test, a consistent amount of fat, 70 to 100 g daily, is given for five days preceding the test. Test diets are not always nutritionally adequate, but this fact is not a matter of concern if they are used for a very brief period.

Quantitative and qualitative diets. An additional diet categorization that is sometimes useful is the division into quantitative and qualitative diets. Qualitative diets are any of those in which the patient may have any amount of the allowed foods that he or she desires. In quantitative diets, the amount of allowed foods is restricted. The diabetic diet and the calorie-restricted diet are the most common of the quantitative diets.

Increasing Nutrient Intake. The primary illness of many patients is accompanied by increased nutrient requirements or depressed appetite or both. A number of techniques are available for attempting to increase intake of routine or modified diets. Not all are applicable to all situations, but approaches may be chosen from the following:[1]

1. Encourage eating at meal time by catering to the patient's preferences, providing a pleasant environment, arranging for assistance in eating if necessary.
2. Increase the number of different foods offered in meals, increase the size of servings, or both, if patient's needs and appetite are increased.
3. Increase the nutrient density of foods by

adding concentrated proteins, fats, or carbohydrates that will not increase total volume. Examples of usable items include skim milk powder, butter or margarine, and sugar. In addition, a number of commercial concentrated nutrient sources can be added to other foods. These products are listed in Appendix G, Table 2. Not all products are suitable for all diets. The clear liquid diet presents a particular problem. Polycose, Citrotein, and Ross SLD are usable in this situation.

4. Increase the frequency of feeding. Patients may be given more frequent feedings, four to six a day being usual. Sometimes, patients are given three regular meals plus "supplementary feedings." Various snack-type foods are sometimes used for this purpose.

Some liquid supplements, such as milk shakes and malted milks, can be prepared from conventional ingredients. In addition, a wide array of commercial products are available. They are listed and described in Appendix G, Table 1. Many of these supplements are intended to provide protein and kilocalories; others are an energy source but are low in protein or are protein-free for patients whose condition requires protein restriction. Some are lactose-free. These products are not intended to replace the diet and, therefore, do not necessarily provide all nutritional requirements. Some of the formulas in Appendix G, Table 3, are also useful for supplementary oral feeding. They are nutritionally complete, but some are not as acceptable in taste; therefore, they must be chosen carefully.

An institution usually does not stock all the products listed. A given purpose may be served by any one of the several products that differ only slightly. Factors that should be considered in choosing items to stock and in choosing a supplement for a specific patient include cost, availability, palatability, composition in relation to the nutrient requirements of the patient, and indications for the use of the product.

Adaptations for Individual Characteristics. In addition to the modifications required for the patient's disease, it is necessary to adapt the diet to the individual characteristics of the patient. Even if a patient is receiving a house diet, personal preferences, habits, and cultural background must be considered if it affects food acceptance.

Vegetarianism. Some patients elect to follow a **vegetarian** diet, and it is necessary for the nutritional care specialist to be familiar with these diets. There are several categories of the more traditional vegetarian diets.[2] Some patients are **partial vegetarians** who elect to use only selected meats. Commonly, partial vegetarians will eat fish and poultry but not beef, pork, or lamb. The **lactoovovegetarian** includes dairy products and eggs in the diet. The **lactovegetarian diet** contains milk products but not eggs, whereas the **ovovegetarian** will eat eggs but not milk. The **vegan** accepts only foods of purely plant origin.

If the patient will eat eggs or milk or both, diets are fairly easy to plan. A modification of the Basic Four for vegetarian diets, suggested by King et al.,[3] includes four servings of milk, two servings of legumes, and one serving of nuts along with six servings of whole grain or enriched cereals. In addition, three servings of vitamin C–rich fruits and vegetables, one and a half dark green vegetables, and three other fruits and vegetables are included, for a total of seven and a half servings of fruits and vegetables.

The vegan diet requires more careful planning. It lacks concentrated sources of proteins of high biologic value and is limited in calcium, iron, riboflavin, and vitamin B_{12}. In order to plan for an adequate supply of amino acids to support normal growth and maintenance, a simplified system has been described.[4] It recommends the use *at each meal* of whole grains and cereals. In addition, at each meal a supplementary protein should be added. This may be provided by legumes or vegetables, or by a combination of nuts and seeds. Enriched grains will provide iron, the absorption of which can be increased by including a source of ascorbic acid in each meal. Dark green vegetables and some nuts provide calcium, and cereal products provide riboflavin. Vitamin B_{12} may be obtained by vegans from B_{12}-fortified soy milk or meat analogs.[5]

In addition to these traditional vegetarians, usually associated with ethnic cultures or religions, there are the **new vegetarians**, a heterogeneous group whose diets include avoidance of other foods and adoption of nontraditional life styles. Some of the groups are easily identified.[5] For many, their diets can be evaluated only after an extensive nutritional history.

Most, but not all, therapeutic diets can be altered to be acceptable to vegetarian patients.[6] The diets of all vegetarians should be monitored carefully in the presence of risk factors such as a history of weight loss, use of laxatives and enemas, fasting, fluid restriction, pregnancy, lactation, or infancy.

Cultural factors. Some patients have eating habits related to their religion, nationality, or ethnic background that affect their nutritional status. The nutritional care specialist must be familiar with these influences[7] and be prepared to integrate them into the total nutritional care of the patient.

For patients who must follow a diet after discharge from the hospital or for those who are being treated on an outpatient basis, ability to prepare the food and availability of required special items must be considered in addition to the economic and cultural factors. The integration of all these factors requires skill, understanding, and patience, as well as a thorough knowledge of the biologic and social sciences.

Tube Feeding

If, over a period of days, the conventionally fed patient's intake is insufficient to meet his or her needs, more active nutritional support may be undertaken. Specific guidelines to determine when patients require alternative nutritional support have not been developed. In general, if the interval of relative or total starvation has been or is expected to be two weeks or longer, or if protein-energy malnutrition is identified at the time of assessment, active nutritional support is indicated. Well-nourished patients with brief intervals of starvation do not require special nutritional support. Up to seven days of relative starvation is well tolerated and is not thought to impair recovery in the initially well-nourished patient. Conditions that may require the use of tube feeding are listed in Table 5-2.

Tube feeding formulas are useful only in those patients who have sufficient gastrointestinal function to digest and absorb their ingredients. A variety of formulations are available (see Appendix G, Table 3). The formula to be used must be chosen carefully with consideration of the factors discussed in the following sections.

Physical Properties of Tube Feeding Formulas

When choosing a tube feeding formula for a specific patient, a number of physical properties of the formula must be considered.

Osmolality. The **osmolality** of the formula strongly influences the patient's tolerance. The lumen of the gut and the extracellular fluid may be considered to be two compartments separated by a semipermeable membrane in the gut wall. When a very hypertonic formula is put into one compartment, the lumen, there will follow a large shift of fluid across the membrane. The increased fluid in the gut can result in diarrhea, and the loss of fluid from the ECF might cause some degree of dehydration. In addition, gastric emptying is delayed by hypertonic solutions, sometimes causing gastric retention, nausea, and vomiting. Vomiting is particularly hazardous in infants, comatose patients, and others who are in danger of aspirating the vomitus.

Table 5-2. Indications for Use of Tube Feedings

Inability to ingest food normally	*Impairment of digestion and/or absorption*
Stupor, unconsciousness, coma	Pancreatic insufficiency; carcinoma, chronic pancrea-
Cerebrovascular accidents	titis
Inflammation in central nervous system	Bile salt insufficiency
Cerebral neoplasms	Bile acid–induced diarrhea: blind loop syndrome, Zol-
Fracture of mandible	linger-Ellison syndrome
Oropharyngeal neoplasms	Short bowel syndrome
Head and neck surgery	Gluten enteropathy (nontropical sprue)
Dysphagia	Crohn's disease
Radiation to head or neck	Disaccharidase deficiency
Chemotherapy	Abetalipoproteinemia
Multiple sclerosis	Radiation damage
Physiologic deterrents to food intake	Whipple's disease
Nausea or vomiting in pregnancy, drug reactions, radia-	Obstruction of lymph flow
tion, or chemotherapy	*Protein-calorie malnutrition*
Dumping syndrome	*Hypermetabolic states*
Obstruction of gastrointestinal tract (if access is below	Burns
obstruction)	Trauma
Esophageal stricture or neoplasm	Surgery
Spasm of pylorus	Fever
Neoplasm, foreign body, or other obstruction of stom-	*Intestinal surgery*
ach or intestine	Preparation for hemorrhoidectomy[a]
Psychiatric illness	Preparation for intestinal surgery[a]
Anorexia nervosa	*Transition from total parenteral nutrition to conventional*
Depression	*foods*[a]
Diversion of flow (fistulas) (?)	*Renal failure*
	Hepatic failure
	Inborn errors of metabolism

Information gathered from *Dialogues in Nutrition* 1(2):1 (tape). Bloomfield, N.J.: Health Learning Systems, Inc., 1976; American Dietetic Association, *Handbook of Clinical Dietetics.* New Haven, Conn.: Yale University Press, 1980; and Rombeau, J.L., and Miller, R.A., *Nasoenteric Tube Feeding: Practical Aspects.* Mountain View, Calif.: Health Development Corp., 1979.
[a] Defined formula diet.

Renal Solute Load. If the renal solute load (RSL) is especially high, a large quantity of water must be provided to excrete it. If this water is not provided, the patient will become dehydrated, with the attendant signs and symptoms described in Chapter 2. Patients receiving formulas with a high RSL must be monitored carefully for signs of dehydration. Patients particularly at risk are infants, those with impaired renal concentrating ability, and those with increased fluid losses from vomiting, diarrhea, burns, and fever.

Residue. A reduction or absence of residue remaining in the intestine is desirable in connection with some diagnostic tests, in some preoperative and postoperative patients, for patients with gastrointestinal disorders such as Crohn's disease or colitis, and for patients in transition between intravenous and tube feeding. These patients may be given low residue or residue-free formulas. On the other hand, the low residue content of many formulas may cause constipation. For such patients, a formula containing fiber may be used if not contraindicated by the patient's condition.

Viscosity. Formulas containing larger molecules, such as whole protein compared to amino acids, and formulas that have a higher caloric content per unit volume tend to be more viscous. The viscosity of the formula and the caliber of the tube used must be compatible. More viscous formulas require a larger tube, but a larger tube is generally less comfortable for the patient.

Ingredient and Nutrient Content

Tube feeding formulas vary in both quantity and type of ingredients. Both must be considered in relation to the specific needs of the patient.

Caloric Density. The amount of energy per unit volume of the formula is its caloric density, measured in kcal/ml. Most tube feedings yield 1 kcal/ml, but 1.5 and 2.0 kcal/ml formulas are also available. These are useful for patients with high caloric needs and limited appetites or volume tolerance. The more calorically dense formulas also have high osmolality and high RSL. Therefore, precautions must be taken to prevent dehydration, and patients must be monitored carefully.

Carbohydrate. Carbohydrate provides about 55% of the energy contained in most tube feedings. The source and form of the carbohydrate contained may be classified as follows:

1. *Polysaccharides:* from hydrolyzed cereal solids, pureed vegetables, modified food starch, tapioca starch.
2. *Glucose polymers:* from hydrolysis of cornstarch (>100 glucose units), glucose oligosaccharides (2–10 glucose units), maltodextrins, corn syrup, corn syrup solids.
3. *Disaccharides:* lactose (from milk), sucrose, maltose (from digestion of starch or oligosaccharides).
4. *Monosaccharides:* glucose (dextrose), fructose.

Several generalizations may be used as guidelines in choosing a tube feeding formula. First, in formulas with equal proportions of carbohydrates, those containing glucose as a monosaccharide will have higher osmolality than those prepared with glucose polymers because they will have more particles. Starch contributes very little to osmolality. Second, carbohydrate in any form other than monosaccharide requires digestion. Formulas containing these products are not tolerated by patients incapable of such digestion. Third, some formulas provide carbohydrate in the form of lactose and are not usable by lactose-intolerant patients. These patients need a lactose-free formula.

A few formulas that contain fiber are available. These are helpful in regulating bowel function. The effects of fiber on the bowel are discussed in Chapter 8.

Fat. Tube feeding formulas contain fat from a vegetable source such as corn, soy, safflower or sunflower seeds, or from butterfat. These lipids contain glycerol and long-chain fatty acids (14 carbons or more) and are called **long-chain triglycerides** (LCT).

Some patients are incapable of digesting and absorbing LCT. For these patients, some formulas contain **medium-chain triglycerides** (MCT) with 6–12 carbon chains. It is often used for infants and adults with malabsorption syndromes and is prepared by fractionating coconut oil. MCT Oil provides 7 kcal/g. Each tablespoon of oil weighs 14 g and provides about 100 kcal.

LCT does not add to formula osmolality, but MCT is hydrolyzed rapidly and increases the osmolality of the formula. MCT also does not contain essential fatty acids, sometimes has side effects such as nausea, vomiting, and diarrhea, and is expensive. For all these reasons, MCT should not be used unless the patient's condition requires it.

All patients must be provided with a source of essential fatty acids (EFA). The amount of EFA required is unknown, and recommendations vary from 2% to 5% of total kilocalories for adults and 1% to 4% of total kilocalories, or 100 mg/kg body weight, in infants.[8-12]

A generous amount of linoleic acid is provided by LCT. For example, linoleic acid contents of commonly used vegetable oils are as follows:

Corn oil	58%
Safflower oil	74%
Sesame oil	74%

Soy oil   51% (not hydrogenated)
                 39% (hydrogenated)
Sunflower oil   66%

Formulas containing MCT, however, must contain some LCT to provide the required essential fatty acids.

A third type, currently under investigation, is called structured lipids. These are processed chemically to contain both LCT and MCT fatty acids in the same molecule. Structured lipids may be useful for those who are LCT and glucose intolerant, such as adults with major stress in the form of burns and multiple trauma and for some infants.[13,14] The lipids are not yet approved for human use. Their clinical usefulness is under investigation.

Protein. The quality of the protein may be expressed in several ways. The **biological value** (BV) indicates the amino acid ratio in protein by measuring the retention of absorbed nitrogen:

$$BV\ (\%) = \frac{N\ retained}{N\ absorbed} \times 100 \qquad (5\text{-}1)$$

The **protein efficiency ratio** (PER) measures growth in relation to protein intake in rats:

$$PER = \frac{weight\ gain\ (g)}{protein\ intake\ (g)} \qquad (5\text{-}2)$$

The reference protein is casein, which has a PER of 2.5. When PER is 2.5 or more, 45 g of the material provides the adult RDA for protein. The **amino acid profile** lists the amounts of the specific amino acids. The list may be obtained from the manufacturer of the formula.

The quantity of protein varies with the patient's needs. Protein content must provide normal needs plus any increase resulting from the illness and must be of sufficiently high biological value to supply all required amino acids. Excess amounts of protein will increase the renal solute load and increase

cost. It is usually recommended that the protein provide no more than 15% of the total calories.

In order that protein not be used as a source of energy, it is common practice for the amount of protein in a formula to be supplied relative to the energy content. This is expressed as the calorie-nitrogen (C:N) ratio. More specifically, it is expressed as a ratio of nonprotein calories (from carbohydrate and fat) to grams of nitrogen (from protein).

The procedure for calculation is as follows:

$$g\ protein \times 0.16 = g\ nitrogen \qquad (5\text{-}3)$$

Example: 100 g protein × 0.16 = 16 g nitrogen

$$\begin{aligned}nonprotein\ kilocalories =\ &(g\ carbohydrate \\ \times\ 4) + (g\ fat \times 9) \end{aligned} \qquad (5\text{-}4)$$

Example: (600 g carbohydrate × 4) + (90 g fat × 9) = 2400 + 810 = 3210 calories

$$\frac{nonprotein}{kcal/N\ ratio} = \frac{\dfrac{nonprotein}{kcal}}{g\ N} \qquad (5\text{-}5)$$

Example: $\dfrac{3210}{16} = 201{:}1$

Some acceptable ratios are

For a normal adult male	300:1
For a critically ill patient	100–200:1
For anabolism	150:1

The protein in tube feeding can be in one of three forms, depending on the amount of digestion required:

1. *Pure crystalline amino acids* require no digestion, but they add markedly to the osmotic load of the formula.
2. *Hydrolyzed proteins* are prepared by enzyme hydrolysis of intact proteins such as whey to produce peptides and some amino acids. Tripeptides, dipeptides, and single amino acids add to the osmotic load.

Recent data have shown that dipeptides and tripeptides can directly cross the testinal mucosa and are more rapidly and efficiently absorbed than are free amino acids.[15] As a result, some new formulations have higher proportions of peptides and lower amounts of free amino acids. As an example, see in Appendix G, Table 3, the composition of Criticare HN compared with Peptamen, Pepti-2000, Reabilan and Reabilan HN. Note particularly the relative amounts of dipeptides and tripeptides that are of small molecular weight ($<1,000$).

Peptide absorption is less severely affected than is absorption of amino acids in some disorders. The peptide-based formulas are useful for patients with impaired protein digestion and absorption with excessive albumin loss in the intestine or with hypermetabolic conditions such as that seen in patients with burns or head injury.[16]

3. *Intact proteins* are in their original natural form and require complete digestion. Some examples are eggs, milk, and meat. Intact proteins separated from the original food are "isolates." Some examples are soy protein isolate, lactalbumin or casein from milk, and albumin from egg white.

Specific Amino Acids. In addition to the above sources of protein, the effects of certain individual amino acids are now under investigation. Recent work has emphasized glutamine.

Glutamine and alanine transport most of the circulating amino acid nitrogen, including that released from skeletal muscles following injury. Despite high levels of release, glutamine muscle stores and blood levels fall after trauma, surgery, sepsis or major burns, indicating increased uptake in other tissues. Uptake is accelerated in the intestinal tract in surgery, infection, and other stresses. There is evidence that glutamine is essential for maintenance of normal structure of the intestine suggesting that glutamine requirement may be increased in critical illnesses. As a consequence, consideration may be given to supplementation with glutamine for patients given tube or parenteral feedings. This supplementation may be contraindicated, however, in patients with liver disease or other disorders with elevated serum ammonia levels. Further study will be necessary before the mechanisms and use of this type of supplementation are understood.[17]

Vitamins and Minerals. Most ready-to-use tube feedings provide the NRC recommended allowances of vitamins and minerals if a sufficient volume of feeding to meet caloric requirements is given. If a patient has an increased requirement consequent to his disease, further supplementation may be necessary. Some formulas do not contain vitamin K, which may need to be provided in a weekly supplement if the formula is used for an extended period and for patients with fat malabsorption.

Products Available

A number of tube feedings, known as **fixed-ratio formulas**, are available and are listed in Appendix G, Table 3. They are ready to use or require only the addition of water in some cases. There are five types of fixed-ratio formulas. Their properties are summarized in Table 5-3.

Some patients have needs which cannot be met by presently available fixed-ratio formulas. For these patients, individual ingredients, called **modules**, may be used to make a specially tailored (**modular**) formula to meet the patient's unique needs. A module may also be added to make some adjustment to a fixed-ratio formula.

The modules provide various protein, fat, and carbohydrate sources and vitamin and mineral supplements. Products available are listed in Appendix G, Table 2.

Evaluation of Tube Feedings

The characteristics of an ideal tube feeding are given in Table 5-4. These characteristics

Table 5-3. Properties of Tube Feedings

Type	Characteristic Ingredients	Properties	Requirements	Where Given
Blenderized	Intact protein, starch, LCT[a]	Moderate osmolality High viscosity Low cost Contain lactose	Normally functioning digestive tract Lactose tolerance	Stomach
Milk based protein isolates	Milk proteins, oligosaccharides, oil, vitamins, minerals	Most palatable High protein High renal solute load Osmolality 500–700 mOsm/kg	Lactose tolerance Normally functioning digestive tract	Stomach or upper duodenum
Non-milk-based protein isolates	Protein isolates (non-milk-based), oligosaccharides, oil, vitamins, minerals	Lactose-free Osmolality 300–400 mOsm/kg 1–2 kcal/ml Low viscosity	Normally functioning digestive tract	Stomach or upper duodenum
Hydrolyzed-protein-based	Amino acids or small peptides; glucose or glucose oligosaccharides; minimum LCT; MCT[b]	Highly osmolar Require minimal digestion Very unpalatable Flavor packets provided, but increased osmolality High cost	Used in malabsorption	Jejunum
Special-purpose formulas	Variable	(Used for patients with renal or hepatic failure, pulmonary disease, or severe metabolic stress)		

[a] Long-chain triglycerides.
[b] Medium-chain triglycerides.

should be considered in choosing items for use. It is interesting to find that taste may be important even when the patient is being fed by tube. Patients frequently state that they can taste a tube feeding and request changes in flavor if it is unpleasant. It has been suggested that some component in the feeding,

Table 5-4. Characteristics of an Ideal Tube Feeding

Limited cost
Uncontaminated
Tolerable osmolality
Caloric density equivalent to 1 kcal/cc
Suitable protein-calorie ratio
Adequate nutrient intake
Balanced nutrient composition, including electrolytes and amino acids
Nutritional adequacy for short-term use or, when indicated, for long-term feeding
Convenience and ease of administration
Suitable viscosity

after absorption, circulates in the blood and is secreted into the saliva.

Techniques of Administration

Routes. The placement of tubes for feeding is shown in Figure 5-2. **Intragastric** (or nasogastric or NG) tubes are used in problems of ingestion such as head and neck surgery. Longer silicon-tipped tubes may be **nasoduodenal** or **nasojejunal**, reducing the incidence of vomiting or aspiration of regurgitated tube feeding into the lungs.

If the condition of the patient is such that access through the nose or mouth is not possible, an artificial opening or **stoma** may be created by the surgeon. The location of the stoma depends on the reason it was created. A **cervical esophagostomy** creates an opening into the esophagus at approximately the shoulder level. It has an advantage in that it does not require the patient to undress for

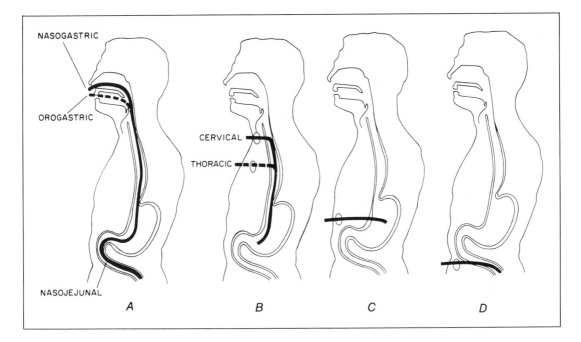

Figure 5-2. Types and sites of tube feeding. A. An intragastric tube, which is passed through nose or mouth into the stomach and secured in place. (A tube passed through the mouth is more correctly called an orogastric tube. An orogastric tube ordinarily is inserted at meal time and removed following the meal.) B. Esophagostomy. A temporary or permanent opening (stoma) is constructed at one of several sites to allow a tube to be introduced through the skin into the esophagus. The feeding tube usually is removed between meals. C. Gastrostomy: A temporary or permanent stoma is constructed allowing food to be introduced through the skin directly into the stomach. D. Jejunostomy: A stoma is constructed that gives direct access to the jejunum. This method of feeding may be used when the stomach must be bypassed. (Reprinted with permission from Suitor, C.W., and Crowley, M.F., Nutrition: Principles and Application in Health Promotion, 2nd ed. Philadelphia: J.B. Lippincott, 1984, p. 391.)

feeding and the opening is easily concealed. Esophagostomies are dependable for long-term use and are easy to handle. A **gastrostomy** provides an opening directly into the stomach. It is created by a surgeon. A related method is the **percutaneous endoscopic gastrostomy (PEG)**, in which the gastrostomy tube penetrates the stomach wall and

the abdominal wall. It is placed under local anesthesia and sedation. A **jejunostomy** creates access directly into the jejunum. A **needle catheter jejunostomy** consists of a catheter implanted into the jejunum for access rather than creating a stoma. The jejunostomy bypasses the duodenum and the duct system that provides bile and pancreatic enzymes. Therefore, a jejunostomy feeding must consist of predigested materials. With a jejunostomy, there is a high incidence of dumping syndrome (see Chapter 7) and diarrhea, and adequate nutrient intake may be difficult to maintain.

Delivery Systems. The method of delivery of the feeding into the tube is very important. In **bolus feeding**, the patient is fed a relatively large amount at stated intervals. For example, a patient receiving 2,000 ml/24 hours in eight bolus feedings would receive 250 ml at each feeding. Each feeding would be given in 5–10 minutes. The method provides a variable rate of delivery and is time-consuming for the busy nursing staff. As a consequence, there is a problem of missed feedings and an increased incidence of intolerance to the feeding. In **intermittent feed-**

ing, the formula is given more slowly than is a bolus feeding, perhaps over a 30-minute period.

In the **gravity drip** method, the feeding in its container is placed above the patient's head and connected to the tube. The flow rate is regulated with a stopcock but is variable, changing with the patient's position and the viscosity of the mixture. It is not usable for very viscous mixtures, but many commercial feedings are packaged so that they can be delivered by gravity drip.

A **peristaltic pump** is essential for feedings that go directly into the intestine and will deliver at a more constant rate at any site. It controls the rate of flow electronically over a 24-hour period. Battery operation makes it possible for the patient to be ambulatory while being fed. Equipment costs are high, but labor cost is reduced, and rate of delivery of the formula is more constant. A **pump** is also necessary to deliver a blenderized diet. Pumps are expensive, but labor costs are reduced with their use.

Types of Tubes. A soft flexible tube is most comfortable for the patient. Polyvinyl and red rubber tubes tend to become hard and be uncomfortable. They may even cause intestinal perforation, esophagitis, or esophageal stricture.[18] Several new types of tubes made from Silastic or polyurethane are available. They are more comfortable and do not harden with use. An enclosed tungsten or silicon weight at the end of the tube assists in insertion and passage into the duodenum. Tubes may be labeled so they are visible on roentgenography to confirm their proper placement.

The quality of feeding tubes has improved greatly in recent years. They are available in various diameters, and a tube must be chosen to suit the size of the patient and the viscosity of the feeding. The patient will be most comfortable with a tube of the smallest diameter through which the feeding will pass. **French** is a scale used to denote the size of catheters and other tubes. Each unit is roughly equal to 0.33 mm in diameter. The French size, however, refers to *outside* diameter (O.D.). For a given O.D., the inside diameter (I.D.) is greater in polyurethane than in Silastic tubes. As a result, there is some variability in the ability to pass formula through the tubes.

As general guidelines, defined formula diets will go through No. 5, 6, or 8 French tubes, and lactose-free formulas, through a No. 5 or 6 Fr. if pumped or No. 7.3 Fr. by gravity drip. Milk-based formulas require a No. 7.3 to 9.6 Fr. by pump or No. 8 to 9.6 Fr. by gravity drip. Blenderized feeding requires a No. 8 to 9.6 Fr. by pump and a No. 12 to 18 Fr. by gravity.[19]

Rate, Frequency, and Concentration of Feeding. If liquids high in osmolality are given rapidly, nausea, vomiting, severe cramping, and diarrhea are likely to occur. The danger of aspiration is increased. Therefore, tube feedings are begun cautiously, allowing an adjustment period.

For feedings into the stomach, hyperosmolar feedings are often well tolerated. Gravity feedings are also well tolerated. If such is not the case, a pump may be used. Bolus feeding should not be used until the patient demonstrates a tolerance to drip feeding.

A common protocol is to begin administration slowly, that is, 50 cc/hr or less of the formula. If no untoward symptoms occur in 8–12 hours, the feeding rate is increased. In some institutions, the formula is diluted at the beginning. However, this procedure increases the risk of contamination and is now done less often.

Gastric residuals, the volume of feeding remaining in the stomach, should be aspirated up the tube and measured every four to six hours or before each bolus feeding. If residuals are more than 100 ml two hours after the last feeding, or if the patient vomits, gastric feeding should be stopped. Nasoduodenal feedings may be necessary in these circumstances.

In gastric feeding, the patient's head should be elevated during and 30 minutes after intermittent feeding to reduce the risk of aspiration. Some institutions do not feed at night for the same reason.

In any type of tube feeding, fluid requirements must be considered. Fluid is particularly important for patients who are unable to communicate. Fluid intake is the sum of the water content of the formula (total volume − [weights in grams of protein + fat + carbohydrate]) along with any other fluid taken. This can include fluid given with medication, any other food or drink that might be given, and the water used to flush the tube after intermittent feedings. The difference between intake and need is provided as free water and is put into the tube.

Tube feedings are usually administered at room temperature. Many believe that chilled formulas cause cramping and diarrhea.

Contraindications to Tube Feeding

The primary contraindication to tube feeding is obstruction, unless access is available below the area of the obstruction. Patients with obstruction of the esophagus, for example, may be fed through a gastrostomy. In cases of **paralytic ileus** (obstruction from inhibition of bowel motility), which is seen for a period following abdominal surgery and also occurs in burn patients, tube feeding should not be instituted until bowel sounds resume.

In addition, a highly osmolar defined formula diet is not used with conditions that cause the patient to be unable to handle a high osmotic load, such as dumping syndrome, jejunal fistulas, and some hepatic and renal diseases. They should not be used for infants and only in very dilute form for small children.

Complications

Complications may be related to the mechanics of the tube feeding process, the patient's gastrointestinal function or metabolic processes, psychosocial factors, or infection. Those which are most likely to involve the

nutritional care specialist are summarized in Table 5-5.

An additional complication, only recently recognized, is bacterial translocation, the migration of bacteria or endotoxin across the intestine to sites outside the intestine. Normally, the intestinal mucosa is a barrier between the bacteria in the gut and systemic organs. However, in immune deficiency, any conditions causing disruption of the mucosa, overgrowth of enteric bacteria, or long-term parenteral feeding, the bacteria may "escape" the intestine and cause a systemic infection. The problem seems to be exacerbated by protein malnutrition. Studies in rats showed that bacterial translocation occurred in 66% of parenterally fed rats and 33% of tube-fed rats, but in none fed a standard rat chow.[20] It has been suggested that glutamine supplementation may reduce the incidence of this complication, and thus reducing the occurrence of endotoxemia and bacteremia.[21-23] Other protective dietary materials may be soluble fiber, a precursor for short-chain fatty acids as the active principle.

Patient Monitoring

Monitoring the tube-fed patient for formula tolerance, hydration status, and nutritional response is the responsibility of the nutritional care specialist as well as that of the physician and nursing staff. The actual volume of intake, as well as the incidence of vomiting, stool frequency or diarrhea, abdominal cramps, or bloating should be observed carefully. Tolerance may also be indicated by an absence of urine glucose or acetone.

It is important to observe the patient for signs of dehydration, particularly if the formula is high in protein or electrolytes. The thirst mechanism may safeguard alert adult patients, but all children and patients who are comatose, very weak, very ill, or have fever or drainage from a fistula should be observed with extreme care. Fluid intake and output and signs of edema and sudden weight gain should be noted. Values on the

Table 5-5. Nutrition-Related Problems in the Tube-Fed Patient

Problem	Possible Causes	Suggested Corrective Measures[a]
Nausea	Improper location of tube tip	Consult with physician or nurse on replacement of tube
	Excessive rate of feeding; excessive volume of feeding	Decrease volume or rate of feeding[a]
	Anxiety	Reassure patient
Vomiting	Excessive formula volume	Reduce volume of feeding[a]
Diarrhea	Very cold formula	Give formula near room temperature
	Too-rapid infusion	Give formula more slowly
	High osmolarity or high concentration of feeding	Adapt patient gradually; start with 1 : 2 – 4 dilution; add applesauce, pectin, banana flakes; add methylcellulose (for bulk); add paregoric, Lomotil, codeine, or Kaopectate to feeding[a]
	Lactose intolerance	Use lactose-free formula[a]
Vomiting *and* diarrhea	Contamination	Check sanitation of formula and equipment; consult with bacteriologist
	Anxiety	Reassure patient; explain purpose and procedures
Constipation	High milk content	Use milk-free formula
	Lack of fiber	Use stool softeners or laxatives in formula
	Inadequate fluid intake	Increase fluid intake
Dehydration	Rapid infusion of carbohydrate leading to hyperglycemia and osmotic diarrhea	Administer tube feeding slowly; physician may prescribe insulin
	Excessive protein or electrolytes or both	Reduce protein, electrolytes, or increase fluid intake
	Inadequate fluid intake	Increase fluid intake
Edema	Excess sodium in formula	Use formula with less sodium
Gradual weight loss	Inadequate calories	Check if patient is receiving prescribed feeding; estimate caloric intake; possibly increase volume per day or concentration
Other signs of undernutrition	Nutrient content of formula inadequate for needs	Discuss appropriate supplements with physician
Gradual gain of excess weight	Excess calories	Dilute formula or decrease volume per day
Obstructed tube	Formula viscosity excessive for tube caliber	Flush tube before and after feeding
	Failure to flush tube	Push obstruction through with syringe Loosen clog with meat tenderizer or Coca-Cola Strain modular formulas Use less viscous formula or larger tube

[a] In consultation with physician or nursing staff if required by the policy of the institution.

patient's chart to be monitored include blood urea nitrogen, glucose, albumin, and electrolyte concentrations in the serum, as well as urinary glucose and specific gravity. An estimate of nitrogen balance should be provided weekly by the nutritional care specialist.

The nutritional status of patients who are tube-fed over an extended period should be assessed at regular intervals, using the methods described in Chapter 3.

Parenteral Feeding

Conventional diets and tube feedings require the use of the gastrointestinal tract. There are circumstances, however, when the patient is unable to absorb nutrients or the gastrointestinal tract is not available. Such patients are then fed directly into the circulatory system.

In the strict meaning of the term, **parenteral nutrition** refers to the provision of nutrients by any route that does not involve the intestinal tract. It includes, for example, intramuscular injections of vitamins. In common usage, however, parenteral nutrition generally refers to the intravenous route. It may be used for partial or total nutritional support for a brief period, for an extended time, or for life. There are three fundamental types of intravenous feeding:

1. Supplemental nutrition into a peripheral vein, as described in Chapter 2.
2. Total nutrition into a central vein.
3. Total nutrition into a peripheral vein.

The amount of energy that must be provided intravenously is crucial in determining the method to be used.

Some patients need more nutritional support than can be provided by supplemental peripheral venous alimentation. For these patients, more aggressive nutritional support has become available in recent years. The procedure is commonly referred to as **total parenteral nutrition** (TPN). As is implied by its name, TPN may be used as the sole means of feeding the patient, or it may supplement enteral feeding.

A major difference between intravenous and enteral feeding is that the intravenous feeding enters the systemic circulation directly, rather than entering the portal circulation and the lymphatic system. However, because the intestinal tract, with its digestive function, is bypassed in intravenous alimentation, the nutrients must be provided in a predigested state. All the effects of this altered route of entry of nutrients have not been determined. It apparently does not affect nutritional requirements, but immune function, integrity of the intestinal mucosa, and a number of functions of the gastrointestinal tract, including exocrine pancreatic function, intestinal mucosal enzyme content, and gallbladder contraction, may be depressed. These changes are believed to be reversible when enteral feeding is resumed, but resumption of enteral feeding should be

done cautiously if the duration of TPN has been prolonged.

Total parenteral nutrition is a complex and expensive procedure with potential risks and complications. Therefore, it should be undertaken only if adequate nutrient intake via the gastrointestinal tract is impossible or inadvisable. A second contraindication to the use of parenteral feeding is the existence of an advanced terminal condition such as advanced inoperable cancer. Examples of conditions in which TPN may be appropriate are listed in Table 5-6.

Most institutions establish a nutritional support service to provide the necessary detailed attention for TPN patients. The professionals involved in the service vary, but a nutritional support service usually consists of at least a physician, nurse, nutritional care specialist, and pharmacist. Sometimes, a so-

Table 5-6. Indications for Use of Total Parenteral Nutrition

Unavailability of the gastrointestinal tract
Short bowel syndrome
Obstruction
Ileus
Malabsorption
Chronic vomiting

To minimize gastrointestinal function
Inflammatory bowel disease
Fistulas
Intractable diarrhea and failure to thrive
Acute pancreatitis

Preoperative repletion of patients who have lost more than 10–15% body weight

Patients who cannot meet energy needs by oral intake
Hypermetabolism: major surgery or trauma, major burns, or sepsis
Protein-losing gastroenteropathy
Extreme weakness
Anorexia and unwillingness to eat: cancer, chemotherapy, radiotherapy, psychological depression, or anorexia nervosa

Disturbances of nitrogen metabolism
Reversible liver failure
Acute and chronic renal failure

Nonterminal coma

Any patient who cannot be fed for more than 7–10 days

cial worker, physical therapist, administrator, and secretary also are included. The nutritional care specialist on the nutritional support service must have a thorough knowledge of nutrition and an appreciation of the methods, problems, and risks involved in TPN. He or she has a particularly important role in monitoring the patient's nutritional status during the course of the TPN feeding and in providing appropriate nutritional support during the weaning process. These subjects will now be described briefly, with emphasis on central venous feeding.

Central Venous Alimentation

Placement of the Catheter. Insertion of the catheter is a surgical procedure. The catheter commonly is placed into the right or left sub-

clavian vein and then threaded into the superior vena cava. Sometimes the internal jugular vein is used as the starting point for catheter insertion. For relatively short-term TPN, a typical line consists of a 16-gauge percutaneous intravenous catheter (Intracath) (see Figure 5-3). Percutaneous stiffer catheters are not suitable for patients requiring TPN for many months or for life because of the danger of thrombosis, erosion of the wall of the vein, and infection. Instead, a silicone catheter is inserted for long-term use. These catheters are less reactive and are soft and flexible. They are approximately 90 cm long. Part of the catheter lies in a subcutaneous tunnel and emerges just lateral to the sternum at approximately the fourth or fifth rib. In this position, the patient can see and care for it, and it does not interfere with clothing.

Figure 5-3. Central parenteral nutrition (CPN) as administered into large veins: superior vena cava and subclavian.

Preparation and Administration of the Solutions. All TPN solutions must be sterile

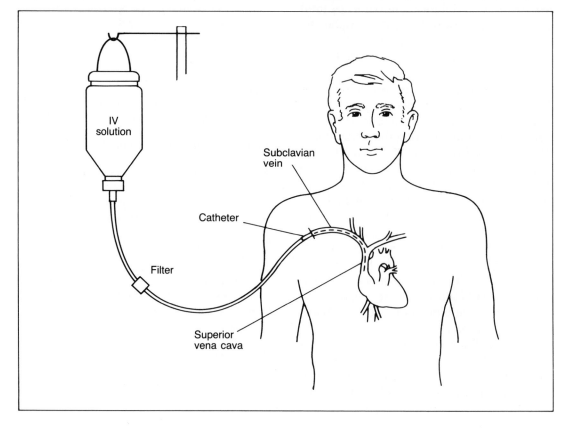

and are prepared in the pharmacy using aseptic techniques. Standard procedure for their administration to the hospitalized patient infuses the solutions steadily over a 24-hour period, beginning with 50 ml/hr the first day, 75 ml/hr the second day, and 125 ml/hr the third day and thereafter. An infusion pump usually is considered preferable to regulate the flow, although gravity drip administration may be used.

Composition of Solutions. To provide a large quantity of nutrients within a volume of fluid that the patient can tolerate, it is necessary to use a hyperosmolar solution that has a higher concentration of the nutrients in a smaller total volume. All required nutrients must be provided in the infusate.

Amino acids. The sources of amino acids used most commonly in TPN are 3.0, 3.5, 5.0, 7.0, 8.5, 10, and 15% solutions of crystalline amino acids. Representative commercially available amino acid mixtures are listed in Table 5-7. The amino acid content of each mixture is available from the manufac-

turer. Those containing all the essential amino acids along with ten or twelve nonessential amino acids similar to egg protein promote best utilization for protein synthesis.[24] The body has a limited capacity to synthesize arginine, so arginine is included in the infusate.[25] Infants require histidine, and premature infants are deficient in cystathionase, the enzyme that converts methionine to cystine; therefore, cystine is essential.[26] Some mixtures are modified to be appropriate for patients with renal or hepatic disease or hypermetabolic conditions; these are discussed in later chapters (see Chapters 9, 13, and 14).

Carbohydrate. Carbohydrate to provide sufficient energy substrate is provided in the form of dextrose solutions available in concentrations of up to 70%. The most commonly used concentration is 50%. Each 10% of dextrose contributes 505 mOsm/L; therefore, osmolality may be estimated as percent dextrose $\times$ 50. The dextrose is in the form of a monohydrate and thus provides 3.4 kcal/g.

Table 5-7. Commercially Available Sources of Amino Acids for Total Parenteral Nutrition

Product	Manufacturer	Amino Acid Concentration (%)
General preparations		
Aminosyn	Abbott Laboratories	3.5, 5.0, 7.0, 8.5, 10.0
Novamine	Kabi-Vitrum	8.5, 11.4, 15
FreAmine III	Kendall-McGaw	3.0, 8.5, 10.0
Travasol	Clintec	3.5, 5.5, 8.5, 10.0
TrophAmine	Kendall-McGaw	6.0 (pediatric)
Vamin	Pharmacia, Canada	7
Special formulations		
Renal[a]		
Aminess	Kabi-Vitrum	5.2
RenAmin	Clintec	6.5
Aminosyn RF	Abbott Laboratories	5.2
NephrAmine	Kendall-McGaw	5.4
Hepatic[b]		
Aminosyn HBC	Abbott Laboratories	7.0
HepatAmine	Kendall-McGaw	8.0
FreAmine HBC	Kendall-McGaw	6.9
BranchAmin	Clintec	4.0 (branched chain only)
Other		
ProcalAmine	Kendall-McGaw	3.0
Aminosyn PF	Abbott Laboratories	7.0, 10.0

[a] Contains only essential amino acids plus histidine.
[b] BCAA-enriched for treatment of hepatic encephalopathy.

Energy sources other than glucose, including fructose (3.75 – 4.0 kcal/g), glycerol (4.32 kcal/g), and alcohol (7 kcal/g), have been used, but no advantage of their use has been established. Amino acids are not considered acceptable sources of energy in the patients being replenished, since the objective is to have these patients retain rather than deaminate amino acids for energy.

Lipids. Lipids may be included at either of two levels, a low level sufficient to prevent essential fatty acid (EFA) deficiency or a larger amount that will contribute significantly to the kilocalorie content of the infusate. Lipids are available as 10% (1.1 kcal/ml) or 20% (2.0 kcal/ml) emulsions of soy or a mixture of soy and safflower oil, in bottles containing 100, 200, 250, or 500 ml. They also contain 1.2% egg phospholipid as an emulsifying agent and 2.2 – 2.5% glycerol to make the mixture isotonic.

If lipids are given only to prevent EFA deficiency, two to four 500-ml bottles (2 to 4 units) of 10% fat emulsion per week are sufficient. If these are not provided, EFA deficiency is seen in the form of circular skin lesions, hair loss, delays in wound healing, and abnormalities in liver function. Changes in the unsaturated fatty acid ratios (triene-tetraene ratio) indicative of deficiency can be seen as early as four days after the use of an EFA-deficient formula.

Lipid can provide up to 60% of the total caloric need. The recommended daily dose is 1 to 2 g/kg/day. It is given in combination with glucose, since lipid alone might maintain body fat while allowing protein loss via gluconeogenesis. The use of lipids as an energy source is somewhat controversial; nonprotein calories are provided primarily as glucose in most large centers. The rationale for the routine infusion of greater amounts of fat in TPN is as follows:

1. Provision of nonprotein calories as glucose and fat most closely resembles a normal diet.
2. The impairment of glucose metabolism induced by catabolic states suggests that a portion of the intake should be substituted with fat.
3. The lipid reduces the osmolality, compared to an equicaloric lipid-free formula.
4. Patients with respiratory failure can benefit from the lower CO_2 production than that seen in glucose oxidation alone.

On the other hand, there are arguments favoring continuation of the predominant use of glucose as the nonprotein energy source in TPN, with limitation of fat intake to amounts sufficient to avoid EFA deficiency. These arguments include the following:

1. There are questions regarding the efficacy of fat as an energy source to support protein metabolism in catabolic patients. Although defects in the complete oxidation of glucose in catabolic states have been identified, studies of the efficacy of glucose and fat in the support of nitrogen balance in catabolic patients have suggested that glucose is more effective. Patients who are not severely catabolic appear to achieve similar nitrogen balance with glucose or with a portion of the intake as fat.
2. Complications specific to the infusion of fat emulsions may include impairment of the diffusion of gas across the alveolocapillary membrane in the lung, impairment of immune function, and impairment of blood coagulation. However, widespread use of currently available fat emulsions is remarkably free of complications.
3. Glucose is an inexpensive energy source. The cost to a hospital pharmacy to prepare an intravenous solution as either 10%, 20%, or 30% glucose varies only slightly. In contrast, the production of infusates containing fat emulsions may be more costly.

Lipid products for parenteral use are described in Table 5-8. Formerly, the lipid was not mixed with the glucose-amino acid solution but was run into a catheter from a sepa-

Table 5-8. Lipid Emulsions for Total Parenteral Nutrition

Product	Lipid Concentration (%)	Osmolarity (mOsm/L)	Kcal/ml	pH[a]	Composition	Fatty Acid Content (%)
Intralipid (Kabi-Vitrum)	10 20	260 350	1.1 2.0	7.5 7.5	Soy oil in water; 1.2% phosphatide; 2.5% glycerol	Linoleic, 55; linolenic, 8; other, 37
IV Fat Emulsion (Kendall-McGaw)	10 20	260 350	1.1 2.0	8.0 8.0	Soy oil in water; 1.2% phosphatide; 2.25% glycerol	Linoleic, 50–55; linolenic, 6–9
Liposyn II (Abbott Laboratories)	10 20	300 340	1.1 2.0	8.0 8.3	50/50 safflower and soy oil in water; 1.2% phosphatide; 2.5% glycerol	Linoleic, 78; linolenic, 0.5
Soyacal (Alpha Therapeutic)	10 20	280 315	1.1 2.0	— —	Soy oil in water; 1.2% phosphatide; 2.2% glycerol	Linoleic, 49–69; linolenic, 6–9; other, 33–49
Travamulsion (Travenol Laboratories)	10 20	270 300	1.1 2.0	5.5–9.0	Soy oil in water; 1.2% phosphatide; 2.5% glycerol	Linoleic, 56; linolenic, 6; other, 38

[a] Adjusted with sodium hydroxide.

137

rate bottle. The separate lines were connected just before they enter the vein. Starting infusion rates might be 1 ml/min. for $\frac{1}{2}$ hour and then be increased to 125 ml/hr. Recently, more stable lipid emulsions have made it possible to prepare **total nutrient admixtures** (TNA), also known as **3-in-1 formulas**, containing dextrose, amino acids, and lipids. The formulas with dextrose and amino acids and no fat are now referred to as **2-in-1 formulas**.

Transient side effects of lipid infusion occur. They include chills, shivering, fever, vomiting, and chest and back pain. Alternative methods of administration may avoid these side effects. It has been claimed that application of corn oil or safflower oil to the skin will supply some of the requirement. For those patients in whom some intake by mouth is possible, 2 to 5 teaspoons of an appropriate vegetable oil taken orally will prevent EFA deficiency.

The **energy-nitrogen ratio** in the final formula is an important consideration. A sufficient amount of energy from nonprotein sources must be provided so that amino acids are used for anabolic processes rather than as a source of energy. There remains some controversy on the best amount to use. A common current practice is to provide a ratio of at least 120 : 1, that is, 120 nonprotein kilocalories per gram of nitrogen. For example, let us assume that a patient is receiving 1 liter of 8.5% FreAmine (see Table 5-7). This would contain 85 g of amino acids, which are 16% nitrogen. The nitrogen content thus is 85 × 0.16 or 13.6 g. In order to receive at least 120 kcal/g of nitrogen, the patient needs 1,632 kcal (13.6 × 120). One liter of 20% dextrose in water (D20W) contains 200 g of dextrose, yielding 3.4 kcal/g or 680 kcal/L. One 500-ml unit of 10% Intralipid contains 450 kcal. Thus the patient might be given 500 ml of 10% Intralipid, which contain 450 kcal, and 2 liters of D20W, which contain 1,360 kcal, to total 1,810 kcal or 133 kcal/g of nitrogen.
Vitamins and minerals. All requirements for **vitamins** must be met, but complete agreement on the amounts to be given has not

been reached. Although it is unclear whether vitamin requirements are increased in stressed patients, patients with surgical or traumatic wounds are assumed to need increased amounts of vitamin C for wound healing. Overdosage with vitamins A and D have led to documented cases of toxicity.

A number of multivitamin products are commercially available for parenteral use, but none provides all the necessary vitamins. In a typical procedure, 10 ml/day of a commercial multivitamin product are added for patients needing maintenance doses. Larger doses may be necessary if the patient is vitamin deficient. Available products are MVI-12 (Armour), Lyphomed 9 + 3 (Lyphomed), Berocca Parenteral Nutrition (Roche), and MVC Plus (Ascot). These are packaged in two vials to separate vitamins that are unstable when mixed. Folacin, biotin, and vitamin B_{12} are segregated into the second container. Typical contents are shown in Table 5-9.

Vitamin K is given as a separate injection, 2 – 5 mg intramuscularly once weekly. It is

Table 5-9. Recommended Parenteral Vitamin Intake

Vitamin and Units	Adults	Pediatrics
Vitamin A, IU	3,300	2,300
Thiamin, mg	3	1.2
Riboflavin, mg	3.6	1.4
Niacin, mg	40	17
Vitamin B_6, mg	4.0	1.0
Pantothenate, mg	15	5.0
Vitamin B_{12}, µg	5	1.0
Ascorbic acid, mg	100	80
Vitamin D, IU	200	400
Vitamin E, IU	10	7
Folate, µg	400	140
Biotin, µg	60	20
Vitamin K, mg	0	0.2

Compiled from Nutrition Advisory Group, American Medical Association, Department of Foods and Nutrition. Multivitamin preparations for parenteral use. A statement by the Nutrition Advisory Group. *JPEN* 3:258, 1987; Moore, M.C., Green, H.L., Phillips, B., Franck, L., Shulman, R.J., Murrell, J.E., and Ament, M.E., Evaluation of a pediatric multiple vitamin preparation for total parenteral nutrition in infants and children. I. Blood levels of water-soluble vitamins. *Pediatrics* 77:530, 1986.

needed particularly by patients receiving oral antibiotic therapy, those with malabsorption syndromes, and those with prolonged prothrombin time. Vitamin K may be eliminated if the patient has a thrombotic tendency or is receiving anticoagulant medications. Serum levels of vitamins should be monitored at intervals, and doses should be adjusted accordingly.

Requirements for **minerals** are not known specifically. Since losses must also be replaced, requirements of individual patients may vary widely. Deficits must be replaced as described in Chapter 2. Approximately 80% of hospitalized patients, however, may be managed with standardized formulations. Some electrolytes are included in the commercial amino acid preparations. Patients receiving antibiotics may receive significant amounts of sodium from that source.[27]

Potassium is the principal intracellular cation that tends to be lost when muscle is catabolized during elevated gluconeogenesis. Potassium deficiency prevents growth,[28] and repletion of 1 kg of lean muscle mass requires 145 to 155 mEq of potassium or 75 mEq/day. Daily urinary potassium excretion of 40 to 60 mEq/day must also be provided for. Therefore, daily needs are 120 to 160 mEq/day, or approximately 50 mEq/L of infusate. Patients with compromised renal function will not tolerate this amount, and so a smaller dose is administered carefully. Potassium is added to the infusate as the chloride, phosphate, or acetate.

Magnesium acts as a cofactor and is taken up intracellularly. At maximum rates of anabolism, 15 to 30 mEq/day have been recommended to meet the requirement.[10,27,28] It is given as the sulfate.

Phosphate is needed for protoplasm formation. A commonly administered amount is 30 mEq/day. It is used for synthesis of membrane phospholipids and high-energy phosphate bonds. It also is important in bone formation. The amount recommended varies widely, with a greater amount required if the patient is very depleted,[10,29] and a lesser amount if renal function is impaired. Phosphate is given as sodium or potassium salt.

Sodium must be provided to replace obligatory urinary losses and to maintain sodium concentration in the ECF. For maintenance, 50 mEq of sodium per liter of TPN infusate usually is sufficient.[27] Since formation of 1 g of protoplasm is accompanied by expansion of 0.8 ml of ECF volume, an additional 70 mEq of sodium is provided during anabolism. Less sodium is given to patients with cardiovascular or renal insufficiency. Sodium is available as the chloride, acetate, phosphate, or bicarbonate.

Chloride balance is maintained if sodium chloride is used. Acidotic patients are given **acetate**,[27] which serves as a bicarbonate precursor, rather than bicarbonate itself, which is not compatible with other ions in TPN solutions. A commonly used protocol specifies a 4 : 1 chloride-acetate ratio. If requirements for chloride are increased in the patient with large losses from a gastrostomy or nasogastric tube, chloride may be given as both sodium and potassium chloride.

Calcium is required to maintain calcium balance, normal parathyroid function, and bone mineralization, but the requirement in TPN is not known. It is provided as calcium gluceptate, chloride, and gluconate in amounts of 200 to 400 mg/day (10 to 20 mEq/day).[30] Immobilization increases urinary excretion of calcium.

Iron may be included at levels of 1 to 2 mg/day,[29] but it is not always added to a TPN solution. Adult males with good iron status and full-term infants have iron stores to last longer than a short course of TPN. Therefore, iron can be omitted for short-term TPN. If a deficiency of iron exists, iron dextran may be added to the formula. The requirement for parenteral iron may be calculated using the following formula:[31]

$$\text{iron (mg)} = 0.3W \times \frac{(100 - \text{Hb})}{0.148} \qquad \text{(5-6)}$$

where W = body weight in pounds; Hb = hemoglobin in g/dl of blood.

Of the trace elements, **zinc** has been studied most extensively. It is necessary as a cofactor for many enzymes. It quickly migrates to rapidly dividing cells, but the mechanism of its action in repair is not known. Nevertheless, low serum zinc levels have been associated with poor repair and chronic skin ulceration (**decubitus ulcers** or "bedsores").

Copper deficiency has been reported in patients on long-term TPN,[32] but exact requirements are not known. Chromium[28] and selenium[33] deficiencies have also been reported.

Addition of 4 mg of zinc (as sulfate) and 1 mg of copper (as sulfate) or more per day often is recommended. It is recommended also that zinc levels be increased up to 300 μg/kg for premature infants. Small bowel zinc losses of 12 mg/L of fluid and diarrheal zinc losses of 17 mg/L of fluid lost must be replaced. Representative trace element solutions also contain 10–12.5 μg of chromium as chloride and 0.4–0.8 mg manganese as a sodium salt. Requirements for other trace elements, including selenium, vanadium, molybdenum, nickel, tin, arsenic, silicon, and cadmium, are not known yet, but deficiencies of these elements in TPN patients have not been reported. Solutions containing trace elements for intravenous use are commercially available. Most institutions have a standard protocol for inclusion of vitamins and minerals in TPN feedings which is used unless there are orders to the contrary.

Osmolarity of the Infusate. The osmolarity of the solution to be infused determines the possible site of infusion. Total osmolarity is calculated by adding the osmolarities of the component parts. The osmolarities can be estimated by multiplying the percentage of dextrose by 50 and the percentage of amino acid by 100. Electrolytes, vitamins, and minerals add 300–400 mOsm/L, and intravenous fat is isotonic at about 300 mOsm/L. Thus a solution consisting of 500 cc of 50% dextrose and 500 cc 8.5% amino acids plus the usual electrolytes, minerals, and vitamins would have an osmolarity of (50 ×

50 × 0.50) + (8.5 × 100 × 0.5) + (300 to 400) = 1,250 + 425 + (300 to 400) = 1,975 to 2,075 mOsm/L. Osmolarity is used, rather than osmolality, since values are given per liter of solution. Osmolarity as high as that in the example must be given in a central vein where it is rapidly mixed into the circulation and diluted.

Estimating Nutritional Needs. The **energy** needs of the patient may be estimated using the methods described in Chapter 3. It is important to make allowance for stress, as represented by the "injury factor" in Equation 3-23. As a general guideline, 30–35 kcal/kg body weight per day or 1.5 times BEE is sufficient for mild or moderate stress. This amount may be reduced for the obese patient. Calories in excess of 40 kcal/kg/day are needed only in some cases of severe burns or extensive trauma.

The first goal is to preserve existing lean body mass. When the patient is more stable, repletion of lost nutrient reserves can then be undertaken.[34] Administration of excessive calories can cause complications including liver and pulmonary dysfunction and osmotic diuresis. Depleted patients, given excess support, may develop a "refeeding syndrome" with hyperglycemia, fluid retention, hypophosphatemia, and cardiac arrest.[35]

The **protein** needs of a patient under mild or moderate stress are 1.2–1.5 grams of protein per kg body weight per day. Extreme stress may increase this rate to 2.5 g/kg/day. A nonprotein kcal/N ratio of 100–150 kcal to 1 g N is needed to promote anabolism.

Dextrose should not be given at a rate greater than 0.36 g/kg body weight per hour. Postoperative surgical patients have been shown to oxidize a maximum of 0.24–0.36 g of intravenous dextrose/kg/hr.[36,37] If an excessive amount of carbohydrate is given, it is used as a substrate for lipogenesis and is thought to lead to fatty liver, liver dysfunction and possibly excess CO_2 production leading to respiratory failure. Minimum carbohydrate requirement is often considered to be 100 g per day, although supporting data are not available.

Fat must be administered at a level to provide at least 2–4% of calories as EFA to prevent EFA deficiency. This may be obtained if 10% of total energy is given as soy or safflower emulsion. The upper limit of fat content is usually set at 60% of total kilocalories as fat. Amounts of fat at the upper end of the range provide greater caloric density in a more nearly isotonic solution. However, excess fat has been associated with dysfunctions in hepatic, renal, cardiac, pulmonary, and neurologic systems.

Electrolytes are usually given in standard solutions unless the patient has special needs. Recommended amounts per day are 60–120 mEq Na, 60–150 mEq K, 60–150 mEq Cl, 80–120 mEq acetate, 20–40 mM phosphorus, 10–15 mEq Ca, and 8–24 mEq Mg. Some amino acid solutions come premixed with standard amounts of electrolytes, and fat emulsions provide some phosphorus.

Vitamins are provided in the multivitamin formulations previously described. They should be added to the mixture just prior to the administration of the formula in order to reduce losses from adsorption to containers and tubes, reactions with other ingredients, or exposure to light.

Trace elements must also be provided. The advent of TPN has increased our knowledge of trace element nutrition, but exact requirements are not known. Several standard solutions are available for addition to the infusate.[38] Amounts per day recommended are 10–20 μg chromium, 0.8–1.5 mg copper, 0.15–0.8 mg manganese, 0.1–0.6 mg molybdenum and 2.5–4.0 mg zinc.[39] Added zinc is given to patients with large losses of fluid from the small bowel (12 mg/L) or large stool losses (17 mg/L). Other recommendations include 2 mg iron for premenopausal women and 1 mg/day for men and postmenopausal women, 0.12 μg iodine, and 0.20 mg or more of selenium.

Procedures for designing a parenteral feeding regimen are described elsewhere and are beyond the scope of this text.[40]

Assuming this type of standard procedure, a TPN order might read, "1 liter of 10% Intralipid and 2 liters of supplemental solution composed of 1 liter of D20W and 1 liter of 8.5% FreAmine amino acid solution per day. IV rate: 83 ml/hr supplemental solution and 42 ml/hr Intralipid."

Complications. There are a number of possible complications of central venous alimentation. A major complication is infection, which can progress from the catheter site and cause general sepsis. Fungal infections, such as *Candida*, and bacterial contamination with *Staphylococcus aureus* or *Staphylococcus epidermidis* occur. Technical complications include **pneumothorax** (air in the thoracic cavity), **hemothorax** (blood in the thoracic cavity), hematoma, embolism, perforation of the vein, air embolus, and injuries to the phrenic nerve or thoracic duct.

Most metabolic complications are avoidable. Hyperglycemia may ensue if the glucose infusion rate is too rapid. It also precedes the onset of sepsis and is seen in patients receiving steroid drugs. Unchecked hyperglycemia may lead to hyperosmolar nonketotic coma (see Chapter 11). This complication is avoidable by diminishing the rate of infusion of glucose or by adding insulin to the infusion if blood glucose measures 250 mg/dl or more.

Hypoglycemia can occur if the infusion rate is decreased too rapidly when the feeding is being discontinued. The infusion should be tapered off slowly over a period of one to two hours, allowing insulin secretion rate to subside. Hypoglycemia can occur also when the infusion stops because of mechanical problems.

Excess energy intake may be detrimental. The development of acute fatty infiltration of the liver associated with mild to moderate hepatic dysfunction has been attributed to excess energy supply. Excess provision of energy as glucose may result in respiratory failure (see Chapter 16). Infused glucose must be cleared from the circulation. Glucose that cannot be oxidized, an amount in excess of 5 mg/kg/minute, must be converted to fat once glycogen stores are saturated. The conversion of glucose to fat yields carbon dioxide as a metabolic by-product, but the reaction does not produce energy. Thus, as increasing loads of glucose are infused, carbon dioxide production divided by oxygen consumption (the **respiratory quotient**) may rise rapidly to values greater than 1. Respiratory failure requiring ventilatory assistance or difficulty in weaning patients from respirators may occur if excess glucose is provided. This complication can be avoided by limiting the kilocalorie content of the infusate to that which covers only the need.

Insufficient or excessive administration of electrolytes also may cause complications. Deficiencies of trace elements, vitamins, and essential fatty acids have been reported, as have overdoses of fat-soluble vitamins and trace elements. These become less common as our knowledge of requirements improves.

Peripheral Venous Alimentation

Indications for TPN by peripheral vein are the same as those for TPN by central vein, but the technique for peripheral venous alimentation avoids the risks of the central route. It also avoids some of the problems of the hyperosmolar solutions, since solutions used in peripheral venous alimentation have lower osmolarity. This lower osmolarity, however, reduces the energy supply per given volume. Thus peripheral venous feeding is usable for patients whose needs are likely to be short term (seven to ten days) and whose requirements are more modest than those that can be met by a central line. The patient must also be able to tolerate a larger fluid load than would be required with central venous alimentation.

It often is recommended that the final concentration of dextrose not exceed 10%. To achieve this, a 20% dextrose solution may be mixed with a 5% crystalline amino acid solution. The osmolarity of this solution is approximately twice that of plasma and will cause phlebitis in 24 to 36 hours.

Two procedures are available to avoid this problem while still providing sufficient energy. One is the use of a fat emulsion, and the other is the use of hydrocortisone plus heparin. A 10% fat emulsion (see Table 5-8) infused along with the dextrose-amino acid solution is reasonably well tolerated. The procedure is diagramed in Figure 5-4. Infusion of 1,500 ml each of dextrose-amino-acid solution and 10% fat emulsion in 24 hours will provide 1,950 kcal, 10 g of nitrogen, and 3 liters of water with a nonprotein calorie-nitrogen ratio of 90:1. This will maintain a stable patient. For malnourished or hypermetabolic patients, a 20% fat emulsion and a large amount of amino acids may meet the need. If this is not the case, a central venous catheter will be required.

An alternative to the use of fat emulsion gives a solution of 2.5% amino acid in 6.5% dextrose with an osmolarity of 900 mOsm, three times normal. To protect the vein, 5 mg of hydrocortisone and 500 units of heparin are added to each liter. In 3 liters of solution, the patient will receive 12.4 g of nitrogen and 780 kcal. This is supportive for the stable patient but is clearly inadequate for the patient with increased needs.

There are several limitations to the use of peripheral venous alimentation for total support. The amount of fat that can be administered is limited to approximately 2 g/kg/day. If this amount is exceeded, the incidence of thrombocytopenia and fat embolism is increased. The total kilocalorie supply thus is restricted.

The administration of 10% glucose plus 5% amino acids provides approximately 500 kcal/L, or approximately 3,000 kcal in 6 liters. With the lipid, a total of 4,500 kcal may be achieved, but the patient must be able to tolerate a large fluid load. This is not the case in patients with renal disease, for example. Patients with respiratory disorders in which pulmonary edema must be avoided also are usually fluid restricted.

Nevertheless, peripheral venous alimentation is useful in several circumstances:

1. For short-term support in patients whose energy needs are moderate.

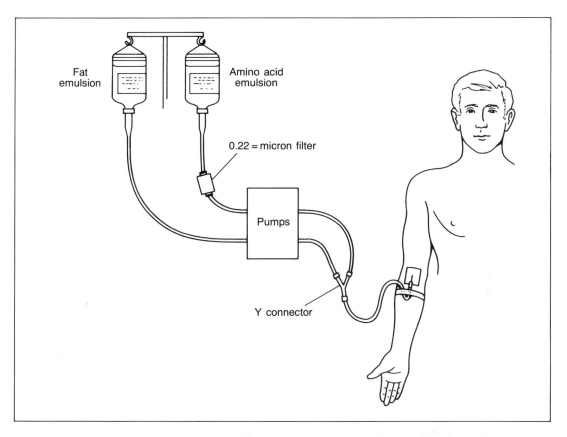

Figure 5-4. Peripheral parenteral nutrition with co-infusion of fat emulsion. If the lipid is mixed with the dextrose-amino acid solution, only one container is used.

2. When risks of central venous TPN are great.
3. When supplemental, rather than total, nutrition is needed.
4. Occasionally, as an intermediate method when weaning a patient from central venous TPN.

Cyclic Parenteral Nutrition

Cyclic parenteral nutrition consists of parenteral feeding a glucose and amino acid solution (2-in-1) for 10 to 16 hours per day. For the remaining 8 to 14 hours, the patient is fed amino acid solution, amino acids plus fat, or nothing at all.

This method provides glucose on a more usual schedule. Serum insulin is reduced when glucose is not fed, and body fat can be used for energy. This has three potential advantages:[41]

1. It provides energy and spares protein.
2. It releases essential fatty acids from stored fat and may prevent their deficiency.
3. It prevents or reduces the tendency to fatty livers.

It is also a convenience when the patient is fed by TPN at home.

Monitoring the TPN Patient

The TPN patient is monitored closely. The nutritional care specialist should observe carefully those items that are relevant to nutrition. Baseline data, preferably obtained before TPN is begun, usually include a complete blood count, blood glucose, serum creatinine, blood urea nitrogen, and serum electrolytes, albumin, transaminases (serum glutamic oxaloacetic transaminase [SGOT] and serum glutamic pyruvic transaminase [SGPT]), calcium, phosphorus, and magnesium.[42] During TPN, blood glucose, electrolytes, and urea nitrogen are obtained three times per week to monitor hydration, renal function, and electrolyte balance. Calcium, phosphorus, and magnesium are monitored until serum levels stabilize. Urine should be checked daily for glucose and acetone to indicate carbohydrate tolerance. Hepatic function is monitored every three to four days by serum bilirubin and the liver enzymes, SGOT or SGPT, lactic dehydrogenase (LDH), and alkaline phosphatase. Plasma triglycerides are used to assess the capacity to clear plasma lipids.

Body weight is obtained daily to check for fluid overload. A weight gain of 1.5 kg/week may occur with intensive nutritional support, but gains above this amount probably indicate water and sodium retention. Once the patient is stable, monitoring once or twice a week is usually sufficient.

Transitional Feeding

The nutritional care specialist plays a particularly important role when the patient progresses from TPN to tube feeding, or from TPN or tube feeding to oral feeding. The patient normally is weaned gradually as enteral intake (by tube or by mouth) slowly increases. Reductions in the rate of TPN infusions are made in appropriate proportion to enteral intake. Total parenteral nutrition has the potential to diminish appetite, but oral intake of food is more often depressed by incomplete recovery from the condition which necessitated the TPN.

Patients who need TPN permanently may manage their condition at home if they are emotionally stable. Patients who are candidates for home TPN are taught catheter care, how to administer the solution, and how to monitor fluid and electrolyte balance.

Study Questions

1. Estimate the amount of water that would be available from a diet containing 70 g protein, 60 g fat, and 200 g carbohydrate.
2. What nutrients are most likely to be deficient in the diet of a vegan?
3. Explain why a vegetarian might refuse the following foods:
   a. Gelatin dessert?
   b. Some ripened cheeses?
4. Why is the osmolality of the formula important in choosing a tube feeding?
5. Explain how a tube feeding can cause dehydration.
6. Why is some long-chain triglyceride included in tube feedings made with MCT?
7. Of the various categories of tube feedings, which would be used if the patient:
   a. Has a jejunostomy tube?
   b. Is lactose intolerant?
   c. Has a gastrostomy tube with intact digestion?
8. List advantages and disadvantages of the following:
   a. Bolus feeding.
   b. Intermittent feeding.
   c. Use of gravity drip feeding.
   d. Use of a peristaltic pump.
9. What is the diameter of a No. 6 French feeding tube?
10. What is the significance of a "gastric residual"? What action would be taken if it is high?
11. A patient is to be given a tube feeding that has a high osmolality. The tube is in the duodenum. The nurse removes the feeding from the refrigerator and hangs it for feeding by gravity drip. It is run at 125 ml/hr at full concentration.

    The patient develops diarrhea and abdominal cramps. What changes would you make in the procedures to avoid this result?
12. Describe in general terms the different circumstances in which tube feeding and TPN would be used.

13. In TPN, what is the usual site of the catheter? Why?
14. What is the difference between a 2-in-1 and a 3-in-1 feeding? What are the relative merits of each?
15. Why is vitamin K omitted from a TPN formula for an adult?
16. How is vitamin K provided? Name some situations where the dose might be reduced or omitted.
17. Estimate the osmolarity of a liter of a mixture of 500 ml of 70% dextrose and 500 ml of 15% crystalline amino acids. How many nonprotein kilocalories are contained in this mixture?
18. When TPN is discontinued, what procedure should be followed? Why?
19. Describe the limitations of peripheral venous alimentation.
20. Why are the following values from the TPN-fed patient monitored?
    a. Blood glucose.
    b. BUN.
    c. Serum electrolytes.
    d. Serum albumin.
    e. Serum transaminases.
    f. Body weight.

References

1. Zeman, F.J., and Ney, D.M. Routine and transitional diets. In *Applications of Clinical Nutrition*. Englewood Cliffs, N.J.: Prentice-Hall, 1988.
2. American Dietetic Association. Position paper on the vegetarian approach to eating. *J. Am. Diet. Assoc.* 77:61, 1980.
3. King, J.C., Cohenour, S.H., Corrucini, C.G., and Schneeman, P. Evaluation and modification of the basic four food guide. *J. Nutr. Educ.* 10:27, 1978.
4. Pemberton, C.M., and Gastineau, C.G., Eds. *Mayo Clinic Diet Manual*. Philadelphia: W.B. Saunders, 1981.
5. Zeman, F.J., and Ney, D.M. Nutritional care of the vegetarian patient. In *Applications of Clinical Nutrition*. Englewood Cliffs, N.J.: Prentice-Hall, 1988.
6. *Diet Manual Utilizing a Vegetarian Diet Plan*. Loma Linda, Calif.: Seventh Day Adventist Dietetic Association, 1989.
7. Zeman, F.J., and Ney, D.M. Cultural factors in nutritional care. In *Applications of Clinical Nutrition*. Englewood Cliffs, N.J.: Prentice-Hall, 1988.
8. National Research Council, Food and Nutrition Board. *Recommended Dietary Allowances*, 10th ed. Washington, D.C.: National Academy of Sciences, 1989.
9. National Research Council, Publication No. 474. *The Role of Dietary Fat in Human Health*. Washington, D.C.: National Academy of Sciences, 1966.
10. Fischer, J.E. Nutritional management. In J.L. Berk, J.E. Sampliner, J.S. Artz, and B. Vinocur, Eds., *Handbook of Critical Care*. Boston: Little, Brown, 1976.
11. Holman, R.T., Castor, W.O., and Wiese, H.F. The essential fatty acid requirement of infants and the assessment of their dietary intake of linoleate by serum fatty acid analysis. *Am. J. Clin. Nutr.* 14:70, 1964.
12. Wiese, H.F., Hansen, A.E., and Adam, D.J.M. Essential fatty acids in infant nutrition. *J. Nutr.* 66:345, 1958.
13. Babayan, V.K. Medium chain triglycerides and structured lipids. *Lipids* 22:417, 1987.
14. Heird, W.C., Grundy, S.M., and Hubbard, V.S. Structured lipids and their use in clinical nutrition. *Am. J. Clin. Nutr.* 43:320, 1986.
15. Sleisenger, M.H., and Kim, Y.S. Protein digestion and absorption. *New Engl. J. Med.* 300:659, 1979.
16. Brinson, R.R., Hanumanthu, S.K., and Pitts, W.M. A reappraisal of the peptide-based enteral formulas: Clinical applications. *Nutr. Clin. Pract.* 4:211, 1989.
17. Souba, W.W. The gut as a nitrogen processing organ in the metabolic response to critical illness. *Nutr. Supp. Serv.* 8(5):15, 1988.
18. Shils, M.E. Enteral nutrition by tube. *Cancer Res.* 57:2432, 1977.
19. Rombeau, J.L., and Miller, R.A. *Nasoenteric Tube Feeding. Practical Aspects*. Mountain View, Calif.: Health Development Corp., 1979.
20. Alverdy, J.C., Aoyo, E., and Moss, G.S. Total parenteral nutrition promotes bacterial translocation from the gut. *Surgery* 104:185, 1988.
21. Fox, A.D., Kripke, S.A., DePaula, J.A., et al. The effect of a glutamine-supplemented enteral diet on methotrexate induced enterocolitis. *JPEN* 12:325, 1988.
22. O'Dwyer, S.T., Scott, T., Smith, R., et al. 5-Fluorouracil toxicity on small intestinal mucosa but not white blood cells is decreased by glutamine. *Clin. Res.* 367A, 1987.
23. Salloum, R.M., Souba, W.W., Klemberg, V.S., et al. Glutamine is superior to glutamate in supporting gut metabolism, stimulating intestinal glutaminase activity, and preventing

bacterial translocation. *Surg. Forum* 40:6, 1989.

24. Bergstrom, K., Blomstrand, R., and Jacobson, S. Long term complete intravenous nutrition in man. *Nutr. Metab.* 14(Suppl.):118, 1972.

25. Shenkin, A., and Wretlind, A. Parenteral nutrition. *World Rev. Nutr. Diet.* 28:1, 1978.

26. Deitel, M., Sauve, Sr. F., Alexander, M.A., et al. A crystalline amino acid solution for total parenteral nutrition. *Can. J. Hosp. Pharm.* 30:175, 1977.

27. Sheldon, G.F., and Kudsk, D.A. Electrolyte requirements in total parenteral nutrition. In M. Deitel, Ed., *Nutrition in Clinical Surgery.* Baltimore: Williams and Wilkins, 1980.

28. Cannon, P.R., Frazier, L.E., and Hughes, R.H. Influence of potassium on tissue protein synthesis. *Metabolism* 1:49, 1952.

29. Meng, H.C. Parenteral nutrition: principles, nutrient requirements, techniques and clinical applications. In H.S. Schneider, C.E. Anderson, and D.B. Coursin, Eds., *Nutritional Support of Medical Practice.* Hagerstown, Md.: Harper and Row, 1977.

30. Deitel, M., and Macdonald, L.D. Current concepts of intravenous hyperalimentation. In H.H. Draper, Ed., *Advances in Nutritional Research,* vol. 3. New York: Plenum Press, 1980.

31. Weinsier, R.L., and Butterworth, C.E., Jr. *Handbook of Clinical Nutrition.* St. Louis: C.V. Mosby, 1981.

32. Karpel, J.T., and Peden, V.H. Copper deficiency in long-term parenteral nutrition. *J. Pediatr.* 80:32, 1972.

33. McClain, C.J. Trace metal abnormalities in adults during hyperalimentation. *JPEN* 5:424, 1981.

34. Goss, J.C., Egging, P., and Dobyns, K. Nutritional support of the stressed surgical patient. *Nutr. Supp. Serv.* 4:28, 1984.

35. Weinsier, R.L., and Krumdieck, C.L. Death resulting from overzealous total parenteral nutrition. The refeeding syndrome revisited. *Am. J. Clin. Nutr.* 34:393, 1980.

36. Wolfe, R.R., O'Donnell, T.F., Stone, M.D., Richmond, D.A., and Burke, J.F. Investigation of factors determining the optimal glucose infusion rate in total parenteral nutrition. *Metabolism* 29:892, 1980.

37. Goodenough, R.O., and Wolfe, R.R. Effect of total parenteral nutrition on free fatty acid metabolism in burned patients. *JPEN* 8:357, 1984.

38. Parenteral nutrition therapy. In D.H. Alpers, R.E. Clouse, and W.F. Stenson, Eds., *Manual of Nutritional Therapeutics.* Boston: Little, Brown, 1983, pp. 233–267.

39. Department of Foods and Nutrition, American Medical Association. Guidelines for essential trace element preparations for parenteral use. *JPEN* 2:263, 1979.

40. Zeman, F.J., and Ney, D.M. *Application of Clinical Nutrition.* Englewood Cliffs, N.J.: Prentice-Hall, 1988.

41. Maini, B. Cyclic hyperalimentation. An optical technique for preservation of visceral proteins. *J. Surg. Res.* 20:515, 1976.

42. Hooley, R.A. Parenteral nutrition — general concepts, part 1. *Nutr. Supp. Serv.* 1:36, 1981.

Bibliography

Rombeau, J.L., and Caldwell, M.D., Eds. *Enteral and Tube Feeding.* Philadelphia: W.B. Saunders, 1984.

Rombeau, J.L., and Caldwell, M.D., Eds. *Parenteral Nutrition.* Philadelphia: W.B. Saunders, 1986.

Silberman, H. and Eisenberg, D. *Parenteral and Enteral Nutrition for the Hospitalized Patient.* Norwalk, Conn.: Appleton-Century-Crofts, 1982.

Truesdell, D.D., and Acosta, P.B. Feeding the vegan infant and child. *J. Am. Diet. Assoc.* 85:837, 1985.

Vyhmeister, I.B., Register, U.D., and Sonnenberg, L.B. Safe vegetarian diets for children. *Pediatr. Clin. N. Am.* 24:203, 1977.

Vyhmeister, I.B. Vegetarian diets — issues and concerns. *Nutrition and the M.D.* 10(5):1–3, 1984.

Zeman, F.J., and Ney, D.M. *Applications of Clinical Nutrition.* Englewood Cliffs, N.J.: Prentice-Hall, 1988.

II. Nutritional Care in Specific Clinical Disorders

6. Nutrition in Diseases of the Immune System

I. The Normal Immune
   System
   A. Components of the
      immune
      system
      1. Mobile cells
      2. Fixed organs and
         tissues
   B. The immune response
      1. Antigens
      2. The humoral
         response
      3. Cell-mediated
         response
      4. Regulation of the
         immune response
         a. effects of cyto-
            kines
         b. nutritional
            modulation

c. genetic regulation
d. local immunity
II. Disorders of the Immune
    System
    A. Immunoproliferative
       disease
    B. Immunologic deficiency
       1. Etiology
          a. viral disease
          b. stress-related
             deficiencies
          c. malnutrition
          d. age-related
             deficiencies
          e. iatrogenic
             deficiencies
       2. Tests for immuno-
          competency
    C. Hypersensitivity
       1. Types

a. immediate (type I)
b. cytotoxic antibody
   (type II)
c. immune complex
   disease (type III)
d. delayed (type IV)
2. Autoimmune
   diseases
3. Graft rejection
4. Food allergy
   a. allergens
   b. mode of contact
   c. clinical manifesta-
      tions
   d. prevention
   e. diagnosis
   f. treatment
      (1) avoidance
          diets
      (2) drug therapy

Malnutrition depresses many aspects of immune function. In addition, it has become evident that the immune responses that have beneficial effects by providing resistance to infection also are capable of causing serious disease. Since nutritional care is important in the treatment of some of these disease states, it is desirable for nutritional care specialists to have an understanding of the principles of immunology.

The objectives of this chapter are three-fold: (1) to provide the basis for an understanding of normal immune responses and, from that perspective, an understanding of mechanisms of immune diseases; (2) to promote understanding of the relationship of immune function, or malfunction, to diseases described in succeeding chapters; and (3) to provide the information fundamental to nutritional care for patients with abnormal immune responses to common foods.

THE NORMAL IMMUNE SYSTEM

The immune system protects the body against "foreign" materials called **immunogens** or **antigens**. These terms are not precisely equivalent in meaning, but they can be used interchangeably for our purposes in this chapter. The immune system, in protecting the body from foreign materials, recognizes materials that are part of "self" and protects us against those materials that are *not* self. The process by which the immune system learns to recognize self is not understood precisely, but recognition apparently develops during gestation and the newborn period.

Resistance to disease can be considered to be either of two types. **Natural, constitutive,** or **nonspecific immunity** consists of mechanisms responsible for nonspecific inflammatory responses to tissue damage, described in Chapter 1. It involves the skin, mucosa, and nonspecific scavenger cells, and does not require recognition of a specific antigen. **Adaptive** or **acquired immunity** is based on the properties of lymphocytes to respond to, or adapt to, specific antigens to produce a permanently altered response to that antigen. When cells are exposed to an antigen a second time, the "memory" cells "remember" that antigen. Their **secondary** or **anamnestic response** is then greater than the primary response. It also occurs more rapidly.

Figure 6-1. Major organs and tissues of the immune system. Only a few of many lymph nodes are shown. Mobile cells are distributed throughout the circulatory system, lymph system, and other tissue.

Components of the Immune System

The immune system comprises a widely scattered group of organs, tissues, and cells. The central system includes the bone marrow, thymus, and tissues that are equivalent to the bursa in birds. The peripheral system comprises the spleen, lymph nodes, and diffuse tissue known as gut-associated lymphoid tissue (GALT) and bronchiole-associated lymphoid tissue (BALT) (see Figure 6-1). These discrete organs are fixed in place and have mostly immunologic functions. Other cells are found as components of organs that have other functions, such as microglial cells in the brain, Kupffer cells in the liver, mesangial cells in the kidney, and synovial cells in the joints. Other components consist of mobile cells and soluble components that the mobile or fixed cells synthesize. They have their origin in various of the fixed tissues and

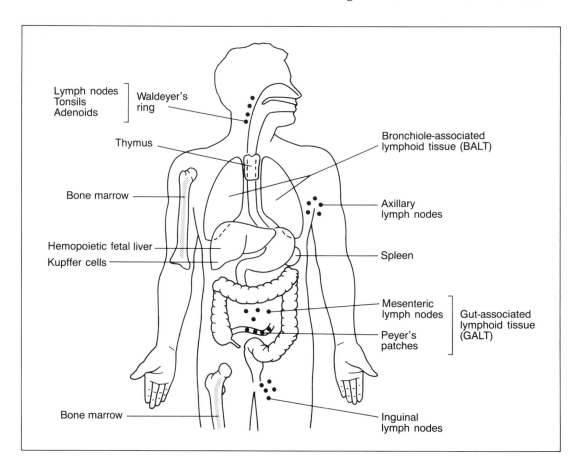

are carried in the blood to the site of their function.

Mobile Cells

The **leukocytes** (white blood cells) are derived from **hemopoietic stem cells**, which are also the source of red blood cells and platelets (see Figure 6-2). Stem cells reside in the bone marrow in adults but are more widely distributed in infants. The mature forms of leukocytes are normal components of the blood; they are present in numbers of 4,000–10,000 cells/μl. They are classified into five groups. Three types of cells, known collectively as **granulocytes** because they contain visible granules when seen under the microscope, are **neutrophils** or polymorphonuclear leukocytes or PMNs (40–75%), **eosinophils** (1–6%), and **basophils** (<1%). The other two groups of leukocytes, categorized together as **mononuclear cells**, are known individually as **lymphocytes** (20–45%) and **monocytes** (2–10%). Cells in all five groups can migrate from blood and lymph into the tissues.

The lymphocytes, which are the principal mediators of the adaptive immune response, are distributed throughout body tissues and fluids. There are several subtypes of lymphocytes. They cannot be distinguished by their appearance under a microscope, but they react and function differently. One type, the **B lymphocyte**, matures to form a **memory cell** as previously described or a **plasma cell**. Plasma cells produce antibodies that interact with antigens. This is called the humoral response because antibodies are carried in the body fluids. The site of transformation of the stem cell to the B cell in humans is not known. In birds, it occurs in the **bursa of Fabricius**—hence, **bursa-dependent** or **B cell**. It has frequently been suggested that, in humans, the equivalents to the bursa are located in the appendix and Peyer's patches of the intestine, or in the liver, spleen, or bone marrow.

The second type of lymphocyte, the **T lymphocyte**, reacts directly with a foreign substance or antigen to produce the **cell-mediated response**. In the formation of T lymphocytes, hemopoietic stem cells from the bone marrow migrate to and mature in the thymus gland and then migrate to other tissues. The cell thus is called a **thymus-dependent** or **T cell**.

T cells have a number of subcategories.[1] Within each subcategory, some cells are **memory cells**, and some are functional or **effector cells**. **Helper/inducer cells** (T_H) abet the transformation of B cells to plasma cells and activate T cytotoxic cells. They are also known as T_4 **cells**. **Suppressor cells** (T_S) inhibit these transformations. **Cytotoxic lymphocytes** (T_C or T_8) are T cells that are capable of causing lysis of cells such as grafted tissue. Of the circulating lymphocytes, 70 to 80% are T cells, and the remainder are B cells.

Null cells are those which do not have characteristics of either T or B lymphocytes. Some null cells destroy certain tumor cells, virus-infected cells, or tissue cells coated with antibody. They are known as **natural killer** (NK) **cells** and are not of thymic origin.

Monocytes and macrophages, highly phagocytic cells derived from monocytes, "process" antigens so they can be recognized by T and B lymphocytes. They also secrete a group of substances collectively known as **cytokines** that regulate the immune response. Monocytes also elaborate a number of other biologically active agents and enzymes. They secrete at least one class of prostaglandins (see Chapter 10), clot-promoting factors, growth factors, angiotensin converting factor and other peptidases. Monocytes are very active phagocytes and contain peroxidase and lysosomal enzymes.

Neutrophils, which are the predominant phagocytic cells found early in localized infections, are part of nonspecific immunity. They engulf bacteria and cellular debris and digest them by means of lysosomal enzymes. The other two granulocytes, the eosinophils and basophils, play a role in a particular type of immune response classified as hypersen-

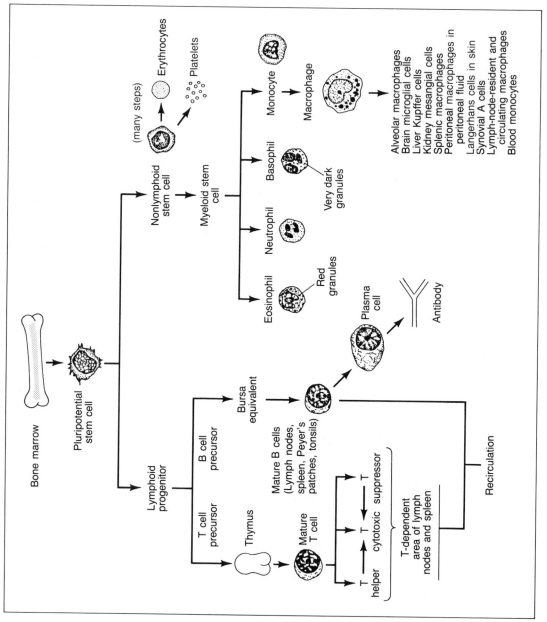

Figure 6-2. Developmental pathways of cell types from the bone marrow stem cell.

sitivities, discussed later in this chapter.[2] Eosinophils detoxify foreign proteins and may participate in dissolving blood clots and antigen-antibody complexes after immune function is complete. They also clean up debris.

Fixed Organs and Tissues

The fixed tissues of the immune system are shown in Figure 6-2. Many of these organs consist of a web of extremely fine (**reticular**) fibers, the meshwork of which supports the **reticuloendothelial cells**. These are fixed phagocytic cells, part of the nonspecific immune system. They form a portion of the walls of the channels of the thymus, spleen, lymph nodes, and liver when mobile monocytes move into these organs and form the macrophages of the **mononuclear/phagocyte system**. Circulating cells such as lymphocytes may enter and be retained by fixed tissues, scattered between the sinusoidal spaces.

The **thymus** is considered to be the "master gland" of the immune system. It is essential for differentiation of the T cells and also produces humoral factors essential for normal immune function. Although the thymus has the highest cell-production rate in the body and produces many lymphocytes, it does not participate directly in immune reactions. Many lymphocytes migrate from the thymus to lymph nodes.

The **lymph nodes** are situated at intervals along the course of the large lymph vessels, mainly at the junctions of major vessels (see Figure 6-1). They contain areas of T cell concentration, and other areas where B cells are concentrated. Lymph nodes also consist of a network of interlacing fibers that act as a filter for the lymph.

The **spleen** contains follicles with B cells as well as areas of T cell concentration. Its reticular network also acts as a filter for the blood. Thus the functional structure of the spleen is similar to that of the lymph node. Both organs create an opportunity for interaction between antigen and lymphocyte by filtering antigens from their respective fluids.

The Immune Response

As previously noted, adaptive immune responses are conventionally divided into two categories known as **cell-mediated** and **humoral** (or **antibody-mediated**) responses. These can be described separately, but it is important to keep in mind that they frequently interact and function simultaneously. In addition, the immune response may consist of a localized nonspecific **inflammatory response**, described in Chapter 1, and a systemic response, often called the **acute phase response**. The symptoms in common of these effects are superimposed on the disease-specified symptoms characteristic of each disorder.

Antigens

An **antigen** or **immunogen** is a substance perceived as foreign to the body that stimulates the immune system to respond specifically to the antigen and not to unrelated substances. The most potent antigens are proteins, but polysaccharides and synthetic polymers also can act as antigens. Lipids, with the exception of phospholipids, are poor immunogens.

The immune response is elicited by a specific chemical configuration of the molecule or one very similar to it called the **antigenic determinant**. The ability of the immune system to react with similar, but not identical, structures of antigens accounts for cross-reactivity.

In general, larger and more complex molecules tend to be more antigenic. Proteins with molecular weights of less than 10,000 and carbohydrates with molecular weights of less than 100,000 are only weakly antigenic. A polymer with a single repeating unit is much less antigenic than is a more complex one with many different units. The presence of aromatic amino acids in the proteins increases antigenicity much more than do aliphatic amino acids. The immune response may vary also with the dose and the route of administration, but this is not always the case.

It is not clear why some antigens elicit a humoral response and others a cell-mediated response. As a general rule, cellular and particulate antigens stimulate a cell-mediated response. Humoral immunity is particularly associated with soluble antigens,[3] but also is associated with cellular antigens.

A wide variety of materials can be recognized as antigenic. These may include infectious organisms, venoms, and tumor cells. Some foods; some pollens, dusts, danders, and molds that a person inhales; plant, animal, or other materials that come in contact with the skin; cells from other humans as in blood transfusions; skin grafts; and organ transplants may be antigenic in the appropriate circumstances. It is even possible for a person's own tissue to be immunologically recognized as foreign. The antisera, hormones, enzymes, diagnostic agents, antibiotics, vitamins, and a variety of drugs used to treat disease may act as antigens. Some antigens are recognized as foreign by everyone. Others are foreign only in certain circumstances categorized as hypersensitivity.

Haptens are not antigenic alone but become antigenic when they complex with another substance. Drug allergies often occur by this means when a drug of low molecular weight complexes with a plasma protein to form a molecule with a sufficiently large molecular weight and foreign structure so that the complex is antigenic.

The Humoral Response

The membranes of B cells contain receptors for specific antigen binding. A simple model, sufficient for our purposes here, states that recognition of a specific antigen by a B cell consists of binding of the antigen to the membrane receptor. The sequence of events thereafter is not entirely clear. It is known that a B cell is stimulated to divide repeatedly, resulting in a population of cells known as **clones**. The cells produced by cloning mature to form **plasma cells**, which then synthesize and release the **antibodies** or **immunoglobulins**. These B cell responses are stimulated by T cell secretions, macrophages, and contact with T helper cells. A deficiency of B lymphocytes is associated with an increased incidence of some bacterial infections and most viral infections.

The antibody synthesized by each plasma cell is specific for the antigen that was initially recognized and bound by the parent B cell. The antibody produced by the plasma cell then binds specifically to the antigen for which it was designed, thus inactivating and neutralizing it. When a virus is bound to an antibody, for example, its virulence and ability to cause disease are decreased. Antibodies also bind to antigenic determinants on foreign cells such as bacteria, tumor cells, or grafts and induce lysis of the cells. Some examples of the types of action of antibodies include **precipitation, agglutination**, and **opsonization**; the last of these is a process by which the cell is made more vulnerable to phagocytosis. In addition, antibodies, by attachment to the antigenic cell surface, may damage it by altering its mobility, metabolism, or physical behavior in fluids. In some cases, the antibody functions via activation, by the antigen/antibody complex, of **complement**, a series of enzymatic proteins found in normal serum. The nine components in this series are symbolized as C_1 through C_9. The component C_1 is a calcium-dependent complex of three proteins designated as C_{1q}, C_{1r}, and C_{1s}, so that there are actually 11 components of complement. They react with each other in a sequence, often called the **complement cascade**, so that one activates the next. The components C_3 and C_5 participate in producing the inflammatory response, while C_1 and C_4 are involved in neutralization of viruses. Some of the effects of various combinations of these components include cell lysis, altered vascular permeability to allow lymphocytes to move to the site of the antigen, increased phagocytosis, opsonization, degranulation of mast cells, and anaphylaxis. Various cells produce complement, including macrophages and the cells of the intestinal mucosa.

Antibody-coated foreign cells are attacked by neutrophils or monocytes. The antigen-antibody (Ag/Ab) complex is phagocytized by neutrophils, macrophages, and monocytes.

Each antibody molecule is made up of a basic unit of two long (**heavy** or **H**) chains and two short (**light** or **L**) chains. These are bound to each other by disulfide bonds in a symmetric structure, as shown in Figure 6-3. There are five classes of immunoglobulins —G, M, A, D, and E, abbreviated as IgG, IgM, IgA, IgD, and IgE, respectively. These are defined by one of the five types of heavy chains. There are only two types of light chains, called kappa and lambda. In each antibody molecule, the two heavy chains are

alike and the two light chains are alike, that is, both light chains are kappa or lambda, but not one of each. Each of these units is made up of an **Fc portion** (fragment, crystallizable), consisting of portions of the two H chains, and an **Fab portion** (fragment, antigen-binding), made up of the two L chains and the remainder of the H chains (see Figure 6-3). The Fc portion binds to the macrophages, lymphocytes, or neutrophils. It also activates complement and releases soluble substances from mast cells.[3]

The Fab portion has a section (shown by the shaded section in Figure 6-3) in which the amino acid sequence is variable. These are the antigen-binding sites, and are the source of the specificity of the antibody for its antigen. This region is identical in all cells of a single clone. Each basic antibody unit can bind with two antigenic sites and therefore has a valence of 2.

Immunoglobulin G (IgG) consists of a single unit, as previously described, with a valence of 2. It comprises approximately 75% of all immunoglobulin. IgG is involved in opsonization and complement fixation. It

Figure 6-3. Typical immunoglobulin G molecule. Constant regions are clear, and variable regions are shaded. Heavy chains are flexible in hinge area. Disulfide bridges bind chains together and also exist within chains.

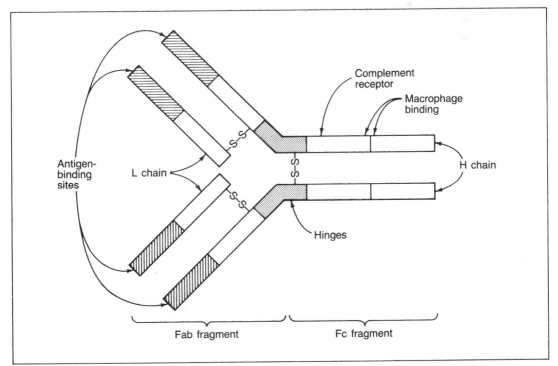

is found in large quantities in the circulatory system and peripheral lymphoid tissue and is the only immunoglobulin capable of crossing the placenta.

Immunoglobulin A (IgA) has two sub-classes, **serum IgA** and **secretory IgA**. Secretory IgA (sIgA) is synthesized by plasma cells in secretory glands of mucous membranes of the alimentary, respiratory, and genitourinary tracts, and the salivary, lacrimal, and mammary glands.[4-7] It occurs mostly in secretions of the mucous membranes and serves as a barrier against environmental pathogens.

The function of IgA in the serum is unknown. It is found in small but significant amounts in the blood and occurs as a **monomer** — that is, with one of the basic units described previously. However, secretory IgA is a **dimer**. Its two basic units are linked by a structure known as a **J** (joining) **chain**, originating in the plasma cell. These then are attached to a glycoprotein known as **secretory piece**, which is synthesized by the epithelial cells.[8-11] Its function may be to facilitate transport of sIgA through the mucosa[3] or to render the IgA resistant to proteolytic enzymes.[12]

Immunoglobulin M (IgM) also occurs as a polymer, usually as a pentamer, with a valence of 10. The units are linked by a J chain, and the molecule also contains secretory piece. Approximately 10% of the immunoglobulins are IgM. Its actions include destruction of antigens on initial exposure, formation of blood group antibodies, and activation of complement. It is very effective in opsonization and effective at neutralizing gram-negative bacteria. It also is antiviral. Immunoglobulin M is found in all body fluids.

Immunoglobulin D (IgD) is found in small amounts in serum and also is associated with IgM on most B cells. Its function is unknown, but it may act as an antigen receptor on the cell surface, and it may be involved in B cell differentiation and memory cells.

Immunoglobulin E (IgE) is found in low concentration in normal serum but in high concentration in the serum of patients with allergies. Immunoglobulin E can attach to cells of the skin, mast cells, basophils, or neutrophils. When IgE attaches, these cells become sensitized to the antigen. The binding of some sensitized cells (usually basophils and mast cells) to the antigen causes the release of pharmacologically active amines known as **mediators**.

There are several mediators known to participate in the humoral response. Of these, **histamine** is probably best known. It occurs in mast cells, basophils, platelets, and perhaps in other cells. It is released when an antigen-IgE antibody complex binds to a histamine-containing cell. It causes vasodilation and increased capillary permeability leading to erythema (redness) and edema in the mucous membranes of the skin.

Cell-Mediated Response

The **cell-mediated immune response** involves primarily the T lymphocytes and operates against bacteria, virus-infected cells, some fungi, tumor cells, and foreign tissue such as transplants. T lymphocytes are responsible for the delayed allergic reactions described later in this chapter.

When T lymphocytes are activated by an antigen, usually on the surface of a macrophage, they are transformed to large **immunoblasts (lymphoblasts)**. These cells divide by mitosis. The daughter cells already are activated and have the same immunologic specificity as the parent cell. As in the case of B cells, the secondary response is stronger and faster than the primary response. The sensitized T cells kill viable antigenic cells by direct attachment. The antigenic cells are lysed and then phagocytized by activated macrophages.

Regulation of the Immune Response

Effects of Cytokines. It usually takes the cooperation of several cells to initiate an immune response. The cells involved either communicate directly with each other or via soluble mediators known as **cytokines**.

There are two subclasses of cytokines. **Monokines** are released from monocytes and macrophages, and lymphocytes produce **lymphokines**. Cytokines have both local effects and hormonelike systemic regulatory effects, that is, the **acute phase response**. A large number of cytokines have been identified, of which three have been studied sufficiently to be considered as regulators of the acute phase response.

Interleukin 1 (IL-1) is a group of proteins released when macrophages are stimulated by phagocytosis or immune complexes. It promotes proliferation and maturation of T cells and induces fever. Under the influence of IL-1, T helper cells are stimulated to secrete **interleukin-2** (IL-2), a lymphokine which activates the proliferation of cytotoxic T cells. It may be the material that promotes proliferation and differentiation of B cells to plasma cells.

Two subcategories are **IL-1α**, which is largely membrane-bound within the original cell, and **IL-1β**, which is released. The cytokine IL-1β is thought to function in systemic regulation. Various activities of IL-1 were indicated by previously used names: lymphocyte activating factor, leukocyte endogenous mediator, endogenous pyrogen, and catabolin.

Tumor necrosis factor (TNF) is also produced by monocytes/macrophages. There is more than one substance in this category also. **TNFα** functions in direct killing of tumor cells. In contrast, **TNFβ**, sometimes called lymphotoxin, has a related structure, but it is a product of activated lymphocytes. These products may have similar effects on metabolic activities of cells outside the immune system. In addition, TNFα is somewhat similar in structure to "cachectin," thought to be a monokine that mediates cachexia.

Interleukin 6 (IL-6, interferon B$_2$, B-cell growth factor, or hepatocyte stimulating factor) is synthesized by stimulated T cells. It also seems to have a role in the acute phase response.

Null cells produce and are activated by **interferon**. Interferons are hormonelike substances with antiviral and antitumor activity. There are a large number of forms which inhibit multiplication of viruses, inhibit cell division, stimulate phagocytosis, and increase cytotoxicity of lymphocytes.

In addition to these substances, there are a number of other materials being studied. More information will be forthcoming on the identity of these materials and their physical characteristics.

A number of metabolic changes are direct effects of the binding of cytokines to target cells. These effects may be mediated by prostaglandins or protein kinases. Alternatively, secondary responses may be induced when a cytokine stimulates the release of a hormone, sometimes by means of an effect on the hypothalamic releasing hormones, or through the release of another cytokine. Information is currently fragmentary, but some generalizations can be drawn from the known biological activities summarized in Table 6-1.

The loss of appetite with reduction of food intake is often included in the immune response. When reduced intake is coupled with the increased resting energy expenditure and increased metabolism accompanying fever, a basis for the severe wasting of the acute phase response is evident.

Other contributors to the fever of the acute phase response include:

- Gluconeogenesis and glycogenolysis to increase glucose production.
- Increased (by 68%) glucose oxidation.
- Increased metabolism to lactate and Cori cycling.
- Decreased fatty acid metabolism.[13-15]

The hypoglycemia produced by these effects is thought not to be the result of cytokinase-induced insulin levels.[16] Interleukin 1 has been shown to increase alanine transport into liver cells and gluconeogenesis for alanine.[17]

The acute phase response is associated with high lipid levels in the blood, mediated by increased liver fatty acid and triglyceride synthesis and reduced clearance by lipoprotein lipase at the adipose tissue. Lipolysis in

Table 6-1. Cytokine Effects on Metabolism[a]

Metabolic Effect	Cytokine[b]				
	IL-1	TNFα	IFγ	TNFβ	IL-6
General effects					
Decreased voluntary intake	X	X			
Increased resting energy expenditure	X	X			
Increased body temperature	X	X	X		
Protein metabolism					
Increased synthesis of acute phase proteins	X	X			X
Increased muscle protein degradation	X				
Glucose metabolism					
Increased oxidation	X	X			
Increased gluconeogenesis	X				
Lipid metabolism					
Decreased lipoprotein lipase activity	X	X	X		
Decreased fatty acid synthesis in adipocytes	X		X	X	
Decreased lipolysis in adipocytes	X	X			
Increased hepatic triglyceride synthesis		X			
Increased hepatic cholesterol synthesis		X			
Mineral metabolism					
Increased hepatic metallothionein synthesis	X				
Increased hepatic ceruloplasmin synthesis	X	X			
Hormone release					
Corticosteroid—increased	X				
Thyroxin—decreased	X				
Glucagon—increased	X	X			
Insulin—increased	X				
Growth hormone—increased	X				

[a] Some effects were shown in vivo only and do not demonstrate effects on target cells.
[b] IL-1 = interleukin 1; TNFα = tumor necrosis factor α; IFγ = interferon γ; TNFβ = tumor necrosis factor β; IL-6 = interleukin 6.

adipose tissue is increased. This is also assumed to contribute to the wasted appearance of many patients.

The effects of protein metabolism lead to the muscle wasting frequently observed.[18-20] There is increased muscle and collagen breakdown and excretion of nitrogen. Amino acids are lost from skeletal muscle and used for energy, gluconeogenesis, synthesis of new leukocytes, immunoglobulins, regulatory proteins, and **acute phase** (AP) **proteins** by the liver. The AP proteins serve a protective role during the acute phase response. They increase the immune response and limit tissue destruction by substances such as proteolytic enzymes released by leukocytes.

Increased serum copper and decreased serum iron and zinc levels are also associated with the acute phase response.[21] The effects of cytokines on carrier proteins involved

with these minerals are a current area of study. Cytokines are also involved in drug detoxification, activation of carcinogens, and local effects on blood flow.

The AP proteins include C-reactive protein (CRP), fibrinogen, orosomucoid, alpha 1 antitrypsin, ceruloplasmin, and some proteins of the complement cascade. This list is not complete, and their effects are not completely understood. Some known or proposed functions of those mentioned are given in Table 6-2. It should also be noted that serum levels of albumin, transferrin, and prealbumin are reduced at the same time.[22,23]

Nutritional Modulation. The possibility of modulating the immune response by alterations in nutrient intake is a recent development. One possible procedure involves the manipulation of polyunsaturated fatty acids

Table 6-2. Functions of Selected Acute Phase Proteins

Protein	Function
C-reactive protein	Activate complement
	Stimulate leucocytic phagocytosis
Fibrinogen	Blood coagulation
	Control of hemorrhage
	Provides a matrix for wound healing
	Promotes leukocyte and macrophage migration
Haptoglobin (Hp)	Binds free hemoglobin (Hb) to prevent renal toxicity
	Peroxidase activity of the HpHb complex
Ceruloplasmin	Maintain serotonin, epinephrine, and ascorbic acid levels in circulation (?)
	Free radical scavenger
	Copper carrier to cytochrome oxidase in electron transport system
	Oxidase ferrous iron to ferric

(PUFA) intake. The mechanisms of PUFA action are not entirely understood, but may include:

1. Interference with function of some enzymes.
2. Changes in lipids in cell membranes with increased PUFA intake leading to alterations in immune cell function.
3. Alterations in active compounds formed from PUFA — prostaglandins, thromboxanes, prostacyclin, and leukotrienes. These compounds are described further in Chapter 10.

The specific consequences of these actions on selected immune reactions are now thought to vary with the amount and kind of the active compounds produced from ingested lipids. As a result, there may be a possibility of immune system modulation by dietary manipulation.

Another possible means of immunomodulation involves provision of increased amounts of arginine to the immunocompromised patient. There is some evidence that additional arginine increases thymus gland weight and T cell response to mitogens.

Addition of nucleotides to the nutrient intake has also been suggested to improve the immune response. T cells may lack the ability to synthesize nucleotides and may thus depend on dietary or salvage pathways for nucleotide sources. Therefore, the addition of nucleotides to enteral and parenteral

feedings that are nucleotide-free has been suggested. One such product containing increased levels of omega-3 fatty acids as a source of PUFA, arginine, and nucleotides is now available. (See Appendix G, Table 3.)

Further research may elucidate in detail the effects of such products and also determine whether other modifications in nutrient intake are appropriate in specific disease states.

Genetic Regulation. The cells of each person's body have protein molecules called **histocompatibility antigens** on their cell membranes, which provide the identity of self. These are called **human leukocyte antigens** (HLA) because they were first discovered on the surface of human leukocytes, but it now is known that they are present on almost all body cells. The specific nature of these antigens in each individual is determined by a cluster of genes on the sixth chromosome pair in an area called the **major histocompatibility complex**. Four loci within this complex have been identified and have been labeled HLA-A, HLA-B, HLA-C, and HLA-D. It is thought that there are others, but they have not been well described.

Each locus in an individual has two alleles. A person inherits one of each pair of alleles in each locus from each parent. A large number of alleles for each gene exist. At present, there are seven known alleles for HLA-C and more than thirty for HLA-B, each identified by a letter and a number, such as HLA-B26. The number of known HLA-A and HLA-D alleles lies between these two extremes. The number of possible combinations in the general population is at least several thousand, but the number in the offspring of a single pair of parents is much smaller.

Near the HLA-D locus, there are **immune response** (Ir) genes believed to have some control over the immune response and the degree of responsiveness in T cells. Other genes appear to control antibody production and macrophage function.

Some HLA antigens have been associated with specific diseases. For example, juvenile diabetes mellitus is associated with persons with HLA-B8. When persons suffering from a given disease have the same antigen, that antigen is a **marker**. It indicates that those carrying that antigen have an increased susceptibility to the disease in question, but they may not actually have the disease unless the necessary environmental conditions also exist. The mechanism of the association of HLA antigens with the occurrence of certain diseases is unknown.

Local Immunity. Nonspecific local defenses exist at surface areas that are exposed to antigens. These barriers to environmental antigens include the skin, respiratory tract, genitourinary tract, eyes, and ears. Some of the mechanisms involved include trapping in mucus; clearance by the cilia; action of digestive enzymes, acids, and alkalis; and a washout action by intestinal motility. Mucous secretions in body openings contain lysozyme and other enzymes that destroy invading bacteria. Specific local defenses include IgA antibody and the large population of lymphocytes in the respiratory and gastrointestinal tracts.

DISORDERS OF THE IMMUNE SYSTEM

Although the purpose of the immune system is protection of the body's cells from foreign materials (**immunity**), it sometimes mal-

functions and may actually cause disease. These diseases are the subject of **clinical immunology**. Diseases of the immune system can conveniently be divided into three categories: (1) excess proliferation of immune cells or their products, (2) deficiency of function, and (3) inappropriate immune response (hypersensitivity). Within each category, there are some conditions in which nutritional care is important. Each category will be briefly described in turn, and those conditions in which nutritional care is of special importance will be described in more detail.

Immunoproliferative Disease

Immunoproliferative disease (excess production of one or more components of the immune system) can affect either the humoral or cellular system. There is a wide spectrum of these diseases. Excesses of B cells are referred to as **gammopathies**. Gammopathies may be produced by one clone only (**monoclonal**) or by more than one (**polyclonal**). There may be high concentrations of the whole antibody or of only the H chain or the L chain. Gammopathies of the latter types are referred to as **heavy chain disease** or **light chain disease**. Monoclonal gammopathy may be benign or malignant, the most common malignant form being multiple myeloma.

One group of immunoproliferative diseases is categorized as **plasma cell dyscrasias**, in which abnormally large quantities of antibodies, especially IgG, are produced. Suppressor T cell excesses contribute to infections. Excesses of phagocytic cells can result in hypersensitivities or autoimmune disorders, discussed later in this chapter. Other categories of immunoproliferative disease are the **leukemias** (abnormal proliferation and accumulation of leukocytes) and the **lymphomas** (solid tumors of stem cells).

Nutritional care is directed primarily toward alleviation of the symptoms produced as a result of the effect of the immune system disease on other organ systems or as a result of the side effects of treatment. The consequences of some of these conditions include renal disease and require some of the nutritional manipulations indicated in other renal diseases (see Chapter 9). Other conditions cause diarrhea, the nutritional implications of which are described in Chapter 8. Leukemia and the nutritional care of leukemia patients are described, along with other forms of cancer, in Chapter 15, where the nutritional implications of some cancer treatments also are discussed.

Immunologic Deficiency

Another group of immune diseases consists of those in which the **immune function is deficient**.

Etiology

Congenital absence or deficiency of humoral or cellular immunity, or both, is seen occasionally in newborns as the results of failure of proper development, but these conditions are rare. More commonly, immune deficiency is secondary to other conditions. One of the most common causes of immune deficiency in developed countries is the result of the use of chemotherapeutic agents in the treatment of cancer. Another is immunosuppression used during organ transplant.

Viral Disease. A recently recognized cause of immunologic deficiency is the viral disease **acquired immune deficiency syndrome** (AIDS), currently an epidemic of major proportions. Although there is some disagreement on this point, it is thought to be caused by a retrovirus known as human immunodeficiency virus (HIV) or human T-lymphotropic virus III (HTLV-III).[24-28]

Retroviruses have RNA as their genetic material. When the virus enters a host cell, this viral RNA is then used as a template to synthesize a viral DNA. A viral enzyme, **reverse transcriptase**, participates in this process.[27] The DNA inserts itself into the host cell DNA and sets the stage for replication of more virus. This process may kill the host cell.

In AIDS, the host cells are mostly helper/inducer T lymphocytes or T_4 cells. The resulting loss of T_4 cells causes, in turn, a major decline in immune function.[15] Patients are then vulnerable to virus-caused cancers and "opportunistic" infections, that is, infections by organisms that are generally present in the environment but that do not usually cause illness. In AIDS patients, there has been a sharp increase in the incidence of Kaposi's sarcoma, carcinomas, and B cell lymphomas. Among infections, pneumocystis pneumonia, caused by *Pneumocystis carinii*, a widespread but usually harmless protozoan, has been prominent. Other common opportunistic infections include herpes simplex, candida, toxoplasmosis, and cryptosporidium.

The virus also affects cells other than the T_4 lymphocyte. It has been found in endothelial cells of the blood and lymphatic vessel walls, the skin and mucous membranes, the glial and nerve cells of the nervous system, and cells of the lining of the intestinal tract.

It has been demonstrated clearly that **malnutrition** depresses immune function. Therefore, it is important that AIDS patients be adequately nourished. In addition, patients often suffer from anorexia and gastrointestinal disorders such as nausea, vomiting, stomatitis, mucositis, malabsorption, and diarrhea as a consequence of the primary disease or secondary to therapy.[28] Nutritional care for these conditions is discussed in later chapters.

Stress-Related Deficiencies. It is also common to find immunologic deficiencies secondary to physical or emotional stress. This condition is called **anergy** (see Chapter 3). The means by which emotional disturbance affects immunity are not clear, but the effect may be mediated via the hypothalamus and, thence, to the pituitary and adrenal glands and by other areas of the brain, mediated by neuropeptides such as the endorphine. Glucocorticoids, produced by the adrenals, are lympholytic and thus might reduce the number of functioning lymphocytes. Increased incidence of infections, increased incidence of cancer, and delayed recovery, all of which are possible consequences of immunodeficiency, have been seen in emotionally disturbed patients.

Physical stresses, including surgery and anesthesia, major burns, neoplasms, and virus infections, also depress immune function. These stresses may function by stimulating the adrenals to produce glucocorticoids. Diabetes mellitus and chronic renal failure also have depressive effects.

Malnutrition. Studies of malnutrition and immune function have shown numerous interrelationships.[29-31] For many years, malnutrition has been associated with increased susceptibility to infection in underdeveloped countries. It is now recognized that the mechanisms involved are not fundamentally different from those seen in malnourished hospitalized patients in developed countries.[32,33]

Immune function has been shown to be adversely affected by every nutritional deficiency that has been investigated. Malnutrition decreases the thickness of the skin and connective tissue and reduces their ability to act as barriers to infection.[34] Protein-energy malnutrition appears to affect cell-mediated and humoral immunity in different ways. The number of T cells, levels of thymic hormones, and production of some mediators are decreased.[35-37] In contrast, the numbers of B cells and plasma cells remain normal and sometimes are increased, but the effects on subclasses of B cells are unknown.[32,38,39] Serum IgE and IgA levels are high, possibly reflecting an increase in the incidence of parasites or a decrease in T cell control.[32,40] Secretory IgA and complement usually are decreased.[39,41-43] Phagocytic cell function has been shown to be significantly abnormal in protein-energy malnutrition.[32,44,45] Other indications of effects of protein malnutrition on immune function include thymus atrophy,[46-48] inability to respond to some antigens with antibody production, and decreased production of some mediators.[49] On the other hand, experiments with animals have shown that moderate energy restriction may be beneficial, provided the intake of nutrients is adequate.[50,51]

Polyunsaturated fatty acids (PUFA) have been shown to depress T cell function. Therefore, it has been suggested that these fatty acids be used in increased quantities in the diet as an adjuvant to immunosuppressive drugs given to transplant patients.[52-54] In contrast, esterified fatty acids increase the **mitogenic** (promoting mitosis) response of the T cells. Therefore, it has been suggested that lipids be included in parenteral feeding to improve the immune response in malnourished patients.[55]

Vitamin A, pyridoxine, zinc, and iron deficiencies also impair cell-mediated immunity.[37,56] Vitamin A deficiency has been associated with reduced antibody formation in animals.[57] Relationships to deficiencies of vitamin B_{12}, folate, pantothenate, thiamine, riboflavin, and ascorbic acid have also been noted, but much more information is needed.[56]

In malnourished hospitalized patients, the malnutrition often is secondary to other conditions. For example, immunoglobulin deficiency may result from excess protein loss from a diseased intestine or kidneys. Nutritional care is important in maintaining adequate nutritional status and preventing anergy in this type of patient, particularly the patient whose disease depresses immune function in addition to causing malnutrition.

Age-Related Deficiencies. The number of T cells declines with age. Although this decrease is apparently inevitable and normal, it may be considered a deficiency because it is associated with an increase in the occurrence of some diseases.

Iatrogenic Deficiencies. Sometimes, the immune deficiency is **iatrogenic**—that is, the result of therapy. In organ transplants, for example, the immune response is deliberately suppressed in order to prevent rejection of the graft. The immune response is often depressed also in the treatment of cancer, either deliberately or as a side effect of treatment.

Obesity, which can also be considered a form of malnutrition, may also affect the immune response. It has been related to changes in T cell function, atrophy of lymphoid tissue, decreased cytotoxicity of granulocytes and decreased lymphocyte proliferation.

It is clear that malnutrition can occur as a significant side effect of other diseases and markedly affects immune function. For those patients, and also for patients who have primary immunodeficiency disease, for the elderly, and for those with iatrogenic immune deficits, it is important to provide an adequate diet to support maximum immune function. In the chapters that follow, nutritional needs in these conditions and procedures for meeting these needs are discussed.

Tests for Immunocompetency

The complexity of the immune system prevents the development of a single test to measure the adequacy of the immune response. The available tests vary from those that are very simple to those that are extremely sophisticated. The most sophisticated tests used in the diagnosis of various immune disorders are not within the scope of this text. They are described in other texts and monographs for those who are interested in further information.[58-60]

Some simple tests of immunocompetency are of interest to nutritional care specialists because they are used in some institutions as an indicator of nutritional status and to identify patients in particular need of nutritional support. Two procedures that are in common use are described in Chapter 3, in the nutritional assessment procedures. Enumeration of **lymphocytes in the peripheral circulation**, a measurement that is affected by many variables, is easily obtained because it is done routinely on almost all patients. **Delayed cutaneous hypersensitivity** (DCH) **skin tests** often are used to indicate the presence of protein-energy malnutrition in hospital patients. The antigens commonly used are purified protein derivative of tuberculin (PPD), histoplasmin, *Candida,* and mumps. The use of these antigens is based on the assumption that DCH is a good indicator of nutritional status. There is evidence that the severity of defective T cell function correlates to some degree with the severity of malnutrition,[35,61,62] but serious questions exist concerning the validity and reliability of these procedures.[63]

Another test of immune function somewhat less frequently used is the determination of T cell blast formation. The uptake by lymphocytes of tritiated thymidine (labeled with ^3H) is used as a measure of the response to **mitogens** (substances that cause cell mitosis). The amount taken up provides some evaluation of the immune system.

The response of an individual to active sensitization can be measured by application of dinitrochlorobenzene to the skin. The procedure is repeated in two to three weeks. If the cellular immunity is intact, the patient develops a lesion at the site.

A great deal more research is needed before the best procedures for evaluating nutritional status with tests of immune function are determined.

Hypersensitivity

Hypersensitivity is a harmful response defined as an adverse immunologic reaction to a substance that is harmless to most people. The term **allergy** is used to refer to a sensitivity to a foreign antigen that does not have a beneficial effect, as does immunity to infection. It is important to remember that allergy is an *immune* response, and, when the term is applied to foods, it must not be confused with food poisoning or with a food intolerance resulting from an enzyme deficiency. In hypersensitivity, the antigen often is called an **allergen**.

Types of Hypersensitivity

The most common classification of hypersensitivity reactions is that of Gell and Coombs,[64] who listed four types. Some diseases may be expressions of two or more types or are variants of these classifications.

Type I. In type I (**immediate, anaphylactic,** or **reagin-dependent**) hypersensitivity, a sensitizing dose is necessary first. Then a specific antibody, usually IgE, is bound to and sensitizes tissue cells such as mast cells and basophils. In following exposures, the antigen seeks out and reacts with the specific antibody at the cell surface. The sensitized cell releases histamine and other mediators. This response is considered immediate, usually occurring in less than 60 minutes. The results of this sequence of events, called **anaphylaxis**, affect organs in which mast cells are fixed. These "shock organs" are smooth muscle in lung and bronchi, endothelial cells of the blood vessels, and associated secretory glands which contain mast cells in large numbers. The response occurs in genetically susceptible individuals who produce IgE antibodies to allergens to which most of the population does not respond.

Some anaphylactic responses are normal in the sense that all individuals will react similarly. Individuals who have abnormal responses, or hypersensitivity, have a genetically based susceptibility. The term **atopy** has been coined to indicate these abnormal responses.

The response may be local or systemic. When the Ag/Ab response is on a mucosal surface, the consequences are fairly mild. This type of response occurs most often to airborne allergens (inhalants) such as pollens, molds, fungal spores, dusts, animal danders, and various substances with volatile components and strong odors. In atopy, allergic rhinitis (hay fever) is, by far, the most common manifestation, usually as a response to seasonal pollens. Bronchial asthma, atopic dermatitis, and gastrointestinal allergy occur less often. Some patients have more than one manifestation of atopy, but not usually at the same time.

The shock organ in atopic individuals varies, but there usually is only one in a given individual. The means by which the symptoms are produced in the shock organ are based on the actions of the mediators. For example, when the allergen-IgE reaction occurs in the nose, release of histamine causes vasodilation and increased capillary permeability. These effects cause leakage of nasal fluid (rhinorrhea). Other factors cause sneezing and nasal itching. The total syndrome is allergic rhinitis or hay fever. In urticaria (hives), involving superficial capillaries, histamine is released locally, causing vasodilation and producing a red flare. The increased permeability of the capillaries allows movement of plasma into the tissue, leading to swelling and formation of a wheal. The raised area plus red flare of hives is referred to as a **wheal-and-flare** reaction. In asthma, the allergen-IgE reaction releases leukotrienes and causes a spasm in the bronchioles of the lung. As a result, the patient has difficulty in breathing.

The systemic response may be more severe. It can occur very rapidly following injection of a drug, insect venom, or foreign serum. The antigen can also be absorbed through the intestinal tract. The possible consequences of systemic anaphylaxis can include bronchospasm and edema of the larynx, sometimes leading to dyspnea, cyanosis, and severe hypotension. If interference with respiration is very severe, it can be life-threatening. This severe form is called **anaphylactic shock**.

Atopic conditions often associated with food allergies include atopic dermatitis, urticaria, and gastrointestinal allergy.

Type II. In type II (**cytotoxic** or **cytolytic antibody**) hypersensitivity, IgG or IgM binds to an antigen on a cell membrane and activates complement, resulting in a toxic effect on the cell or cell lysis. Among the conditions resulting from this type of immune disorder are scleroderma and renal diseases including renal complications of systemic lupus erythematosus. Information on their nutritional care is found in later chapters. Some antibodies stimulate their target cells instead of inhibiting or killing them.[1] This is thought to be the mechanism for thyrotoxicosis.

Type III. In type III hypersensitivity (**immune complex disease**), Ag/Ab complexes deposit in tissues and activate complement, with consequent release of chemotactic factors, cell infiltration, and release of lysosomal enzymes. A chronic inflammatory response follows. When the immune complexes are not cleared in the usual way by the reticuloendothelial system, they continue to circulate and deposit in small blood vessels, producing vasculitis and interfering with blood supply to the tissues. The ability to remove the immune complex depends on the solubility and size of the Ag/Ab particle. When antigen is present in excess, particles are larger and more difficult to remove. The consequences may be systemic (serum sickness) or local (Arthus reaction), occurring at the site of the injection.

The consequences of the disorder vary with the specific organs involved. In some diseases, the association with immune complex disease is suspected but not proved. Some disorders that could be included in this category are of interest to the nutritional care specialist:

In the digestive system, Crohn's disease and chronic ulcerative colitis.
In the kidney, glomerulonephritis and some cases of systemic lupus erythematosus.
In the liver, some cases of hepatitis with cirrhosis.

These conditions are discussed in later chapters.

Type IV. In type IV (**delayed-type** or **cell-mediated**) hypersensitivity, the condition results from the stimulation of lymphocytes specifically sensitized to the antigen. In some cases, it does not involve production of antibodies or complement activation. There is, instead, cytotoxicity from release of lymphokines, which cause the accumulation and activation of monocytes and macrophages.

The response is slower than is the response to type I hypersensitivity. It may occur hours or days after exposure to the antigen. The symptoms are extremely variable and often mimic other disorders. The severity of the symptoms usually is dose-related. Conditions in this category include contact dermatitis, graft rejection, some autoimmune diseases, and some food allergies.

Autoimmune Diseases

When the immune system damages cells of disease-producing organisms, the effect is beneficial, but it is now recognized that the immune system can cause disease by damaging the body's own cells. Conditions known as **autoimmune diseases** are believed to result from the development of an immune reaction to a person's own tissue and may not involve either the humoral or cellular systems. These diseases are particularly difficult because of the constant exposure of the antigen to the antibody or sensitized lymphocyte. Diseases included in this category that have nutritional significance are listed in Table 6-3.

Table 6-3. Some Autoimmune Diseases with Possible Nutritional Care Implications

Active chronic hepatitis
Dermatomyositis
Goodpasture's syndrome
Primary atrophic hypothyroidism
Sjögren's syndrome
Systemic lupus erythematosus
Thyrotoxicosis
Type 1 diabetes mellitus
Ulcerative colitis

At present, autoimmune diseases are classified as type II, III, or IV hypersensitivities, but there also may be other types. In addition, elevated antibody levels have been found in other diseases not currently classified as being of autoimmune origin. Their relationship to autoimmunity is not clear; it is possible that, in some cases, the antibody develops as a consequence, not a cause, of the tissue damage.

There are a number of theories to explain the means by which autoimmunity develops. Three major theories regarding the production of humoral autoimmunity have been proposed.

1. An agent of some type affects a tissue and alters it sufficiently that it is perceived by the immune system as foreign. The types of agents possibly involved are infectious, physical, or chemical, including some drugs. The change is presumed not to be so great that the antibodies produced would attack normal cells.

2. Some constituents of the body normally are isolated from the immune system. Thus during normal development, at the time that the immune system learns to recognize self, recognition is not established. The autoimmune disease process is initiated when one of these "hidden" antigens escapes into an area in which it is not normally found; that is, it is **ectopic**. It comes in contact with the immune system and is perceived as foreign. The consequent immune response to the ectopic antigen causes the disease.

Low concentrations of antibodies to these ectopic materials probably are present normally as a response to the normal turnover of body protein. When large concentrations of tissue debris appear, the formation of antibodies is stimulated. A large number of Ag/Ab complexes are formed, sometimes accompanied by complement fixation. These reactions may lead to further injury of tissue. Immunoglobulin G is believed to be the primary offender in immune complex injury.

Materials that have been proposed as candidates for ectopic antigen status include the protein in the lens of the eye, sperm, thyroglobulin from the thyroid follicle, mitochondria from the inside of cells, molecular DNA, and those forms of RNA normally sequestered within the nucleus. An immune response to one of these substances is thought to cause conditions such as Hashimoto's disease. Immune complex injury also is proposed as the cause of the damage to the kidney in systemic lupus erythematosus.

3. Some cells may be genetically programmed to produce an antibody to self, possibly as the result of a mutation. Normally, these cells would be suppressed. If a disease process interferes with the suppressive mechanism, an autoimmune disease theoretically could result.

Autoimmune disease involving the **cell-mediated system** might be produced by some of the same general mechanisms. In addition, it has been proposed that there are parasites that can live in a cell and alter its surface sufficiently that the cell becomes perceived as foreign. It has been suggested that this mechanism may be responsible for the primary damage in systemic lupus erythematosus, scleroderma, and possibly, rheumatoid arthritis.

Recent studies in inbred strains of mice have suggested that diet may alter the course of autoimmune disease. New Zealand black mice are prone to reduced immune competency and tend to develop an autoimmune hemolytic anemia. This anemia develops earlier in mice fed a low-protein, high-fat diet than in those fed a high-protein, low-fat diet.[65] Also, if these mice are mated with New Zealand white mice, the pups produced tend to develop an autoimmune damage to the kidneys. Caloric restriction prolonged their life span.[66,67] It is not known if such diet alterations would be effective in human patients with autoimmune disease.

Procedures in nutritional care of patients with autoimmune disease are determined by the effects of the disease on damaged organs rather than the effects on the immune system and will be discussed in the chapters on the relevant organ systems.

Graft Rejection

Graft rejection and its nutritional care are of interest in patients with organ transplants and in the treatment of some cancer patients. Currently, almost all grafts are **allografts (homografts)** — that is, grafts between two persons of the same species but differing in genetic constitution. Their differing HLA antigens are called **alloantigens**. When an organ — a kidney, for example — is transplanted from the donor to the host (recipient), some degree of immune response is to be expected, since the kidney consists of a large number of foreign proteins which are the antigens. Specifically, the host reacts immunologically to the histocompatibility antigens on the cells of the donor tissue. This process, called **rejection**, can occur in one of three forms:

1. **Immediate rejection** occurs when the recipient already has antibodies to the donor tissue. The antibodies may have developed as the result of a blood transfusion from the same donor, for example. In these circumstances, the rejection may begin in minutes or a few hours with deposition of Ag/Ab complex in the blood vessels, activation of the complement cascade, and the usual subsequent events. This is a **hyperacute rejection**. An **accelerated rejection** is similar, but the response is somewhat slower because the number of antibodies is lower.
2. **Acute rejection** occurs in a few weeks. It is theorized that donor HLA circulates to lymph nodes and spleen and induces sensitization. Host lymphocytes become sensitized as they circulate to the graft. The cell-mediated response destroys the blood vessels and the kidney tubules by creating an ischemic necrosis. Humoral immunity probably also is involved in acute rejection.
3. **Chronic rejection** may follow in months or years. It appears to be the result of immunoproliferative lesions in the intrarenal arteries, leading to ischemia.

Immunosuppressive drugs are used to prevent transplant rejection. Nutritional care in patients receiving these drugs is described in Chapter 9. Some investigation is beginning on the effects of deficiencies of specific nutrients or modified diets that have an immunosuppressive effect. These might then be used to increase the effects of immunosuppressive drugs.

It seems appropriate here to mention a condition in which, in effect, the graft rejects the host. The immune response is in the opposite direction from that seen in transplant rejection. It occurs in some patients if the host is immuno*in*competent but the donor is immunocompetent. The host may have become immunoincompetent as a consequence of drug treatment or irradiation, or the condition may be genetic. The donor's T lymphocytes will recognize the host as foreign and will mount an immune response against the host. The result is termed **graft-versus-host (GVH) disease**. Signs of GVH disease include diarrhea; skin rash; enlargement of the liver, spleen, and other lymph nodes; weight loss; and death.[58] Nutritional care in GVH disease is described in Chapter 15.

Food Allergy

Hypersensitivity reactions to food are more commonly type I (about 5%) or type IV (about 95%), but types II or III or a combination may also occur.[68] The essential features of types I and IV food allergies are compared in Table 6-4.

Allergens. It is believed that food allergens gain access to the body by absorption from the digestive tract. The majority are plants, and an allergic patient often is sensitive to foods in the same botanical family. Table 6-5 gives the members of various biological classifications of plants, indicating combinations of foods to which a patient might be allergic.

Few animal foods are allergens, but they can be important. The most common food allergens are listed in Table 6-6. Allergies to wheat, cow's milk, and chicken eggs, espe-

Table 6-4. Comparison of Types I and IV Food Allergy Reactions

Immediate (Type I)	Delayed (Type IV)
Not quantitative; all-or-none reaction	Usually dose-related
1–60 minutes	Up to 5 days
IgE-mediated	Cell-mediated
Less common and at times dangerous	Very prevalent
Mortality possible	Morbidity great, but no mortality
Severity predictable; shock-type reaction	Severity cyclic, but morbidity prevalent and chronic
Usually involving one shock organ	Systemic effects
Often permanent	Usually diminishes with prolonged avoidance

Table 6-5. Biological Classification of Foods

Family	Members
Plants	
Apple	Apple (cider, vinegar, apple pectin), crabapple, pear, quince, loquat
Arrowroot	Arrowroot
Arum	Poi, taro
Banana	Banana, plantain
Beech	Chestnut, beechnut
Birch	Filbert, hazelnut, oil of birch (wintergreen)
Buckwheat	Buckwheat, rhubarb
Cactus	Tequila
Carob	Gum acacia
Cashew	Cashew, mango, pistachio
Citrus fruits	Angostura, citron, grapefruit, kumquat, lemon, lime, orange, tangelo, tangerine
Cola nut, cacao	Coffee, chocolate, cola, cola drinks, tea
Cocheospurnum	Guiac gum, guar gum
Composite	Artichoke, chicory, dandelion, endive, escarole, head lettuce, leaf lettuce, oyster plant, sunflower, sesame, safflower, vermouth
Ebony	Persimmon
Fungi	Mushroom, yeast, antibiotics
Ginger	Cardamom, ginger, turmeric
Gooseberry	Currant, gooseberry
Goosefoot	Beet, beet sugar, spinach, Swiss chard
Gourd	Cantaloupe, casaba, citron, cucumber, honeydew, muskmelon, Persian melon, pumpkin, squash, vegetable marrow, watermelon
Grains (grass)	Barley, malt, cane (cane sugar, molasses, corn oil, glucose), corn (cornstarch, corn oil, corn sugar, corn syrup, dextrose, Cerelose, glucose), oats, rice, rye, sorghum, wheat (bran, gluten flour, graham flour, wheat germ), wild rice
Grape	Grape, cream of tartar, raisin
Heath	Blueberry, cranberry, huckleberry, loganberry
Honeysuckle	Elderberry
Iris	Saffron
Laurel	Avocado, bay leaves, cinnamon
Lygethis	Brazil nut
Legumes	Acacia, black-eyed peas, kidney bean, lentil, licorice, lima bean, navy bean, pea, peanut, peanut oil, senna, soybean, soybean oil, stringbean, gum tragacanth
Lily	Aloes, asparagus, chive, garlic, leek, onion, sarsaparilla

(continued)

Table 6-5. (Continued)

Family	Members
Mallow	Cottonseed, okra (gumbo)
Maple	Maple syrup (maple sugar)
Mint	Basil, marjoram, mint, oregano, peppermint, sage, savory, spearmint, thyme
Morning glory	Sweet potato, yam
Mulberry	Breadfruit, fig, hop, mulberry
Mustard	Broccoli, brussels sprouts, cabbage, cauliflower, celery cabbage, collard, cress, horse-radish, kale, kohlrabi, mustard, radish, rutabaga, turnip, watercress
Myrtle	Allspice, bay, cloves, guava, paprika, pimiento
Nutmeg	Nutmeg, mace
Olive	Green olive, ripe olive, olive oil
Orchid	Vanilla
Palm	Coconut, date, sago, palm oil
Papaw	Papaya, papain, pawpaw
Parsley	Angelica, anise, caraway, carrot, celeriac, celery, coriander, cumin, dill, fennel, parsley, parsnip
Pea	Bean, lentil, pea, peanut, soy, alfalfa, clover, licorice, tamarind
Pedalium	Sesame, sesame oil
Pepper	Black pepper, white pepper
Pineapple	Pineapple
Plum	Almond, apricot, blackberry, cherry, nectarine, peach, persimmon, plum (prune), sloe (gin)
Pomegranate	Pomegranate
Poppy	Poppy seed
Potato (nightshade)	Chili, eggplant, green pepper, paprika, pimiento, potato, cayenne pepper, red pepper, tomato
Rose	Blackberry, dewberry, loganberry, loquat, quince, raspberry, strawberry, youngberry
Seaweed	Agar, longan, pulsan
Spurge	Tapioca, cassava
Stercula	Cacao (chocolate), kola bean, gum karaya
Sunflower	Jerusalem artichoke, sunflower seed oil, cardoon, chicory, endive, tarragon
Walnut	Black walnut, butternut, English walnut, hickory nut, pecan
Miscellaneous	Honey
Animals	
Amphibians	Frog
Crustaceans	Crab, crayfish, lobster, prawn, shrimp, squid
Fish (with fins)	Anchovy, barracuda, bass, bluefish, buffalo, bullhead, butterfish, carp, catfish, caviar, chub, codfish, croaker, cusk, corvina, drum, eel, flounder, haddock, hake, halibut, harvestfish, herring, mackerel, mullet, muskellunge, perch, pickerel, pike, pollack, pompano, porgy, rosefish, salmon, sardine, scrod, scup, shad, smelt, snapper, sole, sturgeon, sucker, sunfish, swordfish, trout, tuna, weakfish, whitefish
Fowl	Chicken (chicken eggs), duck (duck eggs), goose (goose eggs), grouse, guinea hen, partridge, pheasant, squab, turkey
Mammals	Beef (butter, cheese, cow's milk, gelatin, veal), goat (cheese, goat's milk), horsemeat, mutton (lamb), pork (bacon, ham), rabbit, sheep (lamb), squirrel, venison
Mollusks	Abalone, clam, cockle, mussel, oyster, scallop
Reptiles	Turtle

Compiled from Collins-Williams, C., and Levy, L.D., Allergy to foods other than milk. In *Food Intolerance,* Ed. R.K. Chandra. New York: Elsevier, 1984; Farrell, M.K., Food allergy. In *Manual of Allergy and Immunology,* ed. G.J. Lawlor, Jr., and T.J. Fischer. Boston: Little, Brown, 1981; Sheldon, J.M., Louell, R.G., and Matthews, K.P., Food and gastrointestinal allergy. In *A Manual of Clinical Allergy.* Philadelphia: W.B. Saunders, 1967; and Monro, J., Food allergy and migraine. *Clin. Immun. Allergy* 2:137–164, 1982.

Table 6-6. Common Food Allergens

Immediate hypersensitivity
Fish
Seafood
Nuts
Legumes (especially peanuts)
Eggs
Salicylates

Delayed hypersensitivity
Milk
Wheat
Chocolate
Cola
Corn
Citrus fruit
Eggs
Beef
White potatoes
Pork
Legumes
Chicken
Oatmeal
Rye
Oranges
Cottonseed
Mustard
Tomatoes
Cucumbers
Garlic

cially if all three are present in the same person, can be particularly troublesome in meal planning.

There is very little cross-reactivity in allergies to animal foods. Patients allergic to eggs are not usually allergic to chicken. Allergies to milk and beef only occasionally occur in the same patient. Of the two, milk allergy is much more common.

Some chemicals used in food processing may be allergens. In some cases, they are haptens. An important group of additives that are considered by some to be causes of atopic reactions are the artificial food colors, but this belief is very controversial. If a diet free of these products is prescribed, certain facts should be kept in mind. Most are petroleum products and are used in very small amounts. Some color is imparted by concentrations of 0.001%. At the other extreme, objectionable overcoloring occurs at approximately 0.008%. Some colors used in foods are Blue No. 1 (brilliant blue), Green No. 3, Red No. 3 (erythrosine), Yellow No. 5 (tar-

trazine), and Yellow No. 6. Orange color is made by mixing red and yellow, and green sometimes is achieved by mixing blue and yellow. Purple is a combination of red and blue. The red, blue, and yellow colors and their derivatives, orange, green, and purple, are found in large quantities in the foods listed in Table 6-7. Brown products, such as root beer and colas, are colored with caramel.

Mode of Contact. Allergens in type I and type IV hypersensitivities often are classified according to their mode of contact. The most common allergens in type I atopy are the **inhalants**. This group comprises pollens, dusts, molds, fungal spores, and other airborne materials. Their primary area of contact is the respiratory tract. Few of these are food-related, but some patients find that strong odors from some foods are antigenic.

Ingestants are substances taken internally as food or drink. Some drugs may be included here, as well as chemical additives and unintentional ingestants such as mouthwashes and toothpastes. The ingestants obviously are of primary interest to the nutritional care specialist.

Contactants are allergenic on direct skin or mucous membrane contact. They may include pollens and food as well as other sub-

Table 6-7. Food Sources of Substantial Amounts of Artificial Colors

Baked goods
Breakfast cereals
Cake mixes
Candies
Carbonated drinks
Cherry pie mix
Colored sugar
Drug syrups (e.g., cough syrup)
Frankfurters
Fruit cocktail, canned
Fruit drinks, artificial
Fruit salad, canned
Gelatin desserts
Gum, bubble
Gum, chewing
Ice creams and cones
Maraschino cherries
Mint jelly
Popsicles

stances in the environment. Contact allergens are type IV hypersensitivities. When a patient is highly sensitive to a specific ingested food, he or she sometimes also develops a contact dermatitis when handling that food. This reaction is not invariable, but the possibility does exist.

Injectants are substances that cause reactions when injected into the body. Injected drugs and sera used in medical treatment as well as insect venoms are in this group.

Clinical Manifestations. With food allergies, the allergen may react with the IgE antibodies locally and produce symptoms in the gastrointestinal tract itself or may affect organs elsewhere in the body. Only when the symptoms occur in the gastrointestinal tract is the condition known as **gastrointestinal allergy**. When organs elsewhere in the body are affected, two possible mechanisms are theoretically possible: (1) the mediators are transmitted systemically and affect the susceptible shock organ; or (2) the antigen itself is absorbed into the systemic circulation and has a direct effect on the shock organ. At the present time, the first of these is more commonly accepted.[69]

Table 6-8 gives a comprehensive list of clinical manifestations that have been suspected to result from allergies to ingested foods. Some of the symptoms in the gastrointestinal tract itself—vomiting, diarrhea, malabsorption, and constipation—are common to many other disorders and therefore are discussed in detail in Chapters 7 and 8.

Anaphylaxis usually occurs promptly after the allergenic food is eaten. Typically, offending foods are legumes, especially peanuts, and also berries, nuts, and seafoods, particularly shellfish. **Urticaria** and **angioedema** are common allergic symptoms to a variety of foods. Atopic dermatitis (**eczema**) occurs frequently from milk, wheat, corn, fish, and legume allergies, but may result from a wide variety of others.[69] Asthma is most often associated with inhalants, but approximately 10% of asthma patients have a sensitivity to aspirin. Cross-reactivity in

Table 6-8. Possible Clinical Manifestations of Food Allergy

Gastrointestinal
Nausea
Vomiting
Diarrhea
Abdominal pain and colic
Loss of appetite
Intestinal hemorrhage
Hepatosplenomegaly
Constipation
Malabsorption
Functional intestinal obstruction
Cheilitis
Stomatitis

Dermatologic
Urticaria
Angioedema
Circumoral rashes
Eczema
Perianal dermatitis
Aphthous ulcers

Respiratory system
Chronic rhinitis
Asthma
Recurrent bronchitis
Recurrent croup
Recurrent otitis media
Chronic coughing
Hemoptysis

Central nervous system
Headache
Insomnia
Irritability
Listlessness
Drowsiness

Hematologic
Anemia
Eosinophilia

Systemic
Anaphylaxis
Failure to thrive
Malnutrition

Other (controversial)
Crib death
Celiac disease
Ulcerative colitis
Tension fatigue syndrome
Hyperkinesia
Migraine
Peptic ulcer
Irritable colon

some of these patients makes them sensitive to some foods and food additives, especially tartrazine yellow.

Feingold[70] has suggested that food additives and **hyperactivity** are related. In particular, he points to tartrazine and salicylates as offenders. His reports have been based on clinical experience, and the concept has not been universally accepted. Controlled studies have been inconclusive.[71]

The immune responses to ingestants obviously are of primary interest to the nutritional care specialist; however, it is important to recognize that individual patients may simultaneously be allergic to inhalants and contactants. Under these circumstances, these allergies have some effect on each other. It has been suggested that each patient has a limit of tolerance or threshold for the appearance of symptoms.[72] Thus some food allergies cause obvious symptoms in the ragweed-sensitive patient only in the season when ragweed is in bloom.

The severity of the clinical manifestations of atopy or delayed hypersensitivity is affected by a number of other factors that add to the patient's **total allergic load**. One of these is the patient's genetic constitution. A tendency to hypersensitivity seems to recur in certain families; however, the specific clinical manifestations may vary within that family. One person might have hay fever, another hives, and so on. An individual's reaction to a given allergen is consistent, though. For example, a person who develops hives from eating strawberries will continue to have hives and will not develop hay fever on the next exposure to strawberries.

In addition to the genetic predisposition, symptoms also tend to be more severe when the patient is physically less well than normal, during emotional stress, and during inclement weather. The question of emotional involvement in allergic patients is a complicated one. The nutritional care specialist should keep in mind not only that emotional stress exacerbates the symptoms, but also that the disease itself may cause emotional problems that must be considered in treatment.

Another important point is that sensitization by one mode of contact may lead to allergic reactions when other means of contact occur. If a patient becomes sensitized to an injected drug, for example, the sensitivity can result in an allergic reaction if that substance or a closely related material is contained in an ingested food. Penicillin sensitivity is an example that will be discussed in more detail.

Prevention. Although most foods are digested prior to absorption, trace amounts can be absorbed in the form of molecules sufficiently large to be antigenic.[73] The prevalence of food allergy is inversely proportionate to age. It is not known whether this relationship results from maturation of the gastrointestinal tract, thus reducing absorption of antigen, or whether an acquired immunity develops.[69] Antigen absorption occurs more commonly in early infancy than in adults, possibly because of low levels of sIgA in the intestine.[74-77]

The infant may also become sensitized to foods that the mother eats in large quantities during pregnancy.[78] Immunoglobulin E does not cross the placenta; therefore, type I allergies are not acquired passively, but foods eaten and absorbed as antigen by a pregnant woman are believed to be capable of crossing the placenta. Antibodies can then be made by the fetus.[79,80] A mixed diet without emphasis on any one food in pregnancy is recommended in families with a genetic predisposition to allergy.

Breast feeding may prevent sensitization in atopic families, since the milk contains less foreign protein.[81] However, some antigens in the mother's diet have been found in the milk.[82] For protection against allergies, long-term breast feeding of the atopic infant and a varied diet for the mother, avoiding large quantities of foods that are common allergens, are recommended.[83] The introduction of new foods to the infant should be delayed as long as possible.

Diagnosis. The occurrence of clinical manifestations of food allergy does not require the presence of antibodies.[84] Delayed sensitivity is not antibody-dependent. Conversely, antibodies can be found before allergic symptoms begin to occur and may be unrelated to current clinical manifestations. As a consequence, measurement of total IgE level in the serum is inadequate for diagnosis. The problem often is approached more indirectly.

The physician is faced with several problems in the diagnosis of food hypersensitivity. One of these is differential diagnosis. For example, some allergic reactions mimic other gastrointestinal diseases such as gluten intolerance and lactose intolerance. It also is important to distinguish hypersensitivity reaction from infections. The problem may be complex, and the diagnosis of hypersensitivity sometimes is made by a process of elimination.

A second problem in diagnosis is the identification of the offending food or other allergens. It is in this process that the skillful nutritional care specialist can be invaluable. The available procedures vary greatly in their innate dependability, and some are more than usually dependent on the skills of the health care professional.

The **diet history** can be important and should be the first procedure used. When allergy is of the immediate reaction type and the response is severe to an obviously present allergen, the patient, or the parent of a child patient, will usually be aware of the identity of the allergen. However, when allergic responses are delayed, are nonspecific in nature, moderate in severity, or result from hidden allergens, skillful and thorough questioning is required. In addition, detailed knowledge of food composition, botanical relationships, and food preparation methods are essential. It is insufficient to ask the patient simply to describe his or her diet. Some useful general lines of questioning are listed here. Judgment must be exercised in choosing questions to ask in specific cases:

What foods were eaten, how often, and in what amounts?

What are the sources of these foods: Home-prepared? Away from home? If away from home, where? Brands? Specific content of mixed dishes? Is the food eaten cooked or raw?

Is chewing gum used? If so, what brand? How often? When?

What is the patient's meal pattern? Time? Amount? Frequency?

Which foods are eaten in especially large quantities compared to normal?

Are there foods eaten to which other members of the family are known to be allergic, particularly parents, grandparents, or siblings?

Do symptoms develop as the result of smelling or handling certain foods?

Do symptoms develop only when exposure occurs in certain locations? Only after certain activities?

Is the patient under emotional stress? Constantly? At recurring intervals?

What cleaning compounds are used? Dishwashing methods?

What drugs, cosmetics, and personal hygiene products are used? Brands? Time and frequency of use? Inquire about aspirin, toothpastes, mouthwashes, throat lozenges, laxatives, and other products in or around the mouth, even if the patient is not conscious of swallowing them.

The answers to these questions may well lead to others.

Another diagnostic method is the **food diary**. Total recall of the diet information in the diet history interview is difficult, if not impossible. Therefore, the patient may be asked to keep a diary for a period of a week or several weeks. The patient will require careful instruction on the information to be entered in this diary and will need encouragement to complete the record carefully and accurately in order for the diary to be useful. The patient should record all food, drink, and other ingestants, along with the time of intake or use, amounts, and preparation methods. Ingredients for all mixtures, as well as the brand names of prepared or packaged items, should be listed. At the same time, the nature, time of onset, and severity of symptoms must be recorded. This information then is examined to detect a relationship between the ingestion of a specific item and the onset of symptoms within approximately three days. A food should be suspected particularly if the interval between ingestion and onset of symptoms is relatively constant.

Cutaneous testing sometimes is used in addition to the history and diary. Specific items that precipitate severe responses may be identified by the history or diary; these should not be the subject for cutaneous testing because the process can be hazardous. However, a list of suspected foods in which the relationship to symptoms is less clear sometimes is also obtained. Cutaneous testing (skin tests) may be used in investigating these suspected allergens. Extracts of suspected offenders are applied to a "scratched" area of the skin or put into areas where the skin is pricked. These epicutaneous tests are known as **scratch** (cutireaction) or **prick tests**. Alternatively, the extract sometimes is injected intracutaneously. Results are interpreted in terms of the size of the wheal-and-flare reactions elicited at each site compared to that produced by administration of the solvent alone or to histamine. Theoretically, a large wheal and flare indicates greater sensitivity. A reaction in 15 to 20 minutes suggests an IgE-mediated reaction. An Arthus-like (type III) reaction is suggested with a reaction in 4 to 8 hours, and a type IV cell-mediated response is probable if the wheal and flare appear in 24 to 72 hours.

The **skin-window test** is also a form of cutaneous testing.[85,86] The surface of the skin is scraped with a blade, a drop of antigen extract is applied, and a microscope slide is taped over the area. The slide is stained and examined for eosinophils and other cells in 24 hours. The test is positive if eosinophils are three times more numerous than in a control area.

Unfortunately, cutaneous testing is not especially reliable in diagnosis of food allergies. Prick or scratch tests often are positive in type I hypersensitivity[87,88] and negative in type IV,[89,90] but there are many false-positive responses, some resulting from nonspecific skin irritation. False-negative responses also are common.[86,91] Intradermal tests are more dependable in type IV sensitivities. One rea-

son for the unreliability of skin tests may be that extracts are made from raw materials and so may not sufficiently closely resemble the cooked items that the patient normally eats. In addition, the allergen may be altered chemically when extracts are prepared or during storage. An additional problem arises in that extracts are not available for every possible antigen. The patient may be allergic to substances not tested. Last, the skin does not always respond in the same way as other shock organs.

Laboratory tests are of limited usefulness but may be used to suggest or confirm the diagnosis. They are not definitive. Increased eosinophil levels in the blood (eosinophilia) suggests allergy,[92] but it occasionally is present in other conditions.[93] Therefore, this test is not useful in differential diagnosis. Increased serum IgE often is seen in type I hypersensitivity, but it, too, is found in other conditions.[91,94] Low serum IgA usually is associated with sIgA deficiency. In the **radioallergosorbent test** (RAST), the amount of the patient's IgE antibody to specified antigens is measured. It therefore tends to be positive in type I sensitivities and negative in type IV.[89,90] The test is expensive; not all antigens are available for use with this method; and it is considered to be less sensitive than intradermal skin testing. Further developments may eventually make this technique more useful.[95]

Diet testing often is of great value, given the limitations of in vitro and skin tests. There are several procedures available for use under appropriate circumstances. One of these procedures is the **restriction of specific foods and diet challenge**. In this procedure, the foods on the suspect list are eliminated from the diet. The patient is given a list of those foods to be eliminated and also a list of foods that may be eaten. Usually, all commercially prepared foods are banned for the duration of the test. The patient should also be advised on meal planning for nutritional adequacy. If the list of foods to be eliminated is long or if many foods in a single group are restricted, the physician may prescribe vitamin and mineral supplementation. It must be remembered that these often contain artificial colors, binders, and other materials to which the patient may be sensitive.

The diet should be followed for three to four weeks. If the patient's symptoms subside, the restricted foods are added to the diet *one at a time*. This challenge test consists of adding the items to the diet in a large serving at each meal for three days. If the symptoms recur during that period, the food item is removed from the diet. The patient uses the previous diet until all symptoms subside and then proceeds to the next test item. A careful food diary is kept by the patient throughout. The procedure is repeated for each item on the suspect list.

Foods added first in the challenge test are those that occur most frequently in the diet and to which patients are most frequently sensitive. Most patients complete this procedure with a very short list of foods to which they are allergic. It may consist of only one or two items. Foods that are shown by this procedure to be allergens should be retested at a later date, perhaps at yearly intervals, since sensitivities sometimes change with time.

A more restrictive or **elimination diet** may be used if specific restriction and diet challenge does not render the patient symptom-free. There are several versions of elimination diets available.[96] Some eliminate foods only in a specific category. Others are much more restrictive and consist only of a limited number of foods, those that past clinical experience has shown to be rarely, if ever, the cause of hypersensitivity responses. Examples of typical diets are given in Table 6-9. The chosen diet is used until all symptoms subside. Then foods are added one at a time at intervals of four or five days, as described previously. The time intervals are important. If the patient does not become symptom-free on one of these diets, another with entirely different components can be tried. Alternatively, the patient may be given a defined formula such as Vivonex.

For small children, an elimination diet may consist of the foods resembling Rowe elimination diet 1, adjusted for age as follows:

Less than three months: milk substitutes.
Three to six months: add rice cereal.
Six to 24 months: add applesauce, pears, carrots, squash, lamb.

If the symptoms do not subside on even the most restricted of the elimination diets, food allergy is an unlikely diagnosis. The patient may, instead, be allergic to an inhalant or other nonfood substances. In some cases, the problem is not an allergy, and the physician must seek the cause elsewhere. The use of elimination diets is hazardous for children if not carefully managed. Such diets may be inadequate for the growing child.

Treatment. Once the foods causing the symptoms have been identified, the most effective treatment is complete avoidance of these foods. In immediate reactions (type I), the immune response is permanent and will recur on reexposure at any time. The avoidance of the allergen, therefore, is needed permanently. In delayed reactions (type IV), a tolerance sometimes develops during a period of abstinence. If, however, the period of abstinence is too short, the recurring symptoms may be more severe.[97]

Avoidance diets. Avoidance of allergens is a simple procedure when the offending foods are eaten only occasionally and if their presence is obvious, but it presents a great problem in sensitivities to foods such as milk, eggs, wheat, corn, and other very common items. Patients, or the parents, must be given lists of foods to be avoided and careful instruction on reading labels to detect hidden sources of the allergen. Copies of diet lists are not always available in institutional diet manuals, since the patients are most often treated on an outpatient basis. Some examples will provide an appreciation of the knowledge required and the dimensions of the patient's problem. Some books on allergy management give diet suggestions but must be modified to the individual needs of the patient.[98–103] The process requires that the nutritional care specialist be very knowledgeable of food composition and processing methods. In many circumstances, the pa-

Table 6-9. Examples of Typical Elimination Diets

Rowe Elimination Diet 1	Rowe Elimination Diet 2	Rowe Elimination Diet 3	Rowe Elimination Diet 4
Cereals			
Rice	Corn	Tapioca	
Puffed Rice	Rye	Breads of any combina-	
Rice Flakes	Corn pone	tion of soy, lima bean,	
Rice Krispies	Corn-rye muffin	potato starch, and tap-	
Tapioca	Ry-Krisp	ioca flours	
Rice biscuit			
Rice bread			
Vegetables			
Lettuce	Beets	White potato	
Chard	Squash	Tomato	
Spinach	Asparagus	Carrot	
Carrot	Artichoke	Lima beans	
Sweet potato		String beans	
Yam		Peas	
Fruit or juice			
Lemon	Pineapple	Apricot	
Grapefruit	Peach	Grapefruit	
Pear	Apricot	Peach	
	Prune		
Meat			
Lamb	Capon (no hens)	Beef	
	Bacon	Bacon	
Other			
Cane sugar	Cane or beet sugar	Cane sugar	Cane sugar
Maple sugar	Karo corn syrup	Maple sugar	Milk
Cane sugar syrup fla-vored with maple	Sesame oil	Cane sugar syrup fla-vored with maple	Cream
Sesame oil	Mazola oil	Sesame oil	Plain cottage cheese
Olive oil	Gelatin, plain or flavored with pineapple	Soybean oil	Tapioca
Gelatin, plain or flavored with lime or lemon	Salt	Gelatin, plain or flavored with lime or lemon	
Salt	Baking powder	Salt	
Baking powder	Baking soda	Baking powder	
Baking soda	Cream of tartar	Baking soda	
Cream of tartar	Vanilla extract	Cream of tartar	
Vanilla extract	White vinegar	Vanilla extract	
Required supplements			
(1) 0.3 ml/day Poly-Vi-Sol	0.3 ml/day Poly-Vi-Sol	0.3 ml/day Poly-Vi-Sol	0.3 ml/day Poly-Vi-Sol
(2) 1 tbsp. b.i.d. Calcium-Sandoz Syrup	1 tbsp. b.i.d. Calcium-Sandoz Syrup	1 tbsp. b.i.d. Calcium-Sandoz Syrup	

tient is allergic to more than one item, and several diets must be combined with great care.

The **milk-free diet** presents special problems when, as is often the case, the patient is an infant. Breast feeding is highly recommended for prevention of the sensitization of infants from families in which allergies are common.[104] If the infant does not tolerate breast milk, the mother's diet should be examined for potential sources of allergens, since some allergens can be secreted into the breast milk. Elimination from her diet of some of the more common allergens, such as eggs, may solve the problem.

Patients who are only moderately reactive to cow's milk may tolerate "superheated" milk that has been boiled 15 to 30 minutes or powdered, evaporated, or lactic-acid-treated milk.[105] Heating probably is most useful to those patients who are allergic to the heat-labile protein in milk, that is, to albumin and gamma globulin. It is not effective in sensitivity to casein.

Approximately 40% of patients sensitive to cow's milk are able to tolerate goat's milk.[72] These patients may be sensitive to lactalbumin, which is species specific. The other protein fractions in milk, such as lactoglobulin, are not species specific. Sensitivity to these fractions will occur with goat's milk as well as cow's milk.

Many milk-sensitive infants are successfully fed formulas using soy protein as the protein source. Several of these are available commercially. Other nutrients are added to make them complete formulas for infant feeding (see Appendix G). These are less successful as milk substitutes for older children or adults, who may find the taste objectionable.

If an infant does not tolerate the soy protein well, other formulations that may be usable include Pregestimil and Nutramigen (Appendix G). The protein in these products is a hydrolysate of bovine casein, filtered to remove large protein molecules. Both products contain corn oil. A meat-base formula, made from beef heart, also is available as a substitute for milk and is sometimes successful.

When solid foods are added to the infant's diet, foods should be chosen that are less often allergens: rice cereal, lamb for meat, applesauce, pears, carrots, and squash. The similarities to the Rowe elimination diet 1 should be clear.

The nutritional care specialist must be prepared to help patients identify hidden sources of milk. Guidelines for a milk-free diet are given in Table 6-10. The patient must also be given suggestions on items that are safe to use. Some margarines sold as Kosher products do not contain milk products but may be colored with tartrazine. Kosher foods in general can be relied on to be milk-free.

Patients must also be given guidance on meal planning for nutritional adequacy. The physician probably will prescribe vitamin and mineral supplements.

The **wheat-free diet** (Table 6-11) presents a difficult problem in the older child and the adult because of the wide variety of foods containing wheat products. All forms of wheat in cereals, flour, bread, and other baked goods must be avoided. Flour must be assumed to be wheat flour unless otherwise stated. The term **graham**, as in graham crackers, refers to wheat. Malt, used in malted products and beer, may be made from wheat or from other cereals such as barley or corn. The term **cereal extract** on a

Table 6-10. Milk-Free Diet

Type of Food	Avoid
Milk	Cow's milk, whole, skim, evaporated, condensed, dried; yogurt; Ovaltine
Soup	Cream soups made with milk, cream, butter, margarine; all canned cream soups
Meat, egg, or cheese	Scrambled egg made with milk or prepared in butter or margarine; egg substitutes; any meat or fish seared in butter or margarine; all cheeses (au gratin); cold cuts; packaged mixed dishes; breaded or creamed meat, egg, fish or poultry
Potato or substitute	Any potato prepared with butter, margarine, milk, cream, cheese (au gratin)
Vegetable	Creamed vegetables; any vegetable seasoned with butter, margarine, milk, cream, cheese
Bread	Any bread made with milk, milk solids, butter, margarine. Read all labels.
Cereal	Any cooked cereal or gruel prepared with milk or cream; high-protein cereals
Fruit and juices	None
Dessert	Puddings made with milk, whipped cream toppings, ice cream and sherbet, cake, cookies, prepared flour mixes, pudding mixes, custard
Beverage	Cream, chocolate or cocoa drink mixes, cocoa made with milk, milk beverages as eggnogs, milkshakes, malted milks
Fat	Butter, margarine churned in milk, salad dressings containing milk products
Sweets	All candy except plain sugar candy
Miscellaneous	Creamed foods, boiled salad dressing, white sauces; all "au gratin" dishes; imitation chocolate chips

Table 6-11. Wheat-Free Diet

Type of Food	Avoid
Soup	Bouillon cubes, all cream soups thickened with flour; all canned cream soups; soups with paste products
Meat, fish, egg, or cheese	Casseroles, croquettes, timbales, meat loaf, patties, hamburgers including bread, flour, or bread crumbs as ingredients; sausage, wieners, cold cuts; soufflés; meat and fish rolled in flour (Swiss steak)
Potato or substitute	Scalloped potatoes, creamed potatoes, au gratin potatoes; paste products; dumplings
Vegetable	Scalloped tomato, French fried vegetable if floured or breaded; vegetable soufflés; casseroles or puddings including flour, bread, or crumbs as ingredients
Bread	White bread, whole wheat bread, rye bread, hot breads, Zweiback, rusk; any foods made with batter, such as griddle cakes, waffles, crackers
Cereal	Any containing wheat, such as Bran Flakes, Krumbles, Crackles, Pep, Pettijohns, Ralston's Farina, Shredded Wheat, Grape Nuts, Muffets, Triscuits, Wheatena, Cream of Wheat, Rice Krispies, Cornflakes, wheat germ, all malted cereals
Fruits and juices	Strained fruits with added cereal
Dessert	Any including flour as an ingredient: cakes, cookies, pastries, doughnuts, ice cream cones, ice cream (thickening), bread pudding; prepared mixes
Beverage	Postum, Ovaltine, malted milk, Cocomalt, malt (beer, whiskies)
Fat	Commercial salad dressings and gravies
Sweets	Chocolate, candy bars
Miscellaneous	Breaded foods; mixtures containing crumbs, flour or bread; mayonnaise (read labels); malt products, gravies, sauces; soy sauce, some yeasts, Accént

label is also a danger signal. Products such as rye bread almost always contain some wheat flour unless labeled "100% rye bread" and packaged in a can. If the product were not canned, it would dry out very rapidly and be inedible. Few breakfast cereals are wheat-free. Cornflakes, for example, almost invariably contain some wheat. Most creamed, thickened, or breaded foods contain wheat. Pasta products such as noodles, macaroni, spaghetti, and similar items are wheat products.

Patients should be given lists of usable commercial products and recipes using alternatives to wheat flour, particularly for baking. Some of these are available from commercial processors of other cereals. Rye, oats, rice, and barley flour may be used in home baking but cannot simply be substituted in recipes for products made with wheat flour. Because of differences in the gluten, special recipes are required, but the products still differ somewhat in texture and acceptability. There is often a cross-reactivity with buckwheat, so buckwheat flour should not be used in these recipes.

The **egg-free diet** (Table 6-12) is some-what more easily managed than those without milk or wheat but still presents some problems. Although eggs in the obvious forms, such as fried or scrambled, are easy to avoid, the hidden forms are difficult to detect. The patient usually is sensitive to the egg white, not the yolk, but precise separation is very difficult.

Some hidden sources of eggs include coffee, wines, root beer, and clear soups that have been clarified with egg white; any product labeled as containing albumin, vitellin, ovovitellin, livetin, ovomucin, or ovomucoid; breads, rolls, pastries with a glazed crust and almost all other baked desserts; and waffles, pancakes, and similar products. Commercial mixtures such as salad dressings, puddings, custards, cookies, some ice cream, sherbet, cake flour, some baking powders, many meat mixtures and prepared meats, many paste products, and some candies may contain egg white.

Patients must be given lists of commercial products known to be egg-free, useful recipes, especially for baking, and guidance in menu planning for good nutrition.

The **corn-free diet** (Table 6-13) is exceed-

Table 6-12. Egg-Free Diet

Type of Food	Avoid
Soup	Bouillons, consommé, or other stock soups cleared with egg; noodle soup, mock turtle soup; egg drop soup
Meat, egg, or cheese	Timbales, croquettes, meat loaves, meatballs, hamburgers, any meat or cheese mixtures containing egg; eggs in any form, yolk or white; powdered eggs; egg substitutes (e.g., Egg Beaters)
Potato or substitute	Noodles, spaghetti, and macaroni unless egg-free; potato dishes with egg (duchess potatoes; potato puffs)
Vegetable	Vegetable soufflés or custards; any combined with egg sauces (e.g., hollandaise)
Bread	Any bread or rolls containing egg or brushed with egg for glazing; griddle cakes; pretzels; waffles; bread crumbs
Cereal	None
Fruits and juices	Fruit whips; any with custard sauce
Dessert	Meringues, cream pies, puddings or gelatin desserts made with egg, cakes, cake flour, cookies, ices, ice cream, icing, egg white, doughnuts, pudding powders, custards, macaroons, fruit whips, sherbet, sauces
Beverage	Coffee cleared with egg, malted drinks, Ovaltine, Ovomalt, wine, root beer, eggnogs
Fat	Mayonnaise; commercial salad dressing; any sauce prepared with egg
Sweets	All candy except hard candies, sugar, honey, jam, jellies
Miscellaneous	Foods made from batter or coated with batter; breaded foods, boiled dressing, baking powder

ingly difficult to manage because many foods contain corn products in hidden forms. Therefore, careful patient instruction is essential. The patient must avoid corn as a vegetable, hominy, grits, cereals containing corn, and popcorn. In addition, products containing corn oil and most cooking oils, cornstarch, corn syrup, corn sugar, dextrose or glucose, dexin, dextrin, dextrimaltose, commercial citric acid, and monosodium glutamate must be eliminated. Malt is often yeast-fermented corn. Commercial fructose may be made from corn. Many cardboard cartons, including milk cartons, are dusted

Table 6-13. Corn-Free Diet

Type of Food	Avoid
Soup	Cream soups, vegetable soup, commercial soups unless corn-free
Meat, egg, or cheese	Cold cuts, ham, wieners, bacon unless corn-free, breaded or fried foods; cheese and cheese spreads unless corn-free; commercial entrees unless corn-free
Potato or substitute	Coated rice, potatoes fried in corn oil
Vegetable	Harvard beets, canned peas, canned vegetables, frozen vegetables in waxed containers, corn, succotash, hominy
Bread	Graham crackers; any bread containing a corn product or baked on a hearth sprinkled with cornmeal; many bakery mixes and finished products; corn fritters, tamales, tacos, tortillas
Cereal	Cornflakes, Rice Krispies, Corn Kix, Post Toasties, cornmeal, Cheerios, hominy grits, presweetened cereals, polenta
Fruits and juices	Canned and frozen fruits and juices with "sugar added"; dates
Dessert	Ices, ice cream, sherbet, gelatin desserts; products containing baking powder, yeast, cornstarch; sauces or toppings; baking mixes; sugar wafers; some brands of flour
Beverage	Milk in waxed paper cartons, chocolate milk, milkshakes, carbonated beverages, soybean milks, sweetened fruit juices, instant tea or coffee; ale, beer, whiskies
Fat	Corn oil or "vegetable" oil, all products made with corn or vegetable oil, salad dressings made with corn oil
Sweets	Powdered sugar, dextrose, glucose, Karo, Cerelose, Cartose, jams, jellies, pancake syrup, many candies
Miscellaneous	Salt, catsup, peanut butter unless corn-free, chewing gum, popcorn, monosodium glutamate, distilled vinegar, vitamin preparations, many medicines, tablets, capsules, and liquids

with cornstarch. Many canned and frozen foods, especially fruits, are sweetened with corn syrup and must be avoided. The phrase "sugar added" on a label often refers to a corn syrup, not sucrose. Cornstarch is a common thickener in a variety of products.

Corn is used in many products in processing or manufacturing and can occur in unexpected places. Some examples are as follows:

Carbonated beverages
Instant tea and coffee
Baked products baked on a hearth sprinkled
    with cornmeal
Frozen vegetables in waxed containers
Gelatin desserts
Salt
Peanut butter
Some brands of flour
Products containing baking powder or yeast
Cold cuts
Distilled vinegar
Beer, whiskey, gin, brandies, and wine

Many vitamin preparations and drugs in tablets, capsules, or liquids contain corn products. Sorbitol usually is made from corn. The patient may also need to be warned of other sources of corn such as breath sprays and drops, many dentifrices, gum on envelopes, labels, stickers, and tapes, chewing gum, and plastic food wrappers.

Some products containing corn are not intended to be ingested but may cause problems if inhaled. These include bath powders, hair sprays, talcum powder, and laundry starch. The cooking fumes from fresh corn are irritants in some patients.

The dimensions of the problem should now be obvious. A list of corn-free products should be given to the patient along with careful counseling on meal planning for good nutrition. Some patients need a combined diet free of wheat, milk, egg, and corn and obviously will need a great deal of assistance.

Other avoidance diets that are encountered less frequently include those that require elimination of soy, cottonseed, linseed, or peanuts. In addition to use in a variety of manufactured foods, these items are found in many industrial products.

Sometimes food restrictions are necessary because the foods contains material not commonly considered to be a food, such as penicillin, salicylates, and a large number of commercial additives. The sensitivity to the antibiotic **penicillin** most commonly develops in the course of drug therapy. It can be very severe, causing anaphylactic shock, and, as such, can be life-threatening. Penicillin once was used widely to treat infections in cows and then appeared in the milk.[106] Most states now require that milk be tested and found to be free of penicillin before it can be sold, but patients with severe penicillin allergies still are reported to have problems occasionally when drinking milk.[101]

Penicillium is a mold found in some cheeses. It is unrelated to the antibiotic penicillin. Patients allergic to penicillin are not necessarily allergic to penicillium, but some patients are allergic to molds and can be expected to react to penicillium.

Salicylates are found in both food and drugs. Allergy to aspirin (acetylsalicylic acid) is fairly common. In addition to aspirin's presence in a long list of over-the-counter and prescription drugs, salicylates occur naturally in some foods (Table 6-14). Salicylates also are used in flavoring materials in processed foods and are found in beer, cider, wine, most distilled beverages, carbonated beverages, and tea. Aspirin sensitivity sometimes is accompanied by a sensitivity to benzoates and tartrazine.[107] The many foods containing these additives must then be eliminated, too. Salicylates also are used in suntan lotions, soaps, and in some other manufactured products. The patient may react to these products and needs careful instruction and a list of aspirin-free substitutes for aspirin.

The diet of the patient with many sensitivities may be very restricted in variety. Foods that the patient has not eaten before often are better tolerated and can provide interesting alternatives. Sometimes items new to the

Table 6-14. Foods Containing Salicylates

Nuts	Almonds
Fruits	Apples, apple cider, apricots, blackberries, boysenberries, currants, gooseberries, oranges, peaches, plums, prunes, raisins, raspberries, strawberries
Vegetables	Cucumbers, tomatoes
Miscellaneous	Cloves, oil of wintergreen, pickles

patient's diet may be obtained in the gourmet section of food stores, health food stores, and from shippers who specialize in special and exotic items. These foodstuffs may be more expensive but, if the patient can afford them, will provide variety in his or her meals.

The patient allergic to food is most frequently a child. The diet must then be adjusted for age and for the physiologic needs of growth. The nutritional consultant must have a knowledge of child development and be able to apply that knowledge in counseling.

Drug therapy. Although allergen avoidance is usually the mainstay of treatment, some drugs may be used. Antihistamines are used to prevent symptoms. Aminophylline (theophylline) or epinephrine are bronchodilators that are commonly used to control symptoms once they occur. Theophylline is a bronchodilator used for relief or prevention of symptoms of asthma. Among its side effects are nausea, vomiting, epigastric pain, hematemesis, and diarrhea. Plasma clearance is decreased by high-carbohydrate diets and depressed in low-carbohydrate and high-protein diets.

Cromolyn sodium is reported to prevent allergic reactions by preventing the release of mediators from mast cell granules by blocking calcium ions from entering the mast cell. It may cause nausea and a bad taste. Prostaglandin synthetase inhibitors (aspirin, indomethacin, ibuprofen) may be useful.

Sometimes corticosteroids and other drugs are prescribed to reduce the response at the target cells. Corticosteroids may inhibit the histidine carboxylase, which functions in the conversion of histidine to histamine. The drug has the potential for a variety of nutrition-related side effects. If it is taken for long periods, the patient should be observed for growth retardation in children, weight gain, gastrointestinal disturbances including bleeding, negative nitrogen balance, negative calcium balance, hyperglycemia, hyperlipidemia, interference with vitamin D metabolism, pancreatitis, fatty liver, and peptic ulcers.

SUMMARY

Immunology is one of the fastest moving and most promising areas of medical research. It may clarify the mechanism of many conditions that are currently poorly understood and thus provide a basis for development of treatment of these disorders. Among these are diabetes, thyroid toxicosis, atherosclerosis, tubular necrosis of the kidneys, and arthritis.

The nutritional care specialist needs a knowledge of the immune system to be able to understand advances in the field of immunology and the interrelationship of these advances to a variety of disorders of other organ systems.

Case Study: Allergy

Mrs. M.R. is a nurse who works the 3 P.M. to midnight shift at your hospital. She has had hay fever for many years. In addition, she develops a severe dermatitis when she eats eggs and gastrointesti-nal upset when eating foods containing wheat. Her father (now deceased) was allergic to milk, and her mother is allergic to shellfish.

The medical history notes milk allergy as an

infant. Patient had a broken arm at age 6 and rubella at age 8. Tests have ruled out gastrointestinal disease, endocrine disease, and malignancy. Nutrition assessment indicates the patient is 10 kg underweight but seems to be otherwise normally nourished.

The allergist refers the patient to the Nutrition Clinic for counseling on diet. In an interview, the patient states that she has recently changed jobs to the afternoon shift and has had difficulty getting food she can eat for her dinner in the hospital cafeteria. In her previous position, she worked days and carried her lunch.

The patient further states that her egg allergy seems to become more severe in the spring and fall of the year. However, it is now midwinter and the problem has suddenly become worse.

Exercises

1. What is the significance of the allergic conditions in the patient's parents?
2. Why might her egg allergy become more severe seasonally?
3. Why might it have become worse at this time?
4. Plan a lunch that this patient might carry.
5. Plan a Sunday dinner for the patient and her husband.
6. How would you modify the meal planned in exercise 5 if the patient's husband were allergic to the following: Corn? Soybeans? Milk?
7. If the patient became pregnant, what advice would you give her concerning diet in pregnancy and lactation to reduce the risk of allergies in the child?

References

1. Ganong, W.F. *Review of Medical Physiology*, 13th ed. Norwalk, Conn.: Appleton & Lange, 1987.
2. Irvine, W.J. *Medical Immunology*. Edinburgh: Teviot Scientific, 1979.
3. Dubiski, S. Diagnostic Immunology. In A.G. Gornall, Ed., *Applied Biochemistry of Clinical Disorders*. Hagerstown, Md.: Harper and Row, 1980.
4. Tomasi, T.B., and Bienenstock, J. Secretory immunoglobulin. *Adv. Immunol.* 9:1, 1968.
5. Heremanns, J.F. Immunoglobulin formation and function in different tissues. *Curr. Top. Microbiol. Immunol.* 45:131, 1968.
6. Crabbe, P.A., Carbonaru, A.O., and Heremanns, J.F. The normal human intestinal mucosa as a major source of plasma cells containing gamma A immunoglobulin. *Lab. Invest.* 14:235, 1965.
7. Bienenstock, J. The significance of secretory immunoglobulins. *Can. Med. Assoc. J.* 103:39, 1970.
8. Halpern, M.S., and Koshland, M.E. Novel subunit in secretory IgA. *Nature* 228:1276, 1970.
9. Mestecky, J., Zikan, J., and Butler, N.T. Immunoglobulin M and secretory immunoglobulin A. Presence of a common polypeptide chain different from light chain. *Science* 171:1163, 1971.
10. Morrison, S.L., and Koshland, M.E. Characterization of the J chain from polymeric immunoglobulins. *Proc. Natl. Acad. Sci. U.S.A.* 69:124, 1972.
11. Tomasi, T.B., Jr., Tan, E.M., Solomon, A., and Prendergast, R.A. Characteristics of an immune system common to certain external secretions. *J. Exp. Med.* 121:101, 1963.
12. Lindh, E. Increased resistance of immunoglobulin A dimers to proteolytic degradation after binding of secretory component. *J. Immunol.* 114:284, 1975.
13. Long, C.L. Energy balance and carbohydrate metabolism in infection and sepsis. *Am. J. Clin. Nutr.* 30:1301, 1977.
14. Wannemacher, R.W., Jr., Beall, F.A., Canonica, P.G., Dingerman, R.E., Hadick, C.L., and Neufeld, H.A. Glucose and alanine metabolism during bacterial infections in fats and rhesus monkeys. *Metabolism* 29:20, 1980.
15. Meszaros, K., Bagby, G.J., Lang, C.H., and Spitzer, J.J. Increased uptake and phosphorylation of 2-deoxyglucose by skeletal muscles in endotoxin-treated rats. *Am. J. Physiol.* 253:E33, 1987.
16. DelRey, A. and Besedovsky, H. Interleukin 1 affects glucose homeostasis. *Am. J. Physiol.* 253:R794, 1987.
17. Roh, M.S., Moldawer, L.L., Ekman, L.G., Dinarello, C.A., Bistrian, B.R., Jeevanandam, M. and Brennan, M.F. Stimulatory effect of interleukin-1 upon hepatic metabolism. *Metabolism* 35:419, 1986.
18. Klasing, K.C. Influence of stress on protein metabolism. In G.P. Moberg, Ed., *Animal Stress*. Bethesda, Md.: American Physiological Society, 1985.
19. Pawanda, M.C. Changes in body balances of nitrogen and other key nutrients. Description and underlying mechanisms. *Am. J. Clin. Nutr.* 30:1254, 1977.
20. Wannemacher, R.W., Jr. Key role of various individual amino acids in host response to infection. *Am. J. Clin. Nutr.* 30:1269, 1977.

21. Klasing, K.C. Nutritional aspects of leukocytic cytokines. *J. Nutr.* 118:1436, 1988.

22. Turner, M.W., and Hulme, B. *The Plasma Proteins: An Introduction.* London: Pitman Medical and Scientific, 1975.

23. Blomback, B., and Hanson, L.A. *Plasma Proteins.* New York: Wiley, 1979.

24. Laurence, J. The immune system in AIDS. *Sci. Amer.* 253:84, 1985.

25. Gallo, R. The first human retrovirus. *Sci. Amer.* 255:88, 1986.

26. Gallo, R. The AIDS virus. *Sci. Amer.* 256:47, 1987.

27. Varmus, H. Reverse transcription. *Sci. Amer.* 257:56, 1987.

28. Garcia, M.E., Collins, C.L., and Mansell, P.W.A. The acquired immune deficiency syndrome. Nutritional complications and assessment of body weight status. *Nutr. Clin. Proc.* 2:108, 1987.

29. Suskind, R.M., Ed. *Malnutrition and the Immune Response.* New York: Raven Press, 1977.

30. Beisel, W.R., Ed. Impact of infection on nutritional status of the host. *Am. J. Clin. Nutr.* 30:1206, 1977.

31. Vitale, J.J. Impact of nutrition on immune function. In J.J. Vitale and S.A. Broitman, Eds., *Advances in Human Clinical Nutrition.* Boston: PSG, 1983.

32. Keusch, G.T. The effects of malnutrition on host responses and the metabolic sequelae of infections. In M.H. Grieco, Ed., *Infections in the Abnormal Host.* New York: Yorke Medical, 1980.

33. Bistrian, B.R. Interaction of nutrition and infection in the hospital setting. *Am. J. Clin. Nutr.* 30:1228, 1977.

34. Schneider, R.E., and Viteri, F.E. Morphological aspects of the duodenojejunal mucosa in protein-calorie malnourished children and during recovery. *Am. J. Clin. Nutr.* 25:1092, 1972.

35. Ferguson, A.C., Lawlor, G.J., Jr., Neumann, C.G., et al. Decreased rosette-forming lymphocytes in malnutrition and intrauterine growth retardation. *J. Pediatr.* 85:717, 1974.

36. Chandra, R.K. T and B lymphocyte subpopulations and leukocyte terminal deoxynucleotidyl transferase in malnutrition. *Acta Paediatr. Scand.* 68:841, 1979.

37. Chandra, R.K. Cell-mediated immunity in nutritional imbalance. *Fed. Proc.* 39:3088, 1980.

38. Bang, B.G., Makalanabis, D., Mukherjee, K.L., and Bang, F.B. T and B lymphocyte rosetting in undernourished children. *Proc. Soc. Exp. Biol. Med.* 149:199, 1975.

39. Stiehm, E.R. Humoral immunity in malnutrition. *Fed. Proc.* 39:3093, 1980.

40. Johnson, S.G.O., Melbin, T., and Vahlquist, B. Immunoglobulin levels in Ethiopian preschool children with special reference to high concentrations of immunoglobulin E (IgE). *Lancet* 1:1118, 1968.

41. Chandra, R.K. Reduced secretory antibody response to live attenuated measles and poliovirus vaccines in malnourished children. *Br. Med. J.* 2:583, 1975.

42. Sirisinha, S., Suskind, R., Edelman, R., et al. Secretory and serum IgA in children with protein-calorie malnutrition. *Pediatrics* 55:166, 1975.

43. Sirisinha, S., Suskind, R., Edelman, R., et al. Complement and C3-proactivator levels in children with protein-calorie malnutrition and effect of dietary treatment. *Lancet* 1:1016, 1973.

44. Douglas, S.D., and Schapfer, K. The phagocyte in protein-calorie malnutrition—a review. In R.M. Suskind, Ed., *Malnutrition and the Immune Response.* New York: Raven Press, 1977.

45. Chandra, R.K., Seth, V., Chandra, S., et al. Polymorphonuclear leukocyte function in malnourished Indian children. In R.M. Suskind, Ed., *Malnutrition and the Immune Response.* New York: Raven Press, 1977, pp. 259–264.

46. Smythe, P.M., Brereton-Stiles, G.G., Coovadia, H.M., et al. Thymolymphatic deficiency and depression of cell-mediated immunity in protein-calorie malnutrition. *Lancet* 2:939, 1971.

47. Watts, T. Thymus weights in malnourished children. *J. Trop. Pediatr.* 15:155, 1969.

48. Mugerwa, J.W. The lymphoreticular system in kwashiorkor. *J. Pathol.* 105:105, 1971.

49. Hoffman-Goetz, L., and Kluger, M.J. Protein-deficiency. Its effects on body temperature in health and disease states. *Am. J. Clin. Nutr.* 32:1423, 1979.

50. McCay, C.M., Crowell, M.F., and Maynard, L.A. The effect of retarded growth upon the length of the life span and upon the ultimate body size. *J. Nutr.* 10:63, 1935.

51. Yunis, E.J., and Greenberg, L.J. Immunopathology of aging. *Hum. Pathol.* 5:122, 1974.

52. McHugh, M.I., Wilkinson, R., Elliott, R.W., et al. Immunosuppression with polyunsaturated fatty acids in renal transplantation. *Transplantation* 24:263, 1977.

53. Mertin, J., and Hunt, R. Influence of polyunsaturated fatty acids on survival of skin allografts and tumor incidence in mice. *Proc. Natl. Acad. Sci. U.S.A.* 73:928, 1976.

54. Broitman, S.A., Vitale, J.J., and Vavrousek-Jakuba, E. Polyunsaturated fat, cholesterol and large bowel tumorigenesis. *Cancer Res.* 40:2455, 1977.

55. Ota, D.M., Copeland, E.M., Corriere, J.N., Jr., et al. The effects of a 10% soybean oil emulsion on lymphocyte transformation. *JPEN* 2:112, 1978.

56. Gross, R.L., and Newberne, P.M. Role of nutrition in immunologic functions. *Physiol. Rev.* 60:188, 1980.

57. Rogers, A.E., Herndon, B.J., and Newberne, P.M. Induction by dimethylhydrazine of intestinal carcinoma in normal rats fed high or low levels of vitamin A. *Cancer Res.* 33:1003, 1973.

58. Benjamini, E., and Leskowitz, S. *Immunology: A Short Course.* New York: Liss, 1988.

59. Roitt, I., Brostoff, J., and Male, D. *Immunology.* St. Louis: C.V. Mosby, 1985.

60. Stites, D.P., Stobo, J.D., and Wells, J.V., Eds. *Basic and Clinical Immunology,* 6th ed. Norwalk, Conn.: Appleton and Lange, 1987.

61. Edelman, R., Suskind, R.M., Olsen, R.E., and Sirisinha, S. Mechanisms of defective delayed cutaneous hypersensitivity in children with protein-calorie malnutrition. *Lancet* 1:506, 1973.

62. Neumann, C.G., Lawlor, G.J., Jr., and Stiehm, E.R. Immunologic responses in malnourished children. *Am. J. Clin. Nutr.* 28:89, 1975.

63. Miller, C.L. Immunological assays as measurements of nutritional status. A review. *JPEN* 2:554, 1978.

64. Coombs, R.R.A., and Gell, P.G.H. Classification of allergic reactions responsible for clinical hypersensitivity and disease. In P.G.H. Gell, R.R.A. Coombs, and P.J. Lachman, Eds., *Clinical Aspects of Immunology.* Oxford: Blackwell Scientific, 1975.

65. Fernandes, G., Yunis, E.J., Smith, J., and Good, R.A. Dietary influence on breeding behavior, hemolytic anemia and longevity in NZB mice. *Proc. Soc. Exp. Biol. Med.* 139:1189, 1972.

66. Fernandes, G., Yunis, E.J., and Good, R.A. Diet and immunity of NZB mice. *J. Immunol.* 116:782, 1976.

67. Fernandes, G., Yunis, E.J., and Good, R.A. Influence of diet on survival of mice. *Proc. Natl. Acad. Sci. U.S.A.* 73:79, 1976.

68. Bahna, S.L. The dilemma of pathogenesis and diagnosis of food allergy. *Immunol. Allergy Clin. North Am.* 7:299, 1987.

69. Terr, A.I. Allergic diseases. In D.P. Stites, J.D. Stobo, and J.V. Wells, Eds., *Basic and Clinical Immunology,* 6th ed. Norwalk, Conn.: Appleton and Lange, 1987.

70. Feingold, B. Food additives and child development. *Hosp. Pract.* 8:11, 1973.

71. Palmer, S., Rapport, J.L., and Quinn, P. Food additives and hyperactivity. *Clin. Pediatr.* (Phila.) 14:956, 1975.

72. Breneman, J.C. *Basics of Food Allergy,* 2nd ed. Springfield, Ill: Charles C Thomas, 1984.

73. Walzer, M. Studies in absorption of undigested protein in human beings. *J. Immunol.* 14:143, 1927.

74. Walker, W.A., Isselbacher, K.J., and Block, K.J. Intestinal uptake of macromolecules: Effect of oral immunization. *Science* 177: 608, 1972.

75. Walker, W.A., Wu, M., Isselbacher, K.J., and Bloch, K.J. Intestinal uptake of macromolecules. III. Studies of mechanisms by which immunization interferes with antigen uptake. *J. Immunol.* 115:854, 1975.

76. Walker, W.A. Host defense mechanisms in the gastrointestinal tract. *Pediatrics* 57:901, 1976.

77. Walker, W.A. Antigen absorption from the small intestine and gastrointestinal disease. *Pediatr. Clin. North Am.* 22:731, 1975.

78. Lyon, G.M. Allergy in an infant of three weeks. *Am. J. Dis. Child.* 36:1012, 1928.

79. Miller, D.L., Hirvonen, T., and Gitlin, D. Synthesis of IgE by the human conceptus. *J. Allergy Clin. Immunol.* 52:182, 1973.

80. Singer, A.D., Hobel, C.J., and Heiner, D.C. Evidence for secretory IgA and IgE in utero. *J. Allergy Clin. Immunol.* 53:94, 1974.

81. Matthew, D.J., Taylor, B., Norman, A.P., et al. Prevention of eczema. *Lancet* 1:321, 1977.

82. Donnally, H.H. The question of the elimination of foreign protein (egg white) in woman's milk. *J. Immunol.* 19:15, 1930.

83. Gerrard, J.W., Ed. *Food Allergy: New Perspectives.* Springfield, Ill.: Charles C Thomas, 1980.

84. Baldwin, J. Some observations of the skin and mucous membrane reactions in hay fever. *J. Immunol.* 13:345, 1917.

85. Galant, S.P., Bullock, J., and Frick, O.L. An immunological approach to the diagnosis of food sensitivity. *Clin. Allergy* 3:363, 1973.

86. Bullick, J.D., and Bodenbender, J.G. A simple laboratory aid in diagnosing food allergy. *Ann. Allergy* 28:127, 1970.

87. Chua, Y.Y., Bremner, K., Lakdawalla, N., et al. *In vivo* and *in vitro* correlates of food allergy. *J. Allergy Clin. Immunol.* 58:299, 1976.

88. Chua, Y.Y., Bremner, K., Llobet, J.L., and Collins-Williams, C. Diagnosis of food allergy by radioallergosorbent test. *J. Allergy Clin. Immunol.* 58:477, 1976.

89. Rowe, A.H. *Food Allergy, Its Manifestations and Control and the Elimination Diets.* Springfield, Ill.: Charles C Thomas, 1972.

90. Speer, F., and Dockhorn, R.J. *Allergy and Immunology in Childhood.* Springfield, Ill.: Charles C Thomas, 1973.
91. Bock, S.A., Lee, W.Y., Remigio, L.K., and May, C.D. Studies of hypersensitivity reactions to foods in infants and children. *J. Allergy Clin. Immunol.* 62:327, 1978.
92. Roth, A. Detection of food allergy. *Postgrad. Med.* 32:432, 1962.
93. Beeson, P.B., and Bass, D.A. *The Eosinophil.* Philadelphia: W.B. Saunders, 1977.
94. Bock, S.A., Buckley, J., Holst, A., and May, C.D. Proper use of skin tests with food extracts in diagnosis of hypersensitivity to food in children. *Clin. Allergy* 7:375, 1977.
95. Bahna, S.L., and Heiner, D.C. *Allergies to Milk.* New York: Grune and Stratton, 1980.
96. Rowe, A.H. *Elimination Diets and the Patient's Allergies.* Philadelphia: Lea and Febiger, 1944.
97. Randolph, T.G. Adaptation to specific environmental exposures enhanced by individual susceptibility. In L.D. Dickey, Ed., *Clinical Ecology.* Springfield, Ill.: Charles C Thomas, 1976.
98. Wood, M. *Gourmet Food on a Wheat-Free Diet.* Springfield, Ill.: Charles C Thomas, 1967.
99. Larson, J., and Nugent, B. *Very Basically Yours.* Chicago: Human Ecology Study Group, 1967.
100. Sheedy, C.B., and Keifetz, M. *Cooking for Your Celiac Child.* New York: Dial Press, 1969.
101. Thomas, L.L. *Caring and Cooking for the Allergic Child.* New York: Drake, 1974.
102. Golos, N. *Management of Complex Allergies.* Norwalk, Conn.: New England Foundation of Allergic and Environmental Diseases, 1975.
103. *Baking for People with Food Allergies.* U.S.D.A. Home and Garden Bull. No. 147. Washington, D.C.: U.S. Department of Agriculture, 1976.
104. Schaeffer, E.B., and Strunk, R.C. Special considerations in allergic children. *Immunol. Allergy Clin. North Am.* 7:331, 1987.
105. Tuft, L. *Allergy Management in Clinical Practice.* St. Louis: C.V. Mosby, 1973.
106. Welch, H. Problems of antibiotics in foods as the Food and Drug Administration sees them. *Am. J. Public Health* 47:701, 1957.
107. Lockey, S.D. Hypersensitivity to tartrazine (FD&C Yellow No. 5) and other dyes and additives present in foods and pharmaceutical products. *Ann. Allergy* 38:206, 1977.

Bibliography

Bowry, T.R. *Immunology Simplified.* Oxford: Oxford University Press, 1984.

Chandra, R.K., Ed. *Food Intolerance.* New York: Elsevier, 1984.

Chandra, R.K. Immunodeficiency in undernutrition and overnutrition. *Nutr. Rev.* 39:225, 1981.

Chandra, R.K., and Newberne, P.M. *Nutrition, Immunity and Infection.* New York: Plenum Press, 1977.

Elwood, P.C. Nutrition and immunology (symposium). *Proc. Nutr. Soc.* 35:253, 1976.

Gershwin, M.E., Black, R.S., and Hurley, L.S. *Nutrition and Immunity.* Orlando, Fla.: Academic Press, 1985.

Grieco, M.H., Ed. *Infections in the Abnormal Host.* New York: Yorke Medical, 1980.

Holborow, E.J., and Reeves, W.G., Eds. *Immunology in Medicine,* 2nd ed. London: Grune and Stratton, 1983.

Kaplan, A.P., Ed. *Allergy.* New York: Churchill Livingstone, 1985.

Kimball, J.W. *Introduction to Immunology,* 2nd ed. New York: Macmillan, 1986.

Lessof, M.H., Ed. *Allergy: Immunological and Clinical Aspects.* Chichester: Wiley, 1985.

Phillips, M., and Baetz, A. Diet and Resistance to Disease. *Adv. Exp. Med. Biol.* 135:1981.

Playfair, J.H.L. *Immunology at a Glance.* Oxford: Blackwell Scientific, 1979.

Speer, F. *Food Allergy.* Boston: PSG, 1983.

Stinnett, J.D. *Nutrition and the Immune Response.* Boca Raton, Fla.: CRC Press, 1983.

Zeman, F.J., and Ney, D.M. *Applications of Clinical Nutrition.* Englewood Cliffs, N.J.: Prentice-Hall, 1988.

Sources of Current Information

American Journal of Clinical Nutrition
Annals of Allergy
Immunology and Allergy Clinics in North America
Journal of Allergy and Clinical Immunology
Journal of Immunology
Journal of Pediatrics
Nutrition Research

7. The Oral Cavity, Esophagus, and Stomach

I. Components of the Alimentary Tract

II. The Oral Cavity
  A. Normal anatomy and physiology
    1. Teeth and mastication
    2. Salivary glands and salivation
    3. Swallowing
  B. Abnormalities of the oral cavity
    1. Effects of malnutrition on oral tissues
    2. Dental diseases
      a. dental caries
      b. acute gingivitis and stomatitis
      c. periodontal disease
      d. the edentulous patient
    3. Jaw surgery
    4. Other problems in chewing and swallowing
    5. Abnormalities of salivary gland function
    6. Loss of taste sensation
  C. Effect of aging on the oral cavity

III. The Esophagus
  A. Normal anatomy and physiology
  B. Esophageal disease
    1. Dysphagia and odynophagia
    2. Disorders of the lower esophageal sphincter
      a. achalasia
      b. stricture of the esophagus
      c. lower esophageal sphincter incompetence
    3. Esophagitis
    4. Replacement of the esophagus

IV. The Stomach
  A. Normal anatomy and physiology
    1. Secretion
    2. Storage and motility
    3. Digestion
  B. Nausea and vomiting
  C. Peptic ulcer disease
    1. Sites of ulcers
    2. Occurrence
    3. Pathogenesis
    4. Clinical manifestations
    5. Treatment
      a. conservative management
      b. surgical treatment
        (1) procedures
        (2) postoperative nutrition
        (3) complications

V. Case Studies

The alimentary tract obviously is of central importance to the maintenance of adequate nutrition. It follows that malfunctions of this system will affect the patient's nutritional status, and so nutritional care specialists have an important role in the management of these conditions.

COMPONENTS OF THE ALIMENTARY TRACT

The components of the alimentary tract and the anatomic relationships to other organs important to digestion are shown in Figure 7-1. Throughout much of its length, the digestive tract has a similar form, which is illustrated in Figure 7-2. The innermost layer, the **mucosa**, consists of three parts, a layer of epithelium supported by an underlying, richly vascularized connective tissue and a thin smooth muscle layer, the **muscularis mucosa**. The next layer, the **submucosa**, is composed of dense connective tissue containing larger blood vessels and a network of nerve cells and their processes called **Meissner's plexus**. The third layer, the **muscle layer**, consists of an inner circular muscle and an outer longitudinal muscle. Another network of nerves, the **myenteric** or **Auerbach's plexus**, lies between them. An outer **serosal layer**, primarily made of connective tissue, surrounds the gastrointestinal tract for most of its length.

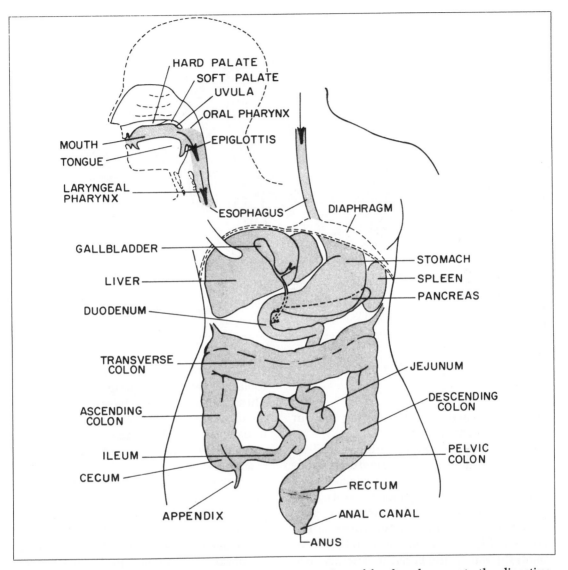

Figure 7-1. The parts of the digestive system. (Reprinted with permission from Ham, A.W., and Cormack, D.H., Histology, 9th ed. Philadelphia: J.B. Lippincott, 1987, p. 476.)

THE ORAL CAVITY

Normal Anatomy and Physiology

The oral cavity consists of the **mouth** and the **pharynx**, a funnel-shaped organ which moves food from the mouth to the esophagus. It is obvious that the primary function of the oral cavity is to provide an opening for ingestion of food and access to the digestive and absorptive organs. Although the oral cavity is simple in concept, it contains many tissues which exist in a complex relationship: teeth, gums (gingival tissue), tongue, taste buds, palate, salivary glands, mucous membranes, and alveolar (jaw) bones.

Teeth and Mastication

The teeth are the major structures for **mastication** (chewing), which reduces food to a size appropriate for swallowing. The tongue also functions in dividing food, by mashing it

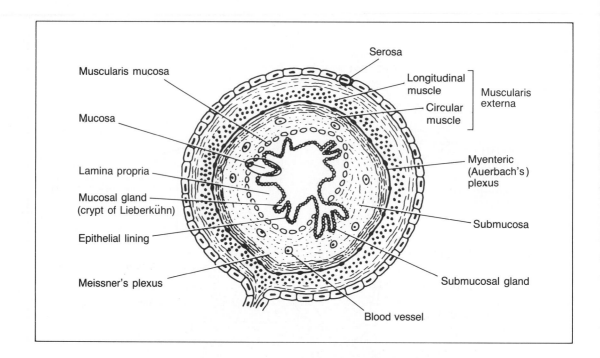

Figure 7-2. General organization of the gastrointestinal tract.

against the palate and by moving food in place for chewing.

The teeth consist of four parts (Figure 7-3). The **enamel**, **dentin**, and **cementum** are calcified tissues. The **pulp** is uncalcified connective tissue containing blood vessels, lymphatics, and nerves that transmit pain sensations only. The enamel, covering the **crown** or exposed portion of the teeth, is the hardest tissue in the body. It contains 96% inorganic matter, mostly hydroxyapatite crystals $(Ca_{10}[PO_4]_6[OH]_2)$, an acid-soluble salt.

The dentin, lying immediately beneath the enamel, is the main component of the teeth. It is similar to bone in composition, containing 10% water, 20% organic matter, and 70% inorganic matter. The organic matter forms a matrix into which the hydroxyapatite is deposited. Dentin does not have a blood supply but is traversed by dentin tubules, a series of microscopic channels coursing through the dentin from the pulp to the enamel. These tubules may have a nutri-

tional function. Dentin is formed by odontoblasts located at the periphery of the pulp. These cells continue to have the capacity to make dentin so that, in a protective response to damage, they form dentin on the border between the pulp cavity and root canal, narrowing the root canal.

Cementum is very much like bone in composition, with 45% inorganic matter. It is deposited in layers over the dentin of the **root** of the tooth and is the site of the attachment of the **periodontal ligament** (or periodontal membrane) that anchors the tooth to the surrounding bone.

The maxilla (upper jaw bone) and the mandible (lower jaw bone) each have a thick projecting ridge called the **alveolar process**, containing sockets or alveoli, one for each tooth. The periodontal ligament extends from the alveolar process into the cementum to hold the tooth firmly in place. In addition to these supporting structures, the **gingiva** surrounds and is attached to the root of each tooth. Near the top of the gingiva, there is a gingival crevice or **sulcus** between it and the tooth. This is a matter of importance in dental disease. The supporting structures sur-

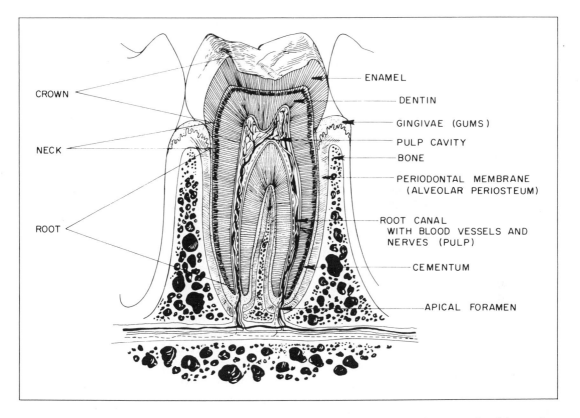

CROWN

NECK

ROOT

ENAMEL

DENTIN

GINGIVAE (GUMS)

PULP CAVITY

BONE

PERIODONTAL MEMBRANE
(ALVEOLAR PERIOSTEUM)

ROOT CANAL
WITH BLOOD VESSELS AND
NERVES (PULP)

CEMENTUM

APICAL FORAMEN

Figure 7-3. Longitudinal section of a molar tooth in its alveolus. (Reprinted with permission from Crouch, J.E., Functional Human Anatomy, *4th ed. Philadelphia: Lea & Febiger, 1985, p. 463.)*

rounding the teeth — the cementum, periodontal ligament, alveolar bone, and gingiva — are known collectively as the **periodontium**.

Salivary Glands and Salivation

The salivary glands consist of three pairs of major glands, the parotid, submandibular, and sublingual glands, and numerous minor (buccal) glands. The parotid glands secrete a **serous** (watery) saliva containing α-amylase (ptyalin), and the sublingual glands, a more **mucous** material which serves primarily as a lubricant.[1] Submandibular secretion is intermediate.

The functions of saliva are digestive or protective and include the following:

1. Moistening and lubricating food for easier swallowing.
2. Holding particles together for easier swallowing.
3. Acting as a buffer (salivary pH is approximately 6.8).
4. Beginning digestion of starch by action of salivary amylase (ptyalin), which continues until stopped by the low pH of the stomach.
5. Promoting some remineralization of the teeth.
6. Enhancing taste by dissolving and washing away food particles on taste buds so the person can taste the next food eaten.
7. Dissolving and washing away food particles between the teeth.
8. Facilitating speech.

Thus malfunction can cause a variety of problems.

The main components of saliva are water, electrolytes (sodium, potassium, chloride, and bicarbonate), enzymes, and other proteins. Potassium and bicarbonate concentrations are high compared to plasma, but the saliva is approximately 50% hypoosmotic. During sleep, saliva secretion is barely perceptible; maximum output may equal 4 ml/min. The usual daily secretion has been estimated to be between 0.5 and 1.5 liters, but others estimate 500 to 600 ml/day.[2] Salivation is reduced by fear, anxiety, and dehydration, and stimulated by smell, taste, or chewing of food. Acidic foods are particularly effective in stimulation. Their effects are mediated via parasympathetic and sympathetic nerves. Hormones have little effect.[1] The high volume and high potassium content are important considerations in patients who have had head or neck surgery and whose saliva is draining externally. In these patients, careful replacement of fluid volume and of electrolytes is needed.

The volume of salivary secretion is controlled by the autonomic nervous system. As a consequence, surgery or trauma in which the nerves are severed has a severe effect on the amount of saliva produced. There is no known hormonal control of salivary volume, but its composition is under both nervous and hormonal control.[1,3]

Swallowing

The act of swallowing or **deglutition** is a process in which related actions of the structures of the mouth, pharynx, and esophagus are carefully integrated (Figure 7-4). The figure legend describes the sequence of events and should be studied carefully.

Abnormalities of the Oral Cavity

Effects of Malnutrition on Oral Tissues

The teeth initially form in the jaws by differentiation of specialized oral epithelial cells. These eventually form an organic matrix beginning at the top of the crown and proceeding toward the root. Calcification closely follows in similar fashion. The earliest differentiation of epithelium occurs in the seven-week embryo. Calcification in the primary teeth begins at four months' gestation and usually ends at 20 to 24 months of age

postnatally. Eruption of primary teeth begins at six to nine months and usually is complete at three years of age. The formation of the organic matrix and calcification of the permanent teeth are almost entirely postnatal, beginning at birth. The process extends to approximately age 25, when the third molar is complete.

From the fourth fetal month to 25 years of age, then, the forming teeth are vulnerable to various insults. The effect of nutrition during pregnancy on tooth development in the fetus has not been studied thoroughly. It appears that a nutritional deficiency must be severe before effects are obvious. The possibility remains, however, that milder deficiencies may cause subtle changes that alter the structure of the teeth and make them more vulnerable to decay.[4] Although the cause of many dental defects is unknown, there is some evidence that deficiencies of vitamins A or D, calcium, or phosphorus, or an imbalance in the calcium-phosphorus ratio interferes with normal development of the teeth.[5]

In experimental animals, prenatal nutritional deficiencies contribute to the incidence of cleft lip, cleft palate, retarded development of salivary glands, and other congenital anomalies.[6] Of course, it is not possible to demonstrate this experimentally in human infants; therefore, the effects in humans are unknown.

After a tooth erupts, it apparently undergoes a maturation process during which its metabolism is different from that of a mature tooth. Saliva may influence the maturation process, but the mechanism is unknown. We do not know whether malnutrition can cause changes in the amount or composition of saliva that could, in turn, affect maturation of the teeth. It does seem clear, however, that the erupted tooth is not so metabolically inert as was once believed.

Nutritional deficiencies are associated with several nonspecific conditions in the oral cavity. These include **gingivitis** (inflammation of the gingivae), **stomatitis** (inflammation of the oral mucosa), **glossitis** (inflammation of the tongue), and **cheilosis** (fissuring and scaling at the angle of the mouth). Their relationship to nutritional deficiency is described in many basic texts on normal nutrition. The nutritional care specialists should be alert to the possibility of oral disease in patients at risk of malnutrition, but it is equally important to realize that, since these conditions are nonspecific, they also occur as a result of nonnutritional factors. Their presence alone does not prove the existence of malnutrition.

*Figure 7-4. Oral and pharyngeal events during swallowing. **A.** The bolus (F) to be swallowed is propelled into the pharynx by placement of the tongue (T) on the roof of the hard palate. **B.** Further propulsion is caused by movement of more distal regions of the tongue against the palate. Contraction of the upper constrictors of the pharynx and movement of the soft palate separate the oral pharynx from the nasopharynx. **C.** Propulsion through the upper esophageal sphincter is accomplished by contraction of the middle and lower constrictors of the pharynx and by relaxation of the cricopharyngeal muscle. Upward movement of the glottis and downward movement of the epiglottis (Ep) seals off the trachea (Tr). **D.** The bolus is now in the esophagus (E) and is propelled into the stomach by a peristaltic contraction. (Reprinted with permission from Weisbrodt, N.W., Esophageal motility. In L.R. Johnson, Ed., Gastrointestinal Physiology, 3rd ed. St. Louis: C.V. Mosby, 1985, p. 24.)*

Dental Diseases

The diseases described in this section can occur in people who are otherwise in good health. They also appear as a complication of existing illnesses and may seriously limit food intake, with a consequent detrimental effect on the patient's nutritional status. The nutritional care specialist must be alert to the possibility of dental disease in patients with unrelated diseases.

There are three types of materials that react with the teeth and supporting tissue and are particularly important in the etiology of dental disease. **Enamel pellicle** is a thin film that adheres to the teeth immediately after cleaning. It is believed to be formed by

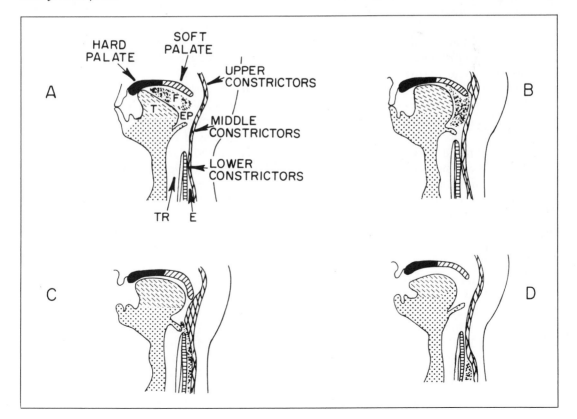

the conversion of glycoproteins in saliva into adhesive polymers by oral bacteria. **Dental plaque** is a sticky, gelatinous material that adheres to the pellicle. It consists of epithelial cells, leukocytes, and bacteria such as *Streptococcus mutans, Streptococcus sanguis,* and *lactobacilli.* The bacterial population varies with the location and age of the plaque, which must be removed mechanically. Plaque should not be confused with food debris. **Dental calculus** is believed to result from mineralization of plaque with minerals from saliva and from fluid in the gingival crevice.

Dental Caries. Dental caries, or tooth decay, refers to the destruction of the enamel, dentin, and sometimes, cementum. It has been reported to be present in 99% of adults by the age of 50. More recently, a 40–60% reduction in the incidence of caries has occurred in the teen-age population. These effects are reported to be the consequence of fluoride in the mouth from fluoridated water and the use of fluoridated dentifrices.[7,8] In another 20%, there is a continuing high decay activity. In the adult population, decay continues to be a problem. The simultaneous presence, over time, of three factors — a susceptible tooth, cariogenic bacteria, and substrates for bacterial action — is considered to be necessary to the **cariogenic** (caries-forming) process.

Conditions in the host that produce susceptible teeth are not entirely understood. The effect of nutrition during gestation may be one of these factors.[9] Nutrients secreted into saliva or entering the tooth via its blood supply may affect resistance to decay in the erupted tooth. These factors need additional study before their role in increasing caries susceptibility can be understood completely.

Cariogenic bacteria, the second requirement for decay, act on monosaccharides or disaccharides, which are the third requirement. Several actions of bacteria may be involved in caries formation. The organism *Streptococcus mutans* is able to synthesize a polysaccharide of glucose, **dextran**, from dietary sucrose. This dextran serves as a matrix that enables the organism to colonize and form plaque on the tooth surface. Various organisms then act on monosaccharides and disaccharides, producing acids that can decalcify the teeth when pH drops from 7.0 to 5.0–5.5 in 15 to 60 minutes.[10]

Because they result in greatest acid formation, the most cariogenic foods are those that are sweet and sticky and tend to adhere to the teeth. Caries formation is influenced also by the frequency of eating. The intake of cariogenic foods at frequent intervals is thought to be more damaging than eating the same amount all at one time.

Some diseases frequently are associated with caries formation, and good nutritional care for these patients includes procedures for caries prevention, combining diet, oral hygiene, and fluoridation. The diet should be adequate, with the preponderance of the carbohydrate in the form of starch rather than sugar. "Sticky" foods should be avoided. Repetitive snacking, especially of refined sugar, resulting in multiple exposures of the teeth to cariogenic foods, should be avoided. Noncariogenic sweeteners have been suggested, but their systemic effects are as yet unknown.

Fluoridation is of most benefit when the teeth are being calcified. It is provided in the drinking water in some communities, at a concentration of 1 mg/L, or 1 ppm. It sometimes is provided in tablets or drops at 0.5 to 1.0 mg/day, in topical gels "painted" on by dentists, or in fluoride-containing mouthwashes and dentifrices. As saliva flows over demineralized teeth, calcium, phosphorus, and fluoride may diffuse back into the tooth and regrow into the carious lesion. This remineralization may be more resistant to further attack if fluoride is available. Thus saliva and fluoride both have a protective effect on the teeth.[11-13]

Rampant caries, extensive caries that worsen rapidly, occur as a complication of other illnesses. The patient requires nutritional management, since rampant caries causes pain and tooth loss. The patient may decrease chewing and swallowing as a result of the pain, thus contributing to nutritional deficiency. It sometimes is necessary to provide the patient with a soft diet to reduce discomfort during an extended period of dental repair. Patients should also be instructed in diet modifications for prevention of future caries.

The **nursing bottle syndrome**, or **bottle caries syndrome**, is another severe problem requiring preventive action. It occurs in young children who habitually are allowed to fall asleep while sucking on a nursing bottle containing fruit juice or a milk formula sweetened with glucose or sucrose. Sucking, swallowing, and salivation decrease during sleep. The liquid then remains in the mouth, and lactic acid formed from the carbohydrate is increased. The acid in fruit juices also contributes to the acidity. The result is extensive decay and loss of many of the primary teeth. There is some evidence that the milk-saliva mixture from such a formula actually prevents decalcification of the teeth.[14] On the other hand, lactose is thought by some to contribute to the decay process. To prevent this syndrome, children should not be put to bed with a bottle. If doing so cannot be avoided, parents are advised that water may be used more safely.

Acute Gingivitis and Stomatitis. **Gingivitis** and **stomatitis** occur as side effects of many other diseases and also can be a consequence of emotional stress. The conditions are seen in mild form in many persons, but gingivitis occasionally occurs in a severe form called **acute necrotizing ulcerative gingivitis** (trench mouth, or Vincent's gingivitis). The direct cause is an infectious organism, but emotional stress, hormone changes, and abnormal diet habits have been implicated as contributing factors.

Early clinical manifestations of gingivitis include easily bleeding gums, a bad taste in the mouth, and fetid breath. The gingivae are red, swollen, and tender. In severe disease, the papillae become ulcerated and necrotic, and the patient suffers from malaise,

fever, and serious loss of appetite. The condition makes the mouth susceptible to colonization by other bacteria and predisposes the patient to periodontitis.

Food intake in the patient with gingivitis may be decreased because of pain, presenting a problem in nutritional care. The patient is given a high-protein, high-calorie liquid diet until the condition of the tissues improves. Then the diet is progressed to a soft diet, taking care to avoid spicy or acidic foods, and later, to a relatively unrestricted diet as tolerated. Vitamin supplements sometimes are necessary. Some patients with severe disease need a pain-relieving mouthwash before eating.

Periodontal Disease. Periodontal disease has been estimated to occur in approximately 65 million adults in the United Sates and to cause loss of teeth in approximately 20 million. It occurs most often in the elderly but is not necessarily related to age; it has been known to begin in children. Periodontal disease tends to occur especially often in patients who are mouth-breathers, or who have diabetes, leukemia, hyperparathyroidism, or hypoparathyroidism. Other factors that contribute to periodontal disease include faulty restorations, missing teeth, misalignment, malocclusion, and the use of tobacco.

It is believed to be a bacterial infection that results in a breakdown of the supporting structures of the teeth. The etiology usually is poor oral hygiene resulting in accumulated plaque and calculus. The gingivae adhere less well to the teeth, and pockets form in which debris collects, causing irritation. The inflammation then spreads into the supporting tissue, resulting in extensive bone resorption and loss of teeth.

The role of nutrition in the etiology of periodontal disease is complex and poorly understood. Squamous epithelium lining the gingival sulcus has a very high turnover rate, being renewed every three to seven days.[15] This fact suggests that gingival tissue is very sensitive to malnutrition. Although periodontal disease is not a primary deficiency disease, the progress of the disease may be affected by the patient's nutritional status via its effect on the patient's immune defenses and on metabolism of oral supporting tissue.[9,16] It is frequently suggested that a 1 : 1 calcium-phosphorus ratio is helpful.[9]

For periodontal disease, the primary preventive measure is removal of plaque, but diet may serve a supporting role. Patients often are advised to reduce the frequency of their intake of fermentable carbohydrates and increase their use of firm fibrous foods, such as raw fruits and vegetables. Fibrous foods are believed to provide stimulation to soft tissue, cleanse the teeth, decrease calculus formation, reduce salivary atrophy, and increase salivary flow rates and protein content of saliva. However, the effectiveness of fibrous foods in prevention of periodontal disease has not been documented adequately.[16]

Good nutrition also contributes to the control of periodontal disease by maintaining normal immune function.[16] There is a constant migration of leukocytes through the gingival epithelium into the gingival crevice. Some of the products of their metabolism may be irritants or a source of nutrients to bacteria. On the other hand, leukocytes also provide antibacterial agents such as lysozyme, complement, and antibodies. Generally, it is believed that the gingival fluid is more protective than damaging, but the effect of nutrition on its composition is unknown.[16]

Nutritional care in the treatment of patients with existing periodontal disease consists primarily of the same procedures described for patients with severe gingivitis.

The Edentulous Patient. Several studies have shown a high incidence of nutritional deficiencies in patients who have no teeth or serviceable dentures or in whom the number and location of teeth are inadequate.[17,18] The condition has been called **masticatory insufficiency**.

Patients who have lost part or all of their teeth may have difficulties with closure of the jaw and with chewing and swallowing. As a result, they may choose soft, low-fiber foods of limited variety and amount. The danger of nutrient deficiency thereby is increased. Those who have dentures sometimes have problems adjusting to the dentures and may respond in similar fashion. Both groups should be monitored for vitamin and mineral status. Bran and wheat germ sometimes are added to the diet to provide fiber until the dental problems are corrected and the patient has adjusted to wearing dentures.

Hospitalized elderly patients sometimes have dentures that are ill-fitting secondary to weight loss. The nutritional care specialist should modify the diet as necessary and attempt to promote weight gain to achieve normal weight in such patients.

Jaw Surgery

A number of patients have surgery of the jaw following injury or disease. Other patients elect to have reconstructive surgery on their jaws. In either case, immobilization of the jaw (maxillomandibular fixation) for five to eight weeks is common, and patients thus require nutritional support.[19] A weight loss of 10% of body weight is common.[20] Thus these patients need nutritional counseling and monitoring of nutritional status, including intake.

The diet may consist of liquids, soups, baby foods, and blenderized regular foods. Nonfat dry milk may be added to these foods. The patient may also need to have formula feedings such as those listed in Appendix G. An increase in the number of meals may also be helpful, as well as vitamin and mineral supplements.

Other Problems in Chewing and Swallowing

Chewing and swallowing can be affected by surgical resection of the tongue, palate, or facial muscles, or by severing the nerves that control these structures. For these patients, it may be necessary to provide all nutrients in liquid form. The types of products and formulations that can be used for this purpose are described in Chapter 19.

Some patients develop a fear of eating (**sitophobia**), because they have pain or discomfort when they eat. This can occur with inflammation, ulceration, or structural defects in the oral cavity or esophagus. Sometimes medication for pain is provided just before meals. In addition, the following procedures may be helpful to modify the diet to the tolerance of the patient:

1. Avoid foods with high acid, salt, or spice content.
2. Avoid very hot foods.
3. Use cold foods if well tolerated. (These may be irritating to some patients.)
4. Use very moist, smooth foods; include liquids with meals.
5. Avoid very dry foods.

Abnormalities of Salivary Gland Function

The symptoms of salivary gland dysfunction are limited in number: swelling, pain, dryness of the mouth (**xerostomia**), and taste abnormalities. These are not the result of primary disease of salivary glands, but rather are secondary to other diseases and their treatment. Nutritional care is important, because these symptoms often cause a decrease in food intake.

A bad taste is most commonly the result of inflammatory conditions in which pus is produced in the mouth. Xerostomia may be the result of mouth-breathing, advanced age, or a number of systemic conditions. A classification of causes of xerostomia is given in Table 7-1, and drugs that induce xerostomia as a side effect are listed in Table 7-2. Nutritional care of patients with xerostomia primarily involves procedures to maintain moisture in the mouth. A glycerin-and-lemon mouthwash often is provided to the patients, and they are advised to increase their fluid intake. In severe cases, an artificial saliva may be used to maintain comfort and promote remineralization of the teeth.[21] Car-

Table 7-1. Etiology of Xerostomia—Classification and Examples

Factors affecting the salivary center
Emotions (fear, excitement, depression, etc.)
Neuroses (endogenous depression)
Organic disease (brain tumor)
Drugs (see Table 7-2)
Factors affecting the autonomic outflow pathway
Encephalitis
Brain tumors
Accidents
Neurosurgical operations
Drugs (see Table 7-2)
Factors affecting salivary gland function
Aplasia
Sjögren's syndrome
Obstruction
Infection
Irradiation
Excision
Factors producing changes in fluid or electrolyte balance
Dehydration
Diabetes insipidus
Cardiac failure
Uremia
Edema

Reprinted with permission from Mason, D.K., and Chisholm, D.M., *Salivary Glands in Health and Disease*. London: W.B. Saunders, 1973, p. 120.

Table 7-2. Classes of Drugs with Xerostomic Side Effects

Analgesic mixtures
Anticonvulsants
Antiemetics
Antihistamines
Antihypertensives
Antinauseants
Antiparkinsonism agents
Antipruritics
Antispasmodics
Appetite suppressants
Cold medications
Decongestants
Diuretics
Expectorants
Muscle relaxants
Psychotropic drugs
    Central nervous system depressants
    Benzodiazepine derivatives
    Monoamine oxidase inhibitors
    Phenothiazine derivatives
    Tranquilizers—major and minor
Sedatives

Reprinted with permission from Bahn, S.L., Drug-related dental destruction. *Oral Surg.* 33:49, 1972.

bohydrate solutions are useful to stimulate salivation but should be recommended only for patients who are edentulous. Xerostomia predisposes the individual to dental caries, since saliva, which has a protective effect on the teeth, is lacking.

It is important to provide adequate nutrition at all times in salivary gland disease. The patient's preferences should be catered to as much as possible.

Loss of Taste Sensation

A description of the anatomic basis for taste sensations and a list of drugs that alter taste sensations and the acceptability of foods are included in Chapter 4. Changes in metabolism and the anatomy in the head area may result in alteration in taste. The palate is most sensitive to bitter and sour. Flavors including these components are altered in patients with upper dentures that cover the palate, with tumors of the palate, or in whom the palate has been surgically removed. Patients with Turner's syndrome, a chromosomal disorder, have highly arched palates and diminished taste perception. Diseases of the tongue may also affect the sense of taste. Some examples are abnormalities affecting the nerves of the tongue, as in Bell's palsy and neuritis, surgical resection of the nerves, and tumors of the tongue. In addition, patients receiving irradiation treatment to the mouth have a decreased sense of taste. Some nervous system conditions, such as multiple sclerosis and head injuries, can have a similar effect. Various metabolic abnormalities altering the sense of taste are listed in Table 4-3.

Since smell and taste interact to a great extent in producing flavor sensations, injury to olfactory nerves or lobes, as from whiplash injury, fracture of the nose, or brain injury, can cause temporary or permanent impairment of olfactory sensation. This may erroneously be perceived by the patient as "taste" impairment.

The nutritional care specialist must be understanding of the problems of lost taste sensation and provide individualized attention to these patients. The patient's preferences should be considered in planning meals. Seasonings may be increased or decreased to conform with the patient's preference in order to make foods more acceptable. Heat tends to increase the sensation of flavor, and cold, to decrease it; flavorings and seasonings should be added with these facts in mind. The sense of taste sometimes varies during the day. If so, the patient can be expected to prefer to eat larger meals when the sense of taste is impaired the least.

Effect of Aging on the Oral Cavity

In the aged, the tongue tends to lose its papillae, and the number of taste bud cells declines, with a consequent decrease in the sense of taste.[22] Both taste bud cells and olfactory receptors are replaced frequently; they have average life spans of 10 days and 30 days, respectively. Structural changes in the taste system and olfactory system in the brain have been observed in the aged.[23] The sense of smell declines, and it has been shown that the aged have a decreased ability to identify tastes.[23] As a result, contrary to common belief, many aging patients find that highly seasoned foods are more acceptable. Enhancement with artificial flavors has been recommended.[23]

Also in elderly patients, the mucous membrane becomes thinner and more susceptible to injury. Consequently, patients may choose soft, easily chewed foods that do not adequately stimulate gingival circulation or saliva flow. At the same time, the cells in the salivary glands atrophy, causing a decrease in salivation and a change in saliva composition. The deficiency of saliva contributes to a dry mucosa and difficulties in chewing and swallowing. Patients may be advised to chew moist foods and sugarless gum to stimulate saliva flow. Lemons also stimulate saliva flow. Patients should be counseled on food choices to meet nutritional needs within the limits of the textures that they can tolerate.

Aging patients sometimes have teeth that are worn and shortened, producing overclosure of the jaws with pain and limitation of jaw movement. For them, a reduction in the intake of very hard foods may be helpful.

THE ESOPHAGUS

Normal Anatomy and Physiology

The esophagus is a tube that carries foods from the pharynx to the stomach. Its structure is similar to that of the intestine, which is shown in Figure 7-2, except that the esophagus has no mesentery or serosa. The mucosa does not absorb as it does in some parts of the alimentary tract.

The **upper esophageal sphincter** (UES) remains closed except during swallowing, preventing the flow of air into the esophagus and into the stomach. At the lower end of the esophagus, there is no obvious sphincter muscle present, but a few centimeters above the entrance of the esophagus into the stomach, the muscle structure functions as if it were a sphincter and therefore is referred to in the literature as the **lower esophageal sphincter** (LES). The LES normally remains contracted, closing the entrance to the stomach and preventing reflux of the stomach contents into the lower esophagus. It opens when swallowed material reaches the bottom of the esophagus, allowing the bolus of material to enter the stomach. Defects of function of the LES may arise from alterations in the smooth muscle, in the innervations of the muscle, or in its hormonal control. The interrelationships of hormone action and sphincter pressure are controversial. Gastrin has a major effect in increasing LES pressure.[24-26] Hormones decreasing pressure include secretin,[27,28] cholecystokinin,[29,30] and glucagon.[31]

The LES contains many drug receptors.[32] Peppermint,[33] spearmint, chocolate,[34] alcohol,[35] and fats,[36] including fat in whole milk, reduces LES pressure. The methylxanthines caffeine and theophylline, contained in cof-fee and tea, have been reported to increase LES pressure by inhibiting phosphodiesterase and thus increasing intracellular concentrations of cyclic adenosine monophosphate in the LES,[37] whereas other reports state that theophylline decreases LES pressure and caffeine has no effect.[36] Coffee is reported to have an effect different from that of pure caffeine. Both caffeinated and decaffeinated coffees were found to cause increased LES pressure in one study.[38] Therefore, some unknown substance in coffee may cause the increase. The mode of action of the carminatives peppermint and spearmint is unknown but is thought to be a local effect.

Since the intake and action of caffeine and related compounds is of concern in several diseases, relevant facts on these substances are outlined in Appendix F.

Esophageal Disease

Disorders of the esophagus compromise the ability to swallow, affecting the ability to consume food. Thus they place the patient at nutritional risk.

Dysphagia and Odynophagia

Dysphagia (difficulty in swallowing) is a complex problem that may be classified in a variety of ways. It may vary in severity from inability to swallow pills or a tendency to drool to the inability to swallow anything including their own saliva without aspirating. The term does *not* include pain. It is not invariably a primary disease of the esophagus, but it will be discussed here for convenience.

The process of swallowing involves oral, pharyngeal, and esophageal phases. Only the oral phase is voluntary, while the others are controlled by reflexes. While the symptoms may localize in any of these tissues, the basic cause may be far removed. Table 7-3 provides a list of conditions which can result in swallowing disorders.

Swallowing involves a sophisticated integration of the function of the nerves and

Table 7-3. Conditions Possibly Leading to Swallowing Disorders

Mechanical disorders (dysphagia for solids greater than for liquids)
Surgical resection or alteration of one or more organs of swallowing necessitated by cancer (intrinsic or extrinsic), trauma, developmental anomalies
Trauma to esophagus with development of internal scar tissue
Inelasticity resulting from repeated inflammation
Development of esophageal ring or web
Tumor in esophagus or adjacent tissue
Aneurysms of aorta
Neuromuscular disorders
Brain stem lesions, cerebral vascular accident, brain tumors
Head injury
Parkinsonism
Bulbar poliomyelitis
Amyotrophic lateral sclerosis
Huntington's chorea
Multiple sclerosis
Diabetic enteropathy
Botulism
Diphtheria
Tetanus
Alcoholic neuropathy
Amyloidosis
Myxedema
Thyrotoxicosis
Dermatomyositis (inflammation of skin, subcutaneous tissue, muscle)
Myotonic dystrophy (stiffening and atrophy of muscles, especially in head and neck)
Myasthenia gravis (progressive paralysis)
Scleroderma
Achalasia
Alcoholic neuropathy

muscles as indicated in Figure 7-4. Even if mechanical disorders, including obstructions, are absent, a wide variety of conditions of the neuromuscular system can lead to swallowing disorders.

Symptoms of dysphagia include drooling, food retention in the mouth, coughing and choking after swallowing, a feeling of a "lump in the throat," frequent throat clearing, and a change in voice quality. Dysphagia may also be characterized by weak or uncoordinated muscles in the mouth, pharynx, or esophagus, and by motor or sensory defects which interfere with chewing or swallowing. Other warning signs include confused mental state, weight loss, and pneumonia. Pain (**odynophagia**) may be present, related to

infections, neoplasms, or mechanical obstructions, but not to dysphagia of central-nervous-system origin.[39] It is not easily distinguishable from coronary artery disease.

The full evaluation of the dysphagia patient requires the participation of a team of health professionals that includes physicians (possibly surgeon, neurologist, ear-nose-throat specialist, radiologist), speech pathologist, nurse, nutritional care specialist, occupational therapist, and physical therapist. The nutritional assessment will include the procedures described in Chapter 3 as well as the following items, which are sometimes obtained directly or from the medical record:

- Medications
- Respiratory status
- Handedness
- Dentition
- Mental alertness, cooperation, emotional state
- Nasal and oral regurgitation
- Pain
- Fatigue
- Reflex and voluntary behaviors, e.g., gag, cough, bite
- Primitive or abnormal reflexes
- Difficulty with liquids, solids
- Facial expression

Cooperation with the speech pathologist is useful in gathering and evaluating this information.

In testing ability to swallow, it is necessary to be certain the patient is able to cough and that personnel necessary in case of aspiration are available. A material may be used initially which is relatively safe if only partially aspirated. A spoonful of crushed ice has been recommended.[39] If successful, this may be followed by a "training period" in which the patient relearns the swallowing process. The positioning of the patient in an upright position is important. Foods used may progress from soft foods such as pudding, custard, gelatin, or ice cream to thickened liquids and then to thinned purees. The next step involving chewable foods might provide diced canned fruits, soft cooked vegetables, and macaroni. Further information on these procedures is contained in Chapter 19.

In summary, the function of the nutritional care specialist in the process can include the following:

1. Consultation concerning the consistency of food.
2. Provision of a variety of foods acceptable to the patient.
3. Recommendations concerning needs for tube feeding or parenteral nutrition (see Chapter 5).
4. Monitoring nutritional status (see Chapter 5).

Disorders of the Lower Esophageal Sphincter

Some special considerations apply for patients with disorders of the LES.

Achalasia. **Achalasia**, also known as **cardiospasm**, is a condition in which the lower esophageal sphincter maintains an excessively high tone while resting and fails to open properly when the patient swallows. In addition, peristalsis in the upper esophagus often is disordered. As a result, the esophagus becomes shaped like a funnel or bag. Symptoms include dysphagia, a feeling of fullness in the chest, and frequent vomiting. The patient loses weight and becomes seriously malnourished if the condition remains uncorrected. Aspiration during the night may lead to pulmonary infection.

At one time, the condition was considered to be emotional in origin. However, there is some evidence that achalasia patients have fewer ganglion cells than normal in the myenteric plexus and vagus nerves.[40] In addition, these ganglion cells are surrounded by inflammatory cells, suggesting a physiologic basis for the condition. A viral agent may be responsible.

Treatment consists of dilating the LES with an air-filled or water-filled bag or partially slitting the muscle surgically (**esopha-** **gomyotomy**). These treatments improve the symptoms of obstruction but do not correct the deficit in peristalsis.

Nutritional care is particularly important in the period prior to dilation or surgical treatment. The major change is usually in the consistency of the diet. Semisolid or liquid foods often are tolerated best, since peristalsis is not required for fluids to move through the esophagus. This and other alterations in the diet that may be helpful in achalasia are given in Table 7-4.

After dilation, the patient is not allowed to eat or drink for at least an hour to avoid spasm of the esophagus. A light meal may be eaten in several hours, and solid foods, the next day.[41]

Postoperative management of the patient with esophagomyotomy often allows oral fluid intake the same day. A normal diet is reinstated as soon as the patient can tolerate it, usually in less than five days. Reflux of gastric contents and the development of esophagitis are possible side effects of the surgery.

Stricture of the Esophagus. A **stricture** is narrowing of the lumen of the esophagus, usually in the lower two-thirds. It most often is due to inflammation from reflux of gastric acid, ingestion of caustic chemicals, a hernia or a tumor in or adjacent to the esophagus. A stricture interferes with food intake in the same way as achalasia. The general ap-

Table 7-4. Nutritional Care in Achalasia

Give semisolid or liquid foods as tolerated.

Provide small, frequent meals as tolerated.

Reduce protein and carbohydrate and increase fat in the diet to promote reduced gastric secretion and a decrease in lower esophageal sphincter pressure.

Avoid temperature extremes in foods.

Avoid foods such as citrus juices and highly spiced foods, which can injure the esophageal mucosa if retained.

Use a low-fiber diet if the patient finds it easier to swallow.

Encourage the patient to eat slowly.

proach to nutritional care is similar to that described for achalasia.

Lower Esophageal Sphincter Incompetence. If the lower esophageal sphincter does not maintain a pressure that is higher than the pressure in the stomach, the contents of the stomach will back up into the esophagus, a condition known as **gastroesophageal reflux**. The wall of the esophagus is not protected from the acid of the stomach and, during reflux, many patients feel a burning sensation behind the sternum that radiates toward the mouth. This condition is known as **heartburn** or **pyrosis**. It is unrelated to disease of the heart.

The hormone gastrin has been shown to cause an increase in LES pressure, as does a high-protein meal. It has been suggested that decreased LES pressure is caused by a deficiency of gastrin. Investigation of gastrin levels in patients, however, shows that there are also other factors in lowered LES pressure. One possibility is an abnormality in the sphincter muscle itself.

Another factor is the presence of a **hiatal hernia**, in which a portion of the stomach protrudes up into the chest cavity through the opening where the esophagus penetrates the diaphragm. At one time, it was thought that hiatal hernia was the cause of gastroesophageal reflux, but surgical repair of the hernia did not always correct the symptoms. Recent evidence suggests that a hiatal hernia is not the major mechanism but may contribute to the symptoms by interfering with the process of clearing acid from the esophagus following reflux, especially if the patient is lying down.

Scleroderma is a connective tissue disease that often involves the gastrointestinal tract. It results in decreased peristalsis and LES pressure, possibly as the result of a neural dysfunction and muscle atrophy.[42]

Estrogen and progesterone have been shown to reduce LES pressure, possibly by diminishing the response to gastrin. This observation offers an explanation for the increase in heartburn in pregnancy and in

women taking contraceptive drugs.[43] Cigarette smoking has a similar effect.

A number of drugs also lower LES pressure. As a result, gastroesophageal reflux and heartburn may occur as a side effect of the drugs used in the treatment of other conditions. Some of these drugs and their uses are listed in Table 7-5. When patients are receiving these drugs, nutritional care specialists should be alert to the development of reduced LES pressure as a side effect, since it may affect food intake.

Drugs and nutritional care are both components of treatment. A mainstay of drug treatment for gastroesophageal reflux is the use of antacids. A mixture of aluminum hydroxide and alginic acid (Gaviscon) floats on top of the gastric contents and reduces the tendency to reflux. Aluminum salts combine avidly with bile salts, which are also irritants. Bethanechol chloride may be used to increase LES pressure in patients who are resistant to antacid and diet treatment. Metoclopropamide may also be prescribed, as well as cimetidine, which decreases acid secretion.

Nutritional care in gastroesophageal reflux includes procedures to (1) increase LES pressure, (2) lessen esophageal irritation, (3) improve clearing of materials from the esophagus, and (4) decrease the frequency and volume of reflux. The general nutritional status of the patient should be monitored. Specific procedures are listed in Table 7-6.

Esophagitis

Chronic esophageal reflux and heartburn can result in esophagitis of the lower esophagus. **Plummer-Vinson syndrome**, inflammation in the upper part of the organ, may result from iron and vitamin B complex deficiency. The nutritional deficiency causes changes in the mucosa, making it more susceptible to damage. A variety of other agents — bacterial, chemical, physical, and traumatic — also cause chronic esophagitis. Nutritional care is generally the same as that for gastroesophageal reflux.

Table 7-5. Drugs That Decrease Lower Esophageal Sphincter Pressure

Drug	Use
Atropine	Anticholinergic; antispasmodic
Diazepam	Tranquilizer
Dopamine HCl	Antiparkinsonism agent
Isoproterenol	Beta-adrenergic agent
Morphine	Narcotic; analgesic
Nitroglycerine	Treatment of symptoms of angina
Nitroprusside	Vasodilator
Phentolamine	Alpha-adrenergic antagonist (shown in animals only)
Theophylline	Smooth muscle relaxant; phospho- diesterase inhibitor

Table 7-6. Nutritional Care in Gastroesophageal Reflux

Increase lower esophageal sphincter pressure
Increase protein in diet
Decrease fat in diet to <45 g/day
Avoid alcohol, peppermint, spearmint
Avoid coffee, strong tea, and chocolate if not well tolerated
Use *skim* milk
Decrease irritation in the esophagus
Avoid irritants: citrus juices, tomato, coffee, spicy foods, carbonated beverages
Avoid any other foods that regularly cause heartburn (*may* include rich pastry and frosted cakes)
Improve clearing of the esophagus
Do not recline for >2 hr. after eating
Elevate head of bed
Decrease frequency and volume of reflux
Elevate head of bed
Do not recline for >2 hr. after eating
Eat small meals, more frequent meals if necesssary
Reduce weight if overweight
Sip only small amounts of fluids with meals
Drink most fluids between meals
Include enough fiber to avoid constipation (straining increases intraabdominal pressure)
Nutritional and other considerations
Monitor effect of citrus and tomato avoidance on ascorbic acid status; supplement as necessary
Monitor effect of antacids on iron status; supplement if necessary
Avoid chewing gum (causes air swallowing)
Avoid smoking immediately following meals

Replacement of the Esophagus

Conditions that may require the replacement of the esophagus include congenital atresia of the esophagus, trauma, stricture, and carcinoma. A portion of the stomach, colon, or jejunum is used as the replacement.

Problems with eating and slow weight gain are common postoperatively. The patient sometimes continues to complain of dysphagia. Solid foods are especially troublesome, but the symptom improves with time. In the interim, suggestions for high-calorie foods to maintain weight are helpful to the patient. Some patients complain that food is tasteless or that there is a constant salty taste in the mouth. This also improves with time. Patients should be encouraged to eat small, frequent meals and to avoid taking solid and liquid foods at the same meal.[44]

THE STOMACH

Normal Anatomy and Physiology

The major parts of the stomach are shown in Figure 7-5. The stomach's functions are storage, mixing, propulsion of its contents into the intestine, and a small amount of digestion. In addition, the stomach exclusively secretes intrinsic factor, gastrin, hydrochloric acid, and pepsinogens. It secretes other materials and substances also formed else-

where: mucus, IgA, histamine, serotonin, and prostaglandins.

Secretion

Important constituents of gastric juices are hydrochloric acid, pepsin, mucus, and intrinsic factor. The usual volume of gastric juice is 1 to 2 liters, but it may reach 8 liters in disease.

Secretion of gastric juice is stimulated by a large number of factors, which are classified as cephalic, gastric, and intestinal. In the **cephalic phase**, the pleasant smell or taste of food, chewing, and swallowing stimulate receptors in the mouth and nose. Impulses travel via the vagus nerves to the stomach, where the release of acetylcholine stimulates mucus, acid, and pepsinogen secretion in the body and gastrin release in the antrum. The response is greater to food the person likes

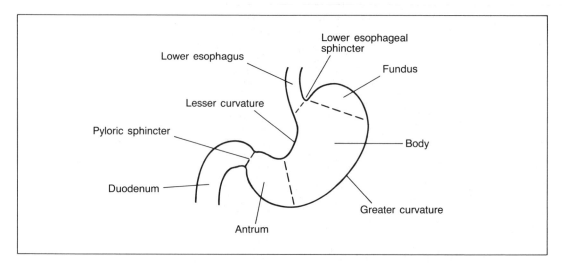

Figure 7-5. Parts of the stomach and duodenum.

and is less marked in response to bland food. These facts should be kept in mind in nutritional care of the anorectic patient. In the **gastric phase**, protein and amino acids in the stomach stimulate secretion by direct contact. Food causes a rise in pH, stimulating the vagus nerves, while distention of the stomach stimulates mechanoreceptors in the mucosa. Calcium and caffeine stimulate acid-secreting cells directly. In the **intestinal phase**, the products of protein digestion stimulate hydrogen ion secretion in the stomach.

Gastric secretion is inhibited by drugs such as atropine and by reflexes initiated by acid, fat, and solutions with high osmotic activity. The hormones cholecystokinin and secretin also inhibit secretion.

The mucosal surface of the stomach is perforated by **gastric pits**. In the proximal two-thirds of the stomach, three to seven gastric glands extend down from the bottom of the pits. These glands contain four types of secretory cells.

Chief or **peptic** or **zymogenic cells** line the walls of the base of the gland in a single layer and secrete pepsinogen into the lumen of the gland. The secretion of pepsinogen is strongly stimulated by acetylcholine, produced as a result of stimulation of the vagus nerves during the cephalic or gastric phase. The acid of the gastric juice also affects the production of pepsin by means of conversion of pepsinogen to pepsin at pH 2, stimulation of secretion of pepsinogen, and enhancement of other stimuli of chief cells.

Oxyntic or **parietal cells** lie between, and also peripheral to, the chief cells. They contain canaliculi (small channels) within the cell and extend between the chief cells to allow their secretions to be discharged into the lumen of the gland. Oxyntic cells secrete hydrochloric acid and intrinsic factor. The acid has many functions. It converts pepsinogen to pepsin, inhibits secretion of gastrin, stimulates secretion of secretin, and has a bacteriostatic effect, preventing infection in the gastrointestinal tract.

Gastric juice also contains a large amount of water and sodium, potassium, and chloride ions. If a patient's gastric contents are being aspirated, the lost fluid and electrolytes must be carefully replaced.

Argentaffin cells also occur in the gastric glands and are responsible for the secretion of histamine, serotonin (5-hydroxytryptamine), and heparin. The cells occur singly between the chief cells and basement membrane.

The **mucous neck** or **mucous chief cells** line the neck of the gland. The neck is that area which extends from the gland to the epithelial cells lining the pit. They secrete mucus, as the name indicates, and are stimulated by the vagus nerves. They also provide replacement cells for surrounding areas.

The mucosal surface and pits in the stomach are covered with **surface mucous cells**. The mucus that they secrete stains differently in the laboratory from the mucus of the chief cells, indicating some difference in its composition. Secretion is stimulated by physical contact with stomach contents and by contact with certain specific materials in the stomach, such as alcohol. Mucus in the stomach and prostaglandins protect the mucosal surface, particularly from autodigestion by gastric secretions. Surface mucous cells occur throughout the stomach.

Glands in other areas differ from those in the body of the stomach. In a band around the cardia, the glands are known an **cardia glands** and contain some oxyntic cells. The **pyloric glands** occur in the distal one-ninth of the stomach. They contain mucous neck cells and a few oxyntic cells.

The mucosa of the antrum includes **G cells**, the source of gastrin, which stimulates acid and pepsinogen secretion. Gastrin also increases gastric blood flow, circular muscle contraction in the stomach, and growth of the mucosa of the stomach and small intestine. Alcohol or meat in the diet stimulates the release of gastrin.

Storage and Motility

The empty stomach has a volume of only 50 ml or so, but it relaxes and enlarges with each swallow. Its maximum capacity has been estimated to be approximately 1,600 ml. As the stomach empties, the **orad** half (closer to the mouth) contracts and maintains the pressure gradient toward the duodenum. There is little mixing of stomach contents in this area, since the fundus and body of the stomach have only weak contractions. Peristalsis begins in the middle of the stomach and progresses toward the duodenum, mixing ingested material and gastric secretions to produce **chyme**.

Peristalsis in the stomach also pushes some chyme into the duodenum. By this process, the stomach is emptied. The time required varies with the nature of the gastric contents and the degree of distention. Solids, lipids, and solutions of high osmotic pressure are emptied from the stomach more slowly than are isotonic solutions. Liquids are emptied more rapidly than solids. In the duodenum, receptors respond to the osmotic pressure, acidity, and lipid content of chyme. The means by which they control gastric emptying are incompletely understood, but some factors involved are gastrointestinal hormones and neurologic reflexes.

The **enterogastric reflex** inhibits peristalsis in the antrum. It is initiated when chyme in the stomach has high or low osmotic activity relative to plasma or when hydrogen ion concentration in the intestine is high. Particle size, viscosity of chyme, and volume of gastric contents also affect emptying time. Emotional stress affects motility by stimulation of the autonomic nervous system.

Digestion

Although some small molecules are absorbed from the stomach, only limited digestion occurs. Pepsin is specific for peptide bonds involving aromatic amino acids. The action of salivary amylase on starch continues when food reaches the stomach until terminated by the low pH of the gastric juice. The stomach produces some gastric lipase, which acts on short- and medium-chain triglycerides. None of these actions are extensive or essential for digestion.

Nausea and Vomiting

Nausea is a feeling of distress with the sensation of the need to vomit. The mechanism by which it is produced is unclear. The vestibules of the ears may be involved, as they are in motion sickness. The nauseated patient has a contraction of the duodenum along with decreased tone and motility in the stomach.

Vomiting or **emesis**, the forceful expulsion of gastrointestinal contents via the mouth, is distinct from **regurgitation**, the slow return of food to the mouth. Vomiting usually is accompanied by nausea but may occur independently. It usually is preceded by activity of the sympathetic nervous system, indicated by sweating, salivation, pallor, dilated pupils, and sometimes retching (involuntary movements of vomiting without expulsion of vomitus). During vomiting, abdominal muscles and the diaphragm contract, increasing pressure in the stomach. The

LES relaxes, allowing expulsion of the gastric contents.

Nausea and vomiting are manifestations of many diseases. They often occur in acute abdominal emergencies such as appendicitis, peritonitis, and intestinal obstruction. In addition, nausea and vomiting are symptoms of diseases of other organ systems. They occur in some cardiovascular diseases such as myocardial infarction and congestive heart failure. Central nervous system disorders, disorders of the labyrinths of the ear, and endocrine disorders, such as diabetic

Figure 7-6. Metabolic consequences of vomiting. ECF = extracellular fluid; Tm = renal tubular maximum. (Reprinted with permission from Fordtran, JS., Vomiting. In M.H. Sleisenger and J.S. Fordtran, Eds., Gastrointestinal Disease, *3rd ed. Philadelphia: W.B. Saunders, 1983, p. 172.)*

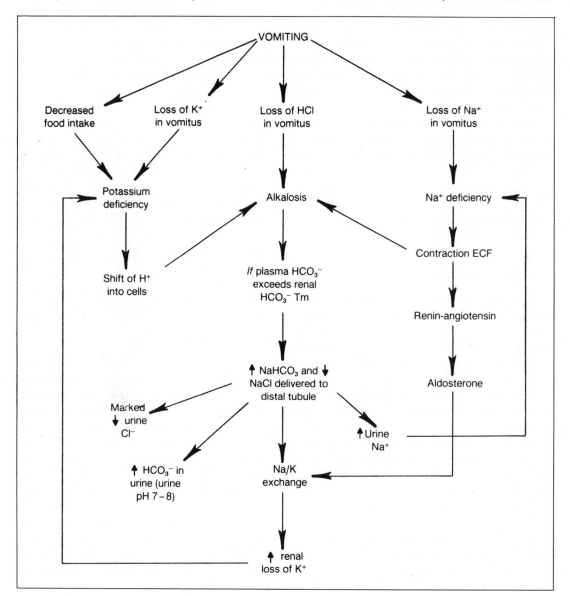

acidosis and adrenal insufficiency, also lead to vomiting. The morning sickness of early pregnancy probably is hormonal in origin. Drugs causing severe nausea and vomiting are listed in Table 4-5.

A brief episode of vomiting is not usually of consequence to the patient's nutrition, but prolonged vomiting may have many deleterious effects. The metabolic effects are diagramed in Figure 7-6. Patients also may have extreme weight loss with deficiencies of many nutrients. The teeth may have an increased incidence of caries. Severe vomiting sometimes tears the junction of the esophagus and stomach (Mallory-Weiss syndrome). Some patients — infants and those in a coma, for example — may aspirate vomitus, producing aspiration pneumonia. Other serious consequences include volume and electrolyte depletion and acid-base imbalance.

Table 7-7. Suggestions for Nutritional Care in Prolonged Vomiting

Recommended foods and foods to avoid

Avoid intake of liquids with meals. Drink liquids between meals, at least 1 hr. before or after meals.

Cold liquids may be tolerated better than those that are hot.

Carbonated beverages sometimes can reduce nausea. Popsicles and gelatin dishes are useful to increase fluid intake.

Eat dry toast, crackers, or dry cereal when feeling nauseated. These sometimes are helpful before arising if morning nausea occurs.

Avoid foods that many persons find difficult to tolerate, including strong-flavored vegetables such as those in the onion and cabbage families, coffee, highly spiced foods, and high-fat and fried foods. Try skim milk in place of whole milk.

Avoid highly acidic foods if they are troublesome; in some cases, tart foods may help to control nausea.

Use cold foods without aromas that may cause nausea. Try sandwiches, fruit plates, or cold meat plates.

Eat frequent small meals. This practice may be helpful to avoid overdistention of the abdomen and, at the same time, avoid having an empty stomach for a prolonged period.

Other recommendations

If vomiting is sporadic and predictable, eat rapidly digested and absorbed foods in the intervals between episodes of vomiting.

Relax, chew foods well, and breathe deeply and swallow when feeling nauseated. Eat and drink slowly.

Stay quiet 1 hr. or more following meals.

Eat whatever will stay down. Cater to the patient's preferences.

Nutritional care of the patient with severe and prolonged vomiting is difficult. In many instances, no food intake is possible, and the patient must be fed parenterally. The techniques in Table 7-7 may be useful if oral intake is possible.

Peptic Ulcer Disease

An **ulcer** is a circumscribed loss of tissue on the surface of the mucosa or skin. In the gastrointestinal tract, an ulcer is distinguished by the fact that it extends through the mucosa, submucosa, and sometimes, the muscle layer. It is distinct from an erosion in which the lesion is superficial and does not extend through the mucosa.

Sites of Ulcers

A **peptic ulcer** can occur in any area that is exposed to pepsin; the tissue must also be exposed to acid. Depending on location, peptic ulcers may be **gastric** (found in the stomach), **duodenal** (found in the duodenal bulb), or **esophageal** (occurring in the lower esophagus as a result of chronic reflux of gastric contents). If the patient's duodenum is surgically removed and the jejunum is joined to the stomach, a peptic ulcer may develop in the jejunum; this is called a **jejunal ulcer**. The creation of a passage between two normally separated organs is an **anastamosis**. Therefore, an ulcer in the area where stomach and jejunum are surgically joined is an **anastamotic ulcer**. Most ulcers occur within 3 cm of the pylorus. Gastric ulcers are located most frequently on the lesser curvature in the antrum where it meets the body of the stomach. Usually, there is gastritis in the surrounding tissue.

Occurrence

Chronic peptic ulcer disease (PUD) has decreased in incidence in recent years. In addition, there is much disagreement on pathogenesis and treatment. Although diet was at one time an important part of treatment, that is no longer the case. Therefore, discussion will be brief.

Pathogenesis

The pathogenesis of PUD is not entirely clear. It is generally agreed that there are parallel increases in acid and pepsin secretion, a decrease in resistance of the mucosa to digestion, or both. However, many questions remain to be answered. High acid production does seem necessary for ulcer formation, but there is great overlap with normal values.

The **Zollinger-Ellison syndrome** (ZES) is the cause of a particularly severe form of PUD. It consists, primarily, of hypergastrinemia and ulcers. One type occurs in later life and is the consequence of tumors of the pancreas or elsewhere. The tumors are usually malignant. Another type is genetic and often presents earlier. It is called multiple endocrine neoplasia – type I (MEN-I). The tumors are more usually benign. Recently, it has been shown that the tumors could make other hormones. In addition, the symptoms can be caused by other mechanisms unrelated to a tumor.[45]

Surgical removal of the tumors is difficult because they are often difficult to find. Instead, a common approach has been removal of the stomach along with any primary tumor that can be found during the surgery. An alternative is medical treatment with cimetidine and anticholinergic drugs.[46]

Clinical Manifestations

The chronic gastric ulcer is characterized by upper gastrointestinal distress and pain that may radiate up the back. Patients with duodenal ulcer complain of epigastric pain when the stomach is empty. In both, pain is relieved by food or antacid medications. Dysphagia and heartburn are characteristic of esophageal ulcers. Jejunal ulcers cause left upper quadrant pain which is not relieved by food intake.

Patients with duodenal ulcers may gain weight from frequent food intake to counteract pain. The loss of weight is more common in patients with gastric ulcers. Duodenal ulcers may be complicated by hemorrhage, perforation, or stenosis (narrowing or stricture of the outlet) causing obstruction. They also tend to recur.

Treatment

Conservative Management. The medical (conservative) management of PUD is a subject of debate. A variety of drugs are available for treatment.

One of the categories of drugs is the **histamine H_2-receptor antagonist**. The mode of action of these drugs is as follows: There are two receptors for the action of histamine. The H_1 receptor controls smooth muscle contractions in the bronchi and gut. The H_2 receptor is believed to affect gastric secretions. Vagal stimulation causes the release of histamine from histamine-secreting cells in the gastric mucosa. The histamine acts on histamine H_2 receptors of the parietal cells, increasing hydrochloric acid production.

Cimetidine and **ranitidine** are two drugs in this category. They accelerate the healing rate and reduce pain. They may also decrease vitamin B_{12} absorption. Therefore, the vitamin B_{12} nutritional status of the patient receiving long-term therapy should be monitored and a supplement provided if necessary.

Antacids may be used in addition to or as an alternative to a histamine H_2 receptor antagonist. They neutralize gastric acid for relief of pain and reduce mucosal damage. They buffer acid for only 30 minutes in an empty stomach but are effective for three to four hours if taken one hour after meals. It seems reasonable to assume that a neutral pH provides an environment that would promote the healing of the ulcer, and there is some evidence that antacids do, in fact, change the rate of healing.[47] There also is some evidence that it is a placebo effect.[48] Therefore, the question remains unresolved. Nutritionally relevant side effects of antacid treatment are listed in Table 7-8. The nutritional management of diarrhea and constipation, which are among the side effects, is discussed in Chapter 8.

Anticholinergic drugs sometimes are used in the management of duodenal ulcers,

Table 7-8. Nutritionally Relevant Side Effects of Antacid Therapy

Side Effect	Types of Antacids and Their Involvement
Disturbed bowel function	Aluminum hydroxide and calcium carbonate cause constipation. Magnesium salts cause diarrhea.
Hypercalcemia and milk alkali syndrome	*Pathophysiology:* Large amounts of calcium in calcium antacids or as milk plus absorbable alkali induce hypercalcemia, reduced parathyroid hormone, phosphorus retention, elevated calcium phosphorus product, and precipitation of calcium.
	Clinical manifestations: Acute manifestations include nausea, vomiting, weakness, mental changes, headache, dizziness, and elevated calcium, blood urea nitrogen, and creatinine, after 1 wk. *Chronic* manifestations include asthenia, muscle aches, polydipsia, polyuria, band keratopathy, and nephrocalcinosis. Acute changes are reversible, but nephrocalcinosis is not. Renal calculi may develop with hypercalciuria.
Sodium retention	Most antacids contain 4–6 mEq of sodium per 100 ml. Riopan contains very little and should be used for patients in whom sodium intake is restricted.
Phosphorus depletion syndrome	Magnesium hydroxide and aluminum hydroxide impair phosphorus absorption, leading to hypophosphatemia, hypophosphaturia, increased calcium absorption, hypercalciuria, resorption of bone phosphorus and calcium, and debility with anorexia, weakness, bone pain, malaise, and involuntary movements.

although there is evidence that they are ineffective.[47,49] They act on the nervous system to block the action of acetylcholine on the nerves and thereby decrease motility and the secretion of pepsin and acid. Side effects include a dry mouth, indicating a need for increased fluids to make the patient more comfortable.

Sucralfate forms a complex that covers the site of the ulcer and protects from attack by pepsin and acid. It does not neutralize the acid, and antacids are sometimes also prescribed. The drug promotes healing, but it does not affect the rate of recurrence.

Prostaglandins are currently being studied as a potential treatment of ulcers.

The use of **diet** in the conservative management of PUD has a long history. Currently, it is believed that only a few diet modifications are helpful in making the patient more comfortable during the healing process, although, as previously stated, they have no effect on the rate of healing. There is some controversy on the best procedure to follow. Patients usually are encouraged to eat any foods not associated with gastric distress.[50] Smaller, more frequent meals may be useful to neutralize acid, but there is some suspicion that frequent meals stimulate further acid secretion. The issue may be decided on the basis of the meal pattern with which the patient is more comfortable.

Patients sometimes are advised to eliminate caffeine and other methylxanthines (see Appendix F). While coffee is a strong stimulant of acid secretion, the caffeine content is apparently not the cause of the dyspepsia that often ensues. Therefore, the use of decaffeinated coffee is also limited. Alcohol, pepper, and aspirin are also eliminated as gastric irritants. Vinegar and mustard are eliminated if the patient finds them irritating. The nutritional care specialist should monitor the diet at intervals to assure that the patient does not restrict the diet excessively and so develop a nutritional deficiency.

Some patients find the elimination of coffee and alcohol a great hardship. Diets for these patients may be modified to allow for a glass of wine with meals and a limited amount of coffee following a meal. There is no specific evidence on this point, but it has been suggested that these practices lead to little acid secretion and little discomfort.[51]

Large amounts of alcoholic beverages without accompanying food or repeated cups of coffee during the day should be avoided. It is important to point out to patients that a combination of alcohol and aspirin is particularly damaging. In addition, patients may be advised to avoid eating before bedtime to avoid stimulation of nocturnal acid secretion.

Surgical Treatment. Gastric retention, hemorrhage, and perforation are often indications for surgical treatment of ulcer disease. However, the specific surgical procedure is also a matter of some disagreement. It will be chosen by the surgeon.

Procedures. **Total gastrectomy** (removal of the whole stomach) may be indicated for gastric malignancy, Zollinger-Ellison syndrome, diffuse gastric polyposis, Menetrier's disease and, sometimes, hemorrhage. **Partial gastrectomy** (removal of part of the

Figure 7-7. Various types of vagotomy. Shading depicts extent of gastrointestinal denervation following each procedure. Disturbances in physiology that may occur relate to some degree to the extent of denervation. (Reprinted with permission from Passaro, E., Jr., and Stabile, B.E., Late complications of vagotomy in relation to alterations in physiology. Postgrad. Med. 63(4):136, 1978.)

stomach) is used in the treatment of peptic ulcers that are resistant to healing during medical management or are complicated by hemorrhage, perforation, or obstruction of the outlet with retention of gastric contents. Surgical removal of a simple ulcer is not effective in place of conservative management, since another ulcer rapidly appears.

The surgical procedures have a common objective, the marked long-term reduction in acid and pepsin content of the stomach. The various procedures from which the surgeon must choose may be associated with different mortality rates, possible complications, and nutritional consequences.

Several surgical procedures include **vagotomy** (severing of the vagus nerves). Vagotomy reduces gastric acid, pepsin, and gastrin production. It also reduces peristalsis in the antrum and thereby controls gastric motility and emptying. There are three main types of vagotomy. In **truncal vagotomy**, the two main trunks of the vagus nerves and any accessory fibers are severed at the level of the hiatus of the diaphragm. Parasympathetic stimulation in the stomach, biliary system, pancreas, and the intestinal tract to the transverse colon is thus halted (Figure 7-7A). In **selective vagotomy**, only the branches to the stomach are severed (Figure 7-7B),

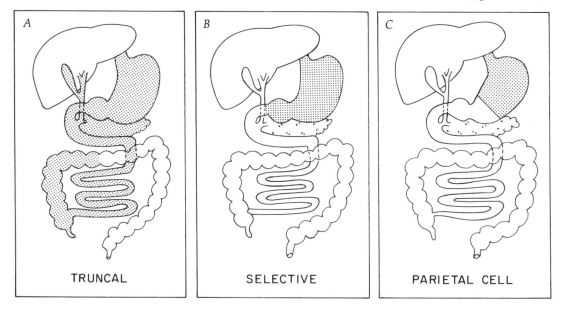

A	B	C
TRUNCAL	SELECTIVE	PARIETAL CELL

Table 7-9. Causes of Postvagotomy Syndromes

Procedure	Mechanism	Consequence	Contributes to			
			Gastric Retention	Dumping	Diarrhea	Duodenogastric Reflux
Denervation of proximal stomach (included in PCV, SV, TV)	Abolition of receptive relaxation → increased intragastric pressure	Accelerated initial emptying of liquids	No	++	++	No
	Early postoperatively: arrhythmia of gastric pacemaker → irregular antral motility	Delayed emptying of solids	+	No	No	No
Denervation of distal stomach (included in SV, TV)	Inhibition of antral motility	Delayed emptying of solids; delayed final emptying of liquids	+++	No	No	+
Intestinal denervation (included in TV)	Alteration of intestinal motility		No	No	+	+(?)
	Interruption of nervous intestinal regulation of gastric emptying	Accelerated emptying of liquids	No	+	+	No
Denervation of biliary tract (included in TV)	Increased capacity of gallbladder	Excessive bile acids in intestine	No	No	+	No
Drainage operation (pyloroplasty, gastrojejunostomy)	Decreased pyloric resistance	Accelerated emptying of liquids and solids	No	++	++	+++

Reprinted with permission from Hoelz, H.R., and Gewertz, B.L., Vagotomy. *Clin. Gastroenterol.* 8:305, 1979.

PCV = parietal cell vagotomy; SV = selective vagotomy; TV = truncal vagotomy; +, ++, +++ = relative severity of effect.

whereas in **parietal cell vagotomy** (also known as **highly selective**, **selective proximal**, or **proximal gastric vagotomy**), the branches to the acid-secreting parts of the stomach are interrupted. The branches to the antrum and pylorus are left intact (Figure 7-7C). The complications of vagotomy are related to the type (Table 7-9); those with nutritional implications will be discussed further.

Truncal and selective vagotomies result in denervation of the gastric antrum and pyloric sphincter. This leads to gastric stasis, since the pump mechanism of the antrum and the valve function of the sphincter are lost. To compensate for this effect, vagotomy often is combined with a "drainage" procedure (Figure 7-8, Table 7-10). Pyloroplasty (Figure 7-8D), the most commonly used procedure, widens the pyloric opening. Gastrojejunostomy (Figure 7-8C), which bypasses the pyloric sphincter, is not used frequently. Parietal cell vagotomy does not denervate the outlet, making concurrent drainage procedures unnecessary.

Resections or **surgical removal** are classified according to the site and extent of resected tissue. Gastric resections include the following:

1. Antrectomy (removal of the antrum), often with vagotomy (Figure 7-8E).
2. Subtotal or partial gastrectomy. The amount removed varies. Vagotomy sometimes is done also (Figure 7-8A and B).
3. Total gastrectomy.

Some of the advantages and disadvantages of various drainage procedures and resections are compared in Table 7-10.

The type of **reconstruction** may be important in nutritional management. Two of these, used in partial gastrectomy or antrectomy, are shown in Figure 7-8A and B. These methods are named after the surgeon who originated them. As indicated in the diagram, the **Billroth I** reconstruction consists of an anastamosis of the proximal end of the

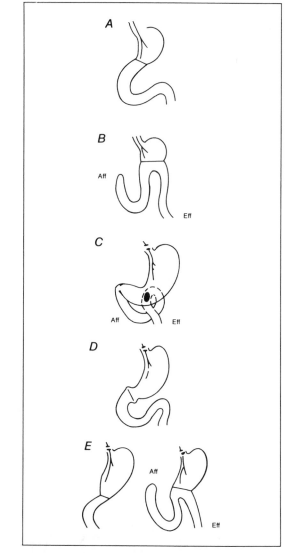

Figure 7-8. Operations for duodenal and gastric ulcers. **A.** Partial gastrectomy with Billroth I reconstruction. **B.** Partial gastrectomy; Billroth II, Polya type reconstruction. **C.** Vagotomy and gastrojejunostomy. **D.** Vagotomy and pyloroplasty. **E.** Vagotomy and antrectomy. Aff = afferent loop; Eff = efferent loop. (Reprinted with permission from Naish, J.M., and Read, A.E., Basic Gastroenterology, 2nd ed. Bristol, Engl.: John Wright & Sons, 1974, p. 77.)

intestine to the distal end of the stomach. The original **Billroth II** reconstruction has been followed by several variations, one of which (Polya's operation) is shown. An im-

Table 7-10. Comparison of Some Surgical Procedures for Gastric and Duodenal Ulcers

Operation	Advantages	Disadvantages
Partial gastrectomy, Billroth I reconstruction (see Figure 7-8A)	Maintenance of normal food pathway guarantees minimum of nutritional disturbances afterward. Less "dumping." Ideal for gastric ulcer.	High rate (6% in men) of recurrent ulceration if done for duodenal ulcer.
Partial gastrectomy, Polya's operation (see Figure 7-8B)	Combines removal of large part of acid-bearing area and antrum with neutralization of anastomotic area by alkaline duodenal juices. Low rate of recurrent ulcer (1–2%).	Poor mixing of food and enzymes. Weight loss and anemia are fairly frequent. "Dumping" symptoms in about 10%. Severe steatorrhea rarely.
Vagotomy and gastrojejunostomy (see Figure 7-8C)	Simple. Low risk. Alkalinization of gastric contents by duodenal juice.	Difficult to make vagotomy complete. Fairly high rate of recurrent ulceration (5–8%).
Vagotomy and pyloroplasty (see Figure 7-8D)	Cuts vagal acid secretion and drains stomach. Low risk. Maintains normal food pathway. Popular at present time.	No alkalinization of gastric contents. Fairly high rate of recurrent ulceration.
Vagotomy and antrectomy (limited resection) (see Figure 7-8E)	Cuts vagally mediated and hormonally mediated (gastrin from antrum) secretion. Low risk.	Removes pH monitoring function of antrum, so gastrin secretion from outside may be permanently high.

Adapted with permission from Naish, J.M., and Read, A.E., *Basic Gastroenterology,* 2nd ed. Bristol, Engl.: John Wright & Sons, 1974, p. 77.

portant feature of this type is the **blind loop** or **afferent loop** created when the stomach is anastamosed to the side of the intestine some distance from its proximal end. The position of the afferent and efferent loops should be observed in the figure. Total gastric resections may simply restore the continuity of the tract, or a larger reservoir may be created using a section of jejunum to make a pouch to provide some space for storage of ingested food.

Postoperative nutrition. The **initial postoperative feeding** is important in preventing complications. Immediately following uncomplicated gastric surgery, the patient is given nothing by mouth (NPO), and a nasogastric tube is inserted. Suction is used to remove gastric contents until peristalsis resumes, and the patient is given fluid and electrolyte therapy to replace what is lost in the aspirate. Sometimes, a tube to be used for feeding is implanted into the jejunum during the surgery. If there are no complications, the typical patient may first be given 2 oz. low-carbohydrate clear liquids plus one-half slice of toast or two crackers every two hours while awake. The clear liquids are chosen from broth, bouillon, decaffeinated coffee, unsweetened gelatin, or unsweetened fruit juice.[52] When gastrointestinal function has returned, a high-protein, low-carbohydrate, moderate-fat diet in small frequent feedings is used. Foods used should be low in fiber. Liquids are included in feedings separate from solid foods. Milk and carbonated beverages are eliminated. The patient may be fed every one to two hours. The purpose of these modifications is to prevent distention of the stomach and development of the dumping syndrome, a complication described later in this section. If no complications occur, other foods are added as tolerated. Some patients are able to have unrestricted intake within two to three weeks.

Sometimes the esophagus is damaged during truncal vagotomy. The patient may have pain and dysphagia for one or two weeks.[53] A soft diet may be helpful.

Complications. Some patients develop complications following gastrectomy, several of which have nutritional implications.

1. **Dumping syndrome** is a group of symptoms that occur after eating in approximately 10% of gastric surgery patients. It has been divided into early and late phases, depending on how soon it occurs after eating.

Early dumping syndrome occurs during the meal or within 10 to 15 minutes after the meal is eaten. It occurs frequently after gastric resection and sometimes in patients in whom a drainage operation has been performed. The patient has a feeling of fullness in the epigastrium, flushing, sweating, weakness, tachycardia (excessive heart rate), diarrhea, and sometimes hypotension. The pathogenesis of early dumping syndrome is not understood entirely, but some facts are clear. The symptoms follow intake of high-carbohydrate foods. The loss of normal sphincter action, whether by resection, bypass, division, or denervation, allows rapid movement of hyperosmolar material from the stomach into the upper small intestine. Fluid is pulled into the intestine, causing intestinal distention and reduced plasma volume. The intestinal distention may cause the diarrhea. It also stimulates the argentaffin cells in the intestinal mucosa to secrete humoral agents such as serotonin, prostaglandins, bradykinin, and enteroglucagon. These may account for the gastrointestinal and vasomotor symptoms,[54-56] but there still is doubt on this point.

The development of early dumping syndrome can often be avoided in gastric surgery patients by cautious postoperative feeding, as described earlier. If dumping syndrome does occur, the treatment is almost exclusively dietary. The rationale and main features of nutritional management are summarized in Table 7-11.

Late dumping syndrome or **alimentary hypoglycemia** develops $1\frac{1}{2}$ to 3 hours after a meal. Patients feel faint and weak and perspire freely. There are varying degrees of effect on the central nervous system, and some patients lose consciousness. There are no gastrointestinal symptoms. The lack of normal pyloric sphincter function allows the

Table 7-11. Nutritional Management of Dumping Syndrome

Individualize the diet to the patient's tolerance. Consult the patient frequently concerning his or her response to individual food items and to portion sizes. The following items are general guidelines.

Reduce intake of carbohydrates to 100–200 g/day. Avoid simple sugars to prevent rapid movement of food into the jejunum with formation of a hyperosmolar solution. Use *unsweetened* fruits.

Increase fat content to 30–40% of calories to retard stomach emptying and to provide calories for weight gain.

Increase protein to 20% of calories for tissue formation and to supply energy. Include some protein in each meal.

Meals should be low in bulk, dry, and frequent: Six or more per day is common. Increase portion sizes as the patient's tolerance increases.

Provide low-carbohydrate fluids between meals, at least $\frac{1}{2}$–1 hr after a meal, to retard gastric emptying. Avoid high-carbohydrate fluids.

All food and drink should be moderate in temperature. Cold drinks, especially, cause increased gastric motility.

Encourage the patient to eat slowly and then lie down for 20–30 min.

Encourage the patient to eat a variety of foods to provide an adequate diet and achievement of ideal body weight. It may be necessary to urge him or her to try foods that were being avoided preoperatively.

The possibility of lactose intolerance exists. Milk should be avoided until it is established that the patient tolerates milk (see Chapter 8).

To progress toward a more normal intake, add moderate amounts of carbohydrate with caution if the patient shows no symptoms of dumping in the first several days. Use sugar in the form of sweetened fruits and fruit juice and desserts such as sponge cake and cookies. If these are well tolerated, add more concentrated carbohydrates and foods at temperature extremes. Fresh fruits and vegetables may be added in 2–3 wk. They should be chewed thoroughly. The diet may be progressed rapidly in some patients and may be lifelong in others.

movement of carbohydrate into the upper small intestine. This carbohydrate is absorbed rapidly and the blood glucose level rises. As a result, a large amount of insulin is released and the blood glucose level falls. The symptoms are characteristic of low blood glucose.

Patients with late dumping syndrome should eat approximately every two hours, avoiding concentrated sweets. However, concentrated sweets should be available at all times and eaten if a hypoglycemic attack begins. Also, if protein foods are taken at this time, they may help to prevent another episode of hypoglycemia.

2. **A change in bowel habits** is common after gastric surgery, especially when vagotomy is included. Bowel function can vary from severe constipation to severe diarrhea. Severe incapacitating diarrhea, usually referred to as **postvagotomy diarrhea**, follows truncal vagotomy, especially if combined with antrectomy, more often than it does the more selective types.[57] It causes severe disability in approximately 2% of patients.

Treatment may include dietary changes as well as antispasmodic and antidiarrheal drugs and cholestyramine. If conservative treatment is unsuccessful, surgical correction may be necessary.

Mild diarrhea may be controlled by the use of small, frequent feedings and limitation of fluid with meals. An increase in dietary fiber may also be helpful.

3. **Weight loss** after subtotal gastric resection occurs in as many as 60% of patients, particularly those with a gastrojejunal anastamosis. Total resection also results in weight loss. The causes are not understood entirely but probably are multiple.

In some patients, weight loss is clearly the result of inadequate food intake. Patients with partial or total gastrectomy have a reduced storage capacity and a rapid development of the feeling of satiety. Those with dumping syndrome sometimes reduce their food intake to avoid the symptoms.

Some patients develop a malabsorption syndrome as a late complication. In the stomach itself, the decreased production of acid and pepsin has an effect, but the significance of this change on overall fat and protein metabolism is not clear. Anatomic changes from surgery sometimes affect the availability of bile and pancreatic enzymes. The digestive and absorptive functions of the intestine are affected if emptying of the stomach and gallbladder and pancreatic secretion are incoordinated. Since many of these changes are similar to those seen in diseases of the intestine, pancreas, and gall-

bladder, their nutritional consequences and management are described in Chapter 8.

4. **Anemia** occurs late as a postoperative complication, sometimes several years later. The incidence varies greatly, depending on the definition of anemia used in the studies that are the source of the data. Several types of anemia are seen.[58] They are described in Chapter 18.

5. **Bezoars** are concretions of various materials sometimes found in the stomach or intestines. They may be formed from a variety of materials. **Phytobezoars** are formed from plant fibers. Trichobezoars may be formed from hair, string, and various textile fibers. Lactobezoars can be formed from milk intake. Other contributing materials are gums, such as chewing gum, and medications, such as aluminum hydroxide gel, cholestyramine, antacid tablets, vitamin C tablets, and iron tablets.[59] Phytobezoars are of greatest concern to the nutritional care specialist. In gastric surgery patients, phytobezoars may form because of reduced gastric motility, decreased mixing and churning in the stomach, delayed gastric emptying, and reduction of gastric secretions. They can also occur in other conditions in which gastric function is compromised, such as diabetes with gastroparesis. Symptoms include anorexia, upper abdominal pain, anemia, and weight loss. In addition, weakness, vomiting, diarrhea, fever, early satiety, dysphagia, hematemesis, constipation and gastric irritation, ulceration, and perforation may be seen. They sometimes can pass from the stomach into the intestine and cause an obstruction.

Gastric phytobezoars can be treated with digestive materials such as papain, cellulase, and pancreatic enzymes using an endoscope. Certain foods seem to be found with some frequency in bezoar formation. These include oranges, persimmons, coconuts, berries, green beans, figs, apples, sauerkraut, brussels sprouts, and potato peelings.[59] Patients with a tendency to bezoar formation should be counseled to avoid these foods.

6. Metabolic **bone disease**—osteomalacia or osteoporosis—occurs as a late compli-

cation of gastrectomy in 1% to 15% of patients.[60] Milder forms are much more common.[61,62] Bone disease has not been observed after vagotomy and pyloroplasty or vagotomy and gastroenterostomy.[57]

Osteomalacia occurs in patients with a Billroth II reconstruction or gastrojejunostomy. It is believed to be the result of malabsorption of fat and fat-soluble vitamins, including vitamin D. Poor dietary intake may be another contributing factor. Patients are treated with vitamin D supplements. **Osteoporosis** occurs 10 to 20 years earlier in gastrectomy patients than in others.[63] There is no specific treatment, but it is reported that most of these patients are malnourished.[64] The following seem to be logical recommendations for nutritional management: Counsel the patient on adequate nutrient intake, and provide supplements if necessary to assure adequate intakes of calcium and vitamin D.

Case Study: Lower Esophageal Sphincter Incompetence

W.M. was first seen at the age of 56 years. He complained of epigastric pain of several years' duration, dysphagia, and belching of uncertain duration. He described the dysphagia as a "feeling of fullness" and food "sticking" in his chest following ingestion of solid food. Sometimes he regurgitated this food but did not vomit. The symptoms were aggravated by lying down or bending over.

Physical examination and the complete blood cell count were normal. He denied any weight loss. X-ray films suggested lower esophageal sphincter incompetence and a sliding hiatal hernia.

The patient was given antacids and referred to the nutritional care specialist for diet counseling.

Subjective:
"I've got to have my morning cup of coffee."

Twenty-four-hour recall:

Breakfast	4 oz. fruit juice
	2 eggs on toast
	Coffee, black
Snack (at work)	Coffee, black
	Sweet roll
Lunch (at work)	Steak sandwich
	French fries
	Tossed salad with French dressing
	Coffee, black
Snack (at work)	Ice cream, 1 scoop
Dinner	12 oz. beer
	Tuna noodle casserole
	Buttered frozen peas
	Fruit salad of canned pineapple, orange
	sections, sliced banana
	8 oz. milk
Snack	12 oz. soft drink
	20 pretzel sticks

Five years later, the patient returned complaining of dysphagia of six months' duration and persistent burning epigastric pain. He was able to eat only soft foods or liquids. His appetite was good, but he had lost 20 lb. Laboratory test values were as follows:

Hematocrit	31%
Hemoglobin	8.1 g/dl
Others	Within normal limits

Esophagoscopy showed a constricting lesion 39 cm from the incisors. A biopsy and esophageal washings showed no tumor cells. Attempts to dilate the stricture were unsuccessful. In the meantime, the patient lost additional weight.

The nutritional care specialist was asked to see the patient and suggest nutritional care necessary to prepare the patient for surgery.

Exercises

1. What clinical manifestations would alert the physician to the possibility of LES incompetence?
2. Evaluate the patient's diet from the 24-hour recall.
3. Describe the nutritional care you would suggest for this patient and explain the rationale.
4. What is the significance of the values obtained for hematocrit and hemoglobin?
5. What preoperative nutritional care procedures would you recommend for the patient?

Case Study: Dumping Syndrome

K.L., a 45-year-old man, was admitted to the hospital for surgery after 15 years of treatment for a gastric ulcer. The ulcer was no longer responding to medical management. Antrectomy with selective vagotomy was performed. Postoperatively, the patient was at first given nothing by mouth. When feeding was begun, he was given low-carbohydrate clear liquids and toast every two hours, and then he progressed to a high-protein, low-carbohydrate diet in six small feedings. Fluids were given at separate feedings.

A week after discharge from the hospital, the patient called his physician complaining of nausea, diarrhea, and abdominal cramping an hour after meals. The physician referred the patient to the nutritional care specialist, who obtained the following 24-hour recall information:

7:00 A.M.	1 cup pineapple juice
	2 slices buttered toast with jelly
	2 scrambled eggs
	Coffee with sugar
10:00 A.M.	Coffee with sugar
	Danish roll

12:30 P.M.	Hamburger on bun
	French fries
	Tossed salad with French dressing
	Lemon meringue pie
	Coffee with sugar
6:00 P.M.	6 oz. pork chop
	1 small sweet potato
	$\frac{1}{2}$ cup peas with butter
	Sliced tomato salad with Thousand Island dressing
	8 oz. milk
	Tea with sugar
9:30 P.M.	12 oz. soft drink
	$\frac{1}{2}$ cup strawberry ice cream

Exercises

1. Explain the rationale for the postoperative diet.
2. What changes in diet (24-hour recall) might be suggested to this patient?
3. Explain the mechanism by which the symptoms of dumping syndrome are produced.

References

1. Sernka, T.J., and Jacobson, E.D. *Gastrointestinal Physiology—The Essentials*, 2nd ed. Baltimore: Williams and Wilkins, 1983.
2. Jenkins, G.N. *The Physiology of the Mouth*, 4th ed. Oxford: Blackwell Scientific, 1978.
3. Mason, D.K., and Chisholm, D.M. *Salivary Glands in Health and Disease*. London: W.B. Saunders, 1975.
4. Kreitzman, S.N. Nutrition in the process of dental caries. *Dent. Clin. North Am.* 20:491, 1976.
5. Gould, R.F., Ed. *Dietary Chemicals vs. Dental Caries*. Washington, D.C.: American Chemical Society, 1970.
6. De Paola, D.P., and Kuftinec, M.M. Nutrition in growth and development of oral tissues. *Dent. Clin. North Am.* 20:441, 1976.
7. Jenkins, G.N. Recent changes in dental caries. *Br. Med. J.* 291:1297, 1985.
8. Fejerskov, O., Thylstrup, A., and Mogens, J.L. Rational use of fluoride in caries prevention. A concept based on possible cariostatic mechanisms. *Acta Odontol. Scand.* 39:241, 1981.
9. Jakush, J.J., Ed. Diet, nutrition and oral health. *J. Am. Dent. Assoc.* 109:20, 1984.
10. Stephan, R.M. Changes in the hydrogen ion concentration on tooth surfaces and in carious lesions. *J. Am. Dent. Assoc.* 27:718, 1940.
11. Silverstone, L.M. The structure of carious enamel, including the early lesion. *Oral Sci. Rev.* 3:100, 1973.
12. Featherstone, J.D.B. Remineralization of artificial carious lesions in vivo and in vitro. In S.A. Leach, Ed., *Demineralization and Remineralization of Teeth*. Oxford: IRL Press, 1983, pp. 89–110.
13. Mandel, I.H. Relation of saliva and plaque to caries. *J. Dent. Res.* 53:246, 1974.
14. Jenkins, C., and Ferguson, D.B. Milk and dental caries. *Br. Dent. J.* 120:472, 1966.
15. Enwonwu, C.O. Role of biochemistry and nutrition in preventive dentistry. *J. Am. Soc. Prev. Dent.* 4:6, 1974.
16. Alfano, M.C. Controversies, perspectives and clinical implications of nutrition in periodontal disease. *Dent. Clin. North Am.* 20:519, 1976.
17. Mann, A.W., Mann, J.M., and Spies, T.D. A clinical study of malnourished edentulous patients. *J. Am. Dent. Assoc.* 32:1357, 1945.
18. Greene, H.I., Dreizen, S., and Spies, T.D. A clinical survey of the incidence of impaired masticatory function in patients of a nutrition clinic. *J. Am. Dent. Assoc.* 39:561, 1949.

19. Martis, C.S. Complications after mandibular sagittal split osteotomy. *J. Oral Maxillofac. Surg.* 42:101, 1984.
20. Kendall, B.D., Fonseca, R.J., and Lee, M. Postoperative nutritional supplementation for the orthognathic surgery patient. *J. Oral Maxillofac. Surg.* 40:205, 1982.
21. Shannon, I.L., Trodahl, J.D., and Starcke, E.N. Remineralization of enamel by a saliva substitute designed for use by irradiated patients. *Cancer* 41:1746, 1978.
22. Arey, L.B., Tremaine, M.H., and Monzengo, F.L. The numerical and topographical relations of taste buds to human circumvallate papillae throughout the lifespan. *Anat. Rec.* 64:9, 1935.
23. Schiffman, S. Food recognition in the elderly. *J. Gerontol.* 32:586, 1977.
24. Castell, D.O., and Harris, L.D. Hormonal control of gastroesophageal sphincter strength. *N. Engl. J. Med.* 282:886, 1970.
25. Lipshutz, W., and Cohen, S. Physiological determinants of lower esophageal sphincter function. *Gastroenterology* 61:16, 1971.
26. Lipshutz, W., Tuch, A., and Cohen, S. A comparison of the site of action of gastrin I on lower esophageal sphincter and antral circular smooth muscle. *Gastroenterology* 61:454, 1971.
27. Cohen, S., and Lipshutz, W. Hormonal regulation of human lower esophageal sphincter incompetence. Interaction of gastrin and secretin. *J. Clin. Invest.* 50:449, 1971.
28. Lipshutz, W., and Cohen, S. Interaction of gastrin I and secretin on gastrointestinal circular muscle. *Am. J. Physiol.* 222:775, 1972.
29. Resin, H., Stern, D.H., Sturdevant, R.A.L., and Isenberg, J.I. Effect of the C-terminal octapeptide of cholecystokinin on lower esophageal sphincter pressure in man. *Gastroenterology* 64:946, 1973.
30. Fisher, R.S., Di Marino, A.J., and Cohen, S. Mechanism of cholecystokinin-induced inhibition of lower esophageal sphincter pressure (abstract). *Clin. Res.* 22(3):358A, 1974.
31. Jennewein, H.M., Waldeck, K., Siewert, R., et al. The interaction of glucagon and pentagastrin on the lower oesophageal sphincter in man and dog. *Gut* 14:861, 1973.
32. Goyal, R.K., and Rattan, S. Neurohormonal, hormonal and drug receptors for the lower esophageal sphincter. *Gastroenterology* 74:598, 1978.
33. Sigmund, C.J., and McNally, E.F. The action of a carminative on the lower esophageal sphincter. *Gastroenterology* 56:13, 1969.
34. Babka, J.C., and Castell, D.O. On the genesis of heartburn. The effects of specific foods on the lower esophageal sphincter. *Am. J. Dig. Dis.* 18:391, 1973.
35. Hogan, W., Viegas de Andrade, S.R., and Winship, D. Ethanol induced acute esophageal motor dysfunction. *J. Appl. Physiol.* 32:755, 1972.
36. Hurwitz, A.L., Duranceau, A., and Haddad, J.K. *Disorders of Esophageal Motility.* Philadelphia: W.B. Saunders, 1979.
37. Harris, J. B., Nigon, K., and Alonso, D. Adenosine 3'5' monophosphate. Intracellular mediator for methyl xanthine stimulation of gastric secretion. *Gastroenterology* 57:377, 1969.
38. Cohen, S., and Booth, G.H. Gastric acid secretion and lower esophageal sphincter pressure in response to coffee and caffeine. *N. Engl. J. Med.* 293:897, 1975.
39. Groher, M.E., Ed. *Dysphagia: Diagnosis and Management.* Boston: Butterworth, 1984.
40. Trounce, J.R., Deuchar, D.C., Kauntze, R., and Thomas, G.A. Studies in achalasia of the cardia. *Q. J. Med.* 26:433, 1957.
41. Ellis, F.H., Jr. Management of oesophageal achalasia. *Clin. Gastroenterol.* 5:89, 1976.
42. Cohen, S., Fisher, R., Lipshutz, W., et al. The pathogenesis of esophageal dysfunction in scleroderma and Raynaud's disease. *J. Clin. Invest.* 51:2663, 1972.
43. Van Thiel, D.H., Gavaler, J.S., Joshi, S.N., et al. Heartburn of pregnancy. *Gastroenterology* 72:666, 1979.
44. Gunning, A.J., and Marshall, R. Replacement of the esophagus. *Clin. Gastroenterol.* 8:292, 1979.
45. Piper, D.W. Antacid and anticholinergic drug therapy. *Clin. Gastroenterol.* 2:361, 1973.
46. McCarthy, D.M. Zollinger-Ellison syndrome. *Ann. Rev. Med.* 33:197, 1982.
47. Peterson, W.L., Sturdevant, R.A.L., Frankl, H.D., et al. Healing of duodenal ulcer with an antacid regimen. *N. Engl. J. Med.* 297:341, 1977.
48. Sturdevant, R.A.L., Isenberg, J.I., Secrist, D., and Ansfield, J. Antacid and placebo produced similar pain relief in duodenal ulcer patients. *Gastroenterology* 72:1, 1977.
49. Ivery, K. Anticholinergics: Do they work in peptic ulcer? *Gastroenterology* 68:154, 1975.
50. Ingelfinger, F.J. Let the ulcer patient enjoy his food. In F.J. Ingelfinger, A.S. Relman, and M. Finland, Eds., *Controversy in Internal Medicine.* Philadelphia: W.B. Saunders, 1966.
51. Taylor, K.B. Gastroenterology. In H.A. Schneider, C.E. Anderson, and D.B. Coursin, Eds., *Nutritional Support of Medical Practice,* 2nd ed. New York: Harper and Row, 1983.
52. Clinical Dietetics Section, Hospital Food Ser-

vice. *Manual of Clinical Dietetics*. Los Angeles: University of California, 1977.

53. Hoelz, H.R., and Gewertz, B.L. Vagotomy. *Clin. Gastroenterol.* 8:305, 1979.
54. Jesseph, J.E. Serotonin and the dumping syndrome. A reappraisal. *Surgery* 63:536, 1968.
55. Thomford, N.R., Sirinek, K.R., Crockett, S.E., et al. Gastric inhibitory peptide. Response to oral glucose after vagotomy and pyloroplasty. *Arch. Surg.* 109:177, 1974.
56. Wong, P.T., Talamo, R.C., Babior, B.M., et al. Kallikrein-kinin system in postgastrectomy dumping syndrome. *Ann. Intern. Med.* 80:577, 1974.
57. Small, W.P. The long-term results of peptic ulcer surgery. *Clin. Gastroenterol.* 2:427, 1972.
58. MacLean, L.D. Nutritional complications in the surgical patient. In C.P. Artz and J.D. Hardy, Eds., *Complications in Surgery and Their Management*, 2nd ed. Philadelphia: W.B. Saunders, 1969, p. 243.
59. Harris, A.I., and Janowitz, H.D. Medical management of problems following peptic ulcer surgery. *Postgrad. Med.* 63:127, 1978.
60. Fourman, P. Effects of gastrectomy on bone. In R.H. Gerdwood and A.N. Smith, Eds., *Malabsorption*. Medical Monographs 4. Edinburgh: University Press, 1969, pp. 59–62.
61. Clark, C.G. Nutritional and metabolic consequences of partial gastrectomy. In A.G. Cox and J. Alexander-Williams, Eds., *Vagotomy on Trial*. London: William Heinemann Medical, 1973, p. 53.
62. Alexander-Williams, J. Some sequelae of gastric operations including the dumping syndrome and metabolic disorders. In R. Maingot, Ed., *Abdominal Operations*. New York: Appleton-Century-Crofts, 1974, p. 491.
63. Nilson, B.E., and Wastlin, L.E. The fracture incidence after gastrectomy. *Acta Chir. Scand.* 137:533, 1971.
64. French, J.M., and Crane, C.W. Undernutrition, malnutrition and malabsorption following gastrectomy. In F.A.R. Stammars and J. Alexander-Williams, Eds., *Complications and Metabolic Consequences*. London: Butterworth, 1963.

Bibliography

Alfano, M.C., and De Paola, D.P., Eds. Symposium on Nutrition. *Dent. Clin. North Am.* 20:441, 1976.

Artz, C.P., and Hardy, J.D., Eds. *Management of Surgical Complications*, 3rd ed. Philadelphia: W.B. Saunders, 1975.

Brooks, F.P. *Control of Gastrointestinal Function*. New York: Macmillan, 1970.

Dworken, H. *Gastroenterology Pathophysiology and Clinical Applications*. Boston: Butterworth, 1982.

Field, M., Fordtran, J.S., and Schultz, S.G., Eds. *Secretory Diarrhea*. Bethesda, Md.: American Physiological Society, 1980.

Guyton, A.C. *Textbook of Medical Physiology*, 7th ed. Philadelphia: W.B. Saunders, 1986.

Irving, M.H., and Beart, R.W., Jr., Eds. Butterworth's International Medical Reviews. Surgery 3. *Gastroenterological Surgery*. London: Butterworth, 1983.

Lifshitz, F., Ed. *Clinical Disorders in Pediatric Gastroenterology and Nutrition*. New York: Marcel Dekker, 1980.

Menguy, R. Surgery of peptic ulcer. In P.A. Ebert, Ed., *Major Problems in Clinical Surgery*. Philadelphia: W.B. Saunders, 1976.

Moody, F.G., Ed., *Surgical Treatment of Digestive Disease*, 2nd ed. Chicago: Yearbook Medical Publishers, 1990.

Newbrun, E. *Cariology*. Baltimore: Williams and Wilkins, 1978.

Nizel, A.E. *Nutrition in Preventive Dentistry: Science and Practice*, 2nd ed. Philadelphia: W.B. Saunders, 1981.

Nord, H.J., and Sodeman, W.A., Jr. The stomach. In W.A. Sodeman and T.M. Sodeman, Eds., *Pathologic Physiology*, 7th ed. Philadelphia: W.B. Saunders, 1985.

Paige, D.M., and Bayless, T.M., Eds. *Lactose Digestion: Clinical and Nutritional Implications*. Baltimore: Johns Hopkins Press, 1981.

Sernka, T., and Jacobson, E. *Gastrointestinal Physiology—The Essentials*, 2nd ed. Baltimore: Williams and Wilkins, 1983.

Skinner, D.B. The esophagus. In W.A. Sodeman and T.M. Sodeman, Eds., *Pathologic Physiology*. Philadelphia: W.B. Saunders, 1979.

Sleisenger, M.H., and Fordtran, J.S., Eds. *Gastrointestinal Disease: Pathophysiology, Diagnosis, Management*, 3rd ed. Philadelphia: W.B. Saunders, 1983.

Vander, A.J., Sherman, J.H., and Luciano, D.S. *Human Physiology: The Mechanisms of Body Function*, 4th ed. New York: McGraw-Hill, 1985.

van der Reis, L., Ed. The Stomach. *Front. Gastrointest. Res.* vol. 6, 1980.

8. The Intestinal Tract and Accessory Organs

I. Normal Anatomy and Physiology
  A. The small intestine
    1. Normal structure
    2. Normal physiology
      a. motility
      b. secretion
      c. digestion and absorption
        (1) triglycerides
        (2) protein
        (3) carbohydrate
        (4) folic acid
        (5) vitamin B_{12}
        (6) other vitamins
        (7) water and mineral elements
      d. protective mechanisms
  B. The biliary tract
    1. Functional anatomy
    2. Normal physiology
  C. The pancreas
    1. Normal anatomy
    2. Normal physiology
  D. The large intestine
    1. Normal anatomy
    2. Normal physiology
II. Conditions Common to Many Gastrointestinal Disorders
  A. Malabsorption syndromes
    1. Pathogenesis of malabsorption
      a. lipids
        (1) pancreatic insufficiency
        (2) intraluminal binding of bile acids
        (3) biliary tract obstruction
        (4) bacterial overgrowth
        (5) reduction of pH of duodenal contents
        (6) ileal dysfunction
      b. carbohydrate
      c. protein
      d. vitamin B_{12}
      e. drug-induced malabsorption
    2. General symptoms of malabsorption
    3. Diagnosis
    4. Treatment
  B. Intestinal antigen absorption
    1. Absorptive mechanisms
    2. Related diseases
    3. Nutritional management
  C. Diarrhea
    1. Pathophysiology and classification
      a. osmotic diarrhea
      b. secretory diarrhea
    2. Diagnosis
    3. Metabolic consequences
    4. Therapy
  D. Protein-losing enteropathies
  E. Intestinal lymphangiectasia
  F. Intestinal fistulas
III. Diseases Affecting Primarily the Small Intestine
  A. Gluten-induced enteropathy
    1. Clinical manifestations
    2. Pathogenesis
    3. Diagnosis
    4. Treatment
  B. Tropical sprue
  C. Inflammatory bowel disease
    1. Crohn's disease
      a. clinical manifestations
      b. causes and predisposing factors
      c. diagnosis
      d. treatment
    2. Chronic ulcerative colitis
    3. Nutritional assessment in IBD
  D. Short bowel syndrome
    1. Etiology
    2. Pathophysiology
    3. Treatment
      a. nutritional management
      b. drug treatment and nutrition
    4. Nutritional assessment
  E. Carbohydrate intolerance
    1. Lactase deficiency
      a. forms of lactose intolerance
      b. diagnosis
      c. nutritional care
    2. Sucrase-isomaltase deficiency
    3. Glucose-galactose malabsorption
  F. Abetalipoproteinemia
  G. Endocrine-secreting tumors of the gastrointestinal tract
    1. Foregut tumors
    2. Midgut and hindgut tumors
  H. Acquired immune deficiency syndrome
    1. Nutritional assessment
    2. Nutritional consequences and care
IV. Diseases of the Gallbladder and Bile Ducts
V. Diseases of the Pancreas
  A. Diagnosis
  B. Acute pancreatitis
  C. Chronic pancreatitis
    1. Pathogenesis
    2. Clinical manifestations

3. Nutritional management
D. Cystic fibrosis of the pancreas
1. Pathophysiology and clinical manifestations
2. Nutritional assessment

3. Diagnosis
4. Treatment
a. nutritional management
VI. Diseases of the Large Intestine
A. Fiber and related substances
B. Intestinal gas
C. Constipation

D. Diverticular disease
1. Clinical manifestations
2. Management
E. Colon surgery
1. Ileostomy
2. Colostomy
F. Rectal surgery
VII. Case Studies

The intestine, exocrine pancreas, and gallbladder are all discussed in the same chapter because they are involved simultaneously in the digestion and absorption of many nutrients. The nutritional consequences of liver disease are described in Chapter 13.

NORMAL ANATOMY AND PHYSIOLOGY

The Small Intestine

Normal Structure

The small intestine is approximately 15 feet long and consists of the **duodenum** (10 inches), the **jejunum** (9.5 feet), and **ileum** (4 feet), in that order. Bile and secretions of the pancreas enter the duodenum through a duct system that penetrates the duodenal wall a few centimeters below the pyloric sphincter.

Three features of the structure of the small intestine increase the surface area that is in contact with the intestinal contents. These are **Kerckring's folds** or **plicae circularis**, the **villi**, and the **microvilli** on the luminal borders of the absorptive cells of the villi. Approximately 20 **crypts of Lieberkühn** lie at the base of each villus and penetrate to a depth of approximately one-quarter of the height of the villus down to the muscularis mucosae. The villi are covered with a single layer of cells, which also extend down into the crypts. Most of the cells in the crypts are undifferentiated and multiply rapidly, maturing as they move up the sides of the crypts

and onto the walls of the villi. The ability of the cells to divide is lost as they leave the crypts. A small number of cells differentiate into **goblet cells**, which secrete mucus, but most become **enterocytes** or **absorptive cells**. As they differentiate, the absorptive cells develop a brush border, enzymes, receptor sites, and carrier proteins, all of which function in digestion and absorption. The cells continue to migrate toward the tips of the villi and, after three to seven days, they are extruded from the tips of the villi into the lumen of the intestine. The intestinal mucosa thus is renewed constantly.

The crypts of Lieberkühn also contain other cells that do not migrate. These include **Paneth cells**, the function of which is unknown, and **enterochromaffin, argentaffin,** or **basal granular cells**. There are several distinct populations within the group of enterochromaffin cells. Some have an endocrine function, but the functions of others are unknown.

In the duodenum, elaborately branched **Brunner's glands** extend down from the mucosal surface. The secretion of these glands is high in mucus and bicarbonate. These substances lubricate chyme and neutralize gastric hydrochloric acid.

The luminal surface of the microvilli is coated with a mucopolysaccharide called the glycocalyx. Several digestive enzymes are located in this area. Above the glycocalyx is a stagnant layer of water, the so-called unstirred layer, through which molecules in the lumen must move to be absorbed.[1,2] The **lamina propria** is the connective tissue layer

Table 8-1. Summary of Digestive Processes

Source of and Stimulus for Secretion	Enzyme	Method of Activation and Optimal Conditions for Activity	Substrate	End Products or Action
Salivary glands of mouth: Secrete saliva in reflex response to presence of food in mouth	Salivary amylase	Chloride ion necessary; pH 6.6–6.8	Starch Glycogen	Maltose plus 1:6 glucosides (oligosaccharides) plus maltotriose
Stomach glands: Chief cells and parietal cells secrete gastric juice in response to reflex stimulation and chemical action of gastrin	Pepsin	Pepsinogen converted to active pepsin by HCl; pH 1.0–2.0	Protein	Proteoses Peptones
	Rennin	Calcium necessary for activity; pH 4.0	Casein of milk	Coagulates milk
Pancreas: Presence of acid chyme from stomach activates duodenum to produce (1) secretin, which hormonally stimulates flow of pancreatic juice; (2) cholecystokinin, which stimulates production of enzymes	Trypsin	Trypsinogen converted to active trypsin by enterokinase of intestine at pH 5.2–6.0; autocatalytic at pH 7.9	Protein Proteoses Peptones	Polypeptides Dipeptides
	Chymotrypsin	Secreted as chymotrypsinogen and converted to active form by trypsin; pH 8.0	Protein Proteoses Peptones	Same as trypsin; more coagulating power for milk
	Carboxypeptidase	Secreted as procarboxypeptidase, activated by trypsin	Polypeptides at the free carboxyl end of the chain	Lower peptides; free amino acids
	Pancreatic amylase	pH 7.1	Starch Glycogen	Maltose plus 1:6 glucosides (oligosaccharides) plus maltotriose

Liver and gallbladder: Cholecystokinin, a hormone from the intestinal mucosa—and possibly also gastrin and secretin—stimulates gallbladder and secretion of bile by liver

Enzyme/Secretion	Conditions	Substrate	Products
Lipase	Activated by bile salts, phospholipids, colipase; pH 8.0	Primary ester linkages of triacylglycerol	Fatty acids, monoacylglycerols, diacylglycerols, glycerol
Ribonuclease		Ribonucleic acid	Nucleotides
Deoxyribonuclease		Deoxyribonucleic acids	Nucleotides
Cholesteryl ester hydrolase	Activated by bile salts	Cholesteryl esters	Free cholesterol plus fatty acids
Phospholipase A_2		Phospholipids	Fatty acids, lysophospholipids
(Bile salts and alkali)		Fats—also neutralize acid chyme	Fatty acid–bile salt conjugates and finely emulsified neutral fat–bile salt micelles

Small intestine: Secretions of Brunner's glands of duodenum and glands of Lieberkühn

Enzyme	Conditions	Substrate	Products
Aminopeptidase		Polypeptides at the free amino end of the chain	Lower peptides; free amino acids
Dipeptidases		Dipeptides	Amino acids
Sucrase	pH 5.0–7.0	Sucrose	Fructose, glucose
Maltase	pH 5.8–6.2	Maltose	Glucose
Lactase	pH 5.4–6.0	Lactose	Glucose, galactose
Phosphatase	pH 8.6	Organic phosphates	Free phosphate
Isomaltase or 1:6 glucosidase		1:6 glucosides	Glucose
Polynucleotidase		Nucleic acid	Nucleotides
Nucleosidases (nucleoside phosphorylases)		Purine or pyrimidine nucleosides	Purine or pyrimidine bases, pentose phosphate

Reprinted with permission from Martin, D.W., Mayes, P.A., and Rodwell, V.W., *Harper's Review of Biochemistry*, 18th ed. Los Altos, Calif.: Lange Medical, 1981, p. 528.

that lies below the epithelium and its basement membrane. It carries blood and lymphatic capillaries close to the epithelial tissue. Absorbed materials thus move from the absorptive cells through the lamina propria and into the blood or lymph.

Normal Physiology

The functions of the intestinal tract include (1) motility to provide mixing and propulsion of intestinal contents, (2) secretion of enzymes, hormones, and other materials, (3) digestion and absorption of ingested materials, (4) protection of other organs' and its own integrity, and (5) excretion of waste products. Simultaneous normal bile production in the liver and normal gallbladder and pancreatic function are essential for normal digestion and absorption.

Motility. Mixing is accomplished mostly by **segmentation**, a kneading action resulting from contractions of circular muscles. **Pendular movements**, longitudinal contractions that shorten the length of the gut, also contribute to mixing. The major function of the wormlike motion known as **peristalsis** is to propel the food through the tract although it, too, may have some mixing effects. Movements of the villi also contribute to mixing and propulsion. Intestinal motor activity is under hormonal and nervous control. Sympathetic nervous system stimulation inhibits propulsive activity and increases sphincter tone.

Secretion. The intestinal mucosa secretes enzymes, hormones, mucus, electrolytes, and water. The enzymes include the **disaccharidases**, such as maltase, sucrase, and lactase, some **peptidases**, and **enterokinase** (Table 8-1).

In addition, the duodenal mucosa secretes gastrointestinal hormones. **Secretin** is released when the low pH of the gastric contents comes into contact with duodenal mucosa. It decreases intestinal motility and stimulates pancreatic secretion of bicarbon-

ate into the duodenum, neutralizing the gastric acidity.

Cholecystokinin-pancreozymin (CCK-PZ) also is secreted by the duodenal mucosa. Its release is stimulated by the presence of fat in the duodenum. Cholecystokinin-pancreozymin increases production of pancreatic enzymes and stimulates contraction of the gallbladder to deliver bile to the intestinal lumen.

Secretion of fluid and electrolytes into the intestinal lumen is greater in magnitude than the movement into any other organ system. The combined volume of ingested and endogenous fluid that reaches the intestinal lumen has been estimated to be approximately 9 liters per day in the average adult, of which approximately 2 liters is exogenous fluid taken in food and drink (see Chapter 2).

Digestion and Absorption. Although digestion and absorption are separate functions in concept, they are somewhat intertwined in fact and will therefore be discussed together.

Most digestion of protein, fat, and carbohydrate takes place in the duodenum and the first 3 feet of jejunum; it involves the action of bile, pancreatic enzymes, and intestinal enzymes. The resulting fatty acids, monosaccharides, peptides and amino acids are absorbed mostly in the first 60 to 100 cm of the jejunum. Materials and vitamins also are absorbed in the duodenum and jejunum, except for vitamin B_{12}, which is absorbed in the ileum. The ileum apparently is capable of absorption of other nutrients, but most are absorbed in more proximal portions of the gut and therefore are not present in the lumen of the ileum. The usual sites of absorption of the various nutrients are shown in Figure 8-1.

Absorption is the translocation of materials from the lumen into the portal and lymphatic systems. The four possible modes by which it is believed to occur are **passive diffusion**, **active transport**, **facilitated transport**, and **pinocytosis**. Following one of these absorptive processes, the material is

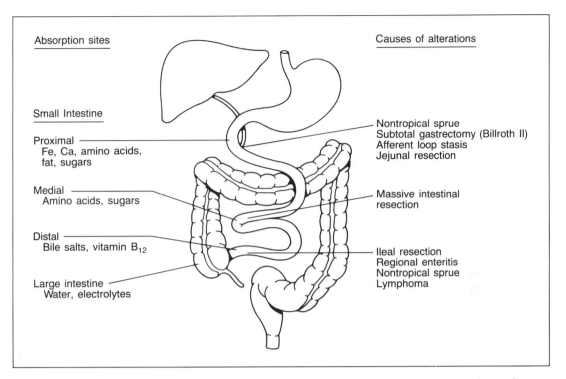

Absorption sites

Causes of alterations

Small Intestine

Proximal
Fe, Ca, amino acids,
fat, sugars

Medial
Amino acids, sugars

Distal
Bile salts, vitamin B_{12}

Large intestine
Water, electrolytes

Nontropical sprue
Subtotal gastrectomy (Billroth II)
Afferent loop stasis
Jejunal resection

Massive intestinal
resection

Ileal resection
Regional enteritis
Nontropical sprue
Lymphoma

Figure 8-1. Nutrient absorption sites.

transported across the cell, is released across the basal or lateral membrane of the cell, crosses the basement membrane, and moves into the capillaries or lacteals.

There is almost total absorption of digested protein, fat, and carbohydrate. Absorption is obligatory; that is, it does not depend on the body's need. Efficiency of absorption of water and of monovalent ions —sodium, potassium, chloride, iodine, and fluoride—also is very high, while absorption of divalent and trivalent ions, including calcium, iron, and zinc, is less complete. It is regulated according to need, thus protecting the body from toxic effects.

Triglycerides. The digestion of triglycerides must be considered in two categories, the digestion and absorption of which differ with the length of the fatty acid chains. One of these categories contains the **long-chain triglycerides** (LCT).

Most dietary fat is triglyceride with smaller amounts of other lipids. The fatty acids present in largest quantity in triglycerides are long-chain fatty acids containing 12 carbons or more. The most common fatty acids, palmitic (C16:0) and stearic (C18:0), are saturated, while the unsaturated fatty acids, oleic (C18:1) and linoleic (C18:2), have one or two unsaturated bonds, respectively.

Pancreatic lipase is required for digestion of these lipids. The action of pancreatic lipase on a triglyceride (**lipolysis**) results in the production of three fatty acids plus glycerol or a β-monoglyceride plus two fatty acid molecules.

When fat enters the intestinal lumen, the action of bile comes into play. Bile, containing bile salts, is secreted by the liver and stored in the gallbladder until needed. Cholecystokinin-pancreozymin stimulates contraction of the gallbladder and increases the delivery of bile to the intestinal lumen. When the bile salts reach the **critical micellar concentration** (0.15 M), they aggregate with the fatty acids and β-monoglycerides to form **micelles**, small particles 3 to 10 nm in diameter with the hydrophilic polar group oriented on the surface. Micelles make it possible for the lipid to be solubilized in the contents of the intestinal lumen, forming a clear aqueous solution. They make enzymatic lipolysis possible in the aqueous environment of the intestinal lumen and increase the rate of lipolysis by removing the end products of the reaction. Micelles also increase the rate at which the lipids can be diffused through the unstirred water layer, preliminary to absorption. Bile acts only in fat digestion and has no role in the digestion of protein or carbohydrate.

The micelle is believed to dissociate at the jejunal cell surface. The fatty acids and β-monoglycerides cross the cell membrane by passive diffusion. The bile salts released from the micelles in the jejunum are carried to the ileum and reabsorbed, creating a cycle known as the **enterohepatic circulation** (Figure 8-2). Approximately 2 to 4 g of bile salts exist in the body pool, but they are recycled six to ten times per day so that the ileum normally is presented with 20 to 30 g to reabsorb. The pool must recycle several times to absorb the lipid in a single meal.[3] The liver synthesizes and the intestine excretes 200 to 600 mg of bile salts daily.

Figure 8-2. The enterohepatic circulation of bile salts. (Adapted from Riley, J.W., and Glickman, R.M., Fat malabsorption—advances in our understanding. Am. J. Med. 67:982, 1979.)

The lipids are reesterified rapidly in the enterocyte (Figure 8-3). The resulting triglycerides become associated with cholesterol, cholesteryl esters, phospholipid, and protein to form **chylomicrons**. The chylomicrons then are released from the cell and enter the lacteal by a process that is not completely understood, possibly by pinocytosis or through gaps at junctions of cells in the wall of the lacteal. The chylomicrons enter the blood by way of the thoracic duct. Their further metabolism and their relationship to cardiovascular disease are described in Chapter 10. Phospholipids and cholesterol also are absorbed by way of the lacteals.

In contrast to the rather complex sequence of events described for long-chain triglycerides, the procedure for digestion, absorption, and metabolism of the **medium-chain triglycerides** (MCT), which contain shorter fatty acids (C6:0 to C12:0), is fairly simple. They are hydrolyzed at lower concentrations of pancreatic lipase to free fatty acids. Very little β-monoglyceride is produced. Furthermore, bile salts apparently are necessary in smaller amounts for micelle formation, and less gallbladder stimulation occurs. MCTs are transported into the capillaries and thence into the portal vein, bypassing the lymphatics, moving directly into the portal vein system. Approximately 30% may be absorbed unchanged. Consequently, medium-

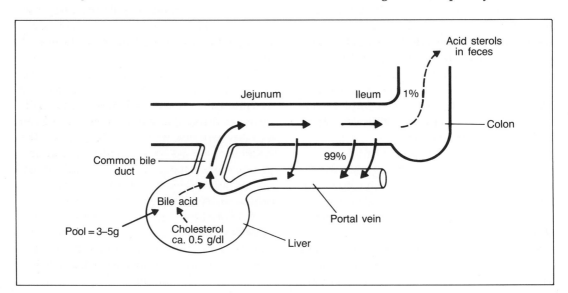

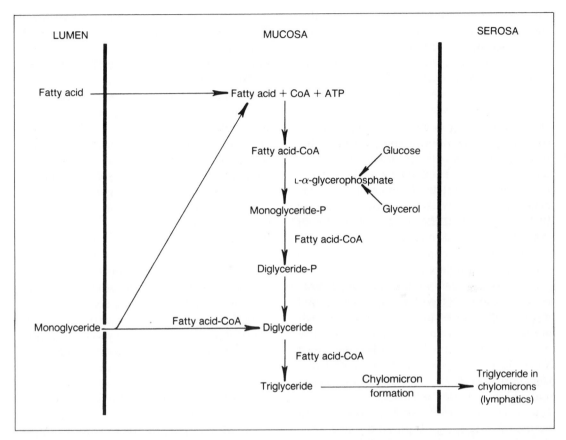

LUMEN MUCOSA SEROSA

Fatty acid ⟶ Fatty acid + CoA + ATP

Fatty acid-CoA

Glucose

L-α-glycerophosphate

Monoglyceride-P

Glycerol

Fatty acid-CoA

Diglyceride-P

Monoglyceride Fatty acid-CoA Diglyceride

Fatty acid-CoA

Triglyceride Chylomicron formation Triglyceride in chylomicrons (lymphatics)

Figure 8-3. Major reactions in mucosal cells during fat absorption. P = phosphate. (Reprinted with permission from Isselbacher, K.J., Biochemical aspects of lipid malabsorption. Federation Proc. 26:1421, 1967.)

chain triglycerides are useful in diseases in which it is difficult to maintain the body weight. These include gastrectomy, extensive ileal disease and resection, obstructive jaundice, premature infants with impaired LCT absorption, lymphangiectasia, lymphoma, Whipple's disease, and selected alterations in lipid metabolism. MCTs also decrease fluid accumulation in chylous ascites. MCTs are also useful in deficiencies of pancreatic enzymes and decreased availability of bile if they cannot be successfully treated otherwise. MCTs are not indicated in diabetes mellitus because they are ketogenic, or in hepatic disease because clearance by the liver is reduced. Their use in nutritional care

in these conditions will be discussed in more detail later in this chapter.

Protein. Protein digestion results primarily from the action of pancreatic enzymes. The site of action of pancreatic proteases, released as a result of vagal stimulation of CCK-PZ action, is not entirely clear. Some hydrolysis of proteins may occur in the intestinal lumen, but some proteases adsorb to the enterocyte membrane and may act at that site. They produce peptides that consist of three to six amino acid residues. **Oligopeptidases** and **tripeptidases**, which have been identified in the brush border, digest the largest molecules to dipeptides and amino acids. There are a number of **dipeptidases**, but their location is not clear. These function in dipeptide hydrolysis to amino acids.

Dipeptides, as well as amino acids, can cross the cell membrane and enter the enterocytes. The nutritional significance of this action is not known. The transport mechanisms involved in amino acid absorption are not understood entirely, but it is known that there is more than one mechanism, affecting various groups of amino acids. The rate of transport can apparently be affected to some degree by dietary manipulation.[4]

Carbohydrate. In the duodenal lumen, pancreatic amylase attacks the 1,4 linkages of starch, producing maltose, maltotriose, and α-dextrins. The α-dextrins contain the branching points with 1,6 linkages and usually consist of approximately eight glucose units. These products of pancreatic enzyme action plus dietary lactose and sucrose are further digested at the surface of the brush border in the intestinal phase. The enzymes, maltases, α-dextrinase, lactase, and sucrase are located in the area of the plasma membrane and glycocalyx. Most of the glucose, galactose, and fructose produced is absorbed into the enterocytes and thence into the capillaries, although a small amount may diffuse back into the lumen. Glucose and galactose are absorbed by a sodium-dependent active transport system. Fructose apparently is absorbed by facilitated diffusion.

Folic acid. Most folic acid in food occurs bound to additional L-glutamic acid residues. It is converted in the small intestine to the free monoglutamate form by the action of **conjugase**, the exact site of action of which is unknown. Absorption of folate occurs in the proximal small intestine, but the mechanism is not clear. Within the enterocyte, it is converted to reduced methylfolate and then is absorbed into the capillaries and carried to the portal vein.

Vitamin B_{12}. Dietary vitamin B_{12} is protein-bound and is released by the action of gastric acid and digestive enzymes. **Intrinsic factor** (IF) is produced by gastric parietal cells, then binds the free vitamin B_{12} to produce a vitamin B_{12}-IF complex. This form is required for the absorption of vitamin B_{12} to occur. Formation of the complex is believed to protect the vitamin from utilization by intestinal bacteria and possibly from digestion.

In the terminal ileum, the complex attaches to receptors in the plasma membrane–glycocalyx. This process is enhanced by calcium ion.[5] The vitamin is released from IF in or on the membrane and is transported into the cell and then into the portal circulation bound to a carrier known as **transcobalamin**. The fate of IF is unknown.

Other vitamins. The processes of absorption of other water-soluble vitamins are largely unknown. Most are believed to be absorbed by simple diffusion, although thiamine, which ionizes slowly, may be poorly absorbed. Absorption of fat-soluble vitamins parallels lipid absorption in general. Bile salts apparently are required for absorption by passive diffusion.

Water and mineral elements. Most of the 9 liters of water presented to the intestine daily are reabsorbed into the portal blood with only 200 ml or so appearing in the feces. Approximately 20% of the ingested water is absorbed per minute.[6] Both passive and active absorption of water are likely, but the driving forces are uncertain. The absorption of water from the intestinal tract is obligatory, as is that of most monovalent ions. Excesses are excreted in the urine, so the kidney, not the intestine, provides the primary homeostatic mechanisms. It is not possible, for example, to cause diarrhea by water intakes in excess of need. Instead, excess water is excreted by increasing urine flow.

Electrolyte transport is an active process. A free exchange of Na^+, H^+, and Cl^- ions occurs across the duodenal mucosa. As a consequence, meals of varying composition are rendered isoosmolar in Na^+ content with plasma, and isotonic and neutral in pH by mechanisms that are not understood completely. Approximately 50% of the water, Na^+, K^+, and Cl^- are absorbed in the jejunum.

In the ileum, Na^+ can be absorbed against a concentration gradient. A model linking exchange of sodium and hydrogen ions on the one hand, and chloride and bicarbonate on the other, has been described by which the ileum absorbs approximately 75% of the load.[7] The colon absorbs the remaining Na^+ and Cl^- into the portal blood against a gradient very effectively, so that normal stools may contain only 1 to 2 mmole/day. Cl^- and HCO_3^- are exchanged. The colonic mucosa is relatively impermeable to the diffusion of Na^+ back into the lumen. It maintains a large negative electric potential that provides a driving force for diffusion of K^+ into the lumen. Monovalent ions, such as sodium and chloride, are absorbed more rapidly than polyvalent ions, such as Ca^{++} and Fe^{++}.

Iron absorption usually is proportionate to the needs of the body. However, ferric iron, commonly found in food, appears to be reduced to the ferrous form before it is absorbed. Following absorption, ferrous iron is oxidized to the ferric form in the mucosal cells and binds to **apoferritin**, a binding protein found in the mucosa. It then crosses the cell membrane and is released into the portal blood. When the apoferritin is saturated with iron, absorption decreases. It has also been observed that certain iron-sugar complexes may move across mucosal cells without binding to apoferritin.

Calcium absorption involves the action of vitamin D metabolite and parathyroid hormone. Approximately 10% to 30% of dietary calcium is absorbed in the acid environment of the proximal duodenum. Details of the complexities of the processes involved in calcium absorption as well as absorption of other mineral elements are found in texts on normal nutrition.

Protective Mechanisms. A number of actions of the intestinal tract serve to protect the intestine itself and other cells of the body from damage. The bactericidal or bacteriostatic effects of saliva and gastric juice have already been described. The normal bacterial flora in the intestine may serve to counteract the growth of pathogenic bacteria, yeasts, and fungi. Vomiting and diarrhea may protect the body by eliminating toxic materials. It is postulated that the intestinal mucosa also serves as a barrier to the absorption of materials that would have a deleterious effect on other cells in the body via the immune system. Several mechanisms protect the integrity of the intestine itself. These include secretion of mucus, dilution, neutralization, and buffering of intestinal contents, and the constant renewal of mucosal cells.

The Biliary Tract

Functional Anatomy

The **hepatocytes** of the liver daily produce 600 to 800 ml of bile from cholesterol. The bile then flows into a duct system that converges to form the **hepatic duct** (Figure 8-4). The **gallbladder** is a hollow, pear-shaped sac with a capacity of 30 to 50 ml. It communicates with the hepatic duct via the **cystic duct**. These two ducts converge to form the **common bile duct**, which conveys bile to the duodenum. **Oddi's sphincter** regulates the flow of bile into the intestine.

Normal Physiology

Bile, synthesized by the liver, contains bile salts, cholesterol, and phospholipids. The primary function of the gallbladder is to concentrate and store bile. The rate at which this concentration occurs is extremely rapid. Almost 90% of the original fluid volume can be reabsorbed in three to six hours. As a result, there is a sharp increase in the concentration of bile salts, cholesterol, and phospholipids. The cells of the gallbladder have an active sodium and chloride transport system, and water is reabsorbed as a consequence of the action of the sodium pump. Thus the concentration of bile may be increased 10 to 15 times, making it possible to store a day's bile production. The compositions of bile as secreted and of bile in the gallbladder are given in Table 8-2.

There are two primary acids (Figure 8-5) that are synthesized in several steps from cholesterol. They are the trihydroxy bile acid, **cholic acid**, and the dihydroxy acid, **chenodeoxycholic acid**. Both conjugate with **glycine** and **taurine**. **Deoxycholic acid**, a "secondary" acid formed from cholic acid, also conjugates with taurine and glycine. **Lithocholic acid** is formed similarly

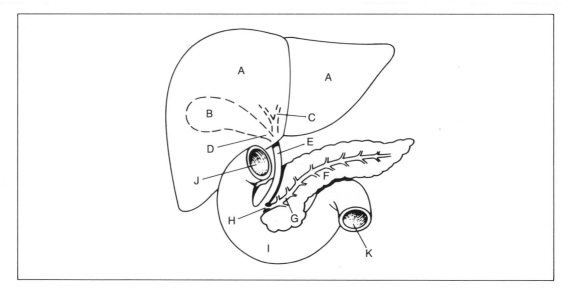

Figure 8-4. Relationship of upper abdominal organs. **A.** *Liver;* **B.** *Gallbladder;* **C.** *Hepatic duct;* **D.** *Cystic duct;* **E.** *Common bile duct;* **F.** *Pancreas;* **G.** *Pancreatic duct;* **H.** *Sphincter of Oddi;* **I.** *Duodenum;* **J.** *Pyloric opening from stomach;* **K.** *Duodenum to jejunum.*

from chenodeoxycholic acid, but in very small amounts. The secondary acids are products of bacterial action and take up approximately 20% of the total pool of bile

Table 8-2. The Composition of Hepatic and Gallbladder Biles

| | Hepatic Bile (as secreted) | | Bladder Bile |
| | % of Total Bile | % of Total Solids | (% of total bile) |
Constituents			
Water	97.00		85.92
Solids	2.52		14.08
Bile acids	1.93	36.9	9.14
Mucin and pigments	0.53	21.3	2.98
Cholesterol	0.06	2.4	0.26
Fatty acids and fat	0.14	5.6	0.32
Inorganic salts	0.84	33.3	0.65
Specific gravity	1.01		1.04
pH	7.1–7.3		6.9–7.7

Reprinted with permission from Martin, D.W., Mayes, P.A., and Rodwell, V.W., *Harper's Review of Biochemistry*, 18th ed. Los Altos, Calif.: Lange Medical, 1981, p. 528.

salts. The bile contains large quantities of Na^+ and K^+, and the bile acids are assumed to exist as bile salts with these cations.

Although bile salts circulate through the intestine over and over again during a day, they are very well conserved (see Figure 8-2). Most are reabsorbed by way of the portal vein and returned to the liver to be secreted again. Only a small fraction of total bile salts is lost each day; however, if the terminal ileum, the main site of bile salt absorption, is removed, the pool is depleted rapidly.

The Pancreas

Normal Anatomy

The pancreas is both an exocrine and endocrine organ, but this chapter will deal only with the exocrine function of the gland. The basic secretory unit of the exocrine pancreas is the **acinus**, a group of cells that form a saclike unit. The apical surfaces of the cells of an acinus share a common lumen into which they secrete the pancreatic enzymes (Figure 8-6). The lumen of the acinus empties into a duct which drains, successively, into the intralobular and interlobular ducts. The ducts actually extend into the center of the acinus. The cells in this portion of the duct are known as **centroacinar cells**. The interlobular ducts ultimately fuse to form the **duct of**

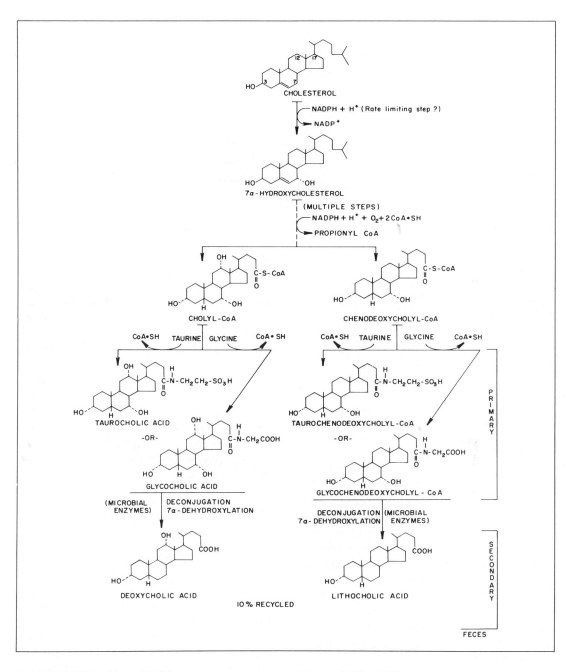

Figure 8-5. Bile acid metabolism.

Wirsung, the main pancreatic duct. Sometimes there is also an accessory **duct of Santorini**. The pancreatic ducts usually drain into the common bile duct but occasionally open into the duodenum directly.

Normal Physiology

The enzymes listed in Table 8-1 are synthesized by the acinar cells of the pancreas into membrane-bound structures called **zymogen granules** and eventually are discharged into the lumen of the acinus. The **duct cells** secrete a thin watery fluid high in bicarbon-

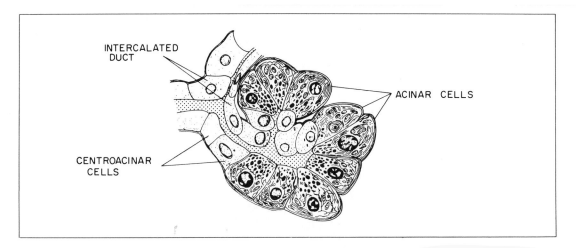

Figure 8-6. The relationship of a terminal branch of the duct system and centroacinar cells to the acinus. (Reprinted with permission from Bloom, W., and Fawcett, D.W., A Textbook of Histology, 10th ed. Philadelphia: W.B. Saunders, 1975, p. 738.)

ate. The pancreatic juice also contains Na^+, K^+, Ca^{++}, Mg^{++}, Cl^-, SO_4^{2-}, HPO_4^{3-}, albumin, and globulin. Daily volume is usually approximately 2 liters.

The Large Intestine

Normal Anatomy

The **large intestine** is approximately 5 feet long, with a diameter greater than that of the small intestine. It attaches to the ileum at the ileocecal valve and consists of the cecum, the ascending, transverse, descending, and sigmoid colon, and the rectum, and ends at the anus (Figure 8-7). Three longitudinal muscles, the **teniae coli**, extend the length of the colon. The wall of the colon forms **haustra coli**, or outpouchings between these muscles. The colonic glands, which extend into the mucosal layer, secrete large quantities of mucus.

Normal Physiology

No enzymatic digestion occurs in the colon, but the large number of bacteria that normally exist in the colon digest some resistant materials. The colon absorbs water, electrolytes, and some vitamins. Sodium ions are absorbed by active transport, and potassium can be excreted. The colon also stores and eliminates wastes as feces. The fecal materials include water, indigestible fiber, dead mucosal cells, bacteria and products of their activity, bile salts, bilirubin, small amounts of unabsorbed nutrients, and nonfood items that may have been swallowed. The fat content of the feces is usually less than 6 g/day.

CONDITIONS COMMON TO MANY GASTROINTESTINAL DISORDERS

The conditions discussed in this section are common to a number of disorders. Specific diseases in which they occur are described in succeeding sections.

Malabsorption Syndromes

The term **malabsorption** often is used to include abnormalities of either digestion or absorption or both. It almost always refers to conditions that cause decreased or inadequate function. As a result, maintenance of good nutrition often is difficult, and patients tend to be undernourished.

The cause of malabsorption may be centered in any organ or tissue that contributes to the digestive or absorptive process — the liver, gallbladder, pancreas, intestinal mucosa, lymphatics, or combinations of these.

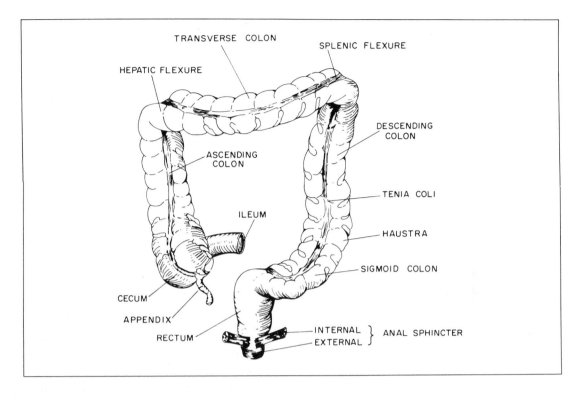

Figure 8-7. The human colon. (Reproduced with permission, from Ganong, WF: Review of Medical Physiology, 13th ed., copyright Appleton & Lange, 1987.)

Sometimes the problem involves a whole organ and, sometimes, only a part or a specific tissue within an organ. On occasion, the problem lies in the duct system. A particular problem may cause malabsorption of one nutrient or of many nutrients. The effects on nutritional status of the patient and the requirements for nutritional care are related to the organ or tissue involved, the extent of involvement, and the nutrients affected.

Many conditions that produce malabsorption are listed in Table 8-3. Although the list is long, the pathologic processes leading to malabsorption are much more limited in number.

Pathogenesis of Malabsorption

Lipids. Malabsorption of lipid occurs more often than with any other nutrient, and the effects are more severe. It can result from abnormalities in any of the steps of fat digestion and absorption and any of the organs and tissues involved in it.

Pancreatic insufficiency. In cases of a deficiency or absence of pancreatic enzymes, most fat is not digested and, therefore, is not absorbed. The lipid then appears in the stools (**steatorrhea**, defined as fecal fat levels greater than 6 g/day). Normal fecal fat is 5 to 6 g/day. The large amounts of fat that appear in the colon in steatorrhea are hydroxylated by the bacteria of the colon. The hydroxylated fats act on the mucosa of the colon, increasing motility and decreasing water and electrolyte absorption in the colon, thus producing **diarrhea**.

Decreased fat absorption in the jejunum may occur under several circumstances. There may be decreased absorptive surfaces such as occurs in damage to absorptive cells from disease, resection of the jejunum, or surgical bypass of the jejunum. Alternatively, disease may cause decreased function of absorptive cells. The failure to absorb fat results in steatorrhea and diarrhea.

Table 8-3. Causes of Malabsorption

Abetalipoproteinemia
Amyloidosis
Bacterial overgrowth
  Blind loops
  Intestinal diverticulosis
  Intestinal motility disturbances
  Strictures
Celiac disease
Dermatitis herpetiformis
Diffuse ileojejunitis
Drug-induced malabsorption
Dysgammaglobulinemias
Endocrine disorders
  Addison's disease
  Carcinoid
  Diabetes mellitus
  Hyperthyroidism
  Hypoparathyroidism
  Systemic mast cell disease
  Zollinger-Ellison syndrome
Enteroenteric fistulas
Gastrectomy (Billroth II)
Intestinal lymphoma
Ischemic bowel disease
  Atherosclerosis
  Polycythemia vera
  Vasculitis
Liver disease
  Extrahepatic obstruction
  Intrahepatic cholestasis
  Hepatocellular disease
Lymphangiectasia
Pancreatic insufficiency
  Chronic pancreatitis
  Cystic fibrosis of the pancreas
  Pancreatic carcinoma
  Pancreatic resection
Parasitic disease
Radiation enteritis
Scleroderma
Short bowel
Tropical sprue
Whipple's disease

Liver and gallbladder function may also be involved in lipid malabsorption, since a number of pathologic processes can cause malabsorption by altering the action of bile:

Intraluminal binding of bile acids. Occasionally, patients are given the resin cholestyramine as a medication. If given in large amounts, the resin binds bile acids and can produce bile acid insufficiency, interfering with micellar formation and lipid digestion.

Steatorrhea and diarrhea can result, as described previously.

Biliary tract obstruction. The obstruction of the bile duct — by a stone or tumor, for example — also produces a deficiency of bile salts. The formation of micelles is compromised, with resultant interference with digestion and absorption. Fecal fat levels may be 25 g/day, accompanied by diarrhea. If the obstruction is also in a position to block the pancreatic duct, there will be a simultaneous deficiency of pancreatic lipase. Lipid digestion then is compromised, and the steatorrhea will be much more severe.

Bacterial overgrowth. The upper part of the small intestine usually contains very few microorganisms, whereas the microbial population of the ileum and the colon is normally very high. The cleansing action of the movement of the intestinal contents normally controls the bacterial population. However, any abnormality that causes stasis or recirculation of intestinal contents may result in bacterial proliferation. Circumstances in which this may occur include structural or postsurgical anatomic defects such as strictures, fistulas, diverticula, and blind loops. For clarification, these are diagramed in Figure 8-8. It may also occur in motor abnormalities such as those which can occur in diabetes mellitus, neuropathy of the autonomic nervous system, and scleroderma. Another cause of bacterial proliferation includes reduced antibacterial capacity.

When bacterial overgrowth in general occurs, there is also an increase in the population of those strains of bacteria that reduce the concentration of conjugated bile salts in the intestinal lumen. The bacteria deconjugate bile salts, and the deconjugated molecules are reabsorbed high in the intestinal tract before they function in fat absorption. Bacterial action also decreases the pH of intestinal contents and reduces the proportion of bile salts that are ionized. Un-ionized salts tend to precipitate out. The resulting decrease in intraluminal concentration of bile salts causes a decrease in micelle formation and thus contributes to fat malabsorption.

Second, under conditions of bacterial

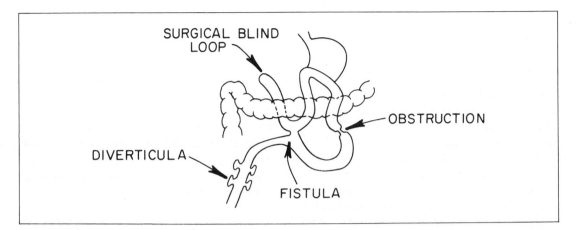

Figure 8-8. Anatomic lesions leading to bacterial overgrowth.

overgrowth, bacterial action can alter the hydroxyl groups at the 3, 7, and 12 positions on the bile salt molecules (see Figure 8-5), converting cholic to deoxycholic acid and chenodeoxycholic to lithocholic acid. It has been suggested that large amounts of deoxycholic and lithocholic acids produced during bacterial overgrowth alter the metabolism of absorptive cells and interfere with their absorptive capacity.

A third means by which bacterial overgrowth may affect fat absorption is through the effect of toxin produced by bacterial metabolism. The toxins may interfere with absorption by direct effects on the enterocytes.

The condition resulting from bacterial overgrowth is known also as **contaminated bowel syndrome**. When it involves stasis of intestinal contents, the terms **intestinal stasis syndrome** or **stagnant loop syndrome** are applied. The syndrome includes other functional impairments as well, although lipid malabsorption usually is most prominent.

Reduction of pH of duodenal contents. In the Zollinger-Ellison syndrome, gastric production of HCl is magnified and may overwhelm the capacity of the duodenum for neutralization. The resulting low pH in the duodenum may also result in precipitation of bile salts similar to that which occurs in bacterial overgrowth.

Ileal dysfunction. The enterohepatic circulation of bile salts depends on their reabsorption in the ileum. If ileal reabsorptive capacity is reduced, bile salts will be excreted in larger quantities. The liver is capable of approximately five times normal production of bile salts, but this capacity may be exceeded if losses are high. The net result, again, is an eventual reduction in bile salt concentration. When the critical micellar concentration is not achieved, leading to deficient micelle formation, steatorrhea and diarrhea result. High losses of bile salts can occur when the ileum is diseased and also when ileal tissue has been surgically removed or bypassed.

When deconjugated bile salts are not reabsorbed, they are carried to the colon where they have a cathartic effect (cholerrheic diarrhea). This is an additional factor contributing to the diarrhea in ileal dysfunction.

Fat malabsorption sometimes is the result of abnormalities in the **lymphatics**, where long-chain fatty acids normally are absorbed. Fat malabsorption may occur in patients with primary intestinal lymphangiectasia (tumor or fibrosis of the lymphatics), Whipple's disease (cause unknown; possibly infection), intestinal lymphoma (tumor), or Crohn's disease.

Carbohydrate. Malabsorption of carbohydrate is less common than fat malabsorption. It can occur when pancreatic exocrine secretion is deficient or absent after pancreatectomy (surgical removal of the pancreas) or because of obstruction of the duct. The digestion of starch is reduced as a result of the absence of pancreatic amylase. A diet low in starch may be used with increased monosaccharides and disaccharides. The diet is difficult to plan satisfactorily. In addition, the patient should be advised on dental care, since the diet will be high in sugar content.

It is more usual for disorders of carbohydrate absorption to be related to deficiencies of intestinal mucosal enzymes, resulting in intolerances to specific oligosaccharides. These are discussed in detail under "Diseases Affecting Primarily the Small Intestine."

Protein. Some degree of protein malabsorption may occur as the result of deficiencies of pancreatic or intestinal enzymes. However, the degree of malabsorption and the severity of the consequences usually are less than those that occur in the case of fat or carbohydrate malabsorption.

Vitamin B_{12}. Malabsorption of vitamin B_{12} may occur for a variety of reasons, most of which can be anticipated based on a knowledge of the steps in normal absorption. Malabsorption of vitamin B_{12} can be expected to follow these conditions:[8]

1. Deficiency of IF, as seen in atrophic gastritis or total gastrectomy, with a reduction in IF-synthesizing cells.
2. Bacterial overgrowth with increased binding or metabolism of the vitamin B_{12}-IF complex by the bacteria.
3. Destruction or absence of ileal receptor sites for absorption, resulting from ileal disease or surgical resection.
4. Intake of certain drugs or toxins, such as neomycin, colchicine, and aminosalicylic acid.
5. Inappropriate pH or ion concentration in the ileal lumen.

Calcium ions are necessary for absorption of the vitamin B_{12}-IF complex at the ileal re-

ceptor site. In chronic pancreatic disease with decreased bicarbonate secretion, calcium soaps are formed in the low pH environment, resulting in decreased availability of calcium. Low ileal pH due to Zollinger-Ellison syndrome has a similar effect.

Drug-Induced Malabsorption. A number of drugs are known to cause malabsorption (see Chapter 4), but those that cause major changes at usual doses are cholestyramine, neomycin, and antacids.

Malabsorption of many nutrients is common in chronic alcoholics.[9] Dietary folic acid and protein deficiency, pancreatic insufficiency, and decreased bile secretion contribute to malabsorption in alcoholics. In addition, alcohol has a direct effect on the

Table 8-4. Factors Contributing to Malabsorption and Diarrhea in Chronic Alcoholics

Factor	Effects
	Mucosal
Folic acid deficiency	Diffuse functional disturbance; morphological changes
Direct alcohol effects	Intestinal damage (cellular and subcellular); altered cellular metabolism (reduced sodium potassium ATPase, ATP); malabsorption (vitamin B_{12}, amino acids, thiamine); inhibition of sodium and water absorption; net secretion of sodium and water; disaccharide deficiency → lactose intolerance
Protein malnutrition(?)	
	Luminal
Pancreatic insufficiency	Due to protein malnutrition and alcohol; alcohol-induced pancreatitis
Liver disease	Decreased bile salt secretion
Increased intestinal motility	

Reprinted with permission from Green, P.H.R., and Tall, A.R., Drugs, alcohol and malabsorption. *Am. J. Med.* 67:1070, 1979.

ATPase = adenosine triphosphatase; ATP = adenosine triphosphate.

intestinal mucosa (Table 8-4). Many of these abnormalities are reversed when the patient's nutritional status is improved, even if alcohol intake continues.[10]

General Symptoms of Malabsorption

Early symptoms of malabsorption include a change in bowel habits, fatigue, apathy, and a smooth surface on the lateral tongue. The patient usually does not seek treatment until the symptoms become more severe. In addition to steatorrhea and diarrhea, the patient frequently has clinical manifestations that are characteristic of specific nutritional deficiencies. These are listed in Table 8-5, with an explanation of the pathophysiology.

Diagnosis

Table 8-6 lists procedures used to diagnose malabsorption. Some tests are useful also in defining the cause of the condition.

The **fecal fat assay** measures the amount of fat that appears in the stool and is a screening test for overall malabsorption syndrome. It is most useful if done in relation-ship to a specified fat intake. Typically, the diet contains 100 g of fat per day. The excretion of more than 6 g of fat per day over a three-day period is considered to indicate fat malabsorption. In some disease states, 40 g of fat per day may be excreted. The test does not distinguish between malabsorption of fat caused by pancreatic disease and that caused by intestinal disease. Simultaneous determination of **fecal nitrogen** suggests pancreatic insufficiency if the content is more than 6 g/day. An acid pH indicates bacterial fermentation of carbohydrates.

Several breath tests are useful. In the **labeled carbon breath test**, the patient is given labeled triolein. Breath samples are analyzed for labeled CO_2. Exhalation of less than normal amounts indicates steatorrhea. Sources of error are obesity or intake of MCT. The **bile acid breath test** requires administration of a labeled bile acid (glycocholic). If the material is not normally reabsorbed in the ileum, it passes into the colon, and increased labeled CO_2 is generated. Sources of error are bacterial overgrowth and abnormal bile salt deconjugation. In the **hydrogen breath test**, malabsorption of carbohydrates and metab-

Table 8-5. Pathophysiologic Basis for Clinical Effects in Malabsorptive Disorders

Pathophysiology	Clinical Effects
Loss of calories	Weight loss and generalized malnutrition
Dihydroxyl bile acids and hydroxyl fatty acids → decreased colonic absorption of sodium and water	Diarrhea
Impaired fat absorption → excess fat content of feces	Bulky, frothy, voluminous stools
Anemia; potassium and magnesium depletion	Weakness and fatigability
Iron, vitamin B_{12}, folate, and other vitamin deficiencies	Glossitis, cheilosis
Vitamin K malabsorption, hypoprothrombinemia	Bleeding problems—oral, genitourinary, gastrointestinal, cutaneous
Calcium malabsorption → hypocalcemia; magnesium malabsorption → hypomagnesemia	Tetany, paresthesias
Vitamin B_{12} deficiency	Peripheral neuropathy
Calcium malabsorption → osteomalacia; protein depletion → osteoporosis; vitamin D malabsorption → impaired absorption of calcium	Skeletal pain
Impaired absorption of amino acids → hypoproteinemia	Edema
Impaired absorption of iron, folate, and vitamin B_{12}	Anemia
Impaired absorption of vitamin A	Night blindness

Table 8-6. Diagnostic Tests for Malabsorptive Disorders

Stool examination for fat malabsorption
  Qualitative
    Neutral fat
    Fatty acid
  Quantitative determination of stool fat
Schilling test for vitamin B_{12} absorption
D-xylose absorption test (25-g dose)
Gastrointestinal roentgenograms of stomach and small bowel
Peroral jejunal mucosal biopsy
^{14}Cr-albumin to diagnose protein-losing enteropathy
Pancreatic function tests
  Secretin test
  Duodenal perfusion with essential amino acids
Hematology, observe for the following:
  Microcytosis
  Macrocytosis
  Hypersegmented polymorphonuclear neutrophils
Blood tests
  Serum iron, ferritin, B_{12}
  Serum calcium
  Serum cholesterol
  Serum albumin
  Prothrombin time
  Serum carotenes
  Serum vitamin A
  Serum 25-hydroxyvitamin D
Urine test: urine 5-hydroxyindoleacetic acid (5-HIAA)
Specialized tests
  Culture of jejunal contents
  Duodenal or jejunal fluid analysis
    Conjugated bile salts
    Unconjugated bile salts
    Micellar lipid
  ^{14}C-glycolic acid breath test
  Breath hydrogen test (after 50 g lactose)

olism by colon bacteria increase breath hydrogen.

The **D-xylose absorption test** is used to distinguish malabsorption caused by intestinal disorders from pancreatic insufficiency. In the test, 25 g of D-xylose, which is not metabolizable, is given orally. Urine is collected for 5 hours and tested for xylose. Normal excretion is 4.5 g every 5 hours. Absorption of xylose does not require pancreatic enzymes or bile. In intestinal malabsorption, xylose concentration in blood and urine is diminished, whereas pancreatic insufficiency does not affect the ability of the enter-

ocytes to absorb xylose. Sources of error include bacterial overgrowth, renal disease, age, edema, and ascites.

The **Schilling test** is of use in differentiating intrinsic factor deficiency from dysfunction in the distal ileum. The patient is given radioactively labeled vitamin B_{12}. Two hours later, a large unlabeled flushing dose is given parenterally. Normally, 10% of the dose will be excreted in 48 hours. A diminished amount of radioactivity in the urine indicates malabsorption. If the vitamin is absorbed normally, ileal disease and pernicious anemia are ruled out. If the vitamin is absorbed only when intrinsic factor is given along with the vitamin, a diagnosis of pernicious anemia is suggested. Patients with severe bacterial overgrowth sometimes fail to absorb the vitamin either with or without intrinsic factor.

Other diagnostic tests include the lactose tolerance test (described on p. 253), tests for pancreatic function, barium studies of the abdomen, computerized axial tomography (CAT) scans, and intestinal biopsy.

Treatment

Any or all of the following may be used as required to treat malabsorption syndromes: surgical resection or repair, and replacement of missing or deficient substances, such as pancreatic enzymes, antibiotics, and antidiarrheal drugs.

Nutritional care can be of great importance. It must be adjusted to the cause, symptoms, and severity of the underlying disease and its clinical manifestation and must be integrated with the other aspects of treatment. The objectives of nutritional care are relief of symptoms with an increase in the comfort of the patient and repletion and maintenance of good nutritional status. Relief of symptoms often involves the use of diets restricting nutrients that cause symptoms when not absorbed. The diet restricted in fat is useful for patients with fat malabsorption. All types of fat are restricted, but the degree of restriction is varied as needed. Useful levels of restriction that have been suggested are as follows:[11]

Mild fat restriction, in which fat comprises 35% to 40% of total kilocalories. (This level exceeds recommended intake, but represents a restriction for some patients.)
Moderate fat restriction, in which fat comprises 25% of total kilocalories.
Severe fat restriction, in which fat comprises 10% to 15% percent of total kilocalories.

The degree of restriction applied to a given patient is related to the severity of the malabsorption. Foods restricted on these diets are listed in the diet manuals of most hospitals.

Some patients with severe steatorrhea and diarrhea are more comfortable if the fiber content of the diet is reduced. Dietary fiber will be discussed later in this chapter.

The maintenance of good nutrition in the patient with malabsorption presents a great challenge to the nutritional care specialist. The following techniques are applied where appropriate:

1. In fat malabsorption, use the highest fat content possible consistent with control of steatorrhea and pain to maintain adequate kilocaloric intake for weight maintenance or gain. Divide the dietary fat equally among the three meals to avoid excessive fat at one meal.
2. Supplement the diet with vitamin and mineral medications. Representative dosages that may be prescribed by the patient's physician are shown in Table 8-7.
3. Add medium-chain triglycerides to the diet of patients with malabsorption of long-chain triglycerides if the fat-restricted diet provides insufficient energy.
4. Use chemically defined diets to supplement or replace the diet.

Medium-chain triglycerides are prepared by steam hydrolysis of coconut oil to separate them from the shorter-chain, more

Table 8-7. Representative Dosages for Agents Used in the Management of Patients with Malabsorption Syndrome

Calcium: Normal replacement is 1 to 2 g/day. Calcium carbonate may be given as Titralac (400 mg calcium per 5 ml) or Os-Cal (250 mg calcium per tablet).

Magnesium: Magnesium gluconate, 500 mg four times daily. Each tablet contains 29 mg of magnesium.

Iron: Ferrous sulfate, one 320-mg tablet four times daily. Each tablet contains 64 mg of iron.

Fat-soluble vitamins
  Vitamin A: 25,000-unit tablets; for severe deficiency, 25,000–100,000 units/day. Maintenance dose is 3,000–5,000 units/day.
  Vitamin D: Initial dose is 50,000 units two to three times per week. Dosage varies considerably, based on patient response as determined by serum and urinary calcium.
  Vitamin K: Vitamin K_1 (water-miscible), 10 mg orally or intramuscularly per day, or vitamin K_3 (menadione), 10 mg orally per day.

Folic acid: 1–5 mg orally per day for 4–5 weeks is adequate to replenish stores and correct anemia. Maintenance dose is 1 mg orally per day.

Vitamin B_{12}: 100–1,000 µg/day intramuscularly for 2 weeks as a loading dose (if required). Maintenance dose is 100–1,000 µg/mo.

Vitamin B complex: Any multivitamin preparation that contains daily requirements (thiamine, 1.6 mg; riboflavin, 1.8 mg; niacin, 20 mg) should be administered twice daily.

Reprinted with permission from Stenson, W.F., Gastrointestinal diseases. In Freitag, J.J., and Miller, L.W., Eds., *Manual of Medical Therapeutics,* 23rd ed. Boston: Little, Brown, 1980, p. 268.

volatile fatty acids. They are available as MCT Oil (see Appendix G).[12] MCT Oil contains C8 (67%) and C10 (23%) fatty acids plus 10% of other lengths. It provides 8.3 kcal/g. It is useful in increasing the available energy in patients with pancreatic lipase and bile deficiencies, deficiencies of chylomicron formation, or abnormalities of lymphatic transport. Some patients find the product somewhat unpalatable. They say it tastes "fishy," and therefore it must be disguised. It can be used only in limited quantities and should be distributed throughout the day, or it will cause diarrhea. MCT Oil does not help meet the need for linoleic acid or fat-soluble vitamins. It may be used in cooking in place of other oils in sauces, salad dressings, and baked goods. It can also be incorporated into milk shakes, casseroles, and juices. The manufacturer provides a recipe booklet that may be helpful to the patient using MCT Oil at home.[13] Other recipes have also been published.[14-17] The development of acceptable methods for its use represents an opportunity for the nutritional care specialist to show imagination and initiative. Since MCT Oil is very expensive, it is not practical to recommend (in the interests of efficiency in food preparation) that it be used for the whole family.

MCT Oil is also available in a variety of casein-based formulas. Information on these products and indications for their use are given in Appendix G.

Intestinal Antigen Absorption

Absorptive Mechanisms

In some diseases, the intestinal mucosa is thought to have lost its ability to act as a barrier to antigens. As a consequence, the patient absorbs toxic amounts of antigens in the diet or toxic products of bacterial metabolism. These may be important in the pathogenesis of disease.

Newborn infants are known to be capable of ingesting macromolecules,[18,19] and there is evidence that some adults normally retain a limited ability to do so.[20] The immunoglobulin A (IgA) antibody in the mucus coating the luminal surface normally complexes with the antigen and prevents its attachment to the membrane and subsequent ingestion. When a small amount of antigen crosses the enterocytes, macrophages and plasma cells in the lamina propria constitute a second line of defense and interact with the antigen, reducing the amount that reaches the general circulation.

In some diseases, excessive quantities of antigen cross the mucosal barrier. Some patients are deficient in secretory IgA, the predominant immunoglobulin in the intestine. In other diseases, the patients are deficient in the secondary defenses. The antigen then may reach the general circulation and cause a toxic or allergic reaction.[21] Patients with combined immunodeficiency disease or with secretory IgA deficiency have been shown to have an increased incidence of malabsorption-related diseases.[22,23] Newborn infants have no antibody in the small intestine or any plasma cells in the lamina propria. Until the immune system in this area matures, they are prone to increased antigen absorption.

Alteration in mucosal permeability also predisposes one to antigen absorption. Inflammation and ulceration are contributing factors. Conditions that enhance adsorption of antigen to the mucosal surface, such as some drugs and some factors in human milk, have been shown in animals to increase antigen uptake.[24,25] The immature enterocytes of the newborn infant have an increased ability to take up antigens by pinocytosis.[26] Patients have an increased number of immature enterocytes following viral gastroenteritis, possibly accounting for their increased antigen uptake.[27]

Lysosomal enzymes sometimes are released inappropriately. Corticosteroids, for example, stabilize the lysosomal membrane.[28] This process could result in decreased antigen breakdown within the cells and an increase in their transport into the general circulation.

In villous atrophy or ulceration, ingested antigens may diffuse across the mucosal barrier. Ionizing radiation, antibiotics, and antimetabolite drugs can alter mucosal function and antigen absorption.

Conditions that increase the concentration of macromolecules in the intestinal lumen may contribute to enhanced antigen absorption. Thus, it has been suggested, but not proved, that pancreatic insufficiency causes increased macromolecule absorption.

Related Diseases

A number of gastrointestinal diseases are suspected to be associated with abnormal antigen absorption. These include gastrointestinal responses to allergy, inflammatory bowel disease, celiac disease, and toxicogenic diarrhea from infection.[28] Those in which nutritional care is important are discussed in this chapter. It is important to remember that the association of these diseases to antigen absorption is somewhat speculative.

Nutritional Management

Prevention of excess antigen uptake in susceptible patients may be beneficial. Procedures suggested to accomplish this objective include encouraging breast feeding in early infancy and decreasing antigen load by using chemically defined formulas based on protein hydrolysates.[28]

Diarrhea

Diarrhea is defined as an increase, as compared to the usual pattern in an individual, in the frequency of bowel movements or excess water content of the stools affecting consistency or volume or both. Usual habits vary, but more than four soft or watery bowel movements per day is considered abnormal in most individuals. Sometimes, the stools are small in volume but frequent. Diarrhea most directly involves the large intestine, but the pathogenesis frequently involves disease of the small intestine, pancreas, or gallbladder. **Acute diarrhea** of bacterial origin is relatively common and often is self-limiting to 3 weeks or less. Specific therapy is not often required, except in infants. The adult patient usually can maintain his or her fluid and electrolyte balance with a clear liquid diet in diarrhea of short duration. A urine flow of 1,500 ml/day indicates adequate fluid intake. **Intractable diarrhea**, chronic or recurrent, has a greater nutritional impact.

Pathophysiology and Classification.

Major mechanisms in the pathogenesis of diarrhea include the presence of excessive amounts of osmotically active substances in the intestinal lumen, secretion into the lumen, and derangement of intestinal motility.

Osmotic diarrhea results from the presence in the intestinal lumen of excessive numbers of osmotically active particles, usually a carbohydrate or a divalent cation. Sources of these include saline laxatives and some antacids. Sometimes these particles are present because of maldigestion or malabsorption of an osmotically active nutrient as a consequence of reduction in a digestive enzyme or reduced absorptive surface. In the presence of these osmotically active nutrients, there is a greater fluid **efflux** (movement of fluid into the lumen) than **influx** (absorption of fluid from the lumen). The total amount of fluid lost can be very great. The patient may have more than 1,000 ml of stool per day. Osmotic diarrhea stops when the intake of osmotically active substances stops. Therefore, osmotic diarrhea subsides during fasting.

Secretory diarrhea occurs when disease causes the secretion of large amounts of fluid into the intestinal lumen even if absorption is normal. This can occur in either the small or large intestine. Two mechanisms may be involved. **Passive secretion**, caused by increased tissue pressure or hydrostatic pressure, is believed to be the cause of increased secretion in obstruction and in intestinal inflammations. The other mechanism postulates a **stimulant** for secretion, which binds to a receptor on the membrane of cells in the crypts of Lieberkühn and stimulates adenyl cyclase. The action of adenyl cyclase increases the production of cyclic adenosine monophosphate (cAMP) in the cell. Cyclic AMP may inhibit sodium absorption by villous cells and induce secretion of the chloride and bicarbonate anions by crypt cells. Sodium, potassium, and water follow the movement of the anions.

An important related issue is the identity of stimulants to secretion. A number of substances are classified as activators of adenyl cyclase. Many of these are enterotoxins, produced by bacteria that colonize in the intestine or have multiplied in food. *Escherichia coli*, causing traveler's diarrhea, and *Vibrio cholerae*, causing cholera, produce enterotoxins in the intestine. *Staphylococcus aureus* causes food poisoning by producing a toxin in the food in which it multiplies.

Prostaglandins have also been shown experimentally to stimulate adenyl cyclase. The diarrhea of some tumors of the intestine may be partly the result of the action of these substances.

Hormone-producing tumors may cause diarrhea. For example, the excess of gastrin produced in Zollinger-Ellison syndrome may stimulate adenyl cyclase. The acid inactivation of lipase leading to steatorrhea also contributes to the diarrhea. Other hormonally mediated diarrheas are the result of VIP-omas and carcinoid syndrome.

Both bile salts and fatty acids stimulate adenyl cyclase. Bile salts are found in the colon when ileal reabsorption is decreased. The fat which then reaches the colon is hydrolyzed by bacteria to produce fatty acids.

Secretory diarrhea causes a greater volume of fluid loss than does osmotic diarrhea and tends to persist during fasting. An exception is the secretory diarrhea resulting from unabsorbed fatty acids and bile salts.

Diarrhea also may result from alterations in intestinal **motility**. Circular muscle contractions normally retard the movement of intestinal contents. Loss of circular muscle tone may then contribute to diarrhea. Increased longitudinal muscle activity, which may occur in intestinal tumors and in emotional disorders, also causes diarrhea.

Sometimes diarrhea is a mixed type that simultaneously involves decreased fluid absorption and changes in secretion and motility. Some diseases of this type are infectious. Organisms involved include viruses, bacteria, protozoa, and helminths in the intestine. Sometimes the basic disease is **idiopathic** (of unknown origin), whereas others are **iatrogenic** (resulting from treatment). Diarrhea can occur as a reaction to medications, (e.g., antibiotics), to poisonings (e.g., by iron or insecticides), to food intolerances, and to a nongastrointestinal infection (e.g., pneumonia, otitis media, and urinary tract infection).

Diagnosis

Many of the procedures described for diagnosis of malabsorption are applicable to the diagnosis of diarrhea in general. Others that may be indicated are listed in Table 8-8.

Metabolic Consequences

With diarrhea, fluid losses may reach 15 liters per day, with accompanying losses of sodium, potassium, and bicarbonate. The pattern of fluid and electrolyte loss is somewhat variable. For example, in osmotic diarrhea, water loss is greater than sodium loss. In persistent mild diarrhea, potassium deficiency can develop. If appropriate replacements are not provided, the patient may develop **dehydration**, **hyponatremia** (low serum sodium), **hypokalemia** (low serum potassium), and **acidosis**.

When diarrhea is a consequence of fat malabsorption, the unabsorbed fatty acids may complex with calcium, magnesium, zinc, manganese, selenium, and chromium, making them unabsorbable. Absorption of fat-soluble vitamins is also reduced.

Table 8-8. Diagnostic Procedures for Diarrhea

Culture for microorganisms

Examinations for ova and parasites

Examination for fecal leukocytes, which are present in colitis if bacterial, ulcerative, or antibiotic-associated

Determination of electrolyte content and osmolality of stool
  If 2 × [sodium + potassium] is approximately equal to serum osmolality, diarrhea is secretory.
  If difference is more than 100, diarrhea is osmotic.
  A pH of less than 5 suggests disaccharidase deficiency.

Proctosigmoidoscopy

Radiologic tests: flat plate of abdomen; barium enema

Biopsy

Serum gastrin, vasoactive intestinal peptide, thyrocalcitonin

Urinary 5-hydroxyindoleacetic acid to detect carcinoid syndrome

Therapy

The first step in treating diarrhea is to correct fluid and electrolyte disturbances (see Chapter 4). These disturbances can be particularly devastating in infants and small children who have limited capacity to control their water balance. There are a number of products available for treatment in these patients (see Appendix G, Table 3). They are known as **oral rehydration solutions**. One of these has been sponsored by the World Health Organization of the United Nations and is useful in underdeveloped countries where gastrointestinal infections in infants are common. It is easily prepared from common ingredients and is especially valuable for that reason. Its ingredients are $\frac{1}{3}$ to $\frac{2}{3}$ tsp. table salt, $\frac{3}{4}$ tsp. sodium bicarbonate, $\frac{1}{3}$ tsp. potassium chloride, and $3\frac{1}{3}$ Tbsp. sugar in 1 liter of *boiled* water. Several commercial preparations are also available. Their compositions are given in Table 8-9.

These formulas have been used on an outpatient basis for infants with less than 5% dehydration, without vomiting. The infants are given these clear liquids only at the rate of 1–2 oz./hour. If this material is not vomited, the amount can be increased to 3–4 oz. every 3–4 hours. If the diarrhea subsides within a day, formula can be reinstated at half strength and advanced to full strength within about two days. Breast-fed infants can continue breast feeding, but should be given added water and juice. Solid food appropriate for age can be reintroduced in one month if the diarrhea has subsided.

If the diarrhea does not subside, a lactose-free formula may be necessary. Infants with more than 5% dehydration should be treated as inpatients. Some patients may need TPN.

Nonspecific antidiarrheal agents may be used but are not appropriate in all conditions. Among the drugs that sometimes are prescribed by physicians are secretory inhibitors such as bismuth preparations, aluminum hydroxide absorbents such as kaolin-pectin compounds and psyllium seeds, narcotic agents such as paregoric or codeine, diphenoxylate hydrochloride with atropine sulfate (Lomotil), and antispasmodics such as belladonna preparations. Some of these may be accompanied by nutritionally relevant side effects:

Paregoric: Dry mouth, nausea, occasional abdominal distension.
Codeine: Nausea, vomiting, anorexia, constipation.
Lomotil: Nausea, vomiting, anorexia, constipation, bloating, dry mouth.

If diarrhea is severe, food may be withheld for 24 hours or restricted to clear liquids followed by a soft diet in frequent small amounts as tolerated. Raw fruits and vegetables, whole grains, and concentrated sweets may be avoided and added as tolerated as the patient convalesces.

Chronic diarrhea leads to nutritional deficiencies if adequate replacement is not provided. High-protein, high-kilocalorie diets and supplements are useful. Patients may need vitamin supplements as well.

Table 8-9. Approximate Electrolyte Content for Oral Rehydration Solutions

Solution (Source)	Calories per Ounce	Carbohydrate (g/dl)	Electrolyte					Osmolarity
			Na^+ (mEq/L)	K^+ (mEq/L)	Cl^- (mEq/L)	Ca^{++} (mEq/L)	HCO_3^- (mmol/L)	
Lytren (Mead Johnson)	9	7.6	30	25	25	4	—	440
Pedialyte (Ross)	6	4.5	30	20	30	4	—	405
Pedialyte RS (Ross)	—	2.5	60	20	50	—	—	290
WHO solution	—	1.8	90	20	80	—	30	331

Protein-Losing Enteropathies

The leakage of protein into the intestine is considered to be a normal event in the metabolism of plasma proteins.[28,29] It has been estimated that 10% to 20% of the normal plasma protein loss occurs by this route. Protein losses may, however, reach excessive proportions in many diseases (Table 8-10),[29,30] and may be the consequence of increased mucosal permeability, inflammatory exudate, excessive turnover of cells, or leakage of lymph from obstruction of lacteals.[31]

Loss of lipid, calcium, iron, and copper also may occur. The patient usually has edema and hypoproteinemia. Clinical signs

Table 8-10. Diseases Associated with Protein-Losing Enteropathy

Cardiac
Congestive heart failure
Constrictive pericarditis
Interatrial septal defect
Primary cardiomyopathy
Tricuspid insufficiency

Gastric
Gastric carcinoma
Giant hypertrophy of the gastric mucosa
Atrophic gastritis
Postgastrectomy syndrome
Benign gastric ulcer

Small intestine
Celiac sprue
Tropical sprue
Regional enteritis
Whipple's disease
Lymphoma
Intestinal lymphangiectasia
Intestinal tuberculosis
Acute infectious enteritis
Scleroderma
Jejunal diverticulosis
Allergic gastroenteropathy
Eosinophilic enteritis

Colon
Colonic neoplasm
Ulcerative colitis
Granulomatous colitis
Megacolon

Miscellaneous
Esophageal carcinoma
Gastrocolic fistula
Agammaglobulinemia
Nephrosis
Thrombosis of inferior vena cava
Pancreatitis

of other deficiencies appear. Increases in protein intake and supplementation with vitamins and minerals often are necessary. Primary treatment, however, is directed to the underlying disease.[31]

Intestinal Lymphangiectasia

Intestinal lymphangiectasia was known formerly as **primary protein-losing gastroenteropathy** and is a prototype for the protein-losing enteropathies. The infantile form may result from a congenital malformation of the lymphatic system. In adults, its occurrence sometimes is secondary to damage from other conditions. The cause is unknown. The disease usually manifests itself in children or young adults.

The patient has severe peripheral edema, which may be asymmetrical, plus hypoproteinemia and lymphocytopenia. Gastrointestinal symptoms usually are mild but occasionally are severe. Most patients have intermittent diarrhea and steatorrhea. A few have severe steatorrhea, nausea, vomiting, and abdominal pain and distension.

Electron microscopy has shown accumulation of lipids in the endothelial cells of the intestinal lymphatics and also in the absorptive cells. The fat malabsorption may be explainable on this basis. Alterations in the endothelial cells and surrounding structure may account for the increased pressure in the lymphatics. This increase in pressure causes a dilation of the lymphatics, which may change the architecture of the villi. With increased pressure, lymph, containing both protein and lipid, is forced into the lumen of the bowel. Peripheral lymphatics are hypoplastic, and the thoracic duct may be tortuous, obstructed, or absent.

The normal lymph flow is approximately 1,500 ml/day and contains 70 g of fat and 50 g of albumin. The presence of long-chain triglycerides stimulates lymph flow. Loss of fat may be as much as 40 g/day. Protein loss into the bowel may account for the hypoproteinemia and related symptoms. The patients also often have vitamin B_{12} malabsorption. Some become hypocalcemic.

The reduction of long-chain fatty acids in the diet reduces the lymph flow and reduces the transudation of protein and lipid into the bowel lumen. Serum calcium levels also improve. The fat level in the diet must be very low, less than 5 g/day. Medium-chain triglycerides may be used to improve the energy content of the diet. For infants, Portagen or Pregestimil may be used as the basis for a formula (see Appendix G).

Intestinal Fistulas

Fistulas are abnormal communications between two epithelial surfaces. They are classified according to their location or volume of output. They may be **internal**, between two hollow epithelium-lined organs, including two loops of intestine (**enteroenteral**) (see Figure 8-8), or **external**, between a hollow organ such as the intestine and the skin (**enterocutaneous**). An intestinal fistula may be congenital or acquired. Acquired fistulas may be spontaneous, resulting from a disease process, or the result of trauma, postoperative, or iatrogenic. Spontaneous fistulas may occur as a complication of peptic ulcers, tumors, inflammatory bowel disease, or trauma.

External gastrointestinal fistulas are classified further by volume of output. **High-output fistulas** produce 200 ml/day or more of effluent. Sometimes total volume is as much as 5 liters. **Low-output fistulas** produce less than 200 ml/day of effluent. Fistulas of the stomach, duodenum, pancreatic duct, or proximal bowel are high-output. Low-output fistulas are in the distal small bowel and colon. They often are created surgically for excretory purposes and are discussed later in this chapter with other conditions affecting the colon.

When a patient has a fistula involving the small intestine, absorptive surface is lost by resection or by short-circuiting. If a fistula is formed between the small intestine and colon, the small intestine may become contaminated with colon bacteria. Fat malabsorption, steatorrhea, extreme weight loss, excessive losses of fluid and electrolytes, and protein-calorie malnutrition can result.

Other consequences are intraabdominal sepsis, wound infection, excoriation of the skin, and hemorrhage.

In gastric, duodenal, or jejunal fistulas, the fluid is isotonic, and a large amount of sodium is lost. In addition to the resulting fluid and sodium depletion, alkalosis may develop if gastric fluid is lost. Loss of duodenal fluid containing bicarbonate can result in acidosis. Jejunal fistulas seldom cause acid-base problems because the fluid lost has a nearly neutral pH. Digestive enzymes in the jejunal effluent can cause digestion of the abdominal wall. Biliary fistulas result in water and sodium loss, but the losses are not severe. Pancreatic fistulas can involve fluid losses of 1 liter per day, acidosis from bicarbonate loss, and autolysis of the abdominal wall, a particularly troublesome complication.

Nutritional management of small bowel fistulas is an important consideration, as well as control of drainage, skin protection, physical therapy, and psychological support. These are managed simultaneously with nutritional care. Nutritional management involves replacement of fluid and electrolyte losses as a first priority of the physician.[32] Beyond this point, adequate nourishment is essential to a positive outcome. Weight loss and decreased serum albumin have been correlated with increased mortality. On the other hand, adequate nutrition correlates with decreased mortality rate and more frequent spontaneous closure of the fistula. The route of this nutritional support does not make a difference in degree so long as the support is sufficient.

The route of feeding depends on the classification of the fistula. Low-output ileal fistulas, for example, can be treated with a complete liquid diet or tube feeding. A chemically defined feeding is useful if a catheter must be in place for a long period because the smaller catheter is more comfortable. In contrast, jejunal fistulas, particularly if high output, are more successfully treated by TPN.[28]

Most external fistulas close spontaneously within one to two months if the patient is well nourished, although some must be closed surgically.[33] Control of sepsis is of primary importance in survival. Factors increasing risk include high output of the fistula, location high in the digestive tract, presence of cancer, complications involving urinary or biliary systems, and age greater than 65 years.

DISEASES AFFECTING PRIMARILY THE SMALL INTESTINE

Gluten-Induced Enteropathy

Gluten-induced enteropathy has also been known as **nontropical sprue**, **celiac sprue**, **celiac disease**, **gluten-induced sprue**, and **idiopathic steatorrhea**. It typically appears in infancy when cereals are added to the diet, or in adults, primarily at 20 to 30 years of age. Sometimes, a child has a remission of the disease in adolescence, and then the disease recurs. It is a lifelong condition. **Gluten intolerance** may also occur as a transitory condition secondary to intestinal damage in other disorders.

Clinical Manifestations

The patient with gluten enteropathy has steatorrhea and diarrhea with frequent, foul-smelling, bulky stools. This is accompanied by failure to thrive in children, and, in both children and adults, weight loss and irritability are typical. The enterocytes are damaged, with a resultant decrease in disaccharidases and a secondary lactose intolerance. The damage to the cell also alters enterocyte permeability, resulting in active secretion of potassium and other electrolytes into the intestinal lumen.

There is a generalized decrease in villus length, so that the mucosa becomes partially or totally flattened. The lamina propria is infiltrated with lymphocytes and plasma cells. The surface epithelial cells become extensively vacuolated and lose their brush border.

Protein, fat, and carbohydrates are malab-

sorbed, as are fat-soluble vitamins. The consequent deficiencies of fat-soluble vitamins can lead to osteomalacia, rickets, tetany, bleeding tendencies, and night blindness. The patient may also have deficiencies of vitamin B_6 and of trace elements. Malabsorption of iron, folate, and vitamin B_{12} may cause microcytic or macrocytic anemia.

Pathogenesis

The small intestinal mucosa is damaged when the patient eats foods containing toxic **gluten**, a protein found in wheat, rye, barley, and possibly oats. Wheat gluten may be fractionated into two parts, **gliadin**, the damaging fraction, and **glutenin**. The basis for the toxicity of gluten in these cereal products is unknown but may be related to their content of amide or bound glutamine and proline. The toxic glutens, for example, have a higher percentage of amide nitrogen than is found in the well-tolerated corn and rice. Wheat gliadin contains a high proportion of glutamine and proline.

The exact mechanisms by which the disease is produced are not entirely clear, but there are several theories.[34] One suggests that there is an enzyme deficiency, allowing toxic products of gliadin degradation to accumulate and damage the enterocytes; however, the enzyme has not been identified. Another theory suggests that the enterocytes have surface receptors that bind to gluten, or gliadin, causing cell death. Third, a large proportion of gluten-intolerant patients have a histocompatibility marker HLA-8 (see Chapter 4); the evidence indicates that immune factors are important. This last theory appears to have the most support at the present time.[35] There is infiltration of the jejunal mucosa with small lymphocytes and plasma cells[36] and changes in serum immunoglobulin concentrations,[37] particularly a reduction in secretory IgA and resulting antigen uptake.[23] Antibodies to gluten are found in the serum of these patients,[38] and many have autoantibodies to connective tissue.[39] There also is some evidence of an abnormal cell-mediated immune response.[40,41]

Diagnosis

There is no specific diagnostic test. In order to establish a definite diagnosis, three criteria must be met:

1. Evidence of malabsorption. For this purpose, tests in Table 8-6 are used.
2. Jejunal biopsy shows blunting and flattening of villi.
3. Use of a gluten-free diet results in clinical, histologic, and biochemical improvement.

If results are not definitive, the patient may be challenged with 30–50 g gluten given orally. Increased steatorrhea and diarrhea after the challenge confirm the diagnosis.

Treatment

The primary treatment of gluten enteropathy is the strict avoidance of gluten in the diet. Foods containing wheat, rye, barley, oats, and perhaps buckwheat must be carefully eliminated. An important function of the nutritional care specialist is to help the adult patient, or parents of a child patient, to identify sources of gluten or its derivatives in foods in which its presence is not obvious. Examples of foods that may contain gluten are meats prepared with cereal fillers, salad dressings, ice cream, candies, gravies and sauces containing fillers, malted milk, beer and ale that are prepared from barley, paste products, and foods containing bran or labeled **graham**, as in graham crackers. Hospital diet manuals usually contain a detailed list of foods to be avoided. Recovery from intestinal damage may take as long as six months. In primary disease, the gluten-free diet is a lifelong requirement. If the patient eats gluten, the symptoms recur. For patients whose gluten intolerance is secondary to another condition, symptoms will not recur if the primary disease no longer exists.

The patient tolerates corn, rice, and millet. Cornmeal and flours from rice, arrowroot, potato, soy, and wheat starch can be used to prepare baked products. However, they can-

not be substituted freely for wheat flour in recipes. As a consequence, special recipes must be provided to the patient.

For several months early in the dietary treatment, a restriction of fat and avoidance of lactose in the diet may be necessary. When the normal villus architecture returns, steatorrhea subsides and the tolerance to lactose returns, making these restrictions unnecessary. In the interim, however, the patient needs assistance in planning an adequate diet in the face of multiple restrictions. Sometimes MCT Oil is prescribed.

Until the villus architecture returns to normal, the patient is likely to require supportive treatment in the form of mineral and vitamin supplements prescribed by the attending physician. Complete reversion to normal is more likely in children than in adults. Residual effects in the adult may require continuing nutrient supplementation.

Tropical Sprue

Tropical sprue is a diarrheal disease that occurs primarily in the tropics. It also is seen in the temperate zone in patients who have visited the tropics. The cause of tropical sprue is unknown; it is believed to be due to microorganisms, but no single organism has been identified. Laboratory tests usually indicate malabsorption of fat, xylose, and vitamin B_{12}. Jejunal biopsy shows shortened and thickened villi, but the changes are nonspecific. The disease responds to antibiotics, vitamin B_{12}, and folate, but it does *not* respond to a gluten-free diet. Nutritional care includes a high-calorie diet to restore and maintain normal body weight, at least 1 g of protein per kilogram of body weight, and replacement therapy, including folate, vitamin B_{12}, and sometimes iron.

Inflammatory Bowel Disease

Two disorders are together classified as inflammatory bowel disease (IBD). They are **Crohn's disease** (CD) or **regional enteritis** and **chronic ulcerative colitis** (CUC). These may be two distinct diseases or different manifestations of the same pathological process. In either case they have much in common. They are compared in Table 8-11, but clear differentiation between them is not possible in 15–20% of the patients. Both diseases are discussed here for convenience. Also, although CUC is largely confined to the colon, it sometimes involves the distal ileum, and some patients with Crohn's disease have involvement of the colon. The cause is unclear in either case.

Crohn's Disease

Crohn's disease can occur at any age but is more common between the ages of 15 and 30 years and between 50 and 60 years. It usually is insidious in onset and becomes chronic and intermittent.

Clinical Manifestations. Patients with Crohn's disease complain of abdominal pain, nausea, and vomiting and have secretory diarrhea with weight loss and fever. There is a chronic inflammation of the affected bowel, often with granulomas. The terminal ileum is typically the primary site, but the colon and rectum are sometimes involved. The involved tissue may be discontinuous, with areas of healthy tissue interspersed among areas of diseased tissue. All layers of the intestinal wall are affected, and the mesentery and the lymph nodes in the area may also be involved. Possible complications include stenosis, mechanical obstruction, ulcers, abscesses, and internal or

Table 8-11. Comparison of Crohn's Disease and Chronic Ulcerative Colitis

Factor	Crohn's Disease	Chronic Ulcerative Colitis
Etiology	Unknown	Unknown
Age of onset	10–30, 50–60	10–30, 50–60
Tissue primarily involved	Mouth to anus Any part of intestinal wall (may penetrate)	Colon and rectum only Mucosa and submucosa only
Intestinal complications	Stricture and obstructions Fistula	Stricture and fistula unlikely

external fistulas. The incidence of colon or rectal cancer is increased. Occasionally, the disease affects other tissues, such as skin, eyes, bile ducts, liver, or joints. There is growth failure in child patients.

Malnutrition frequently accompanies Crohn's disease for several reasons. First, food intake usually is decreased secondary to anorexia, altered taste, abdominal pain, and diarrhea. In addition, malabsorption may result from loss of bowel function due to bacterial overgrowth, inflammation, resection, or bypass surgery. Blood, protein, fat, carbohydrate, water, electrolyte, and vitamin losses are increased. The patient's losses may be increased because of gastrointestinal bleeding, protein-losing enteropathy, and loss of bile salts. There also may be increased requirements because of fever and for repletion of body stores and catch-up growth. Specific effects vary with the site and effect of involvement and may include the following:[42]

- Anemia from iron, folate, and vitamin B_{12} deficiencies.
- Hypoalbuminemia consequent to protein loss, decreased intake, and decreased albumin production in the liver.
- Poor wound healing from vitamin A, E, and C deficiencies and protein-calorie malnutrition.
- Impaired immune response.

Causes and Predisposing Factors. The cause of Crohn's disease is unknown. Genetic, infectious, and immunologic factors have been suggested. No specific pathogenic organism has been identified. Abnormal antigen absorption may be involved in its pathogenesis.[28]

Diagnosis. Careful X-ray examination of the bowel is important in diagnosis. If the colon is also involved, a rectal biopsy is useful. Laboratory values are largely nonspecific, reflecting malabsorption and inflammation.

Treatment. During an acute attack, bed rest is required. The diarrhea and abdominal pain are treated with anti-inflammatory and immunosuppressive medications. Prednisone, a glucocorticoid anti-inflammatory drug, increases absorption but tends to retard growth. It is used when mainly the small bowel is involved. Sulfasalazine, also an anti-inflammatory drug, is useful in colonic involvement, and metronidazole in anal disease. Sulfasalazine is a non-steroid with side effects of nausea and vomiting. It tends to inhibit folate absorption, sometimes creating a need for folate supplementation. Antidiarrheal drugs (e.g., loperamide) are also used. The efficacy of drugs is difficult to evaluate because of the usual fluctuating severity of the disease.

Nutritional management in Crohn's disease is supportive and very important. It must also be individualized. In general, it is recommended that the diet provide 1.5–2.0 g protein/kg body weight for children plus sufficient energy to maintain normal growth. Growth of child patients should be followed on growth charts. Vitamins and minerals at one to five times RDA levels should be given as supplements.

A number of diets have been provided with varying results. Sometimes, patients are given nothing by mouth for short periods to allow the bowel to "rest." For longer periods and for patients in whom medical management fails, TPN may be used. Tube feedings may be used if the feeding can be given below any existing fistula. Lack of nutrients in the lumen tends to decrease villous height and absorptive function. Therefore, enteral feeding should be used if possible. Patients with Crohn's disease generally have a better outcome following TPN than do patients with CUC.

When given conventional feedings, many patients are more comfortable with a diet that is reduced in fiber to reduce fecal output and avoid obstruction. Foods that are known to stimulate peristalsis, such as prunes and coffee, should be avoided. Low-fat meals to reduce steatorrhea, with increased protein and carbohydrate, may be helpful, and patients may better tolerate smaller, more frequent meals.

Vegetables and fruits sometimes are tolerated poorly, especially if raw, and their intake is reduced if the fiber of the diet is restricted. The need for fiber restriction is, however, controversial. The guidelines for restricted fiber diets in many diet manuals list specific fruits and vegetables that may have to be limited in amount. Ascorbic acid and folate intake particularly may need to be supplemented if the diet is fiber-restricted. If the disease especially affects the ileum, parenteral vitamin B_{12} may be needed. Poor absorption of calcium, magnesium, and iron indicates a need for supplements of these elements. If there is a secondary lactase deficiency, lactose should be avoided. If the patient has bile salt deficiency as a consequence of ileal disease, medium-chain triglycerides may be useful.

Between acute attacks, the patient should be encouraged to eat as wide a variety of foods as possible. The intake should be monitored at intervals to assure adequate nutrition.

Surgical procedures usually are reserved for those who have failed medical management and for treatment of complications, since the disease tends to recur in 50–75% of the patients following resections. In preparation for surgery, TPN may be useful to improve the patient's nutritional status. The general nutritional care of surgical patients is described in Chapter 14. The nutritional care of the chronic presurgical patient is continued after surgery in view of the recurrence rate. The care of patients who have had resections of large portions of the bowel is described in the section on short bowel syndrome.

Chronic Ulcerative Colitis

The onset of chronic ulcerative colitis (CUC) usually is slow, but it can be sudden and severe. The disease often is treated on an outpatient basis. It is characterized by remissions and exacerbations, but it can run a severe course in some patients. The patient has a bloody diarrhea and abdominal pain. During acute episodes, 20 to 30 bowel movements per day consisting of a mixture of mucus, blood, pus, and feces may be produced. The mucosa of the rectum is edematous and ulcerated with an exudate of mucus, pus, and blood. There may be fever, negative nitrogen balance, decreased serum albumin, nutritional edema, dehydration, and anemia. The patient often is extremely anorexic. Lesions elsewhere in the body include rash, hives, arthritis, and conjunctivitis, supporting the speculation that the disease is an immune response.[28]

The treatment includes drugs, diet, and sometimes surgery. The anti-inflammatory actions of corticosteroids are useful to bring the disease into remission, and sulfasalazine can prolong the length of the remission. The sulfasalazine is split in the colon into sulfapyridine and 5-aminosalicylic acid (5-ASA). The effect of the drug is believed to be (1) a local effect on the colon and (2) primarily residing in the 5-ASA fraction. The mode of action is not clear. Side effects include anorexia, headache, nausea, vomiting and gastric distress. It is helpful if the drug is taken *after* meals.

The objectives of the diet are (1) to provide adequate nutrition, including nutrients for repair, (2) to reduce stool frequency, and (3) to make the patient more comfortable. A low-fiber diet sometimes is recommended to reduce pain and the number of stools. Elemental feedings are sometimes used. TPN is indicated (1) to prepare patients for surgery, (2) to maintain patients during postoperative complications, and (3) to maintain patients during exacerbations of the disease when other nutrient intake is not possible. The major effort often needs to be expended in dealing with the anorexia and emotional problems of patients. Many patients have been described as hostile, tense, and immature, suggesting an emotional etiology. Special effort should be made to cater to the patient's preferences and provide attractive service in cheerful surroundings to encourage the patient to eat. Small frequent meals often are used.

Possible complications are hemorrhage,

perforation, fistulas, obstruction, and **toxic megacolon**, in which the colon loses tone and dilates. Cancer develops more frequently in chronic ulcerative colitis patients than in the nonaffected population. Surgical resection of the affected parts is required in approximately 25% of the patients. The disease, unlike Crohn's disease, is curable surgically.

Nutritional support is required to prepare the patient for surgery. Depending on the extent and location of the lesion, surgery may result in an end-to-end anastamosis, or the colon may be resected, requiring the formation of an ileostomy or colostomy. Nutritional care of ostomy patients is discussed later in this chapter.

Nutritional Assessment in IBD

Routine anthropometric methods of evaluating body composition and monitoring compositional changes are useful in IBD, as is observation of visceral protein. When patients are children or adolescents, growth should be monitored on growth charts. Patients should also be observed for clinical manifestations of specific nutrient deficiencies. Efficacy of enteral and parenteral feeding may be evaluated by methods described in Chapter 2.

Short Bowel Syndrome

Etiology

The short bowel syndrome (SBS) is created when a large portion of the small intestine is resected. Extensive intestinal resection may be necessary in the following conditions:

1. Crohn's disease (regional enteritis).
2. Thrombosis (formation of a blood clot in a blood vessel) or embolism (transfer of a mass in the vascular system), causing obstruction of the mesenteric artery.
3. Strangulated volvulus of the small intestine (torsion of a loop), causing ischemia and gangrene.
4. Fistula.
5. Neoplasm.

6. Trauma.
7. Intestinal bypass for obesity or hypercholesterolemia (iatrogenic).
8. Radiation injury.
9. Functional disorders such as scleroderma and pseudoobstruction.
10. Congenital atresia (absence of normal diameter lumen at birth).
11. Congenital Peutz-Jehgers syndrome (multiple polyps).
12. Meconium ileus.
13. Necrotizing enterocolitis.
14. Aganglionosis.

Pathophysiology

The consequences of intestinal resection depend on the extent and site of bowel loss, presence or absence of the ileocecal valve, the function of the remaining bowel as well as the function of the remaining digestive tract, and degree of adaptation of the bowel. Resection of small lengths of the jejunum does not result in any significant malabsorption, and resection of 40% to 50% of the small intestine usually is well tolerated if the proximal duodenum, proximal jejunum, distal half of the ileum, the ileocecal valve, and the ascending colon remain. The loss of more than 50% of the small intestine usually produces significant malabsorption, while removal of more than 75% makes survival questionable unless TPN is used. Protein malabsorption and carbohydrate, mostly lactose, malabsorption occur.

The ileocecal valve is important in prolonging intestinal transit time and preventing ileal contamination with colonic bacteria. If the ileocecal valve is removed, even if ileal resection is limited, a severe intractable diarrhea with life-threatening fluid and electrolyte losses can occur.

Removal of the duodenum compromises absorption of calcium, magnesium, and iron. Severe hypocalcemia and anemia may result.

Bile salts and vitamin B_{12} are absorbed in the terminal ileum. With removal of less than 100 cm of terminal ileum, reabsorption of bile salts is reduced. The liver cannot compensate for this loss, and mild steatorrhea (more than 20 g fecal fat) ensues. Unabsorbed bile salts enter the colon, are deconjugated and cause colonic secretion of fluids and electrolytes. The result is a watery **cholerrheic diarrhea**. If more than 100 cm of terminal ileum is resected, the resulting steatorrhea may be severe (more than 50 g fecal fat).[43]

Loss of terminal ileum with reduction of IF-bound vitamin B_{12} can lead to B_{12} deficiency in two to five years. Bacterial metabolism of vitamin B_{12} also contributes to the deficiency. Megaloblastic anemia and peripheral neuropathy may then result, as described previously in this chapter.[44] Divalent ions (Ca, Mg, Zn, Mn, Se, Cr) complex with unabsorbed fatty acids and are not absorbed. Absorption of fat-soluble vitamins is also impaired. Loss of fat-soluble vitamins may result in night blindness, hypoprothrombinemia, and osteomalacia.

The patients also have an increased incidence of gallstones and renal stones. There are no diet modifications that are known to prevent gallstones. Cholesterol stones, associated with SBS, may be secondary to decreased bile salts. Sometimes, during the surgery resulting in SBS, removal of the gallbladder is considered as a preventive measure.

Renal stones are calcium oxalate stones. Calcium and oxalate in the intestine normally bind and are not absorbed. In the SBS patient with diminished bile salts in the intestine, free fatty acids and calcium bind. Oxalates are then unbound and pass into the colon. Oxalates are absorbed and excreted by the kidney. Urinary oxalates bind to urinary calcium to form calcium oxalate stones, which occur in 75% of SBS patients.[42,45] A low-oxalate diet and calcium supplementation may be used as a preventive measure.

An important consideration is the function of the remaining intestinal tissue. Depending on the primary condition that led to the loss of gut tissue, intestinal function may be quite variable. Disease processes involving other organs of the digestive system, such as the pancreas, may also contribute to overall impaired function.

The deficit causing malabsorption in the short bowel syndrome is probably a combination of deficiency of digestion, deficiency of absorbing area, and increase in transit speed, but the relative importance of these factors is unknown.

For several weeks postoperatively, a severe watery diarrhea occurs in about 50% of SBS patients.[46] As a consequence, fluid, electrolyte, and acid-base balances can present problems. The causes of the diarrhea may include any of the following, depending on the site and extent of the resection:

1. The jejunal absorptive surface is reduced, and the transport capacity of the remaining tissue is overwhelmed. Larger amounts of fluid reach the colon. Many patients have partial removal of the colon, reducing its ability to absorb the added load.
2. Nutrients normally absorbed in the jejunum reach the colon. Carbohydrates are metabolized by colonic bacteria to short-chain fatty acids. The increased osmotic load contributes to an osmotic diarrhea. Long-chain fatty acids from the diet inhibit colonic absorption, especially if hydroxylated by bacteria.[47,48]
3. Bile acids normally absorbed in the ileum may alter colonic absorption and induce colonic secretions (cholerrheic diarrhea).[49]
4. The loss of the ileocecal valve may allow bacterial overgrowth in the remaining jejunum.
5. Gastric hypersecretion, which occurs in approximately 50% of the patients,[50] may aggravate the diarrhea by inactivating pancreatic enzymes. Changes in hormones affecting HCl secretion or hyperplasia of HCl-secreting cells may be responsible for this effect.

In time, some adaptive changes occur.[51] Elongation of the bowel, higher villi, and deeper crypts (Table 8-12) provide more

Table 8-12. Intestinal Adaptation After Small Bowel Resection

Structural changes
Increased diameter of intestine
Increase in villus height
Increase in crypt depth
Hyperplasia-increased cell proliferation and migration rate
Increased rate of DNA synthesis; increased total DNA, RNA, and protein concentration

Functional adaptations
Increase in water, electrolyte, and nutrient transport per centimeter of small intestine
Increase in mucosal enzymes per centimeter of small intestine
Changes in tissue metabolism accompanied by regeneration and growth

Reprinted with permisson from Sheldon, G.F., Role of parenteral nutrition in patients with short bowel syndrome. *Am. J. Med.* 67:1026, 1979. (Adapted from Weser, E., *Viewpoints on Digestive Diseases,* No 10. Chapel Hill, N.C.: American Gastroenterologic Association and Digestive Disease Foundation, 1978, p. 1.)

cells, resulting in increased absorptive surface.[52,53] In addition, functional adaptations (see Table 8-12) result in more efficient active transport.[53] The mechanisms of this adaptation are listed in Table 8-13. It is important to note that stimulation by intraluminal nutrients is one of the adaptive mechanisms, providing a rationale for feeding the patient enterally as soon as possible. The total adaptation process takes up to two years.

Treatment

Nutritional Management. The first need in nutritional support is intravenous replace-

Table 8-13. Mechanisms of Intestinal Adaptation After Small Bowel Resection

Stimulation by intraluminal nutrients
Stimulation by bile and pancreatic secretions
Trophic effects of gut hormones
Altered intestinal blood flow
Altered innervation

Reprinted with permission from Weser, R., Nutritional aspects of malabsorption. Short gut adaptation. *Am. J. Med.* 67:1017, 1979.

ment of fluid and electrolytes (see Chapter 2). This is followed by provision of greater amounts of the patient's nutritional needs by TPN for repletion of stores and control of diarrhea and steatorrhea (see Chapter 5). The patient with massive resection of the small bowel usually needs TPN for three weeks to six months, depending on the extent of the resection. When bowel sounds return and diarrhea declines to less than 2 liters/day, enteral feeding can be undertaken.

Oral feeding must be resumed gradually in order to avoid causing diarrhea. In addition, early feeding into the lumen stimulates elongation of the remaining bowel and hypertrophy of absorptive cells. This adaptation is evidenced by decreasing diarrhea, increased urination, and greater fat and lactose tolerance.

Frequently, enteral feedings are begun with the use of a chemically defined diet containing amino acids and small-molecule carbohydrates administered by tube. A pump is used to deliver a constant low volume over the 24-hour period to make maximum use of the remaining absorptive surface. Gradually, these feedings are increased in volume. The diet may then progress gradually to feedings containing polypeptides and starch. Osmolality should be low. Electrolyte and vitamin supplements are taken orally by some patients. The earliest trial of inclusion of lipid in the feeding is often more successful if medium-chain triglycerides are the lipid of choice. As the tube feedings are increased in caloric content, parenteral feedings should be diminished sufficiently so that the combined feedings provide adequate nutrition without loss of appetite.

The transition to conventional feeding may begin with low-fiber foods in small frequent feedings. Lactose restriction is needed if insufficient lactase secretion has resulted from loss of secreting cells. Very hot or cold items or caffeine should be avoided because they stimulate peristalsis. If blood oxalate is increased, foods high in oxalate should be avoided. The size of the meals should be increased as tolerated. A low-fat diet with added medium-chain triglycerides is often helpful if the diarrhea continues to be a problem.[54] The fat content should be as high as can be tolerated without aggravating the diarrhea, usually 30 g or less.[54] As the intake of the foods is increased, the tube-feeding volume is decreased. Supplements taken between meals are helpful in achieving an adequate calorie intake when the patient is no longer being tube-fed.

After several months, the patient may be able to take all of his or her caloric requirements in the form of conventional foods by mouth, but the lactose restriction sometimes is still needed. Six to eight small meals are recommended.

An occasional patient has such extensive resection of the small intestine that maintenance of life with oral intake is not possible. Parenteral nutrition becomes a permanent necessity. With appropriate support, home parenteral nutrition can be maintained by the patient.

Drug Treatment and Nutrition. Drugs that may be prescribed by the physician include antiperistaltic drugs to prolong the time available for absorption. Cholestyramine binds bile salts and reduces the diarrhea-stimulating effect. Broad-spectrum antibiotics — tetracycline, ampicillin, kanamycin, or neomycin — may be prescribed if bacterial overgrowth is found. Cimetidine reduces gastric acid hypersecretion, and pancreatic enzymes are provided for replacement if gastric hypersecretion inactivates the endogenous enzymes. Sometimes antacids are prescribed.

The nutritional care specialist must be alert to drug-nutrient interactions in these patients. In addition, the patients have usually been given narcotics for several months for the purpose of reducing intestinal transit time, and it is important also to be aware of the possibility of drug addiction. Vomiting, poor intake, abdominal distention, and cramping may be the result of narcotic addiction rather than intolerance to the diet.

Nutritional Assessment

The SBS patient will need the usual nutritional assessment prior to surgery and will require frequent monitoring postoperatively. The degree of adaptation of the intestinal tract must be estimated. In the adaptation process, which may continue for years, the following information is useful:[55,56]

Extent and site of intestinal resection: duodenum? proximal jejunum? ileum? ileocecal valve? ascending colon?

Adaptation of remaining intestine: weight maintenance? fat and lactose tolerance? fecal fat? urine production? D-xylose absorption?

Function of remaining bowel, liver, gallbladder, or pancreas: presence of residual disease?

Stool characteristics: frequency? volume? consistency? color? odor? frothy? greasy?

Results of function tests: fecal fat, carotene, cholesterol? bile acid breath test?

Clinical signs of vitamin and mineral deficiencies? (See Chapter 3.)

Evidence of gallstones or renal stones.

Carbohydrate Intolerance

An intolerance to a carbohydrate is most commonly the result of a deficiency of a disaccharidase necessary for digestion of a disaccharide to monosaccharides. Intolerances to monosaccharides do occur, but they are very rare.

Lactase Deficiency

The most common of the carbohydrate intolerances is caused by a deficiency of lactase. In the lactase-deficient patient, lactose taken in the diet cannot be digested to monosaccharides and absorbed. The lactose remains in the intestinal lumen where it has an osmotic effect. It has been estimated that 50 g lactose results in 150 ml of added fluid load. The increased fluid stimulates peristalsis, producing a watery diarrhea in which fluids and electrolytes are lost. It also contributes to a feeling of distention and discomfort. Bacterial action on the lactose in the colon metabolizes lactose to lactic acid and volatile fatty acids. These irritate the intestinal mucosa adding to the osmotic effect and increasing peristalsis. Carbon dioxide and hydrogen are produced, causing bloating and flatulence.

Forms of Lactose Intolerance. Lactose intolerance occurs in several forms, which vary in their severity and incidence. **Congenital lactose intolerance** is present at birth and is severe. It occurs as **Holzel's syndrome** or as **Durand's syndrome**. In both, vomiting and diarrhea begin within a few days after birth. In Holzel's syndrome, lactase activity is approximately 10% of normal. Durand's syndrome is more severe. It differs from Holzel's syndrome in that, accompanying the symptoms previously described, a large quantity of lactose in the urine (**lactosuria**) and usually albuminuria, aminoaciduria, and acidosis are present. Enzymes for digestion of sucrose and maltose are often also absent. The prognosis is poor. Congenital lactose intolerance in either form is rare.

Primary lactose intolerance is more common. Ethnic origin apparently is important in its occurrence, the condition being more prevalent in blacks, Orientals, Jews, and Indians than in whites of North European ancestry.[56] Those of Mediterranean ancestry and Arabs also show an increased incidence. The condition rarely is present at birth but may develop as early as weaning or at various times thereafter.[57] Sometimes, it does not develop until adulthood. The loss of lactase activity is an autosomal recessive trait and is a permanent condition.

Patients who have diseases of the intestinal tract that involve damage or removal of the intestinal mucosa may develop a **secondary intolerance**, the severity of which varies with the severity of the underlying cause. If enterocyte damage is repaired following treatment, secondary lactose intolerance subsides.

In either primary or secondary intolerance, the severity is variable. In patients with primary intolerance, for example, some patients have no symptoms unless lactose intake is very high. Many can tolerate at least 12 g of lactose, the amount in 1 cup of milk.

Diagnosis. Congenital lactase deficiency is diagnosed by intestinal biopsy and enzyme assay. For suspected primary or secondary deficiencies, a **lactose tolerance test** often is used. In this test, 50 g of lactose is given to an adult orally. The dose for children is 2 g/kg. Blood samples are taken at intervals of 1, 15, 30, 60, and 120 minutes. An increase in plasma glucose of 30 mg/dl indicates normal lactase activity in which glucose is produced, whereas an increase of less than 20 mg/dl suggests lactase deficiency, especially if associated with symptoms. Increases of between 20 and 30 mg/dl are questionable.

An even more accurate test is the **breath hydrogen test**. Breath is collected for the measurement of hydrogen content before and after an oral load of 50 g of lactose. In lactase deficiency, some of the unabsorbed lactose is metabolized to hydrogen in the colon. The hydrogen diffuses into the blood and then into the air in the lungs. Breath hydrogen levels greater than 51 ml/4 hr. are indicative of lactase deficiency.

Some physicians simply prescribe a diet free of lactose for a trial period as a diagnostic procedure. If symptoms subside, lactose intolerance is assumed. It is, however, important to distinguish between lactose intolerance and milk intolerance. Milk intolerance is the existence of symptoms following milk intake. It may be due to lactose, to the milk protein, or to drugs or environmental contaminants in milk.

Nutritional Care. The essential aspect of nutritional care is a reduction of lactose intake to the level of tolerance. In congenital deficiency, the infant at birth must be given a formula free of lactose. Some acceptable products are Isomil, ProSobee, Pregestimil, or Nutramigen (see Appendix G). The patients require a lactose-free diet indefinitely, and the nutritional care specialist must in-

struct patients or families carefully on the "hidden" sources of lactose. Most hospital diet manuals include lists of lactose-containing foods to be excluded from the lactose-free diet.

Patients with less severe forms of lactase deficiency may be able to tolerate small to moderate amounts of lactose in the diet. This diet, sometimes called a **lactose-restricted diet**, must be planned for the individual tolerance of each patient. Most patients can tolerate $\frac{1}{2}$ to 1 cup of milk each day without unpleasant symptoms, especially if the milk is taken with meals.[57] Some patients tolerate chocolate milk better than unflavored whole milk, since its higher osmolality delays emptying time. A lactase enzyme (Lact-Aid, SugarLo Company, Atlantic City, N.J.), derived from the yeast *Saccharomyces lactis*, can be used to hydrolyze much of the lactose in milk. The amount of hydrolysis can be varied with the amount of enzyme, the time allowed, and the temperature. One envelope per quart at refrigeration temperature provides 70% conversion in 24 hours. Three envelopes will give 95% conversion. The amount of milk that can be tolerated thus is increased. When the enzyme is used, the resulting milk is higher in osmolality and sweeter but quite acceptable.

Cultured foods (e.g., cultured buttermilk and unfermented acidophilus milk) have been reputed to be more easily digested and absorbed by lactase-deficient subjects than milk. A recent study comparing digestion of yogurt, cultured buttermilk, and sweet acidophilus milk showed that only unpasteurized yogurt enhanced lactose digestion. Pasteurization of yogurt caused an increase in lactose malabsorption, but no increase in gastrointestinal distress.[58,59] Aged cheeses such as Cheddar and Swiss contain markedly less lactose because the lactose has been removed in the whey. The lactose content of cultured buttermilk and yogurt is influenced by the manufacturing methods. In manufacture, buttermilk and cottage cheese are cultured with *Streptococcus lactis* and *Streptococcus cremoris*. The starter culture for yogurt may be *Streptococcus thermophilus* or *Lactobacillus bulgaricus,* and *Lactobacillus acidophilus* is used in sweet acidophilus milk. Yogurt may be well tolerated because the organisms in the culture produce some lactase. On the other hand, dried milk solids are sometimes added in the preparation. Microbial lactase may be destroyed if the yogurt is pasteurized. Only a small amount of lactose is metabolized by the bacteria in buttermilk or in sweet acidophilus milk.

Prolonged use of a milk-free diet has been reported to result in calcium deficiency[60] and possible osteoporosis.[61] Lactose intolerance does not interfere with the absorption of calcium, and dietary sources of calcium that do not contain lactose should be stressed. Calcium supplements, prescribed by the physician, may be required. The effect of lactose intolerance on other nutrients has been investigated. No effect on nitrogen retention, on nitrogen balance, or on fat, phosphorus, or magnesium absorption was seen.[57,62,63]

Sucrase-Isomaltase Deficiency

Congenital **sucrase-isomaltase deficiency** is a rare condition that probably is a recessive trait. The condition can also be **acquired** as a result of mucosal damage or extensive intestinal resection. The deficiency of sucrase usually is more severe than the deficiency of isomaltase. The patient is unable to digest sucrose or dextrins. Starch with a high proportion of **amylopectin** is not well tolerated. Amylopectin is highly branched, and its digestion produces large amounts of isomaltose. Starches with a large proportion of amylose, such as those from corn or rice, produce only small amounts of isomaltose and are better tolerated.

As the result of the presence of sucrose and isomaltose in the intestinal lumen, diarrhea and other clinical manifestations are produced that are similar to those seen in lactose intolerance.[64] The symptoms are more severe in infants and smaller children than in older patients.[65] The condition may be diagnosed by a sucrose tolerance test, intestinal biopsy, and the onset of symptoms when sucrose, dextrins, or starch are fed.

In feeding patients with this condition, the infant formula must be free of sucrose. Lactose or fructose may be used in place of sucrose for the added carbohydrate in commonly used formulas based on diluted evaporated milk. Foods fed in addition to the formula also must be free of sucrose. Sucrose is added to many prepared infant foods; therefore, it may be necessary for the mother to prepare these at home.

Older patients and some infants may be less severely affected. The sucrose content of the diet should be adjusted to the level of tolerance. For those severely affected, a **sucrose-free diet**, eliminating all sources of sucrose, including almost all fruits, vegetables, cereals, and all foods to which sucrose has been added in processing or preparation, must be used. A **sucrose-restricted diet**, allowing limited quantities of fruits, vegetables, and cereals containing very small amounts of sucrose, may be used for less seriously affected patients. Details of the content of these diets are contained in some diet manuals. An enzyme, **glucomylase**, may be prescribed by the physician. Patients taking this enzyme are able to tolerate a higher sucrose content in the diet. Diets low in sucrose usually are low in ascorbic acid, folic acid, thiamine, riboflavin, and iron, and supplements of these nutrients are recommended.

Glucose-Galactose Malabsorption

Glucose-galactose malabsorption is a rare inherited, congenital condition in which the infant has a watery diarrhea and other symptoms seen in disaccharidase deficiency after the intake of sucrose, lactose, glucose, or galactose. The basic defect may be an alteration in the glucose-galactose shared transport system, but the normal process of absorption is not understood entirely; therefore, the specific nature of the defect is unknown.

Infant formulas containing fructose as the carbohydrate or carbohydrate-free formulas are tolerated. Some tolerance for glucose and galactose develops as the child becomes older, but some degree of defect is permanent.

Abetalipoproteinemia

Abetalipoproteinemia (Bassen-Kornzweig syndrome; acanthocytosis) is a rare inherited disorder affecting primarily individuals of Mediterranean or Jewish origin. There is a deficiency of β-lipoprotein. The incorporation of triglycerides and beta-lipoprotein to form chylomicrons is depressed, and lipid accumulates in the enterocytes. It has been suggested that when triglyceride accumulation reaches a certain level in the enterocyte, steatorrhea ensues.[66]

Other clinical manifestations of this progressive disease include **ataxia** (incoordination), intention tremors, absence of reflexes, muscular and skeletal deformities, and retinitis pigmentosa leading to blindness. Often, growth is retarded, and the patient is thin. Plasma cholesterol is less than 80 mg/dl. Serum triglycerides are very low or absent. The relationship between the neuropathy and retinitis, on one hand, and the β-lipoprotein deficiency, on the other, is unknown.

A fat-restricted diet with added medium-chain triglycerides allows some weight gain and reduction of steatorrhea but does not improve the neurologic symptoms. The diet should be supplemented with fat-soluble vitamins. Folate, iron, and linoleic acid supplements may be necessary also.

The prognosis is poor. Patients have progressive disability and many die in childhood, often from congestive heart failure.

Endocrine-Secreting Tumors of the Gastrointestinal Tract

In recent years, there has been increasing recognition of the endocrine functions of the gastrointestinal tract and of the pancreas, biliary tree, and bronchus, all of which are derived embryologically from the same source. When tumors occur in the endocrine cells of these organs, a wide variety of metabolic and nutritional problems ensue. Some cells secrete abnormally large quantities of their usual hormones, whereas others produce **ectopic hormones** (a hormone of a different cell type), making their quantities excessive. These tumors are classified according to their location as foregut, midgut, and hindgut tumors.

Foregut Tumors

One example of the category of diseases known as **foregut tumors** in the stomach, duodenum, pancreas, and biliary tract is the Zollinger-Ellison syndrome, described previously. Another type is a tumor in those cells, located in the pancreas and bronchi, that secrete vasoactive intestinal peptide (VIP). It is thought to cause a condition known as **pancreatic cholera, Verner-Morrison syndrome**, or **WDHA syndrome** (watery diarrhea, hypokalemia, and achlorhydria), although there is some controversy as to the hormone involved. The patient has a massive watery diarrhea and extensive potassium losses.

Midgut and Hindgut Tumors

Midgut and hindgut tumors occur in the appendix, the small intestine, and occasionally the colon, stomach, or bronchi. Tumors of the appendix, however, rarely cause symptoms. Those in the other organs involve the argentaffin cells, which secrete a variety of potent substances including serotonin, histamine, kinins, adrenocorticotropic hormone, and prostaglandins. Thyroid medullary carcinoma secretes serotonin as well as thyrocalcitonin.

Excess serotonin is the most common hormonal abnormality presently recognized. It produces a complex of symptoms known as **carcinoid syndrome** or **APUDoma** (amine precursor uptake and decarboxylation). Its effects on the intestinal tract include malabsorption, diarrhea, hypermotility, nausea, vomiting, abdominal cramps, and sometimes, intestinal obstruction or **intussuscep-**

tion (telescoping of one part of the intestine into an adjoining part).

The simultaneous occurrence of these clinical manifestations and excessive serotonin suggests a causal relationship, but serotonin may not be responsible for all the symptoms. Some symptoms may be attributable to excess secretion of prostaglandins. Carcinoid tumors also produce kallikreins, which lead to an increase in circulating bradykinins and then to flushing. The overall manifestations are summarized in Table 8-14.

Diagnosis of carcinoid syndrome is made by determination of the presence of 5-hydroxyindoleacetic acid, a metabolite of serotonin, in the urine; the normal value is 16 mg/24 hr. For two days prior to the test, foods containing serotonin must be eliminated from the diet. These foods are walnuts, bananas, avocados, mushrooms, shellfish, tomatoes, pineapple, red plums, eggplant, and papaya.

Surgical removal of the tumor and various medications are the primary forms of treatment. Nutritional care is supportive. The clinical course is prolonged, averaging eight years, and nutritional care can make an important contribution to the quality of life during that period.

Table 8-14. Principal Manifestations of the Carcinoid Syndrome

Vasomotor disturbances—cutaneous flushes and cyanosis

Hepatomegaly—large nodular liver

Intestinal hypermotility—borborygmi, cramps, diarrhea, vomiting, nausea

Bronchial constriction—cough, dyspnea, wheezing

Cardiac involvement—endomyocardial fibrosis with valvular deformity

Absence of hypertension—incidences no greater than general population

Prolonged clinical course—patients survive years longer than those with other tumors with metastases

Reprinted with permission from Kowlessar, O.D., The carcinoid syndrome. In M.H. Sleisenger and J.S. Fordtran, Eds., *Gastrointestinal Disease: Pathophysiology, Diagnosis, Management,* 3rd ed. Philadelphia: W.B. Saunders, 1983.

For patients with diarrhea, nutritional support for malabsorption and diarrheal losses is necessary. Vitamin and mineral supplements may be required. In conditions with excess serotonin, niacin supplementation is needed. Some patients complain that milk, cheese, eggs, and citrus fruits cause flushing and diarrhea, and they are more comfortable if these foods are eliminated from the diet. Ascorbic acid, riboflavin, and calcium may be needed as replacements. The patient should be instructed on choosing a nutritionally adequate diet in view of these omissions.

This is an active area of research, and additional information will undoubtedly be forthcoming. The nutritional care specialist should be alert to new developments in this field.

Acquired Immune Deficiency Syndrome (AIDS)

The acquired immune deficiency syndrome (AIDS), first described in 1981, has spread widely since that time. Most health care professionals will likely have some contact with these patients.

Although AIDS is basically an immune function disease, it has a marked effect on gastrointestinal function. Therefore, it is discussed in this chapter.

The course of the disease is currently described by the Centers for Disease Control as occurring in four stages:

Stage I: Primary HIV infection, often appearing to be similar to mononucleosis. Nutritional complications are minimal.

Stage II: An asymptomatic "carrier" state. Nutritional complications are minimal.

Stage III: Persistent, generalized lymphadenopathy. This stage is often called *AIDS-related complex* or ARC. Symptoms occur which affect nutrition. This may include persistent temperature elevation, involuntary weight loss, abdominal discomfort, and diarrhea.

Stage IV: Symptoms as in Stage III. In addition, there may be development of other

Table 8-15. Nutritional Effects of Drugs Prescribed for HIV-Infected Patients

Drug	Indication(s)	Nutrition-Related Effects	Notes
Amphotericin B	Fungal infections of gastrointestinal tract, e.g., *Candida* esophagitis, or of central nervous system, e.g., cryptococcal meningitis	Fever, anorexia, weight loss, dyspepsia, cramping, epigastric pain, nausea and vomiting, hypokalemia. Rare: diarrhea	
Erythromycin	*Campylobacter* infections of colon; other bacterial infections	Abdominal pain and cramping, nausea and vomiting, diarrhea, stomatitis, heartburn, anorexia	Dose-related
Ampicillin	*Shigella* or *Salmonella* infections of colon; other bacterial infections	Nausea and vomiting, diarrhea, glossitis, stomatitis, anemia	
Isoniazid	Tuberculosis; mycobacterial infections	Dry mouth, anorexia, nausea and vomiting	Supplement with vitamin B_6
Trimethoprim-Sulfamethoxazole	Bacterial infections; *Pneumocystis carinii* pneumonia	Fever, nausea and vomiting, hyponatremia, glossitis, stomatitis, diarrhea	Folate supplement
Metronidazole	Parasitic infections of colon; certain bacterial infections	Nausea, anorexia, dry mouth, metallic taste, abdominal discomfort, diarrhea	Prohibit alcohol
Pentamidine isothionate	*Pneumocystis carinii* infection	Nausea and vomiting, hypo-/hyperglycemia, diabetes mellitus, nephrotoxicity	Folate supplement
Bleomycin sulfate	Kaposi's sarcoma	Nausea and vomiting, generalized weakness, anorexia and weight loss, fever, mental confusion	
Vinblastine sulfate	Kaposi's sarcoma	Nausea and vomiting, anorexia, diarrhea, constipation, epigastric and abdominal pain, pharyngitis, stomatitis, vesiculation of mouth, hemorrhagic enterocolitis, rectal bleeding, mental depression, weakness, leukopenia	
Vincristine sulfate	Kaposi's sarcoma	Peripheral and autonomic neuropathies, abdominal cramps, anorexia, nausea, vomiting, constipation, fever, anemia	
Ketoconazole	Fungal infections, e.g., oral thrush	Topical cream: low toxicity Oral tablets: renal and hepatic toxicity	
Nystatin	Fungal infections	Well tolerated	
Clotrimazole	Fungal infections	Well tolerated	
Ganciclovir	CMV[a] infection of esophagus, stomach, colon, retina	Nausea and vomiting	
Zidovudine	HIV infections	Nausea and vomiting, GI/abdominal pain, anorexia, malaise, taste alterations, sometimes weight gain	

[a] CMV = cytomegalovirus

immune deficiency diseases, opportunistic infections, and neurologic diseases such as peripheral neuropathy, myelopathy, and dementia.

Other symptoms of those infected with the human immunodeficiency virus (HIV) include malaise, fatigue, nausea and vomiting, pain, dyspnea, lesions of the skin and mucous membranes. Esophagitis and dehydration are also seen.

Nutritional Assessment

The standard anthropometric measurements may be used with these patients, as well as measurements of visceral protein such as serum albumin, serum transferrin, and total iron-binding capacity. Since AIDS is an immune disorder, total lymphocyte count and delayed hypersensitivity testing are not useful.

Estimates of energy needs must consider the increased needs caused by fever. Vitamin and mineral intake should be assessed because they are important in immune function.

Nutritional Consequences and Care

Patients with AIDS often have a weight loss of 16% or more. This may be the result of malabsorption, altered metabolism, chronic diarrhea, and sometimes simple starvation. A high-protein, high-carbohydrate diet is a routine provision. Restrictions of fiber, lactose, or fat may be helpful if chronic diarrhea exists.

The opportunistic infections and malignancies often associated with AIDS contribute to the nutritional problems. Kaposi sarcoma lesions also occur in the intestine. Malabsorption may involve glucose, xylose, lactose, amino acids, fat, folate, vitamins B_{12} and A, minerals, and trace elements. The diet must be modified depending on the part of the bowel affected.

Kaposi sarcoma and pulmonary infections may interfere with food intake secondary to dyspnea and coughing. Infections such

as candidiasis (thrush), cytomegalovirus (CMV), and herpes, as well as Kaposi sarcoma, infect the mouth and esophagus, resulting in dysphagia and odynophagia. Liquid or soft diets may be needed. Various infections also can invade the intestinal tract.

Although there is no specific medication for AIDS, some drugs are used for symptomatic treatment and must be considered in nutritional care (see Table 8-15). For example, chemotherapy may be used for treatment of the malignancies. Nutritional effects and related care are discussed in Chapter 15. Antibiotic effects on nutrition and food intake are described in Chapter 4. As the search for a cure proceeds, investigational drugs will be seen. These may have nutritional side effects, and the nutritional care specialist will be required to respond to these as they appear.

An additional problem that may arise is the fear that AIDS generates. Generally, no special precautions concerning food service are needed. However, the recommended, desirable procedures concerning food service sanitation and personal hygiene should be followed carefully.

DISEASES OF THE GALLBLADDER AND BILE DUCTS

Abnormalities of the gallbladder and bile ducts are very common. They tend to be seen more frequently in women than in men, particularly those who are middle-aged, obese, and multiparous (having had more than one baby). Diabetes, female hormones, and heredity have also been implicated.

Gallstones (cholelithiasis) usually are formed from cholesterol and bile salts, but some consist of bile pigments or a combination of these. Some stones are asymptomatic; others can cause inflammation of the gallbladder or obstruction of the duct (**choledocholithiasis**).

Cholecystitis (inflammation of the gallbladder) may result from the presence of gallstones or from chemical irritation of the wall of the gallbladder. It formerly was thought to be the result of infection, but no infectious organisms have been found. Symptoms include epigastric pain, vomiting, and flatulence.

Biliary dyskinesia is the result of malfunction of Oddi's sphincter, which controls the opening of the bile duct into the duodenum. If the sphincter is in spasm or simply fails to open, a back pressure into the gallbladder can develop, causing vague discomfort and sometimes pain.

In the treatment of gallbladder or bile duct disease, a low-fat diet sometimes is recommended to give symptomatic relief. Fat tolerance is highly variable, and the diet should be individualized. Some patients report that they are more comfortable if pork, eggs, fried foods, pastries, and other high-fat foods are excluded. Others find it difficult to tolerate spicy foods, onions, cabbage, cucumbers, and a few other vegetables. If the patient is obese, weight reduction is recommended.

In an acute attack, which usually occurs as a result of bile duct obstruction, a clear liquid diet may be used temporarily, with solid foods and fats added as tolerated.

The current primary treatment of gallstones and cholecystitis is surgical removal of the gallbladder, or **cholecystectomy**. A more conservative treatment, dissolving gallstones by medication with chenodeoxycholic acid (CDCA) or lecithin, is promising when stones are small, but the process may take from six months up to two or three years. In addition, the long-term metabolic effects of CDCA administration are unknown. A high-fiber diet is recommended during this period for cholesterol binding and weight reduction.[67]

The postcholecystectomy patient may be more comfortable with a low-fat diet for several weeks or months. Eventually, the bile duct dilates and takes over the function of the gallbladder, and the patient can return to an unrestricted diet. A few patients continue to have unpleasant symptoms, referred to as **postcholecystectomy syndrome**. The etiologies include stones in the common duct, strictures, tumors, stenosis of the biliary tree, and diseases of adjacent organs. A low-fat diet may give these patients some symptomatic relief.

DISEASES OF THE PANCREAS

Various diseases of the exocrine pancreas have pancreatic insufficiency as a common clinical manifestation. As a result, they have common clinical features. Those features of nutritional significance include steatorrhea, increased fecal nitrogen loss, and vitamin B_{12} malabsorption, as described earlier.

Diagnosis

A number of tests are used to assess pancreatic function and diagnose pancreatic disease.[68] **Serum amylase** and **serum lipase** determinations are increased in inflammations of the pancreas, as is **urine amylase**.

The **secretin-pancreozymin test** measures the pancreatic response to these two hormones. The hormones are given intravenously, and secretions into the duodenum are collected. Normal values are as follows:

Secretin response	Volume output, 2.0 mg/kg/80 min. Bicarbonate output, 10 mEq/30 min. Bicarbonate concentration, 80 mEq/L
CCK-PZ response	Amylase, 50 to 175 units/dl serum

In pancreatic insufficiency, both HCO_3^- and enzyme responses usually are reduced.

The **Lundh test meal** or **synthetic tripeptide test** causes an increase in the release of CCK-PZ and then of enzyme output. Other tests include the measure of fecal levels of fat, nitrogen, or pancreatic enzymes, roentgenography, ultrasound, and biopsy.

Acute Pancreatitis

There are many conditions that cause acute pancreatitis. Two of the most common are biliary tract disease and alcoholism coupled with a genetic predisposition to damage. Other common causes include abdominal trauma, peptic ulcer disease that penetrates the organ wall, and cholelithiasis. A variety of infections, drugs, surgical procedures, cancer, and vascular diseases can also cause acute pancreatitis. The mechanism by which the condition is produced is not well understood, however. One scenario suggests that alcohol stimulates secretin release, increasing pancreatic flow while the duct is blocked at the outlet by edema.[69] Gallstones also may block the ampulla of Vater. Given a duct obstructed by one of these mechanisms, the most commonly accepted current theory of pathogenesis of the disease is that of autodigestion. Pancreatic enzymes normally are secreted into the intestinal lumen in proenzyme form and are activated there. In acute pancreatitis, they may begin a sequence of activation of many enzymes, which then accumulate in the pancreas sufficiently to overcome trypsin inhibitor. Trypsin is activated within the pancreas and digests the pancreas itself.

The major symptom is abdominal pain. Nausea, vomiting, fever, edema, and shock are common. When the outflow of amylase and lipase is obstructed by inflammation, cellular debris, and edema, the enzymes diffuse into the blood and blood levels can become very high. Circulating enzymes affect the hormonal regulation of calcium, and hypocalcemia results. Serum calcium levels of less than 7 mg/dl indicate a poor prognosis. Other effects include exudates in the peritoneal and pleural spaces, necrosis of mesenteric fat, and increased permeability of alveoli of the lungs with resultant pulmonary edema. Urinary amylase is increased. The disease is self-limiting in some patients but may progress to chronic pancreatitis in others.

The patient is given nothing by mouth, since all food and drink, even water, stimulates pancreatic secretion and adds to the pain. Fluids, electrolytes, and colloids may be given intravenously. Once the patient improves, oral feeding may begin with a fat-free clear liquid or chemically defined diet. The diet is advanced slowly, providing six small meals of low-fat, high-carbohydrate, high-protein foods. Alcohol is strictly prohibited. Patients with severe protracted pancreatitis require total parenteral nutrition. Also, TPN is used in complications such as fistula formation, abscesses, or pseudocyst.

Chronic Pancreatitis

Chronic pancreatitis is seen most frequently in patients who have a history of alcoholism. Other causes include metabolic diseases, including cystic fibrosis and hyperlipoproteinemia, as well as inflammation or neoplasm of the sphincter of Oddi and hyperparathyroidism. Pancreatic damage may progress without signs or symptoms for a long period, but eventually the damage becomes severe enough that acute attacks occur with periods of increased alcohol intake. The loss of 90% of the pancreatic tissues causes pancreatic insufficiency, with weight loss and steatorrhea.

Pathogenesis

Three types of action of alcohol on the pancreas have been suggested:

1. Direct toxic effects of alcohol on pancreatic cells.
2. Stimulation of pancreatic secretion with simultaneous induction of spasm in the duct system and Oddi's sphincter.
3. Precipitation of protein material, possibly from degenerating cells, in the small ducts. (The large ducts become involved later.)

As a result of these changes, acinar cells atrophy. The pancreas becomes inflamed, necrotic, hemorrhagic, and edematous. Acini may be replaced by fibrotic tissue. The islets of Langerhans, especially beta cells, eventually become involved, and some patients become diabetic.

Clinical Manifestations

Abdominal pain is the chief complaint in chronic pancreatitis. It may be episodic at first but becomes continuous if alcohol intake continues. Vomiting is frequent. Progressive pancreatic insufficiency leads to malabsorption of multiple nutrients, steatorrhea, and the accompanying symptoms. Weight loss and debilitation are severe. Pathophysiological processes are summarized in Figure 8-9.

Serum amylase and lipase are elevated early but may be normal or even low in advanced disease when pancreatic tissue is destroyed. Roentgenography sometimes shows calcification of the pancreas. Other complications include pleural and pericardial effusions, **ascites** (accumulation of fluid in the peritoneal cavity), psychosis, and necrosis of the bone.[70] Glucagon and insulin reserves are decreased.

Nutritional Management

Replacement pancreatic enzymes, taken orally with meals, are the mainstay of the control of maldigestion and malabsorption. Antacids are given simultaneously to reduce inactivation of the enzymes by gastric acid. A diet low in fat and high in protein is helpful. A high-carbohydrate diet may be used unless the patient is diabetic. This diet may be supplemented with medium-chain triglycerides, chemically defined tube feeding, or intravenous feeding. Multivitamin, mineral, and trace element replacements are often indicated. Complete abstinence from alcohol is essential but difficult to achieve.

Cystic Fibrosis of the Pancreas

Cystic fibrosis (CF) is an inherited disorder of the mucus-producing glands in the pancreas, bronchi, intestines, and bile ducts. The condition is an autosomal recessive trait that occurs about once in 2,000 white live births, once in 17,000 black live births, and once in 90,000 Oriental live births. The abnormal gene has recently been found in the long arm of chromosome 7. In CF patients, one of 1,480 amino acids is missing in the protein tentatively called **cystic fibrosis transmembrane conductance regulator.** The absence of this amino acid interferes with normal functions in the pancreas, lungs, and sweat glands.

As a result of this discovery, it may soon be possible to develop screening methods for prenatal diagnosis and for identification of carriers. Further work may then lead to improved therapy and perhaps to a cure. In anticipation of a cure, it is essential that every effort be made to maintain life in these patients and provide the best quality of life possible.

The pancreatic problems are prominent in this disorder and are those most closely related to nutrition; therefore, discussion of the disease is included in this chapter.

Pathophysiology and Clinical Manifestations

The basic metabolic deficit in cystic fibrosis is not entirely clear. Recent research suggests there is a blockage of the channels through which chloride leaves the affected cells, but it is not clear that this is the primary deficit. Chloride is trapped in the cell, and sodium levels consequently are also high. The chloride channel itself appears to be normal, but an abnormality may exist in the mechanism that opens and closes the channel. This mechanism might be a protein in the epithelial membrane of involved cells.[71,72] An abnormally large amount of a very viscid mucus is secreted, and the sweat has three to five times the normal concentration of sodium and chloride.

There are many manifestations of this disease. In the newborn, the meconium tends to be thick and sticky, causing intestinal obstruction known as **meconium ileus.** The in-

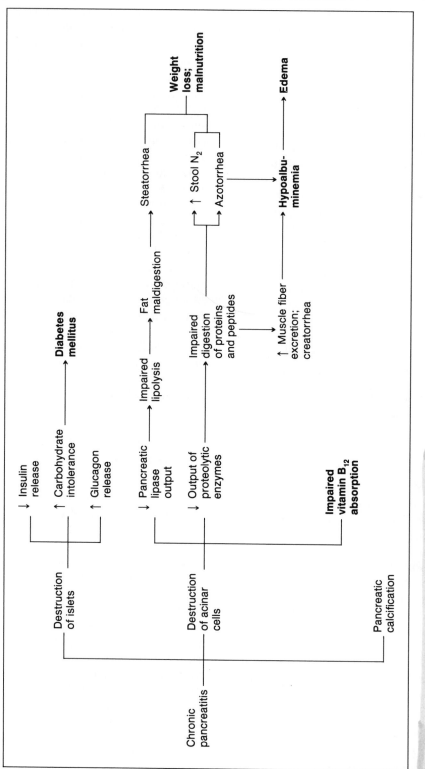

Figure 8-9. Pathophysiology in exocrine pancreatic insufficiency.

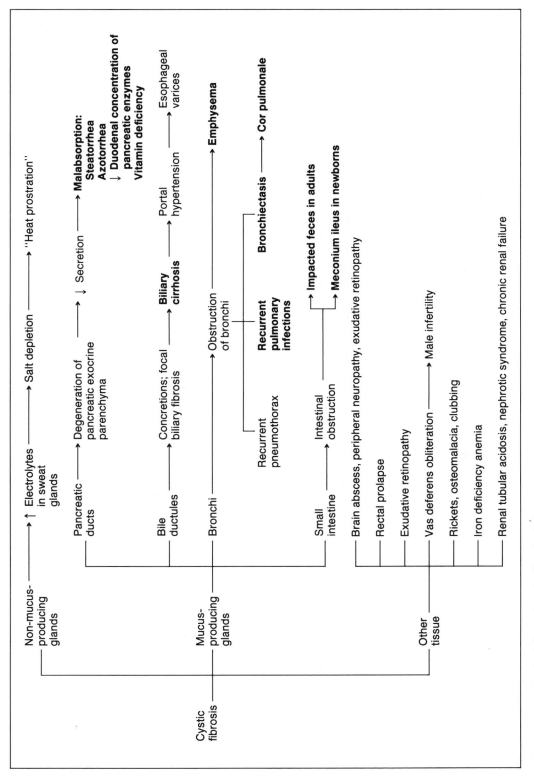

Figure 8-10. *Pathophysiology of cystic fibrosis of the pancreas.*

cidence of volvulus, peritonitis, atresia, obstruction, and rectal prolapse also is increased (see Figure 8-10).

Usually, but not always, pancreatic insufficiency is observed. When it is present, steatorrhea occurs along with maldigestion of protein and carbohydrate. Fat digestion is most severely affected. Assays for pancreatic enzymes show them to be absent or reduced. The resulting malabsorption may be complicated by hepatic abnormalities. Other manifestations are listed in Table 8-16.

The lungs usually are involved, with obstruction of the bronchi and increased incidence of **bronchiectasis** (chronic dilation with coughing and purulent exudate), **atelectasis** (collapsed or airless portions of the lung), and pneumonia. Death often occurs from bronchopneumonia.

CF patients are frequently below standard height, weight, and other anthropometric measures. The extent of the deficit has been correlated with the severity of the pulmonary disease, rather than the degree of malabsorption. Currently, the average life expectancy of a cystic fibrosis patient is about 20 years. Treatment is long-term and requires the cooperation of physicians, nurses, nutritionists, physical therapists, and social workers.

Nutritional Assessment

Since cystic fibrosis affects many organ systems, there are many approaches to nutritional assessment. The growth should be monitored in these children with the use of growth charts for height and weight (see Appendix L). The electrolyte disorders indicate the need to monitor serum sodium, potas-

Table 8-16. *Principal Clinical Manifestations of Cystic Fibrosis of the Pancreas*

Viscid secretions and small duct obstruction	Portal hypertension
Respiratory disorders	Eosphageal varices
Sinusitis	Hypersplenism
Nasal polyps	*Renal disorders*
Atelectasis	Renal tubular acidosis
Emphysema	Nephrotic syndrome
Bronchitis, bronchopneumonia, bronchiectasis	Chronic renal failure
Lung abscess	*Reproductive system disorders*
Aspergillosis	Males: sterility; absent vas deferens, epididymis, and
Respiratory failure	seminal vesicles
Cor pulmonale	Females: decreased fertility, thickened cervical mucus,
Intestinal disorders	pregnancy complications
Meconium ileus	
Intussusception	*Nervous system disorders*
Volvulus	Brain abscess
Appendicitis; peritonitis	Exudative retinopathy, retinal hemorrhage
Ileal atresia	Autonomic nervous system dysfunction
Rectal prolapse	*Skeletal disorders*
Obstruction	Clubbing
Pancreatic disorders	Retardation of bone age
Malabsorption, pancreatic insufficiency	Hypertrophic osteoarthropathy
Steatorrhea, creatorrhea	Demineralization
Diabetes mellitus	Rickets, osteomalacia
Vitamin deficiencies	
Loss of bile salts	*Other disorders*
Recurrent acute pancreatitis	Salt depletion
Hepatobiliary disorders	Heat stroke
Fatty liver	Metabolic alkalosis
Mucous hypersecretion	Salivary gland hypertrophy
Atrophic gallbladder	Hypertrophy of apocrine glands
Cholecystitis; cholelithiasis	Hiatal hernia
Focal biliary cirrhosis	Gastroesophageal reflux
Laennec's cirrhosis	Thyroid amyloidosis
	Iodine goiter

sium, magnesium, chloride, blood pH, pCO_2, and pO_2. The malabsorption suggests observation of albumin, hemoglobin, hematocrit, pancreatic enzymes, white blood cells, fecal fat, serum cholesterol, and serum carotene. Blood glucose is monitored to follow pancreatic islet function.

Diagnosis

Cystic fibrosis varies greatly in the age at which the clinical manifestations become evident. A classic sign in the newborn is meconium ileus, and gastrointestinal and pancreatic manifestations tend to predominate. As the child advances in age, respiratory complications are more likely to predominate.

The diagnosis is often made on the basis of chloride levels in the sweat. Values of 60 mEq/L or more are considered indicative of CF.

Treatment

Aspects of treatment vary with the severity of the disease, the age of the patient, and the specific signs and symptoms. The respiratory signs and symptoms are treated by evacuation of the mucus by postural draining, clapping, and vibrating. Medications indicated by varying degrees of severity include aerosols, bronchodilators, expectorants, corticosteroids, antibiotics, vaccines for respiratory disease, and oxygen. Potassium iodide and mucolytics liquefy secretions.

Nutritional Management. For pancreatic insufficiency, pancreatic enzyme extracts (Cotazyme, Viokase, Pancrease) prescribed by the physician are taken with each meal. The dose is high and may be 0.1 to 0.3 g per kilogram of body weight per day. The patient must be instructed not to chew the material. A low-fat, high-protein (3–4 g/kg), high-carbohydrate diet may be used but varies with the degree of malabsorption. A diet with 30–35% of total calories as protein and 30% of total calories as fat is often useful. Total kilocalorie content of the diet may have to be as high as 200 kcal/kg in infants and 150 kcal/kg in children in order to achieve normal weight. MCT Oil, Polycose, and protein powders (see Appendix G) are added if necessary to provide sufficient energy, with the objective of reaching normal weight for height.[73,74] Appetites sometimes are voracious in the first four years but may diminish later or in response to pain and diarrhea.[75] For infants, Pregestimil may be needed in place of milk or other more commonly used formulas. Portagen, Tolerex, and Nutramigen are often used for children and adults as an alternative to milk. These vary greatly in their acceptability. Total parenteral feeding sometimes is used for infants who are unable to achieve adequate caloric intake orally.[75,76] For older children needing nutritional supplementation, a percutaneous gastrostomy is often recommended.[74] Multivitamin supplements in water-soluble form are necessary and are prescribed by the physician. Twice the recommended allowances of vitamins A, D, and E are added. Additional salt (4–6 g) must be taken in hot weather, fever, or when the patient sweats excessively. Other needed supplements may be iron, vitamin K, and zinc. Fluid intake should be liberal to help liquefy secretions and to prevent dehydration. Some patients do not have pancreatic insufficiency, and so diet modifications are unnecessary.

DISEASES OF THE LARGE INTESTINE

Fiber is considered useful in treatment of diseases of the large intestine, atherosclerosis, diabetes mellitus, and obesity. Prior to a discussion of these conditions in this and succeeding chapters, an understanding of the classification, chemical composition, physical properties, and physiological effects of fiber is necessary.

Fiber and Related Substances

The term **dietary fiber** includes that portion of plant cells that are resistant to digestive enzymes in humans. It consists of a number of substances and has been expanded to include materials such as guar gum, which is used as a food additive but does not occur naturally in food.

Dietary fiber represents a mixture of a number of materials listed in Table 8-17. They are obtained from plants and may be defined as structural polysaccharides (cellulose, hemicellulose, and some pectins), nonstructural polysaccharides (pectins, gums, and mucilages), and structural nonpolysaccharides (lignin).[77] They vary in fermentability and physical properties such as water-holding capacity, viscosity, and adsorption or binding capacity. Fiber can be water-soluble (pectins, gums) or water-insoluble (cellulose, hemicellulose, lignins).

Dietary fiber must be distinguished from **crude fiber**, the residue remaining after plant food has been treated with lipid solvent and dilute acid and alkali. Crude fiber includes only cellulose and lignin. The values for fiber that appear in food composition tables are for crude fiber. Unfortunately, values for dietary fiber, which would be more useful in diet planning, are not available because of a lack of adequate assay methods. It has been estimated that dietary fiber may equal two to six times the amount of crude fiber.

Physiological responses related to dietary fiber include (1) increased fecal bulk, (2) decreased plasma cholesterol, (3) lowered glycemic response, and (4) reduced nutrient availability. Different components of dietary fiber have different effects. Therefore, the use of these materials in pathological conditions should be approached with caution.

A limited amount of digestion of dietary

Table 8-17. Classification of Dietary Fiber by Structure and Human Physiologic Function

Fiber Class	Chemical Structure	Suggested Human Functions
Noncellulosic polysaccharides Gums (secretions)	Galactose, glucuronic acid-mannose, galacturonic acid-rhamnose main chain; xylose or galactose side chain	1. May slow gastric emptying 2. Provide fermentable substrate for colonic bacteria, with production of gas and volatile fatty acids 3. Bind bile acids variably
Mucilages (secretions, plant seeds)	Galactose-mannose, galacturonic acid-rhamnose, arabinose-xylose main chain; galactose side chain	
Algal polysaccharides (from algae and seaweeds)	Mannose, xylose; glucuronic acid, glucose main chain; galactose side chain	
Pectin substances (intercellular cement)	Galacturonic acid main chain; rhamnose, arabinose, xylose, fructose side chain	
Hemicelluloses (from the cell wall of many plants)	Xylose, mannose; glucose main chain; arabinose, galactose side chain	1. Hold water, increase stool bulk 2. May reduce *elevated* colonic intraluminal pressure 3. Bind bile acids variably
Cellulose (principal cell wall constituent)	Unbranched glucose polymer	1. Depending on particle size, holds water 2. May reduce *elevated* colonic intraluminal pressure 3. May bind zinc
Lignin (woody part of plants)	Polymeric phenylpropane, noncarbohydrate	1. Serves as antioxidant 2. May bind metals

Compiled from Mendeloff, A.I., Dietary fiber and health. An introduction. In *Nutrition and Disease: Fiber.* Columbus, Ohio: Ross Laboratories, 1978; and Slavin, J.L., Dietary fiber. Classification, chemical analyses and food sources. *J. Am. Diet. Assoc.* 87:1164, 1987.

fiber does occur. Fermentation by microorganisms produces the volatile fatty acids acetic, propionic, and butyric, as well as hydrogen, carbon dioxide, methane, and ammonia gases.[78,79] Some proposed functions of dietary fiber are also given in Table 8-17.

Despite the limited information available, some manipulation of the fiber in the diet is possible. Generally, diet modifications refer only to **total** fiber in the diet. They are called **high-fiber** or **low-fiber** diets. There is no quantitative definition, but the terms "high" and "low" often are relative only to the patient's previous diet. A diet history for a patient eating a usual Western-type diet will demonstrate an intake of 3–12 g crude fiber or about 20 g of dietary fiber. For such a patient, a high-dietary-fiber diet might contain 30 g of fiber or up to a maximum of 50 g. A low-fiber diet then would contain less than 20 g, perhaps 3–4 g dietary fiber per day.

Some institutions use a **minimal fiber** or **minimal residue** diet containing about 1 g of dietary fiber per day. The excretion of sloughed enterocytes, intestinal bacteria, and mucus results in some residue even if nothing is eaten. Therefore, no diet is "residue-free."

Some guidelines for increasing or decreasing the fiber content are contained in Table 8-18.

Intestinal Gas

Flatulence (excessive formation of gas in the digestive tract) and **eructation** or **belching** have been the basis for humor and social embarrassment. Flatulence also may be the cause of distension, bloating, and pain sufficiently severe to be mistaken for a heart attack. It may signal a serious disorder of the intestinal tract, or it may be benign.

Gas is present normally in the colon, but its volume and composition vary widely. The normal mean volume of gas passed from the rectum is 600 ml/day, but rates from 200 to 2,000 ml have been measured.[80] The amount in the intestinal tract at any one time usually is less than 200 ml.[81,82] The gas present con-

Table 8-18. Guidelines for Increasing and Decreasing Fiber Content of the Diet

Planning a high-fiber diet
Increase fruits, vegetables, legumes, and nuts in the diet.
  Legumes have a significant gum content.
  Increase cabbage-family vegetables, peas, and beans.
  Leave vegetables, such as potatoes, unpeeled.
Emphasize raw, unpeeled fruits and vegetables.
  Emphasize fruits containing skin and seeds.
  Pineapple and rhubarb are higher in fiber.
  Fruit juices are low in fiber.
Use whole-grain bread and cereals in place of refined products.
  De-emphasize "instant" products.
  Oatmeal has a significant gum content.
  Bran (¼–1 cup) may be added to cereals, breads, and casseroles gradually, in divided doses, during the day.
Increase fluid intake.
Planning a low-fiber diet
Use refined breads and cereals; avoid whole-grain products.
Use fruit and vegetable as juices, cooked whole or pureed (depending on degree of restriction).
  Avoid prune juice.
  Avoid fruits with seeds and skins.
Use meat, milk, eggs, any fat.
Use desserts without fruits, nuts, seeds.

sists almost entirely of various proportions of nitrogen, oxygen, carbon dioxide, hydrogen, and methane and is a combination of swallowed air and gas diffused from the blood and from intraluminal production.

The type of gas present suggests its source. Our atmosphere consists of approximately 80% nitrogen and 20% oxygen. These dissolve in the blood and then diffuse from the mucosal blood supply into the lumen. Swallowed air, too, is nitrogen and oxygen. One study indicated that 2 to 3 ml of air reaches the stomach with each swallow.[83] It is believed that most of this material normally is regurgitated, and diffusion from the blood accounts for most of the nitrogen seen in rectal flatus.[84]

Carbon dioxide is produced in large quantities from the reaction of normal gastric hydrogen ion and pancreatic bicarbonate. Most of it is reabsorbed. Hydrogen is produced by bacterial metabolism in the colon,[85] but some bacteria use hydrogen.[85,86] Bacteria also are believed to be the source of carbon dioxide found in the flatus, since increases of both hydrogen and carbon dioxide usually are concurrent. Methane is produced by colonic bacterial metabolism but is not found in all individuals.

Studies have shown that some patients who complain of excess gas actually have a normal volume and composition of gas in the digestive tract.[87] Instead, they may have disorders of intestinal motility and increased sensitivity of the bowel to distension.[88] Disordered motility sometimes is treated with anticholinergics, but their effectiveness is unknown. Nutritional care includes methods to reduce intestinal gas to subnormal levels to avoid the patient's increased sensitivity. Patients can be advised to eat slowly and eat with the mouth closed. A straw should not be used for drinking. Chewing gum and smoking have been assumed to contribute to air swallowing. Although there is no supporting evidence, advice to the patient to eliminate these habits seems a logical step.

Foods reputed to increase intestinal gas may be eliminated. Some foods contain carbohydrates that are not digestible by intestinal enzymes but are digestible by colon bacteria (such as some fruits and vegetables and whole-grain cereals) and provide substrates for gas production; these foods may be eliminated. Beans, which have a well-known reputation, contain the trisaccharide **raffinose** and the tetrasaccharide **stachyose**, both of which serve as a substrate for colon bacteria. Other vegetables reputed to be gas-forming include cabbage, cauliflower, broccoli, onions, turnips, corn, and cucumbers. No studies, however, have established that the reputation is deserved. If a diet history reveals that these foods cause flatulence or that the patients believe they do, they may be eliminated from the diet. Foods that contain large amounts of gas, such as carbonated beverages, whips, and meringues, may be restricted. Sometimes a low-fat diet is useful in reducing the fatty acids that may serve as a source of hydrogen. It is important to monitor the patient's diet to assure adequate nutrient intake.

Some patients are believed to have excessive gas because of **aerophagia** (air swallowing). This often occurs in tense, nervous individuals whose main need is reassurance that there is no organic basis for the condition. Diet modification usually is unnecessary. Some patients may be cautioned against gas-containing foods and chewing gum, and advised to eat slowly with closed mouth.

In those patients whose flatulence results from a malabsorption syndrome, the flatulence usually subsides with treatment of the basic disease. In lactase deficiency, for example, hydrogen is produced when undigested lactose is fermented by colonic bacteria.

Constipation

Constipation consists of the slow passage or retention of fecal matter until feces are too hard to pass easily or other uncomfortable symptoms occur. It can occur alone or as a symptom of other disease. Many drugs induce constipation, such as aluminum hydroxide antacids, anticholinergics, iron supplements, some antihypertensive agents, and some narcotics. Other circumstances that predispose to constipation include diabetes, hypothyroidism, colon cancer, prolonged immobilization, and conditions that cause pain on defecation, such as hemorrhoids and anal fissures.

The usual amount of time that elapses between eating and defecation varies greatly but most commonly is 24 to 72 hours. The normal number of bowel movements also may vary from several per day in some individuals to only once in several days in others. Given this wide variation, it is important to define constipation in terms of the usual habits of the individual and the presence of symptoms.

The types of constipation are categorized as obstructive, atonic, or spastic. **Obstructive constipation** occurs as a result of obstructions caused by adhesions, impaction, or tumors, including cancer. Impacted material may be feces or foreign materials and must sometimes be removed surgically. In preparation for surgery, the patient may need a low-residue chemically defined diet or TPN.

Atonic constipation is more likely to be the consequence of poor health habits. These include diets excessively low in fiber, inadequate water intake, irregular meals, habitually ignoring the defecation reflex, lack of exercise, and habitual use of cathartics. Sometimes atonic constipation accompanies hypothyroidism or the use of medications containing iron, aluminum, magnesium, or calcium compounds. It often occurs in the aged, the obese, and pregnant women. Patients who are confined to bed for long periods may be chronically constipated. Constipation is a frequent problem in handicapped patients (see Chapter 19).

When no organic basis is found for atonic constipation, changes in diet are the primary mode of management. The patient is encouraged to increase his or her intake of fiber-containing foods, fruits, vegetables, and whole-grain cereals. Prunes and prune juice are useful to stimulate peristalsis. The active principle in prunes has been reported to be **dihydroxyphenyl isatin**, but there is some disagreement on this point. An increase in the intake of fluids also is helpful. At least 1 qt./day in fluid form is recommended. Sometimes 2 teaspoons of bran with meals also is recommended. The increased undigested fiber absorbs water to increase the bulk of the intestinal contents and stimulates defecation. Therefore, the patient should be advised to eat breakfast to stimulate the gastrocolic reflex leading to defecation. In addition, the establishment of a regular pattern of food intake and exercise is helpful.

Spastic constipation occurs as one of the symptoms in the **irritable bowel syndrome**, also known as **mucous colitis**, **irritable colon, or spastic colon**. It is one of the most common gastrointestinal disorders presented for treatment. No organic abnormality is known to cause mucous colitis. Therefore, it is regarded as a functional disease and generally is believed to occur as the result of

emotional stress. Other contributing factors that have been suggested include lack of sleep, insufficient fluid intake, excessive use of cathartics, coffee, tea, alcohol, or tobacco, and, sometimes, enteric infections and antibiotics. The condition possibly involves overstimulation of nerve endings, causing disturbances in motility, irregular contractions, and decreased sensitivity to the defecation reflex. The resulting symptoms include abdominal pain, heartburn, flatulence, and constipation, which may alternate with episodes of diarrhea.

Treatment consists primarily of emotional support and establishment of regular habits as described for atonic constipation. The diet may be a basically normal adequate diet with increased amounts of fruits, vegetables, and whole-grain cereals, with 2 teaspoons of unprocessed bran with meals. During diarrheal episodes, avoidance of carbonated beverages and coffee may be recommended. It is not known if the effects of these diet changes are physiologic or psychological.

Constipated patients may be prescribed cathartics. Others will be seen to have acquired a habit of chronic laxative use by self-medication. In either case, the nutritional care specialist needs to be familiar with the major types, modes of action, and side effects of these drugs. Agents that promote defecation are **cathartics**. These may be classified by increasing intensity of their action as **laxatives**, **purgatives**, and **drastics**. They are also classified according to their modes of action.

Emollient laxatives are wetting agents or emulsifying agents that soften the fecal mass by allowing water and fat to penetrate the stool. **Dioctyl sodium sulfosuccinate (Colace)** and **dioctyl calcium sulfosuccinate (Surfak)** may cause nausea, vomiting, anorexia, and sometimes diarrhea. They have a bitter taste and are throat irritants; therefore, they should be taken with milk or fruit juice. Surfak is useful if the patient has a sodium-restricted diet.

Bulk-forming laxatives increase the moisture content of the stool and thus stimulate peristalsis. **Psyllium (Metamucil)** or **methyl-cellulose** should be taken with a large amount of water to guard against formation of phytobezoars and intestinal obstruction. Bulk-forming laxatives may also cause steatorrhea, flatulence, and, if taken chronically, alterations in electrolyte absorption.

There are several **stimulant cathartics** that produce their effect by local irritation or by action on Auerbach's plexus resulting in increased motor activity. **Castor oil** is used in preparation for bowel examination almost exclusively. It is taken with juice on an empty stomach. **Bisacodyl (Dulcolax)** stimulates colon peristalsis. It may cause colic, diarrhea, and hypokalemia. A related compound, **phenolphthalein (Ex-Lax)**, may decrease absorption of fat-soluble vitamins and other nutrients. If use is prolonged, it can cause dehydration and electrolyte imbalance. The incidence of allergy is high (5–7%). **Anthraquinone cathartics**, **extract of cascara**, and **extract of senna (Senokot)** stimulate the colon. They should be taken with meals or with at least 8 oz. of water. Chronic use may cause sodium and potassium depletion.

Saline cathartics are nonabsorbable salts with osmotic activity that causes water retention in the lumen of the colon. **Milk of magnesia**, for example, may cause nausea, colic, polyuria, and diarrhea.

Diverticular Disease

The colon wall consists of the mucosal layer, a layer of circular muscle, and three longitudinal bands, the teniae coli (see Figure 8-7). A **diverticulum** is a common condition in the middle-aged and elderly in which diverticula are present in the intestinal tract. When first formed, the diverticula are reducible when intraluminal pressure falls; therefore, their number varies. In time, they cannot be reduced or expel the feces they contain. The feces becomes **inspissated** (thickened), and the surrounding tissue may become inflamed. Only 10% to 15% of patients with diverticulosis develop diverticulitis.

Epidemiologic evidence indicates that these conditions occur in those eating a refined Western-type diet.[89] In less-developed countries where food is not processed as extensively, the disease is almost unknown. In those countries, the colon tends to be quite enlarged and there is, instead of diverticulosis, a higher incidence of volvulus or intussusception.

One theory for the development of diverticula proposes that there is an increase in intraluminal pressure when the content of the lumen is reduced or the lumen is narrowed and segmentation increases. It has been suggested that these alterations occur more frequently in those eating a highly refined diet. It has also been suggested that sigmoid contractions in response to emotional stress contribute to intraluminal pressure.

Clinical Manifestations

Diverticulosis may be asymptomatic, or the patient may have pain and constipation sometimes alternating with diarrhea. Diverticulitis involves inflammation with fever and pain. Sometimes there is ileus, anorexia, and nausea.

Management

Diet has recently become an important feature of long-term management of chronic diverticular disease. A high-fiber diet increases the bulk of the material reaching the colon. The diameter of the lumen of the colon is enlarged, decreasing the need for excessive segmentation and reducing the symptoms. Sometimes analgesics or tranquilizers are prescribed if the patient is in pain.

Between 10 and 15 g of bran and 200 g of fruits and vegetables are recommended to increase stool weight to at least 150 g/day. This diet is recommended for treatment of chronic diverticulosis but has not been shown to prevent diverticular disease or its symptoms.[90]

In diverticulitis, antibiotics and supportive

therapy for water and electrolyte balance may be required. A liquid diet, used for a short time, is followed by a low-fiber diet as tolerated. When acute symptoms subside, the high-fiber diet for diverticulosis may be used. Surgery occasionally is required, particularly for complications. Complications that sometimes occur include abscesses, peritonitis, fistulas, hemorrhage, or obstruction.[89]

Figure 8-11. Ostomy sites. (Reprinted with permission from Tucker, S. M., Breeding, M.A., Canobbio, M.M., et al., Patient Care Standards, 2nd ed. St. Louis: C.V. Mosby, 1980, p. 242.)

Colon Surgery

A portion or all of the large intestine must sometimes be removed or rested. Diseases that make resection or rest necessary include chronic ulcerative colitis, Crohn's disease, colon cancer, familial polyposis, and birth defects. When part of the bowel is removed, it is sometimes possible to restore the continuity of the remaining bowel with an end-to-end anastamosis. In other cases, the location and size of the resection make that impossible. Then a stoma is made to provide a new exit for the intestinal contents; this stoma is permanent. However, when the

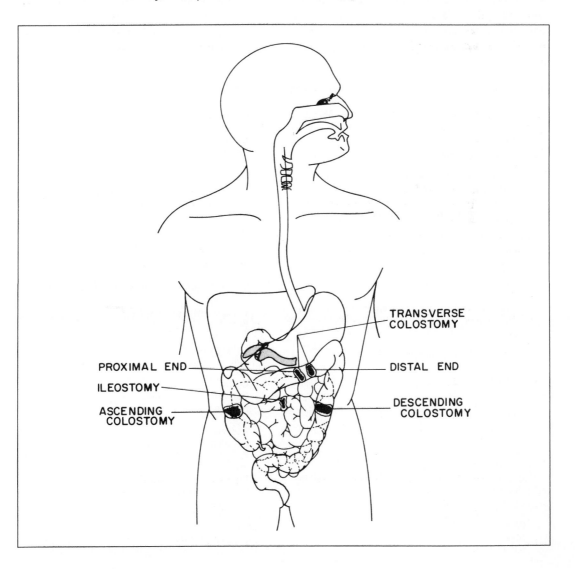

purpose is to rest the bowel, the stoma may be temporary, and the continuity of the bowel may be restored at a later date. Temporary ostomies are closed in weeks, months, or sometimes years.

Ileostomy

An **ileostomy** provides an opening from the distal ileum through the abdominal wall (Figure 8-11). It bypasses the colon, rectum, and anus. The contents of the ileum are very liquid, because the colon's function of reabsorbing electrolytes and water has been lost. The daily loss immediately postoperatively may be 500 ml of water and 30 to 50 mEq each of sodium and chloride in excess of normal.[91] These amounts increase in hot weather, heavy exercise, diarrhea, or vomiting. At one time, all patients with an ileostomy had to wear an "appliance" or **ileostomy bag** into which the ileostomy drained constantly. Now, an internal reservoir may be created surgically. The result is called a **continent ileostomy**. It contains a nipple within the reservoir, formed from a length of ileum intussuscepted back into the reservoir.

Oral feeding postoperatively may begin with a clear liquid diet and progress to a low-fiber diet. Most ileostomy patients eventually can follow a normal diet. The diet they followed preoperatively is no longer needed, but some adjustments may be required to prevent obstruction, watery discharge or an excessively large volume of discharge, and excessive odor and gas. The diet must be ad-

---

Table 8-19. Some Procedures for Nutritional Management of an Ileostomy

Add foods one at a time to progress from a low-fiber diet to the unrestricted diet, so that problem foods can be identified.

To prevent obstruction:
  Increase fluid intake.
  Use prune juice and grape juice to increase liquidity of the effluent.
  Avoid foods high in fiber or with seeds or kernels.
  Chew foods thoroughly; be sure dentures are properly fitted.
  Approach with caution potential problem foods, including
    Corn on the cob
    Celery
    Coleslaw
    Lettuce
    Chinese vegetables, such as bean sprouts and bamboo shoots
    Peas
    Mushrooms
    Citrus fruit membranes
    Nuts
    Coconut
    Peanuts
    Tough meats
    Fruits with seeds
    Raw fruit
    Tomatoes
    Pineapple

To prevent watery discharge:
  Approach with caution potential problem foods, including
    Apple juice
    Prune juice
    Beer
    Milk
    Baked beans

Green beans
Cabbage
Broccoli
Spinach
Highly spiced foods
Raw fruit

When a food causes a problem, it should be eliminated for a period and then tried again later. There is some adaptation in time.

Boiled milk, rice, peanut butter, and potatoes may be used as "binding" foods in some patients.

To avoid flatulence with pain and odor:
  Eliminate gas-producing and odor-producing foods. These should be tried again at intervals:
    Asparagus
    Dried beans and peas
    Beer
    Mustard
    Cabbage family
    Spiced foods
    Fish
    Onions
    Carbonated beverages
    Melons
    Eggs
    Radishes
    Cucumbers
    Fatty foods, such as pastries and deep-fried foods
    Pickles
    Whips and meringues
    Strong-flavored cheeses
  Avoid chewing gum.
  Do not use a straw.
  Chew food with mouth closed.
  Eat regular meals.
  Add cranberry juice, yogurt, and buttermilk.

justed individually. Foods are added one at a time so that problem foods can be identified. A regular diet can usually be achieved in two to three weeks. Suggested procedures and problem foods are listed in Table 8-19.

The ileostomy patient should be advised to increase fluid and salt intake permanently. Salt and water are lost in varying amount when the colon is removed, and dehydration can occur. If the volume of effluent exceeds 1,000 ml/day, the patient probably will need additional intake of fluid and sodium, which often is provided intravenously. If potassium losses are not large, small deficits can be replaced by encouraging the patient to increase intake of orange, grapefruit, or tomato juice, milk, or various beverages advertised for use by athletes. It is important that the ileostomy patient understand that reducing his or her fluid intake causes dehydration, not a reduction in effluent volume. This is especially important when losses by other routes are increased, such as in fever and vomiting. If the patient is chronically dehydrated, urine volume decreases and the incidence of renal stones increases.

Vitamin supplements may be required. If the terminal ileum has been removed, parenteral vitamin B_{12} will be needed. If the patient

also has lost large portions of the small intestine, supplements of fat-soluble vitamins may be necessary.

Common problems occurring a year or more postoperatively are excessive weight gain or weight loss. Long-term nutritional care should include monitoring body weight and giving advice on weight control or gain as necessary. The ileostomy does not preclude participation in active sports, including swimming and other water sports, running, tennis, and similar activities. Some physicians advise against contact sports. The patient also is capable of relatively strenuous work. The patient's activity should be considered in advising him or her on caloric intake.

Colostomy

Colostomies are placed at various locations, depending on the location and amount of colon removed (see Figure 8-11). If the stoma is in the cecum, it is called a cecostomy. Colostomies may be in the ascending, transverse, descending, or sigmoid colons. The solid or liquid state of the effluent depends on the location and has an important effect on management (Figure 8-12).

A right-sided colostomy, in the ascending colon, is near the ileum and has a highly liquid effluent similar to that from an ileos-

Figure 8-12. Alterations of colon content consistency in length of intestine.

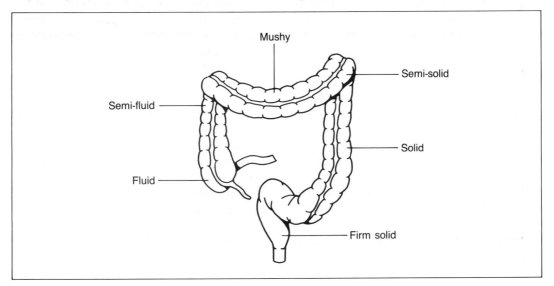

Case Study: Gluten Intolerance

R.M. was admitted to the hospital, complaining of anorexia, weight loss, and abdominal cramps. She reported frequent, foul-smelling, light-colored stools. Physical examination showed a pale, weak, 24-year-old woman, 5 ft. 8 in. tall and weighing 110 lb. The patient said she had recently had an intestinal infection.

A biopsy of the small intestine showed flattened villi. Fecal fat was 18 g/day. The D-xylose absorption test revealed 4 g excretion per 5 hours. Twenty-four-hour recall produced this information:

8 A.M.	4 oz. grapefruit juice
	1 slice white toast with butter
	½ cup bran flakes
	½ cup milk
10 A.M.	Coffee, black
	Sweet roll
12 noon	Chicken noodle soup
	Ham salad sandwich
	Coffee
6 P.M.	4 oz. roast lamb
	½ cup buttered green beans
	Molded fruit salad
	2-in. square devil's food cake
	Tea with lemon

Diagnosis: primary gluten intolerance, with fat malabsorption secondary to it. A gluten-free, low-fat diet was prescribed.

Exercises

1. Explain the rationale for the diet.
2. Evaluate the results of the laboratory tests and explain their significance.
3. Modify the patient's diet as given in the 24-hour recall to conform to the diet prescription.
4. If the patient had pancreatic insufficiency, what change would you expect in the results of the D-xylose absorption test?

References

1. Wilson, F.A., Sallee, V.L., and Dietschy, J.M. Unstirred water layers in the intestine. Rate determinant of fatty acid absorption from micellar solutions. *Science* 174:1031, 1971.
2. Wilson, F.A., and Dietschy, J.M. Characterization of bile and absorption across the unstirred water layer and brush border of the rat jejunum. *J. Clin. Invest.* 51:3015, 1972.
3. Bergstrom, B. On the importance of bile salts. *J. Lipid Res.* 16:411, 1975.
4. Adibi, S.A., and Allen, E.R. Impaired jejunal absorption rates of essential amino acids induced by either dietary caloric or protein deprivation in man. *Gastroenterology* 59:404, 1970.
5. Herbert, V., Cooper, B.A., and Castle, W.B. The site of vitamin B_{12}-intrinsic factor complex "releasing factor" activity in the rat small intestine. *Proc. Soc. Exp. Biol. Med.* 110:315, 1962.
6. Code, C.F., Bass, P., McClary, G.B., Jr., et al. Absorption of water, sodium, and potassium in small intestine of dogs. *Am. J. Physiol.* 199:281, 1960.
7. Turnberg, L.A., Bieberdorf, F.A., Morawski, S.G., and Fordtran, J.S. Interrelationships of chloride, bicarbonate, sodium and hydrogen transport in the human ileum. *J. Clin. Invest.* 49:557, 1970.
8. Corcino, J.J., Waxman, S., and Berbert, V. Absorption and malabsorption of vitamin B_{12}. *Am. J. Med.* 48:562, 1970.
9. Roggin, G.M., Iber, F.L., Kater, R.M.H., and Tabon, F. Malabsorption in the chronic alcoholic. *Johns Hopkins Med. J.* 125:321, 1969.
10. Green, P.H.R., and Tall, A.R. Drugs, alcohol and malabsorption. *Am. J. Med.* 67:1066, 1979.
11. Council on Foods and Nutrition. The regulation of dietary fat. *J.A.M.A.* 181:139, 1962.
12. Losowsky, M.S., Walker, B.E., and Kelleher, J. *Malabsorption in Clinical Practice.* Edinburgh: Churchill Livingstone, 1974.
13. *Recipes Using MCT Oil and Portagen.* Evansville, Ind.: Mead Johnson, 1970.
14. Schizas, A.A., Cremen, A.A., Larson, E., and O'Brien, R. Medium-chain triglycerides—Use in food preparation. *J. Am. Diet. Assoc.* 51:228, 1967.
15. Kalser, M.H. Medium chain triglycerides. *Adv. Intern. Med.* 17:301, 1971.
16. Howard, B.D., and Morse, E.H. Muffins and pastry made with medium-chain triglyceride oil. *J. Am. Diet. Assoc.* 62:51, 1973.
17. Bowman, F. MCT cookies, cakes and quick breads. Quality and acceptability. *J. Am. Diet. Assoc.* 62:180, 1973.
18. Greesky, F.L., and Cooke, R.E. The gastrointestinal absorption of unaltered protein in

normal infants and in infants recovering from diarrhea. *Pediatrics* 16:763, 1955.

19. Rothberg, R.M. Immunoglobulin and specific antibody synthesis during the first weeks of life of premature infants. *J. Pediatr.* 75:391, 1969.

20. Korenblat, R.E., Rothberg, R.M., Minden, P., and Farr, R.S. Immune response of human adults after oral and parenteral exposure to bovine serum albumin. *J. Allergy* 41:226, 1968.

21. Ament, M.E. Immunodeficiency syndromes and gastrointestinal disease. *Pediatr. Clin. North Am.* 22:807, 1975.

22. Crabbe, P.A., and Heremans, J.F. Selective IgA deficiency with steatorrhea. A new syndrome. *Am. J. Med.* 42:319, 1967.

23. Savilahti, E., Pelkonen, P., and Visakorpi, J.K. A clinical study with special reference to intestinal findings. *Arch. Dis. Child.* 46:665, 1971.

24. Hardy, R.N. The influence of specific chemical factors in the solvent on the absorption of macromolecular substances from the small intestine of the newborn calf. *J. Physiol.* (Lond.) 204:607, 1969.

25. Leece, J.G., Morgan, D.O., and Matrone, G. Effect of feeding colostral and milk components on the cessation of intestinal absorption of large molecules (closure) in neonatal pigs. *J. Nutr.* 84:43, 1964.

26. Gitlin, D., Kumate, J., Morales, C., et al. The turnover of amniotic fluid protein in the human conceptus. *Am. J. Obstet. Gynecol.* 113:632, 1972.

27. Kerzner, B., McClung, J., Kelly, M., et al. Intestinal secretion in acute viral enteritis. A function of crypt-type enterocytes? *Gastroenterology* 68:909, 1965.

28. Walker, W.A. Antigen absorption from the small intestine and gastrointestinal disease. *Pediatr. Clin. North Am.* 22:731, 1975.

29. Holman, H., Nickel, W.F., Jr., and Sleisenger, M.H. Hypoproteinemia antedating intestinal lesions and possibly due to excessive serum protein loss into intestine. *Am. J. Med.* 27:963, 1959.

30. Waldmann, T.A., Steinfeld, J.L., Dutcher, T.F., et al. Role of gastrointestinal system in "idiopathic hypoproteinemia." *Gastroenterology* 41:197, 1961.

31. Jeffries, G.H. Protein metabolism and protein-losing enteropathy. In M.H. Sleisenger and J.S. Fordtran, Eds., *Gastrointestinal Disease: Pathophysiology, Diagnosis, Management,* 2nd ed. Philadelphia: W.B. Saunders, 1978.

32. Diehl, J.T., Steiger, E., and Hooley, R. The role of intravenous hyperalimentation in intestinal disease. *Surg. Clin. North Am.* 63:11, 1983.

33. Kaminsky, V.M., and Deitel, M. Nutritional support in the management of external fistulas of the alimentary tract. *Br. J. Surg.* 62:100, 1975.

34. Falchuk, Z.M. Update on gluten-sensitive enteropathy. *Am. J. Med.* 67:1085, 1979.

35. Chandra, R.K., and Sahni, S. Immunological aspects of gluten intolerance. *Nutr. Rev.* 39:117, 1981.

36. Paulley, J.W. Observations on the aetiology of idiopathic steatorrhea. *Br. Med. J.* 2:1318, 1954.

37. Baklien, K., Brandtzaeg, P., and Fausa, O. Immunoglobulins in jejunal mucosa and serum from patients with adult coeliac disease. *Scand. J. Gastroenterol.* 12:149, 1977.

38. Taylor, K.B., Thomson, D.L., Truelove, S.C., and Wright, R. An immunological study of coeliac disease and idiopathic steatorrhoea. *Br. Med. J.* 2:1727, 1961.

39. Seah, P.P., Fry, L., Hoffbrand, A.V., and Holborow, E.J. Tissue antibodies in dermatitis herpetiformis and adult coeliac disease. *Lancet* 1:834, 1971.

40. Bullen, A.W., and Losowsky, M.S. Peripheral blood lymphocyte subpopulations in adult coeliac disease (CD). *Gut* 18:A408, 1977.

41. Allardyce, R.A., and Shearman, D.J.C. Leukocyte reactivity to alpha-gliadin in dermatitis herpetiformis and adult coeliac disease. *Int. Arch. Allergy Appl. Immunol.* 48:395, 1975.

42. Ryan, J.A., Jr., and Beshlian, K. Nutritional significance of the small intestine. In C.E. Lang, Ed., *Nutritional Support in Critical Care.* Rockville, Md.: Aspen, 1987.

43. Hofmann, A.F., and Poley, J.R. Role of bile acid malabsorption in pathogenesis of diarrhea and steatorrhea in patients with ileal resection. I. Response to cholestyramine or replacement of dietary long chain triglyceride by medium chain triglyceride. *Gastroenterology* 62:918, 1972.

44. Allcock, E. Absorption of vitamin B_{12} in man following extensive resection of the jejunum, ileum and colon. *Gastroenterology* 40:81, 1961.

45. Dobbins, J.W., and Binder, H.J. Derangements of oxalate metabolism in gastrointestinal disease and their mechanism. *Prog. Gastroenterol.* 3:505, 1977.

46. Bochenk, W., Rodgers, J.B., and Alaint, J.A. Effects of changes in dietary lipids on intestinal fluid loss in the short bowel syndrome. *Ann. Intern. Med.* 72:205, 1970.

47. Soong, C.S., Thompson, J.B., Paley, J.R., and

Hess, D.R. Hydroxy fatty acid in human diarrhea. *Gastroenterology* 63:748, 1972.

48. Ammon, H.V., and Phillips, S.F. Inhibition of colonic water and electrolyte absorption by fatty acids in man. *Gastroenterology* 65:744, 1973.

49. Mekhjian, H.S., Phillips, S.F., and Hofmann, A.F. Colonic secretion of water and electrolytes induced by bile acids. Perfusion studies in man. *J. Clin. Invest.* 50:1569, 1971.

50. Aber, G.M., Ashton, F., Carmalt, M.H.B., and Whitehead, T.P. Gastric hypersecretion following massive small bowel resection in man. *Am. J. Dig. Dis.* 12:785, 1967.

51. Williamson, R.C.N. Intestinal adaptation. *N. Engl. J. Med.* 298:1393, 1978.

52. Trier, J.S. The short bowel syndrome. In M.H. Sleisenger and J.S. Fordtran, Eds., *Gastrointestinal Disease: Pathophysiology, Diagnosis, Management*, 2nd ed. Philadelphia: W.B. Saunders, 1978.

53. Obertop, H., Nundy, S., Malamud, D., and Malt, R.A. Onset of cell proliferation in the shortened gut. Rapid hyperplasia after jejunal resection. *Gastroenterology* 72:267, 1977.

54. Weser, E. The management of patients after small bowel resection. *Gastroenterology* 71:146, 1976.

55. Weser, E., and Urban, E. The short bowel syndrome. *Gastroenterology* 3:1792–1802, 1985.

56. Granaderos, C. Nutritional assessment and management of patients with the short bowel syndrome. *Dietitians in Nutr. Supp.* 8(6):6, 1987.

57. Committee on Nutrition, American Academy of Pediatrics. The practical significance of lactose intolerance in children. *Pediatrics* 62:240, 1978.

58. Kolars, J.C., Levitt, M.D., Aouji, M., and Savaiano, D.A. Yogurt: An autodigesting source of lactose. *N. Engl. J. Med.* 310:1, 1984.

59. Savaiano, D.A., Abou ElAnouar, A., Smith, D.E., and Levitt, M.D. Lactose malabsorption from yogurt, pasteurized yogurt, sweet acidophilus milk and cultured milk in lactase-deficient individuals. *Am. J. Clin. Nutr.* 40:1219, 1984.

60. Hadley, R.A. Calcium and hypoallergenic diets. *Ann. Allergy* 30:36, 1972.

61. Birge, S.J., Keutmann, H.T., Cautrecasas, P., and Whedon, G.D. Osteoporosis, intestinal lactase deficiency and low dietary calcium intake. *N. Engl. J. Med.* 276:445, 1967.

62. Bowie, M.D. Effect of lactose-induced diarrhea on absorption of nitrogen and fat. *Arch. Dis. Child.* 50:363, 1975.

63. Calloway, D.H., and Chenoweth, W.L. Utilization of nutrients in milk- and wheat-based diets by men with adequate and reduced abilities to absorb lactose. I. Energy and nitrogen. *Am. J. Clin. Nutr.* 26:939, 1973.

64. Bayless, T.M. Disaccharidase deficiency. *J. Am. Diet. Assoc.* 60:478, 1972.

65. Cornblath, M., and Schwartz, R. *Disorders of Carbohydrate Metabolism in Infancy*, 2nd ed. Vol. 3. *Major Problems in Clinical Pediatrics*. Philadelphia: W.B. Saunders, 1976.

66. vanBuchem, F.S.P., Pol, G., de Gier, J., et al. Congenital beta-lipoprotein deficiency. *Am. J. Med.* 40:794, 1966.

67. Tangedahl, T. Dissolution of gallstones— When and how? *Surg. Clin. North Am.* 59:797, 1979.

68. Arvanitakis, C., Cooke, A.R., and Greenberger, N.J. Laboratory aids in the diagnosis of pancreatitis. *Med. Clin. North Am.* 62:107, 1978.

69. Cameron, J.L., Capuzzi, D.M., Zuidema, G.D., and Margolis, S. Acute pancreatitis with hyperlipemia. Evidence for a persistent defect in lipid metabolism. *Am. J. Med.* 56:482, 1974.

70. Greenberger, N.J., and Winship, D.H. *Gastrointestinal Disorders: A Pathophysiologic Approach*, 2nd ed. Chicago: Year Book Medical, 1981.

71. Schoumacher, R.A., Shoemaker, R.L., Halm, D.R., Tallant, E.A., Wallace, R.W., and Frizzell, R.A. Phosphorylation fails to activate chloride channels from cystic fibrosis airway cells. *Nature* 330:752, 1987.

72. Li, M., McCann, J.D., Liedtke, C.M., Nairn, A.C., Greengard, P., and Welsh, M.J. Cyclic AMP-dependent protein kinase opens chloride channels in normal but not cystic fibrosis airway epithelium. *Nature* 331:358, 1988.

73. Holt, P. Medium chain triglycerides. *D.M.* June 1971, pp. 1–30.

74. Gerson, W.T., Swan, P., and Walker, W.A. Nutrition support in cystic fibrosis. *Nutr. Rev.* 45:353, 1987.

75. Schwachman, H. Gastrointestinal manifestations of cystic fibrosis. *Pediatr. Clin. North Am.* 22:787, 1975.

76. Chase, H.P., Long, M.A., and Lavin, M.H. Cystic fibrosis and malnutrition. *J. Pediatr.* 95:337, 1979.

77. Southgate, D.A.T. Definitions and terminology of dietary fiber. In G.V. Vahouny and D. Kritchevsky, Eds., *Dietary Fiber in Health and Disease*. New York: Plenum Press, 1982.

78. Cummings, J.H. Nutritional implications of dietary fiber. *Am. J. Clin. Nutr.* 31:5, 1978.

79. Mendeloff, A.I. Dietary fiber and human health. *N. Engl. J. Med.* 297:811, 1977.

80. Kirk, E. The quantity and composition of human colonic flatus. *Gastroenterology* 12:782, 1949.

81. Bedell, G.N., Marshall, R., Dubois, A.B., and Harris, J.H. Measurement of the volume of gas in the gastrointestinal tract. *J. Clin. Invest.* 35:336, 1956.

82. Levitt, M.D. Volume and composition of human intestinal gas determined by an intestinal washout technique. *N. Engl. J. Med.* 284:1394, 1971.

83. Maddock, W.G., Bell, J.L., and Tremaine, M.J. Gastrointestinal gas. Observations on belching during anesthesia, operations and pyelography; and rapid passage of gas. *Ann. Surg.* 130:512, 1949.

84. Levitt, M.D., and Bond, J.H. Intestinal gas. In M.H. Sleisenger and J.S. Fordtran, Eds., *Gastrointestinal Disease: Pathophysiology, Diagnosis, Management*, 2nd ed. Philadelphia: W.B. Saunders, 1978.

85. Levitt, M.D. Production and excretion of hydrogen gas in man. *N. Engl. J. Med.* 281:122, 1969.

86. Murphy, E.L., and Calloway, D.H. The effect of antibiotic drugs on the volume and composition of intestinal gas from beans. *Am. J. Dig. Dis.* 17:639, 1972.

87. Lasser, R.B., Bond, J.H., and Levitt, M.D. The role of intestinal gas in functional abdominal pain. *N. Engl. J. Med.* 293:524, 1975.

88. Ritchie, J. Pain from distension of the pelvic colon by inflating a balloon in the irritable colon syndrome. *Gut* 14:125, 1973.

89. Painter, N.S. *Diverticular Disease of the Colon.* London: William Heinemann Medical, 1975.

90. Eastwood, M.A. Medical and dietary management. *Clin. Gastroenterol.* 4(1):85, 1975.

91. Phillips, S.F. Absorption and secretion by the colon. *Gastroenterology* 56:966, 1969.

Bibliography

Carey, M.C., Small, D.M., and Bliss, C.M. Lipid digestion and absorption. *Ann. Rev. Physiol.* 45:651, 1983.

Dwyer, J.T., Goldin, B., Gorback, S., and Patterson, J. Dietary fiber and fiber supplements in therapy of gastrointestinal disorders. *J. Maine Med. Assoc.* 69:51, 1978.

Gorman, M.A., and Bowman, C.B. Position of the American Dietetic Association. Health implications of dietary fiber—Technical support paper. *J. Am. Diet. Assoc.* 88:217, 1988.

Lebenthal, E., Ed. *Textbook of Gastroenterology and Nutrition in Infancy*, 2nd ed. New York: Raven Press, 1990.

Lloyd-Still, J.D. *Textbook of Cystic Fibrosis.* Boston: John Wright, PSG, Inc., 1983.

Reisir, S., Ed. *Metabolic Effects of Utilizable Dietary Carbohydrates.* New York: Marcel Dekker, 1982.

Royal College of Physicians of London. *Medical Aspects of Dietary Fiber.* Tunbridge Wells, U.K.: Pitman Medical, 1980.

Sleisenger, M.H., and Fordtran, J.S., Eds. *Gastrointestinal Disease: Pathophysiology, Diagnosis, Management*, 3rd ed. Philadelphia: W.B. Saunders, 1983.

Spiller, G.A., Ed. *CRC Handbook of Dietary Fiber in Human Nutrition.* Boca Raton, Fla.: CRC Press, 1986.

Vahouny, G.V., and Kritchevsky, D., Eds. *Dietary Fiber: Basic and Clinical Aspects.* New York: Plenum Press, 1984.

Vahouny, G.V., and Kritchevsky, D., Eds. *Dietary Fiber in Health and Disease.* New York: Plenum Press, 1982.

Sources of Current Information

Clinics in Gastroenterology
Digestive Diseases and Sciences
Pediatric Gastroenterology and Nutrition
Progress in Gastroenterology
Scandinavian Journal of Gastroenterology

9. The Urinary System

I. The Normal Kidney
  A. Renal anatomy
  B. Renal physiology
    1. Waste excretion and maintenance of homeostasis
    2. Regulation of osmolality and fluid volume
    3. Regulation of sodium balance
    4. Regulation of potassium balance
    5. Regulation of hydrogen ion concentration
    6. Regulation of calcium and phosphate balance
    7. Excretion of metabolic wastes
    8. Endocrine functions
    9. Other metabolic functions

II. Renal Disease
  A. Diagnostic tests
    1. Urinalysis
    2. Blood analysis
      a. serum creatinine
      b. serum urea nitrogen (SUN) or blood urea nitrogen (BUN)
      c. serum uric acid
    3. Renal function tests
    4. Direct examination of kidney tissue

  B. Renal failure
    1. Chronic renal failure
      a. etiology
      b. pathophysiology
      c. natural history
      d. manifestations
      e. metabolic alterations and nutritional care in conservative management
        (1) abnormalities related to protein and amino acids
        (2) energy needs
        (3) abnormalities of sodium balance
        (4) abnormalities of fluid balance
        (5) abnormalities of potassium balance
        (6) acidosis
        (7) calcium and phosphorus
        (8) iron
        (9) zinc
        (10) vitamin needs
        (11) carbohydrate
        (12) lipids
        (13) additional problems
        (14) planning the diet
      f. the dialysis patient
        (1) hemodialysis
        (2) peritoneal dialysis
      g. renal transplantation
      h. nutritional assessment
        (1) modification of routine assessments
        (2) monitoring renal patients

    2. Acute renal failure
      a. etiology
      b. pathogenesis
      c. pathology
      d. pathophysiology
      e. clinical course and prognosis
      f. nutritional management
        (1) sodium and fluid
        (2) protein
        (3) energy
        (4) potassium
        (5) other electrolytes
      g. monitoring the ARF patient
      h. nonoral nutritional support
  C. Glomerulopathy
    1. Etiology and pathogenesis
    2. Pathology
    3. Acute glomerulonephritis
      a. clinical manifestations
      b. treatment
        (1) fluid and sodium
        (2) protein
        (3) potassium
      c. clinical course
    4. Chronic glomerulonephritis
    5. Nephrotic syndrome
      a. definition and etiology
      b. clinical manifestations
        (1) proteinuria
        (2) hypoproteinemia
        (3) edema
        (4) hyperlipidemia
        (5) lipiduria
        (6) other manifestations
      c. treatment
        (1) diuretic drugs
        (2) diet
  D. Diabetic renal disease

III. Case Study

THE NORMAL KIDNEY

Renal Anatomy

The components of the urinary system are the **kidney, ureters, bladder,** and **urethra** (see Figure 9-1). Each kidney is enclosed by a fibrous nonelastic capsule beneath which the renal cortex forms a layer 4 to 6 mm thick in an adult (see Figure 9-2).

The cortex is made up of **renal corpuscles, proximal** and **distal convoluted tubules,** and the upper portions of the **loops of Henle** and **collecting ducts** (see Figure 9-3). The **medulla** lies beneath the cortex and is composed of several **pyramids** containing the remaining portions of the loops of Henle and the collecting ducts. Basement membrane surrounds the tubules and is supported by very delicate reticular fibers. There is very little connective tissue in the kidney.

The functional unit of the kidney is the **nephron** (Figure 9-3). It has been estimated that each kidney contains 1 to 1.5 million nephrons, each of which includes a tuft of approximately 50 capillaries called the **glomerulus.** The glomerulus invaginates a **Bowman's capsule,** a blind-ended epithelial sac, which, with the glomerulus, forms the **renal corpuscle.** Bowman's capsule is continuous with a tubular system, the parts of which are, successively, the proximal convoluted tubule, the loop of Henle, the distal convoluted tubules, and the collecting duct. Urine flows through the collecting ducts to an opening in the **papilla** (the apex of the pyramid) and enters the pelvis of the kidney, which forms the funnel-shaped proximal end of the ureter through which the urine passes into the bladder (see Figure 9-2).

A more detailed knowledge of the structure of the renal capsule is important to the understanding of some renal diseases. Bowman's capsule consists of an outer, **parietal layer,** which is continuous with the tubules. The parietal layer then is reflected back to form the **visceral layer,** which covers the capillaries. The area between the parietal

Figure 9-1. Components of the urinary system.

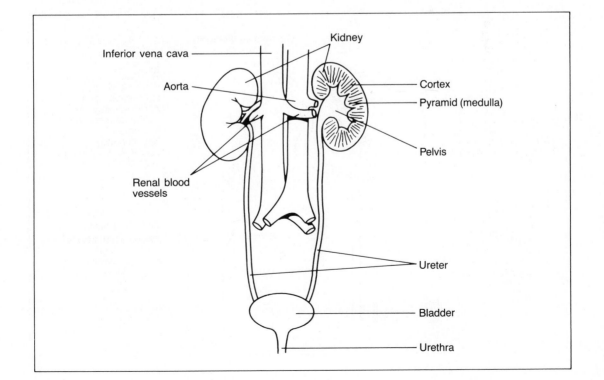

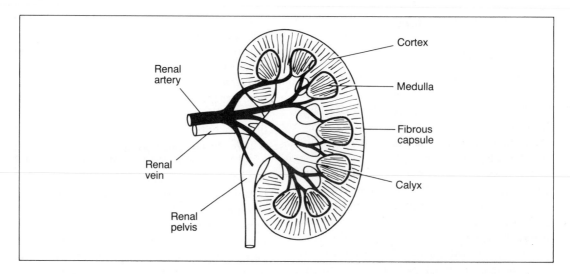

Figure 9-2. Structure of the kidney.

and visceral layers is the **capsular space** (Figure 9-4). The visceral layer is composed of **podocytes**, which have projections called **foot processes**. These are in contact with the

Figure 9-3. Structure of an individual nephron.

basement membrane of the capillary endothelial cells. **Mesangial cells**, which are part of the immune system, are located between the capillaries. Together, they are enveloped by a basement membrane.

Another important feature of the nephron structure is the **juxtaglomerular apparatus**. It contains the **macula densa**, which is composed of specialized epithelial cells located in

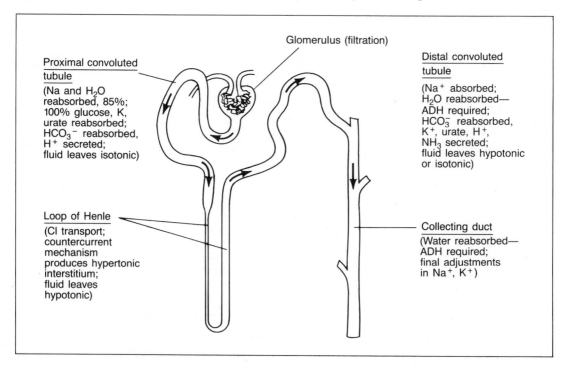

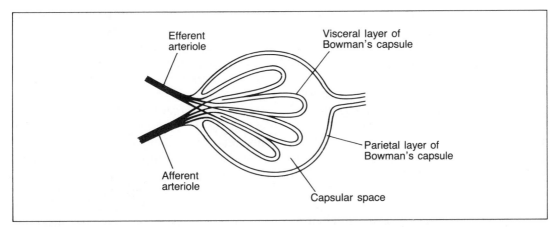

Efferent arteriole

Visceral layer of Bowman's capsule

Parietal layer of Bowman's capsule

Afferent arteriole

Capsular space

Figure 9-4. Invagination of capillary loops into the blind end of a renal tubule.

that part of the distal tubule nearest the afferent and efferent arterioles of Bowman's capsule, and specialized granular cells in the afferent arteriole. The juxtaglomerular apparatus functions in production of the hormone renin, for the control of blood pressure.

Renal Physiology

The kidney has excretory, metabolic, and endocrine functions that have broad systemic effects.

Waste Excretion and Maintenance of Homeostasis

Urine formation consists of three basic processes: glomerular filtration, tubular secretion, and tubular reabsorption. By these processes the kidney regulates the composition of body fluids and removes metabolic wastes.

As blood flows through the glomerulus, water, smaller molecules (mostly those with molecular weight of 5,000 or less), and a small amount of protein are filtered into the capsular space. Blood cells and large protein molecules, collectively called colloids, remain in the capillaries. An adult produces approximately 180 liters per day of glomerular filtrate from the 900 liters per day of

blood that pass through the kidney. Glomerular filtration rate (GFR) is an important indicator of renal function. The normal rate is approximately 180 liters/(24 hours × 60 minutes), or 125 ml/min. The glomerular filtrate has the approximate composition of blood plasma except for the colloids. Tubular secretion and reabsorption change the composition of the filtrate as necessary to maintain body homeostasis and form the final urine.

If all the water, glucose, electrolytes, and other materials filtered were excreted in the urine, the body would become depleted very quickly. Instead, as the glomerular filtrate moves through the tubules, many components needed to maintain homeostasis are reabsorbed. These normally include approximately 99% of the water, all of the glucose, 99.5% of the sodium, 92.5% of the potassium, 50% of the urea, and almost all of the calcium and amino acids. Phosphate and lipid-soluble drugs are also reabsorbed.

Regulation of Osmolality and Fluid Volume

In homeostatic control of osmolality, the movements of sodium and water vary with the cell permeability in the distal tubules and collecting ducts. Permeability is controlled by the effect of antidiuretic hormone (ADH). Changes in plasma osmolality are sensed by receptors in the posterior pituitary gland and hypothalamus, which alter the rate of secretion of ADH by the pituitary gland.

An excess of body water causes a decrease in osmolality and inhibits ADH release. Then, permeability of the distal tubule cells is low, and water is not reabsorbed, increasing both urine volume and plasma osmolality. When body water is decreased, osmolality increases and ADH secretion rises. In the presence of increased ADH, permeability is high and water is reabsorbed, reducing both urine volume and plasma osmolality. Sodium transport is not affected by ADH. These processes, therefore, can result in production of a hypoosmotic or isoosmotic urine. Osmolarity of the urine may be as low as 50 mOsm/L.

By contrast, in order to produce a hyperosmolar urine, a countercurrent system in the loop of Henle is used. It creates an osmotic gradient from the cortex through the medulla to the papilla. The gradient is maintained by the parallel blood vessel structure known as the vasa recta. Water and solutes are reabsorbed from the tubules into the interstitium, then into the vasa recta, and carried into the general circulation. As the fluid flows through the collecting ducts, an osmotic gradient exists between it and the interstitial fluid. If the cells of the collecting ducts are permeable to water as a result of ADH action, water diffuses out of the ducts to equilibrate with the interstitial fluid. The kidney is thus capable of producing a hyperosmotic urine which may reach a maximum osmolarity of 1,400 mOsm/L.

The normal adult body excretes 600 mOsm or more of urea, sulfate, phosphate, and other waste products each day. This solute load (see Chapter 2) increases with increased intake of protein and electrolytes. In order to eliminate a solute load of 600 mOsm, a minimum of 600/1,400, or 0.43 liter per day of water is required. This will be excreted as long as the kidneys function. More water is used to excrete an increased solute load. The amount of water needed to excrete the solute load is the **obligatory water loss**. On the average, of the total 170 to 180 liters of glomerular filtrate, all but about 1.5 liters is reabsorbed.

At the same time as tubular reabsorption is occurring, some substances are secreted into the filtrate by cells of the tubular epithelium. Hydrogen ions, potassium, ammonia, and various organic acids and bases are secreted by the tubules. This process also is necessary to maintain homeostasis. It is important, for example, in acid-base balance (see Chapter 2).

Some substances secreted by the tubules are subsequently reabsorbed. Therefore it is important to distinguish between **secretion** and **excretion**. Excretion occurs only for those materials that are contained in the final urine.

Regulation of Sodium Balance

The excretion of sodium is controlled separately from the regulation of osmolality. Normal plasma sodium concentration is 136 to 146 mEq/L; therefore, 140 mEq × 180 L/day, or approximately 25,200 mEq of sodium are filtered each day. Since daily sodium intake is only a small fraction of this amount, most of the filtered sodium must be reabsorbed. The kidney can conserve sodium very efficiently, so that excretion may be as low as 1 mEq/day. Conversely, if sodium intake is high, large quantities of sodium can be excreted by reducing sodium reabsorption in the tubules.

Most sodium is reabsorbed in the proximal tubules (see Figure 9-5). An important additional factor in control of sodium reabsorption is aldosterone, produced by the zone glomerulosa of the adrenal cortex. Aldosterone stimulates the reabsorption of sodium in the distal convoluted tubules and collecting ducts, providing the "fine adjustment."

Other factors are involved in this complex control system. Prostaglandins and kallikreins synthesized within the kidney also influence sodium and water absorption. The atrial natriuretic factor (ANF) or atriopeptin, secreted in the atrium of the heart, acts as a vasodilator and increases GFR to increase so-

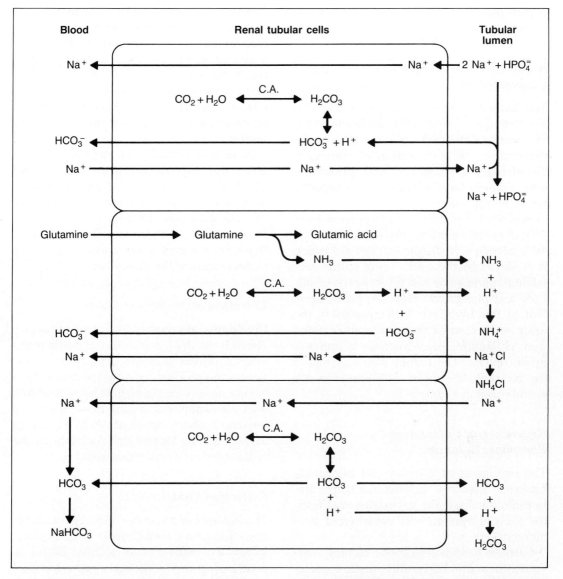

Figure 9-5. Renal tubular function in acid-base balance.

dium and water excretion. It may also inhibit renin, ADH, and aldosterone. There is much yet to be learned concerning control of sodium balance.

Regulation of Potassium Balance

As with sodium, potassium balance is maintained by excretion of the amount ingested daily. Most of this excretion is urinary. Potassium is freely filtered at the glomerulus and is reabsorbed by the tubules. It is actively transported in the proximal convoluted tubules and loops of Henle. When the filtrate enters the distal convoluted tubules, it contains only 10% or less of the original filtered potassium. The distal convoluted tubules and collecting ducts may either reabsorb or secrete potassium. In the distal tubules, in the presence of adequate aldosterone and sodium, potassium is exchanged for sodium. There is a large reserve capacity for potassium excretion; therefore, potassium toxicity is difficult to produce if renal function is normal.

Regulation of Hydrogen Ion Concentration

The kidneys play an essential role in the maintenance of hydrogen ion homeostasis by means of their effects on secretion and excretion or on reabsorption of hydrogen, bicarbonate, ammonium, and phosphate ions. Kidneys have a large reserve capacity for excreting acid.

In a normal person eating approximately 70 g of protein per day, the kidneys excrete 40 to 60 mEq of hydrogen ion, most of which is produced by the oxidation of sulfur-containing amino acids and phosphorus to sulfuric and phosphoric acids. Approximately half of this hydrogen load appears in the urine in the form of ammonium ion created from glutamine. The remainder is buffered by phosphate. The kidney also replenishes the bicarbonate supply. The processes are summarized in Figure 9-5.

Regulation of Calcium and Phosphate Balances

The regulation of calcium and phosphate balances involves interrelationships between the kidney, the gastrointestinal tract, the skeletal system, and parathyroid hormone (PTH).

Calcium functions in blood clotting, nervous system irritability, and muscle contractility. Phosphate is important in the formation of ATP. While these substances have separate functions in general cellular metabolism, they unite in bone to form crystals and provide rigidity if present in appropriate proportions. Thus appropriate concentrations of each must be maintained.

Parathyroid hormone is important in maintaining calcium and phosphorus homeostasis by increasing their absorption from the gut and reabsorption from the bone. In the kidney, approximately 50% of plasma calcium is protein-bound. The remainder is

filtered, of which about 99% is actively reabsorbed. When increased intake causes increased plasma calcium levels, more calcium is filtered, and PTH secretion decreases. As a result, tubular reabsorption of calcium falls and excess calcium is excreted. The action of PTH also reduces renal tubular reabsorption of phosphate, lowering its plasma concentration.

Final hydroxylation of vitamin D to the active hormone occurs in the kidneys and affects the processes of calcium metabolism in which vitamin D participates. These are calcium absorption from the gastrointestinal lumen and bone resorption. These actions of the kidney are of great importance in the maintenance of the skeletal system.

Excretion of Metabolic Wastes

In addition to excretion of excess water and electrolytes, the kidney also must excrete the waste products of metabolism. The elimination of the products of nitrogen metabolism is very important. Creatinine, urea, and uric acid are prominent among these, but there are many others, not all of which have been identified. The kidney also functions in the elimination of drugs and toxins.

Endocrine Functions

The kidney has a number of endocrine functions that have a broad impact on body physiology. The activation of vitamin D and its relationship to the skeletal system have already been described. In addition, the kidney synthesizes **renin**, which functions in the renin-angiotensin system for control of blood pressure. Prostaglandins and kallikreins, which they elaborate, also affect blood pressure (see Chapter 10). The effects of renal prostaglandins are thought to function only within the kidney itself. An additional important renal function includes the maintenance of normal red cell production by stimulation via **erythropoietin**.

The kidney influences the action of other hormones, since it degrades and eliminates circulating peptide hormones including insulin, glucagon, PTH, prolactin, thyrotropin, and growth hormone. Gastrointestinal hormones and vasopressin are also affected, but the mechanisms are unclear.[1]

Other Metabolic Functions

In addition to the functions already described and their effects on metabolism, the kidney also affects other metabolic functions directly. It influences the pattern of amino acid concentrations in the circulation.[2,3] The kidney also synthesizes and degrades glucose and, in starvation, may be a glucose producer.[4] It also degrades choline.[5]

RENAL DISEASE

In the past 30 years, great progress has been made in the treatment of renal disease. Complex and expensive methods, such as dialysis and organ transplants, have extended the lives of patients whose kidneys fail; however, none of these methods is entirely satisfactory.

Most of the renal diseases in which nutritional care is important are those that are progressive and for which there is no available cure. Overall management of the disease is designed to prolong the patient's life and improve the quality of that life. The nutritional care specialist cooperates with other members of the health care team to achieve these objectives.

To a great extent, the purpose of nutritional management is to compensate for the loss of the function of the kidney in maintaining the constancy of the internal environment. Since food and fluid intakes normally make a large contribution to this variability, a major part of nutritional management consists of reducing the intake of substances that the kidney must excrete and providing replacements for those materials lost in abnormal quantities. While these modifications to the diet are being made, the patient must be provided with nutrients to maintain optimum nutritional status in the form of a diet that encourages acceptance by the patient. This represents a challenge to the skill of the nutritional care specialist, since the patient often suffers from anorexia, nausea, and vomiting. In summary, the overall objectives of nutritional care of most renal disease patients are (1) to maintain optimum nutrition, (2) to minimize metabolic disorders and related symptoms, (3) to retard progression of the disease, and (4) to delay the necessity for dialysis.

Diagnostic Tests

In order to understand the patient's needs and the rationale for the diet, the nutritional care specialist must be able to interpret the results of the relevant laboratory tests. This section describes a variety of tests used in the diagnosis of the disease and in the evaluation of its progress.

Urinalysis

The urine may be examined for the presence of materials not normally seen in the urine or for abnormal quantities of substances normally found in the urine. Substances that, when present in the urine, may indicate kidney or urinary tract disease include erythrocytes, leukocytes, microorganisms, glucose, and protein. Measurements of the pH and specific gravity of the urine are sometimes of diagnostic value as well, since they indicate the capacity of the kidney to maintain acid-base balance and a normal osmolality of body fluids.

Abnormal urine color and odor may be indicative of disease. However, ingestion of beets and blackberries are known to color urine, and asparagus provides a noticeable odor in normal kidneys.

Blood Analysis

If the kidneys are not functioning normally, substances usually excreted by the kidneys accumulate in the blood; however, it should be appreciated that the kidney has a large reserve capacity. Up to 50% of renal function may be lost without a change in concentration of many of the substances measured in clinical diagnosis. Nevertheless, many blood analyses are simple and relatively inexpensive and often are useful in evaluating the course of the disease.

Serum Creatinine. Phosphocreatine in muscles is formed from glycine, arginine, and methionine. Creatinine is a degradation product of phosphocreatine. It is produced in an amount proportionate to muscle mass and is excreted in the urine. Normal concentration in the serum is usually 0.6 to 1.5 mg/dl. If the kidney is unable to excrete nitrogenous waste products, the concentration of creatinine will increase in the blood.

Serum Urea Nitrogen (SUN) or Blood Urea Nitrogen (BUN). The deamination of amino acids results in the production of ammonia, a highly toxic substance. In the human liver, ammonia is converted to urea by the urea cycle and then is excreted in the urine. If the kidney is unable to excrete nitrogenous wastes, urea, too, will rise in concentration in the blood. The normal ranges of urea nitrogen concentrations are 5 to 20 mg/dl of blood and 6 to 20 mg/dl of serum.

Serum Uric Acid. Uric acid is a product of purine metabolism and normally appears in the serum in a concentration of 3 to 7 mg/dl in men or 2 to 6 mg/dl in women. Like urea and creatinine, it increases in concentration as renal function diminishes.

Renal Function Tests

Renal function tests evaluate specific aspects of the actions of the nephron, glomerular filtration, tubular function, or renal plasma flow. Several commonly used indicators of various aspects of renal function are listed in Table 9-1. The **creatinine clearance test** is used very frequently in clinical situations. It measures the amount of blood that can be cleared of creatinine per minute. Normal values are 110 to 150 ml/min. for men and 105 to 132 ml/min. for women when corrected to 1.73 m^2 of body surface area.

Direct Examination of Kidney Tissue

A number of means are available for direct examination of the kidney, including the following:

Plain radiography: A roentgenogram will show shadows indicating the size and location of the kidney. Calcified areas and renal calculi will be seen.

Sonography: Ultrasound can be used to show kidney size and the presence of cysts or masses in the kidney.

Intravenous pyelogram (IVP) or excretory urography: A substance that is opaque to X-ray is injected into the vein, and roentgenograms are taken at intervals as the dye is filtered by the kidney.

Isotopic renogram: A radioactive-isotope-labeled material is injected into a vein, and its concentration and excretion are followed.

Renal arteriography: A radioopaque substance injected into the renal artery outlines the vascular system on the X-ray

Table 9-1. Tests of Renal Function

Function	Clinical Tests
Glomerular filtration rate	Blood urea nitrogen; creatinine clearance
Renal plasma flow	Phenolsulfonphthalein excretion; renal scan with isotopes
Transport in proximal tubules	Urinary excretion of amino acids, glucose, phosphate
Transport in Henle's loops and distal tubules	Maximum and minimum urine specific gravity and osmolality
Concentrating and diluting ability	Maximum and minimum urine specific gravity and osmolality

plate and detects abnormalities in renal blood flow.

Renal biopsy: A small core of renal tissue is obtained using a special needle. The tissue then is examined under a microscope.

Computerized tomography (CT) scan: This is a noninvasive procedure used to visualize internal organs and structure, such as tumors.

Renal Failure

Renal failure exists when the kidney is no longer able to maintain the constancy of the internal environment. Chronic renal failure will be discussed first, since nutritional management is of paramount importance in this condition and is now believed to be capable of slowing the progress of the disease. An abbreviated description of acute renal failure, particularly as it differs from chronic failure, will follow.

Chronic Renal Failure

Chronic renal failure (CRF) is an irreversible loss of excretory capacity of the kidney that occurs over an extended period of time, from months to years. Endocrine and metabolic functions also are lost.

Etiology. A variety of renal and systemic diseases, some of which are listed in Table 9-2, can result in chronic renal failure. However, the cause of CRF in some patients is unknown.

Pathophysiology. The loss of nephron function has been shown by Bricker[6-8] to occur in an orderly fashion. Bricker's **intact nephron hypothesis** proposes that most of the nephrons of the diseased kidney in CRF fall into one of two categories. They are either nonfunctioning nephrons, as a result of destruction of any portion of their structure, or they are nephrons that function normally. The changes in renal function occur as the result of a reduction in the number of functioning nephrons.

Table 9-2. Causes of Chronic Renal Failure

Diseases in which kidney involvement is predominant
Glomerulonephritis
Interstitial nephritis
Renal calculi
Congenital nephritis
Polycystic disease
Renal hypoplasia
Renal tubular acidosis
Urinary tract obstructions that may *lead to renal failure*
Prostatic enlargement
Urethral stricture
Bladder neck obstruction
Neurogenic bladder
Malignancy
Conditions that often *cause renal failure*
Malignant hypertension
Periarteritis nodosa
Lupus erythematosus
Analgesic drug abuse
Potassium deficiency
Hypercalcemia
Cystinosis
Primary oxaluria
Lead or cadmium poisoning
Systemic diseases in which renal failure sometimes *occurs*
Benign essential hypertension
Atherosclerosis
Embolism
Gout
Diabetes
Heart failure

The kidneys continue to respond to the needs of the body insofar as they are able to do so. However, as the number of functioning nephrons diminishes, there are adaptations that occur in a regular sequence. First, the remaining functional nephrons increase in size and function. As plasma levels of various materials increase, more is filtered and excreted. In the tubules, there is a reduction in reabsorption of electrolytes or compounds normally excreted and an increase in secretion of those normally secreted. The nature of the adaptive mechanisms varies with the solute that is controlled. The control systems affecting these adaptations are still being investigated but are believed to be those that function in the normal kidney, not new systems produced as a result of the disease process.

Another important consideration is whether the adaptive mechanisms are always of positive value, or whether there sometimes are detrimental consequences. Bricker's **trade-off hypothesis**[9] suggests that some adaptations are detrimental but that they are the price to be paid to correct conditions that are more life-threatening. The body "trades off" one condition for a less serious one. An example is given in the discussion of calcium and phosphorus beginning on page 301.

Natural History. The progression of CRF has been described as occurring in four stages that are not sharply separated but, rather, are phases in a continuing degenerative process with loss of more and more functioning nephrons. The four phases are (1) decreased renal reserve, (2) renal insufficiency, (3) renal failure, and (4) uremia or uremic syndrome.

Given the large reserve capacity of the kidney, at least 55% of normal renal function must be lost before blood urea increases, although there may be some nephron hypertrophy during the first phase of **decreased renal reserve**. The GFR is greater than 55 ml/min., but less than the normal 125 ml/min. At this stage, the patient does not have any symptoms.

In **renal insufficiency**, up to 80% of nephron function may be lost, and the GRF is 30 to 55 ml/min. There is a mild **azotemia** (excessive amounts of nitrogen components in the blood). Serum urea and creatinine are thus above normal. The patient becomes more susceptible to the effects of stresses such as large changes in intake of fluids, protein, and electrolytes. There is some loss of concentrating ability, producing **nocturia** (excessive urination at night). The patient may remain symptom-free if no overwhelming metabolic stress occurs, but symptoms occur if the patient is subjected to a stress such as infection.

In **renal failure**, loss of nephron function may reach 90%. The GFR is 12.5 to 30.0 ml/min. The patient shows moderate to severe azotemia and anemia, decreased concentrating ability, and impaired ability to maintain electrolyte and acid-base balance.

Loss of function in the final phase, **uremia** or **uremic syndrome**, is 90% to 100%. The GFR is less than 12.5 ml/min. The patient is **oliguric** (produces insufficient urine) or **anuric** (produces no urine), with uremic symptoms involving many organ systems.

Therefore, it is the patient with 20% or less of normal renal function who has lost the ability to adjust to the wide variations in fluid and nutrient intake that commonly occur in a healthy person.

Manifestations. The onset of renal insufficiency and renal failure tends to be gradual and insidious. The patient may first present with **polyuria** (increased urine flow) and nocturia with a vague feeling of malaise. Nausea, vomiting, anorexia, and fatigue, possibly related to anemia and retention of organic acids, with some degree of breathlessness may follow. As the kidney function diminishes, many other organ systems become more clearly involved. These are summarized in Table 9-3, which illustrates the extent of the illness.

The development of methods of dialysis and of renal transplantation have revolutionized the treatment of CRF. However, these procedures often follow a long period of slow deterioration of kidney function, during which management is aimed at maintaining homeostasis with maximum possible function of the remaining nephrons. In these patients, it is particularly important that food and fluid intake be correlated with the functional capacity of the kidney. With appropriate treatment, many patients remain almost symptom-free until the GFR decreases to approximately 10 ml/min. When the GFR falls below this level, it becomes very difficult to prevent the onset of severe complications of uremia and to maintain adequate nutrition. At this point, known as **end-stage renal disease** (ESRD), dialysis or transplantation is necessary to prolong life.

Metabolic Alterations and Nutritional Care in Conservative Management. Chronic renal failure is a progressive, terminal disease that, if untreated, continues an

Table 9-3. Signs and Symptoms of Advanced
Chronic Renal Failure

Tissue or Organ	Clinical Effects
Digestive system	Dry mouth, stomatitis, glossitis, uremic fetor Hiccups Nausea, vomiting Parotitis Gastritis; gastroenteritis Malabsorption Paralytic ileus Gastrointestinal bleeding
Integumentary system	Pruritus, dry skin and hair Pigmentation
Cardiovascular system	Arrhythmias, pericarditis, myocarditis Hypertension, dyspnea Congestive heart failure
Respiratory system	Hemoptysis, dyspnea, pleurisy, pneumonitis, pleuritis Pulmonary edema
Hematopoietic system	Anemia Platelet abnormalities, bleeding tendencies, clotting defects
Central nervous system	Peripheral neuropathy; paresthesias, irritability Muscular weakness, atrophy Fatigue, lethargy, apathy, convulsions, coma Abnormal behavior, psychoses Visual disturbances; impaired hearing Insomnia
Skeleton	Poor bone growth; bone pain; joint pain Poor healing Rickets, osteomalacia, osteodystrophy, osteoporosis, tetany
Other	Decreased resistance to infection Impaired wound healing Decreased ovulation, vaginal hemorrhage Decreased spermatogenesis, impotence Vaginal hemorrhage

inexorable course to the death of the patient. Conservative management was at one time the only treatment available. Some relief of symptoms and some prolongation of life were achieved with no change in the inevitable outcome.

With the advent of dialysis and renal transplantation, the role of conservative management with diet modification and medication has changed so that it is now used (1) for relief of symptoms and to improve the quality of life while delaying the necessity for dialysis; (2) to avoid irreversible physiologic changes and maintain the patient in the best possible condition prior to dialysis or transplant; and (3) to relieve symptoms and improve the quality of life for those patients for whom neither dialysis nor transplant is indicated. In order to understand the basis for the diet modifications, it is necessary to have a grasp of the metabolic alterations that occur.

Abnormalities related to protein and amino acids. The diseased glomerulus may be unable to retain serum proteins, which are then lost in the urine (**proteinuria**). The protein lost is primarily albumin, and so the condition frequently is called **albuminuria**. Low serum protein levels occur (**hypoproteinemia** or **hypoalbuminemia**), and **edema** develops as serum protein falls. The triad of proteinuria, hypoproteinemia, and edema constitute the **nephrotic syndrome**. This syndrome occurs in relation to a number of renal diseases and is discussed in greater detail in the section on glomerulopathy (see pp. 329–332).

As the number of functioning nephrons declines, hypertrophy of the nephrons and osmotic diuresis, considered to be adaptive mechanisms, supervene. Serum levels of nitrogen metabolism (such as creatinine and urea) rise, producing **nitrogen retention**, **azotemia**, or **uremia**. It now becomes important to reduce the demands on the remaining nephrons by reducing the amount of material that must be excreted.

The patient seems to feel well despite high levels of nitrogen metabolites until the GFR has decreased to about 15 to 20 ml/min. At the same time, serum creatinine often has risen approximately to 10 mg/dl, and serum urea to above 100 mg/dl. The patient then begins to show signs and symptoms of chronic renal failure (see Table 9-3). Although the severity of many symptoms of renal failure seems to correlate well with blood urea levels, there is no evidence that either urea or creatinine is particularly toxic. Therefore, SUN and serum creatinine are used only as yardsticks to measure the severity of the disease and the effects of treatment.

The patient in advanced renal failure tends to negative nitrogen balance and muscle wasting. Protein metabolism may be affected by the accumulation of nitrogenous metabolites, hormonal derangements, alterations in amino acid metabolism and other nutrients, and anorexia with consequent poor food intake. It is unclear whether there is increased muscle catabolism or decreased anabolism.[10-13]

The effect of insulin, an anabolic hormone, is also unclear. Glucose metabolism is impaired and may thus influence protein synthesis secondarily.[14] However, this insulin resistance may not apply directly to amino acid metabolism.[12,15]

The search for *the* uremic toxin has been long and futile. Many substances that accumulate in the blood of the renal failure patient have been identified. These include phosphate, potassium, amino acids and other organic acids, amines, guanidines, indoles, phenols, myoinositol and other polyols, nucleic acid metabolites, and the "middle molecules." Middle molecules have molecular weights of 350 to 4,000 daltons and include some enzymes, such as transketolase, hormones such as PTH, and some vitamins.[16,17] There is evidence that an increase in PTH in the serum is an important cause of a variety of hematologic, neurologic, and metabolic alterations in CRF.[18] None of these retained materials singly reproduces the usual clinical picture of uremia. It seems more likely that the complex of symptoms is produced by the accumulated disturbances resulting from renal failure and the interactions of these disturbances with one another.

In determining the protein content of the diet, a balance must be sought to reduce the accumulation of nitrogenous end products while maintaining a positive nitrogen balance. Provision of essential amino acids is required. Histidine is an essential amino acid for renal failure patients as well as for infants and must be supplied in the diet.[19]

Some degree of protein restriction is necessary in CRF, but the protein level to be used and the point at which the restriction should begin are matters of some debate. It is now recognized that the protein restriction serves two purposes:

1. To ameliorate symptoms and offer some relief to patients.
2. To slow the degenerative processes in the kidneys.

There are several protocols which have been recommended. Symptomatic relief is achieved by providing a low-protein diet (0.3 g per kg body weight) when GFR falls to 10 ml/minute or less. In order to slow the degenerative process, the protein restriction is instituted earlier in the progress of the disease. A diet containing 0.6 g protein per kg body weight (40 g of protein per day) is initiated when GFR is 50 ml/min. This restriction must be accompanied by adequate energy intake, control of excess serum levels of phosphate and calcium, as described in later subsections, and control of hyperlipidemia (see Chapter 10). In an alternative protocol, if the patient has a normal or increased urine volume, dietary protein usually is not restricted until the patient reaches the stage of renal failure with moderate to severe azotemia. Kopple[20] suggests that protein restriction should begin before the SUN rises to 90 mg/dl or even 60 mg/dl in order to avoid the symptoms that accompany higher levels. Recommended protein restrictions may be 60 to 90 g when the GFR is 20 to 25 ml/min and may be lowered to 40 to 60 g (0.5 to 0.65 g per kg ideal body weight) as the GFR falls to 10 to 15 ml/min. At least 70% of this protein should be of high biologic value in order for the diet to be most effective in reducing SUN.

If the patient has proteinuria, the protein in the diet should be increased sufficiently to provide replacement of the losses. This level of protein intake usually will prevent uremic symptoms until the GFR falls to approximately 4 to 5 ml/min. The diet should be planned for maximum anabolic effects of protein and maximum acceptability. Some general guidelines are given in Table 9-4.

An important element in the total picture of CRF which is of special interest to nutri-

Table 9-4. General Guidelines for the Management of the Protein-Restricted Diet

1. Distribute protein evenly throughout the day to minimize hepatic deamination.
2. Emphasize the use of proteins of high biologic value.
3. Provide energy needs from other sources to avoid the use of protein to provide energy.
   a. Use low-protein pasta products and wheat starch, if necessary, to meet energy needs.
   b. Use low-protein, high-energy supplements if necessary. (See Appendix G for a description of available products.)
4. Use protein "stretchers"—combining protein foods with cereals, vegetables, mayonnaise, and so on. See *The Mayo Clinic Renal Diet Cookbook*[a] or similar volumes for recipes.
5. Use protein exchange lists in planning.
6. Encourage exercise within permissible limits to avoid muscle atrophy.

[a] Margie, J.D. *The Mayo Clinic Renal Diet Cookbook.* New York: Golden Press, 1974.

tionists is the **wasting syndrome**. In wasted patients, body weight, adipose tissue, and muscle mass are decreased. Children are growth-retarded. Serum albumin, transferrin, and some immune system proteins are reduced. Poor dietary intake is believed to be a major cause of wasting, but blood losses and other concurrent illnesses may contribute. In addition to malnutrition, there are indications of other derangements that contribute to wasting and to other symptoms.

There is an increased synthesis and release of alanine and glutamine from skeletal muscles, which contribute to the degradation of skeletal muscles and the wasting syndrome.[21,22] These changes also provide substrates for alterations in carbohydrate metabolism, including increased gluconeogenesis.

Aberrations in serum and muscle amino acid profiles, the significance of which are not entirely understood, have also been found.[23-26] For example, there are increased concentrations of nonessential amino acids and decreased concentrations of essential amino acids. The branched-chain amino acids (leucine, isoleucine, and valine) are among those increased. The tyrosine-phenylalanine ratio is reduced, suggesting diminished activity of phenylalanine hy-

droxylase, which functions in the formation of tyrosine from phenylalanine. At the same time, other metabolites of phenylalanine are increased. The significance of these changes is unknown.

The essentiality of histidine in the uremic adult also indicates an alteration in metabolism. Histidine is important in the structure of hemoglobin, and the reduced plasma histidine may be related to hematologic changes. Supplementation with histidine has been shown to result in increased hematocrit and decreased reticulocytes (immature red blood cells).[27]

The cause of these metabolic alterations is not clear. It is conceivable that uremic toxins affect protein or amino acid metabolism in a variety of ways. High serum urea has been reported to inhibit urea cycle enzymes.[28] The concentration of some urea cycle intermediates may then increase and enter other metabolic pathways. Uremic toxins could also affect membrane transport and other aspects of amino acid metabolism. The various endocrine disorders and their interactions with nutrients may be significant. Alterations in the metabolism of carbohydrate, lipids, and some vitamins and minerals affect protein and amino acid metabolism.

Our knowledge of these matters is sketchy at best. A better understanding may be useful in determining the ideal kind and amount of protein for the uremic patient and the ideal amino acid or analogue supplementation that should be used.[25] The specialist in nutritional care should be alert to new developments in this field.

Energy needs. Sufficient sources of kilocalories must be provided so that body protein is not metabolized to provide energy. The patient's loss of appetite together with the protein restriction tends to present problems in achieving this goal. If intake of sufficient kilocalories is to be achieved, the advice, skill, and encouragement of persons experienced in nutritional care are essential. A number of carbohydrate and lipid supplements intended to increase the caloric content of the diet are available. They are almost protein-free with low levels of electrolytes.

Further information on these products is contained in Appendix G, Table G-2.

Abnormalities of sodium balance. As the number of functioning nephrons decreases, the remaining nephrons hypertrophy to compensate for the loss. Glomerular filtration decreases, but sodium balance is maintained by adaptation of the tubular reabsorption in the remaining nephrons until impairment is significant.[9] As renal function diminishes further, there is usually an impaired ability to conserve sodium. The obligatory loss of sodium may be 20 to 40 mEq/day, but some patients are less able to restrict renal losses of sodium. These so-called "salt-wasters" lose salt as a result of either the osmotic diuresis resulting from the increased solute load (of urea) or specific damage to tubule cells. In addition, some patients lose sodium from vomiting and diarrhea.

Moderate sodium losses are replaced if the patient is given a diet containing 4 to 6 g of salt. When larger amounts of sodium are lost than can be replaced by normal sodium intake, the patient becomes sodium-depleted (**hyponatremia**). Extracellular fluid volume falls as the patient loses water to restore normal osmolality. The reduced plasma volume results in decreased cardiac output, further compromising renal function as blood flow to the kidney diminishes.

The sodium concentration must be maintained in these patients by adequate replacement. Additional sodium is provided in increased quantities of salty foods. If sodium bicarbonate is being used to treat acidosis, it will also provide some of the necessary sodium. Sodium chloride tablets, which might serve as a source of sodium, tend to cause gastric irritation, but some patients will put salt into capsules and take those.

With a further reduction in the number of functioning nephrons, the kidney's ability to excrete sodium is diminished, despite the adaptive mechanisms. Less sodium is filtered for excretion, and sodium retention results. This is accompanied by increased extracellular volume (fluid retention) to restore normal osmolality. The consequences of increased fluid volume may include peripheral edema, hypertension, congestive heart failure, pulmonary congestion, and pulmonary edema. It has been estimated that retention of 20 mEq/day of sodium will cause the retention of 1 liter of fluid per week, causing a weight gain of 1 kg.[28] It then becomes necessary to restrict sodium intake to a degree dependent on the state of hydration and the severity of the hypertension.

The CRF patient is poised precariously between sodium depletion and sodium overload. The amount of sodium in the diet must be determined for each patient. The maximum amount of sodium that the patient can tolerate should be allowed in order to maintain normal extracellular fluid volume and promote the maximum GFR of which the kidneys are capable.

Sodium-restricted diets are used in the nutritional care of patients with fluid retention or hypertension. These conditions are seen frequently, not only in patients with renal disease, but also in cases of diseases of the liver and cardiovascular system. Most institutional diet manuals contain copies of diets restricting sodium to varying degrees of severity. The most **severe** restriction is usually the 250-mg (11-mEq) sodium diet. It requires the substitution of low-sodium milk for regular milk and the limited use of animal protein foods. All foods are prepared without added salt, and all foods with high sodium levels or those in which sodium compounds are added in processing are eliminated. It usually is used for a short period only. Patient compliance is difficult to maintain.

Patients vary in their sensitivity to the taste of salt.[29] Those with reduced sensitivity generally find compliance with salt restriction more difficult. If at all possible, diets with higher sodium levels are used for these patients. The 500-mg (22-mEq) sodium diet (**strict** restriction) is used to reduce edema. In this diet all foods processed with salt or other sodium compounds must be omitted. Milk must be limited, but not necessarily eliminated altogether.

The 1,000-mg (43-mEq) sodium diet (**moderate** restriction) is used to reduce very mild edema, for edema prevention, or for prevention of hypertension. It eliminates highly salted foods and uses no salt in cooking. Other sodium-restricted diets more commonly used contain 2,000–3,000 mg (**mild** restriction) or 4,000–5,000 mg of sodium ("**no added salt diet**"). These are employed to prevent edema or hypertension and for patients receiving steroid therapy. They omit salt at the table but allow a limited amount of salt in cooking.

In choosing the appropriate sodium restriction level, the nutritional care specialist considers the immediate condition indicating the need for sodium restriction but also must take into consideration the need for protein in the diet. Since most protein foods are relatively high in sodium content, the need to increase dietary protein limits the extent to which sodium can be restricted. The patient's living conditions must also be considered in the nutritional care of outpatients. For example, the patient who must eat many meals in restaurants may need a more moderate sodium prescription with increases in drug dosage.

The nutritional care specialist must have a detailed knowledge of the sodium content of foods. Some foods contain significant amounts of sodium, even in the unprocessed state. These include meat, eggs, fish, poultry, milk, and milk products. A few vegetables, such as carrots, beets, greens, turnips, and celery, are also naturally high in sodium content. Other foods may contain appreciable amounts of sodium because salt (sodium chloride) or some other sodium-containing compound has been added in processing or in preparation. Canned vegetables, for example, are salted unless stated otherwise on the label.

Patients must be counseled to read labels carefully and understand the following definitions:

- "Unsalted" or "Having no salt added": Processed without salt in food normally processed with salt. Sodium content must be stated.

- "Reduced sodium": Processed to reduce usual sodium level by 75%.
- "Low sodium": 140 mg or less per serving.
- "Very low sodium": 35 mg or less per serving.
- "Sodium-free" or "salt-free": Less than 5 mg sodium per serving.

The use of baked goods containing baking soda (sodium bicarbonate) or baking powder is limited on the more restrictive diets. Other sodium compounds used in food include monosodium glutamate, sodium nitrate, and sodium benzoate. There are many others, and therefore it is important to read labels carefully.

Drinking water contains appreciable amounts of sodium in some areas. Furthermore, the sodium content of the water in some homes is increased when water is softened. Many softeners act by exchanging the sodium cation for the calcium and magnesium ions that cause hardness, providing 7.5 mg of sodium per quart of water for each grain of hardness per gallon.

Some dentifrices and mouthwashes contain significant amounts of sodium, as do some drugs, including nonprescription drugs. Sodium may be contained in laxatives, cough medicines, and antacids, and the labels must be read carefully by patients.

A severe and prolonged sodium restriction may be harmful if the patient has excessive losses. The patient with renal disease who cannot conserve sodium and excrete a dilute urine is at risk. Patients on diets with severely restricted amounts of sodium should be observed for clinical manifestations of depletion. These signs and symptoms are

Abdominal cramps and aching muscles
Weakness, lassitude
Anorexia and vomiting
Mental confusion

Diet manuals list foods to be eliminated or avoided by patients on sodium-restricted diets. Many contain exchange lists, which are used in a manner similar to the diabetic exchange lists described in Chapter 11. These lists are particularly helpful in planning the more severely restricted diets.

Some special low-sodium products are available to provide additional variety and added nutrients. These include low-sodium milk, low-sodium baking powder, unsalted canned vegetables, unsalted meats and cheese, unsalted bakery products, and unsalted margarine and sweet butter. All tend to be more expensive than their salted equivalents. There are also potassium exchange lists. Eventually, the patients needs to combine protein, sodium, potassium, and fluid restriction. For these patients, many diet manuals contain combined exchange lists which categorize foods according to their protein, sodium, and potassium diets. The various exchanges may be divided in various ways. Commonly used categories are as follows:

- Meat (animal protein): Divided into "high sodium" and "low-sodium."
- Dairy products.
- Fruits and fruit juices: Divided into subcategories according to potassium content.
- Vegetables and vegetable juices: Divided into subcategories according to potassium content.
- Starches: Includes breads. Divided into "salted" and "unsalted" groups.
- Fats: Divided into "salted" and "unsalted" groups.
- "Sweets."
- "Protein-free."
- Low-sodium specialty items: Useful for severe sodium restriction.
- High-salt items: Useful for "salt wasters."

Many commercial salt substitutes are available but should not be used without the consent of the physician. Most contain potassium chloride, which may be harmful to patients with renal disease. Others contain ammonium salts, hazardous in some liver diseases. Most salt substitutes are somewhat unpalatable and, if used, should be tried cautiously at first. The use of products consisting of 50% sodium chloride and 50% other salts must be discouraged unless planned into the diet. Patients should be encouraged to use other spices and flavorings instead. A number of recipe books and meal-planning guides are available for patients who need assistance in preparing palatable and varied menus. Some suggested methods and procedures for management of sodium-restricted diets are listed in Table 9-5.

Compliance with the diet is improved if the patient's food habits and preferences are considered. In the case of sodium restriction, the Orthodox Jewish diet may present a particular problem. Koshering of meat requires the addition of salt to raw meat to promote removal of blood. As a result, the salt content is at least doubled. If beef or veal is soaked for an hour in a large amount of tap water, the added salt will be removed. Chicken requires longer soaking.[30]

Abnormalities of fluid balance. When the number of functioning nephrons has decreased sufficiently to produce renal insufficiency in CRF, the remaining functioning nephrons are presented with a greater solute load, provoking a **solute diuresis**. More fluid must be provided if this load is to be excreted. The maximum efficiency of the kidney in excreting solutes is reached when urine volume is 2.0 to 2.5 liters, requiring an intake of approximately 3 liters of fluid. Polyuria and nocturia result. An increased thirst may provide the stimulus for the necessary water intake, but for some patients a specific intake must be prescribed to assure adequate fluids. The prescription often is written as **force fluids**, **encourage fluids**, or **push fluids**. Obviously, physical force should not be used. A day's fluid intake should be distributed throughout the 24 hours. Beverages should be offered frequently and should be those the patient particularly likes. Frozen and gelatin desserts, soups, and frozen juices are helpful. Small frequent servings usually are more effective than large servings at less frequent intervals.

Table 9-5. Methods and Procedures for Nutritional Care of Patients Requiring a Sodium-Restricted Diet

1. Plan the diet for the individual patient's physiologic needs and life style.
2. Specify amounts for foods that must be limited because of their sodium content.
3. A given level of sodium can be planned in many combinations, especially when the diet is more moderately restricted.
⁕4. All foods should be cooked without the addition of salt in diets allowing less than 1,000 mg of sodium. In diets allowing 500 mg or less of sodium, foods containing high levels of naturally occurring sodium are carefully limited. Diets containing 1,000 mg of sodium may include ¼ tsp. of salt or specific amounts of salted foods. Diets allowing 2,000 mg or more of sodium may include some foods cooked with a limited amount of salt or other added sodium products, but no salt is added during meals.
5. Diet manuals and exchange lists give information on the sodium content of foods in each food group. These should be consulted in detail in diet planning. Outpatients must be instructed carefully about foods to be avoided and the use of exchange lists.
6. Plan the amounts of high-protein foods carefully.
   a. Meats, fish, and poultry that are smoked, cured, pickled, processed with sodium nitrite, or canned with salt must be used with special caution.
   b. In more restricted diets, use unsalted canned meat or fish.
   c. Use low-sodium milk in 250-mg sodium diets. Several products of variable palatability are available. They often are needed in diets of 500 mg or more of sodium. When low-sodium milk is used, serve it very cold, add flavorings that are low in sodium, or incorporate it in cooked dishes. Outpatients should be provided information on the source, cost, and preparation of this product and given recipes for its use.
   d. Kosher meats usually are high in sodium, 200 to 350 mg/oz., and generally must be avoided. Alternatives are meats that are broiled to allow the blood to drip away. Some meats can be boiled in water to reduce sodium content. The water is discarded.
   e. See diet manuals for the sodium content of cheese and cheese products and use them only as permitted by the degree of sodium restriction.
7. Avoid or limit foods containing the following:
   Baking soda or baking powder
   Sodium alginate (in some ice cream and chocolate milk)
   Sodium benzoate (a preservative)
   Sodium propionate (a mold inhibitor)
   Sodium sulfite (a fruit bleach and preservative)
   Sodium phosphate (in some cereals and cheeses)
   Monosodium glutamate (a flavor enhancer)
   Limited amounts of these products are acceptable on more moderately restricted diets.
8. Avoid obviously salty foods, such as potato chips, pretzels, pickles, and sauerkraut.
9. The more restrictive diets require low-sodium bread and sweet butter. The patient should be provided information on sources of these products.
10. Avoid most commercial seasonings, salad dressings, and condiments.
11. Consider the sodium content of drinking water in the area. Avoid locally bottled beverages if the sodium content of the water is high. Question the patient about water softeners in the home. It may be necessary to advise the patient to use distilled or bottled water for cooking and drinking.
12. Instruct the patient carefully on reading labels. Adjust instructions to the level of restriction required. Minor sodium sources may be ignored when the restriction is moderate.
13. Provide encouragement and emotional support. Remember that in some illnesses the patient has a reduced ability to taste salt.
14. Assist the patient in planning for variety in the menu. Provide recipes and information on special products, including low-sodium baking powder. Give instruction and encouragement on the use of spices, herbs, and other alternative flavoring agents.
15. Assist the patient in planning for home-prepared meals in place of presalted convenience foods.
16. Some synthetic detergents contain large amounts of sodium. Dishes should be rinsed carefully to remove the residue.
17. Sodium-restricted diets often are combined with modifications in potassium, protein, or fluid intake.
18. Provide the patient with a list of "free" foods.

As fewer nephrons are available for filtration, the polyuric phase gives way to oliguria. Excess water that is ingested is retained, and the patient becomes overhydrated. Some renal patients eventually become anuric.

If sodium intake is adequately controlled, the thirst mechanism at first serves as a good guide to fluid intake. Eventually, however, fluid taken out of habit and with medications, plus metabolic water, total an amount in excess of excretory capacity. When the GFR falls below 4 to 5 ml/min. and water begins to accumulate, it usually becomes necessary to restrict fluid intake. Fluid overload otherwise leads to hyponatremia and water intoxication, with muscle cramps, weakness, lassitude, anorexia, vomiting, and mental confusion. Fluid overload may also cause hypertension and pulmonary congestion.

To determine the amount of fluid to provide, dehydrated or overhydrated patients must first be brought to normal hydration. Fluid intake in the normally hydrated patient then is limited to an amount equal to the estimated total water loss. This frequently is based on urine volume for the previous day *plus* 500 to 1,000 ml to compensate for nonurinary losses. The estimates vary depending on environmental temperature and humidity, activity, body surface area, and other disease conditions. Body weight is monitored carefully. Sudden weight gain or loss indicates that fluid intake is inappropriate and should be corrected.

Any allotment of fluid of less than 2,000 ml/day is considered to be a restriction. The anuric or severely oliguric patient obviously will require a severe restriction, sometimes to 500 to 600 ml/day. All beverages and liquid foods must be included within the prescribed allotment, including fruit juice, milk, soup, gruels, coffee, tea, soft drinks, and alcoholic beverages. The juice or syrup on fruits must be included as well as all items that are liquid at body temperature, such as gelatin mixtures, frozen desserts, and ice. The fluid content of solid foods is not included unless the fluid restriction is severe.

In the management of the hospitalized patient, conference and cooperation between the nursing service and nutritional care specialist usually are necessary, since fluid is needed for administration of medications. Some patients require fluid between meals because of a dry mouth or an unpleasant taste. Patients should be consulted regarding their preferences on the form in which their fluids are given. Some patients, for example, are willing to make other sacrifices in order to have that morning cup of coffee.

Abnormalities of potassium balance. The distal tubules have an enormous capacity to excrete potassium. Therefore, in renal insufficiency, **hyperkalemia** (elevated serum potassium, greater than 5.5 mEq/L) usually does not occur as long as at least 1,000 ml of urine are produced. Also, fecal excretion of potassium increases in renal insufficiency.[31] The secretion of potassium is increased by the greater aldosterone activity that is seen in some patients. The increased flow rate during polyuria also encourages potassium secretion. As a result, patients maintain serum potassium levels close to normal until late in the course of CRF.

When hyperkalemia does occur in these patients, food usually is not the main source of excess potassium. Instead, potassium accumulates as a result of intercurrent conditions such as hemorrhage, acidosis, blood transfusions, or catabolic stress such as occurs in surgery or trauma. The use of potassium-sparing medications or of salt substitutes containing potassium also can be a precipitating factor. Since potassium is "exchanged" for sodium in the distal tubule, insufficient sodium may decrease potassium excretion with resultant hyperkalemia.

In late renal failure when oliguria supervenes, potassium balance becomes precarious. Control is essential, since high serum potassium levels cause arrhythmias and possible cardiac arrest with disastrous results. Patients may be given ion exchange resins to reduce intestinal absorption of potassium and insulin to reduce release of cellular potassium. If hyperkalemia persists, dietary intake is limited to the extent indicated by serum potassium levels. Restrictions to 2,800 mg (70 mEq) or 2,000 mg (51 mEq) commonly are used, but occasionally, potassium is restricted to 1,000 to 1,500 (25 to 40 mEq) per day. The average daily diet in the United States contains 75 to 100 mEq of potassium, but a 40-g protein diet will include less than 70 mEq of potassium. Hyperkalemia that persists when intake is restricted is an indication for dialysis.

There are many food sources of potassium. It is present in all living cells and thus is found in all plant and animal foods except purified components such as sugar, starch, and oil. Potassium is very water soluble. Therefore, the potassium content of foods can be reduced by boiling them in large amounts of water and discarding the water. Baking, broiling, and frying do not affect the potassium content of foods. Processing also affects potassium content, depending on the amount of water involved. Canned fruits are lower in potassium than fresh fruits if the syrup is not consumed, whereas dried fruits are higher in potassium content for equal weight, since all components are more concentrated. The potassium in cereals is found in the germ and bran. Therefore, highly refined cereal products contain less potassium. Table 9-6 shows the potassium content of various classifications of foods.

In the potassium-restricted diet, intake of almost every food must be controlled, since there are few foods that are potassium-free. Occasionally, a potassium-free diet is required for an anuric patient with high serum potassium. For these patients, the commercial high-caloric, low-electrolyte supplements, such as Cal-Power, Controlyte, and Hy-Cal, may be useful (see Appendix G, Table G-2). They carry with them, however, an appreciable amount of water.

Since dietary potassium is absorbed rapidly, the potassium must be distributed evenly throughout the day when planning the diet so that sharp increases in serum potassium do not occur. Protein and energy intakes must be maintained to levels that prevent tissue catabolism. Inadequate intakes result in tissue catabolism and release of intracellular potassium into the extracellular fluid. At least 40% of the kilocalorie content of the diet should come from carbohydrates. The movement of glucose into cells carries potassium with it. Patients should be encouraged to exercise as much as the physician allows. Exercise prevents muscle breakdown and increases movement of glucose into muscle cells. Both of these actions tend to reduce serum potassium.

Acidosis. In renal insufficiency, as the number of functioning nephrons diminishes, the ability to produce ammonium ion is impaired, and the ability to excrete hydrogen ion thus is reduced. Diminished ability to reabsorb filtered bicarbonate also contributes to hydrogen ion retention. As a result, patients have a metabolic acidosis that develops when GFR is reduced to 25 ml/min. or less.

The excess acid is partially buffered by the bone. This buffering prevents acidosis from becoming severe even if GFR is less than 10 ml/min., but bone buffering contributes to the skeletal abnormalities commonly seen in renal disease. In addition, acidosis causes nausea and fatigue. The patient breathes more deeply and more rapidly and may be breathless on exertion, but **Kussmaul respiration**, seen in diabetic acidosis, is not common because the acidosis is less severe. These changes are compensatory mechanisms that lower the partial pressure of carbon dioxide and restore the bicarbonate-carbonic acid ratio to normal. However, the patient tends to remain in a state of mild acidosis.

Sodium bicarbonate or sodium citrate is given as medication to correct the acidosis. Calcium carbonate, given as part of the treatment of bone disease, also partially corrects the acidosis. Protein restriction reduces

Table 9-6. Food Sources of Potassium

Food	Serving Size	Food	Serving Size
Less than 3 mEq per serving		*Milk and milk products*	
Fruits		Yogurt	½ cup
Apple, fresh	1 small	*Miscellaneous*	
Applesauce	½ cup	Brewed coffee	1 cup
Blueberries, fresh, frozen	¾ cup	Canned soup	6 oz.
Cranberries	1¼ cup	Cocoa powder	2 Tbsp.
Cranberry juice	⅓ cup	Peanut butter	2 Tbsp.
Cranberry juice, low calorie	1¼ cup		
Milk and milk products		**5–10 mEq per serving**	
Cheese		*Vegetables*	
Cottage	¼ cup	Artichoke, fresh, cooked	1
Other	1 oz.	Asparagus, fresh or frozen	½ cup
Miscellaneous		Beans, lima, fresh or frozen, cooked	½ cup
Almonds	6 whole	Beets, fresh, cooked	½ cup
Brazil nuts	2 medium	Beet greens, fresh, cooked	½ cup
Cashews, roasted	4 large	Broccoli, fresh or frozen, cooked	½ cup
Filberts	5	Brussels sprouts, fresh or frozen	½ cup
Hazelnuts	5	Cabbage, raw	1 cup
Mixed nuts	8–12	Carrots, fresh, raw or cooked	½ cup
Pecans	5	Celery, raw	1 cup
Walnuts	4 halves	Chard, Swiss, fresh, cooked	½ cup
Olives		Collard, greens, fresh, cooked	½ cup
Black	5 medium	Corn, fresh 5-inch ear	1 ear
Green	9–10	Cress, cooked	½ cup
Sweet chocolate	1 oz.	Cucumber, raw	1 cup
Tofu	4 oz.	Dandelion greens, cooked	½ cup
Beverages		Eggplant, baked	½ cup
Postum	1 cup	Kohlrabi, cooked	½ cup
Tea	1 cup	Leeks, raw	¾ cup
Lemonade	1 cup	Parsnips, cooked	½ cup
		Peas, dried, cooked	½ cup
3–5 mEq per serving		Potato, boiled, mashed	½ cup
Vegetables		Pumpkin, fresh	½ cup
Alfalfa sprouts, raw	1 cup	Spinach, cooked	½ cup
Bamboo shoots, cooked	½ cup	Squash, winter, frozen, cooked	½ cup
Bean sprouts, cooked	½ cup	Tomato, cooked, canned	½ cup
Cauliflower, cooked	½ cup	Tomato, fresh	1 medium
Chinese cabbage, raw	1 cup	Tomato juice, low-sodium or unsalted	½ cup
Green beans, cooked	½ cup	Turnip greens, cooked	½ cup
Mustard greens, cooked	½ cup	*Fruits*	
Okra, cooked	½ cup	Apple juice, unsweetened	1 cup
Onion, cooked	½ cup	Apricots, fresh	2 medium
Rutabaga, cooked	½ cup	Apricots, canned, unsweetened	½ cup
Squash, summer, cooked	½ cup	Apricots, dried	4 halves
Sweet potato or canned yam, cooked	⅓ cup or ½ small	Banana	1 small
		Blackberries, fresh or frozen	1 cup
Turnip, cooked	½ cup	Cherries	15 large
Yellow beans, cooked	½ cup	Grape juice, unsweetened	1 cup
Zucchini, cooked	½ cup	Grapefruit	
Fruits		Fresh	½
Cherries, canned	½ cup	Canned	¾ cup
Fruit cocktail	½ cup	Grapes, white, fresh	30 small
Mango	½ small	Kiwi	1 large
Peaches, fresh	1 medium	Nectarines, fresh	1
Pears		Orange juice, unsweetened, fresh or frozen	½ cup
Fresh	1 small	Orange or tangerine	1 medium
Canned	½ cup	Papaya	½ medium or 1 cup
Raspberries, fresh	1 cup		

Table 9-6. (Continued)

Food	Serving Size	Food	Serving Size
Peach nectar	½ cup	*Fruits*	
Prune juice, unsweetened, canned	½ cup	Avocado	½
Prunes, dried	3	Cantaloupe, 6-in. diameter	¼
Strawberries, fresh or frozen	1 cup	Honeydew, 7-in. diameter	⅛
Watermelon, raw	2 cups	*Meats*	
Meats		Cod, cooked	3½ oz.
Meat, poultry, cooked	3 oz.	Flounder, cooked	3½ oz.
Salmon, pink, canned	3 oz.	Halibut, cooked	3½ oz.
Shrimp, fresh or cooked	3½ oz.	Salmon, fresh cooked	3½ oz.
Tuna, fresh or canned	½ cup	Scallops, cooked	3½ oz.
Milk and milk products		*Miscellaneous*	
Skim, 2%, or whole milk	1 cup	Peanuts, roasted with skins	45
Miscellaneous		Walnuts	¾ cup
Coffee, instant	1 tsp.	Salt substitute	¼ tsp.
Molasses, Brer Rabbit	5 tsp.		
Chocolate, bitter	1 oz.	**15–20 mEq per serving**	
Low-sodium canned soups	½ cup	*Fruits*	
		Dates, dried	15
10–15 mEq per serving		Figs, fresh	1 large
Vegetables		Nectarine, dried	10 large
Beans, dried, cooked	½ cup	Peach, dried	3
Beet green, cooked	½ cup	Rhubarb, fresh	1 cup
Potatoes, baked or raw	½ cup or 1 small	*Meats*	
		Chicken breast	6 oz.
Soybeans, cooked	½ cup		
Spinach, raw, chopped	2 cups		

the production of acid, but there is no diet modification that is specific for prevention of acidosis. Acidosis frequently is accompanied by nausea, adding to the problems of nutritional care.

Calcium and phosphorus. In renal disease, alterations in vitamin D metabolism and in calcium and phosphorus homeostasis have far-reaching consequences.

The skeletal system is seriously affected. Calcium and phosphate concentrations in the extracellular fluid normally are close to those at which calcium phosphate salts would precipitate (calcium $\times$ phosphate product greater than 70 mg/dl). When the GFR decreases to 25% of normal or less, phosphate is retained, and serum phosphate levels rise. Calcium phosphates are deposited both in bone and soft tissue such as the lung and eye. The deposition reduces the serum concentrations of phosphate and also reduces serum calcium, which was not elevated originally. The depressed serum calcium (less than 8 mg/dl) stimulates secretion of PTH, reducing tubular reabsorption of phosphate and restoring serum phosphate and calcium to normal. A new steady state thus is established until the GFR falls further, but at the price of increased circulation of PTH.[32,33]

As the GFR falls, the process is repeated until the GFR decreases to approximately 20 ml/min. Then phosphate levels increase and remain high, and serum calcium is lower than normal. In an effort to keep serum calcium at normal levels, PTH secretion becomes chronically increased. Decreased renal clearance contributes to the maintenance of the high PTH levels.[32] Serum calcium is increased toward normal, but it remains somewhat depressed. Impaired calcium absorption from the intestine also contributes to the deficit in serum calcium. Intestinal absorption is affected when renal hydroxylation of the 25-hydroxycholecalcif-erol form of vitamin D to the 1,25 form, which stimulates calcium absorption, is de-pressed.

Acidosis, excess PTH, alterations in vita-min D metabolism, and reduced calcium ab-sorption all contribute to the development of bone disease and other pathologic manifes-tations in patients with CRF. According to Bricker's trade-off hypothesis,[9] bone disease may be the price that is paid to maintain serum calcium levels within normal limits.

The bone disease, referred to as **osteodys-trophy**, is a combination of four possible forms in varying proportions:[34]

1. *Osteitis fibrosa cystica:* classic hyperpara-thyroidism.
2. *Osteomalacia:* excessive uncalcified bone matrix.
3. *Osteopenia:* decreased bone mass.
4. *Osteosclerosis:* increased bone density.

The specific clinical features in a given pa-tient depend on which of these four pro-cesses is dominant. The features include bone pain and an increase in fractures.

High serum calcium also has nonskeletal effects. In addition to soft tissue calcification, high calcium levels in the skin cause severe itching. Other symptoms include muscle weakness and a variety of neurologic abnor-malies.[32]

Diet modification in treatment of bone disease is limited in effectiveness. An aver-age adult's diet in the United States has been estimated to contain 1.0 to 1.8 g of phospho-rus per day. In the renal patient with a diet of 40 g of protein per day, phosphorus intake is usually somewhat lower. A low-phosphate diet, with reduced intake of dairy products, provides 600 to 1,200 mg/day. This level alone is not sufficient to reduce serum phos-phate to normal levels, and a phosphate re-striction, superimposed on the other diet modifications, would further reduce the ac-ceptability of the diet and patient compli-ance. In addition, planning for nutritional adequacy becomes exceedingly difficult. A low-phosphate diet also tends to be low in calcium. As a consequence of all these diffi-culties, aluminum gels, which bind phos-phate and prevent its absorption from the gastrointestinal tract, have been used rather than diet to control hyperphosphatemia. The gels are taken *with meals* in the form of alu-minum carbonate or aluminum hydroxide.

Recent work has shown that early use of phosphate binders prevents progression of bone lesions and may be useful in prevention of bone lesion formation.[35] However, there are side effects of the use of phosphate binders. Aluminum is elevated in tissues of patients receiving aluminum hydroxide or aluminum carbonate binders. It has been suggested that accumulation of aluminum in the brain may be related to a "dialysis de-mentia" sometimes seen in dialysis pa-tients.[36] The source of the aluminum is un-certain but may be from water used in dialysis. A second problem consequent to the intake of phosphate binders is the occur-rence of severe constipation and nausea. Products such as Amphojel (an aluminum hydroxide gel) have been incorporated into cookies to make them more acceptable.

Given the side effects and the unanswered question of long-term safety of phosphate binders, some clinics have returned to the restriction of phosphorus intakes[37] along with administration of $CaCO_3$. The objective is a Ca:P product <60 mg/dl. Patients are advised to eliminate foods with high phos-phorus content. These foods are listed in Table 9-7.

With the low-phosphorus diet, calcium supplements usually are given to prevent concurrent hypocalcemia, but serum phos-phorus levels are reduced first to avoid soft tissue calcification. A recommended dose of 1,000 mg of calcium is provided in 2,500 mg of calcium carbonate per day. Vitamin D also is supplemented. The most potent form is 1,25-dehydroxycholecalcerol (calcitriol [Ro-caltrol]). The effects of long-term use of this material are unknown, since it is fairly new.

An alternative use of dietary phosphorus restriction is in a very-low-protein (20–25

Table 9-7. Foods with High Phosphorus Content

Food	Measure	Phosphorus Content (mg)
Dairy products		
Milk		
Whole	½ cup	125
Chocolate	½ cup	125
Evaporated	¼ cup	125
Half and half	½ cup	115
Yogurt, plain	½ cup	165
Pudding	½ cup	130
Custard	⅓ cup	100
Ice Cream	¾ cup	100
Vegetables and fruits		
Peas	½ cup	50
Lima beans	⅓ cup	60
Apricots, dried	10	41
Carrot juice	6 oz.	77
Pumpkin seeds	1 oz.	333
Meats and substitutes		
Liver	1 oz.	130
Fish, bass, mackerel, salmon	¼ cup or 1 oz.	120
Cheese		
Processed	1 oz.	215
Swiss	1 oz.	175
Cheddar, mozzarella	1 oz.	145
Cottage	¼ cup	70
Egg	1	90
Breads and cereals		
Cereals		
100% bran	¾ cup	400
Bran Buds, All-Bran	⅓ cup	265
Bran flakes, Bran Chex	½ cup	150
Cooked	½ cup	135
Bread, whole wheat	1 slice	70
Wheat germ	1 Tbsp.	80
Waffles, frozen	1	135
Fats and oils		
Nondairy creamer	2 Tbsp.	50
Cola beverage	1 cup	30

g/day), low-phosphorus diet with supplementary amino acids or ketoacids. There is some evidence, although it is controversial, that the decline in renal function is slower and the need for dialysis is delayed, particularly if this diet is started early in the course of the disease.[38-43] In addition, symptoms are modulated.[44] The diet is supplemented with B vitamins, calcium, iron, and zinc, which may be deficient.[45] Special attention must be paid to energy intake. In view of the protein restriction, additional energy can be provided with liquid sources of oligosaccharides or specialized low-protein cereals, and baked products.[46,47]

Iron. Anemia is a common finding in uremic patients. The major cause is apparently bone marrow failure due to decreased erythropoietin production in the kidney. Without the stimulation of erythropoietin, the bone marrow fails to produce red blood cells from its stem cells. Reduced iron absorption, gastrointestinal bleeding, and frequent blood sampling also contribute to severe anemia.

Patients are often given blood transfusions, but there are a number of risks to this procedure: Risk of blood-borne infections (including AIDS and hepatitis); toxic accumulations of iron ("iron overload"); and formation of antibodies that reduce possibility of successful transplant. Recently, a human recombinant erythropoietin (epoetin-alfa or Epogen) has been developed. It has made it possible for renal patients to return to more normal activity. This medication must be combined with adequate iron stores in order to be effective. Increased dietary iron is often not adequate, and intravenous iron dextrans may also be needed.

Zinc. Zinc deficiency may be the cause of impaired taste and smell acuity and impaired sexual function in men. It has been suggested that dysgeusia in renal patients be treated with zinc supplements.[48] This may be of some importance in nutritional care, since it can be assumed to affect food intake.

Vitamin needs. CRF patients frequently are deficient in water-soluble vitamins. Anorexia, nausea and vomiting, and restricted intakes are assumed to contribute to these deficiencies. Specifically, pyridoxine, folate, and ascorbic acid tend to be low.

On the other hand, vitamin A tends to be elevated in the serum and liver. Patients may have signs of vitamin A intoxication, such as xerosis and pigmentation. Vitamin A may increase parathyroid secretion and contribute to osteodystrophy.

Thus commonly recommended procedures are to give patients a daily supplement of 1.0 mg folic acid, 100 mg ascorbic acid, 5.0

mg pyridoxine hydrochloride, and Recommended Dietary Allowances of the remaining water-soluble vitamins. Vitamin A supplements are not indicated. Vitamin K sometimes is given. The need for vitamin D is discussed in relation to bone disease.

Carbohydrate. A number of disorders of carbohydrate metabolism are associated with CRF, including fasting hyperglycemia and glucose intolerance similar to that seen in diabetes mellitus (see Chapter 11).[49] Circulating insulin levels are high,[49] and there is evidence of peripheral insensitivity to insulin in most patients.[49-52]

The nature of the defects in the peripheral tissues is not understood completely. The binding of insulin to receptor sites appears to be normal, but there is some evidence that the metabolic steps following binding are abnormal.[51] The presence of circulating insulin antagonists has also been suggested but not proved.[49] The glucose intolerance is not sufficiently severe to present a clinical problem in most CRF patients. They do not develop ketoacidosis.

Lipids. Patients with CRF have hyperlipidemia and elevated triglycerides, usually of the type IV pattern and sometimes type II (see Chapter 10).[53] Uremic patients have a high incidence of atherosclerosis and coronary artery disease, which have been related to high triglyceride levels. Therefore, some attempts have been made to treat hyperlipidemia by diet.[54,55] The effectiveness of these modifications in CRF is unknown. In addition, abnormalities of the apolipoproteins (the protein portion of plasma lipoproteins) have been found in CRF patients.[56] It has been suggested that the hyperlipidemia is a consequence of reduced lipoprotein lipase and other enzymes.[21]

Cardiovascular disease (CVD) is a common cause of death in CRF. Though diet modification to delay or prevent CVD seems to be a logical procedure (see Chapter 10), planning is difficult.

Additional problems. The multiple dietary restrictions imposed on the uremic patient reduce the variety and palatability of the diet. Patients tend to complain that the diet is sweet and greasy. In addition, CRF patients often have ulcers of the mouth, nausea, and vomiting. The fluid restriction leads to thirst. Uremic patients suffer from anxiety, depression, and fear. They may progress to psychosis and coma. Their feelings of frustration may result in noncompliance and antagonism. Under these circumstances, nutritional management of these patients is difficult and requires a great deal of skill. Individualization of the diet is very helpful.

The pediatric (child) patient presents some special problems. A decrease in growth rate frequently occurs when the GRF is 50% of normal or less, and uremia occurs earlier in the progress of the disease than in adults.[57] The child's protein intake per kilogram of body weight should, of course, be higher than in adults in order to support growth. Food to supply the higher energy requirement of the child will carry with it more sodium relative to body weight. Therefore, the use of other sources of sodium, such as salt added to foods, must be more severely restricted under otherwise equivalent conditions. The use of daily multivitamin preparations for pediatric patients is recommended.

Planning the diet. The various nutrient needs of the CRF patient must consider protein, energy, sodium, potassium, and fluid simultaneously. Thus the calculation of the diet becomes complex.

For ease of calculation, "exchange" lists that group foods according to their protein, sodium, and potassium contents have been developed. There are a number of such lists available, which vary slightly from each other. An example of a summary of the exchanges for renal patients is given in Appendix J along with lists of foods commonly included in each exchange.

The following steps may be used in calculating the diet:[58]

1. Calculate the amount of high-biological-value (HBV) protein required.
2. Using the average values for each food group listed in Appendix J, determine the

number of servings of milk, meat, and egg needed to provide the HBV protein. Usually one egg is included because it is especially high in biological value.

3. Using the average values, determine the number of servings of fruits, vegetables, and bread/cereal/starch that will provide the low-biological-value protein, sodium, potassium, fluid, and energy required.

4. Add to obtain the total of protein, sodium, potassium, fluid, and energy. If any values are in excess of the prescription or are insufficient, go back to step 3 and make the necessary adjustments.

5. Add sources of added kilocalories from fat and carbohydrate (miscellaneous list, Table J-15).

6. Add items from the "salt" list (Table J-17) if necessary to reach the prescribed sodium intake (possibly necessary for salt wasters).

7. Add beverages if possible within the fluid prescription.

The Dialysis Patient. **Dialysis** is a process of diffusion and filtration between solutions separated by a semipermeable membrane. In renal disease, blood is circulated on one side of the semipermeable membrane and a cleansing fluid, known as the **dialysate**, on the other. Dialysis has been shown to improve the condition of most patients in end-stage renal disease, but it cannot be used for all patients.

Dialysis is employed in the treatment of both acute and chronic renal failure. In chronic disease, it may be planned to continue indefinitely (maintenance dialysis) or for a short period prior to transplantation. It also is used sometimes after a renal transplant until the grafted kidney begins to function. Indications for beginning its use are hyperkalemia unresponsive to other treatment, severe metabolic acidosis, fluid overload, pericarditis, and uremia. In CRF, the patient usually begins dialysis treatments when the GFR is 5 to 10 ml/min. The patient who is dialyzed for an extended period is of most concern in nutritional care. There are two basic dialysis methods available, hemodialysis and peritoneal dialysis.

Hemodialysis. An "artificial kidney machine," or **dialyzer**, is used in **hemodialysis** to cleanse the blood of undesirable materials. The patient is connected to the dialyzer in such a way that the blood in an artery of an arm or leg circulates through the machine before being returned to the parallel vein.

Various methods have been used to achieve attachment to the machine. Originally, when a **shunt** was used, cannulas were placed surgically into an artery and a vein of an extremity, and the exteriorized ends were connected by a bypass. The machine was connected when the bypass was removed. More recently, subcutaneous **arteriovenous fistulas** have been created surgically. The fistula connects an artery and a vein so that arterial pressure enlarges the vein. This access site is less prone to accidents and provides less access to infection but does require puncture through the skin for each dialysis period. Alternatively, a **graft** of another material (e.g., Gortex) may be used to connect the artery and vein. This also lies under the skin.

Although dialyzers vary in design, all are based on the same fundamental principle. Each machine has a semipermeable membrane that is permeable to water and substances of low molecular weight, such as potassium, sulfates, and the nitrogenous waste products, urea, creatinine, and uric acid. The membrane also is permeable to the middle molecules. Substances of even higher molecular weights, up to approximately 140,000 daltons, cross the membrane slowly. The membrane is impermeable to blood cells and most plasma proteins.

Although the patient's physical condition usually is improved with hemodialysis, dialysis is not a perfect substitute for a normally functioning kidney. It has been suggested that results may be improved by removal of the middle molecules. For this purpose, the use of a more permeable membrane with a larger surface area and slower blood flow has been suggested. Excess water is removed by **ultrafiltration.** The hydrostatic pressure gradient across the membrane is increased with the use of pumps on the inflow of the blood and the outflow of the dialysate. Materials of low molecular weight, such as urea and potassium, that are in high concentration in the blood and low concentration in the dialysate are removed by diffusion across the membrane. At the same time, other substances, also of low molecular weight, may be maintained in the blood or even increased by having a high concentration in the dialysate, so that they diffuse in the opposite direction. Thus the composition of the dialysate is very important. It has approximately the same composition as normal blood serum but with lower potassium and without urea or creatinine. Glucose is not always included in the dialysate, since it can serve as a medium for growth of bacteria.

Hemodialysis may be performed at various dialysis centers, which often, but not always, are located in hospitals. Patients usually must be dialyzed two to three times per week for periods that may vary from 4 to 6 hours. Some patients may be dialyzed at home, but home dialysis requires a high degree of motivation, intelligence, and emotional stability in the patient. It also requires an appropriate home environment and the dedicated help of a family member or other person. Candidates for home dialysis and the persons assisting them must be carefully instructed.

As the availability of hemodialysis increases, there is a continuing tendency to undertake it earlier in the course of the disease to prevent some of the irreversible complications of uremia. This is not a procedure to be taken lightly. The effects on the patient and the patient's family have been vividly described by Campbell and Campbell[59] in a personal account.

Nutritional care is important in maintaining the best possible physical condition in the dialysis patient. The participation of a renal nutritionist is essential. Since hemodialysis is intermittent, the substances nor-

mally excreted by the kidneys will accumulate between dialysis treatments as they did prior to dialysis. Therefore, nutritional management must continue in a supportive role. It usually is possible, however, to liberalize the diet compared with that used in conservative management. The extent to which this may be done is variable. It is influenced by the frequency and effectiveness of the treatments, the amount of residual renal function, if any, and the psychological response of the patient.

Chronic hemodialysis is a catabolic process, and malnutrition is a continuing problem. The patient may lose amino acids, peptides, and some protein during each session, along with an amount of glucose that varies with the glucose content of the dialysate. The **protein** in the form of amino acids lost in hemodialysis, estimated to be 10 to 13 g for each dialysis, must be replaced. In addition, there is some loss due apparently to accelerated protein catabolism resulting from an interaction between blood and the membranes in the dialyzer.[39] A protein intake of 0.75 to 1.4 g/kg body weight has been recommended, at least 70% of which should be of high biologic value.[39] The diet may need to be more restricted if dialysis is limited to twice weekly. The degree of azotemia that develops between treatments will influence the choice.

Intake of sources of **energy** must be sufficient to spare protein and maintain body weight. Commonly recommended levels are 35 to 50 kcal/kg body weight. The hyperlipidemia and cardiovascular disease of renal failure do not respond to hemodialysis or transplantation.[60-62] Therefore, it often is considered desirable to adjust the diet to lessen these tendencies.[63,64] A diet containing 15% of total kilocalories from protein, 35% from fat, and 50% from carbohydrate, primarily polysaccharides, has been recommended. It also has been suggested that a 2:1 ratio of polyunsaturated-saturated fat be included (see Chapter 10), but this issue is controversial.

Cardiovascular disease is a common cause

of death in dialysis or transplant patients.[65] This is believed to be a consequence of the lipid alterations seen in the predialysis period.[66-68] Chronic hypertension is also a risk factor.[69]

Usually **sodium** and **fluid** intakes must continue to be decreased moderately, since the accumulation of large amounts of these materials between treatments leads to hypertension, edema, and congestive heart failure. Sodium intake is restricted to the amount that limits weight gain from edema between dialyses to 0.5 kg/day. Sodium restriction varies from 2 to 4 g/day (85 to 170 mEq), and fluid may be limited to 500 to 1,500 ml in addition to that contained in solid food. Body weight and blood pressure are carefully monitored and used as indicators of the success of the restrictions.

Potassium usually is restricted to 1,600 to 3,000 mg/day (50 to 75 mEq), particularly if the patient is anuric. More severe restrictions are necessary in some patients.

Calcium and **phosphorus** levels should be controlled in the same manner as that used in conservative management. Hemodialysis does not correct the tendency to bone disease.

Water-soluble vitamins also are lost in dialysis, and patients become deficient if they are not given replacements. The permeability of the membrane to the various vitamins varies. Often, supplements of 1 mg of folate, 5–10 mg of pyridoxine, 100 mg of ascorbic acid, and recommended dietary allowances of other water-soluble vitamins are provided.

Anemia generally does not improve when a patient is dialyzed. Therefore, many patients are now given epoetin-alfa.

Dialysis patients may have low **iron** intake secondary to anorexia, nausea, and vomiting. Loss of iron occurs if the patient is taking salicylate medications, from occult gastrointestinal bleeding, and because some blood remains in the dialyzer after each treatment. Iron supplementation may be given, either orally, bound to ascorbic acid, or intravenously. Clearly, it is important that the patient have an adequate diet to avoid increasing the severity of the malnutrition.

Additional problems in nutritional care involve the emotional response of the patient. Some patients become very apprehensive; however, psychological, or even psychiatric, problems often regress as dialysis continues and uremic symptoms subside.

Food intake while dialysis is in progress is treated differently in different centers. Some dialysis centers serve meals during dialysis. Others do not do so because of the risk of hepatitis, but they allow patients to bring in their own food. Some units allow a "treat" the night before dialysis, reasoning that the dialysis will remove unwanted materials. Others expect the patient's diet limitations to be strictly observed or only partially liberalized.

In some patients, complications of hemodialysis must be considered. **Hypertension** is a frequent problem, particularly in patients who have high intakes of water and sodium. In many patients, these excesses can be treated by dialysis along with appropriate dietary sodium and fluid restrictions. It often is a challenge in nutritional care to elicit patient cooperation in these restrictions. On the other hand, dialysis patients seem to be peculiarly sensitive to sodium and volume depletion; therefore, it is important that restrictions not be excessive.

The various forms of bone disease are seen less frequently as we learn more about calcium, phosphate, and PTH metabolism. Parathyroid hormone levels sometimes remain above normal in dialyzed patients and may be reduced by increasing the magnesium levels in the dialysate. If this procedure is ineffective, parathyroidectomy is necessary. The continued use of aluminum gels and restriction of intake of dairy products reduce phosphorus levels. These methods often are necessary because phosphorus removal during dialysis is relatively inefficient. Calcium levels are manipulated by altering calcium concentrations in the dialysate or by regulating calcium intake. Dietary calcium should be at least 800 to 1,600 mg/day, but calcium supplements generally are necessary. A high-calcium diet is not feasible because it would also increase dietary phosphorus.

Other symptoms, such as peripheral neuropathy and central nervous system dysfunction, sometimes continue despite dialysis. Approximately 50–75% of the patients treated for one year or more can become normally productive.[70] Infections and vascular disease cause death in 4–15% of dialyzed patients, and dialysis is unsuccessful in another 10–15% of cases.

For the pediatric patient, **retarded growth** remains a concern. Inadequate protein and energy intake are considered to be the major causes. The diet for pediatric patients on hemodialysis should provide 1.5 to 2.0 g of protein per kilogram of body weight, or 8–12% of the total energy from protein, at least 70% of which should be of high biologic value. Recommended energy intakes are 75 to 100 kcal/kg/day. Recommended energy intakes are 75 to 100 kcal/kg/day. Potassium intake is restricted to 1–3 g/day (25.6–77 mEq). Fluid is restricted to the amount that will limit weight gain between dialyses to 1.0–1.5 kg.

Peritoneal dialysis. An alternative to hemodialysis is **peritoneal dialysis**; it uses the membranes of the peritoneal cavity as the dialytic membrane. The **peritoneum** is the membrane that lines the abdominal cavity and surrounds the abdominal organs, forming a sac. The dialysate enters the sac through a catheter penetrating the abdominal wall (Figure 9-6) and is exchanged 20 to 40 times at 20- to 60-minute intervals. A hyperosmolar solution causes fluid flow into the peritoneal cavity.

This procedure is used for short periods in acute renal failure or in combination with conservative management of chronic renal failure when some reversible event, such as an infection, further reduces the GFR temporarily. It has also been used to maintain a patient who is waiting to enter a chronic hemodialysis program or for a transplant.

For some years, peritoneal dialysis for long-term use was in disrepute, largely because of a high incidence of infection and the hazard of intestinal perforation. The availability of improved equipment providing an automated delivery system, permanent catheters, disposable equipment, and sterile solutions has reduced infections and made peritoneal dialysis earlier and more practical for home use. Peritonitis, however, still occurs, often as a result of bacterial translocation (see Chapter 6). Nevertheless, long-term dialysis is now being used more often. It is considered preferable to hemodialysis in elderly patients, diabetics, patients with systemic diseases, and children, and for home dialysis when the patient does not have adequate help.[71] It also is useful for patients who have exhausted their access sites for hemodialysis. Sometimes it is used for fluid and electrolyte disturbances unrelated to renal disease, such as diuretic-resistant congestive heart failure. The dialysate solution commonly used in uremia contains 1.5 g/dl of dextrose solutions (350 mOsm/L), a concentration that is slightly hypertonic to plasma. If the patient is overhydrated, a dextrose solution with 4.25 g/dl (490 mOsm/L) can be used. Hyperosmolar solutions cause a net flow of water into the intraperitoneal space of up to 300 to 500 ml per exchange. The excess fluid can then be removed. Lactate (35 mEq/L) is included as an alkalinizing agent.[72] A recommended sodium content is 132 mEq/L. Potassium content varies greatly with need.

There are several protocols for peritoneal dialysis. One of these is **intermittent** (IPD), commonly four times a week for 10 hours each, usually at night. Another is **continuous ambulatory peritoneal dialysis** (CAPD). In this procedure, sterile dialysate in a plastic pouch is infused and drained by gravity at 4-hour intervals five times daily, seven days a week.

A third type is **continuous cyclic peritoneal dialysis** (CCPD). The same solutions are used, but a machine delivers three or four

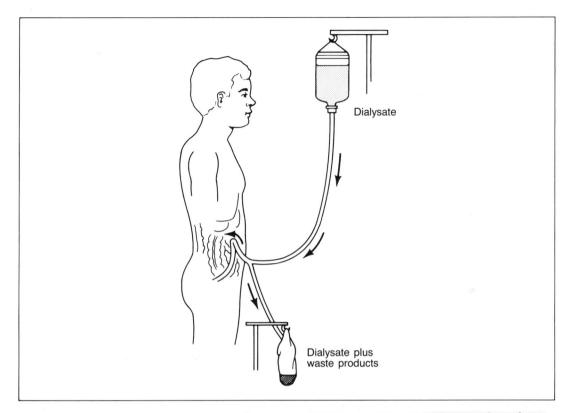

Dialysate

Dialysate plus
waste products

*Figure 9-6. Peritoneal dialysis. Dialysate flows
from the bag into the peritoneum. Waste materials
cross the peritoneal membrane into the dialysate
by diffusion. The dialysate with waste materials
flows back into the same bag, which is then
discarded.*

exchanges of $2\frac{1}{2}$ to 3 hours each at night. About 2 liters of dialysate are left in the peritoneal cavity during the day for 12 to 15 hours.

The nutritional management of the peritoneal dialysis patient is handicapped by limited information. The rationale and current practices have been described by Blumenkrantz et al.[73] Protein losses may be extensive. In peritoneal dialysis, both whole protein and amino acids may be lost. They vary with dialysate volume and dwell time —that is, the time the dialysate remains in the peritoneal cavity. Protein losses in the patient without peritonitis have been estimated to be 5 to 20 g/day,[74] and these increase in patients with episodes of peritonitis.[75] Patients receiving intermittent peritoneal dialysis may have low body weight with decreased body fat, muscle, and serum protein.[76] These parameters do not differ significantly from those seen in hemodialysis patients.[77] Recommendations for protein intake vary but normally are in the range of 1.0 to 1.5 g of protein (largely of high biologic value) per kg body weight per day.

Recommended kilocalorie intake is 35 kcal per kg of ideal body weight per day in IPD and 25 to 35 kcal/kg/day in CAPD and CCPD.[78] These estimates must be adjusted for body size and activity, for concurrent illnesses, and when repletion is desired. As appetite improves in CAPD patients, obesity can occur. Glucose absorbed from the dialysate during CAPD may contribute to the gain. Similar absorption does not occur in IPD because the period of exposure is shorter.[79] An estimation of glucose absorption is sometimes useful in planning for weight gain. An example of the procedure is as follows:[79]

$$y = (11.3x - 10.9) \times \text{vol. (L)} \qquad \text{(9-1)}$$

where y = glucose absorbed (g) per total exchange, and x = glucose (g) per *deciliter* of solution.

The glucose contained in the dialysate is hydrated (see Chapter 3). Therefore, glucose concentrations in dialysate exchange are

1.5% dialysate = 1.3 g/dl

2.5% dialysate = 2.2 g/dl

4.25% dialysate = 3.76 g/dl

If we assume that the patient uses a dialysate with 2.5% glucose (concentration 2.2 g/dl) and four exchanges of 2 liters each are used, then

$$y = [(11.3 \times 2.2) - 10.9] \times 8$$

In this example, the patient would have 112 g glucose in addition to his oral intake.

A simpler method of calculation is

$$y = \text{vol. (ml)} \times \text{glucose concentration} \times 0.8 \qquad \text{(9-2)}$$

where absorption is assumed to be 80%. Therefore, using the same values as for Equation 9-1:

$$8,000 \times 0.022 \times 0.8 = 140.8 \text{ g}$$

Clearly, these methods do not provide equal results, but they do provide reasonable estimates. The true test is the effect on the patient's body weight.

Most CAPD patients have improved amino acid metabolism[80] and protein utilization and achieve positive nitrogen balance readily.[81] For patients who have difficulty eating enough protein, addition of amino acids to the dialysate has been suggested.[78]

Triglyceride levels tend to remain high, for which several explanations have been offered:[77]

1. In the dialysate, an alpha-1-glycoprotein, a cofactor for lipoprotein lipase, is lost.
2. Unlike patients receiving hemodialysis, peritoneal dialysis patients do not routinely receive heparin, which is a clearing factor.
3. Protein losses to the dialysate and increased glucose absorption may contribute to hyperlipidemia.
4. Patients may continue their former high-fat, high-carbohydrate diet.
5. It may be an unexplained side effect of the treatment.

In order to control triglyceride levels, it has been suggested that the carbohydrate in the diet be reduced and the polyunsaturated fat level be increased (see Chapter 10 for the rationale).[76] Other approaches include exercise, drug therapy, an increase in polyunsaturated fats, and the use of amino acids in place of glucose in the dialysate.[82] The effectiveness of these procedures is unknown.

Water-soluble vitamins may be lost in the dialysate. Recommendations for supplements are similar to those for hemodialysis patients.[76,80] **Vitamin D** supplements may also be indicated.

Sodium and **fluid** can be well controlled in peritoneal dialysis. The patient must be individually evaluated. Neither sodium or fluid may need to be restricted. Peritoneal dialysis may remove as much as 5,700 mg sodium and 2 liters of fluid per day.[78] Patients should take their own blood pressure, weigh themselves, and observe for shortness of breath and edema. They should also be aware of symptoms of, and means of avoiding, hypotension.[78]

Potassium may not need to be restricted if intake is distributed throughout the day.[83] **Phosphorus** may need to be restricted. If high protein intake limits effective dietary restriction, phosphate binders may still be needed.[83]

Acid-base balance is almost completely corrected by CAPD. The continuously available lactate in the dialysate can be converted to bicarbonate. Bicarbonate levels are higher in CAPD patients than in patients on hemo-dialysis or IPD.

Renal Transplantation. Transplantation of a healthy kidney from a donor to a patient in renal failure is very desirable for most patients, since the transplanted kidney more adequately performs the excretory and endocrine functions of the kidney than does dialysis. In addition, a transplanted kidney frees the patient from the time-consuming demands of intermittent dialysis. However, not all renal failure patients are candidates for transplants. Risk factors include advanced age, malignancy, and infection. The availability of donor organs also is limiting. The transplanted kidney is implanted into the pelvis, not in the normal location of a kidney.

Donors may be either living relatives or cadavers in the United States. The use of live donors is illegal in some countries. When a transplant is planned, **histocompatibility testing** ("tissue typing") determines the amount of similarity or dissimilarity between the donor's and recipient's antigens. The donor-recipient matches are graded A (best) to E. Grade A indicates **HLA identity**. It is not common but exists in identical twins and sometimes occurs in other siblings. Not all antigens are identified in tissue typing, so it is possible for even a grade A–matched kidney to be rejected.

Failure of a transplant usually is the result of acute tubular necrosis or immune rejection, indicated by increased plasma creatinine, decreased urine volume, proteinuria, and hypertension. Patients are treated with immunosuppressant drugs to avoid rejection. The dose is reduced in time but must be continued for life.

Nutritional care of the transplant patient is divided into four periods: preparation for transplant, care in the early posttransplant period, management of complications of immunosuppression, and long-term posttransplant care.

In preparation for a transplant, it is important to avoid malnutrition during the periods of conservative management and dialysis. General nutritional care for surgery patients in the immediate postoperative period is described in Chapter 14. This liquid-to-solid progression must be integrated with specific needs of the transplant patient, since the patient is undergoing major surgery. Patients usually receive clear liquids for the first meal and progress to solid foods as tolerated thereafter. The specific diet order will depend on how well the transplanted kidney is functioning. The procedures for nutritional care vary from one transplant center to another and may be liberal or conservative. The following guidelines are examples of those in use, giving the liberal approach first, followed by a more conservative policy. The nutritional care specialist will follow the policies of the institution.

If renal function is adequate, as indicated by urine volume and specific gravity, blood levels of nitrogen metabolites, and a renal scan, a **sodium** content of 2 to 5 g may be prescribed. If renal function is poor, because of rejection or acute tubular necrosis, the sodium level is decreased to the extent indicated by increased serum sodium, diminished urine output, and weight gain. **Fluid** intake also is restricted. At more conservative institutions, the protocol provides a more severely restricted sodium intake, perhaps 500 mg, for the first few days. When the graft begins to function, a diuretic phase ensues, and the diet is liberalized as tolerated. Fluid also is restricted to 600 ml plus urine volume until the onset of the diuresis.

Serum **potassium** concentrations are used as guidelines for determining dietary potassium. Potassium is restricted only if serum potassium rises and its urine output decreases below 100 ml/day. In a more conservative approach, potassium intake is limited to 40 to 50 mEq/day until the onset of diuresis and then liberalized. Some patients need potassium supplements if diuresis is severe.

Because of the **protein** catabolism and negative nitrogen balance seen in transplant patients, protein usually is not severely restricted during the posttransplant period, even during rejection or tubular necrosis. Protein restriction may be required, however, if SUN rises and the patient shows symptoms of uremia. A more conservative approach begins with a 40-gram protein diet with 1,500 kcal on the second postoperative day. The diet is increased as tolerated to 40 to 50 kcal per kg of ideal body weight per day and approximately 80 g of protein per day. Under ideal circumstances, this progression takes a week or so, but it is varied with the SUN concentration.

Whether the procedures in a given institution are liberal or more conservative, it is desirable to individualize the diet for each patient. If a transplant patient requires dialysis after surgery, the diet is somewhat more liberal and follows that for the chronic hemodialysis patient.

Over the long term, weight control is stressed because the patients have an increased appetite and a tendency to weight gain and body composition changes. The need for diet modification diminishes as drug dosage is decreased. Many transplant patients eventually need no diet modifications.

Transplant patients are treated with high doses of immunosuppressive agents. A typical procedure includes **prednisone**, a corticosteroid, to suppress the inflammatory response and either **cyclosporin A** or **azothioprine** (Imuran) to reduce the cellular immune response. Table 9-8 lists the immunosuppressants commonly used at present, their modes of action, side effects, and related nutritional care. The suggested nutritional care procedures should be chosen to coincide with the side effects in the individual patient.

Recently, it has been observed that some leukocytes require exogenous nucleotides and that the immune response is suppressed in their absence. As a consequence, some institutions use a nucleotide-free diet to increase the effect of cyclosporin immunosuppression. This diet uses eggs, milk, and cheese as sources of protein and eliminates the following foods:[84]

All meat, fish, and poultry.
Peas, beans, and lentils.
Wheat germ and bran.
Vegetables: asparagus, cauliflower, celery, mushrooms, peas, radishes, spinach.

During periods of rejection, the diet may need to be changed. Monitoring of the biochemical data will indicate the type of diet required. Some rejection episodes are mild and can be treated medically without complete rejection of the kidney.

Table 9-9 provides an example of the guidelines for nutritional care of adult renal patients in one institution. It is important to remember that these are general guidelines only. The diet should be individualized for each patient.

Procedures for nutritional care of infants and children must be modified for differences in metabolic processes and growth. Table 9-10 provides a summary of usual recommendations. The diet must, however, be carefully individualized.

Infection and atherosclerotic disease are the most frequent causes of death in the renal transplant patient. Myocardial infarctions ("heart attacks") are 25 times more frequent than normal, and cerebrovascular accidents ("strokes") are 300 times more frequent. Contributing factors may be preexisting hyperlipidemia (see Chapter 10), corticosteroid therapy, and cyclosporine therapy.

There is some evidence that a diet containing increased fiber (>30 g/1,000 kcal), decreased cholesterol (<300 mg/day) and a polyunsaturated : saturated fatty acid ratio of >1 may increase survival rate. Because these types of modifications are most commonly used for cardiovascular disease, they are discussed in Chapter 10.

Nutritional Assessment. Patients in chronic renal failure have a high incidence of malnutrition. Some causes include altered food intake, blood loss, infections, and amino acid loss in dialysis. Cardiac arrhythmias in these patients result in increased protein catabolic rates. In addition, many pa-

Table 9-8. Immunosuppressants for Renal Transplant Patients: Mode of Action, Side Effects, and Associated Nutritional Care

Immunosuppressant	Mode of Action	Side Effects	Nutritional Care
Azothioprine (Imuran)	Interferes with DNA and RNA synthesis Suppresses cell-mediated hypersensitivity Inhibits cell division Suppresses antibody	Steatorrhea; Infection Mouth ulceration (herpes) Esophagitis Severe bone marrow depression Nausea, vomiting, diarrhea, anorexia	Liquid or soft diet as tolerated Decrease fat intake Increase protein and energy intakes if indicated Isolation techniques
Prednisone	Inhibits antibody formation Anti-inflammatory Suppresses cell-mediated hypersensitivity	Alters carbohydrate metabolism (increased gluconeogenesis; reduced glucose uptake; hyperglycemia; steroid-induced diabetes) Alters lipid metabolism (hypertriglyceridemia; increased serum cholesterol) Protein and nucleic acid degradation Reduced protein synthesis Sodium and fluid retention Pancreatitis Increased gastric HCl production Peptic ulcer Inhibits calcium absorption Increased appetite and weight gain Increased calcium excretion Joint pain Fractures Osteoporosis	Decrease intake of concentrated mono- or disaccharides Decrease intake of saturated fat Limit sodium intake Decrease fat intake Increase high-calcium foods Small, frequent feedings Avoid caffeine, alcohol, pepper Avoid poorly tolerated foods
Cyclosporin A	Paralyzes some lymphocytes (may be replacement for azothioprine) Antibiotic Inhibits cell mediated and humoral immunity Decreases delayed hypersensitivity	Hyperkalemia Hypertension Nephrotoxicity Hypomagnesemia Hyperuricemia Gum hyperplasia Gingivitis Nausea, vomiting, diarrhea, anorexia	Reduce K intake Reduce Na intake Monitor serum Mg Increase protein and energy intake Diet as tolerated
Antithymocyte globulin (ATG)	Inhibit cell-mediated immune response Decrease hypersensitivity reactions Decrease circulating lymphocytes	Nausea, vomiting, diarrhea Stomatitis Fever	Diet as tolerated

tients do not comply well with their treatment regimens. As a result, repeated nutritional assessments are important to evaluate changes in the patient's condition related to the progress of the disease, in compliance with the diet, and in effectiveness of the diet. The procedures for assessment described in Chapter 3 are generally applicable. However, a number of differences make certain adjustments necessary.

Table 9-9. Recommendations for Nutritional Care of Adults in Renal Failure (GFR 4–25 ml/min.)

Nutrients	Predialysis	Maintenance Hemodialysis	Peritoneal Dialysis	Transplant[a]
Protein	0.55–0.60 g/kg/day (70% HBV)[c] or 0.28 g/kg/day plus supplementation with essential amino acid mix or with amino acid + ketoacid mix[d]	1.0–1.2 g/kg IBW[b]	1.2–1.5 g/kg/day (50% HBV)	1.3–2.0 g/kg IBW
Energy	35 kcal/kg/day if at desirable weight 30 kcal/kg if obese 45 kcal/kg if underweight Encourage nonprotein energy sources	35 kcal/kg/day for weight maintenance 40–50 kcal/kg/day for weight gain or repletion 25–30 kcal/kg/day for weight loss	35 kcal/kg/day for weight maintenance 40–50 kcal/kg/day for weight gain or repletion 20–25 kcal/kg/day for weight loss For CAPD or CCPD, include dialysate kcal in total intake	30–35 kcal/kg/day for weight maintenance 40–45 kcal/kg/day for weight gain or repletion 20–25 kcal/kg/day for weight loss
Fat	40–45% of total kcal	40–45% of total kcal	40–45% of total kcal	30% of total kcal
Fluid	Balance with output to avoid edema; often unrestricted	750–1,500 ml/day (to gain 1–2 lb./day between dialyses: 1,000 ml + urine output if any)	Unrestricted (monitor body weight and blood pressure) for CAPD or CCPD For IPD, use amounts for hemodialysis	
Sodium	2,000–3,000 mg/day, or "no added salt" diet More if salt-wasting Calculate Na to ±10% of prescribed	40–120 mEq, usually 90 mEq Calculate Na to ±10% of prescribed	500–1,000 mg/day if blood pressure and weight are elevated CAPD or CCPD: 3,000–4,000 mg IPD: 2,000–3,000 mg	2,000–4,000 mg

Potassium	40–70 mEq/day or 1 mEq/g protein	1 mEq/g protein; usually >60 mEq/day	CAPD or CCPD: restrict only if serum K is high; IPD: 2,000–3,000 mg/day	Not restricted unless K >6 mg/dl
Phosphorus	4–10 mg/kg/day, 600–1,200 mg/day, or 15 mg/g protein prescribed	Depends on K level in dialysate; 8–17 mg/kg day or 15 mg/g prescribed protein	8–17 mg/kg day or 1,200 mg/day	No restriction; may need to supplement
Calcium	1,400–1,600 mg/day; may need $CaCO_3$ supplement	1,400–1,600 mg/day	1,400–1,600 mg/day	
Magnesium	200–300 mg/day	200–300 mg/day	200–300 mg/day	
Iron	10–18 mg/day	10–18 mg/day	10–18 mg/day	
Zinc	15 mg/day	15 mg/day	15 mg/day	
Vitamin supplements[e]				
Vitamin A	None	None	None	None
Vitamin E	15 IU/day	15 IU/day	15 IU/day	
Pyridoxine·HCl	5 mg/day	10 mg/day	10 mg/day	
Ascorbic acid	70–100 mg/day	70–100 mg/day	100 mg/day	100 mg/day
Other				Six small feedings may be necessary

Compiled from Kopple, J.D., Nutrition, diet and the kidney. In M.E. Shils and V.R. Young, Eds., *Modern Nutrition in Health and Disease*, 7th ed. Philadelphia: Lea & Febiger, 1988; Roberts, C., Conservative management–dietary treatment in early stages of chronic renal failure; Harum, P., Nutritional management of the adult hemodialysis patient; McCann, L., Peritoneal dialysis and nutrition considerations; and Shah, R., Nutritional management of renal transplant patients. In *A Clinical Guide to Nutrition Care in End-Stage Renal Disease*, ed. D. Gillit, J. Stover, and N.C. Spinozzi. Chicago: American Dietetic Association, 1987; Urich, J., et al. *Manual of Clinical Dietetics*. Los Angeles: University of California, Los Angeles Medical Center, 1986; and *Mayo Clinic Diet Manual*, 6th ed. Toronto: B.C. Decker, 1988.

[a] CAPD = continuous ambulatory peritoneal dialysis; CCPD = continuous cyclic peritoneal dialysis; IPD = intermittent peritoneal dialysis.
[b] IBW = ideal body weight.
[c] HBV = high biological value (protein).
[d] Or 90 g protein for a GFR of 20–25 ml/min., 70 g for 16–20 ml/min., 50 g for 10–15 ml/min., and 0.6 g/kg/day for a GFR of less than 10 ml/min. (no less than 35–40 g/day).
[e] Supplement all patients with 1.5 mg/day thiamine, 1.8 mg/day riboflavin, 20 mg/day niacin, 5 mg/day pantothenic acid, 3 μg/day vitamin B_{12}, 1 mg/day folate until transplant.

Table 9-10. Recommendations for Nutritional Care of Infants and Children in End-Stage Renal Disease

Nutrients	Predialysis	Maintenance Hemodialysis	Peritoneal Dialysis	Transplant
Infants				
Protein	GFR > 15%, 0–6 months: 2.2 g/kg/day; 6–12 months: 2.0 g/kg/day; GFR < 15%: 1.5–1.6 g/kg/day (70% HBV)	0–6 months: 2.2 g/kg; 6–12 months: 2.0 g/day (50% HBV)	2.5–4.0 g/kg/day	1.3–2.0 g/kg/day
Energy				
Normal body weight	0–6 months: 115 kcal/kg; 6–12 months: 105 kcal/kg	Same	Same	To achieve and maintain ideal body weight
Malnourished	Add 20%			
Fats	55% of total kcal	Same	Same	Limit; give high P/S ratio
Fluid	Urine output + 35 cc/kg insensible losses	Urine output + insensible losses	Not usually restricted	Ad lib
Sodium	1–3 mEq/kg/day	1–3 mEq/kg/day	Not usually restricted	2–3 g (87–130 mEq)
Potassium	1–3 mEq/kg/day when GFR is 10% of normal	1–3 mEq/kg/day	No limit?	Unlimited
Phosphorus	500–1,000 mg/day (limit milk to ½ cup)	500–1,200 mg/day (limit milk to ½ cup)	Minimum possible with adequate protein	Need high intake; supplement if needed
Calcium	0–6 months: 360 mg; 6–12 months: 540 mg	Same	Same	Ad lib; supplement if needed
Vitamins/day	A,E,K not needed; Individualize D; Add 1.5 mg thiamine, 1.8 mg riboflavin, 20 mg niacin, 3 µg vitamin B_{12}, 1 mg folate, 5 mg B_6, 100 mg vitamin C	10 mg B_6; all others same	Same	Supplements not usually required except for D
Other[a]				
Children				
Protein	GFR > 15%: 1–3 years: 1.8 g/kg; 4–6 years: 1.5 g/kg; 7–10 years: 1.2 g/kg; 11–18 years: 1.0 g/kg; GFR < 15%: 1–3 years: 1.0–1.4 g/kg; 4–6 years: 0.9–1.2 g/kg	1–3 years: 1.8 g/kg; 4–6 years: 1.5 g/kg; 7–10 years: 1.2 g/kg; 11–14 years: 1.0 g/kg; 15–18 years: 0.8 g/kg	1–3 years: 2.5–3.5 g/kg; 4–10 years: 2.5 g/kg; 11–18 years: 1.5 g/kg	2–3 g/kg

	7–10 years: 0.8–1.1 g/kg 11–18 years: 0.7–1.0 g/kg (70% HBV for all)	Same		
Energy (normal weight)	1–3 years: 100 kcal/kg 4–6 years: 85 kcal/kg 7–10 years: 86 kcal/kg 11–14 years: 48 kcal/kg (F) 60 kcal/kg (M) 15–18 years: 38 kcal/kg (F) 42 kcal/kg (M)	Same	Same	To reach and maintain ideal body weight
Fats	55% of total kcal; P/S ratio 2.0/1.0	Same	Same	Limit; give high P/S ratio
Fluid	Urine output + 35 ml/kg insensible losses	Same	Same? or ad lib?	Ad lib
Sodium	1–3 mEq/1,000 kcal expended	1–3 mEq/kg/day	Same	If edema and high blood pressure: give less than 1,000 mg, 1–3 years; 2,000–3,000 mg, 4–6 years; 3,000–4,000 mg, 11–18 years
Potassium	1–3 mEq/1,000 kcal expended	1–3 mEq/1,000 kcal expended	1–3 years: 1,000 mg 4–18 years: 1–3 mEq/1,000 kcal expended	Ad lib
Phosphorus	1–10 years: 500–600 mg/day 11–18 years: 600–1,000 mg/day	Same	Same	High intake; supplement as needed
Calcium	1–10 years: 800 mg 11–18 years: 1,200 mg	Same	Same	High intake; supplement as needed
Vitamins	A,E,K not needed Vitamin D: individualize Supplement with 1.5 mg thiamine, 1.8 mg riboflavin, 20 mg niacin, 3 μg vitamin B_{12}, 1 mg folate, 10 mg vitamin B_6, 100 mg ascorbic acid	Same	Same	Supplements not needed

Compiled from information contained in Ulrich, J., et al., *Manual of Clinical Dietetics*. Los Angeles: University of California, Los Angeles Medical Center, 1986; *Manual of Clinical Dietetics*. Chicago: American Dietetic Association, 1988; and Nelson, P., and Stover, J., Principles of nutritional assessment and management of the child with ESRD. In R. N. Fine and A. B. Gruskin, Eds., *End Stage Renal Disease in Children*. Philadelphia: W. B. Saunders, 1984.

[a] Supplement all patients with Zn, Fe, and Cu.

Modifications in routine assessments. Body weights are usually based on dry weight, that is, weight at normal hydration. **Dry weight** is assumed to exist when there is no evidence of edema and when serum sodium and blood pressure are within normal range. In the dialysis patient, dry weight is weight immediately after dialysis. When the dry weight is obtained, it may be interpreted relative to usual weight or optimal body weight prior to illness (see Equation 3-3). Standards for interpretation as percent of usual body weight may be as follows:

Normal or mild deficit	85–95%
Moderate deficit	75–85%
Severe deficit	<75%

Sequential weights may be compared with previous weights to indicate the direction of change in nutritional status. Rapid loss is more significant than slow loss.

A deficit in **height** often occurs in children in renal failure and must be monitored in comparison to standard **height of age**. The height of adults may be measured occasionally since decreasing stature may indicate bone disease.

Standards for **midarm muscle circumference** (MAMC) and **triceps skinfold** (TSF) for renal patients are scant. Some suggested standards are shown in Table 9-11.[85] These standards are not of value if the patient is edematous. In hemodialysis patients, it is often recommended that MAMC be obtained from the nonaccess arm at dry weight. Observing these precautions, these values are useful to indicate directions of change if obtained every two weeks.

Serum albumin and **serum transferrin** may be useful for monitoring over a long period during which directions of change may be observed, but they are influenced by the renal failure and accompanying illnesses unrelated to nutrition. Therefore, they must be interpreted with caution. Suggested standards for interpretation are shown in Table 9-12.[85] Because serum albumin has a long half-life and large body pool, it is less useful. Serum transferrin may be more useful if it is not calculated from total iron binding capacity, which is altered by anemia, low protein intake, amino acid losses in dialysis, and iron medications.

Total lymphocyte counts (TLC) and **delayed cutaneous hypersensitivity** (DCH) are less useful. DCH is decreased in dialyzed patients, and both tests are sensitive to immunosuppressive drugs. High blood urea levels influence the morphology of leukocytes.

A detailed **diet assessment** is important. In addition to the items described in Chapter 3, it must consider fluid, sodium, potassium, and other electrolytes. A three or four day record is more useful than a 24-hour recall. Other needed areas of information are the following:

Use of special dietary products:
    Low protein products? Brand? Amount? Nutritional value?
    Salt substitutes? Brand? Composition? Amount?
    Phosphate binders? Brand? Composition? Amount?
Compliance with diet?
Allergies?

Table 9-11. Suggested Muscle and Skinfold Standards for Renal Patients

Measurement	Moderate Deficit	Severe Deficit
Midarm muscle circumference (cm)		
Men	27	<24
Women	20	<18
Triceps skinfold (mm)		
Men	<8	<5
Women	<18	<12

Table 9-12. Suggested Serum Albumin and Serum Transferrin Standards for Renal Patients

Measurement	Moderate Deficit	Severe Deficit
Serum albumin (g/dl)	2.98–3.5	2.8
Serum transferrin (mg/dl)	150–180	150

Likes and dislikes?
Appetite?
Taste changes?
Who cooks? Where? Facilities?
Number and size of meals?
Activity? Exercise? Employment?
Difficulties with previous diet?

Other factors that must be noted in assessment of the CRF patient include **serum calcium, serum phosphorus, serum vitamin A**, and **serum ferritin**. Serum ferritin has been found to be a better tool for evaluation of iron status than serum iron or transferrin. Ferritin correlates best with iron deposition in the bone marrow.[21]

Monitoring renal patients. In addition to the considerations already discussed, other monitoring procedures may be used to (1) evaluate the efficacy of the nutritional care and (2) evaluate the patient's adherence to the prescribed diet.

Monitoring protein homeostasis is of primary importance. However, special considerations are indicated in renal insufficiency. There are several useful methods. In general, these procedures are based on the use of urea concentrations in the blood and urine to calculate the patient's **protein catabolic rate** (PCR). They are thus known as "urea kinetics."

Serum urea nitrogen (SUN) or **blood urea nitrogen** (BUN) can be used to indicate the extent of renal failure. Increases in SUN can also result from dehydration, catabolic states, intake of catabolic drugs, and gastrointestinal bleeding. However, if the adult patient is nutritionally stable (nitrogen balance = 0), SUN is closely correlated with dietary protein. Levels of 60–80 mg/dl of SUN are acceptable in CRF, since uremic symptoms do not develop until SUN exceeds 80 mg/dl or sometimes 100 mg/dl. Increases are closely associated with dietary protein. On the other hand, if SUN is less than 40 mg/dl, the patient should be checked for malnutrition.

Serum creatinine is used to measure the extent of renal failure and to monitor the

effectiveness of treatment. It is not related to diet unless the diet has a high meat intake, but meat in the diet may add up to 3.2 mg of creatinine per gram of meat intake per day.

Clearances of serum urea and serum creatinine are indicators of glomerular filtration rate. In clinical settings, an average of the two values is often used.

The ratio of SUN to serum creatinine is closely correlated to protein intake in nondialyzed CRF patients because, at a given level of renal function, SUN is related to protein intake, but serum creatinine is not. Using the equation

$$y = 0.13x + 0.77 \qquad \textbf{(9-3)}$$

the **average protein intake** (x) can be estimated if the SUN/serum creatinine ratio (y) is known. For example, if SUN is 80 mg/dl and serum creatinine is 10 mg/dl, the ratio would be 8. Using Equation 9-3, the average protein intake would be about 56 g/day. This equation assumes a stable diet and is for men with normal muscle mass. Under these circumstances, comparison of the estimated protein intake can be compared with the prescribed diet to evaluate compliance. Equation 9-3 does not apply to wasted males, to women, or to children.

Recent protein intake can be assessed, in clinically stable CRF patients, from the urinary urea nitrogen (UUN):

$$\text{recent mean N intake} = \tfrac{10}{9} \times \text{UUN} + 1.8 \qquad \textbf{(9-4)}$$

where all values are given in g/day. The value 1.8 represents fecal, respiratory, and integumental losses. Protein intake is then calculated from 6.25 times the nitrogen.

Alternatively, the following equation may be used in place of Equation 9-4:

$$\text{protein intake} = (7.0 \times \text{UUN}) + 11 \qquad \textbf{(9-5)}$$

where all values are given in g/day.

Urinary area nitrogen as the sole basis for calculation is, however, only useful if the patient is clinically stable — that is, when SUN, body weight, and body water are relatively constant. This is frequently not the case in the renal patient. Therefore, the changes can be taken into account by using calculations for **urea nitrogen appearance** (UNA). This value includes not only the urinary urea nitrogen, but adds the urea accumulated in the body. The amount of urea removed in dialysis is difficult to measure accurately, therefore, these calculations are usually done using data obtained between dialysis treatments. Then UNA per day consists of urinary urea nitrogen excreted per day plus the change in the amount of urea nitrogen in the body per day:

$$\text{UNA (g/day)} = \text{UUN (g/day)} + \Delta\text{SUN (g/day)} \qquad \textbf{(9-6)}$$

The change in urea in the body must take into account the increase or decrease in concentration of urea (SUN) and the change in total amount of body water in which the urea is found. It is assumed that the concentration of urea nitrogen in the serum is the same throughout all body water. Body water is estimated to be 60% of body weight in the adult male (see Chapter 2).

If the SUN rises, the additional urea is calculated as the difference in concentration in 60% of the initial body weight or:

$$\text{UN}_1 = (\text{SUN}_f - \text{SUN}_i) \times (0.6 \times \text{BW}_i) \qquad \textbf{(9-7)}$$

where UN_1 = additional urea nitrogen causing an increased SUN and f and i are final and initial values for the time period used.

If the patient gains weight, it is assumed that the weight gain consists of water and the water contains the same final concentration of urea as is found in other body water. This urea nitrogen must also be included in the UNA. The added weight is multipled by the final SUN:

$$\text{UN}_2 = (\text{BW}_f - \text{BW}_i) \times \text{SUN}_f \qquad \textbf{(9-8)}$$

where UN_2 = urea nitrogen contained in newly retained fluid.

The values obtained in Equations 9-7 and 9-8 are then added to the UUN (if any) to achieve the final equation:

$$\text{UNA} = \text{UUN} + \text{UN}_1 + \text{UN}_2 \qquad \textbf{(9-9)}$$

or

$$\text{UNA} = \text{UUN} + [(\text{SUN}_f - \text{SUN}_i) \times (0.6 \times \text{BW}_i)] + [(\text{BW}_f - \text{BW}_i) \times \text{SUN}_f] \qquad \textbf{(9-10)}$$

UNA is expressed in grams per day. If the initial and final values for SUN and body weight are taken at any other interval, the value should be adjusted accordingly.

As an example of the above calculations, let us assume the patient is an adult male, not edematous, and the data are:

> Initial SUN = 25 mg/dl or 0.25 g/L (postdialysis on Monday)
> Final SUN = 45 mg/dl or 0.45 g/L (predialysis on Wednesday)
> Initial body weight = 60 kg (postdialysis on Monday)
> Final body weight = 63 kg (predialysis on Wednesday)
> UUN = 0.35 g/day
> Time interval = 48 hours

$$
\begin{aligned}
\text{Then total UNA} &= [(0.45 - 0.25) \times (0.6 \times 60)] + [(63 - 60) \times 0.45] \\
&= 0.35 + \frac{0.2 \times 36}{2} \\
&\quad + \frac{3 \times 0.45}{2} \\
&= 0.35 + 3.6 + 0.675 \\
&= 4.625 \text{ g/day}
\end{aligned}
$$

Using the UNA value, total nitrogen output may be estimated with the equation

Total N output (g/day) = 0.97 UNA
   (g/day) + 1.93   **(9-11)**

Total nitrogen intake may be calculated:

Total N intake (g/day) = 0.69 UNA
   (g/day) + 3.3   **(9-12)**

Nitrogen balance may be estimated from the difference between intake and output:

N Balance = N intake − N output   **(9-13)**

To continue with the same example:

Equation 9-12: N intake = (0.69 × 4.625)
                       +3.3 = 6.49 g/day.
Equation 9-11: N output = (0.97 × 4.625)
                       +1.93 = 6.42 g/day.
Equation 9-13: N balance = 6.49 − 6.42
                       = 0.07.

The amount of protein containing 0.07 g of nitrogen equals 0.07 × 6.25 = 0.44 g. Therefore, the patient is approximately in nitrogen balance.

High UNA compared to nitrogen intake obtained from the diet history may indicate increased nitrogen intake, increased protein catabolism, or both. Low UNA compared to nitrogen intake obtained from the diet history may indicate decreased nitrogen intake or increased anabolism (e.g., nutritional repletion, pregnancy, or both). Other interpretations useful in patient counseling are listed in Table 9-13.

An alternative procedure involves the measure of the **protein catabolic rate** (PCR) in the predialysis patient. The PCR equals the dietary protein intake in stable patients and can, therefore, be used to evaluate intake. The procedure can be followed in step-wise fashion as follows:

1. Calculate the patient's residual urea clearance using the equation:

$$KrU = \frac{Uu}{BUN} \times \frac{Uv}{t} \qquad \textbf{(9-14)}$$

Table 9-13. Guidelines for Interpretation of Monitoring Results

Results Observed	Suggested Interpretation
BUN > 100 mg/dl without weight loss	Excess protein intake
Increased BUN, but other values as expected	Excess intake of low-biological-value protein
Increased BUN and phosphate	Excess cheese intake
Increased BUN, K, and phosphate	Excess total protein (probably meat, milk)
High BUN plus weight loss	Protein catabolism
BUN low (for CRF patient) plus low serum albumin	Inadequate protein intake?

where KrU = residual urea clearance (ml/min.), Uu = urine urea concentration (mg/ml), BUN = blood urea nitrogen (mg/ml), Uv = volume of urine collected (ml), and t = time interval of collection (min.).

2. Calculate the **urea generation rate** (Gu) using the equation:

$$Gu = BUN \times KrU \qquad \textbf{(9-15)}$$

where Gu = urea generation rate (mg/min.), BUN = blood urea nitrogen (mg/ml), and KrU = residual urea clearance (ml/min.).

The PCR may then be calculated with the equation:

$$PCR \ (g/day) = (Gu + 1.2)\ 9.35 \qquad \textbf{(9-16)}$$

The **daily protein intake** (DPI) is approximately equal to the PCR in the stable patient.

A proposed alternative calculation of PCR is somewhat simpler. It can be applied to patients in a steady state in a 24-hour period:

$$PCR = 10.7 + \frac{UUN}{0.14} + UPE \qquad \textbf{(9-17)}$$

where UUN = grams of urinary urea in 24 hours, and UPE = grams of urinary protein excretion (if any) in 24 hours.

In monitoring the CRF patient, a number of other items are evaluated at regular intervals, commonly on a flow chart:

1. Body weights, including pre- and post-dialysis, and interdialytic weight gain.
2. Serum sodium and potassium.
3. Serum calcium, phosphorus, and their product.
4. Serum glucose, fasting and nonfasting.
5. Effects of medication.

If serum sodium is in normal range, weight gain indicates sodium intake with reasonable accuracy. A weight gain of 1 kg results from an increase of 1 liter of extracellular fluid and 130–140 mEq of sodium.

The frequency of monitoring varies with the index being monitored and the condition of the patient. One recommended protocol for a CRF patient in a steady state is shown in Table 9-14.[86]

The nutritional care specialist may have a patient load of 150 or more. After the original assessment, patients may be chosen for further consultation based on assessment values. Commonly used guidelines are shown in Table 9-15. In addition, patients should be seen when there is any unex-

Table 9-14. A Recommended Protocol for a Chronic Renal Failure Patient in a Steady State

Variable to Be Monitored	Frequency
Blood chemistries	
Na, K, Cl, CO_2	Every 12–24 hours
Ca, Mg, phosphate	Weekly
Arterial blood gases	As needed
Serum glucose	Every 24 hours
Serum osmolality	Weekly
Nutritional status	
Body weight	Daily
Albumin, transferrin	Weekly
Nitrogen balance	Twice weekly
Renal function	
Urine output	Daily
Creatinine, BUN	Alternate days
Urine osmolality	As needed
Urine creatine and urea (24-hour urine sample)	Twice weekly

Table 9-15. Guidelines to Determine the Need for Further Nutritional Consultation

Variable	Units	Less Than	More Than
Serum sodium	mEq/L	132	148
Serum potassium	mEq/L	3.0	6.0
Predialysis BUN	mg/dl	40	100
Serum creatinine	mg/dl		20
Serum calcium	mg/dl	8.0	11.0
Serum phosphorus	mg/dl		5.0
Serum albumin	g/dl	3.0	
Weight change over longest intradialytic interval	kg		2.0

plained weight change, a new diet order, or expressed patient dissatisfaction.

Acute Renal Failure

A rapid decrease in GFR with accumulation of nitrogenous wastes is known as **acute renal failure**. There is no opportunity for the adaptations seen in CRF. Usually, there is no previous history of impairment of renal function. ARF may, however, be superimposed on chronic renal disease by stress factors such as infection or dehydration. In contrast to CRF, it is reversible in some patients. Alternatively, the primary disease may be far removed from the urinary system. The patient may have a primary disorder involving the cardiovascular, pulmonary, or gastrointestinal system, for example, or have severe burns or sepsis. These are discussed in more detail in Chapter 14.

Etiology. The causes of the ARF itself have been categorized as prerenal, intrarenal, and postrenal. **Prerenal failure**, also known as **functional renal failure**, occurs as a result of a drop in blood pressure and a drop in renal perfusion that may follow shock, hemorrhage, cardiac failure, dehydration, obstruction of renal arteries, use of vasodilating drugs, or abnormal sequestration of large amounts of body fluids. All of these factors decrease blood flow to the kidneys, resulting in a fall in the GFR. In addition, prerenal failure may result from increased production of nitrogenous compounds, for example, from hemoglobin metabolism after gastrointestinal bleeding.

Intrarenal failure, or **parenchymal renal failure**, can occur when the kidney tissue is damaged directly. Damage may be caused by nephrotoxic drugs or other chemicals and by antigen-antibody reactions. Hemolysis of blood, as from a mismatched transfusion, releases hemoglobin, which may precipitate in and injure the renal tubules. Crushing injuries and burns also cause release of hemoglobin and of myoglobin from damaged muscles, adding to the damage from ischemia. The mechanism of hemoglobin and myoglobin damage is not understood entirely. Additional intrarenal causes include acute glomerulonephritis, vasculitis, hypercalcemia, and hepatorenal syndrome, a disease of the liver that also damages the parenchymal tissue of the kidney.

Postrenal failure (obstructive nephropathy) results from obstruction to the excretion of urine. Obstructions may occur as a result of prostatic enlargement in men, calculi (stones), stricture, or malformations. As the hydrostatic pressure rises, it affects the tubule cells directly. It can also compress renal blood vessels, causing ischemia.

When ARF is the result of ischemic or toxic injury, it is called **acute tubular necrosis (ATN)** or **acute tubular insufficiency**. It is commonly seen in postoperative and septic patients. Acute tubular necrosis is accountable for 80% of the cases of ARF.

Pathogenesis. The mechanisms by which ATN is produced are not understood entirely, but several explanations exist. Hypotension causes vasoconstriction in the kidney, particularly in the cortex. This could lead to the fall in the GFR that is seen in ATN. Damage to the tubules may occur as a result of ischemic hypoxia, which might, in turn, cause tubular edema, obstruction of tubules by cellular debris, and increased tubule cell permeability. It has also been suggested that tubular hypoxia results in decreased sodium reabsorption. When the sodium re-

maining in the tubule reaches the macula densa, it stimulates the release of renin and, by means of the renin-angiotensin system, precipitates a severe vasoconstriction and a decline in the GFR with further tubular damage.

Pathology. Two types of structural alterations have been observed. When nephrotoxic damage causes ATN, the proximal tubule cells are damaged, but the basement membrane remains intact. In ATN caused by renal ischemia, there is patchy necrosis of the basement membrane, as well as tubular epithelium, throughout both proximal and distal tubules. Disruptions of the tubule cells result in openings between the tubular lumen and adjacent capillaries, loss of tubular secretory and reabsorptive functions, interstitial edema, and infiltration of inflammatory cells. Recovery is more rapid in nephrotoxic disease in which the basement membrane is intact.

Pathophysiology. Although in ARF there is a significant decline in tubular capacity for sodium and water absorption, oliguria usually is marked. The primary cause is believed to be a decrease in the GFR, which may be as low as 1 ml/min. The cause of the reduced GFR is not understood completely. It may follow vasoconstriction that results in decreased renal blood flow. The renin-angiotensin system possibly plays a role in producing the vasoconstriction, but this theory has not been proved. As a consequence of the low GFR, the patient retains waste products. A few patients produce a normal volume of urine (**high-output renal failure**). This occurs when the GFR is low but water reabsorption is even lower, so that urine volume appears to be satisfactory; however, retention of waste products occurs because the total volume filtered is so small. The prognosis is better in high-output failure than in oliguria.

The onset of ARF follows exposure to the precipitating factor in 48 hours or less. Clinical manifestations include oliguria and sodium, water, potassium, and nitrogen retention. Potassium retention is a particular problem in ARF, an important difference from chronic failure. It is particularly severe in a patient whose renal failure was precipitated by extensive tissue damage with release of intracellular potassium. As the renal failure becomes more severe, clinical manifestations appear in other organ systems, including the central nervous system, gastrointestinal tract, and cardiovascular system. These manifestations are similar to those seen in CRF.

Clinical Course and Prognosis. The overall mortality rate varies greatly depending on the cause of the failure. Patients with ATN from nephrotoxin exposure secondary to dehydration have a mortality rate of 10% to 30%. On the other hand, ATN resulting from septicemia, trauma, or complications of surgery is associated with a mortality rate of 40% to 80%. Mortality rate is reduced in patients who are dialyzed early and frequently. The patient then may recover completely, since renal tubule cells are capable of regeneration. Some patients make a partial recovery but then progress to severe chronic renal disease over a long period.

The clinical course is extremely variable. In ATN, it may be divided into three phases:

1. *Oliguric phase:* The urine volume is 400 to 500 ml/day or less for periods up to several weeks, with hematuria, proteinuria, and isosthenuria.
2. *Diuretic phase:* As the patient begins to recover, he or she progresses to the diuretic phase. Urine flow increases, but the reabsorptive capacity of the tubules may still be depressed. As a result, urea clearance may still be decreased. Serum urea nitrogen and serum creatinine then remain high during part of this period.
3. *Recovery phase:* The patient may have some degree of decreased renal function for months. Others never fully recover.

Nutritional Management. Nutritional requirements in ARF are not clear. Some patients are undernourished prior to the renal failure because of the underlying disease. Many suffer from severe catabolism (see Chapter 14). Patients who are not oliguric tend to be only mildly catabolic and are likely to be able to eat. Those who are oliguric are usually severely anorexic and severely catabolic. They often require parenteral nutrition. The reasons for protein catabolism in ARF are unclear. Some mediators of this catabolic response include the following:

- Insufficient protein and energy intake
- Coexisting catabolic conditions
- Increasing catabolic hormones (parathyroid, adrenal)
- Insulin resistance
- Loss of nutrients during dialysis
- Increased prostaglandin synthesis[70]

Although it seems reasonable to assume that good nutrition will improve the survival rate of ARF patients, there are no unequivocal data to support this assumption. Patients with ARF often are incapable of oral intake and must be fed by tube or intravenously. Special tube feeding formulas, Amin-Aid or Travasorb Renal, are available for patients with renal disease (see Appendix G). If the condition is mild or if dialysis is not available and the patient is capable of oral intake, a more **conservative management** with modification of the diet and fluids can be used. The objectives of nutritional management are

- To achieve and maintain optimum nutrition.
- To reduce or avoid uremic symptoms.
- To maintain normal fluid and electrolyte balance.

Essential features of the diet used in conservative management are discussed in the following paragraphs.

Sodium and fluid. If the patient is dehydrated, normal fluid balance must first be restored (see Chapter 2). As indicated in CRF, fluid intake is limited to the volume of urine output plus 500 ml/day for insensible losses, plus other measurable losses such as from drainage, vomiting, fistula losses, or diarrhea during the oliguric phase. It may also be necessary to include the water of metabolism, 400–500 ml/day in adults, in the calculations. Some fluid must also be reserved for use by the nursing service in giving medications. In the diuretic phase, a large volume of fluid may be needed to provide replacement.

Sodium may be restricted to 20 mEq/day in the oliguric phase but 40, 60, or 90 mEq is more common. Only enough sodium to replace losses is given. If fluid and sodium intake are appropriate, the patient whose caloric intake is severely depressed will lose 0.25 to 0.5 kg of body weight per day, and plasma sodium levels will be normal. The patient should be weighed daily. Weight gain indicates fluid retention and is counteracted with further fluid and sodium restriction to avoid congestive heart failure.

Protein. In the adult who does not have a catabolic condition such as traumatic injury, major surgery, or burns, protein intake may be limited to 0.25–0.5 g per kg of body weight per day to minimize the azotemia.[21] The protein should be of high biologic value. The patient who is severely catabolic, as indicated by an SUN value of 100 mg/day or more plus elevated serum potassium and acidosis, is given more protein. However, the amount and type are still controversial. Many of these patients are fed parenterally. The optimum amino acid content of the TPN formula is unknown, as is the relative desirability of using essential amino acids only versus a mixture of both essential and nonessential amino acids. Recent recommendations suggest a mixture of equal parts of each type.[21]

The amount of protein to be provided may be based on an estimate of protein breakdown obtained from the urea nitrogen appearance:

Normocatabolic: UNA = 4–8 mmol/L representing 30–60 g protein.
Moderately catabolic: UNA = 8–12 mmol/L representing 60–85 g protein.

Hypercatabolic: UNA >12 mmol/L representing >85 g protein.[83]

It has been suggested, for example, that normal catabolic patients may be given a 15–20-g protein diet plus 8–12 g of essential amino acids, including histidine. This diet may prevent uremic symptoms and help to avoid or reduce dialysis treatments.[21] Hypercatabolic patients must be supplied with larger amounts of protein and then dialyzed.

Energy. Ideally, kilocalories are provided in sufficient amounts to prevent protein catabolism and maintain body weight. However, many ARF patients are severely catabolic as a consequence of their underlying disease. When acute renal failure supervenes, it has been assumed that energy requirements increase further. Currently, it is believed that energy needs are not as high as previously thought. It is suggested by some that 30–35 kcal/kg/day is sufficient for most patients.[21] Others recommend 35–60 kcal/kg or BEE × 1.5.[86] The underlying disease may also limit food intake. The tube feeding or TPN formula should provide energy from both carbohydrate and fat. Since insulin resistance is present in uremia, the patient is given a unit of insulin for each 3 to 5 g of glucose. Fat emulsions, 1 g/kg/day, are also included in the TPN formula.[21] The amount of food that can be eaten is often limited by anorexia, nausea, and vomiting in the patient. As a result, the weight loss previously described is a common occurrence. Oral kilocalorie intake is improved with the use of protein-free, low-electrolyte, high-carbohydrate liquid supplements (see Appendix G), hard candy, or "butterballs," a flavored butter and sugar mixture.

Potassium. Hyperkalemia develops rapidly as a result of decreased excretion, increased release of intracellular potassium during tissue breakdown, presence of blood at abnormal sites, and infection. A diet limited to 25–50 mEq of potassium to prevent hyperkalemia until urine volume increases during recovery is needed if the patient is fed orally. An intake of 50 mEq of potassium is the smallest amount compatible with adequate protein. If hyperkalemia occurs despite this limit, it may be managed with glucose, insulin, calcium bicarbonate, Na-K exchange resins, and fluid restriction. Uncontrollable hyperkalemia is an indication for dialysis.

Other electrolytes. An additional diet modification sometimes recommended for patients with ARF is restriction of dietary phosphate. Since a low-phosphorus diet is poorly accepted, phosphate-binding antacids usually are used instead. Medications are commonly used also, instead of diet modification, for treatment of the accompanying hyperuricemia and hypocalcemia.

If the patient is being dialyzed, a more liberal diet is possible. During the diuretic phase, too, the diet is liberalized. Protein should be restricted until serum urea and creatinine fall. Frequently, high potassium intakes are required to replace potassium lost in diuresis. Fluid and sodium may be allowed as desired, since the patient's thirst is a useful guide to fluid and sodium intake during the diuresis phase.

Monitoring the ARF Patient. The ARF patient must be monitored very closely. Many of the procedures are the same as those used for the CRF patient, but are more frequent. Frequency is the greatest in the initial period when the patient is unstable and during the diuretic phase. Urea kinetics are not used because patients are very unstable.

Nonoral Nutritional Support. Acute renal failure may be caused, for example, by a nephrotoxic agent, or it may be associated with pregnancy (**postpartum renal failure**). Nutritional support is not generally required in these cases.

Other conditions, however, may lead to the need for parenteral nutrition. Some of these conditions include short bowel syndrome, inflammatory bowel disease, systemic lupus erythematosus, amyloidosis, radiation enteritis, chronic pancreatitis, AIDS, and cancer of the digestive tract. At the same time, conventional or tube feeding may not be possible. In these circumstances, it is de-

sirable to meet the nutritional requirements of the patient while avoiding exacerbation of the uremia.

The TPN infusion uses an amino acid mixture containing only amino acids if the patient cannot be dialyzed, for example, in extensive burns. If dialysis is possible, a mixture of essential and nonessential amino acids may be used. Useful products are listed in Chapter 5. Lipids are used if tolerated, along with 50–70% dextrose. Electrolytes are adjusted to individual needs.

There is only limited knowledge of vitamin requirements in the parenterally fed patient in renal failure. Requirements differ because there is no gastrointestinal absorption, and the liver is bypassed. Absorption may be impaired in ARF. At the same time, excretion of excess via the kidney does not occur. Removal of an excess may occur during dialysis, and there may be some gastrointestinal excretion.

Current recommendations suggest that the TPN patient in renal failure should have increased amounts of water-soluble vitamins. Since vitamin A accumulates, there is no need to supplement this vitamin. Vitamin D supplements are important. Most TPN lipids are enriched with vitamin E, but the vitamin may adsorb to the plastic bag and tube used in feeding. The need for a supplement is unknown.

Many vitamin supplements contain 500 mg of ascorbic acid per day. This may be metabolized to oxalic acid with soft oxalate deposition in soft tissues. Therefore, a formulation should be used which has lower amounts of ascorbic acid.

In some cases, parenteral nutrition is given during dialysis using a procedure known as **intradialytic parenteral nutrition** (IDPN). Clinical indications usually accepted to justify this procedure include many of the common signs of malnutrition: >10% loss of dry body weight, >50% decrease in TSF or MAMC, <3.5 g/dl serum albumin, and <1,500 total lymphocyte count. The patient also would have an impaired gastrointestinal tract leading to malnutrition to justify use of

IDPN. Every effort should first be made to improve nutritional status with oral supplements or tube feeding.

Other methods are used to control the fluid and electrolyte balance. These are continuous arteriovenous hemofiltration and slow continuous ultrafiltration.

Continuous arteriovenous hemofiltration (CAVH) may be used alone or in addition to hemodialysis to control fluid and electrolyte balance.[87] Some hemodialysis patients suffer from rapid fluid shifts, electrolyte imbalance, and severe hypotension, which limit the fluid removal and the value of the dialysis. ARF patients with multisystem organ failure have high nutrient requirements. Parenteral nutrition in this group may require 3 liters of feeding formula per day. Thus CAVH makes it possible to provide adequate nutritional support within the fluid restriction. It reduces the need for more frequent hemodialysis, which in severe ARF may be needed daily.

In the CAVH procedure, catheters are placed into a large, often femoral, artery and vein. The blood flows through a filtering device. Water and small molecular weight solutes, including urea, creatinine, and electrolytes, are filtered from arterial blood, and a more concentrated blood is returned to the vein. The procedure is powered by the blood pressure. Filtration stops if the patient's blood pressure drops, avoiding the hypotension that may complicate attempts at hemodialysis.

The method may be used for (1) avoidance of hemodynamic instability and high fluid requirements for nutritional support in ARF, (2) correction of electrolyte and acid-base abnormalities, and (3) reduction of fluid overload. This procedure is also useful in cardiogenic shock, pulmonary edema, and acute respiratory failure. In addition to removing the fluid restriction, avoiding electrolyte overload, and avoiding hemodynamic instability, the method allows the use of hyperosmolar solutions and reduces amino acid losses. Total parenteral nutrition may thus be combined with CAVH. The TPN line can be used to provide any replacement fluids that may be needed, or it may be given separately. Nutritional monitoring involves observation of fluid balance. The ultrafiltrate contains electrolytes and vitamins that may need to be replaced.

Slow continuous ultrafiltration (SCUF) is indicated in oliguric acute renal failure requiring TPN or any patient needing daily dialysis plus TPN. It removes more fluid than CAVH with less loss of electrolytes and less loss of amino acids. It can remove two liters of fluid per day. Therefore, TPN can be used without danger of fluid overload. Usually there is also improvement in the nitrogen balance. There is, however, a greater risk of clotting.

Glomerulopathy

The term **glomerulopathy** includes a group of conditions in which the disease process begins in the glomerulus. Glomerulopathies have been categorized on the basis of their etiology when this is known, on the basis of morphological changes seen in biopsy specimens, and according to their symptoms and clinical manifestations. Such methods of categorization have resulted in a number of variable, and sometimes confusing, classifications. Our concern is with those glomerulopathies classified as **glomerulonephritis**, in which nutritional care is of particular importance.

Etiology and Pathogenesis

Glomerulonephritis frequently occurs following an infection and may also occur as part of the total clinical picture of a number of systemic diseases, including lupus erythematosus, Goodpasture's syndrome, hereditary nephritis (Alport's syndrome), and diabetes mellitus.

It is now believed that most, if not all, of the glomerulonephritides are the result of an immune response.[88-90] There are two general types of immune reactions that have been described.[91] In **immune complex glomerulonephritis**, an antibody is formed in the bloodstream in response to a bacterial or viral infection, to a foreign protein, or to the patient's own tissue in an autoimmune disease. An antigen-antibody-complement complex is formed and becomes trapped in the glomerulus when the circulatory system carries it to the kidney. Poststreptococcal glomerulonephritis is the most commonly occurring example of this form of the disease. In a smaller number of patients, antibodies to the glomerular basement membrane (GBM) develop and form a complex with the GBM and with complement. This is called **anti-GBM disease**. The reason for the development of antibodies to basement membrane is unknown. A classic example of anti-GBM disease is Goodpasture's syndrome. In this syndrome, the antibodies also react with basement membranes of alveoli of the lung, which are antigenically similar.

In either type of disease, complement is transformed into a chemotactic factor that attracts neutrophils. The neutrophils attach to the GBM and damage it by releasing proteolytic enzymes and other mediators of inflammation.

Some forms of glomerulonephritis may not involve the immune system but instead may result from coagulation with deposition of fibrin in the capillaries, or from dysfunction of the mesangial cells,[92] metabolic defects, or hereditary factors. Immune complex disease is thought to account for approximately 70% of the cases, anti-GBM disease for approximately 5%, and all other causes for the remaining 25%.

Pathology

The pathologic changes in the glomerulus in acute glomerulonephritis are characteristically (1) **proliferation** of epithelial, endothelial, or mesangial cells, (2) **exudation** of neutrophils in the glomerulus, and (3) **necrosis** of glomerular capillaries. The degree to which each of these appears is variable, as is the location. The lesions may be **diffuse**, involving any glomeruli, or **focal**, involving only some. They also may be **local** or

segmented — that is, involving only parts of the affected glomeruli.

Proliferative changes also are seen in chronic glomerulonephritis. In addition, **membranous** changes, in which the basement membrane becomes thickened, frequently occur. Other chronic lesions include sclerosis, hyalinization, and scarring. Chronic insults may cause tubular damage and scarring in the interstitium (the space between the nephrons).

Acute Glomerulonephritis

Acute glomerulonephritis is most commonly the result of an infection with a type 4 or type 12 strain of *Streptococcus*. There are other causes, including other organisms and hypersensitivity. Sometimes the cause is unknown.

Clinical Manifestations. Clinical manifestations of acute glomerulonephritis include **hematuria**, **oliguria, proteinuria**, **hypertension**, and **edema**. The red blood cells and protein in the urine may coagulate and form plugs or **casts**. These may be washed out in the final urine by the pressure of the filtrate behind them. The presence of casts sometimes is called **cylindruria** because the casts are cylindrical in shape. If a cast does not wash out, the nephron or nephrons "upstream" from it cease to function. The GFR is reduced, and sometimes tubular function also is depressed.

Treatment. No specific treatment is certain to alter the course of the disease. Currently available treatment is intended to maintain the patient until recovery occurs from natural processes. The usual procedures include bed rest during the acute stage, with gradual ambulation during the recovery phase. Drug treatment may include antibiotics given to remove sources of antigen if the etiology of the disease so indicates. Hypertension is treated by the physician with antihypertensive agents that do not reduce renal blood flow. Diuretics and digitalis may be useful in the treatment of edema and congestive heart failure. Glucocorticoids and cytotoxic drugs are used in some forms of the disease. The nutritional care specialist must be alert to possible drug-nutrient interactions when patients are receiving these drugs.

There is some controversy concerning the need for diet modification, but the following procedures sometimes are used.[93]

Fluid and sodium. Fluid retention, indicated by edema formation, oliguria, and weight gain of more than 3 kg, may be treated by restriction of sodium and fluid on the same basis as is used in chronic and acute renal failure. Oral fluids are limited to 500 ml/day plus the volume of urine output for the previous day. Sodium is limited to 500 mg or less.

Protein. Dietary protein restriction does not alter the course of acute glomerulonephritis; however, a moderate restriction, 40 to 70 g/day, for the azotemic patient sometimes is recommended until there is assurance that the patient is not developing renal failure.[91]

Potassium. Potassium restriction occasionally is indicated as a precaution against hyperkalemia when the patient is oliguric.

Clinical Course. Acute glomerulonephritis varies greatly in the severity of the attack and its further consequences. Most children and 50% to 75% of adults have a complete recovery. The course of the disease in the remaining patients appears to follow one of three forms: (1) progression to **chronic glomerulonephritis**, (2) rapid progression to **subacute glomerulonephritis** with nephron destruction and subsequent renal failure in one to two months, or (3) development of **acute renal failure**.

Chronic Glomerulonephritis

Chronic glomerulonephritis may follow as a consequence of acute poststreptococcal glomerulonephritis, but there are other etiologic factors. It is believed that, because it is so diverse in nature, chronic glomerulonephritis is not a single disease but is, instead, a group of conditions with some characteristics in common. Proteinuria and hematuria commonly occur. If proteinuria is not accompanied by symptoms of protein loss, probably no diet modification is needed. Many patients have **nephrotic syndrome** during the course of the disease. Nutritional care in this condition is reviewed in the next section.

There may be a long latent period, but nephron destruction progresses. Chronic renal failure may ensue in ten years or more and is treated as previously indicated (see pp. 314–317).

Nephrotic Syndrome

Definition and Etiology. The nephrotic syndrome is not a single disease but is, instead, a combination of symptoms that occurs in relation to a number of renal and systemic diseases.

Clinical Manifestations. Nephrotic syndrome is commonly defined by the following clinical manifestations and symptoms. Other symptoms also occur, but vary in incidence and nature depending on the etiology.

Proteinuria. Proteinuria is present, with values of 3.5–30.0 g of protein per day. Normal urinary protein is 150 mg/day or less, commonly 40–80 mg. The proteinuria apparently results from an increased permeability of the basement membrane, which allows the loss of protein into the glomerular filtrate. The mechanism of increased permeability is not understood completely, but the size of the protein molecule in comparison to the size of pores through which they are filtered in the glomeruli seems to be of some significance.[92] In renal disease, the pores may enlarge, allowing protein molecules to be filtered; however, additional factors apparently are important.

There is some evidence that abnormal T lymphocytes produce a factor that alters permeability of the glomerulus to protein.[94,95] Alternatively, it has been suggested that negative electric charges exist on the foot processes of the glomerular epithelium,[96,97] the loss of which permits the proteinuria of nephrotic syndrome.[97] Changes in hemodynamics also may cause proteinuria, even in the absence of alterations in glomerular permeability.[98]

Albumin is lost in the largest quantity, with relatively smaller losses of other proteins, such as gamma globulin, transferrin, ceruloplasmin, and thyroxine-binding protein. The protein loss is apparently the primary disease process, and the other abnormalities develop as a consequence.

Hypoproteinemia. Hypoproteinemia can be severe, with the serum protein concentration as low as 1 g/dl. To some extent, this is attributable to the urinary losses. However, the liver has been shown to be capable of synthesizing 50 g of albumin per day. It could provide replacement if urinary loss were the only abnormality. The presence of hypoalbuminemia in patients losing less than 50 g/day suggests that there are other modes of loss. One of these is increased catabolism of protein, which occurs in the tubule cells of the kidney.[99-102] In addition, there is some evidence of loss by migration of protein out of the blood vessels.[103]

Edema. Edema often is the first manifestation noted by the patient and varies from slight to incapacitating. As serum albumin concentration decreases, the colloid osmotic pressure falls, with transudation of fluid from the circulatory system to the interstitial space. The reduction in circulatory volume (**hypovolemia**) decreases renal blood flow and blood pressure, stimulating the renin-angiotensin-aldosterone system and resulting in increased retention of sodium and water by the distal tubules (**secondary hyperaldosteronism**). The retained sodium and water also leak into the interstitial space, aggravating the edema, until the increased hydrostatic pressure limits further edema formation. The mechanism is summarized in Figure 9-7.

The edema appears first in areas of low tissue turgor and is affected by gravity. Although the edema is generalized (**anasarca**), some patients have edema in the face, partic-

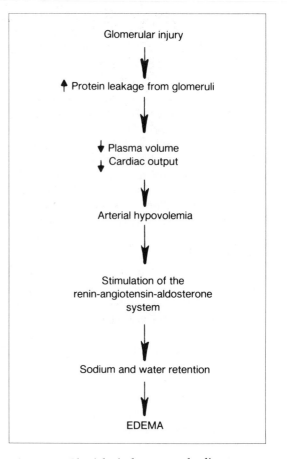

Figure 9-7. Physiological processes leading to edema formation in nephrotic syndrome.

ularly around the eyes (**periorbital edema**), in the morning. Later in the day, the fluid shifts, and the feet and ankles are particularly affected (**pedal edema**). Fluid also accumulates in the pleural cavity, resulting in dyspnea in some patients.

Hyperlipidemia. Hyperlipidemia (see Chapter 10) also occurs commonly in nephrotic syndrome. Its severity is often correlated with the degree of albuminuria. Serum cholesterol levels sometimes are as high as 1,000 g/dl. Phospholipids and triglycerides are elevated. Total serum lipids sometimes reach 5,000 mg/dl. There is also a high ratio of low-density lipoprotein (LDL) to high-density lipoprotein (HDL) (see Chapter 10). It has been suggested that hypoproteinemia enhances hepatic synthesis of lipids, related to decreased serum oncotic pressure, contributing to the lipids in the blood.[104,105] Increased synthesis of lipoproteins by the liver and decreased lipid clearance have been demonstrated in animals.[106,107] The decreased lipid removal may be the consequence of urinary losses of liporegulatory substances.[108] Elevated lipid levels do not always return to normal when the nephrotic syndrome goes into remission.[109] Patients with long-standing nephrotic syndrome have an increased incidence of coronary artery disease to which these alterations in lipid levels may contribute.[110]

Lipiduria. Lipiduria, too, is found in nephrotic patients. The urine contains free fat, oval fat bodies, and fatty casts.

Other manifestations. Other complaints of nephrotic patients include **weakness, anorexia**, and **headaches. Oliguria** is common while edema fluid is accumulating. The protein loss can cause **fatty degeneration of the liver** and **tissue wasting**, especially of muscle and cartilage, but edema may mask the tissue wasting. The loss of protein reduces levels of a number of biologically active proteins and of protein-bound trace elements. The clinical significance of these changes is not known.

Hypocalcemia may also accompany the nephrotic syndrome. Possible contributing causes are hypoalbuminemia, low circulating vitamin D levels, decreased intestinal absorption, and increased losses in the feces.[109] Nephrotic children have been observed to have reduced bone mineralization and retarded growth, but the retarded growth is more likely to result from malnutrition and steroid therapy.[109]

Treatment. The main element of therapy for nephrotic syndrome are diet and the use of diuretic drugs. Some patients receive steroids and other drugs.

Diuretic drugs. Diuretic drugs increase the volume of urine produced by inhibiting tubular reabsorption of filtered sodium. They then induce a contraction of blood volume, which leads to a decrease in renal plasma flow and GFR and an increase in function of the renin-angiotensin-aldosterone system. This counteracts the drug effect, and a new steady state with less fluid is established. The patient is more comfortable, but diuretics are not known to alter the course of the disease.

These drugs are useful in the management of several forms of renal disease, including nephrotic syndrome, renal failure, and renal calculi. In addition, they are of value in the management of other chronic conditions, such as hypertension, chronic congestive heart failure, and cirrhosis of the liver with ascites. Since diuretics are used more frequently in the management of hypertension, details of their action and a list of available drugs is given in Table 10-6.

Moderate sodium restriction often is prescribed for the patient receiving diuretic drugs, but the diet need not be as restricted as it was before diuretics were available. Therefore, the diet now is more acceptable and patient compliance is improved. Moderate salt restriction makes it possible to reduce the drug dosage, thus moderating any side effects of the drug. The use of a severely sodium-restricted diet in combination with a potent diuretic may increase the risk of hyponatremia and ARF.

A side effect of diuretic action is an increase in potassium excretion by one of two mechanisms. Diuretics increase the release of aldosterone, which stimulates potassium excretion, or they increase the amount of sodium reaching the distal tubules and collecting ducts, where it may be exchanged for potassium. Potassium depletion occurs in some patients if dietary intake is inadequate for replacement. Mild symptoms of depletion can often be avoided by increasing the intake of foods high in potassium. Potassium supplements often are given by medication if depletion becomes more marked. The question of supplements versus diet for this purpose is discussed in more detail in the next section.

Diet. The diet should have sufficient **protein** to provide for current needs, including continuing losses.

Compensation for the protein depletion commonly seen in these patients by using a high protein diet has been shown to be unsuccessful. Instead, an increase in protein intake results in increased albuminuria, and increased protein catabolism to urea.[111] Investigations in animal models have demonstrated that intake of a high protein meal is followed by an increase in renal blood flow, hydrostatic pressure, and glomerular filtration rate. These changes may accelerate the progression of renal damage.

Usually 0.8 to 1.0 g protein per kg body weight is recommended.[109] This protein should be of high biologic value to reduce the accumulation of nitrogenous metabolites. It is important that sufficient nonprotein sources of **energy** be supplied so that protein is not catabolized to meet the patient's energy needs, particularly if the patient is azotemic. Provision for 35 to 60 kcal per kg of ideal body weight per day is often desirable depending on the patient's body weight.

If the patient is anorexic, assurance of adequate energy intake becomes a particularly challenging problem. Those patients who are receiving steroid drugs, however, usually have good appetites.

The high levels of serum **lipids** and the increased incidence of cardiovascular disease have led to the suggestion that the diet be modified to decrease the hyperlipidemia (see Chapter 10).[112] Although this seems a logical course of action, there is as yet no evidence that nephrotic patients benefit by such treatment. The effect of another modification on acceptability of the diet and, thus, on protein and energy intake must be considered. Regular aerobic exercise is also recommended.

The comparative values of **sodium restriction** and of the use of diuretic drugs in nephrotic syndrome is a matter of controversy. In general, if the edema is mild or moderate, a moderate sodium restriction of 800 to 1,600 mg, combined with diuretic medication is considered useful. If edema is severe, dietary sodium might theoretically be reduced to as low as 250 mg/day but only at the expense of reduced protein intake, since protein foods contain appreciable quantities of sodium. Generally, if the patient complies with the sodium restriction, no fluid restriction is necessary. High protein and low sodium levels are difficult to plan in the same diet and are incompatible at the extremes. In addition, the diets tend to be unappetizing. Some patients increase their food intake if they are provided with a substitute for salt. When a choice must be made between increasing protein and further restricting sodium, it usually is considered more important to provide sufficient protein in the diet and use diuretics to correct the edema.

Potassium loss and resultant hypokalemia (serum potassium less than 3.5 mEq/L) can result from the use of furosemide and thiazides in renal patients and in patients taking such drugs for other conditions. Hypokalemia can occur, for example, in the many patients taking thiazides for control of hypertension. It is a frequent practice to prescribe potassium supplements as medication for these patients. These supplements have an extremely unpleasant taste and are gastric irritants.

Increased potassium can be supplied by appropriate modification of the diet, as a safe and more palatable alternative. The procedures listed in Table 9-16 are appropriate general guidelines.

Diabetic Renal Disease

It has been estimated that 50% of child diabetics will develop serious renal disease and that renal disease contributes to mortality in 30–40% of maturity-onset diabetes cases.[113] Among dialysis patients, 25% are diabetic. There are 24,000 of these patients.

Diabetic nephropathy is indicated by the presence of proteinuria greater than 0.5 g per day. The proteinuria indicates significant damage to the glomerular filtration mechanism. Some patients have small amounts of low molecular weight albumin, known as *microalbuminemia,* which can be detected in

Table 9-16. Procedures for Planning the High-Potassium Diet

Increase the intake of fruit and vegetables that are high in potassium. These are listed in most diet manuals.

Substitute whole grain for refined cereals.

Increase high-protein foods, particularly milk and fish.

Reduce the servings of refined foods.

Prepare foods to conserve the potassium content. Use small amounts of water or cook with dry heat.

With the physician's concurrence, use a potassium-containing salt substitute.

very sensitive tests. It is currently considered that more than 15 μg albumin per minute indicates progression to future development of renal disease. Patients with less than 15 μg albumin per minute in the urine are considered not to be at risk.

The mechanisms involved in the renal damage is not entirely understood, but some information is available from animal studies. It is postulated that as nephrons are damaged, there develops some hyperfiltration that may reach a GFR of 150 ml/min. The kidney hypertrophies and there is an increase in pressure in the blood vessels in the kidneys. Microalbuminemia appears at first only during periods of poor diabetic control (see Chapter 11). In 10 to 20 years, there develops a reduction of renal function which proceeds to failure in the following five to ten years.

In animals, the degenerative process can be treated with angiotensin-converting enzyme inhibitors and a low-protein diet to prevent the proteinuria and progression of the renal damage. It is not clear whether the same mechanism occurs in human patients and whether other mechanisms also contribute. Some of these other mechanisms could include glycosylation of glomerular tissue, alterations in cell metabolism, and abnormalities in counterregulatory hormones.

At the present time, approaches to prevention and treatment of this condition include:

Careful control of blood pressure (see Chapter 10).

Administration of angiotensin-converting enzyme inhibitors to help slow renal degeneration, although the effectiveness of this drug in incipient nephropathy is unknown.

Careful glycemic control (see Chapter 11).

It is currently recommended that the diet be modified early in those patients who have a tendency to nephropathy. These patients may also need dialysis early in the course of their renal disease than is usual in other patients.

Recommended protein levels are 0.6 g per kg of ideal body weight, low phosphorus, and limited sodium. The protein restriction is often difficult and must be approached in stepwise fashion to improve compliance.

The diabetic diet must be combined with the diet modifications indicated during the period of declining renal function. The reduction of protein intake is accompanied by increases in carbohydrate and fat, a recommendation that many diabetic patients find startling and sometimes disturbing.

As renal function diminishes, the half-life of insulin increases, so that the diabetes becomes less severe. It is believed that this process occurs because the kidney excretes insulin more slowly and because decreased insulinase production by the diseased kidney results in prolonged insulin action and amelioration of the diabetes.

When a patient receives a renal transplant, the insulin requirement increases significantly as corticosteroids are given for immunosuppression. Approximately one year postoperatively, the patient returns to nearly the same severity of diabetes that existed prior to the onset of manifest renal disease. The patient's appetite and activity often increase considerably following transplant.

It is necessary to monitor the nutritional status of the patient frequently during these various stages of his or her disease. The diabetic diet must be adjusted carefully to meet the patient's changing needs related to the severity of both the diabetes and the renal disease.

Case Study: Renal Failure

Mary M., age 12, developed strep throat. A week later her ankles and eyelids were puffy and her urine was reddish brown. She was hospitalized with gross hematuria, 4+ proteinuria, and oliguria of 400 ml/day. Her blood pressure was 155/108, and the hemoglobin was 10.2 g/dl. She was given bed rest and a low-salt diet. In ten days, Mary's blood pressure was 125/87, she had lost 6 kg of body weight, and albuminuria was 1+.

Fifteen years later, Mary noted that she had swollen ankles and felt tired at the end of the day. She had nocturia and had gained 10 pounds in six weeks. Her blood pressure was 150/95. A renal biopsy showed hyalinized and sclerosing glomeruli. Laboratory test results were as follows:

SUN	45 mg/dl
Serum creatinine	2 mg/dl
Creatinine clearance	15 ml/min.
Serum phosphorus	5.9 mg/dl
Serum calcium	8.3 mg/dl
Hemoglobin	9.9 g/dl
Hematocrit	33%
Serum sodium	144 mEq/L
Serum potassium	4 mEq/L
Serum albumin	3.5 g/dl
Urine specific gravity	1.01
Urine volume	1,500 ml/day
Proteinuria	2+

She was given a diet with 40 g of high-biologic-value protein, 2,500 kcal, and 43 mEq of sodium. Furosemide (Lasix) 60 mg per day was prescribed.

After several more years, Mary began to experience headaches, nausea and vomiting, weight loss, hypertension, polyuria, and muscle cramps. The furosemide dosage was increased, and methyldopa (Aldomet), 250 mg three times daily, was added as an antihypertensive agent. A solution of sodium citrate and citric acid was prescribed to correct acidosis. However, the patient became anemic and was weak, irritable, drowsy, and forgetful. Laboratory results were as follows:

SUN	112 mg/dl
Serum creatinine	10 mg/dl
Creatinine clearance	6 ml/min
Serum potassium	5 mEq/L
Serum phosphorus	7 mEq/L
Blood pH	7.35
Proteinuria	3+

Mary was scheduled for dialysis three times per week. A diet with 60 g protein, 2,000 kcal, a sodium intake of 150 mEq/day, 1,500 ml of fluid, and 75 mEq of potassium was prescribed. Folate, pyridoxine, ascorbic acid, water-soluble vitamins, and iron were given as supplements.

Exercises

1. Explain the rationale for the diet modifications used during the original infection.
2. Compare the laboratory results with normal values.
3. Which laboratory values indicate the following?
   a. Problems with solute reabsorption? Problems with excretion?
   b. Problems with protein homeostasis?
   c. Decreasing ability of the renal tubules to regulate fluid balance?
4. Explain the purpose of each medication.
5. Explain the rationale for each diet modification during renal failure.
6. Explain the pathogenesis of the following clinical manifestations in this patient: nocturia; polyuria; anemia; proteinuria; sodium retention; increased serum potassium; decreased creatinine clearance; increased SUN; acidosis.

References

1. Rabkin, R., Glaser, T., and Peterson, J. Renal peptide hormone metabolism. *The Kidney* 16:25, 1983.
2. Kopple, J.D., and Fukuda, S. Effects of amino acid infusion and renal failure on the uptake and release of amino acids by the dog kidney. *Am. J. Clin. Nutr.* 33:1363, 1980.
3. Tizianello, A., DeFerrari, G., Garibotto, G., Furreri, G., and Robaudo, D. Renal metabolism of amino acids and ammonia in subjects with normal renal function and in patients with chronic renal insufficiency. *J. Clin. Invest.* 65:1162, 1980.
4. Owen, O.E., Felig, P., Morgan, A.P., Wahren, J., and Cahill, G.F., Jr. Liver and kidney metabolism during prolonged starvation. *J. Clin. Invest.* 48:574, 1969.
5. Rennick, B., Acara, M., Hysert, P., and Mookerjee, B. Choline loss during hemodialysis. Homeostatic control of plasma choline. *Kidney Int.* 10:329, 1976.
6. Bricker, N.S., Klahr, S., Lubowitz, H., and Rieselbach, R.E. Renal function in chronic

renal disease. *Medicine* (Baltimore) 44:263, 1965.

7. Bricker, N.S. On the meaning of the intact nephron hypothesis. *Am. J. Med.* 46:1, 1969.

8. Bricker, N.S., Bourgoignie, J.J., and Weber, H. The renal response to progressive nephron loss. In B.M. Brenner and F.C. Rector, Jr., Eds., *The Kidney.* Philadelphia: W.B. Saunders, 1976.

9. Bricker, N.S. On the pathogenesis of the uremic state. An exposition of the "trade off" hypothesis. *N. Engl. J. Med.* 286:1093, 1972.

10. Garber, A.J. Skeletal muscle protein and amino acid metabolism in experimental chronic uremia in the rat. *J. Clin. Invest.* 62:623, 1978.

11. Harter, H.R., Karl, I.E., Klahr, S., and Kipnis, D.M. Effects of renal mass and dietary protein intake on amino acid and glucose uptake by rat muscle in vitro. *J. Clin. Invest.* 64:513, 1979.

12. DeFronzo, R.A., Smith, D., and Alvestrand, A. Insulin action in uremia. *Kidney Int.* 24 (Suppl. 16):S102, 1983.

13. Deferrari, G., Garibotto, G., Robaudo, C., Canepa, A., Bagnesco, S., and Tizianello, A. Leg metabolism of amino acids and ammonia in patients with chronic renal failure. *Clin. Sci.* 69:143, 1985.

14. DeFronzo, R.A., Alvestrand, A., Smith, D., Hendler, R., Hendler, E., and Wahren, J. Insulin resistance in uremia. *J. Clin. Invest.* 67:563, 1981.

15. Alvestrand, D. Amino acid metabolism in patients with chronic renal failure. *Clin. Nutr.* 4 (Suppl.):14, 1985.

16. Welt, L.B., Black, H.R., and Krueger, K.K., Eds. Symposium on renal toxins. *Arch. Intern. Med.* 126:773, 1970.

17. Feldman, H.A., and Singer, I. Endocrinology and metabolism in uremia and dialysis. A clinical review. *Medicine* (Baltimore) 54:345, 1974.

18. Avram, M.M. Parathyroid hormone in kidney failure. *Contrib. Nephrol.* 20:1, 1980.

19. Bergstrom, J., Furst, P., Josephson, B., and Noru, L.O. Improvement of nitrogen balance in a uremic patient by the addition of histidine to essential amino acid solutions given intravenously. *Life Sci. (II)* 9:787, 1980.

20. Kopple, J.D. Nutrition and the kidney. In R.B. Alfin-Slater and D. Kritchevsky, Eds., *Human Nutrition: A Comprehensive Treatise,* vol. 4. New York: Plenum Press, 1979, p. 409.

21. Alvestrand, A., and Bergstrom, J. Renal diseases. In J.M. Kinney, K.N. Jeejeebhoy, G.L. Hill, and O.E. Owen, Eds., *Nutrition and Metabolism in Patient Care.* Philadelphia: W.B. Saunders, 1988.

22. Maillet, C., and Garber, A.J. Skeletal muscle amino acid metabolism in chronic uremia. *Am. J. Clin. Nutr.* 33:1438, 1980.

23. Gulyassey, P.F., Avram, A., Peters, J.H. Evaluation of amino acid and protein requirements in chronic uremia. *Arch. Intern. Med.* 126:855, 1970.

24. Young, G.A., Parsons, F.M. Plasma amino acid imbalance in patients with chronic renal failure on intermittent dialysis. *Clin. Chim. Acta* 27:491, 1970.

25. Alvestrand, A., Bergstrom, J., and Furst, P. Plasma and muscle free amino acids in uremia. Influence of nutrition with amino acids. *Clin. Nephrol.* 18:297, 1982.

26. Young, F.A., and Parson, F.M. Impairment of phenylalanine hydroxylation in chronic renal insufficiency. *Clin. Sci. Mol. Med.* 48:89, 1973.

27. Giordano, C., DeSanto, N.G., Rimaldi, S., et al. Histidine for treatment of uremic anemia. *Br. Med. J.* 4:714, 1973.

28. Meneely, G.R., and Battarbee, R.D. Sodium and potassium. *Nutr. Rev.* 34D:225, 1976.

29. Contreras, R.J. Salt taste and disease. *Am. J. Clin. Nutr.* 31:1088, 1978.

30. Burns, E.R., and Neubort, S. Sodium content of koshered meat. *J. Am. Med. Assoc.* 252:2960, 1984.

31. Kopple, J.D., and Coburn, J.W. Metabolic studies of low protein diets in uremia. I. Nitrogen and potassium. *Medicine* (Baltimore) 52:583, 1973.

32. Slatopolsky, E., Caglar, S., Pennell, J.P., et al. On the pathogenesis of hyperparathyroidism in experimental chronic renal insufficiency in the dog. *J. Clin. Invest.* 50:492, 1971.

33. Slatopolsky, E., Caglar, S., Gradowska, L., et al. On the prevention of secondary hyperthyroidism in experimental chronic renal disease using the proportional reduction of dietary phosphorus intake. *Kidney Int.* 2:147, 1972.

34. Hanley, D.A., and Sherwood, L.M. Secondary hyperparathyroidism in chronic renal failure. *Med. Clin. North Am.* 62:1319, 1978.

35. Maschio, G., Tessitore, N., D'Angelo, A., et al. Early dietary phosphorus restriction and supplementation in the prevention of renal osteodystrophy. *Am. J. Clin. Nutr.* 33:1546, 1980.

36. Alfrey, A.C., and Smythe, W.R. Trace element abnormalities in chronic uremia. In B.B. Mackey, Ed., *Tenth Annual Contractors*

Conference of the Artificial Kidney and Chronic Uremia Program of the National Institute of Arthritis, Metabolism and Digestive Diseases (AKCUP-NIAMDD). DHEW Publication no. 77–1442. Bethesda: National Institutes of Health, 1977, p. 37.

37. Pemberton, C.M., Moxness, K.E., German, M.J., Nelson, J.K., and Gastineau, C.F., Eds. *Mayo Clinic Diet Manual,* 6th ed. Toronto: B.C. Decker, 1988.

38. Maschia, G., Oldrizzi, L., Tessitore, N., D'Angelo, A., Valso, E., Lupo, A., Loschiavo, C., Fabris, A., Gammard, L., Rigiu, C., and Penzetto, G. Effects of dietary protein and phosphorus restrictions on the progression of early renal failure. *Kidney Int.* 22:371, 1982.

39. Walser, M. Ketoacids in the treatment of uremia. *Clin. Nephrol.* 3:180, 1975.

40. Barsotti, G., Guiducci, A., Ciardella, F., and Giovanetti, S. Effects on renal function of a low-nitrogen diet supplemented with essential amino acids and ketoanalogues and of hemodialysis and free protein supply in patients with chronic renal failure. *Nephron* 27:113, 1981.

41. Alvestrand, A., Ahlberg, M., Furst, P., and Bergstrom, J. Clinical experience with amino acids and keto acid diets. *Am. J. Clin. Nutr.* 33:1654, 1980.

42. Walser, M. Keto-analogues of essential amino acids. In *Clinical Nutrition Update: Amino Acids.* Chicago: American Medical Association, 1977.

43. Mitch, W.E., Walser, M., Steinman, T.I., Hill, S., Zeger, S., and Tungsanga, K. The effect of a keto acid–amino acid supplement to a restricted diet on the progression of chronic renal failure. *N. Engl. J. Med.* 311:623, 1984.

44. Bergstrom, J., Lindblom, U., and Noree, L.-O. Preservation of peripheral nerve function in severe uremia during treatment with low protein high calorie diet and surplus of essential amino acids. *Acta Neurol. Scand.* 51:99, 1975.

45. Piper, C. Very-low-protein diets in chronic renal failure. Nutrient content and guidelines for supplementation. *J. Am. Diet. Assoc.* 85:1344, 1985.

46. Walser, M., Imbembo, A.L., Margolis, S., and Elfert, G.A., Eds. *Nutritional Management: The Johns Hopkins Handbook.* Philadelphia: W.B. Saunders, 1984.

47. Van Duyne, M.A.S. Acceptability of selected low-protein products for use in a potential diet therapy for chronic renal failure. *J. Am. Diet. Assoc.* 87:909, 1987.

48. Atkin-Thor, E., Goddard, B.W., O'Nion, J., et al. Hypogeusia and zinc depletion in chronic dialysis patients. *Am. J. Clin. Nutr.* 31:1948, 1978.

49. DeFronzo, R.A., Andres, R., Edgar, P., and Walker, W.G. Carbohydrate metabolism in uremia. A review. *Medicine* (Baltimore) 52:469, 1973.

50. Dzurik, T., Niederland, T.R., and Cernacek, P. Carbohydrate metabolism by rat liver slices incubated in serum obtained from uraemic patients. *Clin. Sci.* 37:409, 1969.

51. Lowrie, E.G., Soeldner, J.S., Hampers, C.L., and Merrill, J.P. Glucose metabolism and insulin secretion in uremic prediabetic and normal subjects. *J. Lab. Clin. Med.* 76:603, 1970.

52. DeFronzo, R.A., and Alvestrand, A. Glucose intolerance in uremia. Site and mechanism. *Am. J. Clin. Nutr.* 33:1438, 1980.

53. Bagdade, J.D., Porte, D., Jr., and Bierman, E.L. Hypertriglyceridemia. A metabolic consequence of chronic renal failure. *N. Engl. J. Med.* 279:181, 1968.

54. Lindner, A., Charra, B., Sherrard, D., and Scribner, B.H. Accelerated atherosclerosis in prolonged maintenance hemodialysis. *N. Engl. J. Med.* 290:697, 1974.

55. Bonomini, V., Feletti, C., Scolari, M.P., et al. Atherosclerosis in uremia. A longitudinal study. *Am. J. Clin. Nutr.* 33:1493, 1980.

56. Kleinknect, D., Jungers, D., Chanard, J., et al. Uremic and nonuremic complications in acute renal failure. Evaluation of early and frequent dialysis on prognosis. *Kidney Int.* 1:190, 1972.

57. Holliday, M.A., McHenry-Richardson, D., and Portale, A. Nutritional management of chronic renal disease. *Med. Clin. N. Amer.* 63:645, 1979.

58. Zeman, F.J., and Ney, D.M. *Applications of Clinical Nutrition.* Englewood Cliffs, N.J.: Prentice-Hall, 1988.

59. Campbell, J.D., and Campbell, A.R. The social and economic costs of end-stage renal disease. *N. Engl. J. Med.* 299:386, 1978.

60. Callabresse, J.C., Larson, G., Loomteax, G., et al. Lipids and lipoprotein in chronic uraemia. A study of the influence of regular hemodialysis. *Eur. J. Clin. Invest.* 6:159, 1976.

61. McCask, E.J. Hypertriglyceridemia in patients with chronic renal insufficiency. *Am. J. Clin. Nutr.* 28:1036, 1975.

62. Hussey, H.H. Hyperlipidemia in children following long term hemodialysis or renal transplantation. *J.A.M.A.* 236:1387, 1976.

63. Gokal, R., Mann, D.M., Oliver, D.O., and Ledingham, J.G.G. Dietary treatment of hyperlipidemia in chronic hemodialysis patients. *Am. J. Clin. Nutr.* 31:1915, 1978.

64. Sanfelippo, M.S., Swenson, R.S., and Reaven, G.M. Response of plasma triglycerides to dietary changes in patients on hemodialysis. *Kidney Int.* 14:180, 1978.

65. Brunner, F.P., Brynger, H., Chantler, C., et al. Combined Report on Regular Dialysis and Transplantation in Europe IX. *1978 Proc. Eur. Dial. Transplant Assoc.* 16:3, 1979.

66. Burke, J.F., Francos, G.C., Moore, L.L., et al. Accelerated atherosclerosis in chronic-dialysis patients—another look. *Nephron* 21:181, 1978.

67. Rostand, S.G., Gretes, J.C., Kirk, K.A., et al. Ischemic heart disease in patients with uremia undergoing maintenance hemodialysis. *Kidney Int.* 16:600, 1979.

68. Nicholls, A.J., Catto, G.R.D., Edward, N., et al. Accelerated atherosclerosis in long-term dialysis and renal transplant patients. Fact or fiction? *Lancet* 1:276, 1980.

69. Vincenti, F., Amend, W.J., Abele, J., et al. The role of hypertension in hemodialysis-associated atherosclerosis. *Am. J. Med.* 68:363, 1980.

70. Epstein, F.H., and Merrill, J.P. Chronic renal failure. In G.W. Thorn, R.D. Adams, F. Braunwald, et al., Eds., *Harrison's Principles of Internal Medicine*, 8th ed. New York: McGraw-Hill, 1977.

71. Aeropoulos, D.G. Chronic peritoneal dialysis. *Clin. Nephrol.* 9:165, 1978.

72. Vaamonde, C.A. Peritoneal dialysis. Current status. *Postgrad. Med.* 62:148, 1977.

73. Blumenkrantz, M.J., Roberts, C.E., Card, B., et al. Nutritional management of the adult patient undergoing peritoneal dialysis. *J. Am. Diet. Assoc.* 73:251, 1978.

74. Moncrief, J.W., and Popovich, R.P. Continuous ambulatory peritoneal dialysis. *Contrib. Nephrol.* 17:139, 1979.

75. Giordano, C., and DeSanto, N.G. Dietary management of patients on peritoneal dialysis. *Contrib. Nephrol.* 17:17, 1979.

76. Blumenkrantz, M.J., Kopple, J.D., and V.A. Cooperative Dialysis Study Participants. Incidence of nutritional abnormalities in uremic patients entering dialysis therapy. *Kidney Int.* 10:514, 1976.

77. Coburn, J.W., Blumenkrantz, M.J., and Kopple, J.D. *Controlled Evaluation of Maintenance Peritoneal Dialysis.* Technical Report No. 2, AKCUP-NIAMDD. Bethesda: National Institutes of Health, 1977, p. 120.

78. *A Clinical Guide to Nutrition Care in End-Stage Renal Disease*, ed. D. Gillit, J. Stover, and N.S. Spinozzi. Chicago: American Dietetic Association, 1987.

79. Grodstein, G.P., Blumenkrantz, J.J., Kopple, J.D., Moran, J.K., and Coburn, J.W. Glucose absorption during continuous ambulatory peritoneal dialysis. *Kidney Int.* 19:564, 1981.

80. Bergstrom, J. Introductory remarks. Potential metabolic problems associated with continuous ambulatory peritoneal dialysis. In M. Legrain, Ed., *Continuous Ambulatory Peritoneal Dialysis.* Amsterdam: Excerpta Medica, 1980.

81. Lindholm, B., Aklberg, M., Alvestrand, A., et al. Nutritional aspects of continuous ambulatory peritoneal dialysis. In M. Legrain, Ed., *Continuous Ambulatory Peritoneal Dialysis.* Amsterdam: Excerpta Medica, 1980.

82. Bartlow, B.G. Hyperlipidemia of end-stage renal disease. *Dial. Transplant.* 9:625, 1980.

83. Wells, E. Renal dietitian. Nutritional needs of continuous ambulatory peritoneal dialysis patients. *Dial. Transplant.* 9:988, 1980.

84. VanBuren, C.T., and Kahan, B.D. The renal transplant patient. In J.M. Kinney, K.N. Jeejeebhoy, G.L. Hill, and H.E. Owen, Eds. *Nutrition and Metabolism in Patient Care.* Philadelphia: W.B. Saunders, 1988.

85. Rogen, M., Hull, A., and Davis, M., Eds. *Nutrition Support of the Renal Patient*, 1988.

86. Mirtallo, J.M., Kudsk, K.A., and Elbert, M.L. Nutrition of patients with renal disease. *Clin. Pharm.* 3:253, 263, 1984 (May-June).

87. Kopple, J.D. Nutrition, diet and the kidney. In M.E. Shils and V.R. Young, Eds., *Modern Nutrition in Health and Disease*, 7th ed. Philadelphia: Lea & Febiger, 1988.

88. Unanue, E.R., and Dixon, F.J. Experimental glomerulonephritis. Immunological events and pathogenetic mechanisms. *Adv. Immunol.* 6:1, 1967.

89. McClusky, R.T. Immunologic mechanisms in renal disease. In R.H. Heptinstall, Ed., *Pathology of the Kidney*, 2nd ed. Boston: Little, Brown, 1974.

90. Wilson, C.B., and Dixon, F.J. Diagnosis of immunopathologic renal disease. *Kidney Int.* 5:389, 1974.

91. Dixon, F.J. Glomerulonephritis and immunopathology. *Hosp. Pract.* 2:35, 1967.

92. Schrier, R.C. Glomerular diseases. In G.W. Thorn, R.D. Adams, F. Braunwald, et al., Eds., *Harrison's Principles of Internal Medicine*, 8th ed. New York: McGraw-Hill, 1977.

93. Wrong, O.M. Glomerulonephritis. In P.B. Beeson, W. McDermott, and J.B. Wyngaarden, Eds., *Cecil's Textbook of Medicine*, 15th ed. Philadelphia: W.B. Saunders, 1979.

94. Shalkoub, R.J. Pathogenesis of lipoid nephrosis. A disorder of T-cell function. *Lancet* 2:556, 1974.

95. Giangiacomo, J., Cleary, T.G., Cole, B.R., et al. Serum immunoglobulins in the nephrotic syndrome. *N. Engl. J. Med.* 293:8, 1975.

96. Brenner, B.M., Hostetter, T.H., and Humes, H.D. Molecular basis of proteinuria of molecular origin. *N. Engl. J. Med.* 298:826, 1978.

97. Blau, E.B., and Haas, D.E. Glomerular sialic acid and proteinuria in human renal disease. *Lab. Invest.* 28:447, 1973.

98. Bohrer, M.P., Dien, W.M., Robertson, C.R., and Brenner, B.M. Mechanism of angiotensin II–induced proteinuria in the rat. *Am. J. Physiol.* 2:F13, 1977.

99. Gitlin, D., Janeway, C.A., and Farr, L.E. Studies on the metabolism of plasma proteins in the nephrotic syndrome. I. Albumin, globulin and iron-binding globulin. *J. Clin. Invest.* 35:44, 1956.

100. Kaitz, A.L. Albumin metabolism in nephrotic adults. *J. Lab. Clin. Med.* 53:186, 1959.

101. Jensen, H., Rossing, N., Andersen, S.B., and Jarnum, S. Albumin metabolism in the nephrotic syndrome in adults. *Clin. Sci.* 33:445, 1967.

102. Strober, W., and Waldman, T.A. The role of the kidney in the metabolism of plasma proteins. *Nephron* 13:35, 1974.

103. Walker, W.A., Ulstrom, R.A., and Lowman, J.T. Albumin synthesis rates in patients with hypoproteinemia. *J. Pediatr.* 78:812, 1971.

104. Rosenman, R.H., Friedman, M., and Byers, S.O. The causal role of plasma albumin deficiency in experimental nephrotic hyperlipidemia and hypercholesteremia. *J. Clin. Invest.* 35:522, 1956.

105. Marsh, J.B. Lipoprotein metabolism in experimental nephrosis. *J. Lipid Res.* 25:1619, 1984.

106. Radding, C.M., and Steinberg, D. Studies on the synthesis and secretion of serum lipoproteins by rat liver slices. *J. Clin. Invest.* 39:1560, 1960.

107. McKenzie, I.F.C., and Nestel, P.J. Studies on the turnover of triglyceride and esterified cholesterol in subjects with the nephrotic syndrome. *J. Clin. Invest.* 47:1685, 1968.

108. Staprans, I., Felts, J.M., and Souser, W.G. Glycosaminoglycans and chylomicron metabolism in control and nephrotic rats. *Metabolism* 36:496, 1987.

109. Strauss, J., Zilleruelo, G., Freundlich, M., and Abitol, C. Less commonly recognized features of childhood nephrotic syndrome. *Pediatr. Clin. North Am.* 34:591, 1987.

110. Berlyne, G.M., and Mallick, N.P. Ischaemic heart-disease as a complication of nephrotic syndrome. *Lancet* 2:399, 1969.

111. Kaysen, G.A. et al. Effect of dietary protein intake on albumin homeostasis in enphrotic patients. *Kidney Int.* 29:572, 1986.

Bibliography

Arieff, A.I., DeFronzo, R.A. *Fluid, Electrolyte and Acid-Base Disorders.* New York: Churchill Livingstone, 1986.

Brenner, B.M., and Rector, F.C., Jr. *The Kidney,* 3rd ed. Philadelphia: W.B. Saunders, 1986.

Denny, M.E., Kelly, M.P., and Esrey, T.O. *Pre–End Stage Renal Disease: A Guide for the Professional Nutritionist.* Council on Renal Nutrition, Northern California/Northern Nevada, 1986.

Fine, R.N., and Gruskin, A.B. *End Stage Renal Disease in Children.* Philadelphia: W.B. Saunders, 1984.

Freund, H.R. Renal failure. In C.E. Lang, Ed., *Nutritional Support in Critical Care.* Rockville, Md.: Aspen, 1987.

Guyton, A.C. *Textbook of Medical Physiology,* 6th ed. Philadelphia: W.B. Saunders, 1981.

Kopple, J.D. Nutritional therapy in kidney failure. *Nutr. Rev.* 39:193, 1981.

Kopple, J.D., Massry, S.G., Bonomini, V., and Heidland, A. Symposium on nutrition in renal disease. *Am. J. Clin. Nutr.* 33:1343, 1980.

Legrain, M., Ed. *Continuous Ambulatory Peritoneal Dialysis.* Amsterdam: Excerpta Medica, 1980.

Nissenson, A.R., Fine, R.N., and Gentile, D.E., Eds. *Clinical Dialysis,* 2nd ed. Norwalk, Conn.: Appleton and Lange, 1990.

Nolph, K.D., Gahl, G.M., and Kessel, M. *Advances in Peritoneal Dialysis. Proceedings of the Second International Symposium on Periotoneal Dialysis.* Berlin, June 16–19, 1981. Amsterdam: Excerpta Medica, 1981.

Sources of Current Information

Clinical Nephrology
Contributions to Nephrology
Kidney International
Nephron

10. The Cardiovascular System

Denise M. Ney, Ph.D., R.D.

I. The Normal Circulatory System
   A. Heart
   B. Vascular system
      1. Circulation to specific areas
         a. coronary
         b. cerebral
         c. splanchnic
         d. fetal
      2. Blood Vessels
         a. structure
         b. types
   C. Blood pressure
      1. Cardiac output
      2. Peripheral vascular resistance
      3. Measurement of blood pressure
      4. Regulation of blood pressure
         a. sympathetic nervous system
         b. renin-angiotensin system
         c. kidney
         d. other factors
            (1) eicosanoids
            (2) natriuretic factors
            (3) kinins

II. Hypertension
   A. Classification
      1. Secondary
      2. Essential
   B. Consequences of uncontrolled hypertension
   C. Management
      1. Diet
         a. weight reduction
         b. sodium restriction
         c. alcohol restriction
         d. potassium
         e. other diet components
      2. Drugs

III. Hyperlipidemia
   A. Cholesterol
   B. Lipoproteins
      1. Classification
      2. Metabolism
         a. exogenous transport
         b. endogenous transport
         c. HDL metabolism
   C. Effects of diet on plasma lipids
      1. Cholesterol
      2. Type and amount of dietary fat
         a. fatty acid saturation
         b. fish oil or omega-3 fatty acids
      3. Calories and carbohydrates
      4. Dietary fiber
      5. Alcohol
   D. Classification and treatment
      1. Hyperlipidemia and hyperlipoproteinemia
         a. classification of hyperlipoproteinemia
         b. familial hypercholesterolemia
         c. familial combined hyperlipidemia
      2. Drug management

IV. Atherosclerosis
   A. Etiology
   B. The Lesion
   C. Pathogenesis

V. Coronary Heart Disease
   A. Angina pectoris
   B. Myocardial infarction
      1. Clinical manifestations and diagnosis
      2. Clinical course
      3. Management

VI. Congestive Heart Failure
   A. Pathogenesis
   B. Salt and water retention
   C. Clinical manifestations
   D. Management
      1. Nutritional care
      2. Drugs

VII. Cerebrovascular Disease

VIII. Peripheral Vascular Atherosclerotic Occlusive Disease

IX. Cardiac Cachexia
   A. Clinical manifestations and diagnosis
   B. Treatment

X. Rheumatic Heart Disease

XI. Congenital Heart Disease
   A. Clinical manifestations and pathogenesis
   B. Nutritional management

XII. Heart Disease and Alcoholism

XIII. Case Study

339

Diseases of the cardiovascular system are the leading cause of death in the United States. The etiology of cardiovascular diseases is multifactorial and involves genetic, behavioral, and nutritional components. Nutrition is considered to be a major factor in both the prevention and treatment of cardiovascular disease.

THE NORMAL CIRCULATORY SYSTEM

The cardiovascular system consists of the heart and blood vessels, and it performs three main functions. The heart regulates blood flow to the tissues to deliver the optimal amount of nutrients and retrieve wastes from cell metabolism. The system also serves to regulate body temperature, by alterations in blood flow to the skin. Finally, the cardiovascular system distributes hormones and other endogenous metabolites within the body.

Figure 10-1. The heart and great vessels and the route of blood flow through them. Dark shaded area indicates venous blood flow (low in oxygen). Light shaded area indicates arterial blood flow (high in oxygen). (Reprinted with permission from Memmler, R.L., and Rada, R.B., The Human Body in Health and Disease, *5th ed. Philadelphia: J.B. Lippincott, 1983, p. 172.)*

Heart

The heart is composed of a pair of hollow pumps separated by a **septum**. Each pump consists of an atrium and a ventricle; thus the heart has four chambers. The wall of the heart consists of three layers:

1. The **endocardium**, which lines the interior and forms the valves.
2. The thick muscle layer or **myocardium**.
3. The outer lining or **epicardium**. The epicardium also forms the inner surface of the pericardial sac surrounding the heart.

The route of the blood through the heart is shown in Figure 10-1. Blood enters the heart from the systemic circulation at the right atrium and passes through the **tricuspid valve** to the right ventricle. The tricuspid valve is an atrioventricular (AV) valve. The right ventricle then pumps blood through the **pulmonic valves** (semilunar valves) through which blood flows to the **pulmonary arteries** and then to the lungs. Blood returns from the lungs through the four **pulmonary veins** to the left atrium. It then flows through the **mitral valve**, also an AV valve, into the left ventricle. The left ventricle, in turn, pumps the blood through the **aortic valves** (also semilunar valves) into the

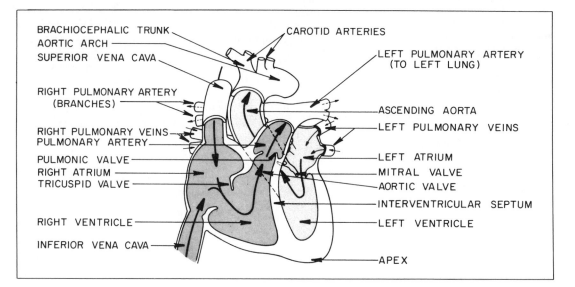

BRACHIOCEPHALIC TRUNK
AORTIC ARCH
SUPERIOR VENA CAVA
CAROTID ARTERIES
LEFT PULMONARY ARTERY (TO LEFT LUNG)
RIGHT PULMONARY ARTERY (BRANCHES)
ASCENDING AORTA
LEFT PULMONARY VEINS
RIGHT PULMONARY VEINS
PULMONARY ARTERY
PULMONIC VALVE
RIGHT ATRIUM
TRICUSPID VALVE
LEFT ATRIUM
MITRAL VALVE
AORTIC VALVE
INTERVENTRICULAR SEPTUM
LEFT VENTRICLE
RIGHT VENTRICLE
INFERIOR VENA CAVA
APEX

aorta and then back into the systemic circulation.

The valves are modifications of the endocardium and are held to a **papillary muscle** by tough connective tissue strands known as **chordae tendinae**. Although attached to muscle, valve movement is dependent on the pressure differences in the two associated heart chambers. Hence, flexibility, which can be affected by some vascular diseases, is crucial for proper valve function.

The contraction of individual cardiac muscle cells produces a rhythmic pumping cycle of the heart as a result of an electrical impulse that spreads through a conduction system in the heart tissue. Innervation serves to regulate the rate and contractile force, but it is not required for the initiation of the cardiac cycle. The impulse begins within the heart in specialized **pacemaker cells** that spontaneously generate action potentials. The **sinoatrial** (SA) **node**, located in the posterior wall of the right atrium, is the normal site of origin for the impulse, and is called the true pacemaker. From the SA node, the impulse travels, by way of the conduction system, through both atria and down the sep-

Figure 10-2. The events of the cardiac cycle illustrating changes in heart sounds, ventricular volume, and the electrocardiogram.

tum to the apex of the heart, and then it spreads through the outer walls of the ventricles. There is a delay in the passage of the cardiac impulse from the atria to the ventricles that allows the atria to contract before ventricular contraction. Atrial contraction, however, normally contributes only slightly to the final phase of ventricular filling. Rather, filling primarily reflects the atrial-ventricular pressure gradient. Atrial contraction may be of more significance during exercise or stenosis. The ventricles are the major pumping chambers of the heart providing the power to move blood through the vascular system.

The **cardiac cycle** is usually defined in terms of four ventricular events, contraction of the ventricle and ejection of blood (**systole**) and then relaxation of the ventricle and filling with blood (**diastole**). Figure 10-2 illustrates the different events occurring during the cardiac cycle. The top curve depicts the heart sounds. The middle curve shows the changes in ventricular volume, and the lower curve indicates the **electrocardiogram** (ECG or EKG) trace.

The ECG detects at the body surface and records the changes in electrical potential that were generated by the spread of the electrical impulse within the cardiac cycle. During a heartbeat, all cardiac cells carry

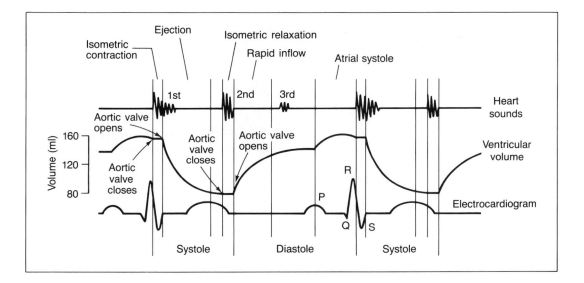

a transmembrane action potential. These summate, creating electrical fields, and are conducted to the body surface through body tissues. Potential differences are generated, since the electrical fields do not simultaneously conduct to all points on the body surface.

The typical ECG is composed of a **P wave** from atrial depolarization, a **QRS complex** from ventricular depolarization, and a **T wave** from ventricular repolarization. Any evidence of atrial repolarization is masked by the QRS complex.

A great deal of information may be ob-

Figure 10-3. The pulmonary and systemic circulations in the adult human. Light shaded areas indicate oxygenated blood; dark shaded areas indicate nonoxygenated blood. Arrows indicate the direction of blood flow. (Adapted with permission from Crouch, J.E., Functional Human Anatomy, *3rd ed. Philadelphia: Lea & Febiger, 1978, p. 404.)*

tained from an ECG. Physiological information may include heart rate, identification of the acting pacemaker, and the conduction pathway. Pathological conditions—including abnormalities of the previously mentioned physiology, chamber enlargement, alterations due to drug action, interstitial ion and fluid changes, and ischemia—may be identified from an ECG trace.

Vascular System

The vascular system is divided into the **systemic** and **pulmonary circulation** as shown in Figure 10-3. In the systemic or major circulation, blood is pumped by the left ventricle through the aorta to the arteries and thence to the arterioles, which branch into a network of capillaries. The capillaries are the functional unit of the vascular system where exchange occurs. Blood then flows through the venules into successively larger veins

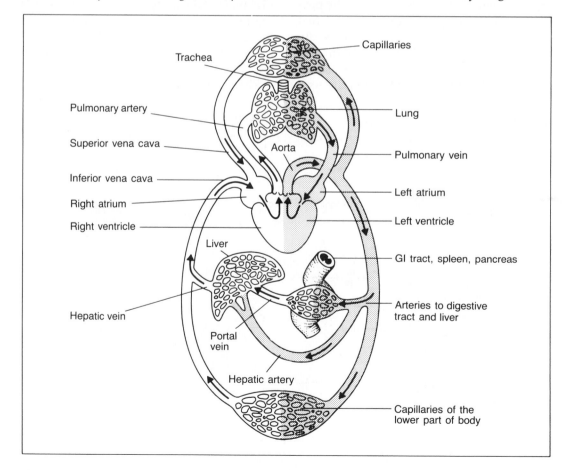

and eventually into the two venae cavae. These then drain into the right atrium. The pulmonary or lesser circulation contains blood pumped from the right ventricle through the pulmonary arteries, arterioles, and capillaries of the lungs and back to the left atrium of the heart through the four pulmonary veins.

Circulation to Specific Areas

The circulation to some organs or areas of the body is of particular importance in understanding cardiovascular diseases. These include coronary, cerebral, and splanchnic circulations. Fetal circulation is also of special concern.

Coronary Circulation. The arteries and veins that feed and drain the heart muscle itself are known as the coronary circulation. As shown in Figure 10-4, the right and left coronary arteries branch off the aorta shortly after the aorta leaves the heart, thus supplying the heart with well-oxygenated blood.

Figure 10-4. The coronary arteries.

The **right coronary artery** circles around the right atrium and supplies the right ventricle and atrium. The left coronary artery splits into two branches, the **circumflex artery** and the **anterior interventricular artery**. The circumflex artery circles the left atrium and supplies the left ventricle and atrium and often the septum. The **anterior interventricular artery** descends between the ventricles to the apex of the heart and then ascends the posterior surface. The major arteries then branch into arterioles and capillaries that rejoin each other in a netlike arrangement. This provides alternate paths by which a region can be supplied with blood.

The coronary veins generally parallel the arteries. Most veins collect into the coronary sinus, which runs across the inferior border of the left atrium along the posterior surface of the heart and drains into the right atrium. Some small veins empty directly into the heart chambers.

The heart receives most of its blood during diastole. Blood flow in the coronary arteries slows during systole due to high pressure in the ventricles. When the heart rate is increased, a condition known as **tachycardia**, the heart spends less time in diastole. Normally, the heart continues to receive ade-

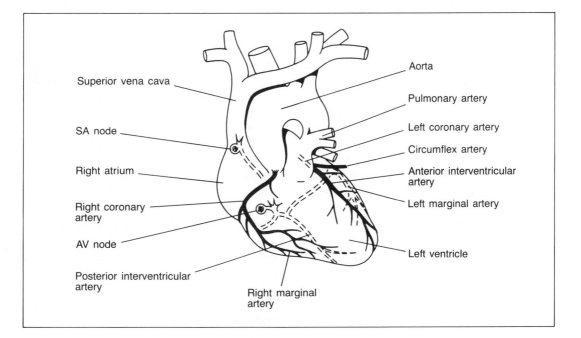

quate blood flow by **autoregulation**, that is, local control of blood flow, as opposed to neural or hormonal control. However, if vessels are occluded, as occurs in atherosclerosis, which will be described later, or if the heart is already providing additional coronary blood flow, as in the case of chronic hypertension, tachycardia may result in inadequate coronary blood supply. The adequacy of the nutrient supply is in part determined by the total mass of myocardial tissue and the diffusion distance from the capillaries to the center of cells. In hypertrophied cells, such as may occur with chronic hypertension, the diffusion distance may be relatively long, resulting in an inadequate nutrient supply.

The autoregulation of coronary blood flow is probably mediated by several metabolites such as adenosine, other nucleotides, prostaglandins, CO_2, or H^+ concentration. Adenosine, which is released in response to an increase in oxygen need, is probably a major factor in coronary autoregulation.[1] Stimulation of the sympathetic nervous system causes coronary vessels to constrict, as in other arteries of the body. However, sympathetic stimulation also increases heart rate and contractility. This, in turn, increases the metabolic needs of the heart muscle, thus causing vasodilation by autoregulation. Norepinephrine, epinephrine, and angiotensin II have a direct effect of vasoconstriction, which is overridden by vasodilation because of increased energy demand.

If an increase in oxygen demand persists in conditions causing hypertrophy of the heart muscle, for example, alternate pathways by which blood can reach an area can develop more fully. These alternate routes comprise the **collateral circulation**. The development of collateral circulation in response to increased nutrient needs is common in individuals with **coronary artery disease**, that is, impairment of blood flow to the heart.

Cerebral Circulation. The blood supply to the brain or cerebral circulation contains approximately 15% of the cardiac output. Blood is supplied to the brain through the **internal carotid** and **vertebral arteries**, which, along with connecting vessels, form an anastamosis known as the **circle of Willis** at the base of the brain. Three trunks, the **anterior**, **middle**, and **posterior cerebral arteries**, arise from the circle of Willis to supply each cerebral hemisphere.

Despite wide fluctuations in blood pressure and activity levels, blood flow to the brain remains quite constant. Regulation of blood flow is affected primarily by the carbon dioxide–oxygen ratio and the hydrogen ion concentration. A relative increase in carbon dioxide or a lowered pH results in increased blood flow.

Splanchnic Circulation. Blood supply to the gastrointestinal tract, liver, spleen, and pancreas is collectively called the **splanchnic circulation**. In this route, venous blood does not return directly to the heart, but instead circulates in a **portal system**, that is, a circulatory route with two capillary networks in series (see Figure 10-3). Splanchnic arteries branch to form a capillary bed in the GI tract, spleen, and pancreas. The venous return collects into the **portal vein**, which enters the liver. In the liver, a second capillary bed forms. The liver is in a prime position to receive blood collected from the digestive system and spleen and perform its major function of detoxification and the initial metabolism of food nutrients. The blood ultimately travels into the hepatic vein and then into the inferior vena cava and to the heart.

The splanchnic circulation can be reduced significantly during exercise when more blood is needed by the heart and skeletal muscles. In contrast, a large increase in blood supply is needed when food is digested. This becomes an important consideration in decisions on feeding patients with failing hearts. The portal circulation and its significance in liver disease are described in Chapter 13.

Fetal Circulation. The fetal blood exchanges nutrients and waste with maternal circulation at the placenta; however, the two blood systems are separated by membranes, and the two blood supplies do not mix. Fetal blood is oxygenated at the placenta rather than in the fetal lungs. The freshly oxygenated fetal blood drains into the umbilical vein to the fetal liver. Most of this blood travels through the liver to the inferior vena cava and thence into the right atrium. Some of the blood bypasses the liver by a shunt called the **ductus venosus** that drains into the inferior vena cava, while a minor portion seeps through the liver tissue.

Both placental blood and systemic venous blood enter the right atrium, but only a small portion is pumped to the right ventricle. Most of the blood passes through the **foramen ovale**, an opening in the septum that leads to the left atrium. The blood that does go to the right ventricle is primarily shunted from the pulmonary artery through the **ductus arteriosus**, which connects directly

to the descending aorta. Thus the pulmonary circulation is bypassed almost completely.

At birth, the ductus venosus constricts because of an absence of blood flow through the umbilical veins. The ductus arteriosus collapses as blood rushes to fill the newly expanded lungs. Pulmonary blood increases the pressure in the left atrium, pressing together the septal folds that close the foramen ovale. Congenital heart disease results when these changes do not occur properly.

Blood Vessels

Structure. A knowledge of the structure of the blood vessels, particularly the arteries, is important to an understanding of some forms of cardiovascular disease. In general, arteries are composed of three layers, the **tunica intima**, **tunica media**, and **tunica adventitia**, as shown in Figure 10-5. The tunica intima is the inner lining of the lumen, and it may be divided into three sublayers. It is composed of an innermost thin layer of

Figure 10-5. Structure of an artery wall. (Reprinted with permission from Luciano, D.L., Vander, A.J., and Sherman, J.H., Human Anatomy and Physiology: Structure and Function, *2nd ed. New York: McGraw-Hill, 1983, p. 469.)*

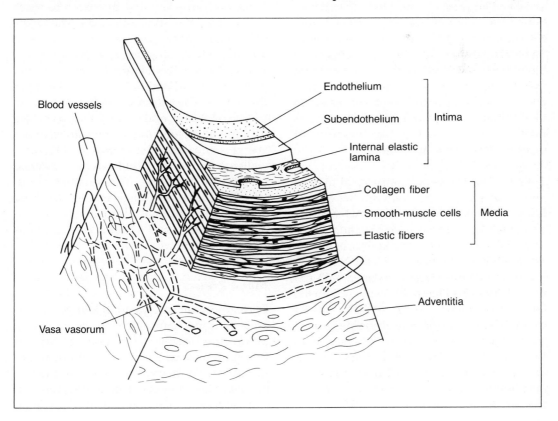

endothelial cells, beneath which there is the **subendothelium**. The subendothelium is composed of a matrix with a layer of loose connective tissue and a few smooth muscle cells. Underneath the subendothelium lies a perforated **internal elastic lamina**. When the blood vessel contracts, this membrane has a scalloped appearance. As an individual ages, smooth muscle cells and matrix accumulate, increasing the thickness of the intima.

The tunica media consists of smooth muscle cells in a spiral arrangement with interposed sheets of fenestrated elastic tissue. The smooth muscle cells are surrounded by collagen and other matrix materials.

The adventitia is composed of elastic connective tissue that fuses with the connective tissue surrounding adjacent organs. Also within the adventitia are fibroblasts, collagen, glycosaminoglycans, glycoproteins, and often an **external limiting membrane**.

The cells of the blood vessels themselves must be nourished. The tunica intima of small and large arteries and the internal portion of the tunica media are nourished from the luminal blood by diffusion. The adventitia of large arteries and veins contains small blood vessels known as the **vasa vasorum** that supply the tissue of those vessels that are too thick to be nourished from the blood in the lumen. Since the blood in veins is poorer in nutrients, the vasa vasorum of veins is more richly branched.

Types. With the general structural plan in mind, we now can consider how various types of blood vessels differ. Arteries are classified according to their size and structure. The large arteries, also known as **elastic arteries**, are the aorta and its large branches. The intima of these vessels is lined with endothelial cells and has a thick subendothelial layer. The media, the thickest layer, consists of a large amount of concentric perforated elastic membrane tissue interspersed with smooth muscle cells and fibroblasts. The adventitia does not have an external limiting membrane. An elastic adventitia is important in the maintenance of blood flow; it

limits the expansion due to systole (contraction of the heart), and the recoil helps to maintain arterial pressure during diastole (relaxation of the heart).

In contrast, small and medium-sized arteries (muscular arteries) have a thick media with more smooth muscle and less elastic material than the large arteries. The adventitia is thicker and has an external limiting membrane. The arterioles are even smaller, usually less than 0.5 mm in diameter. They have endothelium but no subendothelial layer and may lack an internal elastic lamina. The media has only a few layers of muscle cells, and the adventitia is narrow. These vessels are primarily important in monitoring blood flow to capillaries.

The walls of the capillaries are a single endothelial cell in thickness. It is in this area that exchanges between blood and interstitial fluid occur. Most cells are a distance of only 0.1 mm or less from a capillary blood supply.

Veins, in general, follow the routes of arteries and are classified by size into three types, large, medium, and small. The layers of veins are not as conspicuous as those of arteries. When compared to a corresponding artery, the vein has a larger lumen, a thinner wall, and an adventitia that is thicker than the media. The internal elastic lamina may be thin or absent, and the vessel may possess valves. Since blood in the veins flows under low pressure and often against gravity, thick walls are unnecessary, but valves are needed to prevent backflow. The smallest veins, **venules**, consist of a single endothelial layer and a basal lamina. Collectively, the arterioles, capillaries, and venules are known as the **microcirculation**.

Blood Pressure

The cardiovascular system might be considered as a mechanical system containing a pump (the heart), a compression chamber (the elastic arteries), and a variable resistance to outflow (primary arterioles). In order to keep the fluid flowing through the system, it is necessary to maintain a head of pressure.

Blood pressure (BP) is the hydrostatic pressure exerted on the vessel walls by the blood flow. The pressure is primarily a function of the amount of blood present within the systematic circulation, and it is created because the flow of blood from the heart (cardiac output or CO) is pumped into a closed system containing a resistance (R) to outflow. The three variables—cardiac output, blood pressure, and resistance—are interdependent, so that a change in one is reflected in changes in another. The relationship can be expressed mathematically in the following equations:

$$CO = BP/R \qquad (10\text{-}1)$$

or

$$BP = CO \times R \qquad (10\text{-}2)$$

Using this equation, in a situation where cardiac output is constant but the resistance increases, as it does in some vascular diseases, it should be clear that the blood pressure will rise. On the other hand, if resistance decreases, as it does in exercise when blood vessels dilate, cardiac output must rise in order to maintain the blood pressure.

Cardiac Output

The amount of blood pumped to the tissues by the heart, the cardiac output, is expressed as liters of blood pumped per minute. In an average man at rest, cardiac output is typically 5 L/min. It is the product of the stroke volume (SV), the amount ejected from the heart at each beat, and the heart rate (HR) or beats per minute, as follows:

$$CO = SV \times HR \qquad (10\text{-}3)$$

For example, if the stroke volume is 70 ml and the heart rate is 72 beats per minute, cardiac output will be 70×72 or 5,040 ml. The cardiac output can thus be varied by changing either the heart rate or the stroke volume. The heart rate can be increased two to three times by sympathetic stimulation,

whereas parasympathetic stimulation decreases the rate. Both sympathetic and parasympathetic nerve fibers terminate on the SA node. The parasympathetic (vagal) fibers release acetylcholine on the SA nodal cells. Acetylcholine alters the permeability of the membrane and prolongs the time between beats by slowing the rate of membrane polarization, thus slowing the heart rate **(a negative inotropic effect)**. Sympathetic fibers release norepinephrine and increase the heart rate **(a positive chronotropic effect)**. Other factors, including various ions, hormones, and temperature, also influence the heart rate.

When heart rate increases, stroke volume does not decrease because filling of the ventricles is essentially complete by middiastole and emptying is relative complete by midsystole. Thus cardiac output increases when the heart rate rises to 100 to 150 beats per minute.

It is possible to vary cardiac output by changing the stroke volume. Within physiologic limits, an increase in the length of the muscle fibers, and thus an increase in the amount of blood in the ventricle, leads to an increase in the strength of the contraction of the normal heart. Thus the heart adjusts the force of contraction to pump all of the blood that is returned to it by the venous system. This principle is known as the Frank-Starling law. However, there are limitations. A muscle fiber stretched beyond a given point will have weaker, not stronger, contractions. At a given length, increased sympathetic stimulation results in stronger contractions. This reaction is known as an **inotropic response**. On the other hand, increased arterial pressure due to greater resistance tends to cause a decrease in stroke volume.

Peripheral Vascular Resistance

The second factor that determines blood pressure is the amount of friction or resistance to blood flow in the peripheral vessels. Resistance is determined by the viscosity of the blood and the width of the vessels. The viscosity of blood normally does not change, but a high hematocrit due to polycythemia (an excess of erythrocytes) raises blood viscosity and, thus, resistance and blood pressure. The more significant determinant of resistance is vessel width. In fact, resistance is inversely proportional to the radius raised to the fourth power. Thus a small change in the radius of a vessel produces a large change in resistance. At a constant cardiac output, blood pressure will rise as vessels narrow and will fall as vessels dilate. This concept is very important in understanding the effects of atherosclerosis, which will be discussed later in the chapter.

Blood flow through the capillaries is regulated by the contraction and relaxation of the smooth muscle in the arterioles and of the sphincters at the entrance to some capillaries. These muscles always have some tone; that is, they are always partly constricted. By contracting and relaxing certain areas, the arterioles can shunt blood to areas of the body where the need is greatest. For example, more blood is supplied to the skeletal muscle during exercise, to the abdominal organs during digestion, and to the skin when it is necessary to dissipate heat.

Measurement of Blood Pressure

In clinical situations, blood pressure measurements are usually taken on arteries. Pressure is easily measured with a **sphygmomanometer**, which consists of a hollow cuff and gauge that measures the pressure within the cuff. The cuff is wrapped around the arm and inflated to a pressure greater than the arterial pressure during systole. Thus blood flow is completely obstructed. Pressure in the cuff is slowly released, and when it falls to the systolic pressure, atrial pressure at the peak of systole is high enough to force some blood through the now partially obstructed artery. This turbulent pulsatile blood flow can be heard in a stethoscope placed on the artery just distal to the cuff. Thus the pressure at which sound is first heard is noted as the **systolic pressure**. As the cuff pressure is further released, the distinct beats diminish

until a muffled sound is detected. **Diastolic pressure** is recorded as the pressure when the distinct beat first disappears. At lower pressures, laminar flow is reestablished and no sounds are audible.

A measurement of blood pressure is expressed as a fraction with the systolic pressure as the numerator and the diastolic pressure as the denominator, for example, 120/80, which is read "120 over 80." Blood pressure is continuously distributed in a population, but 120/80 is often considered average. Blood pressure drops quickly as blood flows through the arterioles to about 25 mm Hg (also called 25 torr) in the capillaries. It then drops to almost 0 mm Hg as the blood nears the right atrium.

Regulation of Blood Pressure

The homeostatic mechanisms for the control of blood pressure are not completely understood. However, it is clear that pressure is controlled by many complex and interacting systems. The three most important regulators of blood pressure are considered to be the **sympathetic nervous system** (SNS), the **renin-angiotensin system**, and the **kidneys**.[2]

Figure 10-6 shows how the three systems interact to affect cardiac output (CO) and peripheral vascular resistance (PVR), the two factors that determine blood pressure. All three systems affect cardiac output. In addition, the sympathetic nervous system and the renin-angiotensin system also affect peripheral vascular resistance. Note in Figure 10-6 how all three systems affect atrial filling. By constricting or dilating the veins, the SNS and renin-angiotensin systems regulate venous capacity, which affects atrial filling. The kidney affects atrial filling by controlling the total volume of blood in the vessels. Atrial filling, in turn, is one factor that determines stroke volume. Stroke volume affects cardiac output, which, along with peripheral resistance, determines blood pressure.

The regulatory systems work toward short-term and long-term control of blood

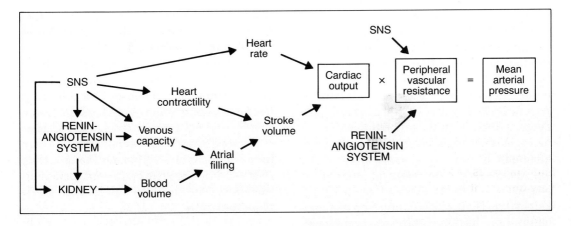

Figure 10-6. Normal blood pressure control—the three major regulation systems. SNS = sympathetic nervous system.

pressure. Short-term regulation is controlled primarily by the sympathetic nervous system, which responds immediately to acute changes in blood pressure, quickly returning pressure to normal levels. If the change in blood pressure persists for days, the short-term controls will adapt and consider this new level "normal." The long-term controls work constantly to define and maintain a normal blood pressure and involve the interaction of the kidneys' regulation of extracellular volume, the renin-angiotensin system, and the sympathetic nervous system. The following sections will look at each of these three systems in detail.

Sympathetic Nervous System. The sympathetic nervous system is the primary short-term regulator of blood pressure. In general, the system consists of three parts: (1) receptors in the body that monitor blood pressure; (2) the **vasomotor center** in the medulla of the brain, which receives impulses from the receptors and sends out impulses to the body; and (3) the tissues that are innervated by sympathetic nerves and act to adjust blood pressure.

The **baroreceptors** are stretch receptors that sense changes in blood pressure. Baroreceptors, located on the carotid arteries in the neck and on the aortic arch, play an impor-

tant role in the reflex regulation of blood pressure. An increase in pressure in these arteries stretches the baroreceptors, thus sending impulses to the vasomotor center. These impulses cause a decrease in vasomotor sympathetic output, resulting in a reduction in blood pressure. When blood pressure drops, the vasomotor center receives fewer impulses from the baroreceptors. This decrease results in greater stimulation of the sympathetic nervous system, which has the overall effect of increasing blood pressure. Specific effects of the SNS that increase blood pressure include (1) secretion of norepinephrine causing contraction of smooth muscle surrounding arterioles and veins, (2) stimulation of the adrenal medulla to secrete epinephrine and norepinephrine into the bloodstream, (3) contraction of skeletal muscles that increases venous return, and (4) stimulation of the posterior pituitary to secrete **vasopressin** (also called **antidiuretic hormone** or ADH). The hormone ADH enhances the ability of the kidney to reabsorb water and also causes vasoconstriction at high concentrations.

In addition, the SNS plays a role in long-term control of blood pressure by innervating the renal vasculature. This innervation, in turn, affects the glomerular filtration rate and the renin-angiotensin system.

Renin-Angiotensin System. The renin-angiotensin system affects the long-term control of blood pressure. Specialized cells of the juxtaglomerular apparatus of the kidney (See Chapter 9) secrete renin into the bloodstream in response to low blood pressure. **Renin** is an enzyme that splits **angiotensinogen**, a protein made in the liver and always present in plasma, to produce **angiotensin I** (Figure 10-7). In the plasma, **converting enzyme**, which is most concentrated in the lungs, cleaves angiotensin I to produce **angiotensin II**. Since converting enzyme and angiotensinogen are always present in plasma, it is the secretion of renin by the kidney that is the rate-limiting step of angiotensin II production. Renin secretion is stimulated directly by a drop in blood pressure in the juxtaglomerular apparatus and also by sympathetic innervation.

Angiotensin II alters blood pressure by its effects on three tissues, as shown in Figure 10-7. Angiotensin II causes the kidneys to decrease sodium and water excretion, the arterioles and veins to constrict, and the adrenal cortex to increase secretion of the hormone aldosterone. **Aldosterone** increases renal sodium reabsorption and potassium excretion. The net effect is an increase in blood pressure.

Kidney. The kidneys regulate blood pressure by altering sodium and water excretion such that extracellular fluid volume remains

Figure 10-7. The renin-angiotensin system and its role in regulation of arterial blood pressure.

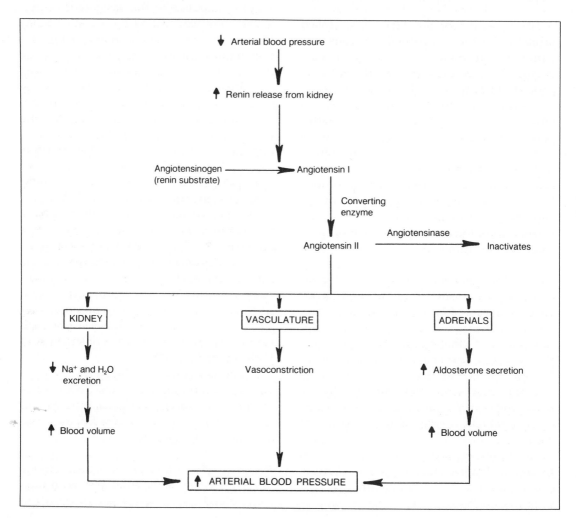

constant despite a wide range of sodium and fluid intake. The hormone ADH plays an important role in this function. It is secreted from the posterior pituitary in response to either high blood osmolarity, as sensed by the hypothalamus, or a drop in blood pressure, as sensed by baroreceptors. The major action of ADH is to increase the reabsorption of water from urine by increasing the permeability of the late distal tubules and collecting ducts to water. The hormone ADH also increases salt reabsorption and, at higher levels, causes vasoconstriction. The net effect of these actions is an increase in extracellular fluid volume and blood pressure.

Other Factors. Eicosanoids are biologically active compounds that are synthesized in most tissues of the body from the 20-carbon, or eicosanoid, unsaturated fatty acids. The term **eicosanoid** encompasses four distinct groups of pharmacologically active compounds: (1) prostaglandins (PG), (2) thromboxanes (TX), (3) prostacyclins, and (4) leukotrienes (LT). The term **prostanoid** includes PG, TX, and prostacyclins.

The prostaglandins affect inflammatory response, reproductive function, gastric secretion, and cardiovascular function. Thromboxanes are synthesized in platelets and, upon release, cause vasoconstriction and platelet aggregation. Prostacyclins are produced by the endothelium of blood vessels and act in antagonism to thromboxanes by causing vasodilation and inhibition of platelet aggregation. The leukotrienes affect immune function, particularly in relation to asthma, allergies, macrophage functions, chemotaxis, and inflammatory responses. Table 10-1 summarizes the actions of these substances.

A balanced production of eicosanoids modulates local responses to injury, perturbation, or infection. The relative quantities of different eicosanoids synthesized depends on the specific tissue and on the physiological state, including the presence of stimulatory events such as infection, trauma, allergy, or toxin exposure. In addition, the type of fat eaten is thought to affect eicosanoid synthesis because membrane phospholipids are the primary substrates for eicosanoid synthesis, and the fatty acid composition of membrane phospholipids reflects, to a certain degree, dietary fatty acid intake.[3,4,5] A review of eicosanoid synthesis is presented, since the eicosanoids have diverse effects on cardiovascular function and blood pressure.[6] Later in this chapter, we will discuss how different types of dietary fat are thought to affect eicosanoid synthesis in regard to blood pressure, hyperlipidemia, and atherosclerosis.

The **omega** or **n-3** and **n-6** families of unsaturated fatty acids are the precursors for eicosanoid synthesis. A summary of the three major families of unsaturated fatty acids is given in Table 10-2. The "n" or "omega" terminology refers to the position of the first double bond as counted from the terminal (omega) methyl carbon of the fatty acid. The n-3 and n-6 families of unsaturated fatty acids are essential fatty acids (EFA) because man cannot synthesize fatty acids with double bonds between the ninth carbon and the terminal methyl carbon of the fatty acid chain. Thus linoleic acid (18:2n6 or 18:2n-6) and alpha-linolenic acid (18:3n3) are EFA that must be provided in the diet. It is generally felt that 1–2% of caloric intake as linoleic acid and less than 0.5% as linolenic acid are sufficient to provide the daily requirements for EFA.[3] Reactions involving elongation and desaturation of dietary EFA result in formation of arachidonic acid from linoleic acid, and eicosapentanoic acid (EPA) and docosahexanoic acid (DHA) from alpha-linolenic acid. There are three series of prostanoids, referred to as PG_1, PG_2, and PG_3, which are synthesized from linoleate, arachidonate, and linolenate, respectively. However, arachidonic acid, derived primarily from dietary linoleic acid, is the major physiological precursor of eicosanoids.

The key steps in the conversion of dietary linoleic acid to arachidonic acid and subsequent synthesis of the 2 series eicosanoids from arachidonic acid are shown in Figure

Table 10-1. Biological Functions of Eicosanoid Compounds

Affected Tissues	Effects	Compounds Involved			
		Prostaglandin	Prostacyclin	Thromboxane	Leukotriene
Circulatory system					
Blood vessels	Vasodilation	X	X		
	Vasoconstriction			X	X
	Permeability				X
Platelets	Adhesion			X	
	Antiaggregation	X	X		
Immune system					
Neutrophils	Adhesion				X
	Chemotaxis/kinesis				X
	Lysozyme secretion				X
Monocytes	Chemotaxis/kinesis				X
Basophils	Histamine secretion				X
Respiratory system	Bronchiole constriction	X		X	
	Bronchiole dilation	X			X
Renal system					
	Glomerular filtration	X	X	X	
	Renin secretion	X	X		
	Naturesis	X	X		
	Diuresis	X			
Gastrointestinal system					
Stomach	Acid secretion	X	X		
Small intestine	Peristalsis	X			
Ileum	Constriction				X
Pancreas	Amylase secretion	X	X		X
Endocrine system					
Pancreas	Insulin secretion	X			
Pituitary	Secretion	X			

10-8. In response to a variety of physiologic stimuli, the enzyme **phospholipase** releases arachidonic acid from membrane phospholipids. Arachidonic acid is then metabolized by one of two enzymes. The first pathway, catalyzed by **lipoxygenase**, leads to the synthesis of LT. Alternatively, **cyclooxygenase** may catalyze conversion of arachidonic acid to unstable endoperoxides, first PGG_2, and then peroxidase catalyzes the formation of PGH_2. One of several **prostanoid synthetases** acts on PGH_2 to form prostacyclin, prostaglandin, or thromboxane. The anti-inflammatory effects of aspirin and indomethacin are attributed to their inhibition of the cyclooxygenase step.

PG, prostacyclin, TX, and leukotrienes have diverse and often antagonistic effects. The net physiological effect of these compounds depends on their relative concentrations in a given tissue, which is thought to be affected by the relative amounts of n-6 and n-3 polyunsaturated fats eaten in the diet.[3] Polyunsaturated fats from the n-3 family, especially EPA and DHA, reduce eicosanoid synthesis by inhibiting both cyclooxygenase and lipoxygenase and by replacing arachidonic acid in phospholipid pools.[3] Eicosanoids synthesized from EPA (3 series prostanoids) also have varying bioactivity compared with those synthesized from linoleic acid (2 series prostanoids). For example, TXA_2 is a potent vasoconstrictor and stimulates platelet aggregation, whereas TXA_3 is inactive and tends to reduce platelet aggregation; PGE_2 mediates inflammation and possesses vasodilation and bronchodilator properties; PGD_2 is a vasoconstrictor; PGF_2 has effects similar to PGE_2 but is a vasoconstrictor; and PGI_2 inhibits platelet aggregation and is a vasodilator.

Natriuretic factors are peptides known to

Table 10-2. Major Families of Unsaturated Fatty Acids

Class Designation[a]	Parent Fatty Acid	Major Metabolites	Principal Sources
n-9	18:1n9 oleic acid	20:3n9 eicosatrienoic acid	Synthesis from acetate; animal and vegetable fats
n-6[b]	18:2n6 linoleic acid	20:4n6 arachidonic acid	Many vegetable oils such as corn, safflower, soybean, sunflower, and cottonseed
n-3[b]	18:3n3 alpha-linolenic acid	20:5n3 eicosapentanoic acid (EPA)	18:3n3—Leafy plant tissues and selected vegetable oils such as rapeseed and soybean
		22:6n3 docosahexanoic acid (DHA)	EPA and DHA—Marine phytoplankton that are consumed by fish resulting in high concentrations of EPA and DHA in fish oils

[a] In the "n" numbering system, the total number of carbon atoms is given first, followed by a colon, the total number of double bonds, "n," and the number of carbon atoms between the terminal methyl group and the closest double bond.
[b] Essential fatty acids.

Figure 10-8. Key steps in eicosanoid metabolism.

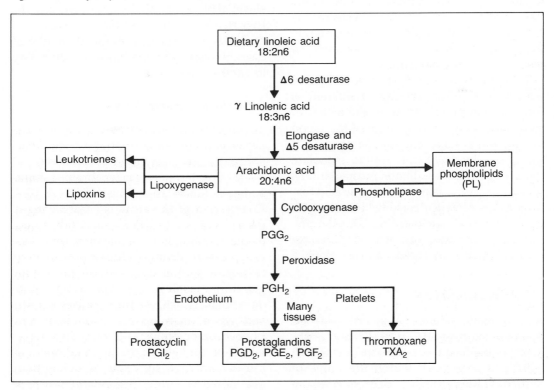

increase urinary salt loss. Currently, there is particular interest in a natriuretic factor secreted by the atrium called the **atrial natriuretic factor** (ANF) or **atriopeptin.** When released, possibly in response to stretch, ANF acts as a vasodilator, and increases renal excretion of sodium and water by affecting the GFR. Apparently, ANF inhibits aldosterone, ADH, and renin. The overall affect of ANF in the bloodstream is to lower blood pressure.[7]

The **kinins** are a group of proteins produced in various tissues that are potent vasodilators and natriuretics.[8] Kinins are cleaved from kininogen by the action of **kallikrein**, and are quickly inactivated by **kininases**. Kininase II is the same as converting enzyme. Thus one substance acts to hydrolyze a vasodilator and form a vasoconstrictor.

Because kinins are inactivated quickly, they are believed to be involved in the regulation of local, rather than systemic, blood flow. Kinins also affect water and electrolyte excretion and capillary permeability, and, in the case of cardiac kinins, they may cause the perception of anginal pain.[9]

The kallikrein-kinin system is integrated with several other systems. Kallikrein is formed from prekallikrein by the action of **Hageman factor**, a component of the blood coagulation system. The release of renin is stimulated by kallikrein. Kinins stimulate the synthesis of vasodilator prostaglandins probably by increasing arachidonic acid formation. The release of renal kallikrein can be stimulated by angiotensin, aldosterone, prostaglandins, and vasopressin. Kinin release is inhibited by adrenal glucocorticoids.

HYPERTENSION

Hypertension is defined as an arterial blood pressure that exceeds an arbitrarily established limit. In adults, a pressure of less than 140/90 is considered within the range of normal.[10] Either systolic or diastolic pressure may be elevated. An increase in diastolic compared with systolic pressure is regarded as a stronger predictor of hypertension-asso-ciated cardiovascular complications. Hypertension is considered to be a major risk factor for coronary heart disease, stroke, congestive heart failure, peripheral vascular disease, and chronic renal failure. Early and aggressive treatment of hypertension has been shown to reduce morbidity and mortality from these cardiovascular diseases.[10] Almost 58 million people, or 25% of the U.S. population, are estimated to have hypertension.[11]

Classification

Hypertension is classified by severity as summarized in Table 10-3. Since blood pressure varies widely under different conditions, including time of day, it is important to base an evaluation on at least two measurements. Hypertension is a symptom associated with a number of conditions and is broadly classified according to etiology. In more than 90% of cases, the etiology of the elevated blood pressure is unknown, and the hypertension is thus classified as **primary** or **essential** hypertension. In less than 10% of cases, the cause of hypertension is secondary to another condition.

Secondary Hypertension

The most prevalent causes of secondary hypertension are chronic renal disease, renal artery disease, coarctation of the aorta, primary aldosteronism, pheochromocytoma, and pregnancy, as outlined in Table 10-4. **Coarctation of the aorta** is a narrowing of the aorta caused by a deformity of the tunica media resulting in a specific increase in systolic pressure. **Primary aldosteronism** refers to any of several disorders of the adrenal gland that result in the hypersection of aldosterone, which, in turn, causes sodium and water retention and potassium loss. **Pheochromocytoma** is a rare disorder in which a tumor on the adrenal medulla causes excessive secretion of epinephrine and norepinephrine. Secondary hypertension is also caused by **Cushing's disease**, the hypersecretion of adrenocorticotropic hormone (ACTH) from the anterior pituitary,

Table 10-3. Classification of Blood Pressures and Follow-up Criteria

Blood Pressures[a] (mm Hg)	Category	Recommended Follow-up
Diastolic		
<85	Normal BP	Recheck within two years
85–89	High normal BP	Recheck within one year
90–104	Mild hypertension	Confirm promptly (within two months)
105–114	Moderate hypertension	Evaluate or refer promptly for care (within two weeks)
≥115	Severe hypertension	Evaluate or refer immediately for care
Systolic		
<140	Normal BP	Recheck within two years
140–159	Borderline isolated systolic hypertension	Confirm within two months
≥160	Isolated systolic hypertension	Confirm promptly (within two months)

Adapted from the 1988 report of the Joint National Committee on Detection, Evaluation and Treatment of High Blood Pressure. *Arch. Intern. Med.* 148:1023, 1988.

[a] In adults age 18 and over. Maximum normal BP is defined in children as a blood pressure at or above the 55th percentile, which is approximately as follows: less than 6 years of age, 110/75; 6–10 years, 120/80; 10–14 years, 125/85; 14–18 years, 135/90.

which results in excess release of cortisol from the adrenal cortex. Treatment of secondary hypertension consists of removal of the underlying cause.

Hypertensive disorders occur in as many as 10% of all pregnancies. The most serious of these conditions is **pregnancy-induced hypertension** (PIH), which was formerly called toxemia of pregnancy. The progression of symptoms from **preeclampsia** to **eclampsia** characterizes PIH. Preeclampsia usually develops after the 20th week of pregnancy and is characterized by hypertension, edema, and proteinuria. If this condition progresses to the more serious stage of eclampsia, convulsions and coma may occur.

Essential Hypertension

By definition, the cause of essential hypertension is unknown. However, epidemiological studies suggest that several factors are associated with an increased incidence of essential hypertension, as summarized in Table 10-5. In general, renal function is thought to play a major role in the etiology of essential hypertension. Some hypertensive individuals show an abnormal control of sodium excretion. In other cases, there appears to be a hyperactive sympathetic nervous system in which plasma norepinephrine is not

adequately suppressed in response to a sodium load. The renin-angiotensin system may be set high; or if there is an abnormally low increase in aldosterone in response to angiotensin II, an excessive amount of angiotensin may be required to produce the proper aldosterone levels. Current research is studying the kallikrein-kinin and prostaglandin systems to determine their roles in the development of hypertension.

In industrialized Western nations, the prevalence of hypertension increases with age. In women, this increase occurs after menopause. Blacks have a higher rate of hypertension than whites; 38% of blacks and 29% of whites demonstrate hypertension.[11] Differences in an individual's genetic background may predispose one to hypertension. Current evidence suggests that the predisposition to hypertension is polygenic and that different genes or gene products are activated or suppressed by single or multiple environmental influences.

Various dietary and behavioral factors are associated with essential hypertension, as outlined in Table 10-5. Alcohol has a significant vasopressor effect, and regular intake is associated with increased blood pressure. In fact, a chronic alcohol intake greater than 1 oz. per day is the most common cause of reversible hypertension among men.[12] Regu-

Table 10-4. Etiologies of Secondary Hypertension

Elevated systolic pressure
Increased cardiac output: aortic valvular insufficiency, arteriovenous fistula–patent ductus, thyrotoxicosis, beriberi
Rigidity of the aorta : atherosclerosis, coarctation of the aorta

Elevated systolic and diastolic pressures
Renal disorders:
  Renal artery disease—atherosclerosis, embolism, traumatic injury
  Renal parenchymal disease—glomerulonephritis, chronic nephritis, polycystic kidneys, connective tissue diseases, diabetic nephropathy, hydronephrosis
Endocrine disorders:
  Adrenal:
    Cortical: Cushing's syndrome, primary aldosteronism, congenital adrenal hyperplasia
    Medullary: Pheochromocytoma
  Thyroid: hyperthyroidism, hypothyroidism
  Acromegaly
  Hypercalcemia
  Tumors: extraadrenal chromaffin, carcinoid
  Exogenous hormones: estrogen glucocorticoids, mineralcorticoids (licorice), sympathomimetics, tyramine-containing foods, and monoamine oxidase inhibitors
Neurological disorders:
  Increased intracranial pressure—brain tumor encephalitis, respiratory acidosis
  Sleep apnea
  Quadriplegia
  Guillain-Barre syndrome
  Lead poisoning
Acute stress: surgery, burns, alcohol withdrawal, hypoglycemia, pancreatitis
Pregnancy-induced hypertension

Based on information in Kaplan, N.M., Systemic hypertension: mechanisms and diagnosis. In E. Braunwald, Ed., *Heart Disease—A Textbook of Cardiovascular Medicine.* Philadelphia: W.B. Saunders, 1988, Table 27-4, p. 822.

Table 10-5. Factors Associated with Etiology of Essential Hypertension

Pathophysiological factors
Abnormal sodium excretion
Hyperactive sympathetic nervous system
Abnormal renin-angiotensin system
Abnormal kallikrein-kinin system (?)
Abnormal prostaglandin synthesis (?)
Genetic factors
Age
Race
Family history of cardiovascular disease
Behavioral factors
Excessive alcohol
Low activity level
Stress (?)
Dietary factors
Obesity
High sodium or high sodium chloride intake
Low potassium, magnesium, or calcium intake
High fat intake, especially saturated fats

lar aerobic exercise has been associated with lower rates of cardiovascular disease. This effect is probably due in part to a lowering of blood pressure. Chronic cigarette smoking is not associated with higher blood pressure levels; however, it is associated with higher mortality rate among hypertensives and is a major risk factor for cardiovascular disease. Caffeine consumption causes a short-term rise in blood pressure but is not associated with chronic hypertension. Mental and emotional socioeconomic stress can cause a temporary rise in blood pressure, but there is no evidence that stresses cause a sustained elevation. Conversely, relaxation and biofeedback treatment techniques lower blood pressure at least temporarily, but their long-term effectiveness has not been adequately evaluated. **Obesity** is clearly related to elevated blood pressure in many patients. Weight loss is usually accompanied by a drop in blood pressure, but even if pressure does not fall, cardiovascular disease mortality and morbidity are reduced.[13]

Numerous epidemiological and experimental studies indicate that the mineral content of the diet affects blood pressure levels. High intakes of sodium, chloride, and cadmium and low dietary levels of calcium, magnesium, and potassium are suggested to contribute to the etiology of hypertension.[14]

Sodium is the major cation in extracellular fluid, and chloride is the major anion. Potassium is the major cation and phosphate the major anion in the intracellular body fluids. The sodium-potassium pump and other energy-requiring pumping systems maintain concentrations of these ions. Calcium is also vital in regulating the movement of sodium and potassium across membranes. Alterations in ion balance within fluid compartments, especially sodium balance, affect total body water balance and blood pressure.

Population studies demonstrate that the prevalence of hypertension is greater in populations with higher sodium intakes. In most studies, there is a subset of hypertensive individuals, referred to as **salt-sensitive**, whose blood pressure responds to changes in sodium intake; however, the mechanism is unclear. Animal models suggest that a high sodium intake may cause hypertension in those instances when an underlying renal defect diminishes the ability to excrete salt rapidly.

Sodium chloride intake is generally restricted in the diet of hypertensive individuals, although, it is currently felt that sodium intake is not the only ion affecting blood pressure. The anionic component of a sodium salt can influence the ability of that salt to increase blood pressure. For example, chloride may play an important role in blood pressure regulation. Sodium salts that do not contain chloride, such as sodium citrate, did not increase blood pressure as sodium chloride did in experiments in men with salt-sensitive hypertension.[15]

Some investigators have suggested that large intakes of potassium may protect from hypertension.[16] Individuals with a low incidence of hypertension, such as vegetarians, often consume relatively low amounts of sodium and high amounts of potassium.[17] In addition, studies with spontaneously hypertensive animal models demonstrate a decrease in blood pressure in animals consuming a high-sodium diet who are given supplemental potassium. Taken together, these observations suggest that the ratio of sodium to potassium in the diet affects blood pressure. Consumption of a safe and adequate range of 1,100–3,300 mg sodium and 1,875–5,625 mg potassium would result in a dietary Na:K ratio of 0.2–1.8, whereas the Na:K ratio of the current average American diet is 1.3–3.9.[18]

Magnesium intake and cadmium intake also affect blood pressure.[14] Diets moderately or severely deficient in magnesium have been associated with increased blood pressure in experimental animals. Some individuals with hypertension demonstrate decreased magnesium levels. Excess cadmium intake in experimental animals adversely affects blood pressure.

Current research suggests that a high calcium intake may protect against hypertension.[19] However, the mechanism of this effect is complex and not understood at this time. For example, a protective role of calcium is difficult to explain in view of the known requirement of calcium for smooth muscle contraction, which determines peripheral vascular resistance, and the effect of drugs known as calcium channel blockers that lower blood pressure. McCarron and Morris[19] suggest that membrane-associated defects of Ca^{2+}-ATPase-dependent calcium transport may account for the failure of hypertensive subjects to defend their calcium balance and thus demonstrate a decrease in blood pressure with calcium supplementation. Resnick[20] and others have demonstrated that hypertensive individuals most likely to respond to calcium supplementation have low serum ionized calcium levels and low plasma renin activity, and they are also salt-sensitive. A decrease in blood pressure with calcium supplementation in these individuals seems to require a decrease in 1,25 vitamin D_3 levels, suggesting that calcium-regulating hormones may mediate the effects of calcium and sodium on blood pressure. Calcium supplementation may reduce blood pressure in the same subset of individuals that show a decrease in blood pressure with sodium restriction.[20] An intake of calcium that provides the RDA should be encouraged in all individuals with hypertension.

Consequences of Uncontrolled Hypertension

Untreated hypertension usually progresses slowly, but is potentially life-threatening. It increases the workload of the heart and often damages the arterial walls. Chronic uncontrolled hypertension is associated with an accelerated development of atherosclerosis and an increased incidence of coronary heart disease and stroke, especially if other risk factors such as smoking and hypercholesterolemia are also present.[10,21]

Uncontrolled hypertension may result in damage to other organs including the brain, kidneys, eyes, and extremities.[2] The heart may suffer congestive heart failure or coronary artery disease. Kidneys can be damaged by renal artery disease or may fail because of nephrosclerosis. Atherosclerosis in the brain can lead to transient ischemic attacks (TIA) or stroke. Microvascular hemorrhage damages the eyes and brain. Atherosclerosis in vessels to the legs may cause claudication or a decreased pulse in the lower extremities.

Stroke and congestive heart failure (CHF) are the most common consequences of hypertension. When the heart compensates for the excessive workload by increasing the size of cardiac cells, leading to hypertrophy of the left ventricle, CHF occurs. Eventually, heart function deteriorates, and the heart fails, as described later in the section on CHF. Stroke occurs when the blood supply to the brain fails. Hypertension can cause damage to arterial walls that accelerates the formation of emboli, thrombi, or atherosclerosis, reducing the size of the lumen. The severity of the damage is determined by the location and extent of the loss of circulation.

In some patients, the blood pressure rises suddenly, representing a change from a slowly progressive benign hypertension to malignant hypertension that has a diastolic pressure greater than 140 mm Hg. Symptoms of progressively increasing blood pressure include headaches, vertigo (dizziness), tinnitus (noise in ears), syncope (fainting), and dimmed vision. Malignant hypertension progresses rapidly and is usually fatal if left untreated.

Management

The management of hypertension has changed over the years from attempts to control hypertension only when it becomes severe to the present policy of aggressively treating fairly mild increases in blood pressure. This policy of early treatment has been promoted by the National High Blood Pressure Education Program (NHBPEP), which was launched in 1972.[10,13] Since the program began, deaths due to coronary artery disease and strokes have declined 25% and 50%, respectively.[10] These statistics support the belief that early treatment of high blood pressure reduces complications and mortality due to hypertension.

Management of hypertension currently includes both nonpharmacological and pharmacological, or drug, treatments. Nonpharmacological methods include weight reduction and other dietary changes, behavior modification to reduce stress, and regular aerobic exercise. In individuals with mild hypertension, that is, a diastolic pressure of 90–104 mm Hg, nonpharmacological methods, especially dietary, are tried first. It is estimated that mild hypertension can be managed without drugs in 40% of such individuals.[22] In those whose diastolic pressure does not fall below 90 mm Hg with nonpharmacological methods, drugs are added to the therapy. It is recommended that hypertensive individuals not smoke, since smoking is a major cardiovascular risk factor.

Diet

Important dietary considerations in the management of hypertension include weight control, restricted sodium intake, assurance of adequate potassium, magnesium, and calcium intake, and restricted alcohol consumption.

Weight Reduction. Weight loss in overweight individuals is considered to be the single most important factor in the control of blood pressure. Thus caloric intake and activity levels should be adjusted to reach ideal body weight (see Chapter 12). Even if the ideal weight is not reached, a partial reduction is advantageous in lowering blood pressure and probably in reducing mortality and morbidity due to cardiovascular disease.

Sodium Restriction. When given a mild sodium-restricted diet of 2–3 g (86–130 mEq) of sodium per day, many individuals with mild hypertension will show a decrease in blood pressure, although the mechanism of this response is unclear. In those who do not respond to a mild sodium restriction, a more severe restriction is unlikely to be effective. However, a mild sodium restriction is still advised because a low-sodium diet will reduce potassium losses due to secondary hyperaldosteronism and allow the use of lower drug doses in most patients taking diuretics. A 2–3 g restriction is significantly lower than the present estimated daily consumption of sodium in the United States of 2,500–8,800 mg (109–383 mEq).[23] It is considered that 1,100–3,300 mg (50–150 mEq) is a safe and adequate sodium intake, and only 200 mg (9 mEq) is required to maintain sodium balance.[18] Thus, in order to control hypertension using a sodium-restricted diet alone, an individual's sodium intake would have to be limited to 250 mg per day, a very severe restriction with which few people can comply. In addition, such a severe sodium restriction may prevent the blood pressure from falling due to marked stimulation of the renin-angiotensin system.[24] With the development of safer, more potent drugs, however, such severe dietary sodium restrictions are rarely used in the management of hypertension.

For use in cardiovascular disease, sodium-restricted diets, described in Chapter 9, are used at the following levels:[23]

1. *Mild* restriction, 2–3 g per day, is used in combination with drugs by patients with moderate heart damage and mild hypertension.
2. *Moderate* sodium restriction of 1 g per day is used to treat mild edema.
3. *Strict* sodium restriction, 500 mg sodium per day, is used for patients who have edema and severe congestive heart failure.

Alcohol Restriction. Chronic consumption of more than 1 oz. of alcohol per day is clearly associated with higher blood pressure in many individuals.[12] However, individuals who abstain from alcohol completely have higher morbidity and mortality due to coronary heart disease than those who drink 0.5 to 1.0 oz of alcohol daily.[12] Thus it is recommended that people at risk for hypertension reduce their alcohol intake to no more than 1 oz. of ethanol per day.[10]

Potassium. A low-potassium intake has been suggested to play a role in the etiology of hypertension; thus hypertensive individuals should be encouraged to consume approximately 1,875–5,625 mg K daily. In addition, the hypertensive patient receiving diuretic medication, especially if the patient's diet is high in sodium, may be at risk of developing a potassium deficiency, or hypokalemia. The concentration of potassium in the extracellular fluid affects the excitability of the myocardium in which conduction and rhythm can be greatly affected. In hyperkalemia, myocardial fibers become less excitable, and the heart may stop in diastole. In hypokalemia, cardiac arrest occurs in systole. Hyperkalemia may be rapidly fatal, whereas hypokalemia has a slower effect.

Patients should be instructed to be alert to symptoms of potassium deficiency, anorexia, malaise, and muscle weakness. Patients at risk may be instructed to increase their intake of potassium-rich foods (see Chapter 9).

Other Diet Components. At this time, there is not enough conclusive evidence regarding the effects of dietary magnesium or calcium to warrant recommending supplements of minerals. However, since evidence suggests that low intake of these nutrients may be associated with hypertension, patients should be encouraged to consume adequate amounts as recommended in the RDA.[14]

Individuals with hypertension may be encouraged to reduce their intake of **saturated fats** because hypertensive patients often have hypercholesterolemia and an increased risk of coronary heart disease. In addition,

Table 10-6. *Drugs Used to Treat Hypertension*

Class	Generic (Proprietary) Names	Primary Action and Use	Nutritional Implications
Diuretics Thiazides	Bendroflumethiazide (Naturetin) Benzthiazide (Exna) Chlorothiazide (Diuril) Cyclothiazide (Anhydron) Hydrochlorothiazide (Esidrix, Hydrodiuril, Oretic) Hydroflumethiazide (Saluron) Methyclothiazide (Enduron) Polythiazide (Renese) Trichlormethiazide (Metahydrin, Naqua)	↓Na reabsorption in loop of Henle and distal tubule. Most act for 12–24 hours.	To prevent hypokalemia: 2–3 g Na diet, high-potassium foods. Low-saturated-fat diet may counteract the hypercholesterolemic effect of diuretics. Other side effects: ↑ Ca reabsorption, hypomagnesemia, hyperuricemia, GI tract disturbances, orthostatic hypotension aggravated by alcohol.
Related sulfonamide compounds	Chlorthalidone (Hydroton) Indapamide (Lozol) Metolazone (Zaroxolyn, Dinlo) Quinethazone (Hydromax)	Same as for thiazides.	Same as for thiazides.
Loop	Bumetanide (Bumex) Ethacrynic acid (Edecrin) Furosemide (Lasix)	↓Na reabsorption in ascending loop of Henle. Short-acting (4–6 hours). Act on large percentage of filtrate; useful in patients with renal insufficiency.	Same as for thiazides.
Potassium sparing agents	Amiloride (Midamor) Spironolactone (Aldactone) Triamterene (Dyrenium)	↓Na reabsorption in distal tubules and collecting ducts. Spironolactone is an aldosterone antagonist; other two directly inhibit Na-K exchange. Often used with a thiazide.	Avoid excess K to prevent hyperkalemia, especially in patients with poor renal function. Low-Na diet ↑effectiveness. Take with food. May cause GI disturbances.
Adrenergic inhibitors Peripheral neuronal inhibitors	Reserpine Guanethidine (Ismelin) Guanadrel (Hylorel)	Inhibits norepinephrine release from peripheral adrenergic neurons.	May cause GI disturbances. Alcohol aggravates orthostatic hypertensive effects.
Central adrenergic inhibitors	Methyldopa (Aldomet) Clonidine (Catapres) Guanabenz (Wytensin)	Stimulation of central alpha-adrenoreceptors reducing sympathetic outflow. Suitable for young, old, blacks, and whites. Methyldopa used for patients with renal insufficiency. Methyldopa and clonidine cause fluid retention, used with diuretic. Safe for diabetics. Methyldopa used in pregnant women.	Dry mouth and GI disturbances may result. May have beneficial effect on blood cholesterol profile.

Category	Drugs	Mechanism/Comments	Notes
Alpha receptor blockers	Phenoxybenzamine (Dibenzyline) Phentolamine (Regitine) Prazosin (Minipress)	↓Total PVR by blocking alpha receptors. Prazosin is most useful. Other two are used primarily with pheochromocytoma. Useful with complicated hypertension, such as with renal insufficiency or diabetes mellitus.	Blood lipid profile may improve.
Beta receptor blockers	Acebutolol (Sectral) Atenolol (Tenormin) Metaprolol (Lopressor) Nadolol (Corgard) Pindolol (Visken) Propranolol (Inderal) Timolol (Blocadren)	Mechanisms unclear. CO and renin↓, but PVR↑. May ↓Ca within cells. Blacks and elderly respond less well. Used for angina. Used with vasodilators to prevent ↑CO.	Some may cause ↓HDL and ↑cholesterol levels. May interfere with insulin secretion; use with caution in diabetics.
Alpha and beta receptor blocker	Labetalol (Normodyne, Trandate)	Mechanisms unclear. Beta-blocking characteristics predominate. Effective in elderly, young, blacks, and whites.	Seems to have beneficial effect on plasma lipid profile. Use with caution in diabetes.
Vasodilators Direct	Hydralazine (Apresoline) Minoxidil Nitroprusside Diazoxide Nitroglycerine	↓PVR by directly relaxing vascular smooth muscle. Hydralazine is used most commonly.	
Calcium antagonists	Diltiazen Nifedipine Verapamil	Vasodilation by blocking Ca entry into smooth muscle cells. Used for angina. Particularly effective in blacks and elderly.	Effectiveness may be reduced by a strict Na restriction. May cause nausea.
Converting enzyme inhibitors (CEI)	Captopril (Capoten) Enalapril (Vasotec)	↓Angiotensin II levels by preventing angiotensin I conversion. May also ↑bradykinin levels, and ↑production of vasodilatory prostaglandins.	Restrict Na. Avoid excess K. May cause GI disturbances. Take captopril 1 hour before meals.
Alpha blockers (see "Adrenergic inhibitors")			

Compiled from The 1988 Report of the Joint National Committee on Detection, Evaluation and Treatment of High Blood Pressure. *Arch. Intern. Med.* 148:1023–1038; *Physicians Desk Reference.* Oradell, N.J.: Medical Economics Company, 1988; Frohlich, E., Essential hypertension. *Med. Clin. North. Am.* 71:935–990, 1987; Braunwald, E., *Heart Disease—A Textbook of Cardiovascular Medicine,* 3rd ed. Philadelphia: W.B. Saunders, 1988.

some antihypertensive drugs may worsen blood lipid profiles. Studies suggest that intake of linoleic acid from polyunsaturated fats tends to reduce blood pressure in animal models and humans with hypertension.[25] This effect of linoleic acid is ascribed to a greater synthesis of vasodilatory prostaglandins in the total body and the kidney as demonstrated by increased urinary excretion of prostaglandin derivatives with increasing levels of linoleic acid intake. A greater total intake of polyunsaturated fat is generally not needed. In studies of hypertensive middle-aged males and females, 5–10% of total kilocalorie intake from linoleic acid was adequate to reduce arterial blood pressure.[25] Intake of omega-3 fatty acids from fish oils may also have an antihypertensive effect due to modulation of eicosanoid synthesis, currently an active area of research.[26]

Drugs

The development of safer, more potent antihypertensive drugs has resulted in less emphasis on severe dietary sodium restriction. In the past, a suitable drug therapy was determined by increasing dosages to their maximum before trying another drug. Now, however, small doses of more than one compound are used in combination in order to take advantage of their synergistic effects and to minimize side effects. All drug therapies should be given against a background of the nonpharmacological treatments discussed previously.

The three major classifications of drugs used to treat hypertension are diuretics, adrenergic inhibitors, and vasodilators. Refer to Table 10-6 for a summary of their actions and nutritional implications. Antihypertensive drugs are generally administered using a "stepped-care" approach that begins with either a diuretic in most cases, a beta-blocker in 15–20% of the cases, or a calcium antagonist or converting enzyme inhibitor (CEI) in 5–10% of cases.[27] This dose is gradually increased to less than maximum. If hypertension is not controlled, either the dose is

increased to maximum, another drug is substituted, or one or more drugs from other classes are added in a stepwise fashion until goal blood pressure is reached.[10] Therapy usually begins with a diuretic that causes substantial urinary sodium and water loss. This initially causes a drop in plasma volume and cardiac output, but eventually sodium balance stabilizes owing to stimulation of the renin-angiotensin system, and cardiac output returns to normal. The net long-term effect of diuretic treatment is a drop in blood pressure due to a decrease in peripheral resistance and a slight decrease in plasma volume.[27] Adherence to diuretic prescription is generally good. Diuretics tend to be especially effective in patients with volume-dependent forms of hypertension, which are common among blacks and people over 50 years of age. There are three major types of diuretics: loop, thiazides and related sulfonamide compounds, and potassium-sparing agents. In the nephron, loop diuretics promote sodium excretion in the ascending limb of the loop of Henle. Thiazides increase sodium excretion at the distal convoluted tubules, and potassium-sparing agents, at the collecting ducts.

If a diuretic alone does not lower blood pressure adequately, an **adrenergic inhibitor** may be prescribed. The **peripheral neuronal inhibitors** block norepinephrine release from peripheral neurons. They are very effective when combined with a diuretic. **Central adrenergic inhibitors** decrease sympathetic outflow from the central nervous system. **Beta blockers** reduce ventricular contractility and heart rate by blocking the beta receptors on the heart. After diuretics, these are the second most popular antihypertensive therapy. **Alpha blockers** act on the neural receptors on vascular smooth muscle to reduce constriction.

The vasodilator class of antihypertensive drugs includes direct smooth muscle vasodilators, converting enzyme inhibitors, and calcium channel blockers. **Direct smooth muscle vasodilators** reduce blood pressure by decreasing peripheral resistance. However, this reduction is accompanied by an increase in sympathetic nervous system activity, renin production, and salt and fluid retention. Thus vasodilators are generally used with diuretics and a beta blocker. **Converting enzyme inhibitors** (CEI) prevent the production of angiotensin II and therefore reduce aldosterone secretion. When starting therapy, CEIs can be used as the first drug, although their activity is enhanced when combined with diuretics. They have few side effects, but can interfere with renal autoregulation. Thus they are contraindicated with some renal disorders. The **calcium channel blockers** cause vasodilation by interfering with calcium transport. Unlike the diuretics, the antihypertensive efficacy of the calcium channel blockers may not be blunted by a high-sodium intake, and strict dietary sodium restriction may actually reduce the effectiveness of calcium channel blockers.[28]

Some antihypertensive drugs affect blood lipid profiles. For example, thiazide diuretics tend to increase triglyceride and total cholesterol, while loop diuretics may decrease HDL cholesterol levels. The significance of these changes will be discussed in the section on hyperlipidemia.

Because loop and thiazide diuretics increase the excretion of potassium as well as sodium, patients are at risk of developing hypokalemia and should be encouraged to increase their dietary potassium intake. Diabetic or elderly patients whose potassium intake may be inadequate are especially susceptible. Serum potassium will be monitored, and if hypokalemia persists, the physician may prescribe a potassium-sparing diuretic in place of or in addition to other diuretics. Patients with left ventricular hypertrophy or coronary artery disease and those who are taking digitalis are at significant risk for ventricular arrhythmias and sudden death at potassium levels less than 3.5 mEq/L and should be monitored closely.[27]

Some diuretics and beta blockers may interfere with the action of insulin. Diabetes mellitus may be aggravated, and insulin-dependent patients may need to adjust their doses.

HYPERLIPIDEMIA

Hyperlipidemia consists of increased levels of cholesterol or triglycerides, the major lipid components in the circulation. The plasma lipoprotein system provides a vehicle for transporting lipids in blood. Defects in lipid metabolism or the plasma lipoprotein transport system may result in elevated blood lipid levels. Hyperlipidemia is associated with increased morbidity and mortality from atherosclerosis and coronary heart disease. The absorption of dietary lipids is discussed in Chapter 8.

Cholesterol

Elevated plasma cholesterol levels, smoking, and hypertension are the three major risk factors associated with the development of coronary heart disease. Because of its association with coronary heart disease, cholesterol metabolism has been the subject of intensive investigation. Cholesterol is an essential metabolite in animal cells, but not plant cells, and performs several important functions in the body. As a structural component of cell membranes, cholesterol modulates membrane fluidity and permeability of the cell to specific compounds; it is also a component of the myelin sheath surrounding the axons of neurons. Cholesterol is a precursor for the synthesis of bile acids and steroid hormones such as cortisone, estrogen, and testosterone. Cholesterol is not essential in the diet because it can be synthesized from acetyl coenzyme A by practically every tissue in the body.

Plasma cholesterol concentration is a function of three factors, dietary intake and absorption, endogenous synthesis, and excretion. The primary route of cholesterol excretion from the body is by biliary secretion and excretion in the feces. Cholesterol is converted to bile acids, followed by biliary secretion of both bile acids and free cholesterol into the small intestine. Approximately 30–60% of biliary cholesterol is reabsorbed with the remaining excreted in the feces as neutral sterols.[29] A small amount of cholesterol is also lost from the body from desquamation of skin. Therapies that increase fecal excretion of cholesterol, such as bile-acid-binding resins that prevent reabsorption of bile acids, are especially effective in lowering blood cholesterol levels.

The total pool of plasma cholesterol largely reflects endogenous cholesterol synthesis and not dietary intake. Endogenous cholesterol synthesis averages 1 g/day for a 70-kg male, which is approximately 1% of the body's total pool of metabolically active cholesterol.[14,29] Average cholesterol intake in the United States is 450 mg/day for men and 300 mg/day for women, of which approximately 50% is absorbed.[14] Therefore, only 20% of the body's cholesterol pool derives from dietary intake, with the rest reflecting endogenous synthesis.

The liver and intestine are the primary sites of cholesterol and lipoprotein synthesis in man. The body normally regulates cholesterol synthesis in response to differences in cholesterol intake or excretion such that a relatively constant concentration of cholesterol is maintained in the blood and different tissues of the body. The principal regulatory site in the cholesterol biosynthetic pathway is the step catalyzed by the enzyme 3-hydroxy-3-methylglutaryl-CoA reductase (**HMG-CoA reductase**). Research by Brown and Goldstein demonstrated the receptor-mediated endocytosis of LDL particles results in feedback control of cholesterol synthesis by means of regulation of the level of HMG-CoA reductase messenger RNA.[30]

Factors that affect the absorption of cholesterol from the intestine, whether derived from the diet or biliary secretion, play an important part in total body cholesterol balance. Cholesterol, which is insoluble in water, must be solubilized in the form of micelles before it can be absorbed (see Chapter 8). The extent to which dietary cholesterol is adequately solubilized and subsequently absorbed depends on a number of factors including the total amount of fat and cholesterol in a meal, bile acid pool size, gut motility, and the presence of plant substances such as plant sterols or dietary fiber that may interfere with cholesterol and bile acid absorption. The absorption of dietary cholesterol is incomplete, ranging from 25% to 75% depending on the factors mentioned.

Transport of cholesterol in aqueous blood is mediated by lipoprotein particles. In order to gain an understanding of cholesterol transport, a knowledge of lipoprotein structure and the dynamics of lipoprotein metabolism is needed.

Lipoproteins

Lipoproteins are complexes of lipid and protein that solubilize hydrophobic lipids, primarily cholesterol and triglycerides, in blood. The function of lipoprotein particles is to transport lipids from the bloodstream to various tissues where they are stored, metabolized for energy, or used for biosynthesis.

Lipoproteins include a heterogeneous group of particles varying in size, composition, and function. The primary structure of a lipoprotein particle consists of a sphere with a hydrophobic core composed of triglycerides and esterified cholesterol, and a hydrophilic surface coat composed of phospholipid, free cholesterol, and specific proteins referred to as apolipoproteins or **apoproteins**. The apoproteins have several key functions besides their structural role, which stabilizes the lipoprotein particles.[31] They serve as activators for enzymes of lipid metabolism and are recognized by membrane receptors, thus mediating uptake of cholesterol and triglycerides by various tissues. The apoproteins direct the metabolism of lipoprotein particles, and thus they are a major determinant of plasma lipid concentrations.

The apoproteins are identified by a lettering and numbering system. The major apoproteins include Apo E, Apo B, Apo A-I, Apo A-IV, and Apo C-I, C-II, and C-III. They range in weight from 6,600 to more than 400,000 daltons.[31] The primary structures of most of the apolipoproteins are known. A greater understanding of the relationship between apoprotein structure and function has recently been aided by identification of genetically determined variants of specific apoproteins that are associated with disorders of lipoprotein metabolism. The function and major apoproteins associated with the classes of lipoproteins are given in Table 10-7. Apo B is not found in HDL; however, the other apoproteins overlap and readily interchange between the lipoprotein fractions as they are metabolized. Apo A-I and A-IV are synthesized primarily by the intestine, and Apo E and the Apo C's are synthesized primarily by the liver. Large and small molecular weight variants of Apo B (B-48 and B-100) are synthesized by the liver and intestine, respectively. Besides its role in cholesterol transport, Apo E has recently been demonstrated to affect many cellular pro-

cesses, including immune function, tissue repair, and modulation of cellular growth.[32]

Classification

Lipoproteins are most commonly divided into five classes based on their size and density as follows: chylomicrons, very-low-density lipoproteins (VLDL), intermediate-density lipoproteins (IDL), low-density lipoproteins (LDL), and high-density lipoproteins (HDL). This terminology reflects the use of ultracentrifugation to isolate the various classes of lipoproteins in the laboratory. Each class of lipoproteins consists of particles of characteristic lipid and protein composition that confer a specific size and density. The properties of the lipoproteins are summarized in Table 10-8. In general, density increases as the proportion of lipid decreases and the proportion of protein increases. Thus chylomicrons are the largest particles that contain the most triglyceride

Table 10-7. Properties of the Apolipoproteins

Apolipoprotein	Location[a]	Tissue Origin	Function[b]
A-I	CM, VLDL, HDL	Intestine, liver	LCAT activator
A-II	CM, VLDL, HDL	Intestine, liver	Unknown
A-IV	CM, VLDL, HDL, free in plasma	Intestine, liver	?LCAT activator
B-48	CM	Intestine	CM secretion, cholesterol and TG transport
B-100	VLDL, IDL, LDL	Liver	VLDL secretion, LDL receptor recognition
C-I	CM, VLDL, HDL	Liver	Inhibits hepatic uptake of lipoproteins
C-II	CM, VLDL, HDL	Liver	Extrahepatic lipoprotein lipase activator
C-III	CM, VLDL, HDL	Liver	Inhibits lipoprotein lipase and premature remnant clearance
E	CM, VLDL, IDL, trace amounts in LDL and HDL	Liver, macrophages, and most tissues except the intestine	Remnant and LDL receptor recognition, immunoregulation, modulation of cell growth
D	HDL	Spleen, liver, intestine, and adrenals	Part of cholesterol ester transfer complex

[a] CM = chylomicron; HDL = high-density lipoprotein; IDL = intermediate-density lipoprotein; LDL = low-density lipoprotein; VLDL = very-low-density lipoprotein.
[b] LCAT = lecithin-cholesterol acyltransferase; TG = triglyceride.

Table 10-8. *Major Classes of Plasma Lipoproteins*

Lipoprotein Class[a]	Density (g/ml)	Electrophoretic Mobility	Size (nm)	Composition (%)					Function	Origin
				Protein	Trigly-cerides	Total Choles-terol	Phospho-lipids		
Chylomicrons	<0.95	Origin	75–1,000	1–2	80–95	2–5	3–6	Transport of dietary lipids.	Intestine
VLDL	<1.006	Prebeta	30–80	5–10	40–80	10–40	15–20	Transport of endogenous and exogenous lipids.	Liver; intestine
IDL	1.006–1.019	Beta	25–30	15	35	33	17	LDL precursor.	VLDL catabolism
LDL	1.019–1.063	Beta	19–25	25	10	45	20	Transport of cholesterol; regulation of cholesterol metabolism.	IDL catabolism
HDL	1.063–1.210	Alpha	4–10	45–50	1–5	20	30	? Reverse transport of cholesterol from peripheral tissues to liver.	Intestine, liver, surface of CM and VLDL remnants

[a] HDL = high-density lipoprotein; IDL = intermediate-density lipoprotein, also called a VLDL remnant; LDL = low-density lipoprotein; VLDL = very-low-density lipoprotein.

and least protein, whereas HDL are the smallest, most protein-dense lipoprotein particle with the least lipid.

Lipoproteins may also be classified according to electrophoretic mobility, since electrophoresis is another laboratory technique used to isolate and characterize the different classes of lipoproteins. Electrophoretic separation of plasma lipoproteins is based on the varying apoprotein content of the lipoprotein classes and the manner in which this affects electrophoretic mobility in relation to migration of the plasma proteins.

Chylomicrons remain at the origin. VLDL migrate beyond the beta-globulins and therefore are referred to as prebeta lipoproteins. LDL migrate along with the beta-globulins and thus are beta-lipoproteins. HDL migrate with alpha-globulins and are referred to as alpha-lipoproteins. IDL migrate to a point intermediate between VLDL and LDL. A summary of the major classes of lipoproteins according to electrophoretic mobility is also included in Table 10-8.

An abnormal lipoprotein, referred to as lipoprotein a, Lp(a), has recently been identified. Lp(a) is a genetic variant of LDL whose presence represents an independent risk factor for coronary heart disease. Lp(a) contains apo B-100 like LDL, but it also contains apo (a) which is attached to apo B-100 by disulfide bridge(s). Due to the additional protein moiety, Lp(a) migrates with prebeta mobility on agarose gel electrophoresis and has a density of 1.050–1.120 g/ml. Lp(a) is not a metabolic product of VLDL, LDL, or CM but appears to be synthesized as a separate lipoprotein. There is a poor correlation between the concentration of Lp(a) and LDL or total cholesterol levels. The atherogenicity of Lp(a) may be due to the fact that apo (a) has a similar amino acid sequence as plasminogen, a protease zymogen that on activation to plasmin promotes the conversion of fibrinogen to fibrin.[33]

The sum of the cholesterol carried by VLDL, LDL, and HDL equals the total plasma cholesterol level. Clinically, the relative amounts of the lipoprotein classes

VLDL, LDL, and HDL are estimated by determining cholesterol content in each of these fractions. HDL cholesterol is determined by automated precipitation methodology. VLDL cholesterol is estimated as 20% of the fasting triglyceride value for levels of triglyceride less than 300 mg/dl, and LDL cholesterol is estimated from the equation

$$\text{LDL cholesterol} = \text{total cholesterol} - (\text{HDL cholesterol} + 0.2\ \text{TG}) \qquad \textbf{(10-4)}$$

Further characterization of the lipoprotein profile using ultracentrifugation and electrophoresis is reserved for individuals with markedly elevated plasma cholesterol and TG levels or an unusual plasma lipoprotein pattern.

The sources and functions of the major classes of lipoproteins vary just as their protein and lipid compositions vary. Chylomicrons and VLDL are both composed primarily of triglycerides. Chylomicrons are synthesized in the intestine and transport most of the dietary triglyceride to peripheral tissues and dietary cholesterol to the liver. VLDL are primarily synthesized in the liver, but may be synthesized in the intestine, and function to transport primarily endogenously synthesized triglycerides to adipose tissue for storage. After chylomicrons and VLDL have been depleted of their triglycerides, the remaining lipoprotein is called a remnant. IDL are referred to as VLDL remnants. IDL serve as precursors of LDL and are believed to be atherogenic.[34] LDL are composed primarily of esterified cholesterol and Apo B-100, as shown in Figure 10-9; LDL function to deliver cholesterol to the liver and peripheral tissues through recognition of Apo B-100 by the LDL receptor. Approximately 75% of the total plasma cholesterol content is located in the LDL fraction, and high serum LDL cholesterol level is a positive risk factor for coronary heart disease. HDL are thought to play a protective role because of their possible function in reverse transport of cholesterol from peripheral tissues to the liver.

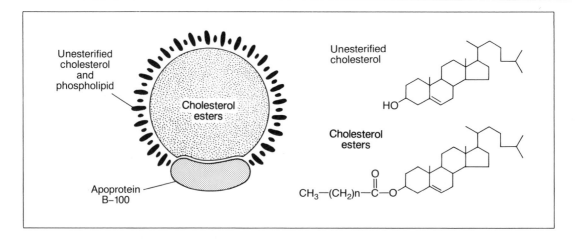

Figure 10-9. Structure of low-density lipoprotein, the primary transporter of cholesterol in human plasma. (Taken from A receptor-mediated pathway for cholesterol homeostasis by Michael S. Brown and Joseph L. Goldstein as published in Science *232:35, April 4, 1986. © 1986 by The Nobel Foundation.)*

Metabolism

The metabolism of the various classes of lipoproteins is a dynamic system that is sensitive to changes in dietary input and hormonal status. The liver and intestine are the principal sites of lipoprotein synthesis and subsequent metabolism. Transport of lipid by lipoprotein particles is often summarized according to exogenous and endogenous pathways, as summarized in Figure 10-10. The exogenous system transports lipids obtained from the intestine, either from the diet or recycled in the enterohepatic circulation, and the endogenous system transports lipids synthesized in the liver.

Exogenous Transport System. After absorption, dietary cholesterol and triglycerides are resynthesized in the intestinal mucosa to chylomicrons, are absorbed into the lymph, and enter the systemic circulation at the thoracic duct (see Chapter 8). In the capillaries of fat and muscle tissue, the chylomicrons bind to the enzyme lipoprotein lipase, which is activated by apoprotein C-II located on the chylomicron. Lipoprotein lipase cleaves the triglyceride's ester bond, freeing the fatty acids to be used by the muscle or adipose tissue. As the triglyceride is removed, the chylomicron shrinks in size, and some of the surface phospholipid and free cholesterol are transferred to HDL. The remaining chylomicron remnant particle contains cholesterol ester, Apo B and Apo E. It is carried to the liver where the remnant receptor recognizes Apo E, thus mediating receptor-mediated uptake of the chylomicron remnant. Within the liver, dietary cholesterol contained in chylomicron remnants is primarily secreted into the intestine, mostly as bile acids, or repackaged with triglycerides in VLDL particles and secreted back into the circulation.

Endogenous Transport System. Hepatic secretion of VLDL initiates the endogenous transport pathway. Like chylomicrons, VLDL triglycerides are removed by the action of lipoprotein lipase in the capillaries of

Figure 10-10. Exogenous and endogenous fat transport pathways are diagrammed. Dietary cholesterol is absorbed through the wall of the intestine and is packaged, along with triglyceride (glycerol ester-linked to three fatty acid chains), in chylomicrons. In the capillaries of fat and muscle tissue the triglyceride's ester bond is cleaved by the enzyme lipoprotein (LP) lipase and the fatty acids are removed. When the cholesterol-rich remnants reach the liver, they bind to specialized receptors and are taken into liver cells. Their cholesterol

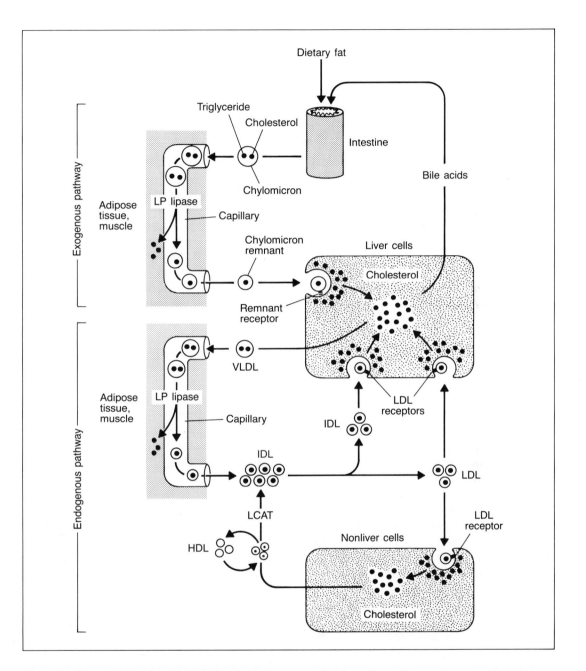

either is secreted into the intestine (mostly as bile acids) or is packaged with triglyceride in very-low-density lipoprotein (VLDL) particles and secreted into the circulation, inaugurating the endogenous pathway. Again the triglyceride is removed in fat or muscle, leaving cholesterol-rich intermediate-density lipoprotein (IDL). Some IDL bind to liver LDL receptors and is rapidly taken up by liver cells; the remainder stays in the circulation and is converted into LDL. Most of the LDL binds to LDL receptors

on liver or other cells and is removed from the circulation. Cholesterol leaching from cells binds to high-density lipoprotein (HDL) and is esterified by the enzyme LCAT. The esters are transferred to IDL and then LDL and are eventually taken up again by cells. (Taken from Michael S. Brown and Joseph L. Goldstein. How LDL receptors influence cholesterol and atherosclerosis. Scientific American 251(5):58–66, 1984. Copyright © 1984 by Scientific American, Inc. All rights reserved.)

adipose and muscle tissues. A cholesterol-rich IDL particle or VLDL remnant results from the action of lipoprotein lipase on VLDL. Some IDL binds to liver remnant receptors and is rapidly taken up by the liver; the remainder is converted to LDL by an unknown mechanism involving loss of most of the remaining triglyceride and almost all of the apoproteins except for Apo B-100. Most of the LDL binds to LDL receptors on liver or other peripheral tissue that recognize Apo B-100 and thus remove LDL cholesterol from the circulation. About two-thirds of LDL is catabolized by the liver.

The LDL receptor is central to understanding how plasma cholesterol levels are regulated.[30] LDL receptors are localized in specialized regions in the plasma membrane called "coated pits" because they are enriched in the protein clathrin. The number of LDL receptors on cell membranes determines LDL uptake from plasma. Once internalized, the LDL dissociates from the receptor, which is recycled to the cell surface. The LDL is delivered to a lysosome, where enzymes break down the apoprotein B-100 into amino acids and cleave the ester bond to yield unesterified cholesterol for membrane synthesis and other cellular needs. An oversupply of LDL cholesterol to cells has three metabolic effects, as shown in Figure 10-11. It inhibits the enzyme HMG CoA reductase, which reduces the rate of endogenous cholesterol synthesis; it activates the enzyme acyl-CoA:cholesterol acyltransferase (ACAT), which esterifies cholesterol for storage; and it inhibits the manufacture of new LDL receptors by suppressing transcription of the receptor gene into messenger RNA. Thus cells regulate their cholesterol level and indirectly affect plasma cholesterol concentration by these three metabolic effects.

HDL Metabolism. HDL metabolism is currently the subject of intense investigation. HDL are thought to arise from at least three sources: hepatic secretion, intestinal secretion, and budding from the surface of chylomicrons and VLDL after triglyceride lipolysis due to lipoprotein lipase. Human HDL represent a heterogeneous population of particles with at least two subpopulations, HDL_2 and HDL_3. The former are associated with a reduced risk of coronary heart disease, whereas HDL_3 are not. Woman and trained athletes such as marathon runners have substantially higher levels of HDL_2, consistent with their lower rates of coronary heart disease.

Newly secreted HDL have a discoidal shape and contain phospholipid, free cholesterol, and Apo A-I. These HDL acquire additional free cholesterol from remnant particles and possibly peripheral tissues, which is then esterified by action of the enzyme **lecithin cholesterol acyl-transferase** (LCAT). The enzyme LCAT circulates in plasma and catalyzes transfer of a fatty acid from the sn-2 position on lecithin to cholesterol. HDL cholesterol is the principle substrate for LCAT, and Apo A-I activates LCAT. Some of the HDL esterified cholesterol is transferred to VLDL, IDL, or LDL by a process catalyzed by **cholesterol ester transfer protein**, while the rest enters the core of the HDL particle causing it to become spherical instead of discoidal. HDL_2 tend to be larger, less dense, and contain more esterified cholesterol than HDL_3. HDL metabolism is extremely complex due to the lability of the functional complexes directing exchange of free and esterified cholesterol.

Epidemiological studies demonstrate a strong inverse relationship between HDL cholesterol or Apo A-I levels and risk of heart disease.[34] An HDL cholesterol level of less than 35 mg/dl is considered a risk factor for coronary heart disease. Researchers have proposed that HDL may leach cholesterol from deposits in the arterial wall and then transport the cholesterol back to the liver for excretion. An alternative explanation is that high HDL levels are merely a reflection of overall healthy lipid metabolism. High HDL are generally considered beneficial, although the mechanism of protection from coronary heart disease is unclear. In inter-

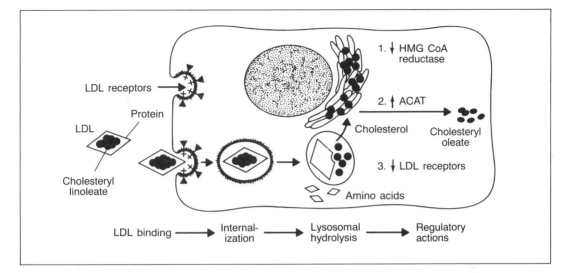

Figure 10-11. Sequential steps in the LDL receptor pathway of mammalian cells. HMG CoA reductase, 3-hydroxy-3-methylglutaryl CoA reductase; ACAT, acyl-CoA: cholesterol acyltransferase. Vertical arrows indicate the directions of regulatory effects. (Taken from A receptor-mediated pathway for cholesterol homeostasis by Michael S. Brown and Joseph L. Goldstein as published in Science *232:34–47, April 4, 1986. © 1986 by The Nobel Foundation.)*

preting clinical information, it is important to realize that high total cholesterol levels are associated with high HDL levels, which may not indicate protection when LDL levels are also elevated. Tables with population percentage values for LDL and HDL cholesterol are contained in Appendix I.

Effects of Diet on Plasma Lipids

Cholesterol

Compared to the effects of the type and total quantity of dietary fat, dietary cholesterol is the least important dietary variable affecting serum cholesterol level.[14] Most of the studies demonstrating a strong positive relationship between cholesterol intake and plasma cholesterol level were conducted using men in a metabolic ward who consumed liquid formula diets to which different amounts of cholesterol were added.[36] Studies using free-living individuals consuming their usual diet

with added amounts of cholesterol from eggs and other typical dietary sources do not demonstrate a significant increase in plasma cholesterol level.[37,38] Current research suggests that most individuals have effective feedback control mechanisms such that little change in plasma cholesterol occurs when dietary cholesterol increases.[37]

The control mechanisms include both a decrease in endogenous cholesterol synthesis and a decrease in the fractional absorption of cholesterol when dietary cholesterol increases. However, research also demonstrates that the response to dietary cholesterol is highly individualized such that some individuals may demonstrate a significant decrease in plasma cholesterol due to dietary cholesterol restriction. In general, the response to an increase in dietary cholesterol is greater when the diet also contains a high proportion of saturated fat.[36–38] In the United States, where the usual daily intake of cholesterol is approximately 450 mg/day,[14] changes in dietary cholesterol intake of 100–200 mg/day may have a relatively small effect on serum cholesterol. For example, only a 4 mg/dl increase in serum cholesterol is projected for an individual consuming 2,500 kcal who increases his cholesterol intake by 100 mg.[39] Although the American Heart Association and the National Cholesterol Education Program recommend an intake of less than 300 mg of cholesterol per day, the 1984 British Committee on Medical Aspects of Food Policy made no recommendation on dietary cholesterol because it judged its effects on plasma cholesterol to be minimal.

The dietary sources of cholesterol are animal foods (Table 10-9). Egg yolk and organ meats such as liver, kidney, and brain are the richest sources. Red meats, dairy products, poultry, and fish also contribute 50–80 mg cholesterol per 3-oz. serving. Improved analytical methods for the determination of cholesterol in food suggest that previous methods have overestimated the cholesterol content of foods. For example, one egg yolk has 208 mg of cholesterol instead of 278 mg as previously reported in U.S.D.A. food composition tables.

Type and Amount of Dietary Fat

Fatty Acid Saturation. Both the type and amount of dietary fat influence plasma lipoprotein composition and the total serum concentrations of cholesterol and triglycerides. Population studies suggest that total fat intake is correlated with serum cholesterol levels and rates of coronary heart disease. Human feeding studies utilizing isocaloric substitution of polyunsaturated vegetable oils for saturated fats such as coconut and palm oils have clearly demonstrated a reduction in total serum cholesterol and LDL cholesterol levels due to polyunsaturated fats. Based on these studies, Keys et al. proposed a formula that quantified the relationship between dietary fatty acid intake and serum cholesterol response.[40] The Keys formula suggests that a decrease in saturated fatty acids is twice as potent in lowering serum cholesterol as an increase in polyunsaturated fatty acids.[14]

Current research suggests that the Keys formula and the concept of the P/S, or polyunsaturated/saturated, ratio of the diet may oversimplify the effects of different types of dietary fats on plasma cholesterol level. Saturated fatty acids with different chain

Table 10-9. Cholesterol Content of Selected Foods

Food	Amount	Cholesterol (mg)
Dairy products		
Milk, skim fluid	1 cup	4
Milk, dry whole	100 g	85
Milk, 2%	1 cup	18
Milk, whole	1 cup	34
Half and half	¼ cup	23
Cheese		
Cheddar	1 oz.	30
Cottage, creamed	½ cup	17
Cream	100 g	120
Ice cream (about 10% fat)	½ cup	30
Meat		
Beef, lamb, pork (lean)	3 oz.	77–79
Veal	3 oz.	129
Liver	3 oz.	270
Sweetbreads, kidneys	3 oz.	329
Heart	3 oz.	164
Brains	3 oz.	1746
Poultry (without skin)		
Chicken	3 oz.	72–80
Turkey	3 oz.	60–72
Fish and shellfish		
Salmon	3 oz.	74
Tuna, light, canned in water	3 oz.	55
Halibut	3 oz.	55
Clams	3 oz.	55
Crab		
Alaskan king	3 oz.	45
Blue	3 oz.	85
Lobster	3 oz.	70
Oysters	3 oz.	92
Scallops	3 oz.	35
Shrimp	3 oz.	130
Other		
Egg, whole	One	208
Egg yolk	One	208
Egg white	One	0
Mayonnaise	1 Tbsp.	10
Butter	1 tsp.	11

Compiled from Briggs, G.M., and Calloway, D.H., *Nutrition and Physical Fitness,* 11th ed. New York: Holt, Rinehart and Winston, 1984; and Report of the National Cholesterol Education Program Expert Panel on Detection, Evaluation and Treatment of High Blood Cholesterol in Adults. *Arch. Intern. Med.* 148:36, 1988.

lengths are not equivalent in their effects on elevating plasma cholesterol relative to polyunsaturates. Palm and coconut oil, which are vegetable sources of 16- and 12-carbon saturated fatty acids, respectively, have a greater hypercholesterolemic effect than saturated fatty acids from beef and butterfat, which contain a greater proportion of 18-carbon fatty acids.[41] In addition, current research suggests that monounsaturated fatty acids such as occur in olive oil are not neutral in their effects on plasma cholesterol as previously suggested. Grundy has demonstrated that high oleic and high linoleic safflower oils produce similar reductions in LDL cholesterol concentration, although the oleic-rich oil did not reduce HDL cholesterol levels as frequently as did the linoleic-rich oil.[42]

Regulation of plasma cholesterol concentration via the LDL receptor may suggest an explanation for the effects of type and amount of dietary fat on plasma cholesterol levels (see Figure 10-12).[30,42,43] A high-fat diet, especially a high-saturated-fat, high-cholesterol diet, may lead to overproduction of VLDL and suppression of LDL receptors leading to an increase in plasma LDL concentration. This would have the effect of increasing IDL and LDL formation owing to a greater quantity of VLDL. It would also increase the proportion of IDL converted to LDL because of a longer residence time for IDL in plasma. Finally, LDL concentration would increase because of decreased LDL uptake by means of the LDL receptor. This theory is supported by evidence from animal and human research suggesting that saturated fats decrease LDL receptor levels.[43,44] The saturated fatty acids may be the real culprit, whereas substitution of polyunsaturated or monounsaturated fatty acids for saturated fatty acids may merely restore LDL receptor activity to normal.

Fish Oil or Omega-3 Fatty Acids. Epidemiologic studies indicate that consumption of fish oils enriched in omega-3 (or n-3) fatty acids is associated with decreased mortality from coronary heart disease. Experimental data suggest that reduced coronary heart disease related to increased fish oil consumption is associated with reduction in both plasma lipids and thrombosis. Fish oils are rich sources of the polyunsaturated fatty acids derived from linolenic acid (see Table 10-2), eicosapentanoic (EPA) acid, and docosahexanoic (DHA) acid. Fish obtain these essential fatty acids by consuming plankton and other plants.

Figure 10-12. Possible consequences of a high-saturated fat, high-cholesterol diet resulting in elevated LDL cholesterol levels. 1. Decreased activity of LDL receptors. 2. Increased VLDL production and altered VLDL composition. 3. Decreased clearance of IDL and LDL. 4. Increased LDL production. (Adapted from Brown, M.S., and Goldstein, J.L., A receptor-mediated pathway for cholesterol homeostasis. Science 232:34–47, 1986.)

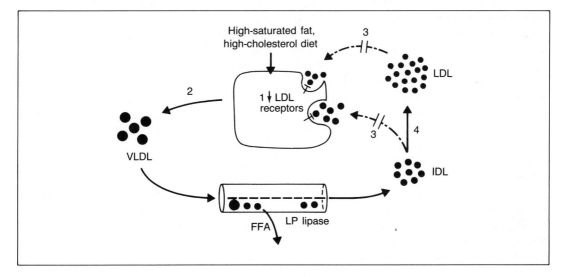

Consumption of fish and fish oils rich in EPA and DHA has been shown to lower serum cholesterol and triglycerides in normal volunteers and in patients with hypertriglyceridemia.[3] In particular EPA and DHA have been reported to inhibit synthesis of the protein and triglyceride components of VLDL.[45] They depress arachidonic acid levels, fatty acid synthesis, and VLDL lipoprotein secretion.[46]

Consumption of fish oils is also associated with reduced platelet aggregation, which may reduce thrombosis, an important factor in initiating a myocardial infarction or a stroke in conjunction with atherosclerosis. The beneficial effects of fish oil consumption are suggested to be associated with alterations in eicosanoid synthesis, as discussed earlier in this chapter. By replacing arachidonate (20:4n6) in phospholipids, dietary n-3 fatty acids may reduce the availability of eicosanoid precursors and thus alter eicosanoid synthesis and the subsequent biochemical events associated with prostanoids and leukotrienes. Reduced platelet aggregation resulting in a favorable antithrombotic status with fish oil consumption is associated with a greater depression in TXA_2 relative to PGI_2 (prostacyclin) levels.

Calories and Carbohydrates

Excessive caloric intake results in obesity, which is often associated with hyperlipidemia, especially elevation in VLDL triglyceride levels. Consumption of excess calories results in storage of the excess calories as fat. This is accomplished by hepatic synthesis of VLDL from carbohydrate and some dietary fat, followed by secretion of VLDL for transport of fat to adipose tissue for storage. Because fat has a higher caloric density than carbohydrate and protein, an increase in total fat intake often leads to obesity and increased VLDL production. Substitution of carbohydrate for fat intake is often associated with an increase in VLDL, although this effect may be only temporary. Populations consuming low-fat, high-carbohydrate

diets tend to have lower HDL levels, but also lower rates of coronary heart disease compared to those consuming higher fat intakes. Caloric restriction is associated with a decrease in VLDL and an increase in HDL levels.

Dietary Fiber

Ingestion of fiber sources containing a greater proportion of the soluble components of dietary fiber, such as oat bran, dried beans, pectin, psyllium, or guar gum, are effective in lowering plasma cholesterol concentration, whereas sources with little soluble fiber, such as wheat bran, are ineffective hypocholesterolemic agents.[47] The addition of 15 to 45 g of soluble fiber to the diet has been noted to reduce total plasma cholesterol by 6% to 19%.[48]

Consumption of 50–100 g of oat bran per day has been reported to decrease serum cholesterol concentration in both normocholesterolemic and hypercholesterolemic subjects, although the decrease is more pronounced in hypercholesterolemic subjects. The hypocholesterolemic effect of oat bran is associated with its content of soluble fiber.[49,50] Ingestion of psyllium hydrophilic mucilloid from the laxative Metamucil also reduces serum cholesterol concentration.[51] The mechanism of the hypocholesterolemic effect of various sources of dietary fiber is unclear; however, enhanced excretion of cholesterol and bile acids and alterations in bile acid and lipoprotein metabolism are thought to contribute in part to this effect. Additional research is needed regarding the composition, physiological effects, and long-term consequences of ingesting increased amounts of various types of dietary fiber.

Alcohol

Alcohol affects lipoprotein metabolism in several ways. It has little effect on LDL cholesterol concentrations, and tends to increase HDL cholesterol and VLDL triglyceride levels. The mechanism of the rise in HDL cholesterol levels is not known, nor is it known whether higher HDL levels due to alcohol consumption are associated with protection from coronary heart disease. The magnitude of these effects varies among individuals depending on the amount of alcohol consumed. Moderate alcohol intake does not appear to have an adverse effect on plasma lipid except in individuals with persistent hypertriglyceridemia, in which case elimination or reduction in alcohol intake may help to reduce VLDL triglycerides and control body weight.

Classification and Treatment

During the past 30 years, an extensive array of research has addressed the questions of how dietary fat affects plasma lipid levels, and whether a decrease in plasma cholesterol level affects the development of atherosclerosis and its progression to coronary heart disease (CHD). More than a dozen randomized clinical trials have studied the effect of lowering LDL cholesterol levels on the incidence of CHD. One of the largest trials, the Coronary Primary Prevention Trial (CPPT), used the drug cholestyramine to reduce LDL cholesterol levels and demonstrated a 2% reduction in the incidence of CHD for each 1% reduction in serum cholesterol level.[52] Based on available evidence, an expert panel of the National Cholesterol Education Program has defined guidelines for the classification and treatment of high blood cholesterol in adults (see Table 10-10).[53] They recommend that fasting serum cholesterol levels be determined at least every five years in all adults 20 years of age and over. Levels below 200 mg/dl are classified as "desirable blood cholesterol." Levels of 200–239 mg/dl are considered "borderline-high blood cholesterol," and those 240 mg/dl and above, "high blood cholesterol." Lipoprotein analysis is also recommended for individuals classified as having high blood cholesterol levels or other risk factors as outlined in Table 10-10. Based on these guidelines, 25% of the adult U.S. population, or approximately 50 million

people, will be assessed as having high blood cholesterol levels and a high risk of coronary heart disease. While most experts agree that individuals with blood cholesterol levels above 240 mg/dl have a considerable risk for developing coronary heart disease, there is controversy in the scientific community regarding the point at which a blood cholesterol level of less than 240 mg/dl poses a significant risk for developing CHD.

Diet is the primary treatment for hypercholesterolemia. The minimal goals of therapy are to lower LDL cholesterol to below 160 mg/dl, or below 130 mg/dl if definite CHD or two other CHD risk factors are present. Dietary therapy is recommended in two steps designed to progressively reduce intakes of saturated fatty acids and cholesterol, and to promote weight loss in those who are overweight (see Table 10-11).

The **Step-One diet** includes a total fat intake of less than 30% of calories, saturated fatty acids less than 10% of calories, and cholesterol less than 300 mg/day (see Table 10-11). The **Step-Two diet** is used if the response to the Step-One diet is inadequate and includes a further reduction in saturated fatty acid intake to less than 7% of calories and in cholesterol to less than 200 mg/day. A minimum of six months of intensive dietary therapy and counseling is recommended before initiation of drug therapy unless LDL cholesterol is severely elevated or CHD is present. Diet therapy should be continued if drug therapy is initiated. A discussion of hyperlipoproteinemias and specific types of drug therapy follows.

Hyperlipidemia and Hyperlipoproteinemia

Hyperlipidemia or hyperlipemia refers to an elevation in blood cholesterol or triglyceride levels, whereas hyperlipoproteinemia (HLP) is a specific term referring to conditions in which the serum concentration of one or more of the classes of lipoproteins is elevated. Primary HLP arises from environmental or genetic factors that affect lipid me-

Table 10-10. *Treatment Recommendations Based on Serum Total and LDL Cholesterol*

Risk Category	Cholesterol (mg/dl)		Recommendations		
	Total	LDL[a]	Diagnosis	Diet	Drugs
Desirable	<200	<130	Remeasure in 5 years		
Borderline					
Without CHD[b] or two other risk factors[c,d]	200–239	130–159	Recheck annually	Initiate diet if LDL ≥ 160	
With CHD or two other risk factors			Lipoprotein assay	Initiate diet if LDL > 130	May initiate drug treatment
High					
Without CHD or two other risk factors	≥240	≥160	Lipoprotein assay	Initiate diet	Initiate drug treatment if LDL ≥ 190
With CHD or two other risk factors			Lipoprotein assay	Initiate diet	Initiate drug treatment if LDL ≥ 160

Adapted from Report of the National Cholesterol Education Program Expert Panel on Detection, Evaluation and Treatment of High Blood Cholesterol in Adults. *Arch. Intern. Med.* 148:37, 1988.

a LDL = low-density lipoprotein.
b CHD = coronary heart disease.
c Risk factors include male sex, family history of premature CHD, hypertension, low levels of high-density lipoproteins, diabetes mellitus, cerebrovascular or peripheral vascular disease, severe obesity, cigarette smoking.
d Children with plasma cholesterol levels exceeding the 75th percentile or 176 mg/dl should be considered for dietary counseling. Drug therapy for hypercholesterolemia in children should only be considered for those children with plasma cholesterol levels exceeding the 95th percentile or 200 mg/dL and only after dietary intervention has been unsuccessful. Committee on Nutrition Indications for Cholesterol Testing in Children. *Pediatrics* 83:141, 1989.

Table 10-11. Dietary Recommendations of the National Cholesterol Education Program

Nutrient	Recommended Intakes	
	Step-One Diet	Step-Two Diet
Total fat	Less than 30% of total calories	Less than 30% of total calories
Saturated fat	Less than 10% of total calories	Less than 7% of total calories
Polyunsaturated fatty acids	Up to 10% of total calories	Up to 10% of total calories
Monounsaturated fatty acids	10–15% of total calories	10–15% of total calories
Carbohydrates	50–60% of total calories	50–60% of total calories
Protein	10–20% of total calories	10–20% of total calories
Cholesterol	<300 mg/day	<200 mg/day
Total calories	To achieve and maintain desirable weight	To achieve and maintain desirable weight

Reprinted with permission from Report of the National Cholesterol Education Program Expert Panel on Detection, Evaluation and Treatment of High Blood Cholesterol in Adults. *Arch. Intern Med.* 148:46, 1988.

tabolism; secondary HLP arises as a result of another disease. Frederickson and Levy proposed a classification system for primary HLP based on five abnormal lipoprotein phenotypes in 1967.[54] Although this classification system is still used clinically, it will eventually be replaced by a more complex classification scheme that more fully reflects the molecular basis of each specific disorder. In this section, the HLP classification system, familial hypercholesterolemia, and familial combined hyperlipidemia will be discussed, as well as drug therapy for disorders of lipoprotein metabolism. Table 10-12 summarizes the features of the Fredrickson and Levy classification system for primary hyperlipoproteinemia phenotypes.

Classification of Hyperlipoproteinemia.

Type I HLP is a rare, autosomal recessive trait that is caused by the absence of the enzyme lipoprotein lipase. The condition is characterized by the inability to clear chylomicrons from plasma, resulting in elevated plasma triglycerides and the presence of chylomicrons in a fasted state, or fasting chylomicronemia. Serum from an individual with Type I HLP usually has a creamy layer of chylomicrons at the top when refrigerated. Type I HLP is usually detected in early childhood and often includes such clinical symptoms as eruptive xanthomas (lipid deposits on the skin which contain primarily cholesterol esters), abdominal pain, recurrent pancreatitis, and lipemia retinalis (a high level of lipids in blood manifested by a milky appearance of the veins and arteries of the retina). The dietary treatment of Type I HLP includes restriction of fat intake to less than 25–35 g per day. Medium-chain triglycerides are used as a fat source in the diet because they do not require chylomicron formation.

Type II HLP is subdivided into two groups, Type IIa, which is characterized by elevated plasma and LDL cholesterol, and Type IIb, which is characterized by elevated plasma cholesterol and triglycerides in conjunction with elevated VLDL and LDL levels. Both Types IIa and IIb are associated with premature atherosclerosis and CHD, and with elevated plasma cholesterol levels, often in the range of 300–600 mg/dl. Type II HLP varies in severity and includes the disorders familial hypercholesterolemia and familial combined hyperlipidemia, which are discussed in the following section. Presenting symptoms include xanthelasma (lipid deposits surrounding the ocular region), xanthomas, and premature corneal arcus (an opaque line partially encircling the margin of the cornea as a result of lipid deposits). Dietary management includes attainment and maintenance of ideal body weight and a low-saturated-fat, low-cholesterol diet as described for a Step One or Step

Table 10-12. Features of the Primary Hyperlipoproteinemias

Type	Defect Terminology	Incidence	Plasma Lipid Levels	Dietary Management
I	Lipoprotein lipase deficiency	Rare	↑TG, fasting chylomicronemia	Low-fat diet, <25–35 g/day; MCT can be used
IIa	Reduced or defective LDL receptors; familial hypercholesterolemia	Common	↑Cholesterol, ↑LDL, normal VLDL	Step one or Step two diet
IIb	Familial combined hyperlipidemia	Common	↑Cholesterol, ↑TG, ↑LDL, ↑VLDL	Weight reduction, Step one or two diet, limit alcohol intake
III	Defective clearance of VLDL remnants; familial dysbeta-lipoproteinemia	Uncommon	↑Cholesterol, ↑TG, presence of β-VLDL	Weight reduction, Step one or two diet
IV	Excessive VLDL synthesis; familial hypertriglyceri-demia	Very common	↑TG, ↑VLDL	Weight reduction, Step one or two diet, limit alcohol intake
V	Unknown	Rare	↑Cholesterol, ↑TG, ↑VLDL, fasting chylomicronemia	Low-fat diet, <25–35 g/day; weight reduction; limit alcohol intake; MCT can be used.

Adapted from Frederickson, D.S., and Levy, R.K. Dietary Management of Hyperlipoproteinemia. Dept. of Health and Human Services Publication No. (NIH) 75-110. Government Printing Office, 1974.

LDL = low-density lipoprotein; MCT = medium-chain triglyceride; TG = triglyceride; VLDL = Very-low-density lipoprotein.

Two diet. Drugs are often required for the management of hypercholesterolemia that is resistant to dietary measures.

Type III HLP or familial dysbetalipoproteinemia is a relatively rare disorder that usually first becomes apparent in early adulthood. It is caused by a defect in the clearance of VLDL remnants that results in elevated serum cholesterol and triglyceride levels and the presence of abnormal beta-VLDL particles. Beta-VLDL are enriched in cholesterol instead of triglyceride and have beta, rather than alpha, electrophoretic mobility. Levels of LDL cholesterol are also elevated. The majority of individuals with Type III are homozygous for a mutant allele of Apo-E termed Apo-E2. Remnants of VLDL with Apo-E2 do not bind normally to LDL and remnant receptors. The incidence of Apo-E2 homozygotes is quite high in the population, from 0.2% to 1.6%. This incidence is much higher than the occurrence of Type III, suggesting that other genetic and environmental factors affect the pathogenesis of Type III. Individuals with Type III HLP often have xanthomas on the bottoms of the feet and palms of the hands, and suffer from premature atherosclerosis, particularly in the peripheral vessels. Dietary treatment usually consists of attainment of ideal body weight and a Step One or Step Two diet.

Type IV HLP or familial hypertriglyceridemia is the most common type of HLP. It is characterized by elevated plasma triglycerides, overproduction of VLDL, and normal to slightly elevated plasma cholesterol levels. Type IV is usually detected in adulthood and is frequently associated with obesity and diabetes mellitus. Alcohol intake, the use of progestational hormones, and perhaps excess intake of simple carbohydrates seem to exacerbate Type IV HLP. Weight reduction and restriction of alcohol intake are very effective approaches for the management of Type IV.

Type V HLP is a rare disorder characterized by elevated plasma levels of cholesterol and triglyceride in conjunction with elevated chylomicrons and VLDL. It is detected in adults and presents with eruptive xanthomas, hepatosplenomegaly (enlarged liver and spleen), abdominal pain, lipemia retinalis, and elevated blood levels of glucose and uric acid.

Familial Hypercholesterolemia. Familial hypercholesterolemia (FH) refers to a common metabolic inherited disorder associated with an increase in LDL cholesterol levels, as occurs with Type IIa HLP, and accelerated atherosclerosis. The cause of FH is a defect in the gene encoding for the LDL receptor such that the receptor is absent, present in reduced number, or nonfunctional.[31] Cells from individuals who are homozygous for FH show little if any LDL binding activity. These individuals have a six- to tenfold elevation in LDL levels and usually die in their teens from CHD. Portocaval shunt and liver transplantation have been used to treat FH homozygotes. Individuals who are heterozygous for FH have a two- to fourfold elevation in LDL levels, possess approximately 50% of normal LDL binding activity, and usually develop CHD during middle age. Familial hypercholesterolemia is a common inherited metabolic disorder in humans; one in 500 individuals are heterozygous for FH. Patients with heterozygous FH rarely respond adequately to dietary therapy alone.

An understanding of the molecular basis of FH has led to the development of effective drug treatment for individuals with heterozygous FH. Therapy with two drugs, a bile-acid-binding resin and an inhibitor of endogenous cholesterol synthesis, has proved to be effective. Resins such as colestipol (Colestid) or cholestyramine (Questran) block the reabsorption of bile acids in the intestine; this blocking results in a decrease in the pool of hepatic cholesterol needed for synthesis of bile acids. In order to provide additional cholesterol, the liver increases cholesterol synthesis via increased HMG-CoA reductase activity. Use of the drug mevinolin (lovastatin or Mevacor) inhibits HMG-CoA reductase activity; this action, in combination with a bile-acid-binding resin, causes the liver to compensate for the deficit in cholesterol by increasing the number of LDL receptors. This increase results in increased LDL clearance and a drop in plasma total and LDL cholesterol levels. A 12-week regimen of lovastatin plus cholestyramine has been noted to produce a 52% drop in plasma cholesterol levels in heterozygous FH patients.[53]

Familial Combined Hyperlipidemia. Familial combined hyperlipidemia (FCHL) is a common inherited disorder that may include the Type IIa, IIb, IV, or V phenotypes. Some FCHL patients have a very high LDL apolipoprotein B concentration with a normal LDL cholesterol level, which is called "hyperapobetalipoproteinemia." The diagnosis of FCHL is made by testing first-degree relatives and by finding multiple lipoprotein phenotypes in a single family. About 5% of people with CHD before 60 years of age have FCHL. Patients with FCHL are at increased risk for CHD regardless of their lipoprotein phenotypes. The underlying metabolic defect in families with FCHL appears to be an overproduction of lipoproteins by the liver with variation in the lipoprotein phenotypes depending on how rapidly these lipoproteins are cleared. Because it represents a heterogeneous group of disorders, FCHL is difficult to treat; however, many patients respond well to weight reduction. Drug therapy is usually needed to manage FCHL, and nicotinic acid is currently the drug of choice.

Drug Management

The decision to initiate drug therapy in individuals with hyperlipidemia requires considerable clinical judgment and a sufficient trial of nonpharmacological approaches to decrease CHD risk, including diet, exercise, and life-style modifications such as quitting smoking. In general, a three-to-six-month trial of intense dietary therapy should be tried first (Table 10-11) before initiating drug therapy. If it is necessary to initiate drug therapy, diet and other life-style modifications should be continued. LDL cholesterol is one of the best parameters to use in deciding when to use drugs and for monitoring the response to drug therapy. Drug therapy is generally indicated when, after a trial of diet therapy, LDL levels are

1. Over 190 mg/dl in patients without CHD or two other CHD risk factors, one of which can be male sex, or
2. Over 160 mg/dl in patients with definite CHD or two other CHD risk factors.[53]

Factors to be considered in the selection of appropriate drug therapy include mechanisms of action and primary effect of the drug, cost, side effects, and data regarding long-term safety and ability to reduce risk of CHD. The five major groups of drugs used to treat hyperlipidemia include bile acid sequestrants (cholestyramine, colestipol), nicotinic acid, HMG-CoA reductase inhibitors (lovastatin), fibric acid derivatives (gemfibrozil and clofibrate), and probucol, as summarized in Table 10-13. The bile acid sequestrants and nicotinic acid are the drugs of first choice, since they have been demonstrated to reduce CHD risk in clinical trials and their long-term safety has been established. The bile acid sequestrants primarily reduce LDL cholesterol levels but are not indicated for patients with concurrent hypertriglyceridemia, whereas nicotinic acid is the preferred drug for patients with both hypercholesterolemia and hypertriglyceridemia. The HMG-CoA reductase inhibitors are a new class of drugs highly effective in lowering LDL cholesterol levels; however, their effect on CHD incidence and their long-term safety have not yet been established. The fibric acid derivatives are primarily effective in

treating hypertriglyceridemia and are currently not approved by the Food and Drug Administration for the treatment of hypercholesterolemia. If the response to single drug therapy is not adequate, combination drug therapy may be used. The combination of a bile acid sequestrant with either nicotinic acid or an HMG-CoA reductase inhibitor has been demonstrated to be particularly effective.

The bile acid sequestrants have the advantages of documented long-term safety and absence of systemic toxicity because they are not absorbed from the gastrointestinal tract; however, their method of administration is awkward and a high frequency of gastrointestinal side effects is associated with intake of these drugs. Cholestyramine and colestipol are both powders that must be mixed with water or fruit juice and taken in two or three divided doses with meals. The choice of a bile acid sequestrant depends on individual preference based on taste and palatability. The most common side effects associated with bile acid sequestrant therapy are gastrointestinal, including constipation, bloating, epigastric fullness, nausea, and flatulence. Bile acid sequestrant therapy is contraindicated in patients with a history of severe constipation. The sequestrants may interfere with the absorption of drugs commonly used by patients with CHD including digitoxin, warfarin, thiazide diuretics, beta blockers, fat-soluble vitamins, and folic acid. Routine vitamin supplementation is not recommended for patients taking bile acid sequestrants.

A water-soluble B vitamin, nicotinic acid, is the least costly of the lipid-lowering drugs, and it has been proven safe in long-term clinical trials. Nicotinic acid lowers total and LDL cholesterol and triglyceride levels and raises HDL cholesterol levels in association with decreased hepatic production of VLDL and subsequent LDL formation. Nicotinamide is not effective in lowering LDL cholesterol and cannot be substituted for nicotinic acid.

Flushing is the primary side effect asso-

Table 10-13. *Features of Drugs Used to Treat Hyperlipidemia*

Drugs	Primary Effects	Adherence	Side Effects	Monitoring
Bile acid sequestrants[a]—cholestyramine (Questran) and colestipol (Colestid)	Increases bile acid excretion, thereby depleting hepatic cholesterol pool and increasing hepatic LDL receptor activity—↓LDL cholesterol 15–30%	Requires education	May ↑VLDL synthesis and plasma triglycerides; not indicated for patients with hypertriglyceridemia. Dose-dependent constipation; GI symptoms; may alter absorption of fat-soluble vitamins, folic acid, and other drugs.	Dosing schedule of coadministered drugs
Nicotinic acid[a]	Decreases hepatic VLDL synthesis and subsequent LDL formation—↓LDL cholesterol 15–30%, ↓TG, ↑HDL	Requires education; least costly of available drugs	Flushing, hyperuricemia, abnormal liver function, hyperglycemia, and GI side effects.	Liver function, blood glucose, and uric acid levels
HMG-CoA reductase inhibitor—lovastatin (Mevacor)	Competitive inhibitor of the rate-limiting step in cholesterol biosynthesis; ↓LDL cholesterol 25–45%	Good, limited long-term safety information	Abnormal liver function, GI side effects, muscle pain, and lens opacities.	Liver function and ocular examination
Fibric acid derivatives[b]—gemfibrozil and clofibrate	Decreases triglycerides with an associated ↑HDL cholesterol, ↓LDL cholesterol 5–15%	Good	May ↑LDL cholesterol in individuals with ↑triglycerides; abnormal liver function; GI side effects.	Hematologic parameters and liver function
Probucol	Decreases cholesterol by 10–15% but may ↓HDL cholesterol by 25%, antioxidant	Good	↓HDL cholesterol, GI side effects, alters EKG.	EKG

[a] Long-term safety and ability to reduce risk of CHD established by clinical trials.
[b] Not approved by the Food and Drug Administration for routine treatment of hypercholesterolemia.

ciated with the use of nicotinic acid. The flushing is mediated by prostaglandins and can be reduced by pretreatment with aspirin or nonsteroidal anti-inflammatory drugs, by slowly increasing drug dosage, and by avoiding administration on an empty stomach. Tolerance to the flushing develops over a period of weeks. Nicotinic acid is initially given as a single dose after the evening meal to reduce flushing during normal daily activities. The number and amount of doses are then gradually increased every four to seven days until a therapeutic dose of 1.5 to 2.0 g/day is reached. Nausea, hyperuricemia, and abnormalities in liver function are other side effects observed in conjunction with chronically high doses of nicotinic acid.

ATHEROSCLEROSIS

The terms **arteriosclerosis** and **atherosclerosis** are currently used interchangeably, although originally their definitions differed. Arteriosclerosis is a general term encompassing several arterial diseases that have the common characteristic of degeneration, thickening, and hardening (sclerosis) of the arterial wall. Atherosclerosis is a disease of the tunica intima of the large and medium-sized arteries, characterized by the development of fibrous, fatty deposits called plaques or atheromas. The atheromas eventually become calcified, resulting in rigidity and narrowing (stenosis) of the arteries. The arteries most commonly affected with atherosclerosis are the aorta, the iliac and femoral arteries (to the legs), and the coronary and cerebral arteries.

Early lesions of atherosclerosis are asymptomatic. Later, as the atheromas develop further, they interfere with the circulation and then cause systemic effects varying with the site of the lesion. Lesions in the coronary arteries result in coronary heart disease, which may lead to **coronary occlusion (myocardial infarction or MI)**. Lesions in the cerebral arteries may lead to a **cerebrovascular accident** (CVA), also known as a **stroke**. Atheromas may interfere with circu-

lation to other organs and structures, such as the legs, kidneys, and pancreas. Congestive heart failure and arrhythmias may also result from atherosclerosis.

Etiology

The etiology of atherosclerosis is unknown but is believed to be multifactorial. Characteristics of individuals who develop CHD, which is believed to be primarily caused by atherosclerosis, have been identified and termed "risk factors." The presence of risk factors is associated with an increase in the severity of CHD and its associated mortality. Most of the evidence relating risk factors to atherosclerotic disease is epidemiologic and therefore consists primarily of statistical evidence for probability of an association. It is important to remember that such evidence does not establish an unequivocal cause-and-effect relationship between a given risk factor and the incidence of atherosclerotic disease.

The three risk factors most consistently associated with an increased incidence of CHD include **hypertension, hypercholesterolemia**, and **cigarette smoking**. Other modifiable risk factors include severe obesity, lack of physical activity, hypertriglyceridemia, and low HDL cholesterol levels (below 35 mg/dl). Modification of these risk factors by diet, drug therapy, or changes in life style is strongly encouraged in an effort to reduce the incidence of CHD. Additional risk factors, which cannot be modified, include male sex, diabetes mellitus, family history of premature CHD, or the presence of definite atherosclerosis. The presence of multiple risk factors is thought to have a synergistic relationship, so that the probability of atherosclerotic disease increases geometrically when two or more risk factors are present.

Expert committees from major scientific associations such as the National Heart, Lung, and Blood Institute and the American Heart Association have concluded from recent clinical trials that a decrease in plasma cholesterol levels will decrease the risk of atherosclerotic disease (the diet-heart hypothesis). However, controversy still exists regarding the efficacy of reducing CHD risk through dietary means because most of the clinical trials demonstrating a decrease in CHD risk in conjunction with lower blood cholesterol levels utilized drugs in addition to diet to achieve a reduction in blood cholesterol levels.

The Lesion

The lesion in atherosclerosis is called an **atheroma** or **plaque**. Fatty streaks are early lesions preceding the most advanced atheroma. The relationship between fatty streaks and fibrous plaques is one of the most controversial aspects of the pathogenesis of atherosclerosis. Both fatty streaks and atheromas consist of cholesterol and cholesterol esters, macrophages, and smooth muscle cells. Four types of cells are involved in the pathogenesis of an atheromatous lesion: endothelium, smooth muscle, platelets, and monocyte/macrophages.[55] The formation of an atheroma is dependent on release by these cells of substances that are chemoattractants or growth factors. Platelet-derived growth factor (PDGF) has been identified as an important mediator of atheroma formation. It is secreted by platelets and many other cells and stimulates arterial smooth muscle cell proliferation in addition to acting as a chemoattractant. The effects of PDGF on cell proliferation appear to result, at least in part, from increased turnover of membrane phospholipids and stimulation of prostaglandin formation.

Fatty streaks consist primarily of macrophages and foam cells. Fatty streaks form in specific locations in the arterial intima as a result of aging and net accumulation of extracellular cholesterol from VLDL and LDL.[56] The cholesterol is stored primarily as cholesterol esters, and when the esters exceed 2–3% of total lipids, they exceed their solubility in membranes and separate into droplets.[57] A cell containing a mass of these cholesterol ester droplets is called a **foam cell**. The formation of cholesterol-supersaturated foam cells from macrophages is a key

prerequisite for plaque formation because these cells lead to precipitation of crystalline cholesterol, causing cell disruption and necrosis.

Advanced atheromatous lesions or fibrous plaques contain a fibrous cap of smooth muscle cells and connective tissue, in addition to macrophages and other types of leukocytes. These lesions have undergone necrosis and degeneration in the deeper region adjacent to the internal elastic lamina and contain a core rich in crystals of free cholesterol. These crystals of cholesterol monohydrate are a hallmark of the advanced atherosclerotic lesion and are quite inert.[57]

Fibrous plaques tend to protrude into the lumen of blood vessels, reducing the size of the lumen. When the atheroma increases in size such that the lumen cross-section is reduced to approximately a third its usual diameter, blood flow to the tissue supplied becomes marginal, and, with exertion and muscular contraction of such tissue, ischemia develops.[57] Ischemia may lead to the clinical symptoms of angina, myocardial infarction, stroke, or claudication. The rough surface of the fibrous plaque also provides a good surface for clot or thrombus formation.

Studies in animal models and man suggest that regression of atherosclerotic plaques can occur. Prolonged periods of low plasma cholesterol result in mobilization of cholesterol, disappearance of foam cells, and dissolving of crystalline cholesterol in plaques from animal models.[55]

The Cholesterol Lowering Atherosclerosis Study (CLAS) compared atheromatous lesions in coronary bypass surgery patients. It demonstrated significant atherosclerosis regression in men whose serum cholesterol levels were lowered by treatment with the drugs colestipol and nicotinic acid, compared with controls.[58]

Pathogenesis

The pathogenesis of atherosclerosis involves the development of an atheroma in the intima of major arteries. Strong support for a causative relationship between hypercholesterolemia and atherosclerosis is suggested by premature atherosclerosis and CHD in individuals with familial hypercholesterolemia, and the fact that atherosclerotic plaques contain large amounts of cholesterol. Animal studies have provided a basis for understanding the sequence of cellular events preceding development of atheromas. Direct information is only recently becoming available regarding how elevated LDL cholesterol levels are related to the cellular events noted in animal models.[55] Current research suggests that oxidation of LDL within the artery wall results in a cytotoxic compound that may initiate atherogenesis.[59]

The current version of the "lipid-infiltration" hypothesis suggests that high plasma LDL levels may be sufficient to account for the development of fatty streaks. Infiltration of the intima by LDL may result in oxidation of LDL in the subendothelial space, resulting in uptake of oxidized LDL by macrophages, release of growth factors and chemoattractants, and formation of foam cells and fatty streaks.[59] A potential linkage between the "endothelial-injury" and "lipid-infiltration"[59] hypotheses has been proposed, as outlined in Figure 10-13. Infiltration and oxidation of LDL in the intima may lead to formation of fatty streaks, and then, through its cytotoxicity, the oxidized LDL may cause the loss of the endothelial cells overlying the fatty streaks. At this point, the events proposed in the "lipid-infiltration" hypothesis could occur, resulting in the progression of the fatty streaks to atheromas.

Another theory, the "endothelial-injury" hypothesis, suggests that atheromas develop in response to injury to a localized area of the artery. The injury results in attraction of platelets and monocytes, release of growth factors, penetration of the subendothelium by cholesterol, and smooth muscle cell migration and proliferation. Injury to the endothelium could be caused by such factors as elevated LDL cholesterol (lipid-infiltration hypothesis), smoking, hypertension, toxins, viruses, or mechanical or immunologic stim-

Figure 10-13. Postulated linkage between the lipid-infiltration hypothesis and the endothelial-injury hypothesis. The lipid-infiltration hypothesis may be sufficient to account for fatty streaks, and the endothelial-injury hypothesis may account for progression of the fatty streak to more advanced lesions. (Taken from Steinberg, D., Metabolism of lipoproteins and their role in the pathogenesis of atherosclerosis. In A.M. Gotto, Jr., and R. Paoletti, Eds., Atherosclerosis Reviews, vol. 18: J. Stokes III and M. Mancini, Eds., Hypercholesterolemia: Clinical and Therapeutic Implications. New York: Raven Press, 1988, pp. 1–23.)

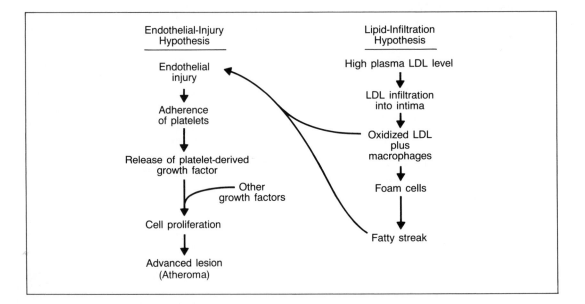

ulation. More recently, this hypothesis has been modified somewhat to suggest that actual disruption of the endothelial surface may not be necessary for atherosclerosis to develop, since loss of endothelial cells does not appear to occur before the appearance of a fatty streak lesion.[55,59] Characterization of the genetic basis underlying the increased susceptibility to atherosclerosis of some individuals with hypercholesterolemia is felt to be critical to understanding why atheromas form.

Another theory of the pathogenesis of atherosclerosis suggests that atheromas originate from the transformation of smooth muscle cells by a mutagen. The mutagen could consist of a toxin such as nicotine from tobacco or a virus. If a mutagen is the critical initiating event, elevated plasma cholesterol levels are still felt to be needed to provide cholesterol, the major lipid component of the atheroma.

CORONARY HEART DISEASE

Coronary heart disease (CHD), also known as **ischemic heart disease** (IHD), **coronary occlusion, atherosclerotic heart disease**, or **coronary thrombosis**, is the most common form of heart disease in individuals older than 40 years and is a leading cause of sudden death. It is a condition in which the oxygen supply to the myocardium is inadequate, usually due to atherosclerosis in the coronary circulation. However, CHD also can result from hypertrophy of the cardiac muscle such as would occur in aortic stenosis (narrowing of the aorta or narrowing of the opening of the heart to the aorta). In addition, it can occur owing to a defect in oxygen binding by hemoglobin, but this is rare.

Coronary heart disease can be divided into two categories, **angina pectoris** and **myocardial infarction**. They differ in degree and in the rate of onset.

Angina Pectoris

Angina pectoris is characterized by precordial pain (pain in the region over the heart and stomach), which may radiate to the neck, jaw, back, abdomen, and arms. Angina is caused by myocardial ischemia and is associated with a disturbance of myocardial function without myocardial necrosis. It is classified into two forms, stable and unstable angina. Stable angina is precipitated by factors that increase the oxygen requirement of the heart, which may include exercise, smoking, eating, anxiety, and exposure to cold. The threshold for stable angina differs among patients and may show little correlation with the degree of coronary atherosclerosis. Unstable angina is characterized by angina at rest as well as with minimal exertion or the occurrence of severe angina superimposed on a normal pattern of stable, exertion-related angina. It is a potentially dangerous condition often requiring hospitalization to diagnose and treat conditions that may be increasing myocardial oxygen demand.

Management of both stable and unstable angina is based on control of myocardial oxygen requirements and reduction of precipitating environmental factors. Rest may be required for the acute phase, but some patients with stable angina will profit from a carefully prescribed and supervised exercise program. Exercise may reduce the heart rate at a given work load and increase the amount of work that can be done before the onset of angina.

Diet modifications as indicated for atherosclerosis (Step One or Two diet) is appropriate for angina patients, especially if hypercholesterolemia is present. Patients should reach and maintain their ideal body weight or be slightly underweight. Drug therapy may also be used (Table 10-6). Drug therapy includes, for acute attacks, the use of nitroglycerine or isosorbide dinitrate (Isordil), which cause vasodilation. Some patients with angina-associated hypertension or heart failure are given digitalis and diuretics. Beta-adrenergic receptor blocking agents are frequently used for those with chronic stable angina as they reduce cardiac response to sympathetic stimulation, thus reducing myocardial oxygen demand during activity or excitement when surges of sympathetic stimulation occur. Propranolol hydrochloride (Inderal), used for this purpose, affects also the smooth muscle receptors in organs other than the heart, including the gastrointestinal tract. Possible side effects include nausea, diarrhea, and fatigue.

Myocardial Infarction

Clinical Manifestations and Diagnosis

In **myocardial infarction (coronary infarction, coronary thrombosis,** or **heart attack),** the ischemia becomes so severe that the cardiac muscle cells become necrotic. Most MIs result from atherosclerosis of the coronary arteries with superimposed coronary thrombosis. There is very little communication between the major coronary arteries, and narrowing of any one artery can result in insufficient blood supply to the portion of the heart that it perfuses, resulting in cell death due to lack of blood supply. The amount of necrotic tissue (the size of the infarct) and the consequences depend on the location of the occlusion. Death can result if, for example, the blood supply to a major portion of the left ventricle is occluded.

Prior to an infarction, patients frequently have nonspecific symptoms, such as fatigue, malaise, insomnia, and flatulence. Angina pectoris usually worsens. The principal symptom of an infarction is precordial pain, which the patient may mistake for severe angina or indigestion.

Both electrocardiography (ECG) and echocardiography are helpful in locating the site of the lesion in myocardial infarction. Changes in serum enzymes are commonly used to diagnose an MI. When cells become necrotic, some enzymes are released and increase in concentration in the serum. Laboratory determination of serum glutamic oxaloacetic transaminase (SGOT), lactic dehydrogenase (LDH), and creatine phosphokinase (CPK) are useful. Elevation of serum CPK is a very sensitive enzymatic detector of MI as CPK peaks within 4–8 hours following an MI and declines to normal within

three or four days. The enzymes SGOT and LDH are also sensitive but more nonspecific than CPK, since false positive elevations occur due to release of these enzymes with disease in other organs. The heart contains principally one of the five isoenzymes of LDH. Demonstration of an LDH_1/LDH_2 ratio greater than 1.0 is a sensitive and specific test for diagnosis of MI.

Clinical Course

Approximately 25% of the first episodes of myocardial infarction result in medically unattended deaths. Most additional deaths occur within the first 24 hours. The immediate objective of management is to recognize and treat arrhythmias, shock, and heart failure. Care of patients with acute MI and other life-threatening cardiovascular diseases is often provided by special units known as coronary care units (CCU).

Management

The primary objectives when the patient is admitted are to prevent death from cardiac arrest or arrhythmia, to increase the oxygen in the blood, and to reduce pain. The surviving patient usually is kept at complete bed rest for at least six to ten days to reduce the work of the heart. Many patients return to normal activity after a convalescence of several months. Those with extensive myocardial damage may progress to cardiac failure.

In nutritional care of patients with myocardial infarction, decisions must be made on when to begin feeding and on the size, frequency, consistency, and temperature of the meals. Factors that must be considered in addition to the diagnosis of myocardial infarction include the use of medications such as digitalis and morphine sulfate, as well as the effects of complications such as nausea, pain, heart failure, or uncontrolled arrhythmias. Nausea may be a side effect of the morphine.

The hypoxia, pain, and anxiety accompanying a myocardial infarction activate the sympathetic nervous system. Epinephrine, norepinephrine, and cortisol are produced in larger quantities. The splanchnic circulation, which receives approximately 25% of the cardiac output in a resting individual, is constricted. Although there is some disagreement on this point, it seems logical to reduce the need for increased splanchnic circulation. To this end, the following guidelines have been recommended for nutritional care of patients in intensive care:

1. Reduce potential arrhythmias by elimination of caffeine and use of a liquid diet in the first 24 hours, when nausea and choking are common.
2. Reduce cardiac work load with small, frequent feedings of soft or liquid foods (800–1,200 kcal/day).[60]
3. Individualize fluid and sodium restriction according to sodium and fluid status.
4. Provide consistent dietary information as a basis for later education for long-term nutritional management.

Little evidence is available concerning the effects of temperature extremes in food. There is evidence both for and against the restriction of the use of very cold foods.[61] Some cardiologists recommend the avoidance of either very hot or very cold foods.[62]

The use of caffeine and other methylxanthines (see Appendix F) also is controversial. Methylxanthines decrease calcium binding at the cell membrane, affecting the action potential and possibly causing ventricular fibrillation. In addition, they stimulate the release of catecholamines from the adrenal medulla. Catecholamines may mobilize free fatty acids, possibly causing arrhythmias. Under these circumstances, methylxanthines may be restricted until later in convalescence.[63]

Sodium restriction may be provided if the patient shows signs of congestive heart failure (described in the next section) or pulmonary edema.[64] The risks of indiscriminate use of sodium restriction, as listed by Goldberger,[65] include (1) the danger of precipitat-

ing shock by reducing the circulating blood volume; (2) excessive sodium loss, since many myocardial infarction patients have disturbances of renal tubular function; and (3) the risk of sodium deficiency in the vomiting patient with myocardial infarction who has lost sodium in the vomitus. Sodium restriction may be used for certain patients for whom it is specifically indicated, but it is not a routine procedure.[62]

Long-term management will require adequate energy intake to maintain ideal body weight. In addition, the patient may require sodium restriction, a fat-controlled diet, or both. Programs promoting rapid weight reduction, that is, weight loss of more than 2 pounds per week, should be used cautiously in the postinfarction period. The elevation in plasma free fatty acid levels that occurs during rapid weight loss can induce cardiac arrhythmias. In addition, the fluid and electrolyte alterations that accompany rapid weight reduction can be particularly dangerous to the post-MI patient maintained on diuretic and digitalis therapy.

The postinfarction patient who has had successful coronary bypass surgery also needs appropriate sodium restriction and adherence to a diet. Atherosclerosis may progress more rapidly in bypass graft vessels than in the native circulation. Patients often consider themselves cured because of dramatic relief of symptoms after bypass surgery and must be carefully counseled on their nutritional needs.

CONGESTIVE HEART FAILURE

Congestive heart failure (CHF) occurs when the heart fails as a pump and cannot deliver an adequate amount of oxygenated blood to body tissues. A failure to deliver enough oxygen **(cardiac decompensation)** may occur at first only during exercise. As the condition worsens, decompensation occurs during normal activity and with meals and, eventually, during bed rest.

It may be caused by a primary disease of

the myocardium or by a disease that affects other cardiac structures, such as the valves, conduction system, endocardium, or pericardium, and then involves the myocardium secondarily. Congestive heart failure also can occur secondary to diseases outside of the heart that cause a great increase in the work load of the heart.

Pathogenesis

Congestive heart failure may occur by three mechanisms. One of these is a **decrease in the number of contractile units**. Myocardial infarction is an example in which heart muscle is destroyed and replaced by scar tissue. Second, there may be a decrease in the **quality of contractile units** (ability to contract). This occurs in **cardiomyopathies** (disorders of heart muscle of unknown cause). Last, the heart may be presented with an **excessive work load**. This increased work load may be a **pressure overload** or a **volume overload**. A pressure overload, also known as **excess afterload**, occurs when the heart must pump blood against an increased pressure. In systemic hypertension or aortic stenosis, the left ventricle is presented with an increased work load to maintain the necessary blood flow. The right ventricle receives a pressure overload in pulmonic or mitral stenosis. A volume overload can occur, for example, when the mitral and aortic valves do not close properly in diastole and blood that has been pumped out regurgitates back into the ventricle. It then has to be pumped out again on the next systole, increasing the total amount of blood that the heart must pump. Other conditions add to the work load of the heart, sometimes by increasing tissue need beyond the capacity of even a normal heart.

In some people, the heart can be damaged but it adjusts to the need (**compensated failure**) by enlarging or increasing the rate,[66] thus increasing output toward normal.[67] If a condition that increases the work load is superimposed, it may precipitate CHF. Some of these precipitating factors are fever, anemia, pregnancy, pulmonary embolism, thyrotoxi-

cosis, or myocardial infarction. Sometimes CHF can be precipitated simply by excess sodium intake.

Congestive heart failure is divided into **left ventricular heart failure** and **right ventricular heart failure**, owing to the double pump structure of the heart. In right ventricular heart failure, there is decreased venous return to the heart and congestion (edema) of peripheral tissues. In left ventricular heart failure, there is pulmonary congestion. As congestion of the lungs becomes chronic, compliance and elasticity of the lungs are decreased.[68] Consequently, there is an increase in energy expenditure by the lungs. Eventually, the failure of one side of the heart affects the other and both will fail. Sometimes CHF also is categorized as **backward** versus **forward failure**, **systolic** versus **diastolic failure**, or **high-output** versus **low-output failure**. Many of these types of failure are the basis for theories explaining salt and water retention. Nevertheless, a thorough explanation of these mechanisms is not yet available.

Salt and Water Retention

In heart failure, blood stagnates in the venous system returning blood to the heart, and venous pressure increases. Fluid diffuses from the blood vessels into surrounding tissues. The reduced cardiac output reduces the renal blood supply and renal blood pressure. This initiates the renin-angiotensin-aldosterone response described previously, causing sodium and water retention. Vasopressin may also be released and stimulates water reabsorption. Other factors probably are involved and may be very important. The net effect of sodium and water retention is edema and congestion in the peripheral tissues.

In moderate failure, the retained fluid increases blood flow to the heart, priming the heart to pump more blood. As failure progresses, the amount of blood increases and stretches the heart muscle so it becomes overstretched, weakens further, and eventually fails completely.

Clinical Manifestations

The signs and symptoms of CHF vary with the degree of congestion and the organs involved. The most common symptom of heart failure is **dyspnea** (respiratory distress). It may occur at first only during activity but steadily worsens until the patient is breathless even at rest. Patients also develop **orthopnea** (dyspnea when recumbent) as the failure progresses. This sensation is relieved when the patient is upright, so that the patient sleeps partly propped up on pillows or bolt upright.

Other symptoms include anorexia, nausea, a feeling of fullness, abdominal pain, malabsorption, enlarged liver, and liver tenderness, related to failure of adequate circulation to the abdominal organs. Patients may be constipated. Decreased blood supply to the brain can result in mental confusion, memory loss, anxiety, insomnia, and headache. Pallor, cool extremities, and sweating also are seen. Additional findings include pulmonary edema, fluid accumulation in the chest cavity (**hydrothorax, pleural effusion), ascites** (fluid accumulation in the abdominal cavity), and **cardiac edema**. Edema appears almost invariably in the legs in ambulatory patients and in the sacral region in recumbent patients.

In advanced CHF, patients may become severely malnourished, a condition known as **cardiac cachexia.**

Management

In the management of CHF, elimination of the basic cause and precipitating factors are essential if possible. In addition, the work load of the heart must be reduced. Reduction of work load is accomplished by providing oxygen, by decreasing physical activity, by diet, and with drugs.

Nutritional Care

In order to reduce fluid retention, the hospitalized patient in severe cardiac failure usually is given a diet containing 500–1,000 mg of sodium per day or less. A higher sodium level in the diet may be tolerated in moderate failure. Some patients may tolerate as much as 1,000–3,000 mg. The need for fluid restriction is an individual matter. For some patients, fluid intake need not be restricted if the patient complies with the sodium restriction. For others, a relatively severe fluid restriction may be necessary.

Potassium balance must be carefully observed. Patients receiving diuretics may require potassium supplements. Calories should be low for several reasons. Obesity must be eliminated. In addition, restricting food intake will decrease the work of the heart. Feedings should be small and frequent, and patients should be instructed to eat slowly. Coffee is a stimulant and can cause increased heart rate and arrhythmias. Thus there is controversy concerning its inclusion in the diet.

Drugs

A number of drugs are used in the treatment of cardiac failure, some of which have side effects of nutritional significance. Drugs are used to increase contractility of the myocardium. Digitalis often is used, but its exact mode of action is unknown. Hypokalemia predisposes the patients to digitalis toxicity and must be prevented. Symptoms of toxicity include anorexia, nausea, vomiting, abdominal discomfort, hallucinations, depression, drowsiness, and cardiac arrhythmias.

Reduction of congestive symptoms is achieved by the use of diuretics in addition to the sodium-restricted diet. Available diuretics and nutritional side effects are given in Table 10-6.

CEREBROVASCULAR DISEASE

Cardiovascular diseases sometimes affect the brain. The effects may take several forms. Some patients have **transient ische-**

mic attacks (TIAs) in which the blood supply to the brain is temporarily inadequate. The symptoms vary with the arteries involved, the area of the brain they perfuse, and the amount of collateral circulation. Treatment of a TIA includes cessation of smoking, treatment of hypertension, and drugs. Nutritional care usually is aimed at lowering the blood pressure and consists of some degree of sodium restriction. Diet modification for atherosclerosis may be added.

A **cerebrovascular accident** (CVA or **stroke syndrome**) often is the consequence of occlusion of the cerebral blood supply from atherosclerosis **(atherothrombotic brain infarct)**. Cerebrovascular accidents may also be caused by a hemorrhage of an artery in the brain. In some patients, an aneurysm, which may be congenital, is the cause of a CVA.

The consequences of a CVA vary depending on the area of the brain involved. Those effects that influence the patient's ability to obtain and prepare food, to feed himself or herself, or even to swallow are of particular relevance to the function of the nutritional care specialist. Since these patients may be left with permanent handicaps, their care is discussed in more detail in Chapter 9.

PERIPHERAL VASCULAR ATHEROSCLEROTIC OCCLUSIVE DISEASE

Peripheral vascular atherosclerotic occlusive disease (PVAOD) is a general term referring to conditions that result from occlusion of peripheral arteries. The typical patient is a man more than 50 years of age who is hypertensive and smokes. If the condition involves the legs, as when femoral arteries are occluded, the patient develops **intermittent claudication.** The legs are comfortable at rest, but there is pain and weakness when walking. This worsens until walking is impossible, but subsides with rest. If the occlusion becomes total, the leg can

become gangrenous and then must be amputated.

Patients should stop smoking. Some patients are treated surgically by an endarterectomy in which the thickened tunica intima of the affected arteries is excised. Portions of affected arteries may also be removed and replaced with an artificial substitute.

Nutritional care of these patients includes weight control and the diet for prevention of further atherosclerotic disease. Care of surgical patients is described in Chapter 14.

CARDIAC CACHEXIA

Clinical Manifestations and Pathogenesis

Some patients with cardiac disease develop a condition known as **cardiac cachexia**. In this condition, there is progressive and extreme loss of both fat and lean tissue in a patient with prolonged myocardial insufficiency.[69] It occurs, for example, in many patients with congestive heart failure. Cachexia also occurs in other conditions (see Chapters 14 and 15). The metabolic basis of cachexia, however, varies with its origin. The cardiac patient with cachexia has cardiomegaly, increased basal metabolic rate, and elevated sympathetic tone, in contrast to starvation cachexia in which there is a decrease in the size of the heart, decreased sympathetic tone, and decreased basal metabolic rate.

The development of techniques for cardiac surgery has created a new group of patients with cardiac cachexia. In these patients, postoperative complications can prevent the usual postoperative food intake.

Four mechanisms have been suggested to produce this condition: anorexia, increased metabolic rate, increased nutrient losses, and impaired delivery of nutrients and removal of wastes. The relative importance of these factors is unknown.[70,71]

Anorexia is suggested to be the most important mechanism. Edema as well as an unpalatable sodium-restricted diet, digitalis intoxication, and opiate use can induce anorexia.[69,70,72] Another explanation for anorexia involves increased sympathetic tone and resulting elevated blood levels of epinephrine or norepinephrine, which have been shown in animal experiments to suppress food intake.

Increased metabolic rate is seen in cachectic patients in congestive heart failure. It is thought to be the consequence of increased metabolic demands of the enlarged heart, the lungs, and bone marrow, elevated body temperature, and hormone changes.[73,74] The demands of the bone marrow may be caused by the stimulatory effects of hypoxia on red blood cell formation. Elevation in body temperature can result from pulmonary congestion, inflammation, and the production of endogenous pyrogens (see Chapter 14). The hormone changes are less well understood but may involve the catecholamines.

There are a number of routes of **nutrient losses**. Iatrogenic losses, especially of protein and iron, can occur when body fluids are removed to reduce edema. Diuretics can cause sodium, potassium, and zinc depletion.[70,72] Protein-losing gastroenteropathy (see Chapter 8) also can occur in congestive heart failure.[72] The total losses by these routes can result in the depressed serum levels of albumin, hemoglobin, potassium, calcium, magnesium, zinc, and iron seen in cardiac cachexia.[70] Fat malabsorption is also noted.

Impaired delivery of nutrients has been suggested as another basis for cardiac cachexia.[70] However, increased nutrient extraction rates may account for decreased nutrient concentration in the blood.[69] **Decreased waste excretion** resulting from reduced renal function may contribute to cachexia by causing anorexia and the retention of pyrogens.[69,73]

Treatment

Treatment of cardiac cachexia involves recompensation of the cardiac status. Restoration of body tissue then follows. Maintenance energy needs may be 1.5 to 2.0 times basal energy expenditure or higher. If the patient is to have major surgery, nutritional support may be required. However, aggressive treatment with parenteral nutrition may be hazardous because fluid intake frequently needs to be limited in these patients. Fluids may be limited to 0.5 ml/kcal/day or 1,000 to 1,500 ml/day. Vitamin and mineral supplements are usually given.

Small frequent meals are preferable to large meals. Large feedings may cause accumulation of carbon dioxide and respiratory failure. If voluntary intake is less than 1,500 kcal, the diet may be supplemented with enteral formula feeding (see Chapter 5). Fat malabsorption may be modified by decreasing long-chain fats in the diet and adding medium-chain triglycerides. Most cardiac cachexia patients are prescribed diets in which sodium is restricted to 500–2,000 mg, depending on individual factors. Caffeine often is restricted.

RHEUMATIC HEART DISEASE

Rheumatic fever is an infection caused by group A beta-hemolytic streptococci. The disease may be self-limiting, but it can lead to **rheumatic heart disease**.

Rheumatic heart disease follows only hypertension and coronary artery disease in incidence. It affects the valves of the heart, resulting in valvular stenosis or insufficiency or both. The mitral and aortic valves are those most frequently involved. Valvular disease can also be caused by syphilis (lues), a dissecting aneurysm of the aorta, aortic atherosclerosis, and hypertension, affecting primarily the tricuspid and pulmonic valves.

In its acute stage, rheumatic fever may lead to myocarditis, pericarditis, or pulmonary embolism. Care is primarily nonnutritional. In the chronic phase, patients may have hypertension, subacute bacterial endocarditis, atherosclerotic coronary heart disease, arrhythmias, and cardiac failure.

Nutritional care requires avoidance of obesity. Sodium intake is limited to 2 to 5 g/day. Usually vitamin supplements are given as a general support measure.

CONGENITAL HEART DISEASE

Clinical Manifestations and Pathogenesis

Infants may be born with defects of the heart known collectively as **congenital heart disease**. Some of the more frequently seen defects are **coarction of the aorta, aortic stenosis,** and **ventricular septal defect** (VSD) in which there is an opening between the right and left ventricles. Some infants have a **transposition of the great arteries** in which the pulmonary artery arises from the left ventricle, and the aorta, above the right ventricle.

Cardiac malformations appear to result from complex interactions between genetic and environmental factors. Maternal rubella (German measles), chronic maternal alcohol abuse, and maternal ingestion of various drugs during early gestation are all environmental factors associated with congenital heart defects. Genetic influences are also apparent, since congenital heart disease occurs with high frequency in patients with chromosomal abnormalities such as Turner's or Down syndromes, connective tissue disorders such as Ehlers-Danlos or Marfan's syndromes, and inborn errors of metabolism such as Pompe's disease or Hurler's syndrome.

The effects of congenital anomalies of the heart vary with the type of defect present. Some patients have pulmonary hypertension or frank heart failure. Cyanosis and tachycardia are also common. Growth failure is a common finding, although the mechanisms causing growth failure are unclear. An increased metabolic rate in addition to poor food intake, tissue hypoxia, and frequent respiratory infections are all contributing factors. The metabolic rates of infants with congenital heart disease are elevated in proportion to their degree of growth retardation and heart failure.[75]

Nutritional Management

It has been suggested that the reduced intake seen in infants may be a protective mechanism that spares the heart. For normal growth rate, however, additional calories above normal requirements are usually needed. The normal infant requires 80–145 kcal/kg of body weight.[18] The infants with congenital heart disease may need as much as 150–175 kcal/kg/day. The child should be in the best possible nutritional state when surgical correction is undertaken, often at 12 to 15 months of age. Nutritional management of infants with congenital heart disease requires careful consideration of renal solute load, fluid intake (see Chapter 9), and caloric density of the formula used. In order to meet higher energy needs and not exceed the tolerance to fluid and renal solutes, it is often necessary to increase the caloric density of an infant formula from the usual 20 kcal/oz. to 24–28 kcal/oz. This is accomplished by the addition of fat or carbohydrate, from sources such as Polycose, MCT Oil, or vegetable oil, to a commercial infant formula. SMA and Ross PM 60/40 infant formulas are frequently used, since these formulas contain less sodium than other standard infant formulas. Special low-sodium formulas usually are not necessary. Vitamin and mineral supplements may be necessary in cases where intake is poor and malabsorption occurs.

Special care must be taken to meet, but not exceed, fluid requirements and still provide adequate energy for growth. Fluid requirements are approximately 100–125 ml of fluid per kilogram of body weight for infants from 1 to 12 months of age, and 60–80 ml/kg for children. The adequacy of formula intake may be assessed by monitoring urine osmolality or specific gravity. Poor growth with a urine osmolality below 300 mOsm/L suggests the need for a formula with a higher caloric density. Poor growth with a urine osmolality of 400 mOsm/L or greater suggests the need for a formula with a lower caloric density.

HEART DISEASE AND ALCOHOLISM

Some alcoholic patients are susceptible to the development of heart disease, whereas others develop liver disease (see Chapter 13).

The most common form of alcoholic heart disease consists of cardiomegaly and failure with arrhythmia. Another consists of cardiomegaly, failure, and electrocardiogram abnormalities. The third, **thiamine-responsive beriberi** or **cardiac beriberi**, responds to thiamine supplementation. Abstinence from alcohol is necessary for all three forms of alcohol-related heart disease, in addition to the usual procedures for patients in heart failure.

Case Study: Acute Myocardial Infarction

Phase 1. Mr. J.R.W., a white 52-year-old man measuring 5 ft. 10 in. and weighing 180 lb., has been under the supervision of a physician for several years for essential hypertension. He has been taking a thiazide diuretic and was advised to reduce his sodium intake to 2,000 mg/day. He did reduce the amount of salt he used but did not follow the diet completely. After approximately nine months, he developed a feeling of fatigue and was quite weak. His serum potassium was 3.4 mg/dl, and he was referred to a nutritional care specialist for counseling on a low-sodium diet and advice on methods of increasing his potassium intake.

Phase 2. Mr. W.'s latest physical examination showed that his blood cholesterol was 330 mg/dl and his fasting blood glucose was 125 mg/dl. Fasting triglycerides were 385 mg/dl. His blood pressure was 135/85. He stated that he "usually" took his antihypertensive medication. Body weight was up to 195 lb. At this time, the patient stated that his father had died of a heart attack at the age of 57 and that his mother has hypertension. He was diagnosed as having Type IIb, or familial combined, hyperlipidemia; essential hypertension; and moderate obesity and was advised to stop smoking and to lose 30 lb. He was also referred to a nutritional counselor for advice on diet for the hyperlipidemia. He was given nicotinic acid when the effect of the diet was unsatisfactory.

Phase 3. On a hot day in the summer, Mr. W. was mowing his lawn when he began to feel a "crushing" pain in his chest. At first, he complained of indigestion. However, when the pain continued, he called his doctor.

An electrocardiogram taken in the emergency room of the hospital was abnormal. The patient was also having trouble breathing and was sweating profusely. He was transferred to the cardiac care unit and a tentative diagnosis of acute myocardial infarction was made. Results of the blood tests showed the following:

Cholesterol	340 mg/dl
SGOT	50 units/ml
CPK	187 units/ml
LDH_1/LDH_2	1.15

Exercises

1. What is the function of the diuretic in the management of essential hypertension?
2. Why was the patient advised to reduce his sodium intake?
3. Describe the mechanism by which the potassium deficiency was produced.
4. What foods are high in potassium?
5. Discuss the relative merits and disadvantage of a high-potassium diet and potassium supplement for this patient.
6. What is the patient's ideal body weight?
7. Discuss the significance of each laboratory test result given.
8. What factors in this patient's history are risk factors for myocardial infarction?
9. What diet would you recommend for this patient during phase 2? Give the rationale.
10. Describe the lesion of atherosclerosis.
11. What are the clinical manifestations of ischemic heart disease?
12. What is the difference between angina pectoris and myocardial infarction?
13. Describe the sequence of diets you would recommend for this patient while he is in the cardiac care unit, assuming he makes an uneventful recovery.
14. What diet might be recommended when this

patient is discharged from the hospital? Give the rationale.

15. The patient also was given the following medications: reserpine; clofibrate; nicotinic acid; hydrochlorothiazide. What is the mode of action and purpose of each?

References

1. Guyton, A.C. *Textbook of Medical Physiology.* Chapter 20: Local control of blood flow by the tissues, and nervous and humoral regulation. Philadelphia: W.B. Saunders, 1986.
2. Somermeyer, M.G., and Davidman, M. *Perspectives in Rational Management: Hypertension.* Cardinal Health Systems, Eden Prairie, Minn., 1986.
3. Kinsella, J.E. Food components with potential therapeutic benefits. The n-3 polyunsaturated fatty acids of fish oils. *Food Tech.* 40:89, 1986.
4. Hwang, D.H., and Carroll, A.E. Decreased formation of prostaglandin derived from arachidonic acid by dietary linolenate in rats. *Am. J. Clin. Nutr.* 33:590, 1980.
5. Adam, O., Wolfram, G., and Zollner, N. Relationship between linoleic acid intake and prostaglandin formation in men. In P.O. Avogaro, Ed., *Phospholipids and Atherosclerosis.* New York: Raven Press, 1983, p. 237.
6. Leaf, A., and Weber, P.C. Cardiovascular effects of n-3 fatty acids. *N. Engl. J. Med.* 318:549, 1988.
7. Needleman, P., and Greenwald, J.E. Atriopeptin. A cardiac hormone intimately involved in fluid, electrolyte and blood pressure homeostasis. *N. Engl. J. Med.* 314:828, 1986.
8. Carretero, O.A., and Scicli, A.G. The renal kallikrein-kinin system in human and experimental hypertension. *Klin. Wochenschr.* 56 (Suppl. 1):113, 1978.
9. Ganong, W.F. Chapter 31: Cardiovascular regulatory mechanisms. In *Review of Medical Physiology,* 13th ed. East Norwalk, Conn.: Appleton & Lange, 1987.
10. 1988 report of the Joint National Committee on Detection, Evaluation and Treatment of High Blood Pressure. *Arch. Intern. Med.* 148:1023, 1988.
11. *The Surgeon General's Report on Nutrition and Health.* Washington, D.C.:U.S. Government Printing Office. Publication No. 88–50210, 1988.
12. Kaplan, N.M. Nonpharmacologic therapy of hypertension. *Med. Clin. North Am.* 71:921, 1987.
13. Final Report of the Subcommittee on Nonpharmacological Therapy of the 1984 Joint National Committee on Detection, Evaluation and Treatment of High Blood Pressure. In "Nonpharmacological Approaches to the Control of High Blood Pressure." *Hypertension* 8:444, 1986.
14. Council for Agricultural Science and Technology. *Diet and Health,* Report No. 111. Ames, Iowa: CAST, March 1987.
15. Kurtz, T.W., Al-Bander, H.A., and Morris, R.C. "Salt sensitive" essential hypertension in man. Is the sodium ion alone important? *N. Engl. J. Med.* 317:1043, 1987.
16. Tobian, L. High potassium diets reduce stroke mortality and arterial and renal tubular lesions in hypertension. AIN Symposium Proceedings, *Nutrition,* 1987, p. 119.
17. Sacks, F.M., and Kass, E.H. Low blood pressure in vegetarians. Effects of specific foods and nutrients. *Am. J. Clin. Nutr.* 48:795, 1988.
18. Committee on Dietary Allowances, Food and Nutrition Board, National Academy of Sciences. *Recommended Dietary Allowances,* 10th ed. Washington, D.C.: U.S. Government Printing Office, 1989.
19. McCarron, D.A., and Morris, C.O. Metabolic considerations and cellular mechanisms related to calcium's antihypertensive effects. *Federation Proc.* 45:2734, 1986.
20. Resnick, L.M. Calcium and vitamin D metabolism in the pathophysiology of human hypertension. *AIN Symposium Proceedings, Nutrition,* 1987, p. 110.
21. Leitschuh, M., and Chobanian, A. Vascular changes in hypertension. *Med. Clin. North Am.* 71:827, 1987.
22. Stamler, R., Stamler, J., Grimm, R., Gosch, F., Elmer, P., Dyer, A., Berman, R., Fishman, J., VanHeel, N., Civinelli, J., and McDonal, A. Nutritional therapy for high blood pressure. Final report of a four-year randomized controlled trial—The hypertension control program. *J.A.M.A.* 257:1484, 1987.
23. Zeman, F.J., and Ney, D.M. *Application of Clinical Nutrition.* Englewood Cliffs, N.J.: Prentice-Hall, 1988.
24. Laragh, J.H., and Pecker, M.S. Dietary sodium and essential hypertension. Some myths, hopes and truths. *Ann. Intern. Med.* 98:735, 1983.
25. Iacono, J.M., and Dougherty, R.M. Dietary polyunsaturated fat and blood pressure regulation. AIN Symposium Proceedings. *J. Nutr.,* 1987, p. 105.

26. Knapp, H.R., and Fitzgerald, G.A. The anti-hypertensive effects of fish oil. A controlled study of polyunsaturated fatty acid supplements in essential hypertension. *N. Engl. J. Med.* 320:1037, 1989.

27. Moser, M. Diuretics in the management of hypertension. *Med. Clin. North Am.* 71:935, 1987.

28. Nicholson, J.P., Resnick, L.M., and Laragh, J.H. The antihypertensive effect of verapamil at extremes of dietary sodium intake. *Ann. Intern. Med.* 107:329, 1987.

29. Steinberg, D., and Olefsky, J.M., Eds. *Hypercholesterolemia and Atherosclerosis: Pathogenesis and Prevention.* New York: Churchill Livingstone, 1987, p. 117.

30. Brown, M.S., and Goldstein, J.L. A receptor-mediated pathway for cholesterol homeostasis. *Science* 232:34, 1986.

31. Mahley, R.W., Innerarity, T.L., Rall, S.C., and Weisgraber, K.H. Plasma lipoproteins. Apolipoprotein structure and function. *J. Lipid Res.* 25:1277, 1984.

32. Mahley, R.W. Apolipoprotein E. Cholesterol transport protein with expanding role in cell biology. *Science* 240:622, 1988.

33. Scanu, A.M. Lipoprotein (a) — A potential bridge between the fields of atherosclerosis and thrombosis. *Arch. Pathol. Lab. Med.* 112:1045, 1988.

34. Mahley, R.W. Atherogenic hyperlipoproteinemia. The cellular and molecular biology of plasma lipoproteins altered by dietary fat and cholesterol. *Med. Clin. North Am.* 66:375, 1982.

35. Castelli, W.P., Garrison, R.J., Wilson, D.W., Abbott, R.D., Kalousdian, S., and Kannel, W.B. Incidence of coronary heart disease and lipoprotein cholesterol levels. The Framingham study. *J.A.M.A.* 256:2835, 1986.

36. Mattson, F.H., Erickson, B.A., and Kligman, A.M. Effects of dietary cholesterol in man. *Am. J. Clin. Nutr.* 25:589, 1972.

37. McNamara, D.J., Kolb, R., Parker, T.S., Batwin, N., Samuel, P., Brown, C.D., and Ahrens, E.H. Heterogeneity of cholesterol homeostasis in man — Responses to changes in dietary fat quality and cholesterol quantity. *J. Clin. Invest.* 79:1729, 1987.

38. Flaim, E., Ferrei, L.F., Thye, F.W., Hill, J.E., and Ritchey, S.F. Plasma lipid and lipoprotein cholesterol concentrations in adult males consuming normal and high cholesterol diets under controlled conditions. *Am. J. Clin. Nutr.* 34:1103, 1981.

39. Hegsted, D.M. Serum-cholesterol response to dietary cholesterol. A re-evaluation. *Am. J. Clin. Nutr.* 44:299, 1986.

40. Keys, A., Anderson, J.T., and Grande, F. Prediction of serum cholesterol response to man to changes in fats in the diet. *Lancet* 2:959, 1957.

41. Keys, A., Anderson, J.T., and Grande, F. Serum cholesterol response to changes in the diet. IV. Particular saturated fatty acids in the diet. *Metabolism* 14:776, 1965.

42. Grundy, S.M. Monounsaturated fatty acids, plasma cholesterol and coronary heart disease. *Am. J. Clin. Nutr.* 45:1168, 1987.

43. Brown, M.S., and Goldstein, J.L. How LDL receptors influence cholesterol and atherosclerosis. *Sci. Am.* 251:58, 1984.

44. Spady, D.K., and Dietschy, J. Dietary saturated triglycerides suppress hepatic low density lipoprotein receptors in the hamster. *Proc. Natl. Acad. Sci., USA* 82:4526, 1985.

45. Nestle, P.J., Connor, W.E., Reardon, M.F., Connor, S., Wong, S., and Boston, R. Suppression by diets rich in fish oil of very low density lipoprotein production in man. *J. Clin. Invest.* 74:82, 1984.

46. Kinsella, J.E. Food lipids and fatty acids. Importance in food quality, nutrition and health. *Food Tech.* 42:124, 1988.

47. Kritchevsky, D. Dietary fiber. *Annu. Rev. Nutr.* 8:301, 1988.

48. Kris-Etherton, P.M., Krummel, D., Russell, M., Dreon, D., Mackey, S., Borchers, J., and Wood, P.D. The effects of diet on plasma lipids, lipoproteins and coronary heart disease. *J. Am. Diet. Assoc.* 88:1373, 1988.

49. Shinnick, F.L., Longacre, M.J., Ink, S.L., and Marlett, J.A. Oat fiber. Composition versus physiological function in rats. *J. Nutr.* 118:144, 1988.

50. Ney, D.M., Lasekan, J.B., and Shinnick, F.L. Soluble oat fiber tends to normalize lipoprotein composition in cholesterol-fed rats. *J. Nutr.,* 118:1455, 1988.

51. Anderson, J.W., Zettwoch, N., Feldman, T., Tietyen-Clark, J., Oeltgen, P., and Bishop C.W. Cholesterol-lowering effect of psyllium hydrophilic mucilloid for hypercholesterolemic men. *Arch. Intern. Med.* 148:292, 1988.

52. Lipid Research Clinics Program: The Lipid Research Clinics Coronary Primary Prevention Trial Results II. The relationship of reduction in incidence of coronary heart disease to cholesterol lowering. *J.A.M.A.* 251:365, 1984.

53. Report of the National Cholesterol Education Program Expert Panel on Detection, Evaluation and Treatment of High Blood Cholesterol in Adults. *Arch. Intern. Med.* 148:36, 1988.

54. Frederickson, D.S., and Levy, R.K. *Dietary Management of Hyperlipoproteinemia.* Dept. of Health and Human Services Publication No. (NIH) 75-110. Government Printing Office, 1974.

55. Ross, R. The pathogenesis of atherosclerosis. *N. Engl. J. Med.* 314:488, 1986.

56. Newman, E.P., III, Freedman, D.S., Voors, A.W., Gard, P.D., Sathanur, S.R., Cresanta, J.L., Williamson, D.G., Webber, L.S., and Berenson, G.S. Relation of serum lipoprotein levels and systolic blood pressure to early atherosclerosis. The Bogalusa Heart Study. *N. Engl. J. Med.* 314:138, 1986.

57. Small, D.M. Progression and regression of atherosclerotic lessions — Insights from lipid physical biochemistry. *Atherosclerosis* 8:103, 1988.

58. Blankenhorn, D.H., Nessim, S.A., Johnson, R.L., Sanmarco, M.E., Azen, S.P., and Cashin-Hemphill, L. Beneficial effects of combined colestipol-niacin therapy on coronary atherosclerosis and coronary venous bypass grafts. *J.A.M.A.* 257:3233, 1987.

59. Steinberg, D., Parthasarathy, S., Carew, T.E., Khoo, J.C., and Witztum, J.L. Beyond cholesterol — Modifications of low-density lipoprotein that increase its atherogenicity. *N. Engl. J. Med.* 320:915, 1989.

60. Bagatell, C.J., and Heymsfield, S.B. Effect of meal size on myocardial oxygen requirements. Implications for postmyocardial infarction diet. *Am. J. Clin. Nutr.* 39:421, 1984.

61. Neill, W., Duncan, D., Kloster, F., and Mahler, D. Response of coronary circulation to cutaneous cold. *Am. J. Med.* 56:471, 1974.

62. Christakis, G., and Winston, M. Nutritional therapy in acute myocardial infarction. *J. Am. Diet. Assoc.* 63:233, 1973.

63. Gould, L., Venkatamaran, K., Goswami, M., and Gomprecht, R. The cardiac effects of coffee. *Angiology* 24:455, 1973.

64. Hemzacek, K.I. Dietary protocol for the patient who has suffered a myocardial infarction. *J. Am. Diet. Assoc.* 72:182, 1978.

65. Goldberger, E. Dangers of a low-sodium diet in the treatment of acute myocardial infarction. *Am. J. Cardiol.* 8:300, 1961.

66. Goss, R.J. Adaptive growth of the heart. In N. Alpert, Ed., *Cardiac Hypertrophy.* New York: Academic Press, 1971.

67. Spann, J.F. Cardiac muscle performance in ventricular hypertrophy and congestive heart failure. In N. Alpert, Ed., *Cardiac Hypertrophy.* New York: Academic Press, 1971.

68. Sahn, S.H., and Levine, I. Pulmonary nodules associated with mitral stenosis. *Arch. Intern. Med.* 85:483, 1950.

69. Pittman, J.G., and Cohen, P. *The Pathogenesis of Cardiac Cachexia.* New York: Grune and Stratton, 1965.

70. Heymsfield, S., Smith, J., Redd, S., and Witworth, H.B., Jr. Nutritional support in cardiac cachexia. *Surg. Clin. North Am.* 61:635, 1981.

71. Blackburn, G., Gibbons, G.W., Bothe, A., et al. Nutritional support in cardiac cachexia. *J. Thorac. Cardiovasc. Surg.* 73:489, 1977.

72. Buchanan, N. Gastrointestinal absorption studies in cardiac cachexia. *Intensive Care Med.* 3:89, 1977.

73. Pool, P.E. Energy stores and energy utilization in the myocardium in hypertrophy and heart failure. In N. Alpert, Ed., *Cardiac Hypertrophy.* New York: Academic Press, 1971.

74. Cohn, A.E., and Steele, J.M. Unexplained fever in heart failure. *J. Clin. Invest.* 13:853, 1934.

75. Butte, N.F. Energy requirements during infancy. In R.C. Tsang and B.L. Nichols, Eds., *Nutrition During Infancy.* Philadelphia: Hanley and Belfus, 1988.

Bibliography

Braunwald, E. *Heart Disease — A Textbook of Cardiovascular Medicine,* 3rd ed. Philadelphia: W.B. Saunders, 1988.

Braunwald, E., Isselbacher, K.J., Petersdorf, R.G., Wilson, J.D., Martin, J.B., and Fauci, A.S., Eds. *Harrison's Principles of Internal Medicine,* 11th ed. New York: McGraw-Hill, 1987.

Committee on Nutrition and Health, Food and Nutrition Board, Commission on Life Sciences, National Research Council. *Diet and Health — Implications for Reducing Chronic Disease Risk.* Washington, D.C.: National Academy Press, 1989.

Ganong, W.F. *Review of Medical Physiology,* 13th ed. Norwalk, Conn: Appleton & Lange, 1987.

Guyton, A.C. *Textbook of Medical Physiology,* 7th ed. Philadelphia: W.B. Saunders, 1986.

Hurst, J.W., et al., Ed. *The Heart,* 6th ed. New York: McGraw-Hill, 1986.

Lands, W.E.M. *Fish and Human Health.* New York: Academic Press, 1985.

Lands, W.E. *Polyunsaturated Fatty Acids and Eicosanoids.* Champaign, Ill.: American Oil Chemists' Society, 1987.

Wyngaarden, J.B., and Smith, L.H., Eds. *Cecil Textbook of Medicine,* 18th ed. Philadelphia: W.B. Saunders, 1988.

Sources of Current Information

American Heart Journal
American Journal of Cardiology
Angiology
Atherosclerosis
Circulation
Circulation Research

Heart and Lung
Journal of Chronic Diseases
Journal of Clinical Investigation
Journal of Lipid Research
Journal of Thoracic and Cardiovascular Surgery
Kidney International
Progress in Cardiovascular Diseases

11. Diabetes Mellitus, Hypoglycemia, and Other Endocrine Disorders

Frances J. Zeman, Ph.D., R.D., and Robert J. Hansen, Ph.D.

I. Diabetes Mellitus
  A. Classification
    1. Primary diabetes
      a. impaired glucose tolerance
      b. insulin-dependent diabetes
      c. non-insulin-dependent diabetes
      d. gestational diabetes
      e. malnutrition-related diabetes
      f. increased risk for diabetes
        (1) previous abnormality of glucose tolerance
        (2) potential abnormality of glucose tolerance
    2. Secondary diabetes
  B. Etiology
  C. Pathology
    1. Anatomic changes
    2. Metabolic alterations
      a. endogenous insulin
      b. carbohydrate metabolism
        (1) glucose utilization
        (2) gluconeogenesis
        (3) glycogen metabolism
      c. lipid metabolism
        (1) fatty acid synthesis and storage
        (2) fatty acid utilization and ketone body formation
        (3) development of ketoacidosis
        (4) loss of body fat
      d. amino acid and protein metabolism
    3. Pathogenesis of clinical manifestations
    4. Complications of diabetes
      a. acute complications
        (1) hypoglycemia
        (2) ketosis and ketoacidotic coma
        (3) hyperosmolar nonketotic coma
        (4) other problems
      b. chronic complications
        (1) metabolic lesions
        (2) anatomic and physiologic lesions
  D. Diagnosis
  E. Nutritional assessment and monitoring of control
    1. Nutritional assessment
    2. Monitoring
      a. urine testing
      b. blood testing
  F. Management
    1. Hypoglycemic drugs
      a. sulfonylureas
      b. insulin
        (1) types of insulin
        (2) modes of insulin administration
          (a) conventional therapy
          (b) intensive therapy
    2. Nutritional care
      a. determining the diet prescription
        (1) estimating total calories needed
        (2) partitioning the calories
        (3) distributing the nutrients among meals and snacks
      b. the diabetic meal plan
      c. planning daily menus
        (1) planning for increased fiber
        (2) weighed, measured, and unmeasured diets
        (3) foods not recommended
        (4) special foods for diabetic diets
        (5) alternative sweeteners
        (6) alcoholic beverages
      d. vitamin and mineral supplements
      e. alternatives to the exchange system
      f. glycemic index
      g. other considerations in nutritional care
      h. adjustments for missed meals or reduced appetite
      i. emotional problems and diabetes

3. Exercise
   a. metabolic effects
   b. establishing an exercise program
   c. exercise in NIDDM
   d. exercise in IDDM
4. Education of the patient
G. Self-management
H. The diabetic child
I. Diabetes and reproduction
   1. The child of the diabetic mother
   2. Pregestational diabetes
   3. Gestational diabetes

4. Self-management in pregnancy
5. Diabetes management during labor and delivery
6. Lactation
J. The diabetic patient in surgery
K. Diabetes and nutritional support
II. Hypoglycemia
   A. Clinical manifestations
   B. Classification
   C. Diagnosis
   D. Nutritional care
      1. Fasting hypoglycemia
      2. Reactive hypoglycemia

   a. Functional
   b. Organic
III. The Adrenal Cortex
   A. Adrenocortical insufficiency
   B. Adrenocortical hyperfunction
   C. Adrenocorticotropic hormone or glucocorticoid therapy
IV. Thyroid Dysfunction
   A. Hyperthyroidism
   B. Hypothyroidism
V. Other Nutrition-Endocrine Interrelationships
VI. Case Studies

The **ductless glands** throughout the body make up the **endocrine system**, the major components of which are shown in Figure 11-1. There are also other endocrine tissues, not shown in the figure, which are widely distributed in nonendocrine organs in the body — for example, in the gastrin-secreting cells in the stomach. Endocrine glands secrete **hormones** which, along with the nervous system, control body functions. These hormones enter into the blood and are carried directly to their **target organs**. The primary effects of hormones are one or more of the following: (1) control of growth and maturation, (2) control of metabolism, (3) control of reproduction, or (4) integration of the physiologic response to stress. Not all existing hormones have yet been identified, nor have the mechanisms of action of all hormones been characterized.

Many hormones influence nervous system function. On the other hand, secretion of some hormones is controlled by the nervous system, whereas secretion of others occurs rhythmically or in response to the blood level of some specific substances such as glucose, sodium, calcium, water, or another hormone. In disease, the amount of a hormone secreted may increase or decrease, so that the effects of the hormone are increased or decreased, but hormones do not develop new effects in disease.

In this chapter, those endocrine abnormalities in which nutritional care is important will be described. The main focus will be on diabetes mellitus, because the number of patients involved is very large and diet is very important in its treatment.

DIABETES MELLITUS

Diabetes mellitus is a heterogeneous group of diseases of the endocrine system with common symptoms. It is characterized by a failure of control of energy production. It is unrelated to diabetes insipidus, a rare disease of the pituitary gland. When the term **diabetes** is used alone, as it will be in this chapter, it always refers to **diabetes mellitus**.

In diabetes mellitus, the cells metabolize glucose ineffectively, with secondary effects on lipid and protein metabolism. The disease is characterized by **hyperglycemia** (elevated blood glucose concentration) that is the result of an absolute or relative deficiency of insulin. Currently, it is believed that the observed hyperglycemia is also the conse-

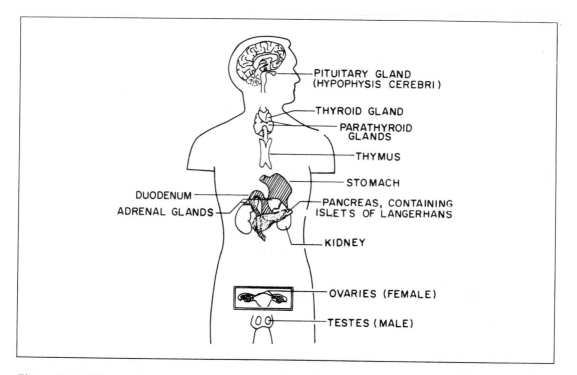

Figure 11-1. Major components of the endocrine system. (Modified with permission from Dean, W.B., Farrar, G.E., Jr., and Zoldos, A.J., Basic Concepts of Anatomy and Physiology. Philadelphia: J.B. Lippincott, 1966, p. 265.)

quence of the hypersecretion of glucagon, epinephrine, glucocorticoids, and growth hormone,[1,2] although this theory has met with some disagreement in the past.[3-5] Diabetes also is characterized by the premature development of generalized vascular disease, especially in small blood vessels.

It is estimated that approximately 3% of middle-aged adults and 6.4% of adults in the 65- to 75-year age group are diabetic, but many are not aware of their disease. In addition, approximately 0.4% of young adults and 0.5% of school-age children are diabetic, but the disease is rare in pre-school-age children.

In the patient population of an acute care hospital, diabetic patients are found in greater number than any other group requiring a modified diet. On the basis of numbers alone, diabetes would be an important problem for nutritional care specialists. In addition, the public health significance of the disease is increased by the fact that it can have serious long-term consequences such as blindness, cardiovascular disease, renal failure, and amputations. Although some diabetics have a normal life span, the average life expectancy is half of normal when onset of the disease is in childhood and two-thirds of normal in adult-onset disease.

Classification

The forms of diabetes are classified on the basis of age of onset, severity, and on the cause when it is known.

Primary Diabetes

Primary diabetes appears spontaneously rather than secondary to another disease. There are several forms of primary diabetes, which may differ in severity, age of onset, and other circumstances. As far as we know, however, the basic metabolic disorders are similar.

Impaired Glucose Tolerance. A condition in which the body has moderate difficulty in metabolizing carbohydrate is classified as impaired glucose tolerance (IGT). About 20% of patients with this condition progress to one of the two forms described in the following sections.

Insulin-Dependent Diabetes Mellitus. Insulin-dependent diabetes mellitus (IDDM) is a condition in which the glucose intolerance is more severe than occurs in the patients with IGT. These patients usually, but not always, are less than 25 years old at onset, are insulin deficient, and are prone to the development of ketosis.

Approximately 5–10% of diabetic patients have insulin-dependent diabetes. The typical IDDM patient is a child or adolescent at the time of onset and is underweight, but some are adults at onset. The disease appears suddenly with severe symptoms but, after the development of the disease, there sometimes is a short period of partial remission. Later, the diabetes worsens and becomes progressively more severe. In the fully developed disease, little or no insulin is produced.

Insulin-dependent diabetes varies in the extent to which it can be controlled. The blood glucose in some patients is reasonably constant with treatment by diet, insulin, and exercise. In others, there are dangerous variations in blood glucose concentrations for unknown reasons, and these are seriously disruptive to the patient's life. This condition is sometimes referred to as **brittle diabetes**.

Non-Insulin-Dependent Diabetes Mellitus. Patients with non-insulin-dependent diabetes mellitus (NIDDM) are usually middle-aged or elderly at onset and are not ketosis prone. They may be subdivided further into obese and nonobese groups.

In the United States and similarly developed affluent societies, 75–90% of diabetic patients are of this type. The classification of a patient as insulin-dependent or non-insulin-dependent is usually obvious but is occa-

sionally difficult. It is based on clinical observation; there is no simple test. The ability of the pancreas to produce and secrete insulin in the NIDDM patient is decreased or delayed but is not absent. In addition, the patient is considered to be insulin-resistant—that is, there is a decreased effectiveness of a given amount of insulin. In contrast to the rapid onset of IDDM, the onset of NIDDM is insidious and may be unnoticed for a long period.

The classification of a patient as IDDM or NIDDM is subject to alteration. Some patients have a stable, mild form of diabetes similar to those with NIDDM, but the hyperglycemia does not respond to other treatment, and insulin must be used. In some patients with non-insulin-dependent diabetes, the disease suddenly becomes more severe. The reason for this change is not always apparent, but sometimes the diabetes worsens temporarily with superimposed stress, such as infection or injury, and then reverts to the milder form when the stress is removed. A comparison of IDDM and NIDDM is given in Table 11-1.

Gestational Diabetes Mellitus. In some women, an abnormal glucose tolerance develops during pregnancy and then subsides postpartum. This condition is classified as gestational diabetes mellitus (GDM) during the pregnancy and will be discussed later in this chapter.

Malnutrition-Related Diabetes Mellitus. While IDDM and NIDDM are the major subclasses in developed countries, the high incidence of diabetes in underdeveloped and tropical countries has led to an additional category, malnutrition-related diabetes mellitus (MRDM).[6,7]

Increased Risk for Diabetes. Some patients are classified as having an increased risk for developing diabetes but are not diabetic at the present time.[6] Those with a **previous abnormality of glucose tolerance (PrevAGT)** have had elevated blood sugar

Table 11-1. Comparison of IDDM and NIDDM

Points of Comparison	IDDM	NIDDM
Former names	Type I Juvenile Growth-onset Ketosis-prone	Type II Adult Maturity-onset Ketosis-resistant
Percentage of diabetics	20%	80%
Age of onset	Any age; usually < 30 years	Any age; usually > 40 years; peak age of onset, 40–50 years
Cause	Deficient or no insulin production	Insulin resistance; insulin levels may be high
Symptoms at onset	Thirst, polyuria, weight loss	Often none; maybe thirst, fatigue, symptoms of vascular or neural complications, visual blurring
Body weight	Normal or thin	Usually overweight; 20% are at normal weight
Serum lipids	Elevated cholesterol	Elevated VLDL and LDL cholesterol
Acute complications	Ketoacidosis	Nonketotic hyperosmolar coma; ketoacidosis not usual
Usual treatment: Medication	Insulin for all; sulfonylureas not useful	Sulfonylurea useful for most; insulin required for 20–30%
Diet	Required	Required; for some, may be used as sole glucose control (no drugs)
Exercise	Recommended; must be integrated with other treatments	Recommended; must be integrated with other treatments

previously as a result of pregnancy (GDM), illness, or other stress. Others have a **potential abnormality of glucose tolerance (PotAGT)**. They have no current evidence of diabetes but have a close relative with IDDM or carry antibodies to pancreatic islet cells.[6,7]

Secondary Diabetes

Diabetes secondary to other conditions can result from pancreatitis, cancer of the pancreas, or surgical removal of the pancreas for any reason, from liver disease, and from chronic administration of some drugs. It also is seen in **hemochromatosis** (excessive iron absorption), **acromegaly** (abnormal growth of face, hands, and feet from overproduction of growth hormone), **pheochromocytoma** (tumor of the adrenal medulla), and **Cushing's syndrome** (overactivity of the adrenal cortex). Glucocorticoids, adrenocorticotropic hormone (ACTH), glucagon, estrogen, vasopressin, and other hormones have a diabetogenic effect whether **endogenous** (produced in the body) or **exogenous** (administered as a

medication). In some cases, diabetes may be reversed if the primary cause is removed soon enough. If the pancreas is removed or if the pancreatic cells are destroyed, the diabetes is permanent and must be treated as IDDM.

Etiology

Primary diabetes is believed to be a genetic disease that becomes evident at varying intervals after birth. The specific nature of the genetic inheritance is unknown but is complex.

The genetic pattern, related to certain HLA antigens, appears to transmit a predisposition to diabetes, rather than the disease itself, with variations in penetrance that are dependent on environmental and other genetic factors.[8] The specific environmental factors affecting penetrance are generally unknown. At one time, it was believed that racial factors, attributable to genetics, were responsible for some of the variation in the incidence of diabetes in different societies, but more recent evidence indicates that economic, social, and cultural factors are more important than race.[9] Viral infections and autoimmune reactions may be important in IDDM.[7]

In NIDDM there is no known association with the HLA system, nor are viral factors thought to be involved.[4,10] In general, the environmental factors are classified as those that increase the demand for insulin, antagonize the action of insulin, or suppress insulin production. The primary defect may lie in the islet cells or in the target cells. Various theories suggest that, if the defect is in the pancreas, there may be an inadequate number of islets of Langerhans, or the islets may be degenerating; they may be unable to recognize a stimulus to secrete or to respond to the stimulus by transmitting the message, or the defect may directly affect the synthesis, storage, or release of insulin. Alternatively, in the target cells, there may be a deficiency of glucose receptors or insulin receptors, abnormal response to hormones antagonistic to insulin, abnormal cellular response to insulin, or an antibody response that has an anti-insulin effect.[11]

Obesity is evidently the most important risk factor in NIDDM. In the United States, 75–80% of persons with NIDDM are reported to be obese, whereas in countries where obesity is uncommon, diabetes is less common.[12] In countries where undernourished populations exist, undernutrition may replace obesity as the risk factor resulting in MRDM. It is postulated that chronic undernutrition results in impaired beta cell function or that the individual becomes more susceptible to other genetic and environmental diabetogenic factors.[13] Another major factor is believed to be exercise. Decreased exercise may increase the penetrance of the gene directly, or it may do so indirectly by contributing to the causes of obesity. Weight loss in obese patients usually causes a reduction in the severity of the disease and sometimes allows it to subside altogether.

Much discussion has centered on the role of specific nutrients in impairing glucose tolerance or damaging the pancreas, apart from obesity. Deficiencies of protein, chromium, zinc, or iron have been implicated in both processes.[14] Epidemiologic and experimental studies have failed to show a relationship between carbohydrate intake and onset of diabetes.[15–21] Increased sucrose intake has been proposed as a factor in genetically predisposed persons,[22–24] but this theory has not been confirmed by other studies.[25,26] Fat has been similarly implicated.[14,18] When intake in various countries is compared, sugar and fat intake are correlated.[27] It now is suggested that the association of high sugar intake and diabetes is explained by an increased risk of obesity.[28]

The extent to which nutritional factors affect the incidence of IDDM in the lean patient is unknown. There are significant differences among different societies that may or may not relate to customary sucrose intake.

Pathology

Anatomic Changes

No pancreatic lesion is pathognomonic for diabetes mellitus. In approximately 40% of the patients, there are no observable anatomic changes. Degranulation of B cells, hyalinization, leukocyte infiltration, hydropic changes, and fibrosis of the pancreas have been seen in some patients at autopsy, but these conditions also occur in nondiabetics.

Metabolic Alterations

Endogenous Insulin. The normal pancreas consists of an exocrine organ, described in Chapter 8, and endocrine tissue, the islets of Langerhans, scattered throughout. There are approximately 2 million islets, which make up about 1% of the weight of the pancreas. The islets of Langerhans contain alpha cells, which produce **glucagon**, beta cells, producing **insulin**, and delta cells, producing **somatostatin**.

Insulin is a polypeptide synthesized in the form of **proinsulin**. The structure of porcine proinsulin is shown in Figure 11-2; human insulin is similar in structure, with some differences in the amino acid sequence. Proinsulin is converted to active insulin by proteolysis, which removes the **C** (connecting) **peptide** to produce a molecule consisting of two chains, the A chain and the B chain, connected by disulfide bonds. The C peptide is apparently inactive, but it remains in the **beta granules** in which insulin is stored in the islets and is released along with the insulin in equimolar quantities. Approximately 250 units of insulin are stored in the human pancreas, of which 20% or so is secreted each day by **emiocytosis** (the opposite of pinocytosis). Calcium is required for insulin release.

Figure 11-2. Proinsulin molecule and insulin structure: Primary structure of porcine proinsulin. The insulin sequence is represented by amino acids (dark circles). Connecting peptides are indicated by light circles. Human insulin is similar in structure, but the amino acid sequence differs somewhat. (From Shaw, W.N., and Chance, R.R. Effect of porcine proinsulin in vitro on adipose tissue and diaphragm of the normal rat. Diabetes 18:737, 1968, modified in Diabetes 21:461, 1972. Reproduced with permission of the authors and the American Diabetes Association, Inc.)

The stimuli to insulin production have been studied extensively and include the hormones glucagon, gastric inhibitory peptide, gastrin, and pancreozymin, as well as dietary glucose and amino acids. In addition, increased serum calcium, acetylcholine, and the administration of sulfonylurea drugs stimulate insulin production. These factors may stimulate the release of stored insulin, a reaction that may occur within seconds, or they may stimulate the synthesis of insulin for release, a process that may require 15 minutes to 2 hours. The response of insulin release to stimulation may thus be biphasic. The half-life of free insulin in blood is 7 to 15 minutes. Insulin is degraded by **glutathione insulin transhydrogenase**, primarily in the liver, kidney, and muscle.[29]

Insulin is the major anabolic hormone secreted in response to feeding. With the secretion of insulin, youngsters can grow, increasing their protein content and storing excess energy as glycogen or triglycerides. If individuals lose the capacity to produce and release insulin, their response to feeding cannot be normal. Indeed, diabetic patients behave metabolically as if they were starved,

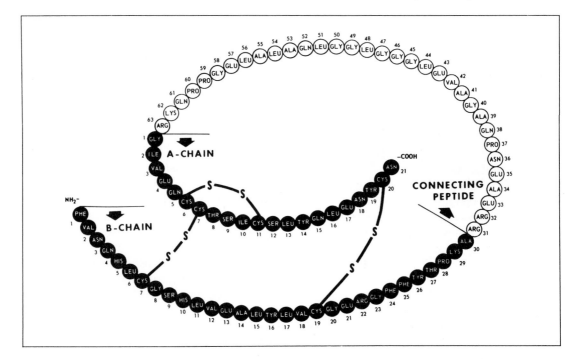

even though they are consuming greater than normal amounts of food. The specific manner or mechanism by which insulin accomplishes its functions is not known, since no unifying hypothesis proposed thus far satisfactorily explains all the changes observed. We are limited by our present knowledge to considering the effects of insulin action or the results of its absence.

To understand better the altered metabolism observed in diabetics, it is necessary to consider some of insulin's actions. Although there are many target cells of insulin, we will consider mainly insulin's effects on the liver, skeletal muscle, and adipose tissue. In general, insulin (1) promotes glucose utilization in tissues and reduces the output of glucose from the liver by glycogenolysis and gluconeogenesis; (2) promotes fatty acid synthesis in the liver and triglyceride storage in adipose tissue; (3) reduces lipolysis in adipose tissue and ketogenesis in the liver; (4) promotes amino acid uptake into muscle and adipose tissue and reduces amino acid catabolism and ureagenesis in the liver; and (5) promotes protein synthesis in muscle, in adi-

pose tissue, and, to a smaller extent, in the liver and reduces protein degradation in all three tissues (Table 11-2).

The most commonly observed action of insulin, lowering blood glucose, is due to three primary actions of insulin: (1) increased transport and utilization of glucose peripherally, mainly in skeletal muscle; (2) reduced gluconeogenesis and glucose release in the liver; and (3) reduced loss of amino acids, major glucose precursors, from peripheral tissues.

In addition to understanding what insulin is doing, it also is necessary to understand the functions of glucagon, adrenal glucocorticoids, and growth hormone, which will loosely be called **catabolic hormones**. These three hormones are antagonistic to almost every action of insulin. According to the definition of diabetes mellitus presented at the beginning of this chapter, the disease is a state caused initially by the absence of insulin activity, but intensified by the hypersecretion of the catabolic hormones. Indeed, if the hypersecretion of the catabolic hormones is prevented in some way, many of

Table 11-2. Metabolic Actions of Insulin, Glucagon, Cortisol, and Growth Hormone

Action	Insulin	Glucagon	Cortisol	Growth Hormone
Blood glucose level	↓	↑	↑	↑
Glucose uptake (M, A)	↑	NE	↓	↓
Glucose utilization (M, A, L)	↑	NE	↓	↓
Glycogenolysis (M, A, L)	↓	↑	↓	NE
Glycogen deposition (M, A, L)	↑	↓	↑	NE
Glycolytic enzyme levels (A, L)	↑	↓	↑	?
Gluconeogenesis (L)	↓	↑	↑	?
Lipolysis (A)	↓	↑	↑	↑
Lipogenesis (A, L)	↑	↓	↓	↓
Protein synthesis: (L)	↑	NE	↑	↑
(M, A)	↑	NE	↓	↑
Amino acid uptake: (L)	NE	↑	↑	↑
(M, A)	↑	NE	↓	↑
Protein degradation: (L)	↓	?	?	?
(M, A)	↓	NE	↑	?
Ureagenesis (L)	↓	↑	↑	↑
Ketogenesis (L)	↓	↑	↑	↑

M = muscle; A = adipose tissue; NE = no effect; L = liver; ↑ = the process is enhanced; ↓ = process is decreased.

the symptoms of the diabetic patient are reduced. The diabetic, then, is in hormonal imbalance: insufficient circulating insulin, the anabolic hormone, coupled with high circulating levels of the catabolic hormones leading to major effects on carbohydrate, lipid, and protein metabolism.

Carbohydrate Metabolism. In describing carbohydrate metabolism, glucose utilization, gluconeogenesis, and glycogen metabolism must be considered.

Glucose utilization. Studies of Levine and Goldstein[30] were the first to demonstrate clearly that insulin stimulated the transport of glucose and some other sugars into skeletal muscle. Subsequent work has shown that insulin also stimulates glucose transport into adipose tissue, fibroblasts, and some white blood cells, but not into liver, intestinal cells, renal tubules, blood vessels, red blood cells, pancreatic islets, the lens of the eye, or most cells of the nervous system. In the absence of insulin, the rate of entry of glucose into insulin-sensitive cells is inadequate.

In addition to stimulating glucose transport, insulin enhances the rate of glucose use in the same tissues and also in the liver. Insulin enhances the activities of many enzymes in glycolysis, in the tricarboxylic acid (TCA) cycle, in fatty acid synthesis, and in glycogen synthesis. Some of the enzymes—pyruvate kinase, pyruvate dehydrogenase, and acetylcoenzyme A (acetyl-CoA) carboxylase—exist in an inactive (phosphorylated) form, and the action of insulin appears to lead to their conversion to the active (unphosphorylated) form. The net result of the changes due to the presence of insulin is that more glucose is converted to carbon dioxide, fatty acids, lactate, and glycogen than when cells do not have insulin present. This process results in a lowering of blood glucose concentration.

In insulin deficiency, then, one of the striking symptoms of diabetes mellitus is hyperglycemia. This hyperglycemia is a consequence of reduced peripheral uptake and utilization of glucose and the increased production of glucose by the liver (Figure 11-3).

Gluconeogenesis. Insulin tends to decrease gluconeogenesis by decreasing the activities of enzymes in the gluconeogenic pathway. These enzymes include pyruvate carboxylase, phosphoenolpyruvate carboxykinase, fructose-1,6-bisphosphatase, and glucose-6-phosphatase. In insulin deficiency and in the presence of glucagon and adrenal glucocorticoids, the production of glucose from glucose precursors such as lactic acid and most amino acids is increased considerably and contributes to the hyperglycemia of diabetes (see Figure 11-3).

Glycogen metabolism. During the postabsorptive state, glycogen in the liver is metabolized to glucose to maintain blood glucose levels. Insulin promotes glycogen formation and reduces glucose release to blood, whereas glucagon increases glycogen breakdown and promotes glucose release. The two controlled enzymes are glycogen synthase and glycogen phosphorylase (see Figure 11-3). If the liver is exposed to high glucagon levels, phosphorylase becomes more active, synthase becomes less active, and glycogen is broken down. The liver puts glucose into the blood, raising the blood glucose level. If blood insulin is high, phosphorylase becomes less active, synthase becomes more active, and glycogen is synthesized, thereby decreasing the blood glucose level.

In normal individuals, insulin and glucagon are secreted as needed, but in untreated diabetic patients, there is a lack of insulin and excess of glucagon. Liver glycogen content is very low in these diabetics and, even though the patient may be eating excess food, little glucose is converted to glycogen in the liver. Instead, glucose remains in the blood, again contributing to hyperglycemia.

In skeletal muscle, insulin has effects on glycogen metabolism similar to those observed in the liver. In the diabetic patient, then, little muscle glycogen is synthesized, also contributing to hyperglycemia.

Lipid Metabolism. Insulin has important effects on synthesis of fatty acids, on triglyceride breakdown, and on the production and utilization of ketone bodies.

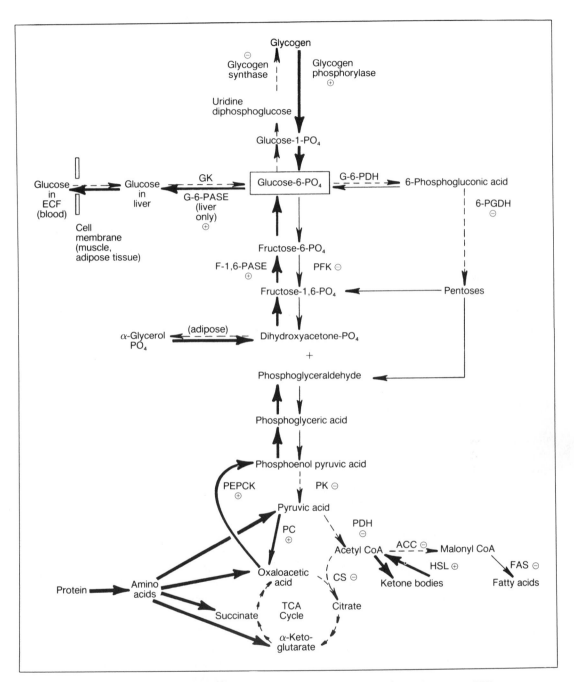

Figure 11-3. Outline of the effects of diabetes mellitus on carbohydrate metabolism. Heavy arrows indicate pathways that are accentuated by the disease, and dashed arrows indicate that the pathway is diminished. Effects of insulin deficiency on enzymes are indicated by + (increase) or − (decrease). GK = glucokinase; HK = hexokinase: G-6-PASE = glucose-6-phosphatase; G-6-PDH = glucose-6-phosphate dehydrogenase; 6-PGDH = 6-phosphogluconate dehydrogenase; PFK = phosphofructokinase; F-1,6-PASE = fructose-1,6-bisphosphatase; PK = pyruvate kinase; PEPCK = phosphoenolupyruvate carboxykinase: PDH = pyruvic dehydrogenase; PC = pyruvate carboxylase; ACC = acetyl-CoA carboxylase; FAS = fatty acid synthetase; CS = citrate synthase; ECF = extracellular fluid; TCA = tricarboxylic acid; HSL = hormone-sensitive lipase.

Fatty acid synthesis and storage. In addition to promoting glucose utilization, insulin promotes the synthesis of fatty acids and their storage as triglycerides. In humans, most of the fatty acids appear to be synthesized in the liver, transported in the blood as very-low-density lipoproteins (VLDLs), and stored in adipose tissue. Insulin has effects on all aspects of this system.

In the liver, insulin stimulates conversion of glucose and precursors such as lactate and amino acids to acetyl-CoA by making pyruvate dehydrogenase, pyruvate kinase, phosphofructokinase, and glucokinase more active. It also stimulates the synthesis of fatty acids from acetyl-CoA by increasing the activities of acetyl-CoA carboxylase and fatty acid synthase. The net effect of insulin, then, is to promote fatty acid synthesis, whereas insulin deficiency reduces synthesis (see Figure 11-3).

Synthesized fatty acids are esterified with alpha-glycerol phosphate (α-GP) to form triglycerides. These are combined with phospholipids, apolipoproteins, and cholesterol to form VLDL and are secreted into the blood. Although very few data are available on this point, it appears that insulin may be necessary for the synthesis of one or more apolipoproteins. In insulin deficiency, with the increased influx of fatty acids from adipose tissue lipolysis and from dietary sources and with a deficit of available apolipoproteins, synthesis and secretion of VLDL are reduced. Abnormally large amounts of triglyceride then accumulate in the liver, resulting in a fatty liver.

In the adipose tissue, when VLDL, as well as chylomicrons from intestinal absorption of triglycerides, reach the tissue, **lipoprotein lipase** hydrolyzes the ester bonds in the triglycerides, thereby releasing glycerol and fatty acids. This enzyme is found in large amounts in capillary beds of adipose tissue when blood insulin levels are high, but it occurs in lower amounts when the ratio of insulin to glucagon changes to favor glucagon. Under the latter circumstances, fatty acids from triglycerides in the blood are not released to enter adipose tissue cells.

Normally, fatty acids enter adipose tissue and again are incorporated into triglycerides for storage. In order to produce these triglycerides, glycerol in the form of α-GP is necessary. Adipose tissue has little glycerol kinase, the enzyme necessary for its production; therefore, glycerol released from VLDL cannot be used. Instead, most of the required α-GP must be derived from glucose by glycolysis to triose phosphate (see Figure 11-3).

When insulin deficiency occurs, glucose transport into adipose tissue cells is reduced, leading to diminished supplies of intracellular glucose. Reduced formation of α-GP results with a consequent decrease in triglyceride synthesis and a resulting elevation in blood lipid levels (**lipemia**).

In addition to lipoprotein lipase in the capillary bed, adipose tissue contains **intracellular triglyceride lipases** that convert stored triglycerides into glycerol and fatty acids. There are two general classes of these lipases. One has a relatively low activity that is uncontrolled, so that there is always some triglyceride breakdown (**lipolysis**). To counteract the effects of these lipases, there is a continuous need for some glucose to provide enough α-GP for reesterification of those fatty acids. The other lipase is hormone-sensitive and can be highly active. **Hormone-sensitive lipase** is activated by glucagon, epinephrine, ACTH, adrenal glucocorticoids, and growth hormone. Conversely, hormone-sensitive lipase is converted to the inactive form by insulin, thereby reducing lipolysis. As with glycogen metabolism, it is clear that the ratio of insulin to catabolic hormone is important. Storage of triglyceride is promoted by insulin, whereas lipolysis and reduced triglyceride storage occur when catabolic hormones prevail. In insulin insufficiency, lipolysis increases and the need for α-GP from glucose increases. The rate of breakdown of triglycerides then exceeds the ability of the adipose cell to obtain sufficient α-GP from glucose to reesterify the fatty acids, and so nonesterified fatty acids (NEFA) are released into the blood in large quantities.

Fatty acid utilization and ketone body forma-

tion. Nonesterified fatty acids are transported in the blood and used for energy by many tissues, such as cardiac muscle and well-oxygenated skeletal muscle. Increased availability of NEFA may be considered both a blessing and a curse. On the one hand, in the presence of adequate oxygen, peripheral cells such as skeletal muscle are able to use NEFA for energy, thereby requiring less glucose to be metabolized. In most tissues that use NEFA for energy, oxidation of fatty acids is carried to completion — that is, to carbon dioxide and water.

On the other hand, in the liver, metabolism can proceed as in other tissues, but, if more acetyl-CoA accumulates than can be used to form citrate for the TCA cycle, the excess acetyl-CoA has a different fate. It is converted to the ketone bodies — acetoacetic acid, beta-hydroxybutyric acid, and acetone — by pathways shown in Figure 11-4.

Normally, the production of ketone bodies is fairly small for two reasons. In the presence of insulin, lipolysis is inhibited, thereby decreasing substrate for ketone body formation. There also is a more direct control in liver cells. **Malonyl-CoA** is a metabolite in the lipogenesis pathway (see Figure 11-3). This pathway is activated by insulin and depressed in its absence. Malonyl-CoA, produced in the presence of insulin, inhibits

Figure 11-4. Formation of ketone bodies. HMG = hydroxymethyglutaryl; β-HBDH = β-hydroxybutyrate dehydrogenase.

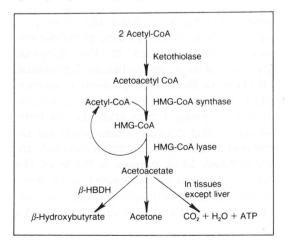

transport of fatty acids into mitochondria and thus prevents their metabolism to acetyl-CoA and to ketone bodies.

Some ketone bodies always are present in blood. Acetoacetic acid, in the presence of oxygen, can be used by any tissue containing the enzyme acetoacetate succinyl-CoA transferase, as shown in Figure 11-4. Liver, however, does not possess this enzyme and, therefore, produces ketone bodies for use by the rest of the body but not for itself.

Although the brain is not able to use NEFA for its energy needs owing to the blood-brain barrier, the brain readily uses ketone bodies. In prolonged starvation, the brain may obtain as much as 30 – 40% of its energy needs from ketone bodies.

Normally, the production and use of ketone bodies are well matched in quantity, but in starvation and in diabetes, when fatty acid catabolism is increased and fatty acid synthesis is depressed, malonyl-CoA levels drop and NEFA more readily enter the mitochondria and are metabolized. The liver thus is provided with vastly more acetyl-CoA than it can use for its own energy needs. The only remaining outlet for liver is to convert acetyl-CoA into ketone bodies. The use of ketone bodies cannot keep pace with their production under these circumstances, and they accumulate in the blood and are excreted in the urine.

Development of ketoacidosis. Of the ketone bodies, acetone is produced in the smallest quantity. It is volatile and may be excreted from the lungs. A fruity odor to the breath may result from excretion of acetone and, perhaps, of some acetoacetate by this route.

When acetoacetic and beta-hydroxybutyric acids are produced by the liver (see Figure 11-4), they are in the acid form. In blood, the ketone bodies dissociate into hydrogen ions and their negatively charged ions. These anions, acetoacetate and beta-hydroxybutyrate, are excreted in urine. To maintain electrical neutrality, a **fixed base** (monovalent cation) must be excreted for each ketone anion. The most prevalent cation in the body is sodium, but normally the kidney can conserve sodium efficiently, excreting potassium and ammonium ions in its place. In insulin deficiency, production of ketone bodies can overwhelm the system, causing depletion of important cations, including sodium.

In addition, the body must deal with the hydrogen ion derived from ionization of ketone bodies. Hydrogen ions in blood are buffered at first by bicarbonate ions and other buffer systems. The lung and kidney excrete excess hydrogen ion as a normal metabolic product. In the uncontrolled diabetic, more hydrogen ion is produced than can be excreted, and the system again is overwhelmed. Blood pH drops, stimulating the respiratory system to excrete more carbon dioxide, resulting from the following reaction:

$$H^+ + HCO_3^- \rightleftharpoons H_2CO_3 \rightleftharpoons H_2O + CO_2$$

Thus blood bicarbonate drops, and blood has less buffer with which to deal with the acidosis. Respiration deepens, then becomes more labored. If this labored breathing is insufficient to correct the pH, then there is a deep, gasping respiration.

Since the kidney does not produce urine with a pH of less than 4.5 to 5.0, there is a limit to the number of hydrogen ions that can be excreted. Continued production of acidic ketone bodies overwhelms the kidney's ability to conserve base, and the body becomes deficient in total fixed base. The inability of the kidney to deal with all the hydrogen ions produced and the loss of bicarbonate from blood results in a drop in blood pH to dangerously low levels.

Loss of body fat. Those who have observed patients with insulin-dependent diabetes are struck by the fact that they are very thin, with virtually no body fat. As discussed earlier, in order to store triglycerides, it is necessary to produce more triglycerides than are being degraded by triglyceride lipases. Recall that in the untreated diabetic there is little or no insulin available to inactivate hormone-sensitive lipase and to promote glucose uptake and use by the fat cells. In addition, there are high blood levels of most of the

hormones that activate hormone-sensitive lipase and inhibit glucose uptake and use. Chronic activated lipolysis, therefore, leads to marked depletion of adipose tissue and weight loss.

Amino Acid and Protein Metabolism. Insulin is necessary for normal growth, development, and maintenance. After the ingestion of a meal, insulin release is stimulated by absorbed glucose and amino acids. Insulin promotes amino acid transport into muscle and adipose tissue cells, promotes protein synthesis in liver, muscle, and adipose tissue, and inhibits protein degradation in all three tissues (see Table 11-3). The mechanism of insulin's actions on these processes is not yet known in full detail. As with carbohydrate and lipid metabolism, insulin enhances uptake of amino acids and synthesis of functional proteins and decreases intracellular degradation of proteins to amino acids.

Insulin does not have the same effect on all proteins but is selective in its actions; in the presence of insulin, a definite profile of proteins is affected. This pattern is comparable to insulin's actions on carbohydrate metabolism, in which the amounts of some enzymes are increased by insulin whereas the amounts of other enzymes are decreased.

In the diabetic, the anabolic actions of insulin on amino acid and protein metabolism are missing, and the catabolic processes promoted by catabolic hormones are enhanced. Amino acid uptake into muscle is depressed, whereas amino acid uptake into liver is accelerated. Synthesis of major classes of proteins, such as myosin, actin, glycolytic enzymes, and enzymes in the lipogenic pathway, is depressed, whereas degradation of many of these same proteins is accelerated, thus providing a greater blood concentration of many amino acids. In the liver, enzymes that degrade amino acids are increased in activity, so more amino acids are catabolized. More glucose is made by the liver cells from the carbon skeletons of amino acids, and more ammonia and urea are produced by amino acid catabolism and the urea

Table 11-3. Interpretation of Oral Glucose Tolerance Tests

Diagnosis	Venous Plasma Glucose [mg/dl (mmol/L)[a]]	Venous Whole Blood Glucose [mg/dl (mmol/L)[a]]
Impaired glucose tolerance[b]		
Fasting	<140 (7.8)	>120 (6.7)
Two-hour post–glucose dose	140–200 (7.8–11.1)	120–180 (6.7–10)
Diabetes Mellitus[b]		
Fasting	≥ 140 (7.8)	≥ 120 (6.7)
Two-hour post–glucose dose	≥ 200 (11.1)	≥ 180 (10)
Gestational diabetes[c,d]		
Fasting	105 (5.8)	
Post–glucose dose		
1 hour	190 (10.6)	
2 hours	165 (9.2)	
3 hours	145 (8.1)	

[a] mmol/L = (mg glucose ÷ 180) × 10.
[b] Shuman, C.R., Diabetes mellitus. In J.M. Kinney, K.N. Jeejeebhoy, G.L. Hill, and O.E. Owen, *Nutrition and Metabolism in Patient Care.* Philadelphia: W.B. Saunders, 1988.
[c] O'Sullivan, J.B., and Mahon, C.M., Criteria for the oral glucose tolerance test in pregnancy. *Diabetes* 13:278, 1964.
[d] WHO criteria are the same as those for diabetes mellitus.

cycle. Even though untreated diabetics are eating, they are in negative nitrogen balance. Lean body mass (muscle) decreases, with progressive weakness and weight loss. Blood proteins, such as albumin, decrease, and, with loss of proteins from the cells, net intracellular charge decreases. Potassium ion is lost from cells, often in exchange for hydrogen ion, and excreted in urine along with ketone body anions.

Pathogenesis of Clinical Manifestations

Having reviewed the biochemical alterations seen in diabetes, we can summarize the sequence of development of clinical manifestations in logical steps. First, there is **hyperglycemia** resulting from the metabolic alterations just described (see Figure 11-3). Kidney tubule cells have a limited capacity to reabsorb glucose. When blood glucose levels exceed this **renal threshold** (160 to 200 mg/dl), the tubules reach their **tubular maximum** for glucose (Tm_G), approximately 350 mg/min. Additional glucose cannot be reabsorbed, and glucose is excreted in urine (**glycosuria**). Urinary glucose has osmotic activity, and additional water remains in

urine, causing increased urine volume (**polyuria**). Glucose osmotic activity in extracellular fluid also causes withdrawal of water from cells. The resulting fluid loss causes dehydration which, in turn, causes thirst, stimulating an increase in water intake (**polydipsia**). Other symptoms of dehydration, when it is severe, include dry skin, sunken, soft eyeballs, decreased tongue size, decreased blood volume, and increased plasma protein concentration. Decreased protein synthesis and increased gluconeogenesis lead to loss of muscle protein and of weight. Glucose and ketone bodies in urine represent a loss of energy, also causing weight loss and a perception by the diabetic that more food must be ingested. Thus the patient develops an increased appetite (**polyphagia**). These, then, are the classic symptoms of diabetes: polyuria, polydipsia, and polyphagia. Increased food intake provides additional carbohydrate, contributing to an even higher hyperglycemia.

Lipemia occurs as the result of two factors. The first is decreased lipoprotein lipase activity, resulting in reduced removal of chylomicrons and VLDLs from the blood following a meal. The second is increased release of NEFA from adipose tissue triglyceride stores.

Liver takes up NEFA at a rate proportional to their concentration and metabolizes them to acetyl-CoA or stores them as triglycerides (leading to fatty liver). Decreased lipogenesis and the limited metabolism of acetyl-CoA in the citric acid cycle causes acetyl-CoA to be diverted to the most readily available pathway—ketone body formation. The body has a limited capacity to metabolize ketone bodies as an energy source. Excess ketone bodies accumulate in blood (**ketonemia**) and are excreted in urine (**ketonuria**). The presence of increased amounts of ketone bodies in the tissue and body fluids is known as **ketosis**.

The ketone bodies, acetoacetic acid and beta-hydroxybutyric acid, ionize, increasing the hydrogen ion concentration in the blood. As blood pH drops, respiration is stimulated (**hyperpnea**) to excrete carbon dioxide and becomes progressively more labored (**dyspnea**) and, eventually, deep and gasping (**Kussmaul respiration**).

The kidney also excretes excess acid. As long as respiratory and renal mechanisms compensate for the increased acid production, blood pH is controlled. This is known as **compensated metabolic acidosis**. Eventually, in the uncontrolled diabetic, these mechanisms become inadequate, and blood pH falls. Sodium, potassium, and bicarbonate ion are lost as respiratory and renal compensatory mechanisms are overwhelmed (**decompensated metabolic acidosis**). The patient now is **ketoacidotic**. Further details concerning acid-base balance are contained in Chapter 2.

Brain function becomes affected. The patient becomes progressively more lethargic, stuporous, and eventually, comatose. There are two theories regarding the cause of **diabetic coma**: decreased nerve irritability as hydrogen ion concentration increases, or dehydration leading to circulatory failure and hypotension, reducing oxygen and energy-producing substrates to the brain. The patient dies if blood pH continues to fall and if dehydration, shock, and renal failure are not corrected.

Complications of Diabetes

The complications of diabetes may be classified as acute or chronic. A few are minor in significance, but many can be life-threatening.

Acute Complications. The acute complications are those that can be reversed quickly with the adjustment of blood glucose level. They comprise situations in which blood glucose is either abnormally high or abnormally low.

Hypoglycemia. Hypoglycemia, usually defined as blood glucose <70 mg/dl, in the diabetic is known also as an **insulin reaction** or **insulin shock**. It occurs when blood glucose concentrations become subnormal. Many other circumstances, unrelated to diabetes, can cause hypoglycemia. These are described later in this chapter.

In insulin-treated diabetic patients, hypoglycemia can occur for a variety of reasons. Among these are (1) failure to eat the prescribed diet, (2) delayed meals following an insulin injection, (3) vomiting, (4) diarrhea, (5) a sudden increase in severe exercise, (6) alcohol, (7) an error in insulin dosage, causing an overdose, (8) weight loss without a concomitant decrease in insulin dosage, and (9) renal insufficiency with decreased renal clearance of insulin.

As blood glucose concentration falls, the patient begins to feel hungry and weak and may become mentally confused and emotionally unstable. As the condition progresses, the patient perspires and has a cold, clammy skin. Central nervous system symptoms become more severe with blurred vision and loss of coordination and orientation. Further progression produces incontinence, paralysis, unconsciousness, and convulsions. The mental symptoms arise from the lack of glucose for brain metabolism. Severe hypoglycemia can be fatal.

The time required for development of the hypoglycemic symptoms is very short, so treatment must be prompt. There is danger of permanent brain damage if the reaction is severe and lasts more than six hours. Repeated severe reactions, even of shorter duration, also can cause brain damage.

Mild reactions can be treated with a quick source of carbohydrate given by mouth. Fruit juice often is used. Other usable items include candy, sugar, honey, molasses, corn syrup, or any other source that can be absorbed quickly. For more severe reactions, injected glucagon may be given along with oral glucose sources to raise the blood glucose level. For unconscious or convulsive patients, glucose may be given intravenously.

Rebound hyperglycemia (the **Somogyi effect**) sometimes follows an episode of insulin-induced hypoglycemia, which has stimulated release of glucagon and other anti-insulin hormones. These hormones stimulate glycogenolysis and gluconeogenesis, causing an elevation in blood glucose. The Somogyi effect occurs most often in insulin-dependent diabetes. It may follow severe exercise but sometimes occurs during the night. It is treated by a 25–30% reduction in insulin dose.

The **dawn phenomenon** also causes early morning hyperglycemia. Insulin sensitivity decreases between 4 A.M. and 9 A.M., possibly because of a surge of growth hormone or glucocorticoids.

Ketosis and ketoacidotic coma. Ketoacidosis and coma account for the deaths of 1–3% of all diabetics. Of those treated for ketoacidosis, 10–15% die; therefore, prevention is very important.

Ketoacidosis occurs in undiagnosed, untreated insulin-dependent diabetes, produced as a result of the metabolic alterations previously described. However, 90% of cases of ketoacidosis involve known diabetics who are being treated. In these patients, the causes include (1) a decrease or omission of insulin dose or error in the type of insulin, (2) failure to follow the diet, with overeating, (3) sudden withdrawal of insulin when starting hypoglycemic agents, and (4) infections, trauma, or other stresses that cause the diabetes to become more severe. Even well-controlled diabetics can become

acidotic during infection, since they become more insulin-resistant. In ketoacidosis, glucagon or glucocorticoids tend to be elevated.

Ketoacidosis may develop slowly or rapidly. In juvenile diabetics, a rapid onset of days or even hours is possible, particularly if there is an infection. In a child, symptoms that can be observed by an adult include

Fatigue, weakness, listlessness
Vomiting (sometimes)
Fruity odor to the breath
Kussmaul respiration and coma in 12 to 24
  hours

In an adult, symptoms are the same as those in the child but usually develop more slowly. The patient may be extremely drowsy but still able to be aroused, rather than being comatose. In both children and adults, comatose or semicomatose states extending for more than 24 hours can result in irreversible brain damage and death.

The ketoacidotic condition varies in severity. One useful classification is shown in Table 11-4. Phases 1 and 2, in particular, are serious medical emergencies. If confused or comatose, the patient is not given food; therefore, treatment is not dietary. In general, treatment consists of large doses of insulin plus intravenous fluid and electrolyte replacement. Blood and urine profiles must be monitored frequently, and treatment must be adjusted as indicated. In addition, artificial plasma expanders sometimes are added to intravenous fluids to treat the hy-

Table 11-4. Classification of the Severity of Ketoacidotic Conditions

Phase	Serum Bicarbonate (mEq/L)	Serum pH	Acidosis
Phase 3: ketosis	20	7.4	None
Phase 2: ketoacidosis	11–20	7.2–7.4	Moderate
Phase 1: diabetic coma	10	7.2	Severe

potension and shock resulting from dehydration. Blood or plasma transfusions can be used, or **dextran**, a glucose polysaccharide with 1,6 linkage, may be added. As blood glucose levels fall, 5% glucose is added to guard against hypoglycemia.

When the patient is fully mentally alert, oral feeding may resume. A common procedure includes the following steps:

1. Use small amounts of fluids to test for nausea and vomiting. Do not feed orally until vomiting stops.
2. Progress to a liquid diet with milk, fruit juice, and broth to provide potassium and phosphate. Milk and fruit juice also provide glucose.
3. Using diabetic diet plans, progress to a full liquid diet, to soft, and then to a regular diabetic diet as tolerated. The diabetes is regulated with regular insulin.
4. When the patient is fully controlled with regular insulin, a partial shift to some longer-acting insulin may be undertaken and the diet adjusted accordingly.

Hyperosmolar nonketotic coma. In some ways, hyperosmolar nonketotic coma is similar to ketoacidotic coma, but it differs in important respects. Hyperglycemia in hyperosmolar nonketotic coma can reach extreme levels, 900 to 3,000 mg/dl, but ketonemia is very mild or absent and acidosis does not develop. The typical patient is more than 50 years old and has mild non-insulin-dependent diabetes. Many are undiagnosed until trauma or development of an unrelated illness precipitates the coma. Some examples of precipitating factors are pancreatitis, myocardial infarction, infection, cerebrovascular accident, renal failure, burns, and gastroenteritis. This superimposed stress causes the diabetes to become more severe. Sometimes, the condition is precipitated by excessive use of diuretics. It also can occur spontaneously.

In the pathogenesis of this condition, increased blood glucose levels develop with increasing severity of the diabetes. Glycosuria and fluid loss occur by the mechanisms already described. The patient may compensate with increased fluid intake at first, but this becomes insufficient and the patient becomes dehydrated. Water loss exceeds glucose loss, and the serum becomes hyperosmolar (350 mOsm or more, compared to a normal value of 285 to 300 mOsm/L). The patient becomes more unresponsive to thirst, causing further dehydration, greater osmolarity, and so on in a vicious circle. However, the patient does not become acidotic, since these patients do have some insulin, which is sufficient to prevent massive fatty acid release but not enough to stimulate entry of glucose into peripheral cells.

Once the patient is in a coma, mortality is 40–70%. Therefore, early treatment before the condition becomes severe is essential. The major features of treatment are insulin administration, potassium replacement, and hypotonic fluid replacement. The hypotonic fluid must be given slowly or the patient may die of cerebral edema when the fluid enters brain cells containing high concentrations of osmotically active glucose.

Other problems. There are several minor complications related to insulin administration that are not easily classified as either acute or chronic. Although they are less serious than the specifically acute or chronic problems, they may be of great concern to the patient; therefore, nutritional care specialists should be aware of them. Some patients may develop **lipomas** (or **lipohypertrophy**), lumpy fat deposits, at the sites of repeated insulin injections. Treatment consists of changing injection sites. Most patients are instructed to do this when they are taught to give themselves insulin. Other patients have **lipoatrophy** (loss of fat around injection sites), producing a depressed area. This is presumed to be the effect of contaminants in the insulin and is less common when purer insulins are used. No diet modification is required; alteration of the fat content of the diet is not effective. Current treatment consists of switching to human insulin and injecting the insulin directly into the atrophied area. It takes 2–4 weeks for improvement.

Chronic Complications. The chronic complications of diabetes are largely the consequence of microvascular lesions. It has been suggested[31] that the incidence of these lesions is genetically determined in some patients (5%) and is unavoidable. These patients perhaps cannot be helped with present methods. In other patients (20–25%), lesions seem to be the consequence of hyperglycemia, that is, the lack of control, but genetic predisposition is so low that they never develop complications. These patients would not need aggressive treatment. In the majority, the development of complications may be a combination of genetic predisposition plus hyperglycemia. It is these patients who may be helped by aggressive treatment. A clinical trial is currently under way to clarify these distinctions.

Metabolic lesions. No single metabolic abnormality accounts for all of the chronic complications. In most cases, the pathogenesis is unknown. A few of the aberrations in metabolism are understood and involve the redirection of glucose metabolism for insulin-sensitive to insulin-insensitive pathways.

One of these is the **sorbitol (polyol)** pathway. In cells that do not require insulin for entry of glucose, intracellular glucose is equal to the glucose levels in plasma. In the hyperglycemic patient, then, glucose concentration in these cells is high. Excess glucose is converted to sorbitol and fructose in the cell. Although glucose has freely entered these cells, sorbitol and fructose cannot readily leave, even if the hyperglycemia subsides. They can accumulate in the cells in concentrations far above normal (20 times normal for sorbitol and ten times normal for fructose), and remain in the cell until metabolized.

The exact mechanism by which sorbitol accumulation contributes to the etiology of complications is not understood entirely.

One line of reasoning suggests that the hypertonicity consequent to sorbitol accumulation causes an influx of sodium and water and a loss of potassium.[32] This, then, is followed by a decrease in amino acid and ATP concentrations and a loss of small peptides, such as glutathione, which participate in cellular metabolism.

Alternatively, it has been suggested that the damage is a consequence of reduction of the oxygen-carrying capacity of erythrocytes.[33] In glycolysis of cells other than erythrocytes, a kinase catalyzes the conversion of 1,3-diphosphoglycerate (1,3-DPG) to 3-phosphoglycerate. In erythrocytes, a different enzyme, **diphosphoglyceromutase**, catalyzes conversion of some of the 1,3-DPG to 2,3-DPG. The affinity of hemoglobin for oxygen is decreased when 2,3-DPG combines with hemoglobin, and oxygen is more easily released for use by peripheral tissues. When sorbitol accumulates, it may displace 2,3-DPG and reduce the release of oxygen to the tissues. It must be recognized that the lowering of blood pH in impending acidosis, rather than increased 2,3-DPG, may be the major mechanism for changes in oxygen release.

A second metabolic alteration leading to chronic complications may involve **glycoprotein formation**. Glycoproteins are proteins with small polysaccharide groups bound to them. In their normal formation, a polypeptide chain, formed on rough endoplasmic reticulum, is **glycosylated** (carbohydrates are attached) in smooth endoplasmic reticulum, and eventually is secreted. In the diabetic, there is increased synthesis of glycoproteins. Some changes in amino acid sequences have also been found, so that the glycoproteins formed may be abnormal. Glycoproteins make up the basement membrane; in the diabetic, basement membranes are thickened and may be abnormal. This fact has particular significance in renal function, leading to increased incidence of renal disease in diabetic patients.

A third possible lesion may involve **muco-**

polysaccharide formation. Mucopolysaccharides have larger proportions of carbohydrates than do glycoproteins. The greater amount of glucose available to their synthetic pathways may cause alterations in their structure. Abnormal mucopolysaccharide structures have been seen in the aorta, kidneys, skin, and retinas of diabetics. Clinical complications also occur in these tissues, but it has not been proved that they are related to abnormal mucopolysaccharides. However, the simultaneous occurrence does suggest that there is a relationship.

The biochemical lesions just described occur most frequently in blood vessels, nerves, kidneys, and eyes of diabetic patients. The consequences of these pathologic alterations seriously impair the general health and shorten the life expectancy of the patient.

Anatomic and physiologic lesions. **Angiopathy** (abnormalities of the blood vessels) accounts for 80% of diabetic deaths. It may be subdivided into **macroangiopathy** (disease in large blood vessels) and **microangiopathy** (disease in small blood vessels).

Disease in the large arteries of diabetics is morphologically identical to that found in the general population except that it occurs earlier, progresses more rapidly, and is more severe. It leads to cerebrovascular accidents of the ischemic occlusive type, myocardial infarctions, senility, congestive heart failure, and other complications of cardiovascular disease (see Chapter 10). One consequence of macroangiopathy deserves special mention in a discussion of diabetes. Severe atherosclerosis in large vessels can occlude the vessels and reduce circulation to a body part. This occlusion occurs particularly in the legs and feet of diabetics, producing **intermittent claudication**. The patients may complain first of pain, coldness, and fatigue in the affected limbs. The limbs become ischemic. In severe cases, wounds and infections do not heal because of poor blood supply. Ulcers and gangrene develop easily (review Chapter 1, if necessary), and amputations are frequent. For this reason, care of the feet is an important aspect of proper treatment of diabetic patients.

Microangiopathy is found in 8% of normal subjects, 53% of prediabetics, and 98% of overt diabetics, and it affects the retina of the eye, the glomeruli of the kidney, and some parts of the nervous system. Since it often occurs before the onset of overt diabetes, it may be the basis for diagnosis. Its manifestations include sclerosis of the arterioles and dilation of the venules with stasis of blood in the venules. The basement membranes around capillaries thicken, contributing to the loss of circulation in the limbs and increasing the susceptibility to infection. It also contributes in important ways to the complications that may occur in kidneys and eyes.

Nephropathy (kidney disease) is responsible for only 10% of all deaths but accounts for 50–60% of deaths of insulin-dependent diabetics. It progresses without symptoms until renal failure is far advanced. Nutritional care must combine that for renal failure described in Chapter 9 and that for diabetes.

Neuropathy (lesions of the nerves) can take many forms. It is less likely to be life-threatening than are angiopathy and nephropathy but can be very distressing to the patient. As in the case of microangiopathy, symptoms sometimes occur prior to the diagnosis of diabetes. Significant nerve damage is thought to occur more frequently if the diabetes is poorly controlled. If the disease is controlled, progress of neuropathy may be arrested but not entirely reversed.

The metabolic lesions that occur in nerves may involve carbohydrate, lipid, or protein metabolic pathways, but they are not understood entirely. The sorbitol pathway may be involved, since sorbitol and fructose do occur in peripheral nerves. Other metabolic aberrations apparently reduce the rate of conversion of glucose to carbon dioxide or fatty acid.

Lipid metabolism of peripheral nerves is generally affected, resulting in differences in fatty acid composition and abnormalities in the formation of fatty acids, cholesterol, glycolipids, and myelin. The formation of protein in myelin is reduced. Inositol metabolism may also be involved.

Neuropathies may occur in either sensory or motor nerves or both. They may affect one nerve or many and they may be one-sided or occur on both sides of the body. Some recovery occurs with control of the diabetes, but it can take months. Depending on the nerves involved, symptoms may include pain, weakness, numbness, and loss of a sense of physical position. Neuropathies may be divided into these subcategories: (1) **polyneuropathy** involving nerve terminals producing sensory loss and pain in hands and feet; (2) **radiculopathy** involving dorsal roots producing sensory loss and pain in the associated dermatomes; (3) **mononeuropathy** in a mixed cranial and spinal nerve to produce sensory loss, pain, and weakness; (4) **amyotrophy** involving a nerve terminal or muscle producing weakness, pain, and muscle atrophy; and (5) **autonomic neuropathy** involving autonomic nerves with various manifestations in viscera.

Neuropathies in the autonomic nervous system can be disabling and occasionally fatal. Some of the clinical manifestations include disorders in the cardiovascular system, bladder disturbances, abnormalities of eye control, and impotence in men. Of particular interest to nutritional care specialists are the gastrointestinal disturbances, including diarrhea, constipation, incontinence, atony of the esophagus with dysphagia, nausea, vomiting, gastric motor disorders, pancreatic enzyme insufficiency, and gallstones, among others. Delayed gastric emptying occurs in **gastroparesis diabeticorum**, in which the action of insulin and absorption of food become unsynchronized. Delay of insulin administration and smaller, more frequent meals may be helpful.[33] Gluten-sensitive enteropathy is associated with diabetes in an unusually large number of cases. Nutritional care for patients with this condition

is described in Chapter 8. Riddle[34] reports that the gastrointestinal symptoms may be caused by hypoglycemia in some patients whose insulin dosage should be reduced.

Retinopathy (disease of the retina) in the diabetic is a common cause of blindness. Patients may complain of blurred vision, double vision, halos, and pain in the eyes. Sometimes these occur prior to the diagnosis of diabetes. Reduction of blood glucose and blood lipids by controlling the diabetes acts as a preventive or at least delays the advance of the disease.

Diagnosis

The detection of the milder forms of diabetes is somewhat difficult. Mild non-insulin-dependent diabetes may be asymptomatic and can exist undetected for many years. Its existence sometimes is first suspected when vascular lesions are seen in the eye, or it may be detected fortuitously during a case-finding survey of the population, during a routine physical examination, or during diagnosis and treatment for another disorder. The major diagnostic tests that have been in use for many years have focused on the effects of diabetes on plasma glucose concentration. There are several of these tests.

In the measurement of **fasting plasma glucose** (FPG) or **fasting blood glucose** (FBG) glucose concentration is determined in venous or capillary blood or plasma from a patient following an eight-hour fast, usually overnight. Normal FPG is less than 115 mg/dl in patients up to age 50. Thereafter, it increases approximately 1% per year. The relationship between plasma and blood glucose levels can be calculated with the formula[7]

$$\text{blood glucose} = (\text{plasma glucose} - 6) \div 1.15 \qquad \textbf{(11-1)}$$

If FPG is greater than 140 mg/dl, a diagnosis of diabetes mellitus can be made. Fasting glucose levels are increased in patients under mental, emotional, or physical stress. As a result, values are not considered truly abnormal unless they exceed 140 mg/dl of plasma or more than 120 mg/dl of whole blood.[35]

A test for glycosylated hemoglobin (HbA$_{1c}$) is used to confirm the diagnosis, particularly if FPG values are borderline. **Hemoglobin A$_{1c}$**, or glycosylated hemoglobin, forms 5% of the total hemoglobin (Hb) in the normal person. It is formed slowly in a non-enzymatic reaction throughout the life of the mature red blood cell by a reaction between the major adult hemoglobin, HbA, and glucose. There are several forms of HbA, depending on the position at which the glycosylation occurs on hemoglobin A. The forms of hemoglobin that migrate most quickly through a chromatographic column of cation exchange resin are "fast hemoglobins," or hemoglobin A$_1$. This is further subdivided into three fractions known as HbA$_{1a}$, HbA$_{1b}$, and HbA$_{1c}$. The HbA$_{1c}$ is mostly closely correlated with blood glucose levels. In hyperglycemia, the rate of formation of HbA$_{1c}$ increases, and levels may reach 15% in uncontrolled diabetes mellitus.[36] The reaction is nearly irreversible, so that a high

HbA$_{1c}$ concentration will fall only as cells die and are replaced by new cells, but will not fall with a temporary decrease in the blood glucose level. The HbA$_{1c}$ concentration, then, reflects the average degree of hypoglycemia over a period of two to three months[37] and can be used as a check on the patient's long-term adherence to the diet as well as serving as a diagnostic tool. Normal HbA$_{1c}$ is 5.4–7.4% in some laboratories. Values above 8.6% suggest a diagnosis. The values vary in different laboratories and must be obtained from the laboratory doing the test.

In order to establish a diagnosis of diabetes or impaired glucose tolerance in asymptomatic individuals whose FPG is between 115 and 139 mg/dl of plasma, a two-hour **oral glucose tolerance test** (OGTT) is sometimes recommended. The OGTT is based on the assumption that a normal person can remove a specified glucose load from the blood within a defined period. Prior to the test, the patient's diet should contain at least 150 g of carbohydrate per day. Usually, this level is achieved with the patient's normal diet, and no special preparation is required. On the day of the test, a urine sample and blood for the FPG are obtained. In a typical procedure, the patient is given a drink, usually containing 75 g of glucose in a 15–25% solution flavored with lemon juice or cola. For children, the glucose dose is 1.75 g/kg up to a maximum of 75 g. The drink must be ingested within 10 to 15 minutes. The glucose content of hourly plasma samples is determined. Figure 11-5 shows a comparison between the normal and diabetic curves. A typical normal curve with affecting factors is shown in Figure 11-6. Although the physiological interactions that contribute to the changes in blood glucose levels are more complex than displayed in Figure 11-6, the figure deals with the major influences of each phase.

Characteristic abnormalities in the glucose tolerance curve that are indicative of diabetes are (1) increased maximum plasma glucose concentration, (2) delayed return to normal plasma glucose concentration, and

Figure 11-5. Normal and diabetic glucose tolerance curves.

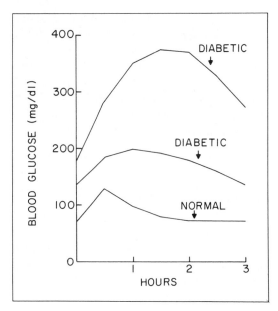

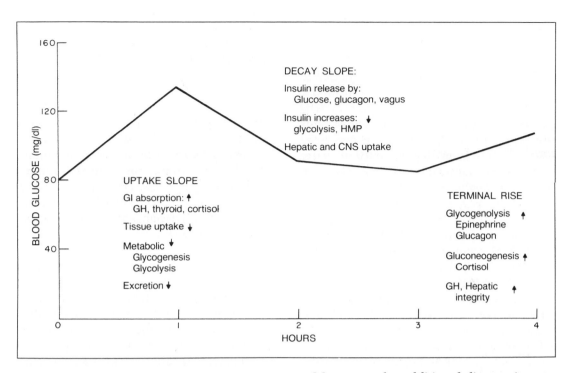

Figure 11-6. Metabolic processes in the normal oral glucose tolerance test. Processes involved in the different phases of the curve are presented. Thick arrows indicate directions of changes in blood glucose levels. HMP = hexose monophosphate (Shunt); GH = growth hormone. (Reprinted with permission from Bacchus, H., Rational Management of Diabetes. Copyright © 1977. University Park Press, Baltimore.)

(3) late hypoglycemia, usually in three to five hours. The specific criteria used to define abnormalities vary, but it is important to remember that many drugs and other illnesses can affect glucose tolerance.

Criteria used for the evaluation of OGTT are summarized in Table 11-3. Prediction of diabetes is best accomplished by interpretation of both fasting and two-hour FPG values. In some instances, further tests may be necessary to confirm diagnosis of diabetes. One of the tests used is a **cortisone OGTT**, where the OGTT is preceded by two doses of cortisone to mimic the effect of stress. The test applies only if the patient is younger than 45 years of age, not pregnant, and has no other diseases.

More recently, additional diagnostic tests have become available. The amount of insulin in the blood is very small, and for many years routine assays were impossible. The development of radioimmunoassay techniques has increased the use of measurement of **blood insulin levels**.

The C peptide, released when proinsulin is converted to active insulin, can be used to measure endogenous insulin secretion even when the patient is receiving exogenous insulin in treatment. The diabetic patient who has no endogenous insulin will have no C peptide. The test is known as the **C peptide chain assay.**[38]

Acid-base balance is important in the differential diagnosis of diabetes, particularly in severe disease. Arterial blood gases (ABGs) and blood bicarbonate are measured. Blood pH is also recorded in the patient's medical record. The gases O_2 and CO_2 are given as partial pressures, labeled as pO_2 and pCO_2. Means and normal ranges are

pH	7.4 (7.35–7.45)
pO_2	90 (80–100) mm Hg

pCO$_2$ 40 (35–45) mm Hg
HCO$_3^-$ 24 (22–26) mEq/L

These values are used by the physician to differentiate among respiratory or metabolic acidosis or alkalosis (see Chapter 2). The metabolic acidosis to which diabetic patients are inclined is demonstrated by depressed pH resulting from depressed bicarbonate and a compensatory decrease in pCO$_2$. Such a patient might have values as follows: pH = 7.2;   pO$_2$ = 90;   pCO$_2$ = 25;   and HCO$_3^-$ = 10. The greater decrease in the bicarbonate (base) compared to the decrease in pCO$_2$ (acid) demonstrates the reason that the condition is called a **base deficit**.

Metabolic acidosis may result from the addition of a strong acid or from gastrointestinal or renal loss of base. These can be distinguished by calculation of the anion gap (see Chapter 2). In diabetic ketoacidosis (DKA), an anion gap > 16 indicates an increase in H$^+$.

Other methods of laboratory evaluation are used to detect complications associated with diabetes. These include a fasting lipid profile with determination of triglycerides and total, LDL, and HDL cholesterol (see Chapter 10).

Nutritional Assessment and Monitoring of Control

Diabetes mellitus is a lifetime disease. Therefore, many of the same evaluation procedures are used for diagnosis, for assessment, and for monitoring of control at various times in the course of the patient's life.

Nutritional Assessment

The procedures described in Chapter 3 are largely applicable to the diabetic patient. The nutritionist should obtain biochemical and anthropometric data from the medical record, as well as the medical and clinical data on both diabetes and any concurrent medical problems. Compliance with the diet is likely to be improved if the diet fits into the patient's current life style. Therefore, detailed information on that life style is needed, requiring a very thorough diet history.[39]

Monitoring

Monitoring is the process of being aware constantly of one's blood glucose level. Its purpose is to provide the information fundamental to procedures for maintaining normal blood sugar levels. There are a number of methods in use, some of which are used primarily by physicians, and others, by the patients themselves.

Urine Testing. To manage their own diabetes, patients must have an indication of their blood glucose status. Although direct measurement of blood glucose seems the logical approach, urine testing for glucose was the method of choice for many years. Patients were taught to test their own urine for glucose and, when necessary, for ketone bodies. The methods are easy, painless, noninvasive, simple, and inexpensive. Urine testing is still being done today, even though there are more informative methods.

The urine test materials consist of the necessary chemicals in a tablet or impregnated on a stick or tape. There are several forms available: Diastix, Chemstrip uG, Clinitest (a tablet), and Tes-Tape. All measure glucose in the urine, although Clinitest also gives a positive reaction to galactose, lactose, fructose, or maltose in the urine. A large amount of ascorbic acid in the urine may interfere with any of the tests.

The tests involve the development of a color, which then is compared with a series of colored standards. Diabetics are taught to test their urine one or more times per day. For some, four times per day — before each meal and at bedtime — is recommended.

There are limitations to urine testing. It gives no indication of levels of blood glucose less than that of the patient's renal threshold. Thus, if the renal threshold is 180 mg/dl, the test will be negative at any value below that level, even though blood glucose may be undesirably high. Urine testing, of course, also gives no warning of impending hypoglycemia. In addition, the amount of glucose in the urine is not always correlated with blood glucose. If urine tests are used, in order to get more current information, a "second voided specimen" is required, particularly in the morning. The urine is voided in the morning and discarded. The testing is done on a urine sample collected half an hour later, the "second voided" sample, which thus reflects more current blood glucose levels.

When urine tests for glucose show an abnormal result, or when feeling ill, the patient may also test for ketone bodies with Ketostix, Acetest, or Chemstrip K. Chemstrip uGK measures both glucose and ketones.

Blood Testing. Logically, a better method of monitoring blood glucose concentrations would be testing of the blood rather than the urine. However, in the past, blood glucose testing was difficult for patients because of difficulties in obtaining blood and because of complex testing methods. Instead, an occasional test was done in the physician's office or clinic. The amount of information obtained was limited because it gave glucose levels only at one time, which might not indicate good control. Good management needs more frequent blood testing or a test indicating long-term control.[40]

Recent developments have provided partial solutions to problems of frequent testing.[41] Single-use lancets are available in order to prick fingers to obtain blood. The blood can be put on a reagent strip (Chemstrip bG, Glucostix, TrendStrips, or Visidex II) that can be read with or without a meter. Better compliance has been reported for patients who monitor their blood glucose.[42,43]

The schedule for self-monitoring is established on an individual basis. When attempting to establish control, blood tests may be done seven times a day: before each meal and at bedtime, and two hours after each meal. Alternatively, patients may test only four times a day, but alternate the time so that, at the end of a week, representative values for all seven times are available. After control is established, the number of tests can be reduced to once or twice daily, alternating the times chosen from the original seven.[40]

In interpretation, desirable or "target" blood glucose levels are approximately as shown in Table 11-5.[7] Patients should keep a record of their blood glucose values so that adjustments can be made to respond to any pattern of hypoglycemia or hyperglycemia that develops. Many patients are instructed to test their urine, in addition. The procedure, in total, is called **self blood glucose monitoring** (SBGM). These records are useful in self-management, described later, and also to members of the health care team. The appearance of high blood glucose levels or glucose in the urine at a given time each day, for example, might indicate to the nutritional care specialist the need to redistribute the meal plan to make the immediately preceding meal smaller. Alternatively, the physician might wish to increase or redivide the insulin prescription.

One problem with the method concerns the reliability of the patient's records. Studies of patients who were provided a monitor with a memory capacity unknown to them showed that a large proportion of patients' records tended to obscure hyper- or hypoglycemia.[44,45]

Hemoglobin A_{1c} is also used as a monitoring tool to indicate the average blood glucose level over the previous two-month period and as a check on the patient's records, but it does not reflect daily fluctuations. Therefore,

Table 11-5. Blood Glucose Levels for Diabetes Patients

Time	Desirable (mg/dl)	Normal (mg/dl)
Before breakfast	70–120	70–105
Before lunch, dinner, or snacks	70–140	70–110
One hour after meals	<180	<160
Two hours after meals	<150	<120
2 A.M. to 4 A.M.	>70	>70

for maximum control, both this test and SBGM need to be used. This method is usually done in the physician's office or clinic, but a method for patient monitoring of HbA$_{1c}$ has been developed.[46] The method is relatively complex but was reported to be effective in reinforcing patient education. Results vary slightly from one laboratory to another, but the values shown in Table 11-6 are useful in interpretation.[7]

Management

Since there is no cure for diabetes, the patient must learn to live with the disease. The overall objectives of treatment are to prolong life and to improve the quality of life as much as possible. Specifically, the treatment is directed toward the following goals:

1. Relieving the symptoms and enabling the patient to live a relatively normal life.
2. Decreasing the severity of the disease by improving the body's ability to metabolize glucose and correcting faulty metabolism so that glucose tolerance is improved and insulin resistance is decreased.
3. Preventing or correcting complications.
4. Assuring adequate nutrition.

These objectives are accomplished by control of the metabolic changes. Control may be measured in various ways. Most commonly, it is measured by the maintenance of blood glucose concentration within normal limits. Other criteria that are sometimes used include absence of symptoms, of glycosuria,

Table 11-6. Hemoglobin Levels in Diabetes Patients and Their Interpretation

HbA$_{1c}$ Level	Control	Average Blood Glucose (mg/dl)
5.4–7.4	Normal (nondiabetic)	70–105
7.4–8.5	Excellent	120–150
8.6–10.5	Good	150–200
10.6–13.0	Fair	200–300
>13.0	Poor	>300

or of hyperlipidemia; normal blood ketoacids; normal hemoglobin A$_{1c}$ values; or normal measurements of function of the eye, kidney, or nervous system.

The successful treatment of the diabetic patient is complex and requires the cooperation of the physician, nurse, nutritional care specialist, and other members of the health care team, but most of all it requires the whole-hearted cooperation of the patient. It commonly is said that, in the final analysis, the diabetic patient is self-treated.

There are four major facets of diabetic care: (1) control of the dietary intake to decrease clinical manifestations while providing for nutritional needs, (2) hypoglycemic drugs, (3) exercise, and (4) education. In addition, the general hygiene and emotional well-being of the patient often must receive attention.

Hypoglycemic Drugs

Although nutritional management of the diabetic patient is the cornerstone of treatment, an understanding of the use and actions of hypoglycemic drugs is necessary to fully understand the rationale for such management. Therefore, we will begin with a discussion of these drugs.

Hypoglycemic or **antidiabetic drugs** are those that lower the blood glucose concentration. Some diabetics do not receive these drugs but are treated by diet alone. Others receive either one of the sulfonylurea drugs or insulin in addition to the diet.

Sulfonylureas. The sulfonylurea compounds are taken orally, and so they often are called **oral hypoglycemic agents** (OHAs). Those available are described in Table 11-7. The second-generation compounds, developed most recently, are more potent, have fewer side effects, and have fewer drug interactions. Tolbutamide and chlorpropamide are those most frequently used in the United States. They are given to almost 50% of diabetic patients, but serious questions have been raised concerning their

Table 11-7. Sulfonylurea Oral Hypoglycemia Drugs

Generic Name	Brand Name	Onset (hours)	Duration (hours)	Recommended Dosage (mg/day)	Doses per Day	Maximum Dose (mg/day)
First generation						
Tolbutamide	Orinase	1	6–12	500–3,000	2–3	2,000–3,000
Acetohexamide	Dymelor	1	12–24	250–1,500	1–2	1,500
Tolazamide	Tolinase	4–6	12–24	100–1,000	1–2	750–1,000
Chlorpropramide	Diabinase	1	Up to 72	100–500	1	500
Second generation						
Glipizide	Glucotrol	1–1.5	10–24	2.5–40	1–2	40
Glyburide	Diabeta, Micronase	2–4	24	1.25–2.0	1–2	20

value, since no long-term benefits of their use over other methods have been documented.[47]

Sulfonylurea drugs stimulate the release of preformed insulin from the pancreas. It has been suggested that their primary mode of action during prolonged use may be to alter cell membranes and increase their responsiveness to insulin, possibly by increasing the number of receptors. A summary of actions outside of the pancreas is given in Table 11-8. Since they act by stimulating formation or release of insulin, they have no effect in the insulin-dependent diabetic who has no endogenous insulin production. They

Table 11-8. Extrapancreatic Effects of Sulfonylurea Drugs

Related to antidiabetes effects
Increased insulin stimulation of carbohydrate transport in skeletal muscle
Increased insulin action on the liver
Decreased triglyceride lipase in liver and adipose tissue
Decreased ketosis
Decreased glucose output from liver
Decreased lipolysis in adipose tissue
Increased uptake and oxidation of glucose in adipose tissue

Side effects
Activation of adenylate cyclase
Decreased adenosine 3′,5′ monophosphate diesterase
Altered rate of amino acid incorporation into protein
Decreased transaminase activity
Reduced intestinal glucose absorption
Decreased insulinases
Increased cardiac contractility
Decreased platelet aggregation

are usable in non-insulin-dependent diabetes, prediabetes, and latent diabetes in an attempt to delay onset of overt disease. They are most effective in patients over the age of 40 whose insulin need is less than 40 units per day.

There are some advantages to the use of sulfonylureas. First, they are taken orally in tablet form rather than by injection, so patient acceptance is high. They may be given to the non-insulin-dependent diabetic who, because of lack of understanding, poor eyesight, or other reasons, cannot safely administer his or her own insulin. There is less danger of hypoglycemia with sulfonylurea use than with insulin use. To the extent that sulfonylureas stimulate insulin production and release by normal pathways, they correct the existing deficiency rather than provide a replacement. Finally, these drugs also provide less potential for allergic reactions because they are not foreign proteins.

Their disadvantages also are important considerations and, in recent years, have been the basis for the reduction in their use in favor of dietary control with or without insulin. It has been suggested, for example, that the use of tolbutamide may increase the incidence and severity of cardiovascular disease.[48] Other side effects of tolbutamide or chlorpropramide include liver toxicity, blood dyscrasias, hypothyroidism, hyponatremia, rash, nausea, vomiting, heartburn, and alcohol intolerance. A major problem from the point of view of the nutritional care specialist is that oral drug treatment is so easy that many patients feel that diet is unimportant.

Insulin. Insulin is given to approximately 25% of diabetic patients. Its use is indicated in diabetic children, all patients with sudden onset diabetes, and underweight diabetics, since these conditions are suggestive of insulin-dependent diabetes. In addition, even if a diabetic has not been treated with insulin previously, it usually is indicated when certain complications such as ketosis, fevers, infections, surgery, burns, or pregnancy occur.

Since insulin is a protein, it would be digested if taken by mouth and therefore must be given parenterally, usually by subcutaneous injection.

Types of insulin. Insulin is most commonly available in vials containing 100 units/ml (U-100). Insulins are also available in U-40 and U-80 concentrations. Each milligram of pure insulin equals 24 units. There are a number of types of insulin available (Table 11-9), classified as rapid-acting, intermediate-acting, or long-acting.[49]

The rapid-acting insulins are Regular insulin and Semilente. Regular insulin is the only insulin produced in solution with no modifying agent. All others are suspensions. Regular insulin is also the only one that can be administered intravenously. Protamine and globin are proteins which, when combined with insulin, slow its rate of absorption. NPH insulin contains protamine and zinc in the suspension. Lente insulin (insulin zinc suspension) is manufactured by a process that produces very large crystals, thus slowing its absorption. It contains zinc but no modifying protein. The long-acting insulins, Protamine Zinc Insulin (PZI) and Ultralente, are rarely used.

Insulin is obtained from three sources — beef, pork, and human. Beef insulin differs from human insulin in three amino acids. It is more antigenic than pork insulin which differs from human insulin in only one amino acid. Beef-pork combinations are also available and is more antigenic than either beef or pork insulin alone.

Human insulin may be **semisynthetic** or **biosynthetic**. Semisynthetic human insulin uses pork insulin as a base. The one differing

Table 11-9. Types of Insulin

Insulin	Onset (hours)	Peak Action (hours)	Peak Duration (hours)	Types Available/Source[a,b,c]			
				Name	Species[d]	Appearance	Modifiers
Rapid-acting	$\frac{1}{2}$–1	2–4	5–7	Regular[a]	b, p, h	Clear	—
	$\frac{1}{2}$	2$\frac{1}{2}$–5	8	Regular[b]	p, h	Clear	—
	$\frac{1}{2}$	1–3	8	Regular[c]	p, h	Cloudy	Zinc
	$\frac{1}{2}$–1	—	12–16	Semilente[a]	b + p	Cloudy	Zinc
	$\frac{1}{2}$	5–10	16	Semilente[b]	p	Cloudy	Zinc
Intermediate-acting	2–4	6–12	18–24	Lente[a]	b + p, h	Cloudy	Zinc
	2$\frac{1}{2}$	7–15	24	Lente[b]	p, h	Cloudy	Zinc
	2–4	6–12	24	NPH[a]	b, p, h	Cloudy	Protamine, zinc
	1$\frac{1}{2}$	4–12	24	NPH[b]	p, h	Cloudy	Protamine, zinc
	1$\frac{1}{2}$	4–12	24	NPH[c]	p, h	Cloudy	Zinc
	$\frac{1}{2}$	4–8	24	Mixtard[c] (30% RI, 70% NPH)	p		
	$\frac{1}{2}$	2–12	24	Novolin 70/30[b] (30% RI, 70% NPH)	h	Cloudy	
Long-acting	2–6	18–24	36+	Ultralente[a]	b + p	Cloudy	Zinc
	4	10–30	36	Ultralente[b]	b	Cloudy	Zinc
	2–6	18–24	36	PZI[a]	b + p		

[a] Eli Lilly.
[b] Squibb–Novo; pork insulin available as standard or purified.
[c] Nordisk–USA.
[d] b = beef; p = pork; h = human; b + p = beef and pork.

amino acid is converted so the molecule is identical to human insulin. Biosynthetic human insulin is made using recombinant DNA and *E. coli.*

Insulins are also classified as "purified" or "improved." Purified insulin is obtained by extraction from beef or pork pancreas, but it contains some impurities. Recent improvements in the technology of insulin purification have led to production of "improved insulins" consisting of monocomponent insulin with few impurities. Using genetic engineering techniques, "human insulin" has been produced. It is hoped that the use of these new insulins will result in fewer side effects of insulin therapy.

The properties of the insulins listed in Table 11-9 should be studied carefully. It is essential that nutritional care specialists be familiar with the speed of onset and duration of action of each of the available insulins, since this information is important in diet planning.

Modes of insulin administration. Insulin administration may be broadly classified as **conventional** or **intensive**. Conventional therapy consists of one, or sometimes two, injections of combinations of regular plus intermediate-acting or long-acting insulins. This is useful for patients whose diabetes is relatively stable. For the unstable diabetic, intensive therapy uses multiple daily injections (MDI) or continuous subcutaneous insulin infusions (CSII) using a pump.

Conventional therapy: Rapid-acting insulin is used when diabetes is being controlled in the newly diagnosed diabetic or following a ketotic episode. It also is used daily by many diabetics to control blood glucose early in the day. If only regular insulin is used, an injection is required before each meal.

To reduce the number of injections, a longer-acting and a rapid-acting insulin are used in combination. They are mixed in the syringe by the patient just before administration. It is not possible to mix them in advance of their use, since they interact and their properties change. A common procedure is to mix the rapid-acting insulin for its effect during the morning with an intermediate-

acting insulin, the activity of which occurs primarily after the noon and evening meals. Commonly used combinations are regular insulin plus either NPH (neutral protein Hagedorn) or Lente insulin. When these combinations are used, it may be possible to control diabetes with only one insulin injection per day, but two or more injections per day provide better control in many patients.

Intensive therapy: In this procedure, blood sugar levels are determined, preferably with a meter, before each meal and at bedtime. In other words, the patient undertakes self blood glucose monitoring. The results are then used to adjust the insulin dosage in order to keep blood sugar as close to normal as possible, providing better control.[50]

The patient on MDI typically has an injection of longer-acting insulin (e.g., Ultralente) once daily and an injection of regular insulin before meals. Administering insulin by CSII, utilizing an infusion pump and indwelling needle, has been gaining increased acceptance by clinicians and patients. This method utilizes regular insulin infused at a constant rate plus a bolus of insulin that the patient adjusts prior to each meal based on the results of self blood glucose monitoring. It is most often recommended to motivated patients who are not able to achieve euglycemia even with multiple daily injections of insulin. However, many physicians offer CSII as an alternative to other methods, leaving the choice of therapy to the patient. Usually, CSII is only recommended to patients when a 24-hour medical facility with a skilled professional team is available to support the patient. These patients use a special preparation of human insulin containing a phosphate buffer to prevent clogging the tubing of the pump.

Problems related to CSII have been relatively few. Failure of the pump to deliver insulin does occur, but with increasing rarity as pumps become more reliable. When a pump fails, immediate medical attention must be sought by the patient. Pumps are designed to signal when they stop or become "runaway," so these problems are held to a minimum. The most common problem encountered in patients using CSII is hypoglycemia, particularly at night when asleep. This problem is usually dealt with by adjusting the rate of delivery of insulin such that the desired minimum fasting blood glucose level (usually around 100 mg/dl) is achieved at 3:00 A.M. rather than after the patient awakens. In comparison to conventional insulin therapy, CSII results in normalization of plasma glucose, lactate, pyruvate, ketone bodies, free fatty acids, and amino acids. It leads to normalization of plasma glucagon, growth hormone, and catecholamine levels. It results in decreases in total plasma cholesterol, total triglycerides, and LDL cholesterol and increases in HDL cholesterol.[51] In addition, CSII has been shown to normalize insulin receptors,[52] which should improve problems in insulin resistance, often observed in diabetics treated by conventional therapy.

In any treatment program, the type of insulin given is important, since the distribution of meals must be planned so there is enough glucose in the blood to prevent hypoglycemia when the insulin reaches its peak action. Patients receiving intermediate-acting insulin often require an afternoon snack in addition to the usual three meals. Long-acting insulins are used much less frequently, but those patients who do use them generally require a snack in the evening to prevent hypoglycemia during the night.

The amount of insulin prescribed by the physician is determined somewhat by trial and error, although there are some general guidelines. The amount prescribed is affected by the diet, the patient's own insulin production (if any), the patient's activity and body weight, the effects of other hormones, and the existence of complications.

Nutritional Care

At one time, a diet restricted in carbohydrate with increased fat was recommended for diabetic patients. In view of the increased incidence of atherosclerotic disease in diabetics, a diet reduced in fat to 30% of total calories

with 50–55% of total calories as carbohydrate is now recommended.[53,54] The American Diabetes Association has made the following recommendations, which are currently followed for most patients:[53]

1. Achieve and maintain ideal weight.
2. Limit protein intake for adults to 0.8 g/kg body weight.
3. Fifty-five percent of total calories should be in the form of carbohydrate.
4. Restrict fat intake to 30% or less of total calories, with saturated fat and polyunsaturated fat comprising 10% or less each and monounsaturated fat the remaining 10% or more.
5. Cholesterol intake should be restricted to 300 mg/day or less.
6. Carbohydrates should be unrefined with fiber to equal up to 40 g soluble fiber per day.
7. Carbohydrates may include "modest" amounts of sucrose only if it can be shown that it does not adversely affect metabolic control or body weight.
8. The use of nutritive and nonnutritive sweeteners is acceptable under the same circumstances as in item 7.
9. Restrict sodium intake to 1,000 mg/1,000 kcal.

The best diet for the treatment of diabetes mellitus has always been a matter of controversy.[55] Broadly speaking, the difference of opinion centers on the amount of control of hyperglycemia that is necessary and how it is to be achieved.

All diabetologists agree that control of significant hyperglycemia is desirable. They also agree that hyperglycemia is preferable to hypoglycemia. On the other hand, experts disagree on the amount of risk of hypoglycemia that is acceptable when aggressively treating high blood glucose levels.

A large body of evidence indicates that even moderate hyperglycemia has a detrimental effect on the incidence of complications and on resistance to infection, but the level of hyperglycemia that has long-term harmful effects has not been firmly established.[56] Thus the recommendations for dietary control, especially for the patient with IDDM, vary from the strict diet, which attempts to control blood glucose levels within very narrow limits, to a more liberal and flexible diet, which allows a higher blood glucose concentration with greater fluctuation. It often is claimed that the strict diet is ineffective, but this may be true because many patients do not adhere to the prescribed strict diet, not because the diet is inherently ineffective. In summary, the emphasis in IDDM is to provide intake to keep plasma glucose and lipid concentrations within normal limits and to maintain consistency of intake to prevent large swings in blood glucose concentration.

There is no controversy on the effectiveness of calorie restriction for the overweight non-insulin-dependent diabetic. Weight reduction controls the disease and may reverse it altogether, with significant clinical benefits.[7]

The basic objective in diet planning in IDDM is consistency of intake from day to day. In NIDDM, the objective is usually weight reduction. In either type of diabetes, there are several additional considerations: (1) all patients must be provided optimal nutrition throughout life; and (2) meal plans should be individualized according to the patient's life style and based on a diet history.

Determining the Diet Prescription. The responsibility for determining the diet prescription is basically the physician's but sometimes is delegated to the nutritional care specialist.

The most commonly used system of planning the diabetic diet is the "exchange system" established by the American Dietetic Association and the American Diabetes Association. Therefore, this method will be described in detail. In general, the procedure involves first estimating the total calorie need, then partitioning the calories among the various nutrients, and finally distributing the calories among the daily meals. This procedure can be used for calculation of a meal plan to initiate treatment. Subsequent adjustments to fit the diet into the patient's life style will promote compliance.

Estimating total calories needed. There are several methods for estimating total calories needed. For lean diabetics, the calculation is based on ideal body weight and the usual intake as determined with the diet history.[39] Alternatively, about 30 kcal/kg of desirable body weight (DBW) are used for a basic figure for maintenance for physically active adult men and 28 kcal/kg DBW for sedentary men, most women, and those over age 55. This value is reduced to about 20 kcal/kg DBW for sedentary women and sedentary adults over age 55.[39] The true criterion of adequate calories is achievement and maintenance of ideal body weight; therefore, the caloric level may be readjusted at intervals as needed.

For children, a common estimate is based on 120 kcal/kg body weight for the first year and 100–80 kcal/kg for ages 1–10 years, with a decline in needs as age increases. The needs for males and females vary during adolescence. The calorie allowance for a large, active, growing adolescent boy may be as high as 50–80 (average 65) kcal/kg between ages 11 and 15. At ages 16–20, after the adolescent growth spurt, 50 kcal/kg for great physical activity, 40 kcal for average activity, and 30 kcal/kg if sedentary will be needed. For the adolescent girl, corresponding values are 35 kcal/kg at ages 11–15 and 30 kcal/kg at ages 16 and up. In children, the emphasis is on **consistency** of intake rather than on restriction of intake. Adequate growth and maintenance of normal weight for height are the criteria for calorie adequacy. Adequacy of growth should be followed on a weight gain chart.

For the obese diabetic, the diet should be reduced in calories to achieve weight loss. Frequently, approximately 20 kcal/kg of ideal body weight are prescribed. If this amount results in a diet with which the patient is unlikely to be able to comply, a higher level may be used. A slow weight loss (1 lb./week) may be achieved with an energy intake 500 kcal/week less than expenditure. Increased exercise is helpful, of course. If and when body weight approaches ideal, the energy content in the diet can be increased to maintenance level. Usually, these diets are at least 1,000 kcal in order that other nutrients can be provided in sufficient amounts.

Partitioning the calories. After total energy need has been determined, the relative amounts of protein, fat, and carbohydrates must be decided. Control can be achieved with various amounts of carbohydrate. For many years, the common practice consisted of providing 40% of the energy from carbohydrate, 40% from fat, and 20% from protein. An 1,800-kcal diet would thus contain 180 g of carbohydrate, 80 g of fat, and 90 g of protein. Carbohydrate was limited to reduce the insulin dosage. When it became evident that diabetics are prone to early severe cardiovascular disease, a diet with less fat and more carbohydrate was recommended.[53,57] It was found that insulin need is more closely related to energy intake than to carbohydrate intake and that diets high in carbohydrate are tolerated well.[58] The increase in insulin dosage as a result of increased carbohydrate in the diet is not as great as had been expected.[55]

The partition of kilocalories should be based, insofar as possible, on the patient's food habits as obtained from the diet history. Compliance with the diet is thus encouraged.

Knowledge of the patient's serum cholesterol and triglyceride levels and the degree of glycemic control HbA_{1c} also should be considered in deciding on distribution of calories.

Distributing the nutrients among meals and snacks. Once the calories are partitioned among the nutrients, the nutrients must be distributed among the daily meals. The resulting pattern should be as close as possible to the patient's habitual meal pattern. For an initial diet, the amount of insulin and the rate and duration of its action may affect the manner in which the nutrients are distributed. For those patients who are controlled by diet alone, by oral hypoglycemic agents, or with fast-acting insulin given before each meal, the carbohydrate often is divided into three equal parts, one-third for each meal. This pattern distributes the carbohydrate evenly and avoids sharp variations in blood glucose. If, however, the patient's FPG tends to be high, less carbohydrate is given at breakfast. The division may be one-fifth for breakfast and two-fifths for each of the other two meals.

When an intermediate- or long-acting insulin is given, its peak activity may be at other than a usual meal time. For good control, it is important that carbohydrate be available when insulin activity is high, and so a snack is given at that time. The patient taking NPH insulin, a morning dose of which reaches peak activity in late afternoon, may have an afternoon snack at 3:30 or 4:00 P.M. Carbohydrate in the diet of a patient receiving protamine zinc insulin, for example, may be divided as follows: one-sixth for breakfast, two-sixths at noon and evening meals, and one-sixth at approximately 8:00 P.M., since peak insulin activity of a morning dose is during the night. This latter snack is called the **HS** (hour of sleep, or **hora somni**) feeding in many hospitals.

The true test is the degree of control that is achieved. Other divisions are possible, if necessary, to achieve this control. Very brittle diabetics, for example, sometimes are given five or even six meals and snacks per day with multiple insulin injections.

The distribution may also be varied to abide by the wishes of the patient, with insulin dosage adjusted as necessary. A patient who prefers a small breakfast and larger dinner, for example, might be given less regular insulin and more intermediate-acting insulin.

Sometimes protein is divided in a similar manner to carbohydrate. The more liberal and current approach is simply to ensure that some protein in the form of milk, meat, or a meat substitute is included in each meal or snack and otherwise to conform to the patient's wishes. Fat exchanges usually are distributed according to the preferences of the patient.

The Diabetic Meal Plan. The written prescription for a diabetic diet, which might read, "Diabetic diet, C-215, P-90, F-55, divide $\frac{1}{6}, \frac{2}{6}, \frac{1}{6}, \frac{2}{6}$," is not understandable to the patient. An important function of the nutritional care specialist is to translate this prescription into terms meaningful to the patient. Since diabetes is a chronic disease, it also is important that the diet plan be one that is acceptable for use over a long period. The **exchange system** of diet planning, which is useful for any category of diabetes, has been used very frequently.[59]

The nutrient contents of the "diabetic exchanges" are provided in Table 11-10, and their use is described in detail. It is essential that the nutritional care specialist know the values in these exchange lists (Tables 11-11 through 11-16) and use them with ease. Table 11-17 lists foods that may be used in

moderate quantities without calculation into the diet. Table 11-18 lists additional foods that may be substituted for the combinations of exchanges indicated. Both lists are useful to provide variety in the diet.

The exchange lists provide an example of a method of diet planning that is useful in the nutritional care not only of diabetics, but also of patients with hypoglycemia and for weight reduction. With different exchange lists, this method may also be used to plan diets with controlled sodium, potassium, and other nutrients.

Exchange lists for the diabetic diet consist of groups of foods that have similar, although not necessarily identical, content of protein, fat, and carbohydrate and that have a similar function in meal planning. It allows the substitution of foods of approximately equal composition and provides for a variety of foods along with consistency of nutrient intake.

The specific foods included in the exchange lists emphasize starch rather than simpler carbohydrates. Starch seems to

Table 11-10. Composition of One Serving in Each Diabetic Exchange

Exchange	Approximate Measures	Weight (g)	Composition			Kilo-calories
			Protein (g)	Fat (g)	Carbohydrate (g)	
Milk, nonfat	1 c.	240	8	Trace	12	90
1%	1 c.	240	8	2	12	100
2%	1 c.	240	8	5	12	120
Whole	1 c.	240	8	8	12	150
Vegetable	$\frac{1}{2}$ c.	100	2	—	5	25
Fruit	Varies	Varies	—	—	15	60
Bread/starch	1 slice (other items vary)	25	3	Trace	15	80
Meat or substitute						
Lean	1 oz.	30	7	3	—	55
Medium fat	1 oz.	30	7	5	—	75
High fat	1 oz.	30	7	8	—	100
Fat	1 tsp. (other items vary)	5		5	—	45

Tables 11-10 through 11-18 are adapted from *Exchange Lists for Meal Planning* (1986) prepared by Committees of the American Dietetic Association and the American Diabetes Association, Inc., in cooperation with the Public Health Service; U.S. Department of Health, Education, and Welfare, *Diet Manual Utilizing a Vegetarian Diet Plan*, rev. ed. Loma Linda, Calif.: Seventh-Day Adventist Dietetic Association, 1975; *Modern Nutrition in Health and Disease*, 6th ed., Ed. M.E. Shils and V. Young. Philadelphia: Lea & Febiger, 1988; *Manual of Clinical Dietetics*. University of California, Los Angeles, 1977: *Mayo Clinic Diet Manual* (6th ed.). ed. C.M. Pemberton. Toronto: Decker, 1988; Franz, M.J. *Exchanges for all occasions.* Wayzata, Minn.: Diabetes Center, 1987; *Ethnic and Regional Practices: A Series.* Chicago: American Dietetic Association, 1989; and Keall, L.P. and Beaser, R.S., *Joslin Diabetes Manual*, 12th ed., Philadelphia: Lea & Febiger, 1989.

Table 11-11. Milk Exchanges[a,b,c]

Type	Amount
Nonfat or very low-fat fortified milk	
Alba 66 or Alba 77	1 envelop
Skim (½%) or nonfat milk	1 c.
Powdered (nonfat dry, before adding liquid)	⅓ c.
Evaporated skim milk, canned	½ c.
Buttermilk (made from skim milk)	1 c.
Yogurt (made from skim milk: plain, un-flavored)	1 c.
1% fat fortified milk	1 c.
Low-fat fortified milk	
Low-fat buttermilk	1 c.
2% fat fortified milk	1 c.
Yogurt (made from 2% fortified milk: plain, unflavored)	8 oz.
Acidophilus 2% milk	1 c.
Canned evaporated 2% milk	1 c.
Whole milk	
Whole milk	1 c.
Evaporated whole milk, canned	½ c.
Buttermilk (made from whole milk)	1 c.
Yogurt, plain, unflavored, made from whole milk	1 c.
Soy milk, unsweetened (add ½ bread exchange)	1 c.

[a] Composition: One exchange of each of the three types of milk includes:

	Carbohydrate (g)	Protein (g)	Fat (g)	Calories
Nonfat	12	8	trace	90
Low-fat (1%)	12	8	2	100
Low-fat (2%)	12	8	5	120
Whole	12	8	8	150

[b] Italic type indicates nonfat.
[c] Contains no dietary fiber.

cause a smaller peak in blood glucose than does an equicaloric amount of dietary glucose and has greater satiety value. The lists also emphasize the use of polyunsaturated rather than saturated fats. The foods in the exchange lists that are particularly useful for planning diabetic diets limited in total fat or in saturated fat, particularly as a precaution against cardiovascular disease, are indicated in italics.

For each diabetic diet, a meal plan is calculated in terms of exchange lists. A sample calculation is shown in Table 11-19. The steps in this calculation are as follows, using the values from Table 11-10:

Table 11-12. Vegetable Exchanges[a,b,c]

Artichoke (½ medium)	*Kohlrabi (⅔ c.)*
Asparagus (5–7 spears)	*Leeks (2 medium)*
Bamboo shoots (¾ c.)	*Mushrooms, cooked*
Bean sprouts	*Okra*
Beets	*Onions*
Broccoli	*Pea pods, snow peas*
Brussels sprouts	*Rutabaga (½ c.)*
Cabbage	*Sauerkraut*
Carrots or juice	*Sprouts, raw (1 c.)*
Cauliflower	*(alfalfa, mung, soy)*
Chayote	*String beans, green, yellow*
Eggplant	*Summer squash*
Green pepper (1 large)	*Tomato, (1 medium)*
Greens:	6 *cherry*
Beet	2 *Tbsp. paste*
Chard	¼ *c. puree*
Collards	⅓ *c. sauce*
Dandelion	½ *c. stewed*
Kale	*Turnips*
Mustard	*Vegetable/tomato juice*
Spinach	*Water chestnuts (5)*
Turnip	*Zucchini, cooked*
Jicama, raw	

Note: Starchy vegetables are found in the bread/starch exchanges. Raw vegetables are found in the free food list (Table 11-17).
[a] One exchange is ½ c. of cooked vegetables or vegetable juice unless otherwise noted. Composition: One exchange = 2 g protein, 5 g carbohydrate, 25 kcal, and 2–3 g of dietary fiber.
[b] Italic type indicates nonfat.
[c] Each serving contains 2–3 g dietary fiber.

1. Estimate the number of milk, fruit, and vegetable exchanges that will fit into the meal plan. To some extent, this is a trial-and-error process, but the following are useful guides, *subject to patient preferences:*
   Nonfat milk: A minimum of two exchanges for adults to a maximum of one exchange for each feeding. Quantities and fat content of milk for children and adolescents are adjusted for age. If the diet history indicates that the patient chooses milk exchanges that contain some fat, 1 g fat can be substituted for the "trace" amounts given.[39]
   Fruits: A minimum of three exchanges, one for each regular meal.
   Vegetables: Two exchanges, one for inclusion at noon and one at the evening meal.
2. Total the carbohydrate provided in the milk, fruit, and vegetable exchange (94)

Table 11-13. Fruit Exchanges[a,b,c]

Fruit	Amount
Apple, 2 in. diam.	1
Applesauce (unsweetened)	$\frac{1}{2}$ c.
Apricots, fresh	4 medium
Apricots, canned, unsweetened	4 halves
Apricots, dried	7 halves
Banana, 9 in.	$\frac{1}{2}$
Berries (raw)	
Blackberries	$\frac{3}{4}$ c.
Blueberries	$\frac{3}{4}$ c.
Gooseberries	1 c.
Loganberries	$\frac{3}{4}$ c.
Raspberries	1 c.
Strawberries	$1\frac{1}{4}$ c.
Cherries, raw	12 large
Cherries, canned, unsweetened	$\frac{1}{2}$ c.
Dates	3 med.
Figs, fresh, 2 in.	2
Figs, dried	$1\frac{1}{2}$
Fruit cocktail, canned, unsweetened	$\frac{1}{2}$ c.
Grapefruit	$\frac{1}{2}$ or $\frac{3}{4}$ c. sections
Grapes	15 small
Kiwi, large	1
Kumquat	5 med.
Mango	$\frac{1}{2}$ small, $\frac{1}{2}$ c. sliced
Melon	
Cantaloupe, 5 in.	$\frac{1}{3}$ melon. 1 c. cubes
Honeydew, Casaba	$\frac{1}{8}$ medium. 1 c. cubes
Watermelon	$1\frac{1}{4}$ c.
Nectarine, $2\frac{1}{2}$ in. diam.	1
Orange, $2\frac{1}{2}$ in. diam.	1
Papaya	1 c., cubed
Peach, $2\frac{3}{4}$ in. diam.	1
Peaches, canned, unsweetened	2 halves
Pear, fresh	1 small or $\frac{1}{2}$ large
Pear, canned, unsweetened	2 halves
Persimmon, native	2 medium
Pineapple, canned, unsweetened	$\frac{1}{3}$ c.
Pineapple, raw	$\frac{3}{4}$ c.

Table 11-13. (Continued)

Fruit	Amount
Plums	2 medium
Pomegranate, $3\frac{1}{2}$ in. diam.	$\frac{1}{2}$ medium
Prunes, uncooked	3 medium
Raisins, uncooked	2 Tbsp.
Tangelo	1 medium
Tangerine, $2\frac{1}{2}$ in. diam.	2

Fruit Juices and Drinks	Amount
Apple juice, unsweetened	$\frac{1}{2}$ c.
Apricot nectar	$\frac{1}{3}$ c.
Cider	$\frac{1}{2}$ c.
Cranberry juice, low calorie	$1\frac{1}{4}$ c.
Cranberry juice, regular	$\frac{1}{3}$ c.
Del Monte fruit drinks	$\frac{1}{2}$ c.
Gatorade	1 c.
Grapefruit or Grape instant breakfast drinks (powder)	3 tsp.
Grapefruit juice, unsweetened	$\frac{1}{2}$ c.
Grape juice, unsweetened	$\frac{1}{3}$ c.
Hawaiian Punch, low calorie	1 c.
Hi-C fruit drinks	$\frac{1}{2}$ c.
Orange juice, unsweetened	$\frac{1}{2}$ c.
Peach nectar	$\frac{1}{3}$ c.
Pear nectar	$\frac{1}{3}$ c.
Pineapple juice, unsweetened	$\frac{1}{2}$ c.
Prune juice, unsweetened	$\frac{1}{3}$ c.
Tang (powder)	3 Tbsp.
Tangerine, unsweetened	1

[a] Composition: One exchange = 15 g carbohydrate, 60 kcal, and 2 g of dietary fiber for fresh, frozen, or dried fruits.
[b] Italic type indicates low fat.
[c] Juice-packed fruit should be drained.

and subtract this total from the amount prescribed (215); that is, $215 - 94 = 121$.

3. Divide the result by the amount of carbohydrate in one bread exchange to find the number of bread exchanges needed: $121 \div 15 = 8$. Again, if the diet history suggests that the patient usually chooses items with > 1 g fat, a fat content of 1 g or more may be included in the original calculation.[39]

4. Total the protein in the milk, vegetable, and bread exchanges (44) and subtract this total from the amount prescribed (90); that is, $90 - 44 = 46$.

5. Divide the result by the amount of protein in one meat exchange (7) to find the number of meat exchanges needed, rounding off fractions: $46 \div 7 = 7$.

6. Subtract the fat in the meat (35) from the amount prescribed (55): $55 - 35 = 20$. If the patient uses meats from all three categories — lean, medium, and high fat — it is usually most convenient to calculate the meal plan using the *medium* fat meat and make adjustments to use other meats when planning daily menus. If, however, the diet history indicates more limited choices, for example, largely from

Table 11-14. Bread Exchanges[a,b] (plus Cereals and Starchy Vegetables)

Food	Amount
Bread	
White (including French, Italian)	1 slice
Whole wheat	1 slice
Rye or pumpernickel	1 slice
Cocktail rye	3 slices
Raisin	1 slice
Bagel, small, 1 oz.	½
Bread sticks, 4 in. × ½ in.	2
English muffin, small	½
Plain roll, bread	1
Holland Rusk	2
Frankfurter roll	½
Hamburger bun	½
Syrian or Pita bread, 6 in.	½
Dried bread crumbs	3 Tbsp.
Tortilla, 6-in., not fried	1
Boston Brown Bread, 3 in. × ½ in.	1 slice
Cereal	
Bran cereals, concentrated	⅓ c.
Flaked bran cereals	½ c.
Unsweetened flaked cereals	½ c.
Puffed cereal (unfrosted)	1½ c.
Shredded wheat	½ c. or 1 biscuit
Cereal (cooked)	½ c.
Grape Nuts	3 Tbsp.
Bulgur wheat, cooked	½ c.
Dried legumes	
Baked beans, no pork (canned)	¼ c.
Beans, peas, lentils, dried	⅓ c.
Starchy vegetables	
Corn	⅓ c.
Corn on cob, 6 in.	1 small
Lima beans	½ c.
Parsnips	⅔ c.
Peas, green (canned or frozen)	½ c.
Plaintain, cooked	½ c.
Potato, white, baked, 3 oz.	1
Potato (mashed)	½ c.
Pumpkin	¾ c.
Winter squash, acorn or butternut	¾ c.
Yam or sweet potato	⅓ c.
Prepared foods	
Biscuit, 2-in. diameter (omit 1 fat exchange)	1
Corn bread, 2 in. × 2 in. × 1 in. (omit 1 fat exchange)	1
Corn muffin, 2-in. diameter (omit 1 fat exchange)	1
Crackers, round, butter type (omit 1 fat exchange)	6
Muffin, plain small (omit 1 fat exchange)	1
Pancake, 5 in. × ½ in. (omit 1 fat exchange)	1

Table 11-14. (Continued)

Food	Amount
Popover, 2–3 inches (omit 1 fat exchange)	1
Potatoes, french fried, length 2–3½ in. (omit 1 fat exchange)	10
Potato, corn or other chips (omit 2 fat exchanges)	1 oz.
Taco shell (omit 1 fat exchange)	2
Tortilla, fried, 7½ in. (omit 1 fat exchange)	1
Waffle, 5 in. × ½ in. (omit 1 fat exchange)	1
Flour, wheat	2½ Tbsp.
Buckwheat flour, dark	3 Tbsp.
Rye flour	3 Tbsp.
Tapioca, dry	2 Tbsp.
Soy flour (omit ½ bread exchange)	¼ c.
Barley, millet	½ c.
Grits, hominy (cooked)	½ c.
Miso	3 Tbsp.
Pasta, cooked (spaghetti, noodles, macaroni, etc.)	½ c.
Popcorn (popped, no fat added, large kernel)	3 c.
Rice, white or brown (cooked)	⅓ c.
Rice, wild	½ c.
Wheat germ	3 Tbsp.
Crackers	
Arrowroot	3
Graham, 2½ in. square	3
Matzo, 4 in. × 6 in.	¾ oz.
Oyster	24
Pretzels, 3⅛ in. long × ½ in. diameter	¾ oz.
Rye wafers, 2 in. × 3½ in.	4
Saltines	6
Other (for occasional use only)	
Cookies, 1¾ in. diam. (omit 1 fat exchange)	2
Frozen fruit yogurt	⅓ c.
Ginger Snaps	3
Granola (omit 1 fat exchange)	¼ c.
Granola bar, small (omit 1 fat exchange)	1
Ice cream, any flavor (omit 2 fat exchanges)	½ c.
Sherbet, any flavor	¼ c.
Vanilla wafers, small (omit 1 fat exchange)	6

[a] Composition: One exchange = 3 g protein, 15 g carbohydrate, a trace of fat, and 80 kcal. Whole grain products average about 2 g of dietary fiber per serving.
[b] Italic type indicates low fat.

Table 11-15. Meat Exchanges (Lean, Medium-Fat, and High-Fat)[a,b]

Type	Description	Amount
Lean Meat (one exchange = 7 g protein, 3 g fat)		
Beef	*Baby beef (very lean), chipped beef, chuck, flank steak, London broil, sandwich steaks, tenderloin, plate ribs, plate skirt steak, bottom round, all cuts rump, spare ribs, tripe*	1 oz.
Pork	*Leg (whole rump, center shank), ham, smoked (center slices), Canadian bacon*	1 oz.
Veal	*Leg, loin, rib, shank, shoulder*	1 oz.
Game	*Opossum, rabbit, squirrel, venison*	1 oz.
Poultry	*Meat (without skin) of chicken, turkey, cornish hen, guinea hen, pheasant*	1 oz.
Fish	*Any fresh or frozen*	1 oz.
	Drained canned salmon, tuna, mackerel, crab, and lobster	$\frac{1}{4}$ c.
	Clams, oysters, scallops, shrimp	5 or 1 oz.
	Sardines (drained)	2 med.
Legumes	*Black-eyed peas, broad beans, garbanzo, kidney, lima, mung, navy, or pinto (omit 2 bread exchanges)*	1 c., ckd.
Cheeses containing less than 5% butterfat		1 oz.
Cottage cheese, dry or 2% butterfat		1 c.
Egg whites		3
95% fat-free cold cuts		1 oz.
Egg substitute with less than 55 kcal per $\frac{1}{4}$ c.		$\frac{1}{4}$ c.
Medium-Fat Meat (one exchange = 7 g protein, 5 g fat)		
Beef	Ground (15% fat), roasts and steaks, corned beef (canned), rib eye, round	1 oz.
Pork	Loin (all cuts tenderloin), chops, roasts, shoulder arm (picnic), shoulder blade, Boston butt	1 oz.
Lamb	Most products	1 oz.
Veal	Cutlet	1 oz.
Poultry	Chicken with skin, duck, goose, and ground turkey	1 oz.
Fish	Tuna, drained, or salmon, drained	$\frac{1}{4}$ c.
	Lox; smoked sablefish	1 oz.
Cheese	Mozzarella, ricotta, farmer's cheese, Neuf-	1 oz.

Table 11-15. (Continued)

Type	Description	Amount
	chatel, Camembert, Edam, Liederkranz	
Legumes	Soybeans	$\frac{1}{3}$ c.
	Soybean curd	$\frac{1}{2}$ block
	Tofu	4 oz.
Liver, heart, kidney, and sweetbreads (high in cholesterol)		1 oz.
Cottage cheese, creamed		$\frac{1}{4}$ c.
Egg (high in cholesterol) (limit to 3 per week)		1
Soy beans		$\frac{1}{2}$ c.
Tofu		4 oz.
High-Fat Meat (one exchange = 7 g protein, 8 g fat)		
Limit choices to 3 times per week		
Beef	Brisket, corned beef (brisket), ground beef (more than 20% fat), hamburger (commercial), chuck (ground, commercial), roasts (rib), steaks (club, rib, Porterhouse, New York strip, T-bone), most prime beef	1 oz.
Lamb	Ground	1 oz.
Pork	Spare ribs, loin (back ribs), pork (ground), country style ham, deviled ham, hocks, feet, sausage, pastrami	1 oz.
Cheeses	Cheddar types, American, blue, Roquefort, brick, gorgonzola, gouda, Gruyère, Limberger, Muenster, Parmesan, Swiss	1 oz.
	Cheese spreads	2 Tbsp.
Peanut butter		1 Tbsp.
Legumes	Peanuts (omit $\frac{1}{2}$ bread, 2 fat exchanges)	1 Tbsp.
	Pumpkin seeds (omit $1\frac{1}{2}$ fat exchanges)	8 tsp.
	Sesame seeds and sunflower seeds (omit $2\frac{1}{2}$ fat exchanges)	4 Tbsp.
	Hummus (omit 1 bread exchange)	4 Tbsp.
	Pignolia nuts (omit $\frac{1}{2}$ vegetable and 1 fat exchange)	6 Tbsp.
Cold cuts, $4\frac{1}{2}$ in. × $\frac{1}{8}$-in. slices		1 slice
Frankfurter (omit additional fat exchange)		1 small

[a] Trim off all visible fat.
[b] Italic type indicates lean (low-fat) meats.

Table 11-16. Fat Exchanges[a]

Fat Source	Amount
Margarine, soft in tub or sticks[b,c]	1 tsp.
Margarine, reduced calorie[c]	1 Tbsp.
Avocado (4-inch diameter)	⅛ (med.)
Oil: corn, cottonseed, safflower, soy, sunflower[c]	1 tsp.
Oil, olive[d]	1 tsp.
Oil, peanut[d]	1 tsp.
Olives[d]	10 small or 5 large
Non-dairy cream substitute, liquid	2 Tbsp.
Almonds[d]	6 whole
Pecans[d]	5 halves
Peanuts[d]	20 small or 10 large
Walnuts	4 halves
Butter[e]	1 tsp.
Bacon fat[e]	1 tsp.
Bacon, crisp	1 strip
Brazil nuts	2 medium
Hazel nuts	5
Pistachios	20
Cashews	4 large
Macadamias	4 medium
Cream	
Light[e]	2 Tbsp.
Sour[e]	2 Tbsp.
Heavy[e]	1 Tbsp.
Cream cheese[e]	1 Tbsp.
French dressing	1 Tbsp.
Italian dressing	1 Tbsp.
Lard[d]	1 tsp.
Mayonnaise	1 tsp.
Salad dressing, reduced calorie	1 Tbsp.
Salad dressing, mayonnaise type	2 tsp.
Salt pork	¼ oz.
Tahini	1 tsp.
Gravy	2 Tbsp.
Wine, sweet kosher	¼ c.

[a] Composition: One exchange = 5 g fat and 45 kcal.
[b] Italic type indicates polyunsaturated fat.
[c] High content of polyunsaturated fat if made with corn, cottonseed, safflower, soy, or sunflower oil.
[d] Fat content is primarily monounsaturated.
[e] Fat content is predominantly saturated.

the lean-meat category, the diet may be calculated accordingly.

7. Divide the result by the amount of fat in one fat exchange (5) to find the number of additional fat exchanges needed: $20 \div 5 = 4$.

When the number of exchanges from each list necessary to meet the diet prescription is

Table 11-17. Free Foods[a]

Condiments	
Catsup (1 Tbsp.)	Flavoring extracts
Horseradish	(almond, butter,
Mustard	lemon, peppermint,
Pickles, dill, unsweet-ened	vanilla, etc.)
Salad dressing, low-calorie (2 Tbsp.)	Garlic, fresh
	Powder
Taco or barbecue sauce (1 Tbsp.)	Herbs
	Hot pepper sauce
Vinegar	Lemon
Soy sauce, regular	Lemon juice
Low sodium ("lite")	Lemon pepper
Wine, cooking (¼ c.)	Lime
Worcestershire sauce	Lime juice
Drinks	Mint
Bouillon or broth	Onion powder
without fat, low so-dium	Oregano
	Paprika
Carbonated drinks, sugar-free	Pepper
	Pimento
Club soda	Spices
Cocoa powder, unsweetened (1 Tbsp.)	*Sweet Substitutes*
	Candy, hard, sugar-free (2–3 pieces)
Drink mixes, sugar-free	Gelatin, sugar-free
Tea/coffee (regular, decaffeinated)	Gum, sugar-free (2–3 sticks)
Tonic water, sugar-free	Jam/jelly, sugar-free (2 tsp.)
Water (carbonated, mineral, regular)	Pancake syrup, sugar-free (1–2 Tbsp.)
Fruit	Sugar substitutes
Cranberries, unsweet-ened (½ c.)	(saccharine, aspar-tame, acesulfame-K)
Rhubarb, unsweetened (1 c.)	Whipped topping, low kcal (2 Tbsp.)
Salad Greens	*Vegetables (raw, 1 c.)*
Endive	Cabbage
Escarole	Celery
Lettuce	Chicory
Romaine	Chinese cabbage (bok choy)
Spinach	Cucumber
Seasonings	Green onion
Basil (fresh)	Hot peppers
Celery seeds	Mushrooms
Chili powder	Radishes
Chives	Sprouts, beans
Cinnamon	Zucchini
Curry	
Dill	

[a] Composition: Contain less than 20 calories per serving. Foods without a specified serving size may be eaten as desired. Foods with a specific serving size should be limited to 2 to 3 servings per day.

determined, the exchanges are distributed among the meals. An example of that process is shown in Table 11-20. In the example, the total carbohydrate (214) is divided ac-

Table 11-18. Combination Foods[a]

Food	Amount	Exchanges
Casserole, homemade	1 cup (8 oz.)	2 starch, 2 medium-fat meat, 1 fat
Cheese pizza, thin crust	¼ of 15 oz. or ¼ of 10-in.	2 starch, 2 medium-fat meat, 1 fat
Chili with beans (canned)	1 cup (8 oz.)	2 starch, 2 medium-fat meat, 2 fat
Chow mein (without noodles or rice)	2 cups (16 oz.)	1 starch, 2 vegetable, 2 lean meat
Macaroni and cheese	1 cup (8 oz.)	2 starch, 1 medium-fat meat, 2 fat
Soups, canned		
Bean	1 cup (8 oz.)	1 starch, 1 vegetable, 1 lean meat
Chunky, all varieties	10 ¾ oz. can	1 starch, 1 vegetable, 1 medium-fat meat
Cream (made with water)	1 cup (8 oz.)	1 starch, 1 fat
Vegetable	1 cup (8 oz.)	1 starch
Spaghetti and meatballs (canned)	1 cup (8 oz.)	2 starch, 1 medium-fat meat, 1 fat
Sugar-free pudding (made with skim milk)	½ c.	1 starch
Beans if used as a meat substitute		
Dried beans, peas, lentils	1 cup (cooked)	2 starch, 1 lean meat

[a] This list gives average exchange values for some typical mixed or combination foods.

cording to the prescription: 214 ÷ 6 = 36. The patient would need a number and variety of exchanges to provide 36 g carbohydrate at breakfast and snack. The remaining exchanges are distributed between lunch and dinner and provide the required 36 × 2 = 72 g carbohydrate, or $\frac{2}{6}$ of the total. Again, it must be emphasized that the meal plan can be altered, along with changes in insulin dosage if necessary, to fit into the patient's life, improve compliance, and thus improve glycemic control.

In order to simplify the use of the exchange system for the patient, the exchanges are not usually subdivided, with few exceptions. Amounts other than whole or half exchanges are difficult for many patients to understand and are not usually recommended. However, milk exchanges (8 oz.) can easily be used as ½ exchanges (4 oz.). An example is given in Table 11-21. Bread exchanges are sometimes assigned to meals as ½ exchanges.

During dietetic counseling, the patient is

Table 11-19. Sample Calculation of a Diabetic Meal Plan Using Exchange Lists

Diet Prescription: P-90; F-55; C-215
Divide $\frac{1}{6}$, $\frac{2}{6}$, $\frac{1}{6}$, $\frac{2}{6}$ with 4 P.M. feeding

Exchange Group	Number of Exchanges	Carbohydrate (g)	Protein (g)	Fat (g)
Milk, nonfat	2	24	16	
Vegetable	2	10	4	
Fruit	4	60		
Subtotal		(94)		
Bread				
(215 − 94) ÷ 15	8	120	24	
Subtotal			(44)	
Meat, medium fat				
(90 − 44) ÷ 7	7		49	35
Fat				
(55 − 35) ÷ 5	4			20
Total		214	93	55

Table 11-20. Diabetic Meal Plan Incorporating Exchanges

Meal Distribution: 215 ÷ 6 = 36. Therefore: 36, 72, 36, 72.

Exchange	*Breakfast* Number of Servings	*Breakfast* Carbohydrates (g)	*Lunch* Number of Servings	*Lunch* Carbohydrates (g)	*Snack* Number of Servings	*Snack* Carbohydrates (g)	*Dinner* Number of Servings	*Dinner* Carbohydrates (g)
Milk, nonfat	½	6	½	6	½	6	½	6
Fruit	1	15	1	15	1	15	1	15
Vegetable			1	5			1	5
Bread	1	15	3	45	1	15	3	45
Meat, medium fat	1		3				3	
Fat	1		1				2	
Total		36		71		36		71

Table 11-21. Sample Diabetic Menus

Food	Exchange Value	Food	Exchange Value
Breakfast		*Breakfast*	
⅓ small cantaloupe	1 fruit	½ c. orange juice	1 fruit
1 egg, poached	1 medium fat meat	1 soft-cooked egg	1 medium fat meat
1 slice wheat toast	1 bread	1 slice white toast	1 bread
1 tsp. margarine	1 fat	1 tsp. margarine	1 fat
½ c. milk, nonfat	½ milk, nonfat	½ c. milk, nonfat	½ milk, nonfat
Coffee or tea, black	Free	Coffee or tea, black	Free
Lunch		*Lunch*	
Spaghetti with meat sauce		½ c. vegetable juice cocktail	1 vegetable
1 c. cooked spaghetti	2 bread	3 rye wafers	1 bread
3 oz. medium-fat ground beef	3 medium fat meat	Sandwich	
½ c. tomatoes	1 vegetable	1 hamburger bun	2 bread
Herbs and garlic	Free	3 oz. sliced chicken (no skin)	3 lean meat
1 slice Italian bread	1 bread	2½ tsp. mayonnaise	1 fat + 1½ fat from meat
1 tsp. margarine	1 fat	Lettuce	Free
Sour pickles	Free	Cranberry garnish, sweetened with saccharine	Free
½ c. diced pineapple	1 fruit	1 medium peach	1 fruit
4 oz. milk, nonfat	½ milk, nonfat	4 oz. milk, nonfat	½ milk, nonfat
Iced tea with lemon	Free	Coffee or tea, black	Free
Snack		*Snack*	
4 oz. plain skim milk yogurt	½ milk, nonfat	4 oz. milk, nonfat	½ milk, nonfat
3 graham crackers	1 bread	3 arrowroot crackers	1 bread
1 small orange	1 fruit	2 medium plums	1 fruit
Dinner		*Dinner*	
Broth	Free	3 oz. sliced leg of lamb	3 meat
3 oz. roast pork loin	3 medium-fat meat	2 small potatoes	2 bread
½ c. mashed potatoes	1 bread	½ c. green peas	1 bread
½ c. green beans	1 vegetable	Sliced tomato salad	1 vegetable
1 plain roll	1 bread	1 Tbsp. French dressing	1 fat
1 tsp. margarine	1 fat	1 tsp. margarine	1 fat
¼ c. strawberries on one 2-in. biscuit	1 fruit 1 bread + 1 fat	4 apricot halves	1 fruit
4 oz. milk, nonfat	½ milk, nonfat	4 oz. milk, nonfat	½ milk, nonfat
Coffee or tea, black	Free	Coffee or tea, black	Free

given this meal plan along with the exchange lists for planning variety into his or her meals and is instructed in their use. The use of a meal plan with the exchange lists eliminates the need for daily calculation of the diet. It also provides the consistency of intake required by the insulin-dependent diabetic and the limitation of calories for the non-insulin-dependent diabetic.

Planning Daily Menus. The use of the exchange system makes it possible to provide variety in meals. Foods essentially free of protein, fat, or carbohydrate may be added to the planned diet at will. The foods listed are not used in the original meal plan. Using the meal plan calculated in Table 11-20, two days' menus are given in Table 11-21 as examples.

Planning for increased fiber. The importance of diets high in carbohydrate and fiber and low in fat in the care and treatment of diabetics has been emphasized by a number of researchers during the past two decades. Feeding diets rich in natural fibers or adding fibers such as guar gum, pectin, or wheat bran to the diet has been reported to result in decreases in fasting blood glucose, urinary glucose excretion, daily insulin requirement, blood cholesterol, and triglycerides, and in improved glucose tolerance.[60-63] In general, individuals with NIDDM respond best to these high-carbohydrate, low-fat, high-fiber diets,[60,64-66] but some studies also indicate similar findings for individuals with IDDM.[67,68] In contrast Hollenbeck et al. found no effects of a high-fiber, high-carbohydrate diet on fasting blood glucose and insulin, 24-hour urinary glucose excretion, or the daily insulin requirement in adult patients with NIDDM.[68,69]

Based on the majority viewpoint, many physicians are advocating diets that are high in carbohydrate, mainly as starch, and high in fiber for their patients with NIDDM and IDDM in order to reduce the insulin requirement and to obtain the other beneficial effects cited here. An intake of 25 g of fiber per 1,000 kcal per day or up to 40 g/day has been suggested. Anderson's group has published reports on the composition and fiber content of many foods commonly used in diets for diabetics in order to help in the selection of foods to be included in the diet of a diabetic patient.[70,71] Although more long-term studies are needed, no serious nutritional side effects have been documented after long-term consumption of high-carbohydrate, high-fiber diets. Certain fibers, especially guar gum and pectin, are poorly tolerated by some patients, possibly precluding their use for those patients.

In choosing foods from the exchange lists for planning meals, it is frequently recommended that fiber intake be increased by choosing whole wheat bread and cereal products, beans, legumes, vegetables, and fruits with increased fiber. Further details on increasing dietary fiber are contained in Chapter 8.

An increase in fiber intake should be approached gradually to avoid abdominal cramping, diarrhea, and flatulence. A concomitant increase in fluid intake is required. SBGM is helpful in control since increased fiber may modulate the postprandial increase in blood glucose and decrease insulin need.

Weighed, measured, and unmeasured diets. At one time, it was thought necessary to weigh all foods for diabetic patients very carefully on a gram scale, but weighing is no longer believed to be necessary for patients using the exchange lists. Instead, a **measured diet** is recommended in which common household equipment, measuring spoons and measuring cups, are used. Since many cuts of meat do not lend themselves to this type of measure, meat portions sometimes still are weighed. Alternatively, the patient may be taught to estimate closely the portion size of meats, using food models.

Foods not recommended. Although some foods are poor choices for a diabetic diet, very few are absolutely forbidden to the diabetic patient. In general, **concentrated sources of simple carbohydrates**, such as candies, cakes with icings, and other sweetened baked goods, are discouraged, since it is assumed that they are rapidly absorbed and tend to cause rapid changes in blood glucose concentrations.[40] Some sugars also may raise serum triglycerides. Under special circumstances — the birthday of a diabetic child, for example — a small serving of birthday cake or other treat is allowed in the meal pattern if the patient or parent is knowledgeable of substitution procedures.

Some useful exchange values are listed at the end of Table 11-14 under the subheading of "other." They should be used only occasionally and only by patients who can maintain good control of their blood glucose.

Mixtures of indefinite composition also may be discouraged for diets using exchange lists because of difficulty in fitting these items into the meal plan. As a result, the use of many commercially prepared convenience foods may be limited. However, some manufacturers of canned soups and other convenience foods have made lists of the exchange values of their products. The nutritional care specialist should keep a library of such lists on hand for the patient who wishes to have a favorite food allowed occasionally in his or her diet. Patients can be taught to substitute these into their meal plan. Making such allowances generally improves compliance with the diet. Since food values change with changes in manufacturing processes, it is necessary to keep the information current. In addition, equivalent dishes can be made in the home where their composition can be controlled. A beef stew, for example, can be made from diced beef (meat and fat exchanges) and onions and carrots (vegetable exchange) or other vegetables. Thickening can be provided with flour (bread exchange), and herbs and spices are free. Other recipes are contained in recipe books for diabetics. The exchange equivalents usually are given with the recipes. Exchanges that may be used for general guidance are contained in Table 11-18.

Special foods for diabetic diets. Some special foods are available for use in diabetic diets. Most foods labeled as "diabetic" or "dietetic" are unnecessary for the diabetic patient, and many are very expensive. In addi-

tion, the patient often believes that they are "free" foods that can be added to the meal plan at will. In fact, they often contain appreciable, but unspecified, amounts of carbohydrate. Their use should be discouraged with the exception of **unsweetened canned fruits**. These have an important place in the diet of the diabetic patient, particularly in those parts of the country and during those seasons when fresh fruits are limited in variety.

The use of **diabetic candy** should normally be discouraged for several reasons. Diabetic candies usually are not calorie-free. Also, with their use, diabetics may develop a taste for sweets and then may substitute the candies for foods of greater nutritive value. It is the opinion of some diabetologists, however, that their limited use for children on very special occasions can be justified.

Alternative sweeteners. Sweeteners that may serve as an acceptable alternative to sucrose are important to some diabetic patients. Such sweeteners are categorized according to their kilocalorie content. One group is known as **nonnutritive sweeteners**. Substances in this group are kilocalorie-free or nearly so. The other group contains an appreciable kilocalorie content. They are classified as **nutritive sweeteners**.

Of the nonnutritive sweeteners, **saccharin** has been used for the longest period. It is 300 to 350 times as sweet as sucrose. About 20 mg equals the sweetness of 1 teaspoon of sugar. Saccharin leaves a bitter aftertaste in solution and therefore is unacceptable to some patients. The use of saccharin is controversial, since its use was reported to be related to an increased incidence of bladder cancer, but it has not been withdrawn from use because of public protests at attempts to do so. Further investigation has since failed to confirm the relationship of saccharin intake to bladder cancer.[72,73] Saccharin is now considered a low-potency carcinogen. It is not metabolized, but is excreted unchanged in the urine in 24–48 hours.

Some patients are very attached to sweetened coffee, tea, and soft drinks and may find saccharin an acceptable substitute for sugar, but it cannot be used as a sugar substitute in baking. Also, it may be added to some foods, such as rhubarb or cranberries, only after cooking, or it will develop a bitter taste. It is sold under various trade names such as Sucaryl, Sugar Twin, Sweet Magic, and Sweet'n Low. Maximum daily intake is recommended to be 1 g/day.[39]

Cyclamates are more acceptable in flavor and are 30 times sweeter than sucrose. They were banned by the U.S. Food and Drug Administration because they were reported to be carcinogenic in animals when given with saccharin[74] but are approved for use in Canada and some European countries. Further studies of the carcinogenicity of cyclamates have been recommended.[75]

Aspartame, 200 times as sweet as sucrose, is a methyl ester of a phenylalanine and aspartic acid combination. Aspartame is used as a sweetening ingredient in commercial food products under the brand name NutraSweet. Equal is a table-top sweetener containing aspartame. It contains a dextrose or lactose carrier and provides 4 kcal per packet.

Aspartame provides a small number of kilocalories because it is metabolized as a dipeptide, but the energy content is so low that it is classed as a nonnutritive sweetener. There is still some concern about the toxic effects of its metabolic breakdown products.[76] Maximum accepted daily intake (ADI) is 50 mg/kg.[39] This would be equivalent to 17 12-oz. cans of soda for a 70-kg man.

Acesulfame-K is a relatively new sweetener approved for use in the United States in 1988. It is sold in packets for table-top use under the brand name Sweet-One. It is also marketed as Sunette for use as a food ingredient.

Its sweetness is about 200 times as sweet as sucrose. It contains no kilocalories and is sodium free. ADI has been set by the Food and Drug Administration at 15 mg/kg body weight. This amount provides sweetness equivalent to twice the daily per capita sugar intake in the United States. The manufac-turer states that it has no lingering aftertaste, an excellent shelf life in liquids, high stabilizing in cooking and baking, and is stable when contained in products that are pasteurized or sterilized.

Some **carbohydrate** and **polyol sweeteners** with appreciable kilocalorie contents have been approved as substitutes for sucrose and glucose. These nutritive sweeteners must be calculated into the diet if they are to be used. Usually, it is advisable to discourage their use.

Fructose sometimes is suggested as a sweetener, since it is 70% sweeter than sugar and can thus be used in smaller quantities.[77] When fructose is absorbed, it is metabolized by the liver, and it provides 4 kcal/g. Insulin is not required for its entry into hepatic cells nor for the steps in its metabolism to trioses. The trioses can then enter the glycolytic pathway or be used to synthesize glucose and triglycerides, pathways which are regulated primarily by glucagon and insulin. In nondiabetic individuals and in well-controlled diabetics receiving sufficient insulin, most of the glucose formed from fructose is stored as glycogen and has little effect on blood glucose concentration. If, however, the patient is severely deficient in insulin, the glucose is released, and plasma glucose rises. In patients who are mildly insulin-deficient or who have insulin-independent diabetes, the rise in plasma glucose is less than that resulting from intake of an equivalent amount of sucrose, glucose, and sometimes starch.[78,79,80] These results are seen over the short term. If taken in amounts in excess of 75 g/day, it may also cause osmotic diarrhea.[81]

The long-term effects of fructose feeding are less well known. A recent study of fructose feeding for six months or more in combination with a high-carbohydrate, high-fiber diet demonstrated no effect on plasma glucose, glycosylated hemoglobin, serum cholesterol, and triglycerides. However, the patients ingested more kilocalories and gained weight. Adherence to the prescribed dietary fat and carbohydrate was improved. The authors suggested that fructose intake is "safe and acceptable" if total caloric intake is controlled to maintain desirable body weight.[82]

High-fructose corn sweetener (HFCS) is a related product composed of "corn sugar" (primarily glucose) and fructose.[83] It is more reasonable in cost as a sweetener in manufactured foods. However, HFCS contains 42%, 55%, or 90% fructose. The remainder in each case is predominantly glucose. Since it is perceived as being sweeter than sucrose, it may be used in smaller quantities. Recent work indicates that the action of high-fructose corn syrup on plasma glucose and insulin is the same as that of sucrose.[83] Therefore, it is not recommended as an alternative sweetener to sucrose.

Some **sugar alcohol** or **polyol sweeteners** have been approved for use in foods, but their kilocalorie content makes them of questionable value for diabetics.

Sorbitol and **mannitol** are sugar alcohols widely used as sweetening agents. Sorbitol is converted to fructose and thus provides 4 kcal/g but is only 60% as sweet as sucrose. Mannitol is also converted to fructose but is only partially metabolized, providing 2 kcal/g. It is 50% as sweet as sucrose. Both are poorly absorbed from the gastrointestinal tract and thus may cause an osmotic diarrhea if amounts in excess of 10 to 30 g/day of sorbitol or 10 to 20 g/day of mannitol are used. Sorbitol is not involved in complications of diabetes related to sorbitol accumulation.[84] Most diabetic children tolerate sorbitol well with no glycosuria or change in the blood glucose concentration,[85] but large doses can cause gastrointestinal distress. Overall, moderation is recommended in the use of both nutritive and nonnutritive sweeteners.[86]

Alcoholic beverages. If it becomes clear that the patient intends to drink alcoholic beverages occasionally, it is best to give some guidance in its management. The procedure recommended depends on the insulin dependency of the patient.

In an NIDDM patient, alcoholic beverages are usually substituted for fat exchanges since they are high in kilocalories.[39,87] For ease of incorporation, an alcohol equivalent has been established.[39] It is equal to two fat exchanges (90 kcal). One equivalent equals the amount of alcohol in

12 oz. beer
4 oz. dry wine, 12%
1½ oz. 80-proof distilled whisky, scotch, vodka, gin, rum, dry brandy

The kilocalorie content of any mixers used must also be calculated into the diet.

Oral hypoglycemic agents, particularly chlorpropramide or tolbutamide, taken by NIDDM patients may produce a disulfiram reaction (see Chapter 4). This does not occur with second-generation sulfonylureas.[39]

In the IDDM patient, alcohol-induced hypoglycemia may occur because alcohol is not converted to glucose and insulin is not required for its metabolism.[87] Therefore, no food should be omitted if alcohol is taken.

Vitamin and Mineral Supplements. Some patients inquire about their need for vitamin and mineral supplements. With few exceptions, they are not needed by the patient with uncomplicated diabetes who adheres to the prescribed diet. Occasionally, a financially very poor patient is given a diet with minimum protein levels to reduce cost; such a patient may profit from iron and calcium supplements. Very obese patients on severely calorie-restricted diets also may require supplements. If the patient has diarrhea secondary to neuropathy or pancreatitis, supplements may be necessary. Supplements of thiamine and vitamin B_{12} have been tried in the treatment of neuropathy and were found to be ineffective.

Alternatives to the Exchange System. The exchange system for meal planning is the most widely used system for diabetics. However, many patients have difficulty with learning or following this method or prefer less structured procedures. In order to improve patient understanding and patient compliance, a number of methods have been used either alone or in combination with the exchange system. These methods have been categorized as follows:[88,89]

1. Basic nutrition guidelines
   a. Dietary Guidelines for Americans (USDA-HHS)
   b. Basic Four Food Groups (USDA)
2. Basic diabetes guidelines
3. Exchange system planning
   a. Exchange Lists for Meal Planning (ADA-ADA)
   b. High carbohydrate–high fiber (HCF and HFM)
   c. Good health eating guide (GHEG)
4. Counting systems for meal planning
   a. Calorie counting
   b. Carbohydrate counting
   c. Total available glucose (TAG)
   d. Point system
5. Food choice plan (FCP)

Any of these methods may be used alone or in combination if the resulting procedure leads to adequate control. In some cases, the methods may be used in sequence, starting with the simplest method. Based on assessment of the patient, the nutritional care specialist chooses the method most effective in the circumstances.

The **basic nutrition guidelines** were developed to guide all individuals in the populations in choice of foods for promotion of health and avoidance of chronic disease. The **Basic Four Food Groups**, the milk, meat, fruit-vegetable, and grain groups, can be used as a basis for diet evaluation and counseling on needed changes in diet.

The more recent **Dietary Guidelines for Americans** provides the following advice:

- Eat a variety of foods.
- Maintain desirable weight.
- Avoid too much fat, saturated fat, and cholesterol.
- Eat foods with adequate starch and fiber.
- Avoid too much sugar.
- Avoid too much sodium.

- If you drink alcoholic beverages, do so in moderation.

Either of these sets of basic guidelines is useful as a first step in counseling patients in diet changes and may also be combined with more structured methods. They also may be used for patients who cannot deal with more complex diets. On the other hand, they may not be as effective as other methods in achieving glucose control.

The **basic diabetes guidelines** may provide a more individualized approach and more guidance to patients. At the same time, they remain useful for patients who need a simplified regimen or who have limited motivation for change. The counseling consists of giving the patients some general guidelines based on the diet history. The patient selects a daily menu that he or she finds most suitable, and alterations from this base are suggested, encouraging complex carbohydrate and fiber and limiting fat, cholesterol, and simple sugars. An example of this type of diet planning is the American Dietetic Association and American Diabetes Association's **Healthy Food Choices**.[88]

The **exchange system of planning** prepared by the American Dietetic Association, American Diabetes Association, and U.S. Public Health Service includes the exchange lists that are described at the beginning of this section. An alternative to this set of exchange lists is the **high carbohydrate–high fiber (HCF)** lists that contain the exchanges given in Table 11-22.[90] The HCF diet is designed primarily for hospital use and consists of about 70% carbohydrate, 20% protein, 10% fat, and 30 g fiber/day. For longer term use, a **high-fiber maintenance (HFM) diet** with 55% carbohydrate, 20% protein, 25% fat, and 25 g fiber is considered to be more practical.

These methods require an understanding of the exchange concept. In addition, they may be too structured for patients with irregular activities. The HCF diet requires a more vegetarian diet, sometimes promotes gastric distress from increased fiber intake, and re-

Table 11-22. Composition of Exchanges for the High-Carbohydrate, High-Fiber Diabetic Diet

Exchange	Approximate Measures	Weight (g)	Protein (g)	Fat (g)	Carbohydrate (g)	Kilo-calories	Fiber (g)
Milk, nonfat	1 cup	240	8	0.5	12	85	0
Vegetables	½ cup	100	1	0	5	25	2
Beans	½ cup, cooked		7	0	17	95	5
Fruit	1 small or 1 small serving	Varies	0	0	15	70	2.5
Cereals	1 oz.	30	3	0	20	90	4
Starches							
Bread	1 slice						
Pasta, grains, starchy vegetables	½ cup						
Rice	⅓ cup						
Crackers	2–4	100	2	0	15	70	2
Protein foods							
Red meats, poultry, cheese	1 oz.	30					
Fish	2 oz.	60					
Tofu	2½ oz.	75	8	2	0	50	0
Fats							
Oil, margarine	1 tsp.	5					
Salad dressings	2 tsp.	10	0	5	0	0	0

quires a great deal of structure in the diet planning. The most recent issue of the exchange lists given in Tables 11-11 to 11-17[59] has increased the emphasis on fiber intake and on limitations of salt and fat so that these lists differ less than was once the case.

Another exchange system is the **good health eating guide (GHEG)**, used widely in Canada. The Canadian Diabetes Association uses six food groups: protein foods, starchy foods, milk, fruits and vegetables, fats and oils, and free foods. The combined fruit and vegetable group contains 10 g carbohydrate and 1 g protein per serving. Other values are the same as in the U.S. system.

The **counting approaches** to meal planning are relatively structured systems. In the **calorie counting** system, the patient is provided with lists of kilocalorie contents of foods. A record form is provided on which the patient may record food and kilocalorie intake. This method is considered to be appropriate for obese NIDDM patients. The patient and counselor agree on a kilocalories-per-day objective that would provide slow weight loss, and the patient chooses foods to reach that objective. This method may also be used by patients using an insulin pump (CSII). The insulin to be used might be calculated with the equation

$$\text{insulin (U)} = \frac{\text{blood glucose} - 100}{25} + \frac{\text{kcal}}{100}$$
$$(11\text{-}2)$$

where blood glucose is given in mg/dl.[91] The patient needs to keep records of insulin dosages, blood glucose monitoring values, and exercise logs. The method is therefore cumbersome and also requires a highly literate patient.

Carbohydrate counting is a similar procedure requiring calculation of carbohydrate intake, rather than intake of total kilocalories. It is reputed to be of value for patients with a pump (CSII) or those who have difficulty with control. It tends to be used for IDDM patients who do frequent self blood glucose monitoring and are willing to spend the time required.

The amount of insulin suggested is 2.6 U regular insulin (RI) per 20 g carbohydrate at breakfast and 1.6 U RI for every 20 g carbohydrate at subsequent meals and snacks.[92]

The **total available glucose** (TAG) counting method requires calculation of the assumed total glucose obtained from the protein, fat, and carbohydrate content of foods eaten using the equation

$$\text{TAG (g)} = 100\% \text{ g carbohydrate} \\ + 58\% \text{ g protein} + 10\% \text{ g fat} \qquad \textbf{(11-3)}$$

The 58% of the protein represents the glucogenic amino acids, and 10% fat represents glycerol in the triglycerides. The method is considered to be suited to insulin-dependent patients who are highly motivated to have excellent control. In addition, it is sometimes used for providing meal replacements on sick days or for making adjustments in insulin in anticipation of larger than normal meals at parties or on holidays.

The **point system** is a simplified method for counting the amount of a nutrient. One point equals 75 kilocalories. Therefore, a 1,200 kcal diet equals 16 points. The patient's diet states the total points per day and may state points for each meal or snack. The patient is also given a reference book of foods and food groups with points for each.

The **food choice plan** requires the planning of three days' menus. The menus and serving sizes are approved by a nutritional care specialist. The patient uses the three-day rotation for about two weeks. Foods eaten and blood glucose levels are recorded. The patient then returns for evaluation and menu adjustment.

Glycemic Index. Glycemic index refers to the effect on the blood sugar level of equivalent amounts of carbohydrate contained in different foods. It has long been known that different carbohydrate foods will produce different glycemic responses even though there is no difference in their macronutrient composition. Differences in rates of digestion of foods of similar macronu-

trient composition appear to produce differences in blood glucose and blood insulin responses to meals.[93,94] Since it became difficult to compare results from one laboratory to another because of lack of standardization, Jenkins and associates proposed the concept of the "glycemic index" as a method of assessing and classifying the glycemic response to carbohydrate foods.[95] The glycemic index classified individual foods by the extent to which they increase blood glucose compared to a reference carbohydrate feeding. The reference is an equicarbohydrate portion of white bread. A substantial number of foods have now been classified.[96] In Table 11-23, the comparative glycemic re-

Table 11-23. Glycemic Index of Selected Foods

Food	Glycemic Index
Grains and cereal products	
White bread	100
Whole wheat bread	99
Rye bread	96
Breakfast cereals	
Cornflakes	119
Shredded wheat	97
All-Bran	73
Oatmeal	85
Fruits	
Banana	79
Orange juice	67
Orange	66
Grapes	62
Apple	53
Grapefruit	36
Plum	34
Vegetables	
Potato, baked	135
Potato, instant	116
Peas, frozen	74
Legumes, dried	
Beans, canned, baked	60
Beans, kidney	54
Lentils	43
Dairy products	
Ice cream	52
Yogurt	52
Milk, whole	49
Milk, skim	46
Sweeteners, nutritive	
Maltose	152
Glucose	138
Honey	126
Sucrose	86
Fructose	30

sponses to various foods are given, setting the response to 1 slice of bread as equal to 100.

The glycemic index may be related to the form in which a food is eaten, its fiber content, the presence of protein and fat, food processing and preparation methods, and rate of food intake, digestion, and absorption.[95-101] In addition, the patient's severity of glucose intolerance and degree of blood glucose control affects the glycemic response.[101] Further study and use of classifications of food on the basis of a glycemic index is needed. Data now available are largely based on tests with single foods. On the other hand, foods with high glycemic indexes do not affect the glycemic response when given in mixed meals.[98,102-105] In addition, a comparison of responses to meals with the same exchanges but different glycemic indexes shows that blood glucose did not differ as much as the differences in glycemic index would suggest.[106] At present, the glycemic index is not incorporated into exchange lists. It does suggest the value of choosing a variety of foods and also the value of self blood glucose monitoring.

Other Considerations in Nutritional Care. In addition to the items already described, there are a number of other factors that must be considered in the nutritional care of the diabetic patient, because the diabetic diet must become a permanent part of the patient's life. Information on these items should be obtained during the nutritional assessment. Compliance will be improved if the diet is compatible with the patient's previous habits and preferences. Under these circumstances, the diet must be tailor-made for each patient. The following are some of the factors that must be considered:

1. *Financial resources:* Many diabetic patients are elderly and living on small fixed incomes. Some are receiving public aid. The existence of diabetes causes additional expense.
2. *Local markets and availability of food:* It is

especially necessary to ascertain that unsweetened canned fruit is available.
3. *Social life of the patient:* Instruction should be given, if necessary, on the limited use of alcohol and the substitution of snack foods into the meal plan.
4. *Work situation and type of activities:* The patient's working hours and level of activity from day to day, or even within a day, must be considered. Also important is how meals generally are provided (e.g., whether lunch is carried to work or purchased there).
5. *Family group and the home:* If someone other than the patient prepares meals, that person should be instructed along with the patient. The facilities available for food preparation must also be considered.
6. *Meal habits of the family:* The diet should be compatible with the number, time, and size of family meals. Necessary changes in insulin dosage or time of injection must be discussed with the physician.
7. *Ethnic food habits, food preferences, and dislikes:* If a patient usually eats certain foods that are not included on the exchange lists, these foods should be added. Supplements to the *Exchange Lists for Meal Planning*[59] are available to adjust to Jewish, vegetarian, Oriental, Indian, and black American food habits. Various lists of Japanese, Chinese, and Mexican foods also are available for this purpose from state and local dietetic associations. If a patient adamantly refuses to eat the foods in one of the exchange lists, the diet must be planned without it. Some examples that may be encountered are the lactose-intolerant patient and the patient who refuses to eat vegetables.
8. *Possible mechanical difficulties:* This consideration most often involves the condition of the patient's teeth. Occasionally, the diabetic diet must be combined with nutritional care for patients with pathologic conditions of the head and

neck (see Chapter 8) if the patient has infection, trauma, or surgery in this area.

9. *Pathologic conditions in addition to diabetes:* Many patients have other conditions that require diet modifications. These must be combined with the diabetic diet, and the exchange lists must be altered accordingly. Modified exchange lists are available for low-sodium and low-fat diabetic diets. Also important is whether the patient has a handicap that interferes with shopping for food or meal preparation.

10. *Intelligence, education, eyesight, and language difficulties and the psychological response of the patient* are additional important factors in instructing the patient.

Adjustments for Missed Meals or Reduced Appetite. Other problems that arise occasionally are missed meals or episodes of reduced appetite. The patient at home may suffer minor illnesses that reduce appetite and may experience delays in meals for reasons such as social occasions. Carbohydrates should be carried by the patient for use on these occasions. Hard candies are useful.

The patients can be advised to follow these procedures if blood glucose is < 70 mg/dl:

1. Eat 15 g carbohydrate (e.g., 1 bread or fruit exchange).
2. Wait 15 minutes and retest for blood glucose.
3. If result is still < 70 mg/dl, eat another 15 g carbohydrate.
4. Repeat until blood glucose is in target range.
5. Eat another 15 g carbohydrate if next meal is not scheduled within one hour.

Patients with IDDM should always have available a glucagon kit so that the glucagon can be injected for treatment of a severe reaction. A family member or friend must know how to use the kit.

In the hospital, if a patient receiving insulin misses or refuses to eat part of a meal, a common practice is to attempt to replace the food with one of equivalent value within a three-hour period. If complete replacement cannot be accomplished, replacement of as much of the carbohydrate as possible should be attempted. Protein and fat usually are not replaced. Fruit juices, regular soft drinks, candy, sweetened gelatin, or sweetened tea are used for the purpose of replacing the carbohydrate. If carbohydrate replacement, too, is impossible, the physician is notified, and the patient is carefully observed for signs of hypoglycemia. The patient can be injected with glucagon to potentiate glycogenolysis. If this procedure is ineffective, glucose can be given intravenously. If food intake is reduced for longer periods, the prescribed calories and insulin may be reduced temporarily. Replacement is *not* necessary for patients who are controlled by diet alone.

In some illnesses, especially infections, the patient becomes more insulin-resistant. Even though food intake is decreased, blood glucose may rise. It should be monitored at least four times a day, and the urine should be tested for ketones if blood glucose is > 240 mg/dl. Thus it is important that the insulin dosage be continued. Patients should be carefully instructed that they should not eliminate their insulin if they are not well enough to eat, since they may actually need more insulin when ill. The diabetic diet can be planned as a liquid diet if necessary. This may be a useful procedure in case of sore throats, tooth extractions, or similar events. Intake should include 8–12 oz. of fluid per hour. This need can be incorporated into the liquid diet with added water, tea, and broth as necessary.[39]

In the patient with chronic complications or other accompanying pathologic conditions, other diet modifications may be combined with the diabetic diet. In the patient with advanced nephropathy, for example, diets appropriate for chronic renal failure may be planned in combination with the diabetic diet. Since the diabetic diet is very flexible, there are few diets with which it cannot be combined.

Emotional Problems and Diabetes. The emotional state of the patient may have a profound effect on his or her ability to be educated in self-care and on the control of the diabetes. Sometimes, the first duty of the nutritional care specialist is to calm fear in the patient or parents. This must be done before any meaningful instruction can occur. Here are some examples of problems that may be encountered:

The emotionally upset patient who is hyperglycemic from stresses such as family or job problems.

The child who tries to control parents by refusing to eat.

The adolescent who refuses to adhere to any treatment plan in order to assert independence.

The counseling skills of the nutritional care specialist are important in these and similar situations.

Exercise

Exercise in diabetes has the same positive effects as in the nondiabetic population, but in diabetics it also provides further benefits. Exercise tends to increase sensitivity to insulin, improve glucose tolerance, and thus decrease blood glucose. Less insulin is needed to stimulate glucose uptake by a working muscle than by a resting muscle.[107-109] In total, exercise may allow a reduction in the insulin dose.

Exercise reverses the insulin resistance seen in obesity. It also is an adjunct to calorie restriction for weight control. Exercise improves cardiovascular fitness, improves blood pressure control, and decreases cardiovascular disease risk factors, such as elevated triglycerides, VLDL, and cholesterol, as well as increasing HDL (see Chapter 10).

To be most effective, diet and hypoglycemic agents must not only be adjusted in relationship to each other, but both must be adjusted in relation to the patient's activity. On the other hand, if improperly handled, these relationships may increase the risks.

Metabolic Effects of Exercise. Exercise requires rapid mobilization of metabolic fuels in order to supply adequate energy to the muscles. In the resting state, muscles depend on oxidation of fatty acids from fat stores. In the nondiabetic individual, when exercise begins, the primary fuel is glucose derived from the breakdown of muscle glycogen. This is followed, after five or ten minutes, by a combination of glucose from glycogen and circulating glucose derived from hepatic glycogenolysis (70–75%) and by gluconeogenesis (25–30%) from pyruvate, lactate, amino acids, and glycerol. After 40–60 minutes of moderate exercise, utilization of plasma free fatty acids (FFAs), derived by lipolysis of adipose tissue, increases, and glucose use subsides. As exercise continues further, liver glycogen is depleted, gluconeogenesis increases, and after about two hours, fatty acid oxidation becomes the principal source of energy.[109] Uptake of FFAs by muscle is not insulin-dependent, but it is proportional to plasma concentration of FFA. After exercise, replacement of muscle and hepatic glycogen occurs in 24–48 hours. The uptake of glucose in this period results in improved glucose tolerance. The replacement of muscle glycogen is insulin-dependent. Thus postexercise replacement is handicapped if insulin is deficient. Exercise has different effects in IDDM and in NIDDM. The effects also vary if the diabetes is well controlled or poorly controlled and with the type of exercise. In diabetic subjects, if control is poor, glycogen storage will be reduced, since it is determined by the availability of insulin. The individual is then more susceptible to hypoglycemia. Since uptake and oxidation of FFAs are increased, ketone body production may increase, resulting in hyperketonemia.

Conditioning (endurance) exercises (e.g., walking, bicycling, or swimming) may lower blood glucose for up to 12 hours. Therefore, these are among recommended choices. On the other hand, flexibility exercises have few effects on blood glucose levels, while strengthening exercises (e.g., weight training) will often increase catecholamine output and thus increase blood glucose.

Establishing an Exercise Program. In discussing a proposed exercise program with a client, the nutritional care specialist must first assure that medical clearance has been obtained. This is particularly important for those over age 30 or those who have had diabetes for ten years or more.

It is then appropriate to discuss the type of activity and the duration that would be enjoyable and effective. The exercise is not required to be strenuous and exhausting. An exercise program may begin with five minutes of a conditioning activity three times a week and increase gradually to 30 minutes five or six times a week.

An additional consideration is the intensity of the exercise. Clients can be taught to monitor their pulse rate. The pulse at the wrist (radial pulse) is counted for 6 seconds and multiplied by 10 to give rate per minute. The activity should be vigorous enough to raise the heart rate to 60–85% of maximum heart rate. In general, the figures given in Table 11-24 can be used as guidelines.[108]

Table 11-25 lists a graded series of exercise levels which differ in intensity, duration, and frequency. The patient should be advised to start at the sedentary level, and then increase frequency and duration gradually.

The "training" period with pulse rate at 100–120 should be preceded by a warm-up period containing mild stretching and range-of-motion exercises, working up to the training level of the activity. It should also be followed by a cool-down period when activity is returned to resting level.

Exercise in NIDDM. In the NIDDM patient, exercise after meals tends to moderate the postprandial rise in blood glucose, ap-

Table 11-24. Pulse-Rate Guidelines for Exercise

Exercise	Pulse Rate
Too light	60–80
Marginal	80–100
Appropriate intensity for most	100–120
Appropriate for the young and those in "good shape"	120–140
Marginally excessive	140–160
Excessive!	160–200

Table 11-25. Levels of Activity

Activity Level	Pulse Rate	Frequency per Week	Duration (min.)
Sedentary	100–120	4–6	10–20
Somewhat active	100–130	4–6	15–30
Moderately active	110–140	3–5	30–45
Very active	120–160	3–5	30–60

parently by decreasing insulin resistance.[109] Thus, a 30-minute walk after meals is often recommended. More strenuous exercise, if reached gradually, may be helpful in patients at risk of cardiovascular disease, but an exercise program must be continued to remain effective.

Exercise in IDDM. In the IDDM patient, control is more complex because the exercise response varies with the relationship of the exercise to the times of insulin administration and food intake. Exercise increases glucose utilization and may result in hypoglycemia.[110,111] Theoretically, this may be approached by reducing insulin dose or increasing food intake. For intense and regular exercise in the well-regulated patient, the insulin dose may be reduced. For sporadic exercise, it is easier to recommend increased food intake in the form of snacks. The amount of food must be related to the intensity and duration of the exercise. About 15 g of carbohydrate may be taken prior to light exercise. Adjustments for moderate and strenuous activity vary with blood sugar levels (see Table 11-26). In prolonged exercise, additional carbohydrate may be required at intervals and also in the postexercise period, since the increased rate of metabolism continues.[112,113]

Exercising tends to increase the rate of insulin absorption. Therefore, exercise should not begin immediately after an injection. An interval of 40 minutes after regular insulin injection and $2\frac{1}{2}$ hours after intermediate-acting insulin is sufficient to avoid the effect.[7] Exercise should also be avoided at the time of peak insulin effect. It is better scheduled at the usual time of appearance of glycosuria.[114] On the other hand, strenuous ex-

Table 11-26. Recommendations for Increases in Carbohydrate Intake and Adjustment of Insulin for Diabetic Control in Exercise

Activity	Blood Sugar (g/dl)			
	<80–100	100–180	180–300	>300
Low to moderate activity (e.g., slow walking, bicycling, ½ hr.)	Add 10 to 15 g	No food increase	No food increase	No food increase
Moderate activity (e.g., 1 hr. swimming, cycling, jogging)	Add 30 g or 10–15 g/hr.	Add 10–15 g/hr.	No food increase	Discontinue exercise
Strenuous activity (e.g., racquetball, football)	Add 45 to 50 g + SBGM	Add 30–40 g	Add 15 g/hr.	Do not exercise
Extended activity (e.g., backpacking, skiing) Half day	As above. Also decrease insulin dose by 10% of total dose.			
All day	As above. Also decrease insulin dose by 20%.			

Compiled from Franz, M.J., Exercise and the management of diabetes mellitus. *J. Am. Diet. Assoc.* 87:872, 1987; Krall, L.P., and Beaser, R.S., *Joslin Diabetes Manual*, 12th ed. Philadelphia: Lea & Febiger, 1989; Powers, M.A., Ed., *Nutrition Guide for Professionals: Diabetes Education and Meal Planning.* Alexandria, Va.: American Diabetes Association, and Chicago, Ill.: American Dietetic Association, 1988.

ercise should not be undertaken under the following circumstances:

- Patients in poor control (blood glucose over 240 mg/dl) to avoid worsening the hyperglycemia.
- Patients with retinopathy to avoid increased pressure in the eye leading to further eye damage.
- Jogging or running of patients with sensory neuropathy in feet to avoid damage to the feet.

SBGM is very valuable to the exercising IDDM patients, who can monitor their blood glucose before, during, and after exercise for maximum control.

In contrast to the well-regulated diabetic, in the patient with hyperglycemia and ketonuria, exercise makes the diabetes worse. The insufficient insulin indicated by the hyperglycemia results in decreased glucose use by muscles. The liver releases more glucose in an attempt to make up for the deficit, raising blood glucose level further. Exercise increases the secretion of the insulin antagonists glucagon and growth hormone.[113,114]

The presence of ketonuria indicates that the body lacks insulin and is breaking down fat. Exercise will exacerbate the process. Therefore, diabetes should be regulated before an exercise program is undertaken.

In summary, the following are safety rules for the IDDM patient related to exercise:[115]

1. Test blood glucose before exercising.
2. Before exercise, eat a snack that was not already included in meal planning.
3. Carry sugar to treat hypoglycemia.
4. Restore control before exercising if hyperglycemia or ketonuria is present.
5. Exercise with someone else.
6. Decrease insulin dose for prolonged activity (i.e., swimming) when extra food is not desirable.

Education of the Patient

The health care team cannot control diabetes without the cooperation of the patient, and, to be able to participate fully in his or her own care, the patient must be well informed and well motivated. Unfortunately, patient education has been, and often still is, seriously neglected. It should begin as soon as the disease is diagnosed and should continue throughout the life of the patient. In addition, education must include those people closely associated with the diabetic: the parents of child patients, the families of all patients, teachers, and associates at work and at recreation.

The list of items that must be taught to the diabetic patient and members of the family is long. The following are items of information needed by all patients:

The basic concepts of the disease and methods for controlling it.

Principles of dietary management, including procedures for following the meal plan, the use of exchange lists or other procedures, diet during minor illnesses, and adjustments for changes in exercise.

Urine and blood testing — why it is important, how to do it, how to interpret results, and record keeping.

Knowledge of acute complications — how to prevent them and how to recognize them.

Knowledge of chronic complications — how to recognize them and what therapy to institute.

Personal hygiene.

Exercise.

Social problems, including employment, licenses, and insurance.

In addition, some patients will need to know about the following, depending on the nature of their particular disease, the therapy used, and their other needs:

How to use insulin, including the kind of insulin, dose, syringe care, prevention of infection, adjustment of the dose in special situations, and its relation to blood or urine testing.

The type, dose, and possible complications of oral hypoglycemic agents.

Family planning, genetic counseling.

Camp and school.

Community resources and other sources of information.

Effects of other medications on diabetic control.

Education of the diabetic requires a careful and very detailed nutritional history. After an individualized treatment plan is made and goals are set, education begins with consideration of the information necessary for basic survival. This is followed by in-depth education that provides the patient with enough understanding so that he or she can manage the disease in such a way to provide maximum flexibility in life style.[39]

It should be obvious that effective patient education requires the effort of the entire health care team. It also requires individualization. There is no packaged program that can be applied to all patients, but there are many helpful teaching aids. Among them are pamphlets (used almost invariably), programmed teaching machines, demonstrations, food models, slides, and movies. Although individual instruction is important, diabetic patients can productively be taught in classes in ambulatory care centers and in hospitals. Bed patients, as well as ambulatory patients, may be gathered for class, complete with wheelchairs and stretchers if necessary. The patients often profit from association with other diabetics. Nutritional care specialists should be familiar with the teaching materials available for both individual and class use and should be expert in applying them and aware of their limitations.

Other information is available to diabetic patients. Many patients subscribe to a magazine published six times yearly.[116] In some communities, there are local diabetes associations with groups for professionals and groups for patients. There are also books available for patients, giving information on the disease in general.

Self-Management

When the IDDM patient has been adequately educated, the patient may be ready to undertake self-management. This procedure is for patients who are alert, highly motivated, and careful and who are trained in SBGM.

The objective is, of course, to maintain the blood glucose levels within normal range. For some patients, blood glucose patterns tend to be quite stable with only occasional slowly developing shifts outside the normal range. Most NIDDM patients are in this group. For some others, usually in the IDDM group, the blood glucose concentrations may vary rapidly and markedly. It is patients in this group who can profit from learning to adjust their insulin dosage to smooth out the pattern of change of glucose concentration.

The patient must keep a logbook of results of SBGM and a record plus notes on factors that affect the values obtained. These include aberrations in the prescribed diet, exercise, and illness. From these data, the patient can be taught to make changes in the diet or insulin and will get immediate feedback on their effects.[40]

The general principles of adjusting insulin dosages are given in Table 11-27 using a typical dosage schedule of regular plus NPH or Lente insulin in the morning and NPH or Lente in the evening. In general, adjustments are made only when blood or urine values are too high or too low for three days. Blood glucose which is "too high" may be defined by the physician. Often it is set at > 120 or 140 mg/dl. "Too low" may be defined as any value < 60 mg/dl or indicated by the occurrence of a hypoglycemic reaction. Urine glucose is too high if it is 1% or more, but cannot be too low since zero is normal.

Insulin dosages to adjust for abnormal blood glucose levels are increased or decreased by no more than 2 units at a time. It is important to proceed cautiously in order to avoid sudden changes and rebounds such as the Somogyi effect.

Table 11-28 gives some examples of the types of adjustments that can be made by patients with common insulin types and dosage schedules. Some general guidelines are as follows:[7]

1. When test results are too high or too low before supper, adjust the intermediate insulin dose taken before breakfast by 2 units.
2. When test results are abnormal before bedtime, adjust the dose of regular insulin taken before supper by 2 units. If no regular insulin has been prescribed, adjust the intermediate insulin dose taken before breakfast.
3. When test results are abnormal before breakfast, adjust by 2 units the intermediate insulin dose before supper or at bedtime. If no insulin dose is scheduled at these times and tests are high, the physician should be notified to consider adding an evening dose.
4. When test results are abnormal before lunch, alter by 2 units the regular insulin

Table 11-27. Example of Recommended Insulin Adjustments in Self-Management of Patients Receiving Regular[a] Plus NPH[b] or Lente[b] Insulins

Time of Poor Test	Time of Change	If Blood Glucose Is > 120 mg/dl, *Increase* Insulin by 2 Units	If Blood Glucose Is < 60 mg/dl, *Decrease* Insulin by 2 Units
Fasting	P.M.[c]	NPH or Lente	NPH or Lente
Before lunch	A.M.[d]	Regular	Regular
Before dinner	A.M.	NPH or Lente	NPH or Lente
Before bedtime or two hours after dinner	P.M.	Regular	Regular

[a] A short-acting insulin.
[b] Intermediate-acting insulin.
[c] The insulin dose of the immediately previous afternoon or evening (on the fourth day after three days of abnormal values).
[d] The insulin dose in the morning of the fourth day.

Table 11-28. Examples of Insulin Adjustments for Patients Receiving Various Dosage Schedules of Insulin if Tests Are Poor Three Days in a Row at the Dosage Time Given[a]

Time of High Results	Dosage Schedule				
	Intermediate Insulin Once a Day before Breakfast	Regular and Intermediate Insulin Once a Day before Breakfast	Intermediate Insulin before Breakfast and before Supper or at Bedtime	Regular and Intermediate Insulin before Breakfast and Intermediate Insulin before Supper or at Bedtime	Regular and Intermediate Insulin before Breakfast and before Supper
Before supper	Increase NPH or Lente 2 units before breakfast of day 4	Increase NPH or Lente 2 units before breakfast of day 4	Increase NPH or Lente 2 units before breakfast of day 4	Increase NPH or Lente 2 units before breakfast of day 4	Increase NPH or Lente 2 units before breakfast of day 4
Before bedtime	—	—	Increase NPH or Lente 2 units before breakfast of day 4	Increase NPH or Lente 2 units before breakfast of day 4	Increase regular insulin 2 units before supper on day 4
Before breakfast	Notify M.D. (may need to add P.M. insulin dose)	Notify M.D. (may need to add H.S. insulin dose)	Increase NPH or Lente dose 2 units in evening of day 4	Increase NPH or Lente dose 2 units in evening of day 4	Increase NPH or Lente dose 2 units in evening of day 4
Before lunch	Notify M.D. (may need to add regular insulin before breakfast)	Increase regular insulin 2 units before breakfast of day 4	—	Increase regular insulin 2 units before breakfast of day 4	Increase regular insulin 2 units before breakfast of day 4

[a] Blood glucose higher than 120 mg/dl for previous 3 days.

451

dose taken before breakfast. If no RI has been prescribed, notify the physician. It may need to be added.

These guidelines are based on the assumption that the patient has been following the prescribed diet and there is no other change that could account for the results, such as infection or major alterations in exercise. It is important also to avoid routine increases in insulin dosage to reduce excess blood glucose. If such increases are made, the patient will become obese. Instead, it may be necessary to reduce the carbohydrate intake.

The Diabetic Child

Approximately 4% of diabetics are children, or more than 100,000 in the United States alone. Important precipitating factors are infection, trauma, and possibly puberty. Obesity is not common. Peak ages of onset are 13 years for boys and 10 years for girls.[8]

The syndrome is typical insulin-dependent diabetes with sudden onset and temporary remission of weeks or months, followed by the onset of overt diabetes that usually becomes total in two to six years. Since no insulin is produced in the usual child patient, insulin is essential in treatment. The typical dose is 0.5–1.0 U/kg/day, but this must be adjusted by monitoring blood sugar levels, and it may reach 1.5 to 1.75 U/kg/day. Insulin is frequently given in divided doses, but the regimen must be individualized for each child.

The diet must provide adequate energy to support growth. Growth should be monitored carefully; therefore, the energy limitations often seen in diets for adults are not appropriate for most children. There are those who suggest that the variation in activity and varying growth rates in children require that the child's appetite serve as the primary guide to food intake. On an unmeasured diet, the child usually receives at least three meals and a bedtime snack, but there may be six or more meals per day in very brittle diabetes. This does not mean, how-

ever, that all control should be abandoned. At the very least, commercial influences, such as advertisements on television, and social influences on food intake should be minimized.

General recommendations for an unmeasured diet for the diabetic child are as follows:[117–119]

1. The child should eat something at each meal, plus one or two small snacks as necessary. The foods on the exchange lists should be used as a guide to meal planning.
2. Concentrated sugar should be used only during vigorous athletic events and for treating hypoglycemia.
3. Meals should be provided at approximately the same time each day.
4. The child's appetite should determine the amount eaten, but meals must not be omitted.
5. Since the child is at risk of developing hypertension and cardiovascular disease later in life, salt and cholesterol intake should be reduced.

Strict diet control often is considered preferable for prevention of acute and chronic complications.[8] However, complications of diabetes are rarely seen in preadolescent children. There is a sharp increase in retinopathy in mid-adolescence, **regardless of the duration of the diabetes**. It has been suggested, therefore, that total duration of diabetes is less important than **duration after puberty**.[119] Delayed nerve conduction velocity also is reputed to worsen during adolescence. These factors demonstrate the importance of careful control of hyperglycemia during this period. Older adolescents and young adults can be taught SBGM and self-management so that they can adjust insulin and diet to changing circumstances.

Diabetes and Reproduction

Ovarian and placental hormones decrease sensitivity to insulin. Therefore, pregnancy is considered to be "diabetogenic." The nondiabetic woman meets this challenge with increased insulin production. However, some women are incapable of such an increase and may experience some difficulties with the pregnancy. These pregnant women may be divided into two categories. Those who are diabetic and later become pregnant are classified as **pregestational diabetics**. During pregnancy, their diabetes becomes more severe. Those who develop carbohydrate intolerance that is first recognized during the pregnancy are considered to have **gestational diabetes mellitus**. These two conditions have much in common but are not identical.

Both pregestational and gestational diabetes mellitus are considered high-risk pregnancies and require special consideration. Maternal ketonemia, hypoglycemia or hyperglycemia, premature labor, nephropathy, and cardiovascular problems are risk factors that must be avoided in order to achieve a successful pregnancy.

The Child of the Diabetic Mother

In the infants of diabetic mothers (IDM), a number of complications can occur. Many of these are listed in Table 11-29, but often can be avoided if maternal diabetes is under "tight" control.

The mechanism by which these problems can occur is not yet entirely clear. White's classification of diabetes in pregnancy, shown in Table 11-30, indicates a relationship to age of onset, duration of diabetes, and existence of complications. More specifically, IDM morbidity and mortality has been related to hyperglycemia as indicated by elevated hemoglobin A_{1c}.[120-124] It has also been suggested that the incidence of complications might be related to ketosis, acidosis, compromise of circulation, decreased fetal zinc or manganese uptake,[125] B-hydroxybutyrate,[126] or disruption of arachidonic acid[127] or glycolytic pathways.[128]

Pregestational Diabetes

It is recommended that diabetic women considering pregnancy establish a high degree of

Table 11-29. Complicatons in the Offspring of Uncontrolled Maternal Diabetes in Pregnancy

Macrosomia (may lead to cesarean section)
Increased muscle
Increased adiposity
Organomegaly
Birth injury
Intrauterine growth retardation
Respiratory system
Asphyxia neonatorum
Respiratory distress syndrome
Hypoplastic lungs
Cardiovascular system
Heart failure
Situs inversus
Cardiac anomalies
    Transposition of great arteries
    Ventricular septal defect
    Atrial septal defect
    Single ventricle
    Hypoplastic left ventricle
Blood
Increased blood volume
Polycythemia
Hyperviscosity
Renal system
Ureter duplex
Renal agenesis
Cystic kidney
Transient hematuria
Digestive system
Small left colon syndrome
Situs inversus
Anal/rectal atresia
Hyperbilirubinemia
Skeletal and spinal disorders
Sacral dysgenesis (caudal dysplasia)
Central nervous system
Neurologic instability
Hydrocephalus
Anancephaly
Open spina bifida
Holoprosencephaly
Encephalocele
Meningomyelocele
Metabolic
Hypocalcemia
Hypomagnesemia
Hypoglycemia
Fetal death

control of the diabetes *prior to* conception. However, advanced complications of diabetes in the mother tend to worsen when metabolic control is restored rapidly. Therefore, improved control should be achieved with some deliberation.[129]

In some centers, diabetic women who have not established good control are hospi-

Table 11-30. White's Classification of Diabetes in Pregnancy

Classification	Age of Onset (years)	Duration (years)	Insulin Need	Description
A	Any	Any	No	Diet alone; any duration or age of onset
B	20	<10	Yes	
C	10–19	10–19	Yes	
D	<10	>20	Yes	Also background retinopathy or hypertension (not preeclamptic)
R	Any	Any	Yes	Proliferative retinopathy or vitreous hemorrhage
F	Any	Any	Yes	Nephropathy with proteinuria
RF	Any	Any	Yes	Combination of R and F criteria
H	Any	Any	Yes	Clinical evidence of arteriosclerotic heart disease
T	Any	Any	Yes	Prior renal transplant

talized as soon as possible. It is imperative to maintain blood glucose at the levels found in nondiabetic pregnant women:[39]

Fasting and premeal plasma glucose	70–90 mg/dl
1-hour postprandial plasma glucose	<140 mg/dl
2-hour postprandial plasma glucose	<120 mg/dl

Treatment to achieve control must be individualized. Some methods that may be used include the following:

In the diet, provide *at least* three meals and a snack. Three meals and three snacks may be necessary to establish sufficient control. Energy intake should be 30 kcal per kg ideal body weight per day in the first trimester and 38 kcal per kg ideal body weight per day thereafter. The recommended division of total calories is 50–60% carbohydrate, 20–37% fat, and 12–20% protein. The diet should contain 200 g carbohydrate or more and 1.5–2.0 g protein per kg body weight per day.

Use combinations of intermediate and regular insulins. Long-acting insulins are usually avoided.

Give insulin at least twice daily. Sometimes three or more injections per day are used. CSII is frequently recommended. NIDDM patients are given insulin when they become pregnant.

Use SBGM if possible. Test blood before each meal, at bedtime, and again if hypoglycemia is suspected. Once a week, test one hour after each meal for one day.

Monitor urinary ketones in the first morning sample and whenever premeal capillary blood glucose is >140 mg/dl. Since there is evidence of fetal brain damage in ketosis, it should be avoided carefully.

Measure HbA$_{1c}$ when treatment is initiated and monthly thereafter.

Weight gain should be the normal gain expected of non-diabetic women if the diabetic woman is at normal weight at the beginning of pregnancy:[39]

First trimester	2–4 lb.
Second and third trimesters	25–32 lb. (0.8–0.9 lb./week)

Overweight women are usually advised not to gain as much weight. A gain of 15–24 pounds has been recommended.[7] Weight loss is not recommended.

Gestational Diabetes

Because gestational diabetes (GDM) increases perinatal losses, it is considered a major public health problem. Therefore, screening for GDM between the 24th and 28th week of pregnancy is included in standard obstetrical care. In the screening test, the patient is given a 50 g oral load of glucose. If plasma glucose an hour later is 140 g/dl or more, a full oral glucose tolerance test (OGTT) is given.

In the OGTT, a load of oral glucose is given after an 8–14 hour fast. Plasma glucose is measured at 0, 1, 2, and 3 hours. A diagnosis of GDM is made if any two of the following are met or exceeded:[129]

Fasting 105 mg/dl
1 hour   190 mg/dl
2 hours 165 mg/dl
3 hours 145 mg/dl

The treatment of GDM is similar to that for pregestational diabetes. Some patients are given insulin, but others can be controlled by diet alone. Sulfonylurea drugs, which may be teratogenic, are not given to GDM patients.

Many GDM patients are obese, and the appropriate energy intake is a matter of some discussion. There is general agreement that pregnancy is not the time for zealous weight reduction. However, a diet providing 38 kcal per kg body weight may represent a significant reduction in intake in the very obese.

Patients with GDM will need extensive counseling, since they have not had the counseling typical of patients who were diabetic prior to pregnancy. They are likely to need follow-up postpartum.

In most GDM patients, diabetes management is not needed during labor or postpartum.[129] There is a high incidence of impaired glucose tolerance in these patients, however, and it is recommended that these patients be monitored.[129]

Self-Management in Pregnancy

Self-management is a valuable procedure for the pregnant diabetic. In principle, it is the same as the procedures given in Table 11-28. However, greater caution is observed to avoid hypoglycemia, hyperglycemia, and ketonemia.

SBGM is highly recommended. The guidelines for insulin adjustment given in Table 11-28 are usually useful, but postmeal glucose levels are also monitored. Guidelines for high postmeal glucose levels are given in Table 11-31.[7] The changes indicated are made after two days of abnormal values instead of three.[7]

Ketoacidosis can be very harmful to a fetus. Therefore, monitoring for urine ketones is important and should be done each morning. If ketones are present when blood sugar is relatively normal, the patient may be having hypoglycemia during the night. A larger evening snack may be necessary.

Monitoring for ketones should also be done if blood glucose is > 240 mg/dl and in cases of even minor illnesses.

Diabetes Management during Labor and Delivery

The various protocols for management of the diabetes during labor and delivery are similar in principle. A mother who is having a cesarean section or whose labor is prolonged usually has both glucose and insulin infused intravenously. In routine vaginal deliveries, blood glucose is monitored at intervals, and intravenous glucose and subcutaneous insulin are given as indicated by the results.[130]

Women in premature labor may be given salbutamol to inhibit uterine contractions, but salbutamol can precipitate ketoacidosis and hypokalemia. They may also be given dexamethasone to promote maturation of fetal lungs (see Chapter 16). These medications, in combination, can lead to severe hyperglycemia. The patients are then given insulin infusions, sometimes in very large doses. Serum potassium must be monitored every four hours and supplemented as necessary.[130]

Lactation

Very little information is available on the impact of lactation on diabetes. Nevertheless,

Table 11-31. Examples of Insulin Adjustments for Pregnant, Diabetic Patients Receiving Various Dosage Schedules of Regular (RI), NPH, or Lente Insulin

	Dosage Schedule				
Time of High Results	Intermediate Insulin Once a Day before Breakfast	Regular and Intermediate Insulin Once a Day before Breakfast	Intermediate Insulin before Breakfast and at Bedtime	Regular and Intermediate Insulin before Breakfast and Intermediate Insulin before Supper or at Bedtime	Regular and Intermediate Insulins before Breakfast and before Supper
Before breakfast or before taking insulin	Notify M.D. (may need to add P.M. dose)	Notify M.D. (may need P.M. dose of NPH or Lente	Increase next P.M. NPH or Lente dose 2 units	Increase NPH or Lente 2 units in P.M.	Increase NPH or Lente 2 units in P.M.
Two hours after breakfast	Notify M.D. (may need to add RI in A.M.)	Increase RI 1–2 units next A.M.	Notify M.D. (may need to add RI)	Increase RI 1–2 units next A.M.	Increase RI 1–2 units next A.M.
Two hours after lunch	Increase NPH or Lente 2 units next A.M.	Increase NPH or Lente 2 units next A.M.	Increase NPH or Lente 2 units next A.M.	Increase NPH or Lente 2 units next A.M.	Increase NPH or Lente 2 units next A.M.
Two hours after supper	Increase NPH or Lente 2 units next A.M.	Increase NPH or Lente 2 units next A.M.	Increase NPH or Lente 2 units next A.M.	Notify M.D. (may need to add P.M. dose of RI)	Increase RI 1–2 units next P.M.

breast feeding is not considered to be contraindicated. It is necessary for nutrient intake to be sufficient. One recommendation is 38 kcal per kg ideal body weight.[129] Snacks before nursing may be necessary to prevent hypoglycemia.[7]

The Diabetic Patient in Surgery

Diabetic patients require surgery for cardiovascular disease, gallbladder disease, cancer of the pancreas, and amputations somewhat more often than does the nondiabetic population. They also may require other types of surgery at the same rate as the rest of the population.

Anxiety, anesthesia, and the surgical procedure itself are stress factors that may cause an increase in catecholamine and cortisol production. This tends to cause a reduction in diabetes control. Patients controlled with oral hypoglycemic agents are given a small dose of insulin prior to surgery. For insulin-dependent patients, the insulin dose is reduced. Patients are given intravenous glucose the day of surgery to prevent hypoglycemia and starvation ketosis. Insulin may be included in the intravenous solution.[131]

Postoperatively, the patient is returned to the previous diet and insulin as rapidly as possible. Regular insulin often is used for faster control. The diabetic diet can be incorporated into liquid, soft, and most other diets as necessary. The principles of nutritional care of the surgery patient in general are discussed in Chapter 14 and apply equally to the patient who is diabetic.

Diabetes and Nutritional Support

Diabetic patients who need tube feedings or TPN may be divided into three groups:[132]

1. Patients with impaired glucose tolerance (IGT) who need insulin only when receiving I.V. glucose.
2. NIDDM patients managed by diet and possibly with oral hypoglycemic agents.
3. IDDM patients.

In these patients, glycemic control must be added to the usual considerations involved in the nutrition support procedures. Although care must be individualized, some general guidelines can be used as a starting point.

For NIDDM patients receiving continuous enteral feedings, 5 to 10 units of NPH or Lente insulin is given every 12 hours. The IDDM patient, by contrast, may be given 25% of the usual daily dose of NPH or Lente insulin every 12 hours. Blood glucose is monitored, and additional insulin is given on a sliding scale as necessary. A common protocol is the addition of 5 units of regular insulin for each 50 mg blood sugar per dl between 200 and 400 mg/dl. Blood sugar levels over 400 mg/dl should be referred to the attending physician for more rigorous treatment. When the tube feeding is discontinued, it may be followed by infusion of 5% or 10% dextrose to prevent hypoglycemia until insulin dosage can be adjusted.[132]

One commercial tube feeding called Glucerna (see Appendix G) has recently become available for use by diabetic patients. It is restricted in carbohydrates, has elevated fat content, and contains fiber. The clinical usefulness of a high-fat, low-carbohydrate formula for tube feeding of diabetic persons remains to be seen.

The patient with IGT or NIDDM who is parenterally fed commonly receives no more than 250 g glucose in the first 24 hours. Blood glucose is monitored every six to eight hours, and human insulin is provided as necessary on the sliding scale described previously.

After 24 hours, if the insulin needed exceeds 20 units, $\frac{2}{3}$ of the amount needed is added as regular insulin to the next infusion bottle. The amount of insulin is increased until control is reached since as much as half of the insulin may adhere to the infusion equipment and be lost. Once the blood glucose levels are consistently less than 250 mg/dl, the amount of glucose per day can be increased. Fat emulsion can be added to further increase energy content, but should not exceed 30% of the solution.

The IDDM patient is approached more slowly. During the first 24 hours, a maximum of 150 g of glucose is given, and insulin is added to the infusion bottle. A recommended procedure is the use of 1.5 times the patient's usual daily dose times the fraction of the patient's energy requirement supplied in one bottle of infusion. For example, if a patient took 40 units of insulin daily and 25% of his energy requirement is provided in one bottle, the insulin added would be $(40 \times 1.5 \times 0.25) = 15$ units.

If this amount of insulin does not provide glycemic control, $\frac{2}{3}$ of the amount indicated on the sliding scale is added to the original amount. This total is then added to the next infusion bottle. For example, if the patient has a blood sugar of 350 mg/dl and the sliding scale amount is 15 units, the amount of insulin added to the second bottle is then $15 + (15 \times \frac{1}{3}) = 15 + 10 = 25$ units.

When the patient is weaned from TPN, it is generally believed that it must be done gradually to avoid hypoglycemia. There is, however, some disagreement on this point. As is true of many aspects of the treatment of diabetes, a great deal of research is still necessary.

HYPOGLYCEMIA

In addition to diabetes mellitus, there are many other disorders in which derangements of carbohydrate utilization occur. Hypoglycemia is a clinical manifestation of many of these disorders. Since nutritional care is important in hypoglycemia, the pathologic conditions in which it occurs are described. It is important to remember that hypoglycemia is a manifestation of disease; it is not the disease itself.

Hypoglycemia usually is defined as a blood glucose concentration lower than 45 to 50 mg/dl; however, the onset of symptoms occurs at varying levels in different individuals. In adults, symptoms usually occur when blood glucose is 40 mg/dl or less. Infants can tolerate lower levels, sometimes 30 or even 20 mg/dl.

Clinical Manifestations

The signs and symptoms of hypoglycemia vary somewhat with the rate of fall of the blood glucose level. When the rate of fall is rapid, the secretion of epinephrine is stimulated in an attempt to restore normal glucose levels. The symptoms are those that result from an increase in circulating epinephrine: sweating, weakness, hunger, and **tachycardia** (increased heart rate).

On the other hand, if blood glucose falls slowly—that is, over many hours—the major effects are on the brain, since the brain uses mainly glucose as a fuel and hypoglycemia deprives it of fuel.[133] The effects include headache, blurred vision, **diplopia** (double vision), incoherent speech, and mental confusion. If the hypoglycemia persists over a long period, there may be sensory or motor deficits in the limbs, hemiplegia, and psychiatric problems. Permanent brain damage can occur. The condition can also progress to convulsions, coma, and death.

Classification

Hypoglycemia has been categorized in many ways. One useful classification is given in Table 11-32. It differentiates between **exoge-**

Table 11-32. Classification of Hypoglycemia

Spontaneous hypoglycemia
Fasting
Pancreatic beta cell tumor, functioning
Nonpancreatic tumor associated with hypoglycemia
Liver disease: acquired (diffuse liver disease) or congenital (glycogen storage disease, galactosemia)
Alcoholism and poor nutrition
Endocrinopathies: hypofunction of anterior pituitary gland, adrenal cortex, thyroid, pancreatic alpha cells
Reactive (postabsorptive)
Functional reactive
Reactive secondary to early diabetes
Dumping syndrome
Leucine sensitivity
Hereditary fructose intolerance
Exogenous hypoglycemia (insulin or sulfonylureas)
Iatrogenic (resulting from treatment by physician or surgeon)
Factitious (artificial—may be self-administered)
Homicidal
Suicidal

nous hypoglycemia, resulting from administration of hypoglycemic drugs, and **spontaneous hypoglycemia**, in which the cause is endogenous. Spontaneous hypoglycemias can be divided into two groups — **reactive** or **postabsorptive**, in which the symptoms occur within one or two hours after eating, and **fasting hypoglycemia**, which occurs approximately eight hours following the last meal. Another classification has two useful divisions — **organic**, in which there is an identifiable anatomic lesion, and **functional**, in which no recognizable anatomic lesion can be found. Some organic lesions cause fasting hypoglycemia and some cause the reactive type. Functional disorders generally are reactive.

Diagnosis

To treat hypoglycemia, it is necessary to know the etiology. Therefore, diagnostic procedures must be used not only to establish the existence of the condition, but also to pinpoint its cause. There are a number of procedures available.

Fasting blood glucose will assist in distinguishing reactive from fasting hypoglycemia. It is low in the fasting type but normal in the reactive type.

The **oral glucose tolerance test** will differentiate early diabetic from functional hypoglycemia.[134] The test must be conducted for the full five hours. Comparative oral glucose tolerance test curves in various hypoglycemic syndromes are shown in Fig. 11-7.

Intravenous glucose tolerance tests can confirm a diagnosis of dumping syndrome (see Chapter 7), since hypoglycemia will not occur in these patients if the glucose is not taken orally.

A **prolonged fast** of 48 to 72 hours is considered the ultimate test to detect organic hyperglycemia. A person with a functioning islet cell tumor usually develops symptoms in 24 hours, whereas a normal person can have 40 to 50 mg/dl of blood glucose within 48 hours and remain symptom-free. If no symptoms occur in 72 hours, the patient is

exercised carefully and a blood sample is taken. A normal person will show a rise in blood glucose following exercise, but a patient with an islet cell tumor will have a further decrease. Symptoms also may occur at this time.

The **intravenous tolbutamide response test** sometimes is used in place of the prolonged fasts. The patient is given an intravenous dose of tolbutamide, and the blood glucose concentration is determined at intervals. Following an overnight fast, a 30-minute test can be used to aid in the diagnosis of diabetes,[135] or a three-hour test may differentiate fasting hypoglycemia.[136]

In the **leucine sensitivity test**, a leucine load is given intravenously or orally, and blood samples are collected every 10 minutes for one hour. A fall to at least 40 mg of glucose per deciliter of blood indicates idiopathic sensitivity, functioning islet cell tumor, or factitious hypoglycemia due to sulfonylurea.[137]

The **fructose loading test** is conducted with a procedure similar to the GTT. Blood samples are analyzed for glucose, fructose, and phosphorus. An abnormal rise in fructose and rapid fall in glucose and serum inorganic phosphorus suggest hereditary fructose intolerance.

Serum insulin levels are used to distinguish a functioning islet cell tumor from a nonpancreatic tumor, which usually does not cause elevated insulin levels.

Circulating antibodies to insulin, if found, are useful in detecting the individual who has **factitious hypoglycemia** following self-administration of insulin.

Nutritional Care

Nutritional care of the hypoglycemic patient depends on the cause of the condition and on other treatments involved.

Fasting Hypoglycemia

In those patients whose hypoglycemia is the consequence of a tumor, the treatment of

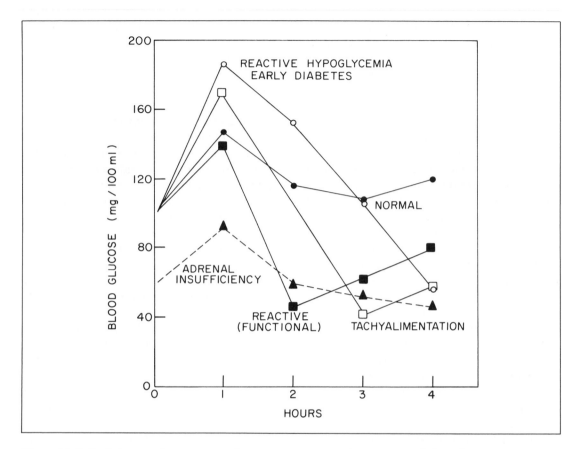

Figure 11-7. Oral glucose tolerance curves in hypoglycemic syndromes. A representative normal curve is presented for comparison. Note that in functional reactive hypoglycemia the one-hour glucose level is lower than in the curve of tachyalimentation and in early diabetes. (Reprinted with permission from Bacchus, H., Rational Management of Diabetes. Copyright © 1977, University Park Press, Baltimore.)

choice is, of course, the surgical removal of the tumor. In **insulin-producing islet cell tumors**, the patient secretes insulin during exercise or fasting, often showing symptoms before breakfast, when meals are delayed, and sometimes as early as two to three hours following a meal. Usually, the patient will already have begun a schedule of eating at regular and frequent intervals, a process that sometimes, but not always, results in massive obesity. Frequent feeding must continue until surgical removal of the tumor. Pancreatic tumors may be difficult to find. If the

surgery is unsuccessful or if the condition is inoperable, the frequent feeding must continue. The patient may be given steroid drugs. Nutritional care for patients given these drugs is discussed on page 313. If the pancreas is removed totally, the patient is diabetic and must be treated accordingly.

Nonpancreatic tumors associated with hypoglycemia are of various types and thus produce the hypoglycemic effect by more than one mechanism. When the tumor is removed, the hypoglycemia disappears. If the condition is inoperable, the diet used for functional hypoglycemia (see the next section) may be helpful in conjunction with an antihypoglycemic drug such as diazoxide. Additional aspects of nutritional care of patients with carcinoid syndrome or Zollinger-Ellison syndrome are discussed in Chapter 8. Other disorders causing hypoglycemia in association with fasting are discussed in detail elsewhere.

Reactive Hypoglycemia

There are five types of reactive hypoglycemia. In the nondiabetic population, the most common is the functional form.

Functional Reactive Hypoglycemia.
Functional reactive hypoglycemia often is associated with anxiety, tension, and emotional upsets. There is some discussion as to which is cause and which is effect and whether some of the patients are actually hypoglycemic. Many seem to develop symptoms at levels tolerated well by normal persons. The glucose tolerance curve begins at normal levels and tends to be rather flat. The blood glucose then subsides to hypoglycemic levels with a spontaneous rebound.

The condition tends to be self-limiting in months or years. In the meantime, a modified diet is helpful. One diet that has been recommended is the high-protein, low-carbohydrate diet, which has the following features:[138]

Kilocalories: To maintain normal weight. The basis for estimation is the same as that described for diabetic patients.
Carbohydrate: Limited, to reduce stimulation of insulin release, to 75 to 120 g, usually at least 100 g. Free sugars are avoided.
Protein: Increased, commonly to 120 to 140 g, to provide a source of glucose without stimulation of insulin release.
Fat: To provide the remaining kilocalories.
Division into meals: Carbohydrate *and protein* are divided as equally as is feasible among multiple feedings. Some patients require as many as six equal feedings per day.
Other restrictions: Alcohol should be avoided as it interferes with gluconeogenesis. Some institutions recommend the avoidance of caffeine-containing substances (see Appendix F).

For example, assuming an 1,800/kcal diet, the distribution might be 100 g of carbohydrate, 140 g of protein, and 95 g of fat. If the patient requires six meals, the division should aim for 16 g of carbohydrate and 23 g of protein in each. Fat is distributed as desired. The patient may need calcium and riboflavin supplements, since milk often cannot be included in the diet.

An alternative approach to diet modification is based on the assumption that restriction of slowly absorbed carbohydrate, such as starch, does not relieve the symptoms. Therefore, only free sugars are restricted; the diabetic diet is used as a general guide, sometimes with division into five or six feedings.[139]

Given the variability of patient needs and responses to diet modification, the nutritional care specialist should be prepared to work with the patient to determine the modifications needed within general guidelines.

Organic Reactive Hypoglycemia.
Organic reactive hypoglycemias comprise four conditions. **Dumping syndrome** is described in Chapter 7. Hypoglycemia also occurs in **early diabetes** (Figure 11-7). **Hereditary fructose intolerance** is a congenital metabolic disorder (see Chapter 17). The remaining entity is **leucine sensitivity**, which occurs almost exclusively in infancy and is thought to be a sign of immature development. The symptoms of leucine sensitivity commonly appear first after ingestion of milk, and treatment consists of restriction of sources of leucine, including milk. The condition is self-limiting and usually disappears by six years of age.

THE ADRENAL CORTEX

Adrenocortical Insufficiency

Adrenocortical insufficiency may be a chronic primary disease (**Addison's disease**), or it may result secondarily from tumors, infections, pituitary hypofunction, or surgical removal. Under these circumstances, **glucocorticoids** and **aldosterone** become deficient.

A deficiency of aldosterone causes a decrease in sodium reabsorption in the renal tubules, an increased loss of sodium, chloride, and water, potassium retention, and a decrease in blood volume and cardiac output. If untreated, the patient may enter a potentially fatal **addisonian** crisis within a few days.

A concomitant deficiency also occurs in glucocorticoid hormones, which function in carbohydrate metabolism. As a result, gluconeogenesis is depressed and blood glucose falls between meals, producing a mild hypoglycemia. The patient may also have nausea, vomiting, diarrhea, anorexia, and weight loss.

The primary treatment for most patients is hormone replacement with medications. Sometimes, increased sodium chloride is given to reduce the need for the costly drug. The patient can then be advised to eat salty foods, salt his or her food generously, and take salt tablets. Patients may carry foods with carbohydrate, protein, and salt as a precaution. Cheese and crackers or salted nuts are useful for this purpose. The patient should also strive to maintain normal weight.

Adrenocortical Hyperfunction

Cushing's syndrome is due to excessive adrenocortical activity resulting from lesions in the hypothalamus or pituitary gland, which control adrenal function, or from lesions of the adrenal gland itself. It can also result from idiopathic hyperplasia of the adrenal cortex or excess corticosteroid medication.

The excess glucocorticoid causes increased gluconeogenesis, and the patient may become protein-depleted. Blood glucose levels may rise. All patients have abnormal glucose tolerances, and 20% develop diabetes mellitus. There are abnormal fat deposits, particularly in the face and over the clavicle. Excess aldosterone causes sodium and water retention and depletion of potassium. A high-protein, sodium-restricted diet sometimes is used for symptomatic relief; however, the main treatment is surgical resection of the adrenal glands. This procedure produces Addison's disease, which is easier to treat.

Adrenocorticotropic Hormone or Glucocorticoid Therapy

Adrenocorticotropic hormone (ACTH), which stimulates glucocorticoid production, or the glucocorticoids themselves are used in the treatment of many disorders. They are given particularly for their antiinflammatory and antiimmune effects and may be used for long periods in chronic inflammatory and autoimmune disorders and in transplant patients.

Over the long term, glucocorticoids stimulate gluconeogenesis, causing negative nitrogen balance with muscle wasting. At the same time, these drugs decrease insulin sensitivity and therefore are diabetogenic. A diet containing 1 g of protein per kilogram of body weight with liberal carbohydrate for protein sparing is recommended. Given the reduced insulin sensitivity, concentrated simple carbohydrates should be avoided.

Increased hydrochloric acid secretion may cause peptic ulcer; therefore, frequent small meals may be preferable. Antacids sometimes are recommended.

Water and electrolyte changes are variable. The patients receiving the drugs as replacement therapy may need added salts and fluid, as previously noted. Others may retain sodium and fluid and lose potassium, making sodium restriction to 1,000 mg/day helpful. Potassium intake may be increased with medication or high-potassium foods.

THYROID DYSFUNCTION

The thyroid gland secretes the hormones **triiodothyronine** (T_3), **thyroxine** (T_4), and **thyrocalcitonin**. These hormones control the metabolic rate, regulating carbohydrate and lipid metabolism and stimulating oxygen metabolism. They also control or promote growth and skeletal maturation, protein anabolism, and hematopoiesis. These effects result in increased heart rate and cardiac output and also increased mental acuity.

Hyperthyroidism

Hyperthyroidism (also known as **exophthalmic goiter, thyrotoxicosis, Graves' disease,** or **Basedow's disease**) may be an autoimmune disease. It can be treated by surgical excision of the thyroid gland, antithyroid drugs, or radioactive iodine.

Until such time as the hyperthyroidism is controlled, there are some metabolic effects that require nutritional care. In particular, the patients have an increased metabolic rate. If other fuels are not available, they will metabolize body protein, with a resulting negative nitrogen balance and muscle loss. They require a high-calorie diet which may reach 5,000 kcal, depending on the severity of the condition. Protein should be provided for maintenance plus replacement of any losses, usually 1 to 2 g per kilogram of body weight. High levels of carbohydrate should also be provided for protein sparing. Fortunately, these patients usually have a ravenous appetite. Mineral and vitamin supplements may be needed in proportion to the increase in the metabolic rate. Stimulants such as beverages containing caffeine and alcoholic beverages are restricted.

Hypothyroidism

A deficiency in activity or secretion of T_3 or T_4 or both is known as **hypothyroidism, Gull's disease, myxedema** (if advanced), or **Hashimoto's thyroiditis** in women. It can be caused by inadequate iodine, increased intake of goitrogens, an inborn error of metabolism, or idiopathic atrophy of the thyroid.

Hormone replacement by medication is the main feature of treatment. Some of the clinical manifestations also suggest the need for nutritional care. The metabolic rate decreases, and the patient may gain excess weight. A reduced-calorie diet then is indicated. Not all patients gain weight, since appetite may be depressed. The blood cholesterol level rises consequent to a decreased cholesterol breakdown. Reduction in dietary cholesterol may be useful. Lastly, patients often have decreased intestinal peristalsis with resulting constipation. A high-fiber diet with generous amounts of fluids is helpful.

OTHER NUTRITION-ENDOCRINE INTERRELATIONSHIPS

Almost every step in the body's handling of nutrients is affected by one or more hormones. Conversely, a person's nutritional status can have important effects on endocrine function. Only those circumstances in which nutritional care is of particular importance were discussed in this chapter. It is not possible to describe all the interrelationships that might occur. The nutritional care specialist should, nevertheless, be alert to the need for nutritional intervention in patients with other endocrine disturbances. It also is important to realize that the nutritional deprivation that occurs as a consequence of many disorders may seriously affect endocrine function.

Case Study: Insulin-Dependent Diabetes Mellitus

Debbie T., a 13-year-old girl, was admitted to the hospital with chief complaints of weight loss, thirst, and urinary frequency. Her mother reported that the child had lost approximately 9 lb. in 4 weeks. Thirst and frequent urination were particularly noticeable for the past week.

Examination revealed the following:

Weight	90 lb.
Height	62 in.

Urine glucose	4+
Urine acetone	Positive
Blood glucose	670 mg/dl

The following was written in the patient's chart:

S: Pt. C/O thirst, urgency, generally "feels bad."
O: BS = 670 mg/dl; U/A = 4+ glucose, large acetone
A: DM

P: Give RI until stabilized. Then adjust to NPH. Diet as recommended by dietitian.

An interview by the dietitian elicited the following 24-hour recall:

Breakfast	½ c. orange juice
	¾ c. cereal with ½ banana
	½ c. milk
Lunch	½ c. tuna salad
	2 slices bread
	1 peach
	½ pint milk
Snack	12 oz. soft drink
	"A few" potato chips
Dinner	Small hamburger with catsup
	⅓ c. buttered green beans
	⅙ apple pie
Snack	12 oz. soft drink

Exercises

1. Explain the reasons for the symptoms observed.
2. Why was the patient's blood glucose level elevated?
3. If the patient had not been treated promptly, how would her disease have progressed?
4. What diet would you recommend for this patient during her hospitalization?
5. Make a diet plan and write one day's sample menu.
6. How should the patient's diet be adjusted when she is discharged from the hospital? (Note: She swims daily from 4:00 to 5:00 P.M.)
7. Outline the information that the patient and her parents need to know to maintain her in good health.

Case Study: Diabetes Mellitus in the Elderly

(Adapted from a case study provided by Mary Ellen Collins, R.D., of Brigham and Women's Hospital, Boston, Mass.)

Millie R. is a 75-year-old woman living with her 80-year-old sister, for whom she is caring. They live in a low-income urban community in a third-floor walk-up apartment. Millie comes regularly to the Medical Clinic. She complained at her most recent visit of blurred vision, symptoms of polydipsia and polyuria, and a weight loss of 6 lb. in the past two weeks.

On admission to the hospital, her blood glucose measured 888 mg/dl. A diagnosis of urinary tract infection and nonketotic hyperglycemia was made.

You obtain the following information from her chart:

Medical history	Hypertension, congestive heart failure, asthma
Family history	Sister has had non-insulin-dependent diabetes mellitus for ten years
Current medications	Digoxin, furosemide (Lasix), hydrochlorothiazide, propranolol hydrochloride (Inderal), prednisone
Height	4 ft. 11 in.
Weight	119 lb. (usual weight 125 lb.)
Cholesterol	380 mg/dl

Subjective: "I'm the thinnest I've ever been and I'm too old to lose weight. I can't be more active because my asthma kicks up. I know about diabetes. My sister has it and she eats the way I do."

On questioning, the following 24-hour recall information was obtained:

Breakfast	2 large shredded wheat biscuits
	1 c. whole milk
	1 slice toast with margarine, jelly
Snack	½ grapefruit, 1 tsp. sugar
Dinner	1 pork chop, approximately 4 oz., with fat
	1 c. rice or potato with gravy
	Greens with salt pork
	2 slices bread with margarine
Snack	½ grapefruit, 1 tsp. sugar

Exercises

1. Explain the mechanism by which the patient's blood glucose level could become so high without producing ketosis.
2. If this patient were not treated, how would you expect her disease to progress?
3. Evaluate the patient's diet, based on the 24-hour recall.
4. What diet would you recommend for this patient?
5. Make a meal plan and write one day's menu.
6. Which items in her present diet would you like to replace with foods more appropriate for this patient?
7. What problems would you anticipate in instructing this patient on her diet?

References

1. Cryer, P.E., and Gerich, J.E. Relevance of glucose counterregulatory system to patients with diabetes. Critical role of glucagon and epinephrine. *Diabetes Care* 6:95, 1983.
2. Cryer, P.E., and Gerich, J.E. Glucose counterregulation, hypoglycemia and intensive insulin therapy in diabetes mellitus. *N. Engl. J. Med.* 313:232, 1985.
3. Gerich, J.E., Lorenzi, M., Karam, J.H., et al. Abnormal pancreatic glucagon secretion and postprandial hyperglycemia in diabetes mellitus. *J.A.M.A.* 234:159, 1975.
4. Unger, R.H., and Orci, L. Role of glucagon in diabetes. *Arch. Intern. Med.* 137:482, 1977.
5. Felig, P., Wahren, J., Sherwin, R., and Hendler, R. Insulin, glucagon, and somatostatin in normal physiology and diabetes mellitus. *Diabetes* 25:1091, 1976.
6. *Report of a WHO Study Group: Diabetes Mellitus.* Technical Report Series 727. Geneva: World Health Organization, 1985.
7. Krall, L.P., and Beaser, R.S. *Joslin Diabetes Manual*, 12th ed. Philadelphia: Lea & Febiger, 1989.
8. Bacchus, H. *Rational Management of Diabetes.* Baltimore: University Park Press, 1977.
9. West, K.M. Epidemiological evidence linking nutritional factors to the prevalence and manifestations of diabetes. *Acta Diabetol. Lat.* (Suppl.) 9(1):405, 1972.
10. McDevitt, H.O., and Bodmer, W.F. HL-A immune response genes, and disease. *Lancet* 1:1269, 1974.
11. Friedman, G.J. Diet in the treatment of diabetes mellitus. In R.S. Goodhart and M.E. Shils, Eds., *Modern Nutrition in Health and Disease*, 6th ed. Philadelphia: Lea and Febiger, 1980.
12. Kannel, W.B., Pearson, G., and McNamara, P.M. Obesity as a force of morbidity and mortality in adolescence. In F.P. Heald, Ed., *Adolescent Nutrition and Growth.* New York: Appleton-Century-Crofts, 1969.
13. Rao, R.H. The role of undernutrition in the pathogenesis of diabetes mellitus. *Diabetes Care* 7:595, 1984.
14. West, K.M., Oakley, E.L., Sanders, M.E., and Rubenstein, A.H. Nutritional factors in the etiology of diabetes. In H. Keen, Ed., *Epidemiology of Diabetes.* London: World Health Organization, 1977.
15. Cohen, A.M., Bavly, S., and Posnamski, R. Change of diet of Yemenite Jews in relation to diabetes and ischaemic heart disease. *Lancet* 2:1399, 1969.
16. Campbell, G.D. Diabetes in Asians and Africans in and around Durban. *S. Afr. Med. J.* 37:1195, 1963.
17. Reig, J.M., Fullmer, S.D., Pettigrew, K.D., et al. Nutrient intake of Pima Indian women. Relationships to diabetes mellitus and gallbladder disease. *Am. J. Clin. Nutr.* 24:1281, 1971.
18. West, K.M., and Kalbfleisch, J.M. Influence of nutritional factors on prevalence of diabetes. *Diabetes* 20:99, 1971.
19. Cohen, A.M., Briller, S., and Shafrir, E. Effect of long-term sucrose feeding on the activity of some enzymes regulating glycolysis, lipogenesis and gluconeogenesis in rat liver and adipose tissue. *Biochim. Biophys. Acta* 279:129, 1972.
20. Anderson, J.W., Herman, R.H., and Zakim, D. Effect of high glucose and high sucrose diet on glucose tolerance of normal men. *Am. J. Clin. Nutr.* 26:600, 1973.
21. Brunzell, J.D., Lerner, R.L., Porte, O., and Bierman, E.L. Effect of a fat free, high carbohydrate diet on diabetic subjects with fasting hypoglycemia. *Diabetes* 23:128, 1974.
22. Hildebrand, S.S., Ed. Is the risk of becoming diabetic affected by sugar consumption? *Proceedings of the Eighth International Sugar Research Foundation Conference.* Bethesda, Md.: International Sugar Research Foundation, 1974.
23. Campbell, G.O., Batchelor, E.L., and Goldberg, M.D. Sugar intake and diabetes. *Diabetes* 16:62, 1967.
24. Cohen, A.M. Environmental aspects of diabetes. *Isr. J. Med. Sci.* 18:358, 1972.
25. Kahn, H.A., Herman, J.B., Medalie, J.H., Neufeld, H.N., Ress, E., and Goldbourt, U. Factors related to diabetes incidence. A multivariate analysis of two years' observation on 10,000 men. *J. Chron. Dis.* 23:617, 1971.
26. Keen, H., Thomas, B.J., Jarrett, R.J., and Fuller, J.H. Nutrient intake, adiposity and diabetes. *Br. Med. J.* 1:655, 1979.
27. Wretlind, A. World sugar production and usage in Europe. In H. Sipple and K.W. McNutt, Eds., *Sugars in Nutrition.* New York: Academic Press, 1974.
28. Finter, N. Sugar substitutes in the treatment of obesity and diabetes mellitus. *Clin. Nutr.* 4:207, 1985.
29. Tomizawa, H.H. Mode of action of insulin degrading enzyme of beef liver. *J. Biol Chem.* 237:428, 1962.
30. Levine, R., and Goldstein, M.S. On the mechanism of action of insulin. *Recent Prog. Horm. Res.* 11:343, 1955.
31. Raskin, P., and Rosenstock, J. Blood glucose

control and diabetic complications. *Ann. Intern. Med.* 105:254, 1986.

32. Gabbay, K.H. Hyperglycemia, polyol metabolism and complications of diabetes mellitus. *Ann. Rev. Med.* 26:521, 1975.

33. Molitch, M.E. Complications of diabetes mellitus. In M.A. Powers, Ed., *Handbook of Diabetes Nutritional Management.* Rockville, Md.: Aspen, 1987.

34. Riddle, M.C. Relief of gastrointestinal symptoms by correcting insulin excess. *Diabetes Care* 4:296, 1981.

35. Shuman, C.R. Diabetes mellitus. In J.M. Kinney, K.N. Jeejeebhoy, G.L. Hill, and O.E. Owen, *Nutrition and Metabolism in Patient Care.* Philadelphia: Saunders, 1988.

36. Koenig, R.J., and Cerami, A. Hemoglobin A_{1c} and diabetes mellitus. *Ann. Rev. Med.* 31:29, 1980.

37. Gonen, B., Rubenstein, A.H., Rockman, H., et al. Haemoglobin A_1: An indicator of the metabolic control of diabetic patients. *Lancet* 2:734, 1977.

38. Block, M.B., Rosenfield, R.L., Mako, M.E., et al. Sequential changes in beta-cell function in insulin-treated diabetic patients assessed by C-peptide immunoreactivity. *N. Engl. J. Med.* 288:1144, 1973.

39. Powers, M.A., ed. *Nutrition Guide for Professionals: Diabetes Education and Meal Planning.* Alexandria, Va: American Diabetes Association, and Chicago, Ill.: American Dietetic Association, 1988.

40. Beebe, C.A. Self blood glucose monitoring. An adjunct to dietary and insulin management of the patient with diabetes. *J. Am. Diet. Assoc.* 87:61, 1987.

41. Jovanovic, L., and Peterson, C.M. Is home blood glucose monitoring for you? *Diabetes Forecast* 33(4):30, 1980.

42. Peterson, C.M., Forhan, S.E., and Jones, R.L. Self-management. An approach to patients with insulin-dependent diabetes mellitus. *Diabetes Care* 3:82, 1980.

43. Schneider, J.M., Huddleston, J.F., Curet, L.B., and Menzel, D.L. Pregnancy complicating ambulatory patient management of diabetes. *Diabetes Care* 3:7, 1980.

44. Ziegler, O., Kolopp, M., Gott, I., Genton, P., Debry, G., and Dronin, P. Reliability of self-monitoring of blood glucose by CSII-treated patients with type I diabetes. *Diabetes Care* 12:184, 1989.

45. Gonger-Frederick, L.A., Julian, D.A., Cox, D.J., Clarke, W.L., and Carter, W.R. Self-measurement of blood glucose. Accuracy of self-reported data and adherence to recommended regimen. *Diabetes Care* 11:579, 1988.

46. McDermott, D., Cooks, M., and Peterson, C.M. Patient-determined glycosylated hemoglobin measurements. An aid to patient education. *Diabetes Care* 4:480, 1981.

47. Lebovitz, H.E., and Feinglos, M.N. Sulfonylurea drugs. Mechanism of antidiabetic action and therapeutic usefulness. *Diabetes Care* 1:189, 1978.

48. American Diabetes Association. The UGDP controversy. *Diabetes Care* 2:1, 1979.

49. Levine, R., and Smith, M. Antidiabetic drugs. In W. Modell, Ed., *Drugs of Choice 1976–1977.* St. Louis: C.V. Mosby, 1976.

50. Skyler, J.S., Seigler, D.E., and Reeves, M.L. Optimizing pumped insulin delivery. *Diabetes Care* 5:135, 1982.

51. Raskin, P. Treatment of type I diabetes with portable insulin infusion devices. *Diabetes Care* 5(Suppl. 1): 48, 1982.

52. Lecavalier, L., et al. Effects of continuous subcutaneous insulin infusion versus multiple injections on insulin receptors in insulin-dependent diabetes. *Diabetes Care* 10:300, 1987.

53. American Diabetes Association. Nutritional recommendations and principles for individuals with diabetes mellitus, 1986. *Diabetes Care* 10:126, 1987.

54. Special Report Committee, Canadian Diabetes Association. Guidelines for the nutritional management of diabetes mellitus. *J. Can. Diet. Assoc.* 42:110, 1981.

55. Nuttall, F.Q. Diet and the diabetic patient. *Diabetes Care* 6:197, 1983.

56. Godine, J.E. The relationship between metabolic control and vascular complications of diabetes mellitus. *Med. Clin. North Am.* 72:1271, 1988.

57. Bierman, E.L., Albrink, M.J., Arky, R.A., et al. Special report. Principles of nutrition and dietary recommendations for patients with diabetes mellitus. *Diabetes* 20:633, 1971.

58. West, K.M. Diet therapy of diabetes. An analysis of failure. *Ann. Intern. Med.* 79:425, 1973.

59. American Diabetes Association and the American Dietetic Association. *Exchange Lists for Meal Planning.* Chicago: American Dietetic Association and American Diabetes Association, 1986.

60. Spiller, G.A., and Kay, R.M., Eds. *Medical Aspects of Dietary Fiber.* New York: Plenum, 1980.

61. Vinik, A.I., and Jenkins, D.J.A., Dietary fiber in the management of diabetes. *Diabetes Care* 11:160, 1988.

62. Anderson, J.W. Fiber and Health. An overview. *Am. J. Gastroenterol.* 81:891, 1986.

63. Anderson, J.W. Dietary fiber. Diabetes and obesity. *Am. J. Gastroenterol.* 81:898, 1986.

64. Brunzell, J.D., Lerner, R.L., Hazzard, W.R., et al. Improved glucose tolerance with high carbohydrate feeding in mild diabetes. *N. Engl. J. Med.* 284:521, 1971.

65. Kay, R.M., Grobin, W., and Track, N.S. Diets rich in natural fiber improve carbohydrate tolerance in maturity-onset, non–insulin dependent diabetes. *Diabetologia* 20:18, 1981.

66. Jenkins, D.J.A., Leeds, A.R., Gassull, M.A., Cochet, B., and Alberti, K.G.M.M. Decrease in postprandial insulin and glucose concentrations for guar and pectin. *Ann. Intern. Med.* 86:20, 1977.

67. Anderson, J.W. Dietary fiber in nutrition management of diabetes. In G.V. Vahouny and D. Kritchevsky, Eds., *Dietary Fiber in Health and Disease.* New York: Plenum, 1986, pp. 343–360.

68. Hollenbeck, C.B., Coulston, A.M. and Reaven, G.M. To what extent does increased dietary fiber improve glucose and lipid metabolism in patients with noninsulin-dependent diabetes (NIDDM)? *Am. J. Clin. Nutr.* 43:16, 1986.

69. Hollenbeck, C.B., Coulston, M.S., and Reaven, G.M. Glycemic effects of carbohydrates. A different perspective. *Diabetes Care* 9:641, 1986.

70. Anderson, J.W., Lin, W.-J., and Ward, K. Composition of foods commonly used in diets for persons with diabetes. *Diabetes Care* 1:293, 1978.

71. Anderson, J.W., and Bridges, S.R. Dietary fiber content of selected foods. *Am. J. Clin. Nutr.* 47:440, 1988.

72. Kessler, I.I., and Clark, J.P. Saccharin, cyclamate and human bladder cancer. *J.A.M.A.* 240:349, 1978.

73. Morrison, A.S., and Buring, J.E. Artificial sweeteners and cancer of the lower urinary tracts. *N. Engl. J. Med.* 302:537, 1980.

74. Egeberg, R.O., Steinfeld, J.L., Frantz, I., et al. Report to the Secretary of HEW from the Medical Advisory Group on Cyclamates. *J.A.M.A.* 211:1358, 1970.

75. National Research Council. *Evaluation of Cyclamate for Carcinogenicity.* Washington, D.C.: National Academy Press, 1983.

76. American Dietetic Association. Appropriate use of nutritive and non-nutritive sweeteners: Technical support paper. *J. Am. Diet. Assoc.* 87:1690, 1987.

77. Brunzell, J.D. Use of fructose, xylitol or sorbitol as a sweetener in diabetes mellitus. *Diabetes Care* 1:223, 1978.

78. Brunzell, J.D. Use of fructose, sorbitol, or xylitol as a sweetener in diabetes mellitus. *J. Am. Diet. Assoc.* 73:499, 1978.

79. Bohannon, N.V., Karam, J.H., and Forsham, P.H. Advantages of fructose ingestion over sucrose and glucose in humans. *Diabetes* 27(Suppl. 2):438, 1978.

80. Crapo, P.A., Kolterman, O.G., and Henry, R.R. Metabolic consequence of two-week fructose feeding in diabetic subjects. *Diabetes Care* 9:111, 1986.

81. *The Physician's Guide to Type II Diabetes (NIDDM): Diagnosis and Treatment.* Alexandria, Va.: American Diabetes Association, 1984.

82. Anderson, J.W., Story, L.J., Zettwoch, N.C., Gustafson, N.J., and Jefferson, B.S. Metabolic effects of fructose supplementation in diabetic individuals. *Diabetes Care* 12:337, 1989.

83. Akgun, S., and Ertel, H.H. The effects of sucrose, fructose and high-fructose corn syrup meals on plasma glucose and insulin in non-insulin-dependent diabetic subjects. *Diabetes Care* 8:279, 1985.

84. Gabbay, K.H. The sorbitol pathway and the complications of diabetes. *N. Engl. J. Med.* 288:831, 1973.

85. Steinke, J., Wood, F.C., Domenge, L., et al. Evolution of sorbitol in the diet of diabetic children at camp. *Diabetes* 10:218, 1961.

86. American Dietetic Association. Position of the American Dietetic Association. Appropriate use of nutritive and non-nutritive sweeteners. *J. Am. Diet. Assoc.* 87:1689, 1987.

87. Walsch, D.H., and O'Sullivan, D.J. Effects of moderate alcohol intake on control of diabetes. *Diabetes* 23:440, 1974.

88. Green, J.A., and Holler, H.J. *Meal Planning Approaches in the Nutrition Management of the Person with Diabetes.* Chicago: American Dietetic Association, 1987.

89. Green, J.A. Meal planning approaches for nutritional management of diabetes. In M.A. Powers, Ed., *Handbook of Diabetes Nutritional Management.* Rockville, Md.: Aspen, 1987.

90. Anderson, J.W., Gustafson, N.J., Bryant, C.A. and Tietyen-Clark, J. Dietary fiber and diabetes. A comprehensive review and practical application. *J. Am. Diet. Assoc.* 87:1189, 1987.

91. Schade, D.S., et al. Future therapy of the insulin-dependent diabetic patient—The implantable insulin delivery system. *Diabetes Care* 4:319, 1981.

92. Hamet, P., et al. Patient self-management of continuous subcutaneous insulin infusion. *Diabetes Care* 5:485, 1982.

93. Crapo, P.A., Insel, J., Sperling, M. and Kolterman, O.G. Comparison of serum glucose, insulin and glucagon responses to different types of complex carbohydrate in non-insulin-dependent diabetic patients. *Am. J. Clin. Nutr.* 34:184, 1981.

94. Jenkins, D.J.A., Wolever, T.M.S., Thorne, M.J., Jenkins, A.L., Wong, G.S., Josse, R.G., and Csima, A. The relationship between glycemic response, digestibility and factors influencing the dietary habits of diabetics. *Am. J. Clin. Nutr.* 40:1175, 1984.

95. Jenkins, D.J.A., Wolever, T.M.S., Taylor, R.H., Barker, H.M., Fielden, H., Baldsin, J.M., Bowling, A.C., Newman, H.C., Jenkins, A.L. and Goff, D.V. Glycemic index of foods. A physiological basis for carbohydrate exchange. *Am. J. Clin. Nutr.* 34:362, 1981.

96. Jenkins. D.J.A., Wolever, T.M.S. and Jenkins, A.L. Starchy foods and glycemic index. *Diabetes Care* 11:149, 1988.

97. Collier, G., and O'Dea, K. Effect of physical form of carbohydrate on the post-prandial glucose, insulin and GIP responses in Type II diabetes. *Am. J. Clin. Nutr.* 36:10, 1982.

98. Wong, S., and O'Dea, K. Importance of physical form rather than viscosity in determining the rate of starch hydrolysis in legumes. *Am. J. Clin. Nutr.* 37:66, 1983.

99. Jenkins, D.J.A., Wolever, T.M.S., Taylor, P.H., Ghafari, H., Jenkins, A.L., Barber, H., and Jenkins, M.J.A. Rate of digestion of foods and post-prandial glycaemia in normal and diabetic subjects. *Brit. Med. J.* 2:14, 1980.

100. Jenkins, D.J. Lente carbohydrates. A newer approach to the dietary management of diabetes. *Diabetes Care* 5:634, 1982.

101. Jenkins, D., Wolever, T., Wong, G.S., Kenshole, A., Josse, R.G., Thompson, L.U., and Lam, K.Y. Glycemic responses to food. Possible differences between insulin-dependent and non–insulin dependent diabetics. *Am. J. Clin. Nutr.* 40:971, 1984.

102. Coulston, A.M., Hollenbeck, C.B., Swislocki, A.L.M., and Reaven, G.M. Effect of source of dietary carbohydrate on plasma glucose and insulin responses to mixed meals in subjects with NIDDM. *Diabetes Care* 10:395, 1987.

103. Bantle, J.P., Laine, D.C., Castle, G.W., Thomas, J.W., Hoogwerf, B.J., and Goetz, F.C. Post-prandial glucose and insulin responses to meals containing different carbohydrates in normal and diabetic subjects. *N. Engl. J. Med.* 309:7, 1983.

104. Coulston, A.M., Hollenbeck, C.B., Liu, G.C., Williams, R.A., Starich, G.H., Massaferri, E.L., and Reaven, G.M. Effect of source of dietary carbohydrate on plasma glucose, insulin, and gastric inhibitory polypeptide responses to test meals in subjects with non-insulin-dependent diabetes mellitus. *Am. J. Clin. Nutr.* 40:965, 1984.

105. Nuttall, F.Q., Mooradian, A.D., DeMarais, R., and Parker, S. The glycemic effect of different meals approximately isocaloric and similar in protein, carbohydrate and fat content as calculated using the ADA exchange lists. *Diabetes Care* 6:432, 1983.

106. Laine, D.C., Thomas, W., Levitt, M.D., and Bantle, J.P. Comparison of predictive capabilities of diabetic exchange lists and glycemic index of foods. *Diabetes Care* 10:387, 1987.

107. Berger, M., Hagg, S., and Ruderman, N.B. Glucose metabolism in perfused skeletal muscle. *Biochem. J.* 147:231, 1975.

108. Franz, M.J. Exercise and the management of diabetes mellitus. *J. Am. Diet. Assoc.* 87:872, 1987.

109. Bogardus, C., Ravussin, E., Robbins, D.C., Wolfe, R.R., Horton, E.S., and Sims, E.A.H. Effects of physical training and diet therapy on carbohydrate metabolism in patients with glucose intolerance and non–insulin dependent diabetes. *Diabetes* 33:311, 1984.

110. Saltin, B., Lindgarde, F., Houston, H., et al. Physical training and glucose tolerance in middle-aged men with chemical diabetes. *Diabetes* 28:30, 1978.

111. Ruderman, N.B., Ganda, O.P., and Johansen, K. The effect of physical training on glucose tolerance and plasma lipids in maturity-onset diabetes. *Diabetes* 28:89, 1978.

112. Leon, A.S. *Nutrition and Athletic Performance.* Palo Alto, Calif.: Bull Publishing, 1981.

113. Berger, M., Berchtold, P., Cuppers, H.J., et al. Metabolic and hormonal effects of muscular exercise in juvenile type diabetes. *Diabetologia* 13:355, 1977.

114. Wahren, J., Felig, P., and Hagenfeldt, L. Physical exercise and fuel homeostasis in diabetes mellitus. *Diabetologia* 14:213, 1978.

115. Betschart, J. Exercise. *D.C.&E. Newsletter* 8:3, 1987.

116. American Diabetes Association. *Diabetes Forecast.*

117. Schmitt, B.D. An argument for the unmeasured diet in juvenile diabetes mellitus. *Clin. Pediatr.* (Phila.) 14:68, 1975.

118. Malone, J.T. Nutrition and childhood diabetes. In L.A. Barness, Ed., *Nutrition in Medical Practice.* Westport, Conn.: AVI, 1981.

119. Thorp, F.K. Infants and children. In M.A. Powers, Ed., *Handbook of Diabetes Nutritional Management.* Rockville, Md.: Aspen, 1987.

120. Miller, E.M., Hare, J.W., Cloherty, J.R., et al. Major congenital anomalies and elevated hemoglobin A_{1c} in early weeks of diabetic pregnancy. *N. Engl. J. Med.* 304:1331, 1981.

121. Reid, M., Hadden, D., Harley, J.M.G., et al. Fetal malformations in diabetics with high haemoglobin A_{1c} in early pregnancy, letter. *Br. Med. J.* 189:1001, 1984.

122. Ylinen, K., Aula, P., Stenman, U.-H., et al. Risk of minor and major malformations in diabetics with high haemoglobin A_{1c} values in early pregnancy. *Br. Med. J.* 189:345, 1984.

123. Fuhrmann, K., Reiher, H., Semmler, E., et al. Prevention of congenital malformations in infants of insulin-dependent diabetic mothers. *Diabetes Care* 6:219, 1983.

124. Ruhrmann, K., Reiher, H., Semmler, K., et al. The effect of intensified conventional insulin therapy before and during pregnancy on the malformation rate in offspring of diabetic mothers. *Exp. Clin. Endocrinol.* 83:173, 1984.

125. Eriksson, U. Diabetes in pregnancy. Retarded fetal growth, congenital malformations and feto-maternal concentrations of zinc, copper, and manganese in the rat. *J. Nutr.* 114:477, 1984.

126. Sheehan, E.A., Beck, F., Clarke, C.A., et al. Effects of beta-hydroxybutyrate on rat embryos growth in cultures. *Experientia* 41:273, 1985.

127. Goldman, A., Baker, L., Piddington, R.L., et al. Hyperglycemia-induced teratogenesis is mediated by a functional deficiency of arachidonic acid. *Proc. Natl. Acad. Sci. USA* 82:8227, 1985.

128. Freinkel, N., Lewis, N.J., Akazawa, S., et al. The honeybee syndrome. Implications of the teratogenicity of mannose in rat-embryo culture. *N. Engl. J. Med.* 310:223, 1984.

129. Powers, M.A., Metzger, B.E., and Freinkel, N. Pregnancy and diabetes. In M.A. Powers, Ed., *Handbook of Diabetes Nutritional Management.* Rockville, Md.: Aspen, 1987.

130. Hollingsworth, D.R. *Pregnancy, Diabetes and Birth.* Baltimore: Williams and Wilkins, 1984.

131. Gaare, J.M., and O'Sullivan-Maillet, J. Surgery and surgical nutrition in diabetes. In M.A. Powers, Ed., *Handbook of Diabetes Nutritional Management.* Rockville, Md.: Aspen, 1987.

132. Michael, S. R., and Sabo, C.F. Management of the diabetic patient receiving nutritional support. *Nutr. Care Practice* 4:179, 1989.

133. Lefebver, P.J., and Luyckx, A.S. Spontaneous and insulin-induced hypoglycemia. In K. Sussman and R. Metz, Eds., *Diabetes Mel-litus,* 4th ed. Philadelphia: W.B. Saunders, 1975.

134. Freinkel, N., and Metzger, B.E. Oral glucose tolerance curve and hypoglycemias in the fed state. *N. Engl. J. Med.* 280:820, 1969.

135. Unger, R.H., and Medison, L.L. Comparison of response to intravenously administered sodium tolbutamide in mild diabetic and non diabetic subjects. *J. Clin. Invest.* 37:627, 1958.

136. Fajans, S.S., Schneider, J.M., Schteingart, D.O., and Conn, J.W. The diagnostic value of sodium tolbutamide in hypoglycemic states. *J. Clin. Endocrinol. Metabol.* 21:371, 1961.

137. Fajans, S.S. Leucine-induced hypoglycemia. *N. Engl. J. Med.* 272:1224, 1965.

138. Conn, J.W. The advantage of a high protein diet in the treatment of spontaneous hypoglycemia. *J. Clin. Invest.* 15:673, 1936.

139. Pemberton, C.M., and Gastineau, C.F. *Mayo Clinic Diet Manual.* Philadelphia: W.B. Saunders, 1981.

Bibliography

Borensztajn, J., Ed. *Lipoprotein Lipase.* Chicago: Evener, 1987.

Brownlee, M., Ed. *Handbook of Diabetes Mellitus,* vols. 1–5. New York: Garland STPM Press, 1981.

Brudenell, M., and Doddridge, M. C. *Diabetic Pregnancy.* Edinburgh: Churchill Livingstone, 1989.

Ellenberg, M., and Rifkin, H., Eds. *Diabetes Mellitus: Theory and Practice,* 3rd ed. New York: Medical Examination Publishing, 1983.

Fain, J.N. Mode of action of oral hypoglycemia drugs. *Fed. Proc.* 36:2712, 1977.

Horton, E.S., and Terjung, R.L., Eds. *Exercise, Nutrition and Energy Metabolism.* New York: Pergamon Press, 1989.

Schade, D.S., Eaton, R.P., Alberti, K.G.M.M., and Johnston, D.G. *Diabetic Coma.* Albuquerque: University of New Mexico Press, 1981.

Williams, R.H. *Textbook of Endocrinology,* 7th ed. Philadelphia: W.B. Saunders, 1985.

Zeman, F.J., and Ney, D.M. *Applications of Clinical Nutrition.* Englewood Cliffs, N.J.: Prentice-Hall, 1988.

Sources of Current Information

Diabetes
Diabetes Care
Diabetologia
Journal of Clinical Endocrinology and Metabolism
Recent Progress in Hormone Research

12. Disorders of Energy Balance and Body Weight

I. Adipose Tissue
II. Some Definitions of Terms
III. Control of Energy Balance
  A. Control of food intake
    1. Central controls
    2. Peripheral control mechanisms
      a. gastrointestinal factors
      b. liver metabolism
      c. adipose tissue
      d. endocrine factors
      e. sensory factors
      f. cortical factors
  B. Control of energy expenditure
    1. Types of energy expenditure
      a. obligatory thermogenesis
        (1) resting metabolic expenditure
        (2) endothermic thermogenesis
      b. facultative thermogenesis
        (1) thermic effect of exercise
        (2) thermic effect of feeding
        (3) adaptive thermogenesis
    2. Mechanisms of control
IV. Obesity
  A. Diagnosis
    1. Research methods
    2. Comparison with tables of ideal weight
    3. Triceps skinfold
    4. Height-weight ratios
    5. Bioelectrical impedence
    6. Rapid self-assessment methods
  B. Classification of obesities
    1. Classification according to pathogenesis
    2. Etiologic classification
      a. genetic factors
      b. hypothalamic obesity
      c. endocrine disorders
      d. physical inactivity
      e. nutritional factors
      f. overfeeding of children
      g. physiologic and psychic trauma
      h. environmental factors
      i. factors of psychological origin
    3. Anatomic classification of fat distribution
      a. localized fat accumulations
      b. generalized fat distribution
        (1) somatotypes
        (2) gynecoid versus android distribution
        (3) hyperplastic versis hypertrophic obesity
    4. Classification by age of onset
  C. Hazards of obesity
  D. Metabolic alterations in obesity
    1. Effects of increased adipose cell size on its metabolism
    2. Effects on metabolism in general
    3. Physiologic responses to energy deficit during weight loss
    4. Immune factors in obesity
  E. Treatment
    1. Dietary treatment
      a. conventional restricted-calorie diet
      b. formula diets
      c. fasting or starvation
      d. packaged food programs
      e. fad diets
        (1) low-carbohydrate or no-carbohydrate diets
        (2) diets emphasizing few foods
        (3) interference with digestion, absorption, or metabolism
    2. Other aids to weight reduction
      a. exercise
      b. behavior modification
      c. group counseling
      d. drugs
        (1) anorectics
        (2) bulking agents
        (3) metabolic affectors
      e. acupuncture
      f. surgery
        (1) lipectomy and liposuction
        (2) intragastric balloon therapy
        (3) bypass procedures
        (4) gastric restrictive surgery
        (5) jaw wiring
      g. psychotherapy

h. hypnosis
3. Most highly
recommended
therapy for obesity
F. Psychological factors
in obesity
G. Aspects of nutritional
assessment and
monitoring
H. Prevention of obesity

I. Effects of repeated
cycles of weight loss
and gain
V. Underweight
A. Underweight in general
1. Etiology
2. General effects
3. Treatment
B. Anorexia nervosa
1. Etiology

2. Clinical manifesta-
tions
3. Nutritional Assess-
ment
4. Treatment
C. Bulimia nervosa
1. Effects
2. Nutritional Assess-
ment
3. Treatment
VI. Case Studies

Increased and decreased body weights are of concern if either is extreme. In terms of numbers of patients, excess body weight is the more common problem presented to the nutritional care specialist and is considered one of the most prevalent public health problems in the United States. Whereas many people maintain normal body weight with little effort, many others struggle to lose or gain weight to bring their body weights within the limits that are considered desirable in American society. In this chapter, problems characterized by excess or insufficient body weight — that is, obesity and underweight — will be explored first by presenting some general principles and then by a discussion of the etiologies, effects, and various approaches to treatment of obesity and underweight.

Energy intake may consist of food or infused nutrients, and total energy expenditure is the sum of energy used for resting metabolism, physical work, maintenance of body temperature, and thermogenic effects of food. The laws of thermodynamics that govern the universe also apply to human beings and other animals. If a person has an energy intake that is greater than his or her output, he or she is in **positive energy balance** and will store energy and gain weight, primarily as fat. If energy use is greater than energy intake, a person will be in **negative energy balance** and will lose weight. The principle is very simple, but difficulties arise in understanding why some people cannot maintain weight within normal limits.

We do not understand the reasons for the positive energy balance in overweight patients, whether it be the consequence of excess food intake or decreased activity. It is no more helpful to say that a person is fat because he or she eats too much than to say a person is an alcoholic because he or she drinks too much, although we have tended to simplify the problem in this manner. Because our understanding of the control mechanisms is limited, excess body weight can be a problem that is resistant to known methods of treatment.

ADIPOSE TISSUE

Since energy is conserved, that energy which is consumed in excess of requirement will be stored as chemical energy. In the adult, the major storage form of this energy is triglyceride. The tissue that stores body fat is known as **adipose** (fatty) **tissue** and the individual cells are **adipose cells**. In many other chapters of this text, we discussed diseases of a specific organ or organ system. In this chapter, we will consider the adipose tissue as an organ or perhaps as an organ system that is distributed at a number of sites throughout the body, as is the immune system.

There are two types of adipose tissue, white and brown. **White adipose tissue** (WAT) differentiates at three to four months of gestation from mesoderm and is a form of connective tissue. It is located predominantly around the kidneys and in the abdominal cavity (omental fat), under the skin, and between skeletal muscle fibers. Its primary function is to store energy.

Each cell of white adipose tissue contains a thin layer of cytoplasm surrounding triglyceride in a single droplet (**monolocular**), the size of which determines the size of the cell. The cell nucleus lies in the thin layer of cytoplasm so that a cross section of a lipid-filled cell that passes through the nucleus looks like a signet ring.

Brown adipose tissue (BAT) is located between the muscles of the neck and back, in the **axillae** (armpits) and groin, and around the viscera of the abdomen and thorax. In the cells of brown adipose tissue, the fat exists as multiple droplets (**multilocular**). The cells are only approximately 10% of the size of white adipose tissue cells, but they have larger mitochondria in greater numbers.

Brown fat is well developed in newborn infants and will oxidize its fat during exposure to cold in order to produce heat (**nonshivering thermogenesis**). The large mitochondria are important in this process. The heat warms nearby tissue and is carried elsewhere in the body by the circulation. The thermogenesis apparently is accomplished by means of a futile cycle in which triglycerides are hydrolyzed to fatty acids, then to their coenzyme A derivatives, and back to triglycerides. In this process, high-energy phosphate is expended. ATP is hydrolyzed to AMP and inorganic phosphate and then regenerated. The net result is the combustion of fuel that generates heat but accomplishes nothing else. As a consequence, BAT metabolism is currently under investigation as a means by which excess calories might be dissipated as heat rather than stored as adipose tissue.

There is some dispute on the question of whether BAT and WAT differentiate from the same or two different precursor cells, whether they are two entirely separate categories of cells or the two extremes of a continuum of types, whether one type can be transformed to the other, and, if so, what are the control mechanisms involved.[1-3]

Nonshivering thermogenesis is easily demonstrated in newborn infants. Some brown adipose tissue has also been shown, by histologic methods, to be present in adult men and women.[4] Its metabolism in the adult is under investigation.

A 70-kg man contains, on the average, 9 to 13 kg of adipose tissue, of which approximately 80% is triglyceride. However, the total weight of adipose tissue has been reported to be capable of varying as much as a thousandfold, a change which is greater than that of any other organ in the body while still being compatible with life. The amount varies normally with sex. In proportion to body weight, it is greater in women than in men. It also varies with age. It comprises approximately 28% of body weight at birth and 20% at one year of age. It then tends to remain constant until puberty when there may be another period of increase in girls. Usually in boys, there is a decrease at puberty.

The increase in adipose tissue can occur, as it does in other organs, by an increase in the number of cells or an increase in the size of the cells or both. However, it currently is believed that a decrease in "adipose organ" size occurs only by a decrease in the size of adipose cells, not by a decrease in the number of cells.

At one time, adipose tissue was considered to be a rather static, nonreactive tissue that provided padding and insulation from cold and was a passive recipient of excess calories. It now is appreciated that adipose tissue is in a continuous state of flux and is important in many metabolic processes.

Adipose cells form and store triglycerides and also release fatty acids for energy. When the body is not in a fed state, the supply of carbohydrate for energy is depleted in a matter of hours (see Chapter 11). Thus adipose tissue serves an important function in making us independent of food intake, which otherwise would have to occur every few hours.

Theoretically, the adipose cell can acquire fatty acids by three routes. They are acquired primarily after release from lipoproteins, a reaction catalyzed by lipoprotein lipase. In addition, fatty acids may be synthesized within the adipose cell from excess glucose.

In the presence of insulin, glucose entry into cells and synthesis of fatty acids from glucose are increased. Fatty acids may also be acquired from those circulating in the plasma bound to albumin.

Adipose tissue has two lipase systems, each with its own regulatory system. **Lipoprotein lipase** (LPL) catalyzes the reactions by which plasma triglyceride is metabolized to free fatty acids for triglyceride synthesis within the adipose cell. Lipoprotein lipase activity is increased following food intake, possibly owing to increased insulin levels. Thyroid hormone also increases in activity. In humans, the adipose cell is believed to get most of its fatty acids by esterifying preformed fatty acids, and very little by synthesis from glucose within the cells.

The other lipase, **hormone-sensitive lipase**, catalyzes the metabolism of triglyceride within the adipose cell for release of free fatty acids into the plasma. It is inhibited by insulin. Details of the reactions involving these lipases and their control are given in Chapter 11.

SOME DEFINITIONS OF TERMS

Before we consider body weight control mechanisms, some definitions are necessary. **Hunger** is defined as a craving that arises physiologically from the body's need for food. The sensations usually are unpleasant. Hunger occasionally is used to refer to a craving or need for other materials, such as "air hunger," but this use of the term is less common. In contrast to hunger, **appetite** is a natural desire for a specific food that is stimulated by the sight, smell, and thought of food. It is strongly influenced by memory and other associations. **Satiety** refers to the complete absence of hunger. It occurs very rapidly. **Anorexia** is the abnormal absence of a desire for food at a time of physiological need for food and when the desire for food would be expected.

The energy content of food is measured most commonly in **kilocalories**, often loosely called **calories**, particularly in the popular literature. A proposal to convert units of energy from calories or kilocalories to joules and kilojoules has received some attention. To review, the **joule** is the **work** done in moving a mass a distance of 1 m against a force of 1 newton. A newton is the force that will move a mass of 1 kg with an acceleration of 1 m/sec/sec. The **kilocalorie** (kcal) is the amount of **heat** required to raise the temperature of 1 kg of water 1°C from 14.5° to 15.5°C. There are 1,000 calories in a kilocalorie. The kilojoule is equal to 0.239 kcal, or a kilocalorie equals 4.184 kJ. The conversion can thus be made by applying the formula

$$kJ = kcal \times 4.184 \qquad \text{(12-1)}$$

In the calculation of the energy of nutrients, then, we have:

Carbohydrate	1 g = 4 kcal	= 17 kJ
Protein	1 g = 4 kcal	= 17 kJ
Fat	1 g = 9 kcal	= 37.6 kJ
Alcohol	1 g = 7 kcal	= 29.3 kJ

Most patients will not be familiar with joules but will have some concept of a calorie. Therefore, it is necessary for the nutritional care specialist to continue to use this term in contacts with patients. On the other hand, the joule is increasingly used in the scientific literature, and so the nutritional care specialist must understand its meaning to read the professional literature. Because tables of food values and estimations of energy expenditure useful to the nutritional care specialist give values in kilocalories, that is the term used in this text.

CONTROL OF ENERGY BALANCE

There is evidence that a control mechanism exists for the maintenance of a normal proportion of adipose tissue, estimated to be approximately 120 g/kg of body weight in men and 260 g/kg of body weight in women. Since energy balance relates energy intake to energy expenditure, it is intake and use that, in the final analysis, are the possible points of regulation.

Control of Food Intake

The central nervous system (CNS) integrates the overall control of food intake. To understand the control processes completely, we would have to know three things. First, we would need to know how the central nervous system is informed of the nutrient status. Second, we would need to know how that information is integrated with information on nutrient needs, previously learned knowledge of specific foods, and other related matters. Last, the process by which the decision to eat is translated into eating activity in a given environment would have to be understood. At the present time, we do not have a complete knowledge of any of these phases of food intake control. However, some facts are known, and theories are plentiful. The control mechanisms are considered

Figure 12-1. Cross section of rat brain showing location of paired ventromedial hypothalami, lateral hypothalami, and paraventricular hypothalami, along with selected surrounding tissues.

to be divided into central and peripheral effects, although the distinction is not always clear.

Central Controls

Experiments with animals have demonstrated that central influences on eating activity involve many areas of the brain. Among these, the hypothalamus, an area at the base of the brain that serves as the main controlling center of the autonomic nervous system (Figure 12-1), has been studied extensively. Within the hypothalamus, there are cell aggregations that participate in the control of food intake. The **ventromedial nuclei** or **ventromedial hypothalami** (VMH) have been considered to act as a center for satiety. Nearby on either side are another pair of centers, the **lateral nuclei** or **lateral hypothalami** (LH). Normally, when the VMH is stimulated, it inhibits the LH. The animal will continue to eat unless the VMH turns off the LH system.

If the fiber tracts lateral to the VMH are destroyed, the inhibition of LH is removed, and a laboratory rat will overeat (**hyperphagia**).[5] Destruction of the VMH itself is associated with hyperinsulinemia and hypothalamic obesity. Destruction of either the VMH or associated fiber tracts is associated with hyperactivity of the vagus nerve. In contrast,

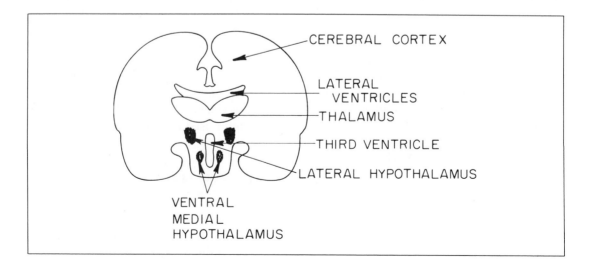

CEREBRAL CORTEX

LATERAL VENTRICLES

THALAMUS

THIRD VENTRICLE

LATERAL HYPOTHALAMUS

VENTRAL MEDIAL HYPOTHALAMUS

if the LH is destroyed, a rat will stop eating (**aphagia**). In people in whom the VMH or LH has been damaged by a tumor or trauma, the response has been shown to resemble that seen in the rat, with the hypothalamus serving as an integrating and relay station for food intake control.

In addition, the **paraventricular nuclei** (PVN) lie anterior and dorsal in the medial hypothalamus and are believed to act as integrators of influences on satiety. Laterally, a **perifornical region** (PFR) of the hypothalamus integrates the influences on feeding.[6] The fornix is a nerve tract of the hippocampus. It arches over the thalamus and terminates mostly in the mammillary bodies of the hypothalamus. A diagram of a medial

Figure 12-2. Medial view of the human brain showing structures involved in control of food intake. **1.** *Mammillary body;* **2.** *Fornix;* **3.** *Thalamus;* **4.** *Corpus callosum;* **5.** *Hypothalamus;* **6.** *Paraventricular nucleus;* **7.** *Dorsomedial nucleus;* **8.** *Ventromedial nucleus.*

view of the hypothalamus and surrounding tissue shows the location of these structures (Figure 12-2).

The question then arises regarding how these impulses are transmitted. Recent investigations of CNS functions in food intake control have centered on the biochemical messengers known as neurotransmitters that function in impulse transmission. Catecholamine (CA) neurotransmitters involved in control of feeding include norepinephrine (NE), epinephrine, and dopamine (DA). Injections of norepinephrine into the PVN stimulate feeding. Conversely, injection of epinephrine and DA into the PFH are inhibitors. Therefore, a current hypothesis states that these catecholamines modulate feeding and satiety.[6] Other neurotransmitters also are apparently involved. **Serotonin** has an inhibitor effect at medial hypothalamic sites on feeding and antagonizes NE-induced feeding with an effect on the PVN. **Endorphin** and **dynorphin** in the PVN stimulate feeding. In the brain there is an extensive integration of the effects of these materials.

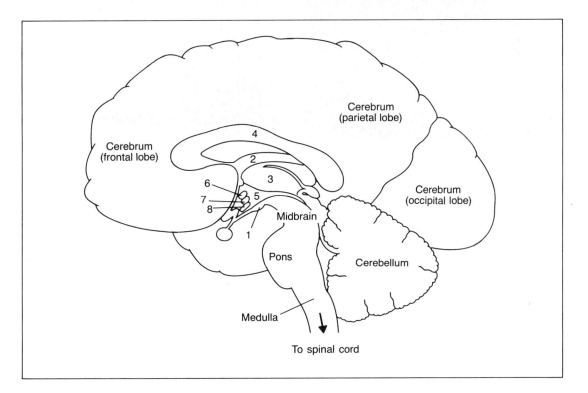

Peripheral Control Mechanisms

There are apparently a number of peripheral factors that provide information to the central control. The control produced may be short-term or long-term. It generally is believed that medium-term and long-term controls are more precise. Although food intake may vary greatly from day to day, the long-term control normally will maintain body weight within very narrow limits. Control mechanisms are not well understood and are obviously complex.

Gastrointestinal Factors. The gastrointestinal tract may provide signs related to meals. Stomach distension may be one of these, signaling satiety. It has been suggested that gastric receptors signal caloric content of meals, and the process of gastric emptying is signaled by feedback from the intestine.[7,8]

In the small intestine, there is some evidence of receptors for different nutrients and properties of food. These may include osmoreceptors that sense tonicity, tension receptors sensing intestinal distension, chemoreceptors sensing specific nutrients, and possibly a calorie sensor.[9-11]

Transmission of these signals to the brain may be by the vagus nerve. In addition, endocrine factors may be involved. These include cholecystokinin (CCK), bombesin, somatostatin, glucagon, and neurotensin, all of which may be signals of satiety.[10,12-14]

Liver Metabolism. The liver has been suggested to be another source of signals monitoring food intake by sensing changes in the liver's metabolic status.[15] It has been suggested that there are glucose receptors in the liver that respond to liver glycogen or portal vein glucose or both.[10] An alternative "hepatostatic" theory postulates that food intake is controlled by sensing increased pyruvate levels from glycolysis or pyruvate deficit, indicating glycogen breakdown.[16]

Adipose Tissue. Signals for longer-term controls may be derived from the adipose tissue itself. The nature and source of such signals, which reflect the size of adipose tissue stores, are unknown. It has been suggested that the signals are derived from blood levels of glycerol and free fatty acids or adipose cell size and number.[6,17-19]

Endocrine Factors. Hormones also affect food intake. **Insulin** may serve as a signal for long-term control, since circulating insulin levels are proportional to adipose tissue mass. Increased insulin may be sensed as an indicator of increased adipose tissue and promote reduction of feeding.[20]

In addition, an alteration in the interaction among the nervous system, selected hormones, and peripheral metabolism may influence the tendency to obesity. The hypothalamus influences insulin release, hepatic glycogen synthesis, and fatty acid mobilization by way of the splanchnic and vagus nerves. It also influences the turnover of norepinephrine in peripheral tissues. In the obese, these factors are altered so as to favor lipid deposition.[21]

An alternative theory suggests that hypothalamic dysfunction results in oversecretion of insulin. The resulting metabolic abnormalities then produce obesity.[22]

The **catecholamines**, described in relation to central controls, affect nerve fibers known as **adrenergic fibers**. The contradictory actions of catecholamines on adrenergic fibers have been explained as responses to two different receptors, called **alpha** and **beta**. In general, norepinephrine is believed to have a strong alpha, but weak beta, effect. Norepinephrine has been found both in the hypothalamus and in sympathetic nerves. Therefore, it has both central and peripheral effects.

Epinephrine responses may have a strong beta, but also some alpha, effect. Isoproterenol, a synthetic analog of epinephrine, has a strong beta and weak alpha effect.

In the control of food intake, norepinephrine and related compounds, called **alpha agonists**, largely promote eating. This effect can be antagonized by **alpha-blocking** agents such as phentolamine. On the other hand, isoproterenol is a **beta stimulator** or **beta agonist** and inhibits feeding. Amphetamines are believed to function as beta agonists, but other interpretations have been presented.

Prostaglandins have also been shown to inhibit eating. The prostaglandin PGI_1 appears to block the effects of norepinephrine; that is, it is an alpha receptor blocker. This effect is inhibited by **polyphoretic phosphate** (PPP). Thus drugs may be used to block the tendency to feeding or to satiety, and are useful in studying the effect of hormones on food intake.

Glucagon and **growth hormone** are also involved in hunger and satiety. The overall effect of the hormone balance on food intake is far from clear. Further research is needed to clarify the role of each hormone before the effects of their interaction can be studied.

Sensory Factors. Taste, smell, and texture of food may influence food intake by their effects on the brain, with responses being based on previous experiences. By means of the autonomic nervous system, these factors can elevate insulin secretion and intestinal motility in preparation for food intake.

Cortical Factors. Some emotional reactions also influence food intake. Unpleasant situations may interfere with eating, whereas pleasant sensations can cause a person to eat past the point of satiation. For example, people may eat until uncomfortably full on holidays and during other celebrations.

Control of Energy Expenditure

Types of Energy Expenditure

Energy expenditure may be divided into **obligatory** and **facultative** categories. **Obligatory thermogenesis** (heat production) is the heat produced to maintain the basal state. A major portion is the **resting metabolic expenditure** (RME), the energy expended to

support normal body homeostasis and function plus a small amount for sympathetic nervous system (SNS) activity. It is slightly higher than basal metabolic rate and equals 60–75% of the total, or about 1,500 kcal/day in a 70-kg man, but it can be altered by age, gender, body composition, thyroid function, and nutritional state. An additional part of RME is **endothermic thermogenesis**, the energy required to maintain normal body temperature. It is largely controlled by thyroid hormone.[23]

Facultative thermogenesis encompasses the heat produced by factors added to the basal state. It includes several categories, each of which is highly variable in size. The **thermic effect of exercise** (TEE) is the additional energy expenditure for muscular activity and also includes shivering and "fidgeting." It often accounts for 20–30% of total energy requirements, but may vary from <100 kcal/day for the sedentary to >1,000 kcal/day for the active person. It is generally believed that exercise added to caloric restriction will increase fat loss, help preserve lean body mass, and limit the decrease in RME following low-energy diets.

There is some evidence that exercise does not increase weight loss. It may, instead, promote a further decrease in RME.[24] In contrast, it has been suggested that exercise may (1) increase RME after an exercise period, (2) increase RME response to food intake in the postexercise period, and (3) have a physical conditioning effect if exercise is regular.[25] Others have found that metabolic rate falls quickly after exercise.[26,27] It has been suggested that RME is increased only if the exercise is severe and prolonged.[25] Studies of training for physical fitness were also inconsistent in results. Clearly, the relationship of exercise, energy expenditure and weight loss needs further study.

Thermic effect of feeding (TEF), or **diet-induced thermogenesis**, is the increment to RME following food consumption and includes the energy needed for food absorption, metabolism, and storage. It equals 5–15% of the daily expenditure, and has been subdivided into **obligatory** and **facultative** categories. Obligatory TEF provides energy for absorption and transport of foods and for protein, fat, and carbohydrate synthesis. Facultative TEF is an amount that may be mediated by SNS activity and cycling of substrates. Total TEF is influenced by genetic factors, nutritional status, previous diet, and the composition and caloric content of individual meals. It is not correlated with body size or body composition.

When a person is placed in a negative energy balance, as with a low-kilocalorie diet, there is a fall in expenditure for RME and TEF.[28] This can be frustrating to the individual trying to reduce body weight, since it requires a further reduction in intake to remain in negative energy balance. Conversely, energy expenditure appears to increase with overfeeding, but the weight gain may not be proportional to the excess energy. It has been suggested that there is an "energy wasting" mechanism that limits weight gain and causes an increased caloric requirement to maintain the excess weight. The effect of overfeeding is still considered controversial.[25,29,30]

Adaptive thermogenesis (AT) is referred to in animals as **nonshivering, facultative**, or **regulatory thermogenesis**. It is the alteration in RME, TEF, or both that occurs as a result of environmental influences such as adaptation to cold, composition and quantity of diet, hormonal effects, and responses to drugs. It may equal 10–15% of total energy expenditure at most, but it can have a significant cumulative effect over a long period. Its contribution to energy expenditure in man is controversial.

Nonshivering and diet-induced thermogenesis are sometimes categorized together as **chemical thermogenesis**.

Mechanisms of Control

If excess energy can be dissipated, obesity can be avoided. On the other hand, if energy dissipation is defective, the individual will have a tendency to gain weight. In addition, decreased dissipation of energy will be antagonistic to weight loss.[31]

The processes by which chemical thermogenesis might be controlled are currently being studied. One suggested mechanism involves the **sympathoadrenal system**, which consists of the adrenal medulla and the sympathetic nervous system. In animals, stimulation of the SNS increases heat loss by nonshivering thermogenesis. Free fatty acid release from adipose tissue and increased hepatic glucose release provide energy for this process. The process is believed to be the same as that which occurs in exposure to cold. Animals exposed to cold have an enhanced response to norepinephrine, an effect localized in the brown adipose tissue. It has been demonstrated in the rat that SNS activity is also increased in overfeeding and may thereby increase diet-induced thermogenesis.[32]

A high-energy mixed diet and increased carbohydrate intakes without an increase in total energy content have been shown to increase SNS activity in both rodent and human subjects.[33-38] Increased fat has a similar effect in rodents, but the effect in humans is unclear. In total, the data suggest that the stimulatory effect of overfeeding may allow the use of excess energy as heat. In the laboratory rat, the heat is produced by BAT, but in the human body the role of BAT is also not understood.[31] Elevated **glucocorticoids** may impair the sensitivity of BAT to diet-induced stimulation of the SNS in animals. Their role in pathogenesis in human obesity is unknown.[39]

The role of insulin is also unclear. While obesity is often associated with increased serum insulin levels and insulin resistance, the primary defect is unknown. Suggested mechanisms include a decreased number of insulin receptors, a defect in intracellular insulin metabolism, or decreased hepatic insulin clearance.[40-42] Insulin action is apparently related to sympathetic nervous system activity, since the response to norepinephrine is decreased in diabetic animals.[43] Conversely, insulin has been shown to stimulate the SNS in humans and cause an increase in heat production.[44,45]

Growth hormone levels are depressed in the obese,[46] but the physiological effects are not entirely understood. Linear growth is normal in obese subjects,[47] but growth hormone may increase glucose intolerance and insulin resistance.[48]

Thyroid hormone is the main regulator of obligatory thermogenesis, but it may also be involved in SNS-induced facultative thermogenesis. As such, a defect in thyroid hormone's effects on heat production may predispose to weight gain. This effect has been shown in the genetically obese mouse, which also shows an improved response when exogenous thyroid hormone is given.[23] However, thyroid hypoactivity is rare in obese human subjects.[47]

It is possible, therefore, that reduced SNS and thyroid hormone activity, impaired insulin-mediated thermogenesis, and hyperinsulinemia stimulating lipogenesis may contribute to the pathogenesis of obesity. When energy intake is restricted in affected individuals, metabolic rate might be depressed, reducing the effectiveness of the diet.[31]

Another question related to the role of energy expenditure in the regulation of energy balance asks whether changes in food intake influence physical activity. There is good evidence that they do in some circumstances. Some laboratory animals and humans, when underfed, will reduce their physical activity.[49] On the other hand, underfed rodents increase their activity. It is not known whether overfeeding will stimulate an increase in activity. The insistent demand of small children for physical activity may indicate that such an effect does exist. But there is no concrete supporting evidence.

The thermogenic response after feeding arises partly from the increased rate of synthetic reactions, but this does not account for all heat. After exercise, oxygen is consumed at an accelerated rate. It is proposed that this oxygen is used in replenishing phosphocreatine, reoxygenating myoglobin and hemoglobin, converting lactate to glucose and glycogen, and stimulating futile cycles. This latter might persist for hours and add considerably to the total energy expenditure. Stress is thought to increase the activity of cycles for mobilization and the use of glucose and fatty acids, by pathways involving epinephrine and glucagon. James et al.[50] proposed an interaction between dietary fat intake and brown fat metabolism as well as differences in dietary thermogenesis. Current research is investigating the possibility of differences in these metabolic processes in obese and nonobese individuals.[50]

OBESITY

Obesity is defined as an excessive accumulation of body fat, but the proportion of fat is difficult to determine. As a consequence, we commonly use body weight in relation to height to define obesity. On that basis, obesity is defined as body weight 20% or more above desirable levels in women and 25% or more above desirable levels in men. When equipment is available to determine body fat content itself, a body fat level above 25% in young men and 30% in young women is defined as obesity.

Morbid obesity refers to a degree of obesity that clearly correlates with excess morbidity and mortality. Frequently, 45.4 kg (100 lb.) of excess weight or an overweight of 100% is used as a standard, although these definitions are arbitrary.

Diagnosis

Research Methods

The definitions just given suggest that obesity is defined on the basis of body weight compared to a standard. Although that usually is the case, such an approach is limited in that it does not provide a measure of body fat. Methods that provide a basis for estimates of body fat are available for research purposes. These include measurements of body density or specific gravity and measurements of body water using radioactive or stable isotopes or measurement of radioactive potassium. A recent method is measurement of body conductivity. Other relatively new methods include computed tomography (CT scan), nuclear magnetic resonance imaging (NMRI), neutron activation analysis, and whole body photon absorptiometry. These methods require sophisticated equipment and are expensive. For most clinical purposes, simpler and less expensive methods are used.

Comparison with Tables of Ideal Weight

The most widely used method of determining obesity is to compare an individual's body weight with that listed on height-weight tables for a person of the same height and sex.

Over the years, a number of tables have been issued. They have purported to give average, desirable, recommended, or ideal weights. Often they were based on mean weights at age 20 to 29 years and later increases were assumed to be undesirable.[51] They are generally based on assessment of body fatness in populations and vary slightly. As described in Chapter 3, it is important to observe whether the person measured is barefoot or wearing shoes and the height of the heel.

The tables issued by the Metropolitan Life Insurance Company, based on life insurance mortality statistics (see Table 3-3), are widely used. These tables consider sex, height, and frame size. A method for frame size estimation is given in Table 3-4. The values given in the tables are for individuals aged 25 to 59 years. For young women 18 to 24 years old, 1 lb. is subtracted for each year younger than 25. The weights are given assuming that indoor clothing, weighing 5 lb. for men and 3 lb. for women, and shoes with 1-inch heels are worn.

A rapid estimate of ideal weight consists of calculating weight from height with Equations 3-4 and 3-5 given in Chapter 3. A somewhat more generous estimate that takes frame size into consideration provides 105 to 110 lb. for the first 5 ft., 5 lb. for each added inch *plus* 5 lb. for medium frame or 10 lb. for heavy frame.

Whether tables of ideal weight or one of these rapid calculations is used, a useful means of expressing overweight is as a percentage above ideal:

$$\frac{(\text{present weight} - \text{ideal weight}) \times 100}{\text{Ideal weight obtained from a table}} = \% \text{ overweight} \qquad (12\text{-}2)$$

This is not very exact, but errors are not large, and it has the advantage of being easily understood by most patients.

Another data base, which comes from the National Center for Health Statistics (NCHS), is based on a representative sample of the American population. The NCHS defines overweight persons as those in the 85th percentile or more of weight for height, using the weights of those 20 to 29 years old as the reference. Severe overweight is defined as the 95th percentile or more.[52]

Separate tables are used for children. The NCHS[53] has issued growth charts for children aged 0 to 36 months and 2 to 18 years. These are divided according to sex. Obesity can be detected using these charts. If a child is in the 50th percentile for height and the 80th percentile for weight, obesity is probable.

Triceps Skinfold

The method of diagnosing obesity by measuring the triceps skinfold is described in Chapter 3. Measurements greater than 18.6 mm in men and 25.1 mm in women indicate obesity. Skinfolds are used also to indicate fat distribution.

Height-Weight Ratios

Several ratios of height and weight have also been used to diagnose obesity. In order of preference, according to Keys et al.[54] they are as follows: **Body mass index (obesity index; Quetelet index):**

$$\frac{W \text{ (kg)}}{H^2 \text{(m)}} \qquad \text{(12-3)}$$

Simple ratio:

$$\frac{W}{H} \qquad \text{(12-4)}$$

Ponderal index:

$$\frac{H \text{ (cm or in.)}}{\sqrt[3]{W} \text{ (lb. or kg)}} \qquad \text{(12-5)}$$

where W = weight and H = height. A more complex system, the **adiposity index**, uses skinfold measurements as well as height and weight:

Men:

$$0.34 + 222 \frac{W}{H^2} + (0.00740 \times \text{[subcapsular}$$
$$+ \text{ triceps skinfold in mm]}) \qquad \text{(12-6)}$$

Women:

$$0.34 + 242 \frac{W}{H^2} + (0.00571 \times \text{[subcapsular}$$
$$+ \text{ triceps skinfold in mm]}) \qquad \text{(12-7)}$$

The body mass index (BMI) is widely accepted because it is independent of height. Of those ratios given, it correlates best with independent measures of body fat. One mode of interpretation grades the severity of obesity as shown in Table 12-1.[55]

This method makes no adjustment for age or sex, nor does it provide any indication of the amount of risk. Therefore, other tables providing interpretations have been developed. Table 12-2 indicates acceptable range and evaluation of risk in 19–24-year-olds and gives adjustment of acceptable range for age.

A ponderal index (PI) of 12 or less, calcu-

Table 12-1. The Body Mass Index (BMI) and a Suggested Interpretation

Obesity Grade	BMI	Suggested Treatment
0	20–24.9	Normal; assess basis for anxiety if necessary
I	25–29.9	Community-based group therapy
II	30–40	Individualized counseling
III	>40	Surgery or other special measures

lated using height and the cube root of weight, is also considered to indicate obesity. This measure has not been commonly used, possibly because the necessity to obtain the cube root of the weight presents difficulties. An isogram graph is now available from which the PI can be obtained using the height in inches or centimeters and weights in kilograms or pounds.[56]

Since adiposity has been related to cardiovascular risk, there have been attempts to develop equations which would predict risk. It has been found that a ratio of waist circumference to hip circumference (**abdominal-to-gluteal circumference**, or AGR) is a strong predictor of stroke and myocardial in-

Table 12-2. Health Risks Indicated by Body Mass Index

Risk	Age	Body Mass Index
Acceptable	19–24	19–24
	25–34	20–25
	35–44	21–26
	45–54	22–27
	55–65	23–28
	>65	24–29
Low	19–24	25–30
Moderate	19–24	30–35
High	19–24	35–40
Very high	19–24	>40

Based on data from Committee on Diet and Health, Food and Nutrition Board, National Research Council, *Diet and Health, Implications for Reducing Chronic Disease Risk.* Washington, D.C.: National Academy Press, 1989.

farction in both sexes and of total mortality rate in women. When the ratio exceeds 1.0 in men and 0.8 in women, the risk rises steeply.[57]

When attempts were made to relate the predictive power to the volume of visceral adipose tissue, it was found that waist circumference was a better predictor for visceral fat and that waist/hip ratio predicted cardiovascular risk better.[58]

Bioelectrical Impedence

This method is based on the principle that electrical resistance in the body is inversely proportional to total body water. From the value obtained, lean body mass is calculated. The measurement is obtained with a device with electrodes placed on the patient's hand and foot.[59] This method has not yet been validated for use on children.

Rapid Self-Assessment Methods

A number of simple self-assessment methods, which are imprecise but sometimes useful, have been listed by Stern and Kane-Nussen.[60] With these methods, excess fatness is "probably indicated" as follows:

Belt test: Circumference at navel exceeds circumference at nipples.
Broca index: Weight in kilograms is greater than height in centimeters minus 100. Used extensively in Europe.
"Magic 36" test: Height in inches minus waist circumference in inches equals less than 36.
Ruler test: When lying flat, a ruler parallel to the vertical axis of the body cannot touch both ribs and pubic bone.
Pinch test: A pinch of skin and subcutaneous fat on back of upper arm, side of lower chest, and just below shoulder blade in back exceeds 1 in.
Mirror test: Self-assessment of excess fat while nude before a mirror (except when the person has an abnormal body image, as in anorexia nervosa).

Classification of the Obesities

For many years, obesity was treated as a psychological problem, often with moral overtones. Obese individuals were considered to lack self-control, to be gluttons and social deviants, and to have personality disorders of varying degrees of severity. Although these attitudes still are somewhat common, recent research has indicated the complexity of the problem so that the obesities now are recognized as multiple. They have been classified in several ways, to facilitate understanding of their etiology and pathogenesis.

Classification According to Pathogenesis

Obesity has been classified as **exogenous** (regulatory) or **endogenous** (metabolic). This early classification proposes that exogenous obesity involves an impairment of the central regulation of food intake.[61] Metabolism of other tissues is considered to be normal, but there is evidence that inactivity is characteristic of the individual and often precedes the development of obesity. The inactivity contributes to the positive energy balance by reducing the output of energy.

Metabolic or endogenous obesity has been defined as the type in which overeating is the consequence of abnormal fat and carbohydrate metabolism or some other disorder.[61] A major difficulty with this type of classification is that it tends to obscure the fact that a positive calorie balance is necessary for weight gain in either case.

Etiologic Classification

Classification of obesity according to etiology is more recent and somewhat more useful than pathogenetic classification. Many factors have been shown to be involved in the etiology of obesity.

The involvement of **genetic factors** has been shown clearly in laboratory and farm animals.[62] Genetic effects in most cases of human obesity are less firmly established, but there is evidence of genetic factors obtained from studies of twins[63] and of various ethnic groups.[64] In addition, in a study of adopted children, Stunkard[65] showed a correlation of body weights with those of biological parents but not of adoptive parents.

Also, there are five inherited syndromes that involve obesity among their manifestations.

The **Prader-Willi syndrome** is characterized by mental retardation and the onset of obesity at age 2 or 3 years. Nutritional care of Prader-Willi patients is described in more detail in Chapter 19. This syndrome generally is believed to be genetically transmitted, although the evidence is weak.

The evidence is stronger for genetic transmission of the other four syndromes. The manifestations of the **Laurence-Moon-Biedl syndrome** include mental deficiency, obesity, retinal degeneration leading to blindness in adulthood, **polydactyly** (extra fingers and toes), **hypogonadism** (lack of sexual development), and sometimes congenital heart disease and kidney disease. The **Alstrom syndrome** is characterized by obesity, retinal degeneration leading to blindness in childhood, nerve deafness, and diabetes mellitus. This condition is rare.

Hyperostosis frontalis interna (Morgagni-Stewart-Morel syndrome) usually first appears in women at age 20 to 60 years. Manifestations include obesity and **virilism** (development of masculine physical and mental traits in a woman). The term **hyperostosis frontalis interna** refers to the formation of new bone that protrudes in patches on the internal surface of the forehead. The condition may be accompanied by mental slowness, loss of memory, headache, irritability, and other neurologic symptoms. The syndrome is exceedingly rare.

The last of the four syndromes discussed here actually may be three syndromes with similar manifestations. Collectively they have been called **triglyceride storage diseases**. Little is known of these conditions since they have been identified in only a few families. On the basis of studies of these patients, the three types may be[66]

Type 1, resulting from a defect in the activation of adenyl cyclase complex, producing decreased levels of cyclic AMP in adipose tissue.

Type 2, resulting from failure of activation of hormone-sensitive lipase by cyclic AMP.

Type 3 (also known as **primary familial xanthomatosis**), resulting from a defect of a lipase.

Hypothalamic obesity has been clearly demonstrated in both animals and humans after the hypothalamus has been injured, as in the case of an encroaching tumor. It is very rare.

Endocrine disorders also cause obesity, although perhaps not as often as many would like to believe. Obesity occurs in cases of excess corticosteroids (**Cushing's syndrome**), insulin excess, castration, or alterations in the levels of progesterone or estrogen (**Stein-Leventhal syndrome**). Pregnancy frequently is followed by weight gain.

Physical inactivity is a clear cause of weight gain in patients whose activity is restricted by injury (see Chapter 19). It has also been documented to contribute to other forms of obesity, even though it may not be obvious to the casual observer.[67,68]

Nutritional factors may play a role in the development of obesity in animals and humans. Variation in protein intake affects the amount of energy storage, although the mechanism is not clear. Thus it appears that diet composition affects obesity. High-fat diets and high-sucrose diets are used to produce obesity in animal experiments, but the mechanism may be based on palatability.

Overfeeding of children may be especially important in causing childhood obesity. It has been suggested that overfeeding of infants may "program" the child for obesity later.

The use of some **drugs** can also cause obesity. Cyproheptadine, tricyclic antidepressants, and the phenothiazines are those particularly associated with weight gain (see Chapter 4).

Physiologic and psychic trauma can contribute to the etiology of obesity in animals. In humans, the relationship is less obvious; however, emotional stress has been associated with the onset of obesity in some cases.[61]

Environmental factors such as cultural food habits also can contribute to the development of obesity.[61,62]

Two types of obesity sometimes are classified as of a special psychological origin. One results from the **night-eater syndrome** in which the patient has insomnia and hyperphagia in the evening along with anorexia in the morning. It has been associated with stress and has a poor prognosis unless the stress can be removed. The other type of patient, also reacting to stress, is the **binge eater**. This person may be one who progresses to anorexia nervosa.

In the final analysis, all the factors just listed result in an intake of energy in excess of output. Thus it is necessary to remember that positive energy balance is the only fundamental cause of obesity.

Anatomic Classification of Fat Distribution

There are several means of classifying fat accumulations based on their distribution within the body. This distribution may be generalized or localized.

Localized Fat Accumulations. A number of conditions cause localized fat accumulations. These are not considered obesity but are given here to provide an overall perspective:

Lipomas, associated with other diseases (see Chapter 11).
Dercum's disease (adipose dolorosa), a disease with painful fat accumulations and nerve lesions.
Weber-Christian disease, a nodular pannicu-

litis (inflammation of subcutaneous fatty tissue).
Liposarcomas (see Chapter 15).
Lipid storage disease.

The nutritional care specialist should be aware of the existence of these conditions, but they will not be discussed further in this chapter.

Generalized Fat Distribution. One descriptive system of generalized fat distribution refers to **somatotype** (body build) that has been related to the incidence of obesity. Body build has been classified into three groups. **Ectomorphs** are described as those individuals who are linear in build, appear fragile, and have a large relative surface area, thin muscles, and a thin layer of subcutaneous fat. **Mesomorphs** have a preponderance of muscle, connective tissue, and bone, with a rectangular outline. **Endomorphs** have large digestive viscera, accumulations of fat, and a soft, rounded appearance with large trunk and thighs and tapering extremities. In a study of adolescent girls, obesity occurred most often in endomorphs, less often in mesomorphs, and least often in ectomorphs. The relationship was less clear-cut in adults, but the trend was similar.[69] These constitutional factors may provide a predisposition to obesity and cause body weight to vary somewhat from the ideal because of heavy bone and muscle structure. Endomorphs have a higher incidence of obesity.

Another system of anatomic classification of obesity uses the terms **gynecoid** and **android**. A gynecoid (femalelike) distribution of fat refers to fat accumulation particularly around the hips and lower abdomen. It also is referred to as **lower body obesity**. The android (malelike) type describes fat accumulation over chest and arms (upper body) rather than the lower trunk and is known as **upper body obesity**. Despite the terms used, each of these types can occur in either sex. The differences in fat distribution have been related in insulin-glucose metabolism.[70] It has been hypothesized that insulin resistance is related to upper body obesity.[71]

The relative amounts of adipose tissue deposited in the upper and lower trunk have been quantitated by Vague et al.[72] The method requires measurement of skinfold thickness and circumference (see Chapter 3 for the procedure) of the mid-upper arm over the biceps and of the midthigh (femoral). The **adipomuscular ratio** (AMR) then is calculated:

$$AMR = \frac{\text{skinfold thickness}}{\text{circumference}} \qquad (12\text{-}8)$$

Typical gynecoid values are 0.48 for biceps AMR and 0.63 for femoral AMR. Thus the ratio of biceps AMR to femoral AMR is much less than 1. By contrast, typical android values are 0.21 for biceps AMR and 0.19 for femoral AMR. Thus the ratio is greater than 1. This calculation, then, provides a quantitative definition of the android and gynecoid fat distributions that may affect the chances for success in weight reduction. The mechanisms are unknown, but the gynecoid type is considered to be more difficult to treat successfully.

Obesity has also been divided into two categories indicating the overall location of body fat. In **visceral fat obesity** (VFO), the fat level in the abdominal viscera (mesentery and omental sites) tended to be increased, while in **subcutaneous fat obesity** (SFO), fat deposits were most extraabdominal. A V/S ratio of >0.4 was defined as VFO, and <0.4 as SFO. Intraabdominal fat (VFO) was correlated with disorders of glucose and lipid metabolism.[73]

Another anatomic classification of the obesities is based on the number and size of adipose cells. Obesity has been classified as **hypercellular** or **hyperplastic** (containing an increased number of cells) or as **hypertrophic** (containing larger fat cells) with a more nearly normal number of fat cells (**normocellular**). It is possible to have a mixture of types. Nevertheless, this classification currently is considered useful because there is some evidence that cellularity is based on age of onset of obesity and has prognostic value.

Classification by Age of Onset

The last classification divides obesities into **adult-onset** and **juvenile-onset** conditions. Most obese persons (90–95%) are of the adult-onset type in whom obesity develops slowly, beginning at approximately age 25 years and progressing until age 55 or so. The adult-onset obese person is expected to have a hypertrophic obesity. There is evidence that the juvenile-onset obese person, in whom obesity began in childhood, has a greater number of fat cells—that is, hyperplastic obesity.[74] The juvenile-onset category has been further subdivided into types 1 and 2. In **type 1**, onset is in infancy and the condition is characterized by hyperphagia. In **type 2**, onset is in childhood and the imbalance results from decreased energy expenditure.

Increased organ or tissue size during growth may be the consequence of an increase in the number of cells, an increase in the size of cells, or both. It is postulated that, in humans of normal weight, there are two periods in which adipose tissue cells multiply: in infancy up to the age of two years and during puberty. The stimuli to the increases are unknown but probably are genetic, endocrine, nutritional, and environmental in some combination. In very obese children, the numbers of fat cells may continue to increase between age 2 and puberty, a time when fat cell number is stable in children of normal weight. There is some question on this point. The development of fat cells cannot be studied prior to the time that they contain fat, since we have no satisfactory techniques to identify them. The increase in numbers of cells in obese infants is postulated to stem in part from early overfeeding and the early introduction of solid foods.[75]

The prognosis for successful weight reduction often is estimated on the basis of the android/gynecoid and age-of-onset classifications. Current opinion holds that juvenile-onset hyperplastic obesity with gynecoid distribution of fat is exceedingly difficult to treat successfully.

Hazards of Obesity

In American society, the obese or overweight individual often is stigmatized, and the psychological effects and social rejection are important among the hazards of obesity. There are many other risks, and it generally is agreed that obesity is detrimental to one's well-being.

Obesity has been associated, particularly, with increased incidences of hypertension, hyperlipidemia, congestive heart failure, and diabetes. Other conditions shown to occur with greater frequency in obesity include cerebrovascular accidents, cancer, accidents, renal disease, gallstone disease, some respiratory diseases, osteoarthritis, endometrial carcinoma, and some skin disorders.[60] In obese surgery patients, anesthesia dosages may be difficult to determine,[76] and the incidence of postoperative sepsis and wound rupture are increased. It is controversial whether obesity increases the mortality rate from these conditions. The **Pickwickian syndrome (obesity hypoventilation syndrome)** is the only condition in which excess adipose tissue can lead to death without any other contributing factor (see Chapter 16). It is not clear whether, once an obesity-related disease is established, it can be ameliorated by weight reduction.

Metabolic Alterations in Obesity

Many alterations in metabolism have been observed in the person who is obese. These may be discussed in terms of (1) effects on the adipose cell in particular, (2) effects on metabolism in general, and (3) the response to the energy deficit when the individual is dieting.

Effects of Increased Adipose Cell Size on Its Metabolism

As it enlarges, the adipose cell adapts metabolically, with progressive inhibition of lipogenesis and inhibition of pentose shunt enzymes. As fat cells become larger, they also become insulin-resistant. Among other consequences, they have a decreased number of receptor sites on their cell membranes. Insulin promotes fat storage; therefore, as the cell enlarges and becomes resistant, additional storage becomes more difficult. These reactions may provide a limit to the development of larger cells and also may be a mechanism for maintenance of a set point.

It formerly was suggested that the number of cells did not increase in adult-onset obesity and that the cells only got larger as they filled with lipid. More recent work on rats has suggested that, in the adult, once fat cells have achieved maximum size, further increase involves an increase in cell number if energy intake continues.[77] Some indirect evidence suggests that a similar phenomenon occurs in obese humans.[78]

In weight reduction, as the cell size is reduced and insulin sensitivity is increased, mobilization of triglyceride could become more difficult. Studies suggest that some regulatory mechanism prevents the decrease of body fat below a certain level related to the size of fat cells.

Weight loss apparently causes a decrease in cell size but not in cell number in either juvenile-onset or adult-onset obesity. This fact may provide an explanation for the difficulty in weight reduction experienced by many individuals. If a person with large numbers of fat cells reduces his or her weight, that person may have symptoms of hunger equivalent to those felt by starving nonobese people.[79]

Although largely speculative, the distinction between hyperplastic and hypertrophic obesity might account for the greater difficulty in weight reduction reported in patients with childhood obesity. Investigation has revealed that the patient with hyperplastic obesity whose weight is reduced will maintain the weight a shorter time and experience a higher relapse rate.

The existence of a messenger between adipose cell size and regulation of energy balance is proposed, but its identity is unknown. Those described earlier in the discussion of endocrine factors in weight control (p. 478) are possible candidates.

These theories of the effects of adipose cell size on metabolism require further investigation. However, present knowledge suggests that obesity prevention is greatly preferable to treatment of existing obesity.

Effects on Metabolism in General

A variety of biochemical abnormalities may be present in the severely obese, but none has persisted when body weight was reduced. Therefore, it appears that they are the result, not the cause, of excess body weight. Some of these abnormalities include (1) an abnormal glucose tolerance test, (2) increased fasting levels of plasma glucose and plasma insulin, and (3) increased insulin response to a glucose load and other cues for insulin release. The relationship of insulin to hyperphagia is receiving much attention because it has been shown that the hypothalamus can stimulate increased insulin release from the pancreas by way of the vagus nerve. Other biochemical abnormalities in the obese include hypertriglyceridemia, elevated fasting levels of free fatty acid, and elevated plasma ketones.

Physiologic Responses to Energy Deficit During Weight Loss

When dietary sources of glucose are inadequate, the body's stored glucose reserves are used up in a few hours. Glucose must then be supplied from glucogenic amino acids and from glycerol to those tissues for which it is essential. If the deficit continues, as it would in an obese person who is dieting successfully, the body adapts to conserve its amino

acids. A major energy source is adipose tissue from which the liver produces large amounts of ketones. This adaptive process is described in detail in Chapter 14 and is diagramed in Figure 14-2.

Immune Factors in Obesity

Recent investigation has shown that adipocytes secrete **adipsin** into the bloodstream. Adipsin has activity similar to factor D in the complement cascade. It is deficient in several animal models of obesity, and it has been suggested that adipsin and factor D function in energy balance. The possible relevance in human subjects is still under investigation.[80]

Treatment

In view of the hazards associated with obesity, weight reduction is recommended for those who have body weights of 20% or more above the desirable weights in the Metropolitan Life Insurance Company tables.[81] The midpoint of the range for a medium-build person is used as the baseline. The 20% above desirable weights are equivalent to body mass index values of 27.2 for men and 26.9 for women.

Treatment of obesity is aimed toward weight loss. It has taken many forms, including diet, drugs, surgery, exercise, and behavior modification. Unfortunately, most individuals using standard treatments do not lose any appreciable amount of weight,[82] much less achieve a permanent cure.[83] Those individuals who do achieve permanent weight loss are generally those in whom the amount of excess weight was small.[84] The successful treatment of obesity presents a major challenge to the nutritional care specialist.

Before treatment is undertaken, careful consideration should be given to whether weight reduction is in the best interests of the patient. At one time, weight loss was recommended almost automatically to every patient who was overweight. More recently, consideration is given to the following questions:

1. Is there a serious health condition that makes weight reduction advisable? How much weight loss is necessary?
2. Is the patient well adjusted to his or her weight? Is he or she motivated to change? If so, are the patient's objectives realistic?
3. Has the patient's weight been stable?
4. Will a reduced weight be compatible with the patient's important relationships with others (spouse, close friends)?

The answers to these questions may reveal that attempts at weight reduction are not the most advisable course. If, however, the decision is made to attempt weight reduction, the following procedures may be considered.

Dietary Treatment

To be successful, any treatment must produce and maintain an intake of energy that is less than output so that the individual must draw on his or her body fat stores to supply his or her energy needs. The various means by which this has been proposed to be accomplished are described here.

Conventional Restricted-Calorie Diet.

Many physicians and nutritional care specialists recommend a restricted-calorie diet plan, often based on the same food lists used for planning diabetic diets (see Chapter 11) and planned in such a way as to establish a pattern for lifetime eating behavior. Permanent successful weight reduction is rare with this classic approach, which is regarded as the safest method of reducing. Nevertheless, since the diet is used extensively and there is no effective alternative, its planning will be described.

Step 1: Establish kilocalorie content of the diet. The amount of energy that will maintain weight must be estimated before the caloric deficit can be established. A simple procedure is based on measures of caloric use during starvation. The energy used during star-

vation is taken as the minimum amount necessary to maintain weight. Bray[85] has found that this quantity exceeds 1,000 kcal in adults. Thus any patient whose intake is 1,000 kcal or less will lose weight. This procedure is, of course, very imprecise. It makes no allowances for normal differences in body size or differences in activity.

To individualize the kilocalorie prescription, a second, more desirable approach may be used. The basal requirement for weight maintenance may be estimated by assuming 1 kcal/kg of body weight per hour. Thus a man weighing 90 kg would have a basal requirement of $90 \times 1 \times 24$ or 2,160 kcal. To this figure, an increment for activity is added. Usual additions are 30% of basal for sedentary activity, 50% for light activity, 75% for moderate activity, and 100% for the very active person. Thus our 90-kg man, if he had sedentary activity, would require $2,160 + 648$ or 2,808 kcal to maintain his weight.

A somewhat more exact system involves the use of a nomogram by which surface area is obtained from the body weight and height. The surface area, age, and sex then are used on the nomogram to arrive at basal energy expenditure. An increment for activity must again be added to obtain the maintenance energy level.

Once the maintenance energy level has been estimated, an appropriate diet may be established. Commonly used diets for weight reduction for the average adult contain 1,000 or 1,200 kcal/day. Sometimes diets of 800 kcal are used for the patient who has a small surface area, or for an elderly or handicapped person whose activity is limited. Generally, diets containing even fewer calories are not as effective as might be assumed. Some adaptation to conserve energy may occur[84] so that little more fat is catabolized.[86,87] The mechanism for this conservation of energy is unknown, but Bray[85] suggests that if a diet is more severely limited, little additional weight loss results.

Some patients can reduce body weight while eating diets containing higher calorie levels, such as 1,500 or 1,800 kcals, if they are active or normally have a large body size. A man 6 ft. 6 in. tall who does hard physical labor, for example, would lose weight on an 1,800-kcal diet.

The energy content of body fat is approximately 3,500 kcal/lb. This value may be used to estimate the rate of weight loss. If a patient's intake were 1,000 kcal less per day than his or her need for maintenance, that patient could lose 2 lb./week for the total deficit of 7,000 kcal. Let us assume that our 90-kg (198-lb.) man has an ideal weight of 70 kg (154 lb.). Since he is 44 lb. overweight, he must maintain his daily 1,000-kcal deficit for 22 weeks to reach ideal weight.

This method for estimating weight loss is useful but tends to oversimplify. As patients lose weight, BMR may decrease. If energy intake is not reduced also, the rate of loss decreases. Our 90-kg man, for example, might begin his diet at 1,800 kcal. When his body weight reaches 80 kg, weight maintenance needs could be 2,500 kcal. Under these circumstances, a 1,000-kcal deficit would require a 1,500-kcal diet. There is some evidence that an even lower figure will be required if the loss is to be maintained. In addition, other physiologic changes may help the obese patient maintain weight. Each 100 g of fat produces 112 g of water when it is oxidized. This water must be excreted before weight loss is observed.

When our patient reaches his ideal weight of 70 kg, his weight maintenance need, if activity has not changed, will be 70×1 (maybe) $\times 24$, or $1,680, + 504$, or $2,184$ kcal. A diet of approximately 2,180 kcal might maintain him at ideal weight, but there is some evidence that his basal requirement falls to less than 1 kcal/kg/hr., although the metabolic basis for this change is unknown. At 2,180 kcal, then, it is possible that he will gain weight. If he returns to his previous diet of 2,800 kcal or more, he will surely regain his lost weight.

In determining kilocalorie levels for control of obesity in children, care must be taken to allow for normal growth and develop-

ment. Lean body mass must be preserved carefully; therefore, restrictions are moderate. At ages 1 through 5 years, a restriction of 10% of kilocalories sometimes is recommended. After age 5, a restriction of 10% to 25% may be used to maintain a stable weight while growth in height occurs. Alternatively, weight loss of 0.5 lb./week may be the objective.

Step 2: Distribute kilocalories among protein, fat, and carbohydrate. Having established the desired energy content of the diet, the nutritional care specialist must distribute those kilocalories among protein, fat, and carbohydrate. As a general guideline, protein is provided generously, usually 0.8 to 1.5 g/kg of body weight, and sometimes more. One objective is to prevent loss of lean body tissue. In addition, animal foods have high satiety value, and their generous use may increase compliance with the diet. The nutritional care specialist must remember, however, that their high cost presents a hardship for some patients.

The remaining energy in the diet is distributed between carbohydrate and fat. The merits of a high-fat, low-carbohydrate diet compared to an equicaloric low-fat, high-carbohydrate diet have been debated for decades. Some studies have shown extra weight loss on the low-carbohydrate diet over the short term, but these effects are believed to be related to changes in water balance.[88] Studies over longer periods have not shown any differences in weight loss between a low-calorie, high-fat diet and an equicaloric high-carbohydrate diet.

In summary, weight loss occurs if there is a caloric deficit regardless of the source of the calories contained in the diet. There is no evidence that weight reduction is altered when the source of nonprotein calories is changed. Therefore, plan a diet that is compatible with the patient and to increase compliance, and plan a diet that will help to redefine the patient's eating habits to increase the possibility of long-term maintenance of the weight loss.

Step 3: Establish frequency of meals. The number of meals per day must also be established and has been another area for debate. The effects of meal-eating once or twice daily compared to nibbling at more frequent intervals have been investigated in animals. Rats fed by a stomach tube twice daily had more body fat than those allowed to nibble ad libitum.[89] Epidemiologic and clinical studies have shown that obese individuals tend to eat most of their food in one or two meals per day.[90-92] This pattern of food intake also has a detrimental effect on serum cholesterol and glucose tolerance.[90-93] Nevertheless, the frequency of meals does not affect the overall rate of weight change in subjects on kilocalorie-deficient diets.[94,95] A regimen of three meals or more per day generally is recommended, not for increased weight loss but to modulate serum cholesterol changes and improve glucose tolerance. However, this matter still is the subject of controversy. In planning for the individual patient, it seems logical to use the meal pattern that makes it easiest for the patient to comply with the kilocalorie restriction.

Step 4: Plan for adequate vitamins, minerals, and fluid. The diet is intended to be used for a long period and should be planned carefully to include adequate amounts of vitamins and minerals. Supplements should be given with all diets containing less than 1,200 kcal.

Even if the patient adheres carefully to the diet, weight usually is not lost in a straight linear progression. Water balance is influenced by the carbohydrate content of the diet, and water balance may not be reached for approximately ten days after the diet is instituted. In that time, weight loss may be substantial. At other times, the weight may plateau for ten days or so because of some fluid retention, even though the amount of adipose tissue is decreasing. Unless the patient has a complicating condition affecting water balance, fluid retention is a transient effect and is not a justification for fluid restriction. If this phenomenon is explained to patients, it may help to prevent a feeling of discouragement and defeat and the use of

harmful medications. The use of diuretics for weight reduction should be discouraged.

Step 5: Plan the diet. A common procedure for diet planning is the same as that used in planning the diabetic diet from the exchange lists (see Chapter 11), although a little more flexibility usually is allowed in the calorie distribution. If the patient requires a diet containing 1,000 kcal, the prescription might specify 80 g of protein, 30 g of fat, and 110 g of carbohydrate to provide 1,030 kcal. Using the same method described in Chapter 11, this diet, which is an example of a low-fat diet, might contain the following exchanges:

Food	Exchanges
Milk, nonfat	2
Vegetables	2
Fruit	3
Bread	2
Meat, lean	7
Fat	2

With these exchanges, the diet would contain 78 g of protein, 31 g of fat, and 109 g of carbohydrate, for a total of 1,027 kcal.

Alternatively, a more generous fat allowance could be provided at the expense of carbohydrate by providing 79 g of protein, 39 g of fat, 94 g of carbohydrate, and 1,043 kcal, as follows:

Food	Exchanges
Milk, nonfat	2
Vegetables	2
Fruit	3
Bread	1
Meat, lean	8
Fat	3

Patients are advised to distribute all the foods in somewhat equal proportion among the three meals.

As is true with the diabetic diet, the patient needs information on the use of "free" foods, methods for accurate determination of portion size, and, sometimes, the energy content of alcoholic beverages and snack foods. Practice in estimating portion size is especially important for obese patients, many of whom tend to underestimate portions and thus continue to overeat even though they are attempting to comply with the diet.

Another consideration is the use of fat substitutes with no or few calories. Two products of this type have been developed and research is under way to find others.

Olestra, a product of Proctor and Gamble, is a sucrose polyester (SPE) that is a molecule of sucrose with fatty acid side chains substituted on seven to ten of the hydroxyl groups. It is not absorbed by the body and is therefore calorie-free. It is not degraded by heat and thus may be used in cooking oils and shortenings. It would presumably give the effect of fat on the flavor and texture of a food without the calories. The manufacturer proposes to substitute Olestra for part of the fat in its products.

Simplesse, a NutraSweet Company product currently approved for use in frozen desserts, is made from milk and egg white protein with a change in physical form. It coagulates in cooking and therefore cannot be used in baking, frying, or other heating methods, but can be used in ice cream, cheese, and uncooked salad dressings. It contains $1\frac{1}{3}$ kcal/g.

The use of fat substitutes is unlikely to solve the obesity problem, although they may be helpful. Continuation of diet control is likely to be necessary.

Formula Diets. Formula diets, in the form of liquids, powders, wafers, or bars, become popular at regular intervals. They generally supply approximately 900 kcal from 20% protein (45 g) and 50% carbohydrate. For long-term use, they do nothing to retrain the patient in his or her eating habits. It sometimes is necessary to explain to a patient that the formula is to be taken *in place of,* not in addition to, a meal.

These diets may be useful for a person who wishes to lose just a few pounds or for the person who needs to lose weight quickly in anticipation of surgery. They may be convenient for one meal per day, usually breakfast or lunch, for the long-term dieter. The formula diets do not provide the "miracle cures" for which many patients are looking and may actually contribute to defeat because of their monotony.

Fasting or Starvation. A third type of dietary treatment of obesity involves fasting. This is a severe treatment which should be used only if the patient is hospitalized. It should not be used if the patient has a history of gout or of cardiovascular, renal, or hepatic disease.

In some institutions where this type of treatment is employed, the patients are allowed small amounts of black coffee, tea, or fruit juices and raw vegetables with high water content such as lettuce and tomatoes. The patient receives a liberal amount of water and vitamin supplements and is encouraged to exercise normally. It is claimed that a major advantage of this method is that the patient becomes ketotic and feelings of hunger subside; however, there is some evidence that this is not true.[96]

Other effects of fasting are summarized in Figures 14-1 and 14-2. As these figures indicate, fasting is accompanied by a rapid nitrogen loss at first, followed by an adaptation to a slower, steady rate of loss.

A variation of the starvation regimen is the **very low calorie diet** (VLCD). The diet commonly contains 500 kcal per day or less. Although these diets vary somewhat in composition, they usually include, at least theoretically, enough high biological value protein to prevent loss of lean body mass. This may consist of 30 to 70 g. They may also contain two or three grams of fat or none at all, and enough carbohydrate to avoid severe ketosis and provide the total of 400–500 kcal. Vitamins and minerals are added to provide RDA levels. Patients are advised to drink $1\frac{1}{2}$ to 2 liters of water per day. They are also often advised to avoid strenuous exercise.

There is a great deal of disagreement on the safety and efficacy of such programs.

The relative amounts of loss of lean body mass, fat, water, and potassium are highly variable and not completely understood.[97] The length of time the diet can be used safely also is unknown.[97] Others claim that the diet is safe and has been quite effective.[98,99] However, prior to the availability of the current formulas, liquid formulas containing low-quality protein resulted in several deaths and have encouraged great caution in the use of these diets.

A number of commercial formula products are currently available which appear to be safer than the previous formulations (e.g., Modifast, Optifast, Nutroclin VLC). Use of such products are often part of a program which includes medical supervision, patient support sessions, and advice concerning a maintenance program following weight loss. In addition, certain categories of clients are usually excluded: those less than 16 years of age, pregnant women, or patients with serious disorders other than diabetes mellitus. These factors are assumed to contribute to efficacy and safety. The commercial formulas are not required to prepare a VLCD. The diet can be composed of natural foods, but it is clear that such a restricted diet should not be undertaken without close medical supervision. However, the use of the protein-sparing modified fast has been questioned, since it does nothing to correct the patient's eating habits.

Packaged Food Programs. Some programs (e.g., Jenny Craig Weight Loss Centers and Nutri/System) prepare and package a menu which they sell to dieters. The client supplements this food with skim milk, fresh vegetables, and fruit. Both programs encourage some exercise and provide some counseling and group support sessions. The programs are expensive and do little to help establish more effective eating habits. The foods can also be obtained more cheaply by using items routinely available in grocery stores. However, some clients find the programs helpful because the dieter does not need to make decisions concerning food intake.[102]

Fad Diets. A variety of fad diets have succeeded one another over the years and probably will continue to do so. Many promise miracle cures and easy weight loss without dieting. In fact, any success achieved is usually the consequence of reduced energy intake because the diet is boring or unpalatable.

One type that is regularly resurrected is the **no-carbohydrate** or **low-carbohydrate diet**, which contains high protein plus high or moderate amounts of fat. Like the starvation diet, it tends to cause ketosis. The diet may cause rapid weight loss for a week or so, largely as a result of water loss. In addition, the diet usually is low in calories because of the difficulty in planning for enough calories from protein and fat alone. However, this is yet another diet that does nothing to change faulty eating habits, and the patient usually regains the weight lost.

Another type of diet often presented with great fervor is the one that **emphasizes one or a few foods** that are proposed to have miraculous properties—for example, the grapefruit, or bananas and milk, ice cream, yogurt, lecithin/B_6/apple cider vinegar/kelp or candy ("lollipop") diets. Unfortunately, many are inadequate and most do little to establish better food habits. Some may be downright dangerous.

Another variation on the theme was diets that alternated a very-low-calorie diet (e.g., 600 kcal) with a more generous ration (e.g., 1,800 kcal). A study of the effects of such a diet with behavior modification, and with or without exercise, showed that the diet effects were the same as those seen in controls with a diet equivalent to the mean intake of the experimental subjects. Only exercise resulted in a greater reduction of body weight.[101]

At intervals, a weight reduction scheme is promoted in which it is claimed that some substance will interfere with digestion, absorption, or metabolism of food, thus causing weight loss without calorie restriction. One of these was the so-called starch blocker. It was claimed that this substance, a protein from kidney, northern, or other beans, blocks the action of alpha-amylase and thus interferes with the digestion of starch. Each pill was advertised as interfering with the digestion of 400 to 750 starch calories, depending on the brand. One of its leading proponents advocated that the starch blocker be taken with a diet providing 700 kcal of starch and 500 kcal from other sources. With a 1,200-kcal diet, most patients would lose weight, and attributing the loss to the starch blocker would be unjustified. Nevertheless, starch blockers were selling very well at $10 to $20 per bottle until further sales were banned in the United States by the Food and Drug Administration (FDA) pending evidence that the product was safe and effective. The FDA had received complaints from users of nausea, vomiting, diarrhea, flatulence, and abdominal pain. If starch blockers worked as advertised and undigested starch reached the colon, microbial metabolism of starch could cause flatulence, abdominal cramps, and diarrhea.

Other Aids to Weight Reduction

It has been obvious to nutritional care specialists for many years that simply teaching an obese patient the mechanics of an energy-restricted diet usually does not lead to permanent weight reduction. In view of this fact, a number of other procedures are used in combination with or as a substitute for calorie restriction. Primary among these are exercise programs, behavior modification, group therapy, drugs, and surgery.

Exercise. The amount of exercise required to use excess kilocalories generally is regarded to be very great. Examples of common snack foods and their caloric equivalents in exercise as usually stated are given in Table 12-3. There is some evidence, however, that exercise increases resting and basal metabolic rate for a period of time that exceeds the duration of the exercise itself. This still is controversial, but if true, the energy cost of exercise would be greater than the values indicated by Table 12-3, and thus exercise would be recognized as being of greater value in weight reduction than has commonly been believed. Still, the amount of time required to "work off" the effects of a single milk shake in excess of need, for example, should make clear the advantage of prevention of excess intake.

Given the existence of obesity, though, exercise should be a part of any obesity treatment program, since exercise reduces body fat, regardless of weight. Studies of obese infants,[103] adolescent girls,[104] and adult women[105] indicate that, in all three groups, activity was less even though their food intake was not necessarily greater than that of their lean counterparts. It is difficult to motivate obese individuals to exercise, and careful monitoring or a structured program of exercises may be helpful.

Table 12-3. Energy Equivalents of Selected Snack Foods and Activities

Snack Food	Kcal	Activity (minutes)				
		Walking	Bicycling	Swimming	Running	Reclining
Beer, 1 glass	114	22	14	10	6	88
Cake, two-layer, $\frac{1}{12}$	356	68	43	32	18	274
Carbonated beverage, 1 glass	106	20	13	9	5	82
Doughnut	151	29	18	13	8	116
Ice cream, $\frac{1}{8}$ qt.	193	37	24	17	10	148
Ice cream soda	255	49	31	23	13	196
Malted milk shake	502	97	61	45	26	386
Milk shake	421	81	51	38	22	324

Based on data in Konishi, F., Food and energy equivalents of various activities. *J. Am. Diet. Assoc.* 46:187, 1965.

Exercise may help to decrease food intake, even though many individuals believe that it will increase appetite.[106,107] On the contrary, Mayer[108] has shown that, in both rats and humans, food intake actually is increased when the body is very *inactive*. Food intake decreases with light activity and rises in those with greater activity. The increase with heavy activity was proportionate to expenditure and did not lead to obesity.[108]

The amount and type of exercise should be chosen with care. Complicating conditions, such as cardiovascular disease and degenerative joint disease, must be taken into consideration, especially in the morbidly obese. The nutritional care specialist should work with others (the physician and physical therapist) on the health care team in coordinating kilocalorie intake with an exercise program.

The energy cost of exercise varies with the type of activity, the amount of participation, duration of activity, and the body weight of the individual.[60] According to many tables, a person who weighs 200 lb. might expend only 350 kcal in playing golf or as much as 1,042 kcal in judo or karate in 1 hour. Some activities lend themselves to great variation in the amount of effort expended. Our 200-lb. obese individual might expend, in 1 hour, 304 kcal bicycling at 5 miles per hour, 600 kcal at 10 miles per hour, and 868 kcal at 13 miles per hour. These expenditures would double if he or she continued the activity at the same pace for another hour. The heavier the individual, the greater the weight loss for a given activity. For example, if a man were swimming at a moderate pace of 45 yd./min., approximate expenditure might be 522 kcal/hr. if he weighed 150 lb., 696 kcal/hr. at 200 lb., and 870 kcal/hr. at 250 lb. It is important to remember that these examples are estimations only and are influenced by an individual's skill in a given activity as well as the environmental temperature and consequent need to maintain body temperature.

There is no evidence that exercise is useful in "spot reducing" of subcutaneous fat. It may, in certain activities, lead to muscle development in some areas of the body.[109]

Behavior Modification. The procedures used in modifying eating behavior may vary with the concept of the problem as perceived by the nutritional therapist. One view is to consider problem eating as a sign of personality dysfunction. A more recent concept holds that eating behavior is learned and that poor eating practices can be unlearned. Problem eating is seen as the problem itself, not as a sign of another problem.

The theory behind behavior modification is based on principles of learning that are applied to normal behavior. Three types of learning principles will be described.

Observational or imitation learning requires observation of the behavior of another person who serves as a model. It can be very effective in children, for example, particularly if their behavior is reinforced.

Conditioning (classic conditioning, Pavlovian conditioning, or stimulus-response learning) has also been attempted to modify eating behavior. In general principle, the method involves pairing a stimulus that elicits a given response with a neutral stimulus that does not elicit the response. Eventually, the neutral stimulus alone will elicit the response. It may be used in combination with the third method.

Operant conditioning or **trial-and-error learning** is, to a large extent, the basis for behavior modification techniques used in nutritional counseling and will therefore be described in more detail. It is based primarily on the assumption that behavior is controlled by the consequences that follow it. The behavior to be modified, the **target behavior**, is followed by a consequence known as a **reinforcer**. Reinforcers that increase the frequency of a target behavior are called **positive reinforcers** or **rewards**, whereas those that increase the behavior when removed are **negative reinforcers** or **aversive stimuli**. Negative reinforcers are presented before the desired response begins and are removed when it does begin. Negative reinforcement has been used in obesity therapy by subjecting the patient to unpleasant stimuli such as foul-smelling odors or electric shock prior to presenting problem foods. The method has suffered from a high dropout rate and has been successful primarily only over a short term.[110]

Another aspect of operant conditioning involves the process of **extinction**. It is based on the principle that if reinforcement of behavior is removed, the behavior will decrease. It requires the identification of and removal of reinforcers, processes that may be difficult.

Difficulty in therapy also arises if the desired behavior does not occur and therefore cannot be reinforced. Under these circumstances, a process known as **shaping** can be used. Some part or approximation of the desired behavior can be reinforced and then changed, at intervals, to approach the desired behavior. A patient might first decrease the intake of only one food, or agree to forgo one part of a meal, for example. The desired diet might then be approached and reinforced in stepwise fashion.

In behavior modification programs for weight reduction, a variety of procedures based on the previously listed learning principles has been used. In general, the program begins with a diagnostic period to attempt to identify the factors that cause the maladaptive eating behavior. The patient is asked first to keep a diary of the type and amount of foods eaten and the circumstances of eating such as time, place, position, associated activities, others present, degree of hunger, and emotional state. From this record, the patient and therapist identify problem areas leading to overeating. Some problem areas might include eating leftovers from family meals to avoid waste, snacking while watching television, or eating very rapidly. Once problem areas are identified, the patient and nutritional care specialist together initiate desired changes. The shaping process might be very appropriate here.

Techniques for modification of eating behaviors include the following:

1. **Contingency contracting** consists of a signed agreement between the patient and therapist, which specifies behaviors to be changed and the rewards or penalties to be applied. One example required the patient to deposit specified valuables with the therapist to be "earned" back by weight loss.

2. **Positive reinforcement** can involve earning a reward for certain behaviors — that is, specified weight loss. Spouses have been enlisted to provide rewards in the form of encouragement and approval.

3. **Stimulus control and environmental management** procedures have received a great deal of attention. They seek to modify the environment that supports the overeating behavior.[111] This must be a cooperative procedure, involving both the therapist and patient, and requires imagination. Stuart[112] has suggested some procedures that he found to be useful in suppressing cues to eating:

Eat in one room only.
Do nothing else while eating.
Clear dishes from a meal directly into the garbage.
Make only the proper foods available by shopping from a list and only after a meal.
Prepare and serve small quantities only.
Eat only with utensils.
Chew food slowly.
Set utensils down between bites of food.

4. **Self-monitoring** includes calorie-counting from a chart, keeping a weight chart on a line graph, and writing down the amount of everything eaten. It provides the patient with feedback on progress but has not been successful unless combined with other techniques.

Behavior modification was reported to be very successful when first presented,[113] but subsequent investigation has moderated the original enthusiasm for the method.[114] The weight loss five years after treatment was not significantly better than that seen in patients treated by traditional methods.[114] Nevertheless, if weight loss is to be maintained, eating behavior must be modified; therefore, it is logical to continue to attempt modification by some method.

Group Counseling. Sometimes obese patients are treated in groups rather than individually. Some studies have indicated little or no difference in the effectiveness of long-term group therapy, individual therapy, and no therapy,[115,116] but others report better results with group therapy.[117] For short-term use, at least, group treatment appears to be more effective than individual treatment.

A number of self-help groups have been established, often using behavior modification as part of their program. Examples of this type of program include Weight Watchers, Inc., TOPS (Take Off Pounds Sensibly), Diet Workshop, and Overeaters Anonymous. Little data are available on the effectiveness of these groups. A few limited studies suggest that they are not helpful in the long term for the vast majority of patients.[85] The dropout rate has been reported to be 95%, but the groups may be successful in the remaining 5%.

Summer camps for obese children are numerous, providing programs for kilocalorie restriction, exercise, and nutrition education. Their effectiveness has not been evaluated.

Drugs. The lack of success in treatment of obesity by dieting had led to a search for drugs that might be helpful. The ideal antiobesity drug has been described as one that will (1) provide reduction of fat stores while sparing protein, (2) prevent weight gain after ideal weight is reached, (3) improve compliance with a diet and exercise program, and (4) have no adverse side effects or abuse potential.[118] Although no drug meets all these criteria, a number of drugs have been used. Potential sites and modes of action of drugs in use include the following:

- Decrease food intake, gastric emptying, or intestinal absorption.
- Decrease pancreatic insulin.
- Decrease liver lipid synthesis.
- Increase adipose tissue lipolysis.
- Increase brown adipose tissue thermogenesis.
- Increase energy utilization by muscle or other tissue.[118]

Currently available drugs focus primarily on reducing energy intake. The most commonly used drugs for obesity are appetite depressants or anorectics. A few are variations on amphetamines (Table 12-4). There are various contraindications to their use. They are addicting, tend to increase blood pressure, and may alter insulin action in diabetics. They may affect central nervous system function. They should not be used by patients taking monoamine oxidase inhibitors (see Chapter 19). Other anorexic drugs are not amphetamines, but they also have cardiovascular and central nervous system side effects. Both types of drugs include products containing coloring agents to which patients may be sensitive. These drugs are not recommended for children or pregnant women.

The modes of action of anorexic drugs are not entirely understood. Their side effects also vary. **Amphetamine**, which might be considered the parent compound, may act by an effect on the lateral hypothalamus.[119] It has been suggested that amphetamine causes a stimulation of dopaminergic and beta-adrenergic receptors by causing a release of dopamine and norepinephrine in the LH.[120] By contrast, fenfluramine is postulated to cause the release of serotonin from other central sites.[121] In addition to their modification of central systems in the brain involved with food impulse regulation, some anorexics (e.g., fenfluramine and mazindol) also produce changes in energy metabolism.[122] In animals, triglyceride absorption was reduced and glucose uptake by human muscle and adipose tissue was increased. It is not known yet whether these changes are involved in the production of anorexia or are side effects.

Over the short term (a few weeks), anorectics increase weight loss, but long-term follow-up is difficult to evaluate because of a high dropout rate in the subjects of the studies. As a result, the use of anorectics is controversial and is complicated by their involvement in drug abuse.

Bulking agents, materials such as meth-

Table 12-4. Anorexic Agents Used in Weight Reduction

| Drugs | Dry Mouth | Unpleasant Taste | Gastrointestinal Side Effects[a] | | | | Addictive Classification[b] |
			Nausea	Abdominal Discomfort	Constipation	Diarrhea	
Amphetamines							
Benzphetamine · HCl (Didrex)	X	X	X	X	—	X	III
Dextroamphetamine sulfate (Dexedrine, Obetrol)	X	X	—	X	X	X	II
Methamphetamine · HCl (Desoxyn)	X	X	—	X	X	X	II
Nonamphetamines							
Diethylpropion · HCl (Tenuate, Tepanil)	X	X	X	X	X	X	IV
Fenfluramine · HCl (Pondimin)	—	X	X	X	X	X	IV
Mazindol (Sanorex, Mazanor)	X	X	X	X	X	X	IV
Phendimetrazine tartrate (Plegine, Bontril, Melfiat)	X	—	X	X	X	X	III
Phenmetrazine · HCl (Preludin)	X	X	X	X	X	X	II
Phentermine (Fastin, Ionamin, Adipex-P)	X	X	—	—	X	X	IV

[a] X = present; — = incidence less than with placebo.
[b] Classification of degree of addiction; IV is the least addictive drug.

ylcellulose and guar gum, have been added to food or dietetic candy with the intent to fill the stomach with inert, nondigestible material. The hope is that the obese person then will eat less. Unfortunately, clinical trials do not indicate that the method is effective, and flatulence is a problem.[123]

Another category of drugs used as weight-reducing aids have been categorized as **metabolic affectors**. Some deserve particular mention. **Thyroid hormone** has been used for many years on the assumption that it would stimulate oxygen consumption and increase fuel use. Unfortunately, in addition to fat consumption, protein loss increases.[124] These protein losses can be minimized by increasing dietary protein,[125] but the results of thyroid medication are no better than with diet alone.[85] The use of exogenous thyroid hormone also causes side effects including increased myocardial irritability; therefore, its use rarely is indicated.

Injections of **human chorionic gonadotropin** (HCG) are used in many clinics along with a very-low-calorie (500-kcal), low-fat diet. The originator of this treatment method claims that it "melts away" fat and reduces hunger.[126] Carefully controlled clinical trials indicate that HCG neither reduces hunger nor promotes weight loss beyond that which would be obtained by diet alone.[127–129]

Human growth hormone, another metabolic affector, has been used recently in the treatment of obesity. It depletes body fat, and limited trials indicate that it may be effective. However, the hormone is in short supply. If more becomes available, additional research may be possible.

Other drugs are currently under study. Some are appetite suppressants, and other inhibit gastric emptying, reduce availability of carbohydrate, inhibit lipid synthesis, or promote oxidation, or promote thermogenesis.[130,131]

Acupuncture. In this method, metal staples are placed in the ears. Wiggling the staples is supposed to eliminate hunger. A 400-kcal diet is also given. The method works if the low-kilocalorie diet is followed. One must then ask if the acupuncture increases the effect of the diet.

Surgery. Surgical treatments for obesity have been developed largely because of the poor response to less drastic measures. However, only 5% of patients treated surgically maintain their decreased body weight for several years.[132] In addition, not all patients are appropriate subjects for surgical treatment.

Criteria for choosing patients who are candidates for surgical treatment include the following:[133]

1. *Morbidity.* The association with obesity-related diseases, such as cardiovascular disease, and the effect on the quality of life should be considered. Since quality of life, in particular, is difficult to quantify, there are no established objective standards.
2. *Weight.* Only the morbidly obese should be considered for surgery.
3. *Age.* Growing children and elderly patients are not considered to be good candidates.
4. *Cooperation.* Patients must indicate a willingness and ability to cooperate in a life-long follow-up. Alcoholism and psychiatric disease are considered to be contraindications, but this opinion is not unanimous.
5. *Other diseases.* Many diseases are favorably influenced by weight loss, if the patient is in good condition for surgery. If, on the other hand, a disease tends to cause obesity but is treatable, surgery is contraindicated.

Lipectomy and liposuction. It might seem logical to ask why obesity could not be treated by **adipectomy** or **lipectomy** (surgical removal of adipose tissue) or by **liposuction** (in which fat tissue is suctioned out). Since the number of fat cells is thought to be reduced during weight loss, the surgical removal of numbers of cells might be postulated to make it easier for patients to maintain their loss. There are few studies of the effects of such treatment. However, the little evidence available demonstrated in three patients that lipectomy did not prevent regaining lost weight, although the adiposity did not recur at the same sites.[134] These results suggest that it is the mass of adipose tissues or cell size that is controlled rather than the number of cells. This type of surgery sometimes is undertaken for cosmetic reasons, but it is not considered a primary treatment. In addition, **panniculectomy** (surgical removal of excess abdominal skin and fat) after large weight losses sometimes is done for cosmetic purposes.

Intragastric balloon therapy. Most morbidly obese patients fail to achieve or maintain weight control, and other methods may be added. One of these is the insertion of a balloon or "bubble" that takes up space in the stomach to promote a feeling of satiety and suppress appetite.

The device, which is FDA-approved for use in the United States, is the Garren-Edwards Gastric Bubble, a polyurethane cylinder with a hollow central channel. It is introduced by mouth under sedation and topical anesthesia and inflated when it is in the stomach.

After the bubble is implanted, a full liquid diet with 500 to 700 kcal is given for three to seven days. This is followed by an 800 to 1,200 kcal diet and behavior modification therapy. Contraindications to its use are active peptic ulcer disease, large hiatal hernia, and prior gastric or intestinal surgery. Because of the incidence of peptic ulcer in these patients and the tendency of the bubble to cause gastritis, patients are frequently advised to avoid caffeine, alcohol, highly spiced foods, and aspirin. Antacids and histamine blockers are sometimes prescribed.

It is recommended that the bubble be removed in three months because there is an increased tendency for it to deflate after that time, move into the intestine, and cause obstruction. One study reported complications to include persistent epigastric pain (36%), persistent nausea and vomiting (9%), gastritis (58%), and spontaneous balloon deflation (56%).

This method is currently in use as an adjunct to diet and behavior modification. However, studies have indicated that weight loss has been disappointingly small. Instead of developing a feeling of satiety, the stomach enlarges to provide for more intake. Regain of weight is usual. Therefore, the use of the bubble is recommended only for temporary weight loss to improve surgical risk.[135]

Bypass procedures. Surgical procedures to bypass various parts or lengths of the digestive system have in common the creation of a malabsorption syndrome analogous to that seen in short bowel syndrome. They include jejunoileal, jejunocolic, and biliopancreatic bypasses. See Figure 12-3A, B, and C. The first two were accompanied by a number of serious complications including diarrhea, malnutrition, liver disease, and renal stones. As a consequence, they are much less often done, and many have been reversed by subsequent surgery. The biliopancreatic bypass is newer and is still being evaluated.

Diarrhea occurs in all jejunoileal bypass patients postoperatively.[136] It is important, especially during the first month, to prevent excessive food intake for the size of the remaining bowel, or the patient will vomit, causing loss of protein, electrolytes, and fluid. Approximately 30% of weight is lost in the first year,[137] and the weight stabilizes after approximately two years with weight maintenance at approximately 62% of maximum.

A number of serious side effects may occur. Patients may develop such severe electrolyte imbalances as to require hospitalization.

Progressive liver disease occurs in some intestinal bypass patients, with inflammation and fibrosis, sometimes progressing to cirrhosis.[137,138] The etiology of the liver condition is not clear. Experiments with animals suggest that the hepatic lesion is caused by toxins produced by bacterial overgrowth in the bypassed intestine.[138] Others have suggested that liver failure may be the result of nutritional deficiency.[139]

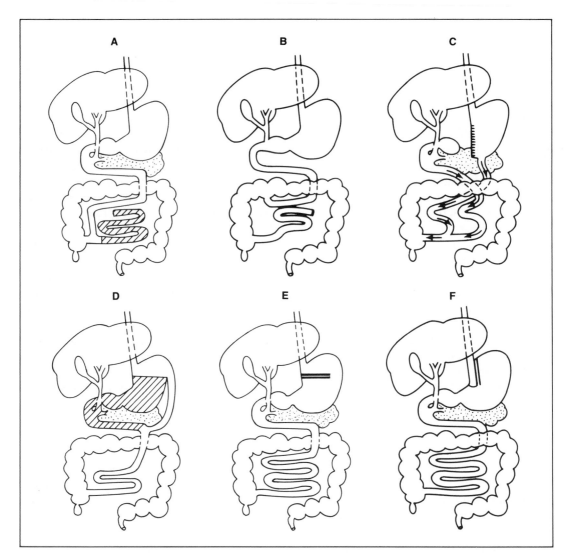

Figure 12-3. Surgical treatment for obesity. A. Jejunoileal bypass. Anastamosis of jejunum and ileum may be end-to-end or end-to-side; B. Jejunocolic bypass; C. Biliopancreatic bypass. The duodenal stump is closed and 75% of the stomach is removed. The small intestine is divided 250 cm from the ileocecal valve. The distal segment, or alimentary limb, is anastamosed to the remaining part of the stomach. It is about 50% of the normal length of the alimentary tract. The proximal stump, or biliopancreatic conduit, is anastamosed to the terminal ileum 50 cm from the ileocecal valve; D. Gastric bypass; E. Horizontal gastroplasty; F. Vertical banded gastroplasty. The staple line creates a small pouch, often with a 20-ml capacity. The band maintains an outlet diameter of 1 cm.

Other complications include death in 0–6% of patients, wound infection in 2–5%, thromboembolism in 1–5%, and renal failure in 3%.[134] A small number of patients develop severe psychiatric problems. Complications are life-threatening in approximately 4% of patients, and the normal intestinal continuity must be reestablished.

Jejunoileal bypass has been done extensively in the past, and some of these patients may come to the attention of the nutritional care specialist postoperatively. The patients should receive potassium supplements, particularly when diarrhea is severe. Potassium-rich fruits and vegetables should be emphasized when the postoperative patient recovers sufficiently to eat them. Supplements of calcium, magnesium, and all vitamins may be required.

A **high-protein** diet to protect the liver and **low fat** to reduce steatorrhea, provided in **small meals**, may be helpful. Alcohol should be avoided for at least a year and preferably permanently to avoid overtaxing the liver. Pregnancy should be avoided while weight loss is occurring.

It is important that patients having their bypass surgery reversed have good protein nutrition prior to surgery. Ideally, restoration is done before the patient is seriously protein-depleted. For protein-depleted patients, Mason[140] recommends the use of hyperosmotic amino acid and glucose infusions through a central vein (see Chapter 5). The patient is given 3 to 4 L/day. One of these infusions is glucose-free to mobilize fat from the liver. The central line is left in place for feeding after surgery, since these patients have a prolonged ileus. Most patients return to their original obese weight after bypass reversal. The most commonly held current opinion is that the risks of this type of surgery are not justified by the benefits.

Biliopancreatic bypass patients rarely have fluid and electrolyte imbalances because they do not usually have diarrhea. Hepatic abnormalities are not seen, and serum lipids tend to normalize. About 3% of these patients have developed renal stones. There is a tendency to hypoproteinemia and anemia. Patients are lactose-intolerant and should be given Lactaid or other assistance. Supplements should be provided for fat-soluble vitamins in water-soluble form, along with vitamin B_6, calcium, and iron.

Gastric restrictive surgery. Restriction of gastric capacity is currently more frequently used than are intestinal bypass procedures. There are a number of possible approaches. The **gastric bypass** and **gastroplasty** ("gastric stapling") are the most common current practices (see Figure 12-3D, E, and F). Gastric bypass is associated with a greater weight loss than that seen in gastroplasty.

The pouch created in gastroplasty has a maximum capacity of 50 ml, but it may be as little as 10 ml, and the opening past the staple line may measure 1.2 cm. This opening must be reinforced to prevent dilation, and sometimes the stomach is wrapped to prevent enlargement. Vertical banded gastroplasty is currently more common than horizontal stapling, since it seems to be associated with fewer complications.

Patients with gastric restrictive procedures require both pre- and postoperative nutritional counseling and intervention if the procedure is to have any chance of success. The purposes are to decrease risk of the surgical procedure and increase potential for postoperative weight loss. Surgical risk may be decreased by an initial weight loss in an amount determined by the surgeon. When weight is reduced, a decrease in dosage of insulin or antihypertensive drugs is desirable. The patient is also advised to stop smoking.

The weight loss is approached preferably with a low-kilocalorie diet combined with behavior modification. The diet must be individualized, but an example from one institution included 1,200 kcal with 1.2 to 1.5 g protein per kg ideal body weight, 100 g complex carbohydrate included in the 1,200 kcal, and only the amount of fat contained in the protein sources.[141] Diabetic exchange lists (see Chapter 11) are used for calculation of the diet. Anticipated weight loss is 1 kg/week.

If weight loss is insufficient, the protein-sparing modified fast, carefully supervised by a physician, may be used. Some patients have a gastric bubble implanted.

The diet following gastroplasty must be progressed with caution. Throughout, kilocalories are severely restricted. A protocol from New England Deaconess Hospital suggests the following:[141]

Stage 1: 30–60 ml hourly of water. Begin when bowel sounds are heard and continue 1–2 days.

Stage 2: Three meals of three servings of 30 ml of dietetic gelatin or bouillon plus 60–90 ml hourly *between meals* of water or decarbonated diet ginger ale (allow to go flat). Carbonation causes discomfort. IV fluids, electrolytes, and amino acids are also usually given.

Stage 3: Three meals per day of three portions with 2 oz. pureed lean meat, fish or poultry, and 1 oz. pureed fruit and/or vegetables. No concentrated sweets or fruit juice are given. Also, give 90–120 ml hourly between meals of clear liquids to total 1,500 ml/day. Include 1½ cup skim or 1% fat milk. Plain coffee or tea may be added. Follow this diet for two months.

Stage 4: Three meals per day of three items each chosen from 2 oz. lean meat, poultry, or fish and 1 oz. unsweetened fruit or vegetable. Include 1 oz. complex carbohydrate per day in place of one fruit or vegetable. Add 120 ml/hour *between meals* of clear liquids and 1½ cups skim or 1% fat milk to total 1,500 ml/day. This diet is to be followed indefinitely.

The volume of food must be carefully limited and eaten slowly. If a greater volume of food is routinely taken, the pouch can be dilated, defeating the purpose of the procedure. The danger of disrupting the staple line is also increased.

Patients are advised to eat the protein-rich foods first and to eat very slowly to avoid stretching the outlet from the small pouch. For the same reason, liquids are taken between meals, not at meals. A chewable multivitamin plus mineral supplement and four Tums for calcium are given. These are crushed or chewed to avoid obstructing the outlet.

Three 20-minute aerobic exercise sessions per week are also included. Expected weight loss is 1% of body weight per week. Patients are followed in the outpatient clinic.

The bypassed portion of the stomach can be restored to continuity if necessary. There are fewer complications, but weight loss is less than that following intestinal bypass. The loss is greatest in young patients. Dumping syndrome, steatorrhea, and gallstones sometimes are complications.[142]

Other techniques of gastric restrictive procedures include gastric banding, similar in concept to belt tightening, and gastric wrapping.

A number of metabolic complications are associated with gastric restrictive procedures. The altered physiology of the gastrointestinal system may lead to anemia, dumping syndrome, and deficiencies of calcium, iron, folate, and vitamin B_{12}. All restrictive procedures can result in vomiting, impaired immune function, gallstone formation, hair loss, and protein and vitamin malnutrition. Thiamine deficiency can result in neuropathy and encephalopathy. Complications of biliopancreatic bypass also may include deficiencies of fat-soluble vitamins and metabolic bone disease.

Jaw wiring. Jaw wiring, or maxillomandibular fixation, consists of wiring the upper and lower jaws together so that intake of liquids is possible but eating solid foods is almost impossible. Weight loss, in one study, averaged 25.3 kg in six months, an amount similar to that seen in intestinal bypass patients.[143] Most regained some of the weight once the wires were removed. Possible complications include dental caries and deterioration of muscle function in the jaw. Patients are advised to carry wire clippers to remove the wire in case of vomiting to avoid choking.

Nutritional care should include counseling on the variety of liquid and semiliquid food that can make up the diet. Particular attention should be paid to ensure that the diet is adequate in protein, minerals, and vitamins without providing excess calories.

Psychotherapy. Psychiatric treatment is not often successful in the treatment of obesity unless the patient has a treatable psychiatric disorder and the obesity is of recent development as a consequence. Some cases of depression are associated with weight gain. Unfortunately, the tricyclic antidepressants also cause weight gain.

Hypnosis. Hypnosis has been used only occasionally, and its long-term effectiveness is unknown. Some techniques reported include posthypnotic suggestion, substitution of gum chewing for eating, substitution of physical activity for eating, and hypnotic anesthesia to control hunger pangs.

Most Highly Recommended Therapy for Obesity

It must be recognized that the causes of obesity are poorly understood and the treatments available at present are largely ineffective and sometimes hazardous. However, almost any treatment will give some short-term results. Given these limitations, the most highly recommended therapy consists of individualized treatment coupled with group counseling, using restriction of calorie intake, increased physical activity, and instruction in behavior modification to change eating behavior permanently. For maintenance of weight loss, the patient may need to remain in treatment almost indefinitely. Successful weight reduction remains a challenge and a source of frustration to the nutritional care specialist. One should remember that a great service is being performed for the patient if he or she is helped to achieve a stable weight and prevent further weight gain.

Psychological Factors in Obesity

The nutritional care specialist must be sensitive to the psychological factors involved in treating obesity, which can be divided into (1) factors causing obesity, (2) those that result from the existence of the obesity, (3) those that arise from attempts to lose weight, and, occasionally, (4) factors that arise from successful weight loss.

Some, but by no means all, patients become obese as a consequence of a psychiatric disorder. No single disorder has been identified as being involved in the etiology of obesity, but when one does exist, it must be treated before nutritional treatment for weight reduction can be undertaken.

The stigma attached to obesity in our society may be the cause of emotional disturbance. The obese person can develop a syndrome of low self-esteem, depression, and hostility.[144] Treatment is thought to require raising the self-esteem. The attitude of health professionals toward the obese can be very important in this regard. Health professionals whose attitude toward the obese is to stigmatize them are unlikely to be helpful.

Other obese patients have problems that are not severe enough to be classified as psychiatric problems but for which their overeating compensates, including emotional problems such as depression, frustration, worry, hopelessness, isolation, guilt, or shame. Social factors are important. Meal size tends to increase as the number of persons present increases.[145] A person who gains weight after giving up smoking may be substituting one method of relieving tension for another. It has been suggested that the effect is mediated by corticosteroid hormones. On the whole, however, the mechanisms relating emotional factors and obesity are unknown.

Emotional problems sometimes arise during or following weight loss. The reasons for this are not always clear. Patients with juvenile-onset obesity in one study showed frequent symptoms of anxiety and depression and viewed the process of weight loss as severe starvation.[146] They had disturbances in body image and continued to see themselves as fat even after weight loss.

Problems may arise for the occasional patient who successfully loses weight. Some patients adjust to the stigma of obesity by developing friendships with other obese individuals. For others, obesity is an important component in maintaining their relationships with spouses. Weight loss sometimes can disrupt these relationships.

Aspects of Nutritional Assessment and Monitoring

In addition to evaluation of the extent of the obesity, it is useful to know of medical and social problems faced by the patient. A history of the patient's previous efforts at weight reduction is also helpful. Information on the following may be elicited, largely by interview. The emphasis of the questions may be altered with the type of treatment being considered.

How long has the patient been overweight?

List all the diets tried.

List weight loss clinics attended.

List exercise program attended.

Exercise tolerance?

Grip strength?

What pills or other injections have been tried?

Has the patient tried acupuncture? Hypnosis? Other? Name them.

Does the patient have problems with shortness of breath? Joint pain? (Name the joint.) Blood pressure problems? Diabetes? Vein Problems? Hiatal hernia? Rashes or other problems under folds? Between thighs? Urinary incontinence? Other? (Name them.)

Are there problems finding clothes? Fitting into chairs?

Describe other social problems.

List previous operations and medical history.

Other desirable information (especially useful after surgery for obesity) includes:

Anthropometric: skinfolds; waist-to-hip circumference ratio.

Assessment of malnutrition: physical examination for clinical signs of malnutrition.

Laboratory methods: serum albumin or transferrin, hemoglobin, lymphocyte count, skin testing.

Factor-increasing needs: excessive losses (vomiting, diarrhea); infection; pregnancy; use of catabolic drugs (e.g., steroids).

Prevention of Obesity

The best "treatment" for obesity is prevention. In contacts with obese patients, the nutritional care specialist sometimes will have an opportunity to influence the parents to prevent obesity in their children. Fomon[147] has suggested some procedures:

1. Encourage mothers to breast-feed their infants.
2. Educate parents on the dangers and problems of overfeeding and on the influence of childhood eating patterns on later nutritional status.
3. Instruct parents to delay introduction of solid food in their child's diet until the child is four to six months old.
4. Promote physical exercise.
5. Encourage parents to develop facilities for year-round physical activity.
6. Instruct parents to use more smaller meals rather than fewer larger meals, but do not increase kilocalories in the process.
7. Give special help and counseling to parents who are obese.

Effects of Repeated Cycles of Weight Loss and Gain

The fact that most obese individuals regain their weight after a weight loss has raised the question of the effect of such "cycling." In a study of the metabolic effect of cycling in rats, it was demonstrated that there was an increase in feed efficiency (weight gain per kilocalorie of intake). These data suggest that repeated weight losses and gains might make subsequent weight loss even more difficult to achieve.[148] However, this question has not been studied in human subjects.

UNDERWEIGHT

A much smaller number of people have a problem in gaining weight rather than in losing weight. These patients are classified as **underweight** (15–20% or more below ideal weight).

Underweight in General

Etiology

A number of conditions can cause a person to be underweight. Poor absorption and utilization of foods was discussed in Chapter 8. Some patients are underweight because they have a wasting disease such as cancer (see Chapter 15). Others are underweight because of psychological or emotional stress or abnormality. Others take in an inadequate quantity or quality of food. If the patient has a disease that causes the underweight condition, the nutritional needs relevant to that disease must also be considered when planning the diet. Thus combinations of several diet modifications may be necessary.

General Effects

Underweight patients have decreased resistance to infection, increased sensitivity to cold, and weakness. Undernutrition can cause depressed function of the pituitary, adrenal, and thyroid glands and the gonads. Growth is retarded in children.

Treatment

Although obese patients may find it hard to believe, it frequently is very difficult for an underweight person to gain weight. In order to increase his or her weight, a person must have an energy intake that is in excess of output. The basic need for the underweight patient is, therefore, a high-calorie diet. Current energy needs must be met plus an additional 500 to 1,000 kcal per day. Food intake may be increased gradually to prevent gastrointestinal disorders. The additional kilocalories may be provided in any of three ways: (1) extra portions of usual foods at regular meals, (2) more concentrated foods, or (3) between-meal snacks. The procedures used should conform to the patient's preferences.

The protein allowance is maintained at a generous or high level, 100 g or more. Protein will be needed for repair and replacement. As the energy level of the diet increases, protein also increases if the planned diet contains normal foods, since most high-carbohydrate foods contain some protein.

The carbohydrate and fat content of the diet must, of course, be increased to achieve the positive calorie balance. The distribution between the two can be made largely on the basis of the patient's preferences. More concentrated sources of kilocalories are advised to reduce the total bulk of the diet.

Vitamins and minerals should be provided at optimal levels. Increased intake of food will increase intake of micronutrients, but supplementation of B vitamins sometimes is needed as kilocalorie intake is increased. Their appetite-stimulating effect may also be helpful.

The patient should be involved in planning the diet. Behavior modification techniques are used as they are for changing the eating habits of obese patients.

Anorexia Nervosa

Anorexia nervosa is a disorder in which underweight can become severe to the point of being life-threatening, with a mortality rate of 6%. It represents a special form of undernutrition that must be differentiated from other causes of weight loss. The condition is difficult to diagnose. The American Psychiatric Association has published criteria for diagnosis of anorexia nervosa and its subgroups and for differentiation from bulimia, described later (see Table 12-5).

More than 90% of anorexia nervosa patients are adolescent girls at onset of the disease. The condition usually first appears shortly after puberty, but occasionally there is prepubertal or late adolescent onset. It was formerly found in the middle and upper classes of affluent societies, but is also now seen in lower socioeconomic groups. First described in 1868, it was long considered a very rare condition. In recent years, however, the incidence is believed to be increasing, although few epidemiologic data are available. It is possible that the change may

Table 12-5. Diagnostic Criteria for Anorexia Nervosa and Bulimia Nervosa

Anorexia Nervosa	Bulimia Nervosa
1. Weight low; emaciation resulting from loss of at least 15% of original body weight (grade 1) or at least 25% of original body weight (grade 2).	1. Normal or overweight.
	2. Intense fear of fatness.
2. Intense fear of becoming obese even though underweight.	3. Awareness that eating pattern is abnormal.
3. Behavior directed to weight loss.	4. Recurring episodes of binge eating[a] at least once a week for the previous four weeks with at least three of the following:
4. Amenorrhea in female—absence of at least three consecutive menstrual cycles.	a. Consumption of high-calorie, easily ingested food during a binge.
5. No known physical illness that accounts for weight loss.	b. Inconspicuous eating binge.
6. Subgroups:	c. Termination of bingeing by abdominal pain, sleep, social interruption, or purging.[b]
a. Restrictor (60%)—bingeing absent and purging usually absent.	d. Repeated attempts to lose weight by purging.
b. Bulimic (40%)—bingeing and purging usually present.	e. Frequent weight fluctuations > 10 lb. because of alternating binges and purges.

Compiled from *Diagnostic and Statistical Manual of Mental Disorders III, 3rd ed.* Washington, D.C.: American Psychiatric Association, 1987; *Diagnostic and Statistical Manual of Mental Disorders, 3rd ed., revised.* Washington D.C.: American Psychiatric Association, 1987; and Hsu, L.K.G., Classification and diagnosis of eating disorders. In B.J. Blinder, B.F. Chaitin, and R. Goldstein, Eds., *The Eating Disorders.* New York: PMA Publishing, 1988.

[a] Bingeing—rapid consumption of a large amount of food in a short period, usually < 2 hours.
[b] Purging—self-induced vomiting or use of cathartics or diuretics.

be due largely to changing standards for diagnosis or to increased awareness.

Etiology

Anorexia nervosa has been classified as primary or atypical. Atypical forms may be secondary to other conditions such as schizophrenia, depression, or hysteria.

The cause of primary anorexia nervosa is uncertain, but the opinion held by most of those who have studied the disease is that anorexia nervosa is psychological in origin. The typical patient is described as highly intelligent, introverted, overly sensitive, perfectionist, and compulsive, with serious deficits in personal development. A deep-seated feeling of ineffectiveness and inadequacy is a common finding. The disease has been proposed to arise from disturbed family relationships in which the patient does not develop a sense of autonomy and effectiveness.[149]

Alternatively, it has been proposed that anorexia nervosa is a disease in which there is immature functioning of the hypothalamus that interferes with normal maturation at puberty.[150] However, this theory does not explain the occurrence of the disease only in developed countries.

It has also been suggested that the pathologic family situations are not the cause of the disease. Rather, they may arise as a result of the stresses created by the disease in one of its members.

Clinical Manifestations

The outstanding feature of anorexia nervosa is severe weight loss that occurs in the absence of organic disease. A weight loss of at least 25% of normal body weight is considered a prerequisite for diagnosis. The patient who loses weight from organic disease typically is aware of the loss, worries about it, and regards it as undesirable. By contrast, the anorexia nervosa patient defends her right to lose weight and complains of being too fat, even when she is seriously emaciated. Only a few known cases were obese before they began dieting. The patients have a **distorted body image** and seem to enjoy and take pride in the progressive weight loss. They often will claim that they do not need to eat and seem to regard their bodies as not their own.

The anorexia nervosa patient **refuses to eat** or eats only a minuscule amount. Bruch[149] tells of one patient who described breakfast saying, "I ate my Cheerio." Patients have been described as spending several hours eating minute amounts of food and complaining of feeling full after only a bite or two. Others have occasional **eating binges** which are **followed by self-induced vomiting** or the use of diuretics, enemas, or large doses of laxatives. There is a great feeling of guilt for losing control.

Many patients are reported to have been somewhat athletic prior to their illness. However, as the disease progresses, the activity tends to change from team sports to those activities that can be performed alone, such as jogging, running, swimming, or calisthenics. The activity takes on a frantic character. Along with the **hyperactivity**, the patient often becomes obsessed with attaining perfection in academic performance. She denies feelings of fatigue despite her various activities and little sleep. Social contact becomes less frequent until the patient is well isolated.

The name of the disease indicates loss of appetite; however, this is apparently a misnomer. Recovered anorexics have reported that they suffered greatly from hunger but somehow obtained great satisfaction from not "giving in." Some patients spend much time preparing food for others to eat, although they refuse to partake themselves. Some collect recipes, walk around food stores, and spend much time in other activities that indicate their minds are consumed with thoughts of food.

As the weight loss progresses, other clinical manifestations appear. They are thought to be the consequence of the malnutrition, since many of these same manifestations have been seen in victims of famine.

There are no definitive laboratory tests for diagnosis. There are a variety of hormone imbalances. Amenorrhea (failure to menstruate) is invariable in girls. Reduction in gonadotropic hormone levels (luteinizing hormone [LH] and follicle-stimulating hormone [FSH]) and alterations in growth hormone and insulin also are found. Neurohormones affecting eating behavior — norepinephrine, dopamine, and serotonin — also regulate insulin, growth hormone, LH, and FSH, and it has been suggested that an alteration of hormone balance in these patients constitutes a biologic predisposition to the disease.[151] However, these changes usually are regarded as the consequence rather than the cause of anorexia nervosa. It is not known whether they precede or follow the onset. Hormone levels do not necessarily return to normal when weight is normalized.

Other manifestations include lowered basal metabolic rate, poor thermoregulation, cold intolerance, anemia, pallor, dry skin, constipation, abdominal pain, hypotension, bradycardia, growth of downy hair (**lanugo**) over the body, and sleep disturbances. Laxative and diuretic abuse can cause electrolyte imbalances and dehydration. The dehydration can produce a reduced production of saliva which is also more viscid. The mouth may be very acidic, caused by vomiting or the use of acid fluids such as fruit juice for thirst. The changes in saliva and the acid pH cause an erosion of the teeth called **perimololysis**, in which the substance of the teeth is lost and many caries appear at atypical locations.[152,153]

As the disease and its attendant weight loss progress, the psychological effects of starvation appear, making the illness even more difficult to treat. The weight lost includes not only body fat but also muscle protein. The biologic effects are those of starvation. Mortality has been reported to vary from 5% to 20%. The cause of death is usually the result of starvation. Suicide is reported in 2–5% of these patients.

Nutritional Assessment

The nutritional care specialist who is to participate in the care of the patient with anorexia nervosa needs detailed information on the eating behaviors and energy expenditure patterns of the patient. Information which may be helpful in nutritional care planning is listed in Table 12-6.

Treatment

The anorexia nervosa patient is very ill, and treatment is urgent. Sometimes, fluid and electrolyte therapy is needed as a life-saving measure. Serum potassium levels may need particular attention. Some physicians recommend the use of TPN, but this is controversial. Longer-term treatment designed to get at the root of the problem consists of a combination of psychotherapy and nutritional rehabilitation.

If the disease is mild, it may be possible to treat the patient on an outpatient basis.

Table 12-6. Information Needed for Nutritional Care Planning in Anorexia Nervosa

Weight history
History of weight change
Ideal weight
Family attitude toward weight

Dieting behavior
Age when dieting began
Method of dieting
Types and amounts of foods eaten
Feelings and beliefs about foods and dieting
Estimation of calorie and protein intake

Eating patterns
Diet prior to disorder
Detailed diet history (number and content of meals and snacks)
Perception of current eating habits
Family eating pattern
Food likes, dislikes, preferences, aversions
Vitamin and mineral supplements
Motivation to change

Exercise pattern
Exercise prior to disorder
Current exercise: type, frequency, duration
Feelings about exercise and energy expenditure

Compiled from Huse, D.M., and Lucas, A.R., Dietary treatment of anorexia nervosa. *J. Am. Diet. Assoc.* 83:687, 1983.

Sometimes, these patients will eat spontaneously when the foci of conflict are resolved. For those with more advanced disease, hospitalization often is recommended, and the patient is placed in a nonstress environment. Psychotherapy is the most important aspect of treatment to address the central problems, but some weight gain prior to the initiation of psychotherapy may be necessary.

Various procedures have been recommended to increase food intake. A goal weight should be established in conference with the patient. One recommended procedure suggests starting with a diet consisting of the calculated requirement for BMR. These patients usually have had a decline in BMR. Therefore, the calculated amount may be sufficient to stop further weight loss, at least. The diet plan should include foods from each food group. It is planned from exchange lists similar to those for diabetic diets plus lists for desserts and for sugars and sweets. There is, however, no need to avoid simple carbohydrate, as in sweetened fruit. In addition, it is helpful to reduce the bulk content of meals by feeding more concentrated foods with less fiber. In this way, counseling can be quite specific. Portions may be weighed or measured at first to be sure they are large enough.[154,155]

Meal plans should include three meals and may include between-meal snacks. Patients' likes and dislikes should be considered.

In counseling, the discomfort following eating must be described with assurance that the patient will be more comfortable as her capacity increases. It is helpful if the patient keeps a diet record. The patient should also be warned that a rapid weight gain will occur with early refeeding. The gain is the consequence of water and electrolyte retention and an increase in liver and muscle glycogen. She must be assured that this gain will resolve if she continues to eat the prescribed diet.

Constipation may occur as a result of the small volume of food intake and reduced gut motility. As caloric intake increases, there may be diarrhea.

The diet is progressed slowly as the patient adjusts. At first, an increase of 200 kcal per day is reasonable, but it must be synchronized with psychological changes. Larger increases can be provided later. It is important that the increases represent a challenge, but not be so overwhelming as to be demoralizing.[154,155]

When the patient reaches her goal weight, a maintenance diet should be designed. The diet and the patient's weight should be monitored at intervals. Monitoring provides support for the patient while she gains more confidence in her ability to eat spontaneously and still control her weight.[154,155]

Patients often require several years of treatment. They are considered recovered if they eat a reasonable diet that maintains a stable weight within reasonable limits, menstruate regularly, and have interpersonal relationships appropriate for age.

Bulimia Nervosa

Bulimia nervosa has only recently been recognized as a separate and definable disease. There are some similarities to anorexia nervosa and also some important differences (see Table 12-5).

Effects

The bulimia nervosa patient, generally female, has episodes of insatiable appetite in which she goes on an eating binge and can consume 10,000 to 20,000 kcal/day. Foods eaten during a binge are frequently easily ingested foods, such as cookies, ice cream, candies, and pastries.[156] The binge is followed by purging by self-induced vomiting and use of laxatives and diuretics. While the anorexia nervosa patient may break off fasting with an occasional binge, the bulimia patient has repeated binges.

Bulimia nervosa is more likely to develop in adults than in adolescents. The typical patient, as in anorexia nervosa, is a perfectionist with low self-esteem and a distorted body image. She is disgusted by fat but preoccupied with food. The bulimia patient, however, may be of normal weight and described as slim. She often is attractive, successful, and extroverted. The food binges and purges are hidden and eventually interfere with other aspects of her life, leading to isolation.

Hazards include electrolyte and fluid imbalances, anemia, tears in the lower esophagus, difficulty in swallowing, swollen and infected salivary glands, and dental problems.

Table 12-7. Information Needed for Nutritional Care Planning in Bulimia Nervosa

Weight history
History of weight change
Weight range and fluctuations
Ideal weight
Events associated with weight changes
Family attitudes toward weight

Dieting behaviors
Age when dieting began
Methods of dieting
Types and amounts of foods eaten
Feelings and beliefs about foods and dieting

Binge eating
Define "binge" for this patient
Frequency and duration
Nature and severity of bingeing
Precipitating incidents and feelings
Feelings during and after a binge
Motivation to change
Efforts to stop or prevent binge

Purging
Frequency
Method (vomiting, laxatives, diuretics)
Longest intervals between purges
Efforts to stop or prevent purging

Eating patterns
Diet prior to eating disorder
Detailed diet history
Perception of current eating habits
Family eating patterns
Food preferences and aversions
Vitamin and mineral supplementation
Motivation to change

Exercise patterns
Exercise prior to eating disorder
Current exercise type, frequency, and duration
Feelings about exercise and energy expenditure

Compiled from Story, M., Nutrition management and dietary treatment of bulimia. *J. Am. Diet. Assoc.* 86:517, 1986.

Nutritional Assessment

A wide variety of information is needed by the nutritional care specialist participating in the care of the bulemic patient. Useful information to be obtained in the assessment procedure is listed in Table 12-7.

Treatment

Treatment consists of psychotherapy, often in groups. Nutritional care is supportive. The nutritional care specialist sometimes can help the patient control the binges. Many of the techniques of behavior modification have been used. For example, patients can be advised to keep a diary to identify and then avoid circumstances that precipitate a binge. Another technique is to set time limits on binges with a kitchen timer. The clock can be set for five minutes for the binge period and then reset for an hour later when another five-minute binge is allowed. This procedure may help the patient achieve some measure of control. Food should not be eaten out of the original container, but a small portion should be put on a plate and eaten in a dining room, a procedure that might interfere with eating whole bags of cookies, gallons of ice cream, loaves of bread, and similar amounts of food. These techniques at least may help to reduce the number of binges and amounts of food consumed and thus reduce the necessity for purging. The potential for cure is unknown.

A recommended diet plan consists of three meals per day with one or two snacks. These are planned using the exchange lists for diabetic diets. The diet should be planned to maintain current weight and should be at least 1,200 kcal/day. Foods that are used for binge eating should be avoided at first, but added as treatment progresses.[157]

Case Study: Obesity

D.N. was a chubby baby and was considered to be "a little overweight" as a child. During her adolescent years, she continued to gain weight at a rapid rate. She had two children while in her twenties and added 15 pounds to her weight after each. By the time she was 30 years of age, she was 80 pounds overweight.

During a routine physical examination, it was learned that she was becoming hypertensive. Her physician referred her to a weight loss program, and she lost 50 pounds.

Five years later, she had regained the lost weight plus an additional 20 pounds. In addition, her hypertension had become more severe, and she was diabetic. She was then referred to a surgeon for consideration for gastric stapling.

Exercises

1. What are the hazards of obesity in this patient?

2. Assume you are the nutrition counselor in the weight loss program to which this patient was referred. Describe the nutritional assessment procedures you would use.
3. The patient is 5 ft. 3 in. tall when you first see her and weighs 195 lb. Her activity is described as sedentary. Describe the diet you would suggest for her.
4. The patient asks you about a "protein modified fast." How would you respond to her question?
5. When the patient is referred for consideration for gastric stapling, what criteria are used by the surgeon to decide if the surgery should be done?
6. The surgeon agrees to do the gastric stapling. Describe the diet to be used following the surgery.
7. What complications might occur following the surgery over the long-term?

Case Study: Anorexia Nervosa

S.H. is a 17-year-old girl in her last year of high school. She considers herself overweight, and has dieted sporadically for a number of years. She runs and swims for exercise.

S.H. has been steadily losing weight until her weight is now 20 pounds below the level consid- ered desirable for her weight and height. Her family becomes very concerned about her dieting and insists that she see the family physician. Attempts to deal with the problem on an out-patient basis are unsuccessful, and S.H. is admitted to the eating disorders unit of a nearby medical center.

Exercises

1. What physical complications might be evident in this patient?
2. Describe the nutritional assessment procedure you would use.

3. The patient is 5 ft. 8 in. tall, weighs 105 pounds, and is still losing weight. She and her family are counseled by a psychiatrist. You are asked to provide some nutritional counseling. Describe the procedure you would use.

References

1. Ashwell, M., Stirling, D., Freeman, S., and Holloway, B. Transformations within the continuous spectrum of the adipose tissue. In E.M. Berry, S.H. Blondheim, H.E. Eliahou, and E. Shafrir, Eds., *Recent Advances in Obesity Research, V.* London: John Libbey, 1987.
2. Nechad, M., and Cannon, B. Control of brown adipocyte differentiation. In E.M. Berry, S.H. Blondheim, H.E. Eliahou, and E. Shafrir, Eds., *Recent Advances in Obesity Research, V.* London: John Libbey, 1987.
3. Ailhaud, G., Amri, E., Barbaras, R., et al. Adipose cell differentiation. Differential expression of specific mRNAs and protein markers in cells from white and brown adipose tissues. In E.M. Berry, S.H. Blondheim, H.E. Eliahou, and E. Shafrir, Eds., *Recent Advances in Obesity Research, V.* London: John Libbey, 1987.
4. Heaton, J.M. The distribution of brown adipose tissue in the human. *J. Anat.* 112:35, 1972.
5. Sclafani, A., and Berner, C.N. Hyperphagia and obesity produced by parasagittal and coronal hypothalamic knife cuts. Further evidence for a longitudinal feeding inhibitory pathway. *J. Comp. Physiol. Psychol.* 91:1000, 1977.
6. Vasselli, J.R., and Maggio, C.A. Mechanisms of appetite and body-weight regulation. In *Obesity and Weight Control,* ed. R.T. Frankle and M.-U. Yang. Rockville, Md., Aspen, 1988.
7. Deutsch, J.A. The stomach in food satiation and regulation of appetite. *Prog. Neurobiol.* 10:135, 1978.
8. McHugh, P.R., and Moran, T.H. Calories and gastric emptying. A regulatory capacity with implications for feeding. *Am. J. Physiol.* 236:R254, 1979.
9. Houpt, K.A. Gastrointestinal factors in hunger and satiety. *Neurosci. Biobehav. Rev.* 6:145, 1982.
10. Mei, N. Sensory structures in the viscera. In *Progress in Sensory Physiology.* ed. D. Ottoson. Berlin: Springer-Verlag, 1983.
11. Novin, D., and VanderWeele, D.A. Visceral mechanisms in feeding. There is more to regulation than the hypothalamus. In *Progress in Psychobiology and Physiological Psychology,* ed. J. Sprague and A.N. Epstein. New York: Academic Press, 1976.
12. Gibbs, J., and Smith, G.P. Satiety. The roles of peptides from the stomach and the intestine. *Fed. Proc.* 45:1391, 1986.
13. Smith, G.P. The therapeutic potential of cholecystokinin. *Internatl. J. Obes.* 8:35, 1984.
14. Morley, J.E., Gosnell, B.A., Krahn, D.D., et al. Clinical implications of neurochemical mechanisms of appetite regulation. *Psychopharmacol. Bull.* 21:400, 1985.
15. Friedman, M.I., and Stricker, E.M. The physiological psychology of hunger. A physiological perspective. *Psychol. Rev.* 83:409, 1976.
16. Russek, M. Current status of the hepatostatic theory of food intake control. *Appetite* 2:137, 1981.
17. Bray, G.A., and Campfield, L.A. Metabolic factors in the control of energy stores. *Metabolism* 24:99, 1975.
18. Faust, I.M., Johnson, P.R., and Hirsch, J. Surgical removal of adipose tissue alters feeding behavior and development of obesity in rats. *Science* 197:393, 1977.
19. Vasselli, J.R. Patterns of hyperphagia in the Zucker obese rat. A role for fat cell size and number? *Brain Res. Bull.* 14:633, 1985.
20. Woods, S.C., and Porte, D., Jr. The central nervous system, pancreatic hormones, feeding and obesity. *Adv. Metab. Dis.* 9:283, 1978.
21. Bray, G.A. Integration of energy intake and expenditure in animals and man. The autonomic and adrenal hypothesis. *Clin. Endocrinol. Metab.* 13:521, 1984.
22. Jeanrenaud, B. An hypothesis on the aetiology of obesity. Dysfunction of the central nervous system as a primary cause. *Diabetologia* 28:502, 1985.
23. Himms-Hagen, J. Thyroid hormones and thermogenesis. In *Mammalian Thermogenesis,* ed. L. Girardier and M.J. Stock. London: Chapman and Hall, 1983.
24. Phinney, S.D., LaGrange, B.M., O'Connell, M., and Danforth, E., Jr. Effects of aerobic

exercise on energy expenditure and nitrogen balance during very low calorie dieting. *Metabolism* 37:758, 1988.

25. Poehlman, J.E.T., and Horton, E.S. The impact of food intake and exercise on energy expenditure. *Nutr. Rev.* 47:129, 1989.

26. Freedman-Akabos, S., Colt, E., Kissileff, H.R., and Pi-Sunyer, F.X. Lack of sustained increase in VO₂ following exercise in fit and unfit subjects. *Am. J. Clin. Nutr.* 41:545, 1985.

27. Pacy, P.J., Barton, N., Webster, J., and Garrow, J.S. The energy cost of aerobic exercise in fed and fasted normal subjects. *Am. J. Clin. Nutr.* 42:764, 1985.

28. Keys, A., Brozek, J., Hanschel, A., Mickelsen, O., and Taylor, H.C. *The Biology of Human Starvation.* Minneapolis: University of Minnesota Press, 1950.

29. Sims, E.A.H., Danforth, E., Jr., Horton, E.S., Bray, G.A., Glennon, J.A., and Salans, A.B. Endocrine and metabolic effects of experimental obesity in man. *Recent Prog. Horm. Res.* 29:457, 1973.

30. Sims, E.A.H. Energy balance in human beings. The problems of plenitude. *Vit. Horm.* 43:1, 1986.

31. Krieger, D.R., and Landsberg, L. Role of hormones in etiology and pathogenesis of obesity. In *Obesity and Weight Control*, ed. R.T. Frankle and M.-U. Yang. Rockville, Md.: Aspen Publishers, 1988.

32. Danforth, E., Jr., and Landsberg, L. Energy expenditure and its regulation. In M.R.C. Greenwood, Ed., *Obesity*. New York: Churchill-Livingstone, 1983.

33. Young, L.B., Saville, M.E., Rothwell, N.J., et al. Effect of diet and cold exposure on norepinephrine turnover in brown adipose tissue in the rat. *J. Clin. Invest.* 69:1061, 1982.

34. O'Dea, K., Esler, M., Leonard, P., et al. Noradrenaline turnover during under- and over-eating in normal weight subjects. *Metabolism* 31:896, 1982.

35. Young, J.B., and Landsberg, L. Effect of diet and cold exposure on norepinephrine turnover in pancreas and liver. *Am. J. Physiol.* 236:E524, 1979.

36. Rappaport, E.G., Young, J.B., and Landsberg, L. Impact of age on basal and diet-induced changes in sympathetic nervous system activity of Fischer rats. *J. Gerontol.* 36:152, 1981.

37. Young, J.B., and Landsberg, L. Stimulation of the sympathetic nervous system during sucrose feeding. *Nature* 269:615, 1977.

38. Walgren, M.C., Kaufman, L.N., Young, J.B., et al. The effects of various carbohydrates on sympathetic activity in heart and inter-

scapular brown adipose tissue (IBAT) of the rat. *Metabolism* 36:585, 1987.

39. York, D.A., Holt, S.J., and Marchington, D. Regulation of brown adipose tissue thermogenesis by corticosterone in obese fa/fa rats. *Internatl. J. Obes.* 9:89, 1985.

40. Olefsky, J.M. The insulin receptor. Its role in insulin resistance of obesity and diabetes. *Diabetes* 25:1154, 1976.

41. Crettaz, M., and Jeanrenaud, B. Postreceptor alterations in the states of insulin resistance. *Metabolism* 29:467, 1980.

42. Smith, U. Regional differences in adipocyte metabolism and possible consequences *in vivo*. In *Recent Advances in Obesity Research, IV*, ed. J. Hirsch and T.B. Van Itallie. London: John Libbey, 1983.

43. Rothwell, N.J., and Stock, M.J. A role for insulin in the diet-induced thermogenesis of cafeteria-fed rats. *Metabolism* 30:673, 1981.

44. Rowe, J.W., Young, J.B., Minaker, K.L., et al. Effect of insulin and glucose infusions on sympathetic nervous system activity in normal man. *Diabetes* 30:219, 1981.

45. Bennett, T., Gale, E.A.M., Green, J., et al. The influence of beta-adrenoreceptor antagonists on thermoregulation during insulin-induced hypoglycemia. *J. Physiol.* 308:26P, 1980.

46. Glass, A.R., Burman, K.D., Dahms, W.T., et al. Endocrine function in human obesity. *Metabolism* 30:89, 1981.

47. Foster, D.W. Eating disorders. Obesity and anorexia nervosa. In *Williams' Textbook of Endocrinology*, ed. J.D. Wilson and D.W. Foster. Philadelphia: W.B. Saunders, 1985.

48. Rivlin, R.S. Drug therapy. Therapy of obesity with hormones. *N. Engl. J. Med.* 292:26, 1975.

49. Hervey, G.R., and Tobin, G. The part played by variation in energy expenditure in the regulation of energy balance. *Proc. Nutr. Soc.* 41:137, 1972.

50. James, W.P.T., Trayhurn, P., and Garlick, P. The metabolic basis of subnormal thermogenesis in obesity. In P. Bjorntorp, M. Cairella, and A.N. Howard, Eds., *Recent Advances in Obesity Research, III*. London: John Libbey, 1981.

51. Weighley, E.S. Average? Ideal? Desirable? A brief overview of height-weight tables in the United States. *J. Am. Diet. Assoc.* 84:417, 1984.

52. Abraham, S., Carroll, M.D., Najjar, M.F., and Fulwood, R. *Obese and Overweight Adults in the United States*. Vital and Health Statistics, Ser. 11, No. 230. DHHS Publ. No. (PHS) 83–1680. National Center for Health Statistics, Public Health Service, U.S. De-

partment of Health and Human Services, Hyattsville, Md., 1983.

53. National Center for Health Statistics. NCHS Growth Charts, 1976. *Monthly Vital Statistics Report* 25(3), Suppl. (HRA) 76–1120. Rockville, Md.: Health Resources Administration, 1976.

54. Keys, A., Fidanza, F., Karvonen, M.J., et al. Indices of relative weight and obesity. *J. Chron. Dis.* 25:329, 1972.

55. Garrow, J.S. *Energy Balance and Obesity in Man.* New York: Elsevier, 1978, p. 171.

56. Flewellen, E.H., and Bee, D.E. Ponderal index. Quantifying obesity. *J.A.M.A.* 241:884, 1979.

57. Larsson, B., Suardsudd, K., Welin, L., et al. Abdominal adipose distribution and risk of cardiovascular disease and death. A 13-year follow-up of participants in the study of men born in 1913. *Br. Med. J.* 288:1401, 1984.

58. Sjostrom, L. New aspects of weight-for-height indices and adipose tissue distribution in relation to cardiovascular risk and total adipose tissue volume. In E.M. Berry, S.H. Blondheim, H.E. Eliahou, and E. Shafrir, Eds., *Recent Advances in Obesity Research, V.* London: John Libbey, 1987.

59. Segal, K.R., Van Loan, M., and Fitzgerald, P.I. Lean body mass estimation by bioelectrical impedence analysis. A four-site cross-validation study. *Am. J. Clin. Nutr.* 47:7, 1988.

60. Stern, J.S., and Kane-Nussen, B. Obesity. Its assessment, risks and treatments. In R.B. Alfin-Slater, D. Kritschevsky, and R.E. Hodges, Eds., *Human Nutrition—A Comprehensive Treatise,* vol. 4. New York: Plenum, 1979.

61. Mayer, J. *Overweight: Causes, Cost and Control.* New York: Prentice-Hall, 1968.

62. Mayer, J. Genetic, traumatic and environmental factors in the etiology of obesity. *Physiol. Rev.* 33:472, 1953.

63. Bourchard, C. Genetics of body fat, energy expenditure and adipose tissue metabolism. In E.M. Berry, S.H. Blondheim, H.E. Eliahou, and E. Shafrir, Eds., *Recent Advances in Obesity Research, V.* London: John Libbey, 1987.

64. Modan, M., Lubin, F., Lusky, A., Chetrit, A., Fuchs, Z., and Halkin, H. Interrelationships of obesity, habitual diet, physical activity and glucose intolerance in the four main Jewish ethnic groups. In E.M. Berry, S.H. Blondheim, H.E. Eliahou, and E. Shafrir, Eds., *Recent Advances in Obesity Research, V.* London: John Libbey, 1987.

65. Stunkard, A., and Thorkild, I.A., et al. An adoption study of human obesity. *N. Engl. J. Med.* 314:193, 1986.

66. Galton, O.J., Gilbert, C., Reekless, J.P.D., and Kaye, J. Triglyceride-storage disease. A group of inborn errors of triglyceride metabolism. *Q. J. Med.* 43:63, 1974.

67. Ravussin, E., Lillioja, S., Knowles, W.C., Christin, L., Freymond, D., Abbott, W.G.H., et al. Reduced rate of energy expenditure as a risk factor for body weight gain. *New Engl. J. Med.* 318:467, 1988.

68. Roberts, S.B., Savage, J., Coward, W.A., Chew, B., and Lucas, A. Energy expenditure and intake in infants born to lean and overweight mothers. *N. Engl. J. Med.* 318:461, 1988.

69. Seltzer, C.C., and Mayer, J. Body build (somatotype) distinctiveness in obese women. *J. Am. Diet. Assoc.* 55:457, 1969.

70. Kissebah, A.H., Peiris, A., and Evans, D.J. Mechanisms associating body fat distribution with the abnormal metabolic profile in obesity. In E.M. Berry, S.H. Blondheim, H.E. Eliahou, and E. Shafrir, Eds., *Recent Advances in Obesity Research, V.* London: John Libbey, 1987.

71. Bjorntorp, P. Adipose tissue distribution and morbidity. In E.M. Berry, S.H. Blondheim, H.E. Eliahou, and E. Shafrir, Eds., *Recent Advances in Obesity Research, V.* London: John Libbey, 1987.

72. Vague, J., Rubin, P., Jubelin, J., et al. Regulation of the adipose tissue mass. Histometric and anthropometric aspects. In J. Vague and J. Boyer, Eds., *The Regulation of Adipose Tissue Mass.* Amsterdam: Excerpta Medica, 1974.

73. Matsuzawa, Y., Fujioka, S., Tokunaga, K., and Tarui, S. A novel classification. Visceral fat obesity and subcutaneous fat obesity. In E.M. Berry, S.H. Blondheim, H.E. Eliahou, and E. Shafrir, Eds., *Recent Advances in Obesity Research, V.* London: John Libbey, 1987.

74. Iverson, F. Psychogenic obesity in children. I. *Acta Paediatr. Scand.* 42:8, 1953.

75. Sonne-Holm, S., and Sorensen, T.I.A. Postward course of the prevalence of extreme overweight among Danish young men. *J. Chron. Dis.* 30:351, 1977.

76. Warner, W.A., and Garrett, L.P. The obese patient and anesthesia. *J.A.M.A.* 205:102, 1968.

77. Faust, I.M., Johnson, P.R., Stern, J.S., and Hirsch, J. Diet induced adipocyte cell number increase in adult rats. A new model of obesity. *Am. J. Physiol.* 235:E279, 1978.

78. Hirsch, J., and Batchelor, P.R. Adipose tissue cellularity in human obesity. *Clin. Endocrinol. Metab.* 5:299, 1976.

79. Nisbett, R.E. Hunger, obesity and the ventromedial hypothalamus. *Psychol. Rev.* 79:433, 1972.

80. Rosen, B.S., Cook, K.S., Yaglom, J., Groves, D.L., Volanakis, J.E., Damm, E., White, T., and Spiegelman, B.M. Adipsin and complement factor D activity. An immune-related defect in obesity. *Science* 244:1483, 1989.

81. National Institutes of Health Consensus Development Conference. Health implications of obesity. *Ann. Intern. Med.* 103:1073, 1985.

82. Stunkard, A.J., and McLaren-Hume, N. The results of treatment of obesity. A review of the literature and report of a series. *Arch. Intern. Med.* 103:79, 1959.

83. Hollenberg, C.H. The fat cell and the fat patient. *R. Coll. Phys. Surg. Can.* 8:119, 1975.

84. Bray, G.A. The myth of diet in the management of obesity. *Am. J. Clin Nutr.* 23:1141, 1970.

85. Bray, G.A. *The Obese Patient.* Major Problems in Internal Medicine, vol. 9. Philadelphia: W.B. Saunders, 1976.

86. Buskirk, E.R., Thompson, R.H., Lutwak, L., and Whedon, G.D. Energy balance of obese patients during weight reduction. Influence of diet restriction and exercise. *Ann. N.Y. Acad. Sci.* 110:1918, 1963.

87. Blondheim, S.H., Kaufman, N.A., and Stein, M. Comparison of fasting and 800–1000 calorie diet in obesity. *Lancet* 1:250, 1965.

88. Russell, G.F.M. The effects of diets of different composition on weight loss and sodium balance in obese patients. *Clin. Sci.* 22:269, 1962.

89. Cohn, C., Joseph, D., Bell, L., and Allweiss, M.D. Studies on the effects of feeding frequency and dietary composition on fat deposition. *Ann. N.Y. Acad. Sci.* 131:507, 1965.

90. Fabry, P., Fodor, J., Hejl, Z., et al. The frequency of meals. Its relationship to overweight, hypercholesterolemia and decreased glucose-tolerance. *Lancet* 2:614, 1964.

91. Huenemann, R.L. Food habits of obese and non-obese adolescents. *Postgrad. Med.* 51:99, 1972.

92. Young, C.M. Scanlan, S.S., Topping, C.M., et al. Frequency of feeding, weight reduction and body composition. *J. Am. Diet. Assoc.* 59:466, 1971.

93. Young, C.M., Hutter, L.F., Scanlan, S.S., et al. Metabolic effects of meal frequency on normal young men. *J. Am. Diet. Assoc.* 61:391, 1972.

94. Bortz, W.M., Wroldsen, A., Issekutz, B., and Rodahl, K. Weight loss and frequency of feeding. *N. Engl. J. Med.* 274:376, 1966.

95. Finkelstein, B., and Fryer, B.A. Meal frequency and weight reduction in young women. *Am. J. Clin. Nutr.* 24:465, 1971.

96. Silverstone, J.T., Stark, J.E., and Buckle, R.M. Hunger during total starvation. *Lancet* 1:1343, 1966.

97. Garrow, J.S. Are liquid diets safe or necessary? In E.M. Berry, S.H. Blondheim, H.E. Eliahou, and E. Shafrir, Eds., *Recent Advances in Obesity Research, V.* London: John Libbey, 1987.

98. Howard, A.N. Safety and efficacy of the Cambridge diet. In E.M. Berry, S.H. Blondheim, H.E. Eliahou, and E. Shafrir, Eds., *Recent Advances in Obesity Research, V.* London: John Libbey, 1987.

99. Kirschner, M.A., Schneider, G., Ertel, N., and Gorman, J. A very-low-calorie formula diet program for control of major obesity: an 8-year experience. In E.M. Berry, S.H. Blondheim, H.E. Eliahou, and E. Shafrir, Eds., *Recent Advances in Obesity Research, V.* London: John Libbey, 1987.

100. Cronin, B.S., and McDonough, A.B. Nutrition management of morbid obesity in conjunction with surgical intervention. *Topics Clin. Nutr.* 2(2):59, 1987.

101. Hill, J.O., Schlundt, D.G., Sbrocco, T., Sharp, T., Pope-Cordle, J., Stetson, B., Kaler, M., and Heim, C. Evaluation of an alternating-calorie diet with and without exercise in the treatment of obesity. *Am. J. Clin. Nutr.* 50:248, 1989.

102. Anonymous. Packaged food weight loss programs. *Nutrition and the M.D.* 15(11):3, 1989.

103. Rose, H.E., and Mayer, J. Activity, caloric intake, fat storage and the energy balance of infants. *Pediatrics* 41:18, 1968.

104. Bullen, B.A., Reed, R.B., and Mayer, J. Physical activity of obese and non-obese adolescent girls appraised by motion picture sampling. *Am. J. Clin. Nutr.* 4:211, 1964.

105. Stunkard, A. Physical activity, emotions and human obesity. *Psychosom. Med.* 20:366, 1958.

106. Edholm, O.G., Fletcher, J.G., Widdowson, E.M., and McCance, R.A. The energy expenditure and food intake of individual man. *Br. J. Nutr.* 9:286, 1955.

107. Crews, E.L., III, Fuge, K.W., Oscai, L.B., et al. Weight, food intake and body composition. Effects of exercise and protein deficiency. *Am. J. Physiol.* 216:359, 1969.

108. Mayer, J. Why people get hungry. *Nutrition Today* 1:2, 1966.

109. Gwinup, G., Chelvam, R., and Steinberg, T.

Thickness of subcutaneous fat and activity of underlying muscle. *Ann. Intern. Med.* 74:408, 1971.

110. Ley, P., Bradshaw, P.W., Kincey, J.A., et al. Psychological variables in the control of obesity. In W.L. Burland, P.D. Samuel, and J. Yudkin, Eds., *Obesity Symposium.* Edinburgh: Churchill Livingstone, 1974.

111. Bernard, J.L. Rapid treatment of gross obesity by operant techniques. *Psychol. Rep.* 23:663, 1968.

112. Stuart, R.B. A three-dimensional program for the treatment of obesity. *Behav. Res. Ther.* 9:177, 1971.

113. Stuart, R.B. Behavior control of overeating. *Behav. Res. Ther.* 5:357, 1967.

114. Levitz, L.S., and Stunkard, A.J. A therapeutic coalition for obesity. Behavior modification and patient self-help. *Am. J. Psychiatry* 131:423, 1974.

115. Bowser, L.J., Trulson, M.F., Bowling, R.C., and Stare, F.J. Methods of reducing. Group therapy vs. individual clinic interview. *J. Am. Diet. Assoc.* 29:1193, 1953.

116. Munves, E.D. Dietetic interview or group discussion-decision in reducing. *J. Am. Diet. Assoc.* 29:1197, 1953.

117. Howard, A.N. Dietary treatment of obesity. In I. McLean-Baird and A.N. Howard, Eds., *Obesity: Medical and Scientific Aspects.* Edinburgh: E. and S. Livingstone, 1969.

118. Sullivan, A.C. Drug treatment of obesity. A perspective. In E.M. Berry, S.H. Blondheim, H.E. Eliahou, and E. Shafrir, Eds., *Recent Advances in Obesity Research, V.* London: John Libbey, 1987.

119. Blundell, J.E., and Leshem, M.B. Central action of anorexic agents. Effects of amphetamine and fenfluramine in rats with lateral hypothalamic lesions. *Eur. J. Pharmacol.* 28:81, 1974.

120. Leibowitz, S.F. Amphetamine. Possible site and mode of action for producing anorexia in the rat. *Brain Res.* 84:160, 1975.

121. Sullivan, A.C., and Cheng, L. Appetite regulation and its modulation by drugs. In J.N. Hathcock and J. Coon, Eds., *Nutrition and Drug Interrelationships.* New York: Academic Press, 1978.

122. Sullivan, A.C., and Comai, K. Pharmacological treatment of obesity. In G.A. Bray, Ed., *Obesity: Comparative Methods of Weight Control.* Westport, Conn.: Technomic Publishing, 1980.

123. Duncan, L.J.P., Rose, K., and Meiklejohn, A.P. Phenmetrazine hydrochloride and methylcellulose in the treatment of refractory obesity. *Lancet* 1:1262, 1960.

124. Bray, G.A., Melvin, K.E.W., and Chopra, J.J.

Effect of triiodothyronine on some metabolic responses of obese patients. *Am. J. Clin. Nutr.* 26:715, 1973.

125. Lamki, L., Ezrin, C., Koven, I., and Steiner, F. L-Thyroxine in the treatment of obesity without increase in the loss of lean body mass. *Metabolism* 22:617, 1973.

126. Simeons, A.T.W. The action of chorionic gonadotropin in the obese. *Lancet* 2:946, 1954.

127. Hastrup, F., Nielson, F., and Skouby, A.P. Chorionic gonadotropin and the treatment of obesity. *Acta Med. Scand.* 168:25, 1960.

128. Young, R.L., Fuchs, R.J., and Woltjen, M.J. Chorionic gonadotropin in weight control. A double-blind cross-over study. *J.A.M.A.* 236:2495, 1976.

129. Carne, S. The action of chorionic gonadotropin in the obese. *Lancet* 2:1282, 1961.

130. Sullivan, A.C., Nauss-Karol, C., and Cheng, L. Pharmacologic treatment. II. In M.R.C. Greenwood, Ed., *Obesity.* New York: Churchill Livingstone, 1983.

131. Arch, J.R.S., Piercy, V., Thurlby, P.L., Wilson, C., and Wilson, S. Thermogenic and lipolytic drugs for the treatment of obesity. Old ideas and new possibilities. In E.M. Berry, S.H. Blondheim, H.E. Eliahou, and E. Shafrir, Eds., *Recent Advances in Obesity Research, V.* London: John Libbey, 1987.

132. Randall, S., and Zeffiro, W.W. Surgical management of the morbidly obese. *Topics Clin. Nutr.* 2(2):55, 1987.

133. Kral, J.G. Surgical therapy. In M.R.C. Greenwood, Ed., *Obesity.* New York: Churchill Livingstone, 1983.

134. Montorsi, W., and Doldi, S.B. Surgical treatment of obesity. In G. Enzi, G. Crepaldi, G. Pozza, and E.A. Renold, Eds., *Obesity: Pathogenesis and Treatment.* London: Academic Press, 1981.

135. Lieber, C.P., Seinige, U.L., Sataloff, D.M., Blake, H.A., III, and Rovito, P.F. Intragastric balloon. In M. Deitel, Ed., *Surgery for the Morbidly Obese Patient.* Philadelphia: Lea & Febiger, 1989.

136. MacLean, L.D., and Shibata, H.R. The present status of bypass operations for obesity. *Surg. Ann.* 9:213, 1977.

137. Bleicher, J.E., Cegielski, M., and Saporta, J.A. Intestinal bypass operation for massive obesity. *Postgrad. Med.* 55(4):65, 1974.

138. Hollenbeck, J.I., O'Leary, J.P., Maher, J.W., and Woodward, E.R. An aetiological basis for fatty liver after jejunoileal bypass. *J. Surg. Res.* 18:83, 1975.

139. Moxley, R.T., Pozefsky, T., and Lockwood, D.H. Protein nutrition and liver disease after jejunoileal bypass for morbid obesity. *N. Engl. J. Med.* 290:921, 1974.

140. Mason, E.E.: *Surgical Treatment of Obesity.* Philadelphia: W.B. Saunders, 1981.

141. Cronin, B.S., and McDonough, A.B. Nutrition management of morbid obesity in conjunction with surgical intervention. *Topics Clin. Nutr.* 2(2):59, 1987.

142. Mason, E.E. From giant hernias to gastric bypass. In W.L. Asher, Ed., *Treating the Obese.* New York: Medcom Press, 1974.

143. Rodgers, S., Burnet, R., Goss, A., et al. Jaw-wiring in the treatment of obesity. *Lancet* 2:1221, 1977.

144. Flack, R., and Grayer, E.A. Consciousness-raising group for obese women. *Soc. Work Health Care* 20:484, 1975.

145. de Castro, J.M., and de Castro, E.S. Spontaneous meal patterns of humans. Influence of the presence of other people. *Am. J. Clin. Nutr.* 50:237, 1989.

146. Grinker, J. Behavioral and metabolic consequences of weight reduction. *J. Am. Diet. Assoc.* 62:30, 1973.

147. Fomon, S.J. *Nutritional Disorders of Children: Prevention, Screening, and Follow-up.* D.H.E.W. Publication No. (HSA) 77–5104. Washington, D.C.: U.S. Department of Health, Education, and Welfare, 1977.

148. Brownell, K.D., Greenwood, M.R.C., Stellar, E., and Shrager, E.E. The effects of repeated cycles of weight loss and regain in rats. *Physiol. Behav.* 38:459, 1986.

149. Bruch, H. *Eating Disorders.* New York: Basic Books, 1973.

150. Katz, J.L., and Weiner, H. A functional anterior hypothalamic defect in primary anorexia nervosa. *Psychosom. Med.* 37:103, 1975.

151. Halmi, K.A. Anorexia nervosa. Recent investigations. *Annu. Rev. Med.* 29:137, 1978.

152. Hellstrom, I. Oral complications in anorexia nervosa. *Scand. J. Dent. Res.* 85:71, 1977.

153. Schleimer, K. Anorexia nervosa. *Nutr. Rev.* 39:99, 1981.

154. Huse, D.M., and Lucas, A.R. Dietary treatment of anorexia nervosa. *J. Am. Diet. Assoc.* 83:687, 1983.

155. Lucas, A.R., Duncan, J.W., and Piens, V. The treatment of anorexia nervosa. *Am. J. Psychiatry* 133:1034, 1976.

156. Kirkley, B.G. Bulimia. Clinical characteristics, development and etiology. *J. Am. Diet. Assoc.* 86:468, 1986.

157. Story, M. Nutrition management and dietary treatment of bulimia. *J. Am. Diet. Assoc.* 86:517, 1986.

Bibliography

Bates, G.W., Ed. Symposium. Body weight and reproductive function. *Clin. Obstet. Gynecol.* 28:569, 1985.

Beaumont, P.J.V. *Handbook of Eating Disorders, Part 1: Anorexia Nervosa and Bulimia Nervosa.* New York: Elsevier, 1987.

Berry, E.M., Blondheim, S.H., Eliahou, H.E., and Shafrir, E. *Recent Advances in Obesity Research, V.* London: John Libbey, 1985.

Bjorntorp, P., Cairella, M., and Howard, A.N. *Recent Advances in Obesity Research, III.* London: John Libbey, 1981.

Bjorntorp, P., Vahouny, G.V., and Kritchevsky, D., Eds. *Dietary Fiber and Obesity.* New York: Liss, 1985.

Blinder, B.J., Chaitin, B.F., and Goldstein, R.S., Eds. *The Eating Disorders: Medical and Psychological Bases of Diagnosis and Treatment.* New York: PMA, 1988.

Bray, G.A., LeBlanc, J., Inoue, S., and Suzuki, M., Eds. *Diet and Obesity.* Basel: S. Karger AG, 1988.

Brownell, K.D., and Foreyt, J.P., Eds. *Handbook of Eating Disorders: Physiology, Psychology and Treatment of Obesity, Anorexia and Bulimia.* New York: Basic Books, 1986.

Buchwald, H., Ed. Symposium on morbid obesity. *Surg. Clin. North Am.* 59(6):961, 1152, 1979.

Cauwels, J.M. *Bulimia: The Binge-Purge Compulsion.* Garden City, N.Y.: Doubleday, 1983.

Greenwood, M.R.C., Ed. *Contemporary Issues in Clinical Nutrition,* vol. 4: *Obesity.* New York: Churchill Livingstone, 1983.

Gross, M., Ed. *Anorexia Nervosa.* Lexington, Mass.: Collamore Press, 1982.

Hirsch, J., and Van Itallie, T.B., Eds. *Recent Advances in Obesity Research, IV.* London: John Libbey, 1985.

Sources of Current Information

International Journal of Obesity
Nutrition and the M.D.
Obesity and Bariatric Medicine

13. Liver Disease and Alcoholism

I. Normal Anatomy and Physiology of the Liver
 A. Normal liver structure
  1. Blood supply
  2. Hepatocytes
  3. Drainage of bile
  4. Units of structure
 B. Functions of the liver
  1. Metabolic functions
   a. carbohydrate
   b. protein
   c. lipids
   d. vitamins
   e. minerals
   f. alcohol
  2. Protective and detoxification functions
  3. Digestion and excretion
  4. Circulatory and other functions
II. Diagnosis of Liver Disease
III. Hepatitis
 A. Clinical manifestations
 B. Treatment
 C. Nutritional Care
 D. Complications
IV. Jaundice
V. Alcoholism and Alcoholic Liver Disease
 A. Alcohol intake
 B. Absorption and distribution
 C. Metabolism and excretion
 D. Mechanism of injury
 E. Nutritional status of the alcoholic

  1. Food intake and alcoholism
  2. Effects of alcohol on digestion and absorption
  3. Effects of chronic alcoholism on nutrient metabolism
 F. Acute adverse effects of alcohol intoxication
 G. Alcoholic liver disease
  1. Steatosis
  2. Alcoholic hepatitis
  3. Alcoholic cirrhosis
 H. Nutritional care of alcoholics
 I. Fetal alcohol syndrome
VI. Cirrhosis
 A. Classification
 B. Clinical manifestations
  1. Portal hypertension and ascites
  2. Varices and hemorrhage in the digestive system
  3. Alterations in protein and nitrogen metabolism
   a. protein synthesis
   b. urea and ammonia metabolism
   c. amino acid metabolism

   d. protein metabolism and hepatic encephalopathy
  4. Alterations in carbohydrate metabolism
  5. Alterations in lipid metabolism
  6. Effects on vitamin metabolism
  7. Effects on fluid, electrolyte, and acid-base balance
  8. Other effects
 C. Care of the cirrhotic patient
  1. General nutritional support
  2. Esophageal and gastric varices
  3. Ascites and edema
  4. Hepatic encephalopathy
  5. Feeding techniques
 D. Specific forms of cirrhosis
  1. Laennec's cirrhosis
   a. etiology
   b. clinical manifestations
   c. nutritional care
  2. Postnecrotic cirrhosis
  3. Biliary cirrhosis
  4. Wilson's disease
VII. Nutrition Support in Hepatic Failure
VIII. Nutritional Assessment
IX. Liver Transplant
X. Case Study

The liver has a central function in nutrition and metabolism. Consequently, its malfunction has far-reaching effects. Malnutrition can be both a cause and a consequence of liver diseases, and nutritional care is important in their overall management.

NORMAL ANATOMY AND PHYSIOLOGY OF THE LIVER

The liver is the largest gland in the body, weighing 1 to 1.5 kg in an adult. It lies in the right upper quadrant of the abdominal cavity immediately below the diaphragm and against the right kidney and adrenal gland, lower esophagus, stomach, and intestine. Its relationship to the vasculature of these organs is particularly important in the complications of some liver diseases.

Normal Liver Structure

The liver has two lobes whose surfaces are closely apposed. They are enclosed in a common connective tissue capsule so that the separation of the lobes is not visible externally.

Blood Supply

The blood vessels carrying blood to the liver enter from below at the **porta hepatis** or **hilus hepatis**. There are two blood supplies to the liver. The largest portion of blood (80%) enters the liver through the **portal vein**, which branches from the mesenteric vein. This drains nutrient-rich blood from the intestine, and the splenic vein drains blood from the spleen and stomach. The **hepatic artery** carries the remaining 20% of the blood but 50% or more of the liver's oxygen supply. It usually is a branch of the celiac trunk, which arises from the aorta.

At the hilus, the connective tissue of the liver capsule extends up into the parenchyma of the liver and branches very much like the branches of a tree. The portal vein and hepatic artery follow the path of this connective tissue, also branching. At the ends of the branches, the blood from both sources flows into and merges in the **sinusoids**, capillary-like structures that are larger and more porous, thereby allowing protein to cross their walls. They are lined by endothelial cells but have no basement membrane. The sinusoids also have **Kupffer cells** attached to their interior walls. These are phagocytic cells of the immune system (see Chapter 6).

After the blood flows through the sinusoids, it is collected into the **central veins** of the liver. These drain into progressively larger veins and thence into the hepatic veins, which leave the back of the liver to connect with the inferior vena cava.

The average rate of blood flow through the liver is 1,400 ml/min. There normally is very little resistance to blood flow through the liver; hepatic vein pressure is 0 mm Hg and portal pressure is approximately 8 mm Hg. Alterations in these pressures are significant in some liver conditions.

Hepatocytes

The parenchyma of the liver consists primarily of cells called **hepatocytes**. They exist in sheetlike **plates** that are two cells thick. When cut in cross section, they appear under the microscope as rows of cells called **hepatic cords**. The sinusoids exist on either side of the two-cell-thick structure. Thus, the blood is in intimate contact with the hepatocyte (Figure 13-1). The Kupffer cells also are considered parenchymal but are present in much smaller numbers.

Drainage of Bile

Since bile is secreted by the liver, provision must be made for its drainage. For this purpose, very small ducts (**bile canaliculi**) exist between the two cells that represent the thickness of the hepatic plate. The bile is secreted into the canaliculi, which drain successively into **canals of Hering, bile ductules**, and **bile ducts** in the portal tract. These structures compose the **biliary tree**,

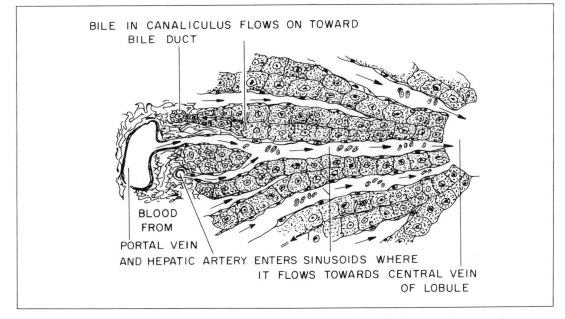

BILE IN CANALICULUS FLOWS ON TOWARD
BILE DUCT

BLOOD
FROM
PORTAL VEIN
AND HEPATIC ARTERY ENTERS SINUSOIDS WHERE
IT FLOWS TOWARDS CENTRAL VEIN
OF LOBULE

Figure 13-1. The flow of blood (indicated by arrows) from the portal vein and the hepatic artery (left) into sinusoids, lined by reticuloendothelium, that lie between hepatic cords; blood empties into the central vein (right). Also shown is the way that bile travels in the opposite direction in canaliculi to empty into bile ducts in portal areas. (Reprinted with permission from Ham, A.W., and Cormack, D.H., Histology, 8th. ed. Philadelphia: J.B. Lippincott, 1979, p. 704.)

which follows the same course as the branching of the hepatic artery and portal vein. The flow, however, is in the opposite direction (see Figure 13-1). Thus, the connective tissue, hepatic artery, portal vein, and bile ducts follow the same path. These are known as **portal tracts**, and they also contain lymphatics and nerves.

Units of Structure

The basic unit of liver structure, which is easily seen with a microscope, is a **liver lobule**. It is roughly hexagonal and consists of a central vein surrounded by the hepatic plates, with three to six portal tracts visible at its edges (Figure 13-2). An alternative structural unit is the **portal lobule**, which is visualized as a triangle with the portal tract in the center and a central vein at each angle (Figure 13-2).

From a functional point of view, the liver can better be divided conceptually into **acini**, although an acinus is more difficult to see with a microscope. In concept, the central structure is the blood supply rather than the central vein that accommodates drainage. The parenchyma consists of those cells supplied by one portal tract (see Figure 13-2); a central vein thus may receive blood from more than one acinus. The acinus is a useful concept, since there are differences in the adequacy of the blood supply at various sites. Those cells closest to the central vein are exposed to blood with the least oxygen and the most carbon dioxide, whereas those closest to the smallest vessels of the blood supply prior to its entrance into the sinusoids are exposed to the freshest blood. The hepatocytes are unequal in other ways. They contain varying amounts of enzymes and so, presumably, they vary in their function. Hepatocytes nearest to the portal tract have high concentrations of glycolytic enzymes, whereas those near the central vein contain more enzymes involved in lipid metabolism. When hepatocytes are damaged, the damage can vary with the location of the cells.

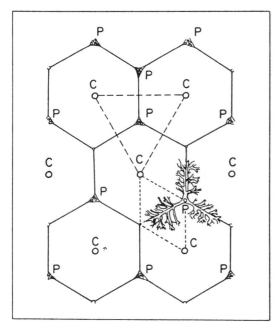

Figure 13-2. The hepatic lobules. The classic liver lobule is outlined with solid lines, the portal lobule with interrupted lines, and the liver acinus or functional unit with a dotted line. The branches of a portal vein and a hepatic artery from one portal area are shown at lower right. P = portal areas; C = central veins. (Reprinted with permission from Leeson, T.S., and Leeson, C.R. Histology, 4th ed. Philadelphia: W.B. Saunders, 1981, p. 391.)

Functions of the Liver

The liver has a variety of important functions. It controls the concentrations of many nutrients and disposes of waste products in the bile. It also prepares materials for disposal in the urine. The liver synthesizes many substances and, through them, has extensive effects on digestion, colloid osmotic pressure, transport of metabolites, and blood coagulation. It also is an important storage depot.

Metabolic Functions

The liver receives directly from the intestine most of the absorbed nutrients that are products of digestion except for those absorbed into the lymphatic system (see Chapter 8).

Thus the liver is important in the metabolism of most nutrients. These metabolic processes are only summarized here. Further details were studied in your biochemistry courses and may be reviewed in elementary biochemistry textbooks.

Carbohydrate. The liver is the main, and sometimes the only, site of several aspects of carbohydrate metabolism. It receives almost all absorbed carbohydrate in the portal circulation. It stores glucose as glycogen (**glycogenesis**) and also breaks down glycogen to form glucose (**glycogenolysis**). It can form glucose from some amino acids (**gluconeogenesis**), metabolizes hexoses other than glucose, and synthesizes various compounds from carbohydrate intermediates. These processes serve to provide a constant glucose supply to extrahepatic tissues, even though the exogenous supply of glucose is intermittent. By taking up glucose, the liver also prevents sudden changes in osmolality of body fluids following meals. In addition, it uses carbohydrates in the synthesis of mucopolysaccharides and synthesizes important metabolites by means of the hexose monophosphate shunt.

Protein. From the intestine, the liver receives amino acids, the sources of which are the diet, desquamated cells, and intestinal and pancreatic enzymes. The liver also receives endogenous amino acids in the blood. It extracts amino acids from the blood to varying degrees. Alanine uptake is very effective, and the glucogenic amino acids, in general, are taken up efficiently. The branched-chain amino acids — leucine, isoleucine, and valine — are not extracted by the liver but are allowed to enter the systemic circulation. The enzymes necessary for the metabolism of branched-chain amino acids are in the skeletal muscle, kidney, adipose tissue, brain, and other peripheral tissue, but not in the liver.[1] This fact is important as a theoretical basis for one suggested method of feeding liver failure patients to be discussed later.

The liver forms new nonessential amino acids by **transamination** and synthesizes a number of compounds containing nitrogen. Some of these are purines, pyrimidines, creatine, choline, coenzyme A, glutathione, porphyrins, glutamine, taurine, and carnosine. It degrades amino acids by **oxidative deamination**, producing alpha-keto acids and ammonia. **Urea synthesis**, which removes and detoxifies ammonia, occurs *only* in the liver.

The liver synthesizes structural and enzyme protein for liver function and is the source of much of the plasma protein. It is the only source of albumin and, as such, functions in the control of the colloid osmotic pressure. It is the principal site of synthesis of transferrin for iron binding and is the source of at least some ferritin. It also is the source of many factors necessary for blood coagulation, including prothrombin, fibrinogen, and factors V, VII, IX, and X.

Lipids. Lipids (fatty acids, triglycerides, phospholipids, cholesterol, and cholesteryl esters) normally make up approximately 5% of the weight of the liver. The liver is capable of synthesizing fatty acids, but most fatty acids are obtained from the diet or by release from adipose tissue. Regardless of the source, the liver is capable of using them to form triglycerides or phospholipids or to esterify cholesterol, which it can synthesize from acetate.

The liver exports triglyceride to other tissue, a process that requires synthesis of apolipoproteins (see Chapter 10). This fact explains why liver protein metabolism is important in lipid release from the liver. The liver also oxidizes fatty acids to produce energy. In this process, it may produce large amounts of ketone bodies (see Chapter 11).

Vitamins. The liver has important functions related to many of the vitamins. Vitamin A is stored in the liver. When it is released, it is bound to retinol-binding protein, which is synthesized in the liver. The liver is also the site of conversion of carotene to vitamin A.

One of the steps in the activation of vitamin D_3 occurs in the liver. Vitamin D then is released attached to a binding globulin and is circulated to the kidney (see Chapter 9) where it is metabolized further. Through its action on vitamin D, the liver is important in the metabolism of calcium and phosphorus. It stores vitamin D and also functions in its disposal. Vitamin E and a small amount of vitamin K also are stored, as are some of the water-soluble vitamins for a short period.

Minerals. The liver stores iron and copper and recovers iron from discarded red blood cells (see Chapter 18). In addition, the liver is known to influence the metabolism of sodium, potassium, calcium, and chloride.

Alcohol. The liver is of major importance in the metabolism of alcohol. Because of the relationship between alcoholism and liver disease, alcohol metabolism will be described in detail under "Alcoholism and Alcoholic Liver Disease" (p. 526).

Protective and Detoxification Functions

The liver is associated with a number of processes by which it protects the body from deleterious substances. The phagocytic action of Kupffer cells has already been mentioned. The liver has a key role in the detoxification of exogenous and endogenous substances such as drugs, endogenous hormones, and toxins. The processes by which this is accomplished are described in Chapter 4. The removal of ammonia and the formation of urea may also be included among the liver's detoxification functions.

Digestion and Excretion

Since it synthesizes bile, the liver can be considered to have a role in digestion. The function of bile in digestion and absorption is described in Chapters 7 and 8. The bile is the vehicle for excretion of cholesterol and fat-soluble foreign materials. Bilirubin, the product of the breakdown of heme when red blood cells are discarded, also is excreted in bile.

Circulatory and Other Functions

The liver has the capacity to serve as a reservoir for blood. It usually contains approximately 650 ml of blood but can expand or contract to alter its blood volume. The controlling mechanisms are not clear. The liver is a major source of lymph, producing lymph with a high protein content. It also serves as a hematopoietic organ in the fetus, but this function is confined to the bone marrow in the normal adult.

DIAGNOSIS OF LIVER DISEASE

As is the case with the kidney, the liver has a great reserve capacity. In the liver function tests described, 75% of function is lost before organ failure is *clinically* evident. Therefore, hepatic failure is defined as loss of 70% or more of hepatic function. There are numerous tests used to evaluate the various functions of the liver. However, they are not specific for liver disease, and the results of many of these tests are influenced by extrahepatic factors. The picture is complicated by a large functional reserve of the liver and the liver's ability to regenerate.

The tests may require analysis of blood, feces, or urine. They differ in their usefulness: some simply indicate the presence of disease or liver damage; others define the extent of the diseases; and still others may assist in defining specific effects on hepatic function. Normal values are given in Appendix C. Biochemical tests of liver function include tests for carbohydrate, lipid, and protein metabolism, detoxification, and excretion. For example, when the damaged hepatocytes are unable to synthesize and secrete its protein products, compounds such as albumin decrease in concentration in the serum. Table 13-1 summarizes many of

these tests but does not exhaust the possibilities.

A few tests are commonly associated with specific liver functions. The **sulfobromophthalein** (Bromsulphalein; BSP) **retention test** measures the ability of the liver to concentrate and secrete the BSP dye. It is used as an overall assessment of liver function. Sulfobromophthalein is injected parenterally and then is bound to albumin, taken up by the liver, conjugated, and excreted in the bile. Increased retention indicates disease of the liver or biliary tract but does not differentiate between them. Normal retention is less then 5% of the dose in 45 minutes but may be higher in obesity, old age, pregnancy, and fever.

Another frequently used test is that for **serum bilirubin concentration**. Approximately 200 mg of bilirubin is formed daily from heme breakdown, and a small additional amount is obtained from myoglobin, cytochromes, and catalase. The bilirubin is attached to albumin and carried to the liver from its site of origin. After uptake by the liver, it is conjugated with glucuronic acid, a reaction catalyzed by glucuronyltransferase, and excreted in the intestine in the bile. The serum concentration of bilirubin rises when the liver is unable to conjugate and excrete it.

Serum bilirubin is measured by **van den Bergh's test**, which measures conjugated (**direct**) bilirubin and total bilirubin. Unconjugated (**indirect**) bilirubin then is obtained indirectly by subtraction. It is helpful in diagnosis to have both values to differentiate between biliary obstruction and hepatocyte disease. For example, increased unconjugated bilirubin indicates that the hepatocytes are decreased in number or incapable of normal conjugation. If the serum bilirubin is increased with proportionately more of the conjugated form, the hepatocytes must be capable of conjugation but the biliary tract may be obstructed, interfering with normal excretion.

Another function test is for **prothrombin time**, a measure of blood clotting ability. When synthesis of clotting factors is im-

Table 13-1. Tests of Hepatobiliary Disease

Function	Test	Comments
Carbohydrate metabolism	Glucose tolerance; glycogen reserves	Usually normal until disease is advanced; not helpful in differentiating between malfunction in carbohydrate metabolism in liver and other diseases
	Galactose tolerance	Sometimes useful; measures ability to clear galactose from circulation
Lipid metabolism	Serum triglycerides; phospholipids	
Cholesterol metabolism	Serum cholesterol and cholesterol esters	Total falls in severe injury; proportion of esters decreases; increases are seen in bile tract obstruction
Ketone formation	Serum ketones	
Protein metabolism	Blood urea nitrogen	Concentration decreases if liver cannot produce urea from ammonia
	Blood ammonia	Increase occurs late in liver disease
	Serum protein concentrations (albumin, globulin, transferrin, total protein)	Decreased in liver or renal disease, protein-calorie malnutrition, protein loss from malnutrition, protein loss from gastrointestinal tract
	Serum protein electrophoresis pattern	Changes may be useful in differential diagnosis of liver disease
	Prothrombin time	Depends on concentration of various clotting factors; increases if liver cannot synthesize fibrinogen or prothrombin
Formation and excretion of bile	Van den Bergh, icterus index, urine bilirubin, urobilinogen, fecal urobilinogen	Measure of combined abilities to synthesize bile acids and clear them from blood
Detoxification and excretion	Bromsulphalein (BSP) retention	Used as overall assessment of liver function; measures ability to concentrate and secrete injected BSP; increased retention occurs in liver or biliary disease
	Indocyanin green	Alternative to BSP retention test
	Antipyrine, phenylbutazone, or labeled carbon dioxide for aminophenazone metabolism	Measures ability to produce enzymes for metabolism of these drugs
	Gamma-glutamyl transpeptidase	Elevated in severe liver or biliary tree disease; induced by drugs or alcohol (?); useful to monitor abstinence
Enzyme synthesis	Serum alkaline phosphatase (ALP)	Normally high in bile duct epithelium; serum levels increase in bile duct obstruction; also elevated in bone disease
	Serum aminotransferases (transaminases) (AST or GOT, ALT or GPT)	Increased in hepatocyte damage; also elevated in muscle disease and hemolytic disorders
	Serum gamma-glutamyl transferase (GGT)	Increased in alcoholic hepatitis and obstructive jaundice
	Serum 5'-nucleotidase (NTP)	Elevated in obstructive biliary disease

Compiled from Price, C.P., and Alberti, K.G.M.M., Biochemical assessment of liver function. In R. Wright, K.G.M.M. Alberti, S.Karran, and G.H. Millward-Sadler, Eds., Liver and Biliary Disease. London: W.B. Saunders, 1979; Mezey, E., Diagnosis of liver disease by laboratory methods. In J.A. Halsted and C.H. Halsted, Eds., The Laboratory in Clinical Medicine, 2nd ed. Philadelphia: W.B. Saunders, 1981; Byrne, C.J., Saxton, D.F., Pelikan, P.K., and Nugent, P.M., Laboratory Tests: Implications for Nurses and Allied Health Professionals. Menlo Park, Calif.: Addison-Wesley, 1981; and Kapland, A., and Szabo, L.L., Clinical Chemistry: Interpretation and Techniques, 2nd ed. Philadelphia: Lea & Febiger, 1983.

GOT = serum glutamic oxaloacetic transaminase; GPT = serum glutamic pyruvic transaminase.

paired in the diseased liver, the prothrombin time increases. This test is, however, not specific to liver disease.

When the liver cells are damaged, **changes in enzyme concentrations** appear in the blood. These changes may be the consequence of (1) an alteration in liver cell activity, (2) leakage from the cell, or (3) alterations in the rate of disappearance from the cell. No tests for serum enzymes are specific for detection of liver disease, but there are several that are reasonably useful. Table 13-1 lists a number of enzyme assays with some notes on the significance of the results. A frequently used screening test uses an assay for serum glutamic-oxaloacetic transaminase (SGOT). If the damaged hepatocytes are unable to transaminate amino acids, SGOT rises.

Other useful diagnostic procedures include visualization of the liver after administration of a radioisotope that would concentrate in the liver (**scintiscan**) or visualization by **ultrasound** or **computerized tomography.**[2] **Angiography** visualizes the circulation. The procedure for visualizing the bile ducts and gallbladder is a **cholangiogram**. The physician may see some structures, particularly of the bile duct, by **endoscopy**.

HEPATITIS

Hepatitis is an inflammation of the liver that is second to alcoholism in frequency of incidence as a cause of hepatic failure. Some of its origins are viral and occur in several forms:

Hepatitis A or **infectious hepatitis** is a viral disease transmitted mostly by a fecal or oral route. There is approximately a 30-day (15–50 days) incubation period. The disease is usually mild but occasionally causes severe hepatic necrosis (**fulminant hepatitis**).

Hepatitis B or **serum hepatitis** is also viral. It may be transmitted parenterally or orally. The incubation period is about 90 days (40–180). The disease is usually more severe and prolonged than hepatitis A.

Hepatitis C, formerly called non-A, non-B hepatitis is an acute, viral hepatitis that is serologically different from type A or B. Fulminant, sudden, and intense hepatitis is more likely to occur following types B or C than in type A hepatitis.

There are other causes and forms of hepatitis. Following are some examples:

Cholangiolitic, cholangitic, or **cholestatic hepatitis** consists of an inflammation of the bile ducts in the liver. It is also viral in origin or may occur in reaction to drugs such as estrogen or chlorpromazine (an antipsychotic and antiemetic).

Neonatal hepatitis is of unknown cause, appearing in infants in the first few weeks. It may be infectious, but is sometimes familial.

Chronic active hepatitis is a chronic inflammation usually following an acute B or non-A, non-B infection in 5% to 10% of cases. It also may be a drug reaction, congenital, or an autoimmune reaction. It can result from exposure to toxins such as carbon tetrachloride or can be secondary to Wilson's disease or Budd-Chiari syndrome (interference with outflow of hepatic blood). Excess intake of alcohol is an important cause of hepatitis (see the section "Alcoholism and Alcoholic Liver Disease," p. 526). Chronic active hepatitis is characterized by necrosis of hepatocytes in the periphery of the hepatic lobules.

Clinical Manifestations

Clinical manifestations of the various forms of viral hepatitis are similar but vary in severity. At first, there is a **prodromal period** (indicating the approach of the disease) in which the patient is easily fatigued and has anorexia, nausea, and vomiting. Some cases go unrecognized throughout, but others progress to clinical jaundice (see next section). With the onset of jaundice, prodromal symptoms often subside.

In acute fulminant hepatitis, hepatic failure is indicated by the following:

- Decreased gluconeogenesis leading to hypoglycemia.

- Fluid and electrolyte imbalance indicated by decreased serum sodium and potassium.
- Decreased synthetic function shown in prolonged prothrombin time following vitamin K therapy.
- Impaired bilirubin excretion with serum bilirubin > 20 mg/dl.
- Decreased levels of consciousness (precoma or coma).

Nutritional care in hepatic failure is discussed later in this chapter. Patients who advance to the recovery period from hepatitis may have fatigue, malaise, lassitude, and depression for weeks or months.

Treatment

Treatment consists of bed rest, diet, and corticosteroid drugs. Hepatotoxins should be avoided to prevent further injury. There are no specific antiviral agents for hepatitis.

Nutritional Care

The basic care of hepatitis consists largely of avoidance of further damage and maintenance of good nutrition to provide for regeneration:

1. Provide energy generously, usually 3,000 to 4,000 kcal for an adult. Such care requires careful attention because patients often are anorexic and nauseated. If the patient is vomiting, intravenous dextrose solutions are used. Sometimes amino acids are included.
2. Include 300 to 400 g of carbohydrate and 1.5 to 2.0 g of high-quality protein per kg of body weight to spare the liver and provide for repair.
3. Restrict fat only if it causes nausea or anorexia. Otherwise, a moderate amount of fat to make the diet acceptable is permitted. The generous intake of energy and protein is more important than fat restriction.

4. Provide fat-soluble vitamins in water-soluble form at two times RDA levels.
5. Cater to the patient's preferences in order to increase intake.
6. Take precautions against the spread of infection to others by way of the patient's tray.
7. Perhaps, advise the patient to avoid alcohol during the acute stage. The effect of alcohol during the convalescent period is controversial.

Complications

In fulminant hepatitis, an attempt is made to manage the major complications, hoping that hepatic regeneration will occur. The major complications include hepatic encephalopathy (see pp. 535–537), respiratory failure (see Chapter 16), coagulopathy with bleeding, renal failure, and cerebral edema.

Coagulopathy consists of the following:

1. Reduction of coagulation factors (fibrinogen or factor I, prothrombin or factor II, and factors V, VII, IX, and X). They are synthesized by the liver only and are therefore not easily replaced.
2. Depressed plasminogen and plasminogen activator.
3. Reduced number and function of platelets.
4. Increased fibrinolysis with intravascular coagulation (rare).

Treatment consists of parenteral vitamin K, plasma, and platelets. Diffuse intravascular coagulation, which also may occur, may be prevented by avoiding triggering factors, sepsis, administration of concentrates of clotting factors, or the use of hemoperfusion (see Chapter 9).

Renal failure as a complication of hepatic disease is often the result of volume depletion or ATN. It is important to restore intravascular volume.

Pathogenesis of **cerebral edema** is not known. There is no known specific and effective treatment.

JAUNDICE

Jaundice occurs in a variety of liver and biliary conditions, one of which is hepatitis. Therefore, it will be discussed here, but this knowledge must also be applied in later considerations of other liver diseases.

The urine becomes dark yellow or brown. In liver disease, hepatocyte damage results in reduced conjugation of bilirubin and a resultant rise in bilirubin levels in the blood. There is visible yellowing of the skin and sclerae of the eyes as the bilirubin concentrations rise.

There are three categories of causes of jaundice: hemolytic, obstructive, and hepatocellular. **Hemolytic jaundice** consists of excessive destruction of erythrocytes leading to an increase in bilirubin formation and anemia. When bilirubin production overwhelms the liver's ability to handle the load, usually above six times normal load, bilirubin accumulates in plasma. This may occur in infections, as a result of action of some drugs, or from the action of antibodies to erythrocytes such as those obtained in a mismatched transfusion. Some congenital defects cause the red cells to be very fragile and thereby increase the load. These defects include sickle-cell anemia, thalassemia, and spherocytosis.

Obstructive jaundice occurs as a result of a block in the biliary system, producing stasis of bile flow in dilated bile ducts. The obstruction may be outside the liver, as from impacted gallstones, strictures secondary to trauma or inflammation, or tumors in the pancreas pressing on the ducts, or it may be intrahepatic from lesions affecting the small biliary vessels, or **cholangioles**. In obstructive jaundice, the bile salts are also retained and cause severe pruritis. Though the urine is dark, as in hemolytic jaundice, the stools are abnormally pale because they do not contain bilirubin. Attacks may be intermittent.

Hepatocellular jaundice is associated with hepatocytes that have been damaged, often by toxins or by infections such as viral hepatitis. The uptake, conjugation, and excretion of bilirubin are compromised. The effects are variable with dark urine and pale stools, plus anorexia and malaise.

The most common cause of jaundice is obstructive. If the obstruction is not corrected, the condition can progress to biliary cirrhosis, described later.

Nutritional care consists of a diet with a generous supply of carbohydrates and high-quality protein. The diet is usually low in fat because of the restricted bile flow. If the obstruction is sudden, the patient has colic, vomiting, and fever. Under these circumstances, a liquid diet may be needed. If the jaundice continues more than a few days, the patient should be given a parenteral supplement of vitamins A, K, and possibly E. If it continues for a longer period, vitamin D and calcium should also be supplemented. In very-long-term obstruction, the condition leads to hepatic failure.

ALCOHOLISM AND ALCOHOLIC LIVER DISEASE

Alcoholism affects 9 million to 11 million people in the United States and has a number of social, economic, and physiologic consequences. Serious liver disease is among its effects; therefore, it will be discussed in some detail.

Alcohol Intake

Ethyl alcohol or **ethanol** (CH_3CH_2OH) is widely used as a social beverage, but its abuse is a major problem. **Alcoholism** is the excessive consumption of alcohol accompanied by alcohol dependence. Its effects may be divided into **acute effects** — that is, those resulting shortly after intake — and **effects of chronic abuse**.

The same dose-response relationship exists for alcohol as for other drugs (see Chapter 4). There is a minimum dose below which there are no observable effects, whereas at higher doses, effects are dose-related. Effects depend on the amount of the drug at the receptor site which, in turn, is a function of the magnitude and frequency of the dose. When speaking of alcohol intake, the effect depends on the alcohol content of the beverage a person drinks, how much, and how often.

Alcoholic beverages may be divided, for purposes of this discussion, into three categories — beer, wine, and distilled liquor. From a practical point of view, their consumption can be considered in terms of "drinks." In addition to their differences in taste and kilocalorie content, they also differ in alcohol and water content.

Some average figures can be used to illustrate the usual method of estimation of alcohol content. The alcohol content of beer may be given in a percentage of weight to volume. Let us assume that a person is drinking a typical 12-oz. can of beer. Beer is, on the average, 3.8% alcohol. For ease of calculation, we also assume 30 ml/oz. Thus one can of beer will contain 360 ml $\times$ 0.038 or 13.7 g of alcohol. If alcohol is considered as a percentage of volume to volume, the percentage of alcohol usually is approximately 4.5–5%.

The alcohol content of unfortified wine is 12–14%. This percentage also indicates weight per volume. A typical drink of wine might be 5 oz. or 150 ml. Thus 150 ml $\times$ 0.12 = 8.0 g of alcohol. Fortified wines — that is, sherry or port — are prepared by the addition of brandy, so that their alcohol content may be 20% or more. Among so-called skid row alcoholics, a variation of fortified wines is popular. When these sweet wines are prepared, fermentation of the sugar is halted by the addition of concentrated alcohol. The wine thus has both a high sugar and a high alcohol content that often is substituted for food almost completely. However, it has no protein and essentially no vitamin or mineral content.

The alcohol content of distilled beverages, such as whisky, rum, gin, or brandy, is more variable. It is measured in **proof degrees**, the definition of which varies from one country to another. In the United States, 1 proof equals 0.5% alcohol. Therefore, 80-proof

whisky contains 40% alcohol. Other distilled beverages vary from 35% to 50% alcohol or 70 to 100 proof. The customary measure is a jigger, the content of which is $1\frac{1}{2}$ oz. or 45 ml. Thus a jigger of 80-proof whisky taken as is or in a mixed drink would contain 45 ml $\times$ 0.40 or 18 g of alcohol.

Absorption and Distribution

Alcohol is a small, un-ionized molecule that is completely miscible with water and also somewhat fat soluble. Its absorption and distribution follow the usual principles that apply to drugs with similar properties (see Chapter 4). It crosses membranes by diffusion, dependent on the concentration gradient. It is absorbed largely from the stomach and more rapidly from the upper small intestine. The rate of absorption from the stomach can be influenced by the presence of food or water in the stomach and by the stomach emptying time.

Most alcohol is carried in the body water. As a consequence, blood alcohol content is used as a basis for calculation of the content in tissue, in which it exists in proportion to the water content of the tissue.

Metabolism and Excretion

Approximately 5% of ingested alcohol can be excreted from the body in urine, expired air, feces, sweat, and milk. The remaining 95% is first oxidized to acetaldehyde by one of at least three pathways.[3]

1. The enzyme **alcohol dehydrogenase** (ADH) is used in the *ADH system* in the reaction:

$$CH_3CH_2OH + NAD \xrightarrow{\text{alcohol dehydrogenase}}$$
(ethanol)
$$CH_3CHO + NADH + H^+ \quad \textbf{(13-1)}$$
(acetaldehyde)

This reaction occurs almost entirely in the liver and is the rate-limiting step in the metabolism of alcohol. Approximately 15 mg of ethanol can be metabolized per hour, a rate reached when blood alcohol is approximately 10 mg/dl.

2. The **microsomal ethanol oxidizing system** (MEOS) also converts a portion of the ethanol to acetaldehyde using a cytochrome protein.[4] The overall reaction is

$$CH_3CH_2OH + NADPH + H^+ + O_2 \xrightarrow{MEOS}$$
$$CH_3CHO + NADP^+ + 2H_2O \qquad \text{(13-2)}$$

Like other microsomal oxidizing systems, this system seems to be inducible — that is, it increases in activity in the presence of large amounts of alcohol.[5] It may become of greater significance in chronic alcoholism.

3. The third system uses **catalase** as an enzyme in the presence of hydrogen peroxide by the following reactions.[6]

$$CH_3CH_2OH + H_2O_2 \xrightarrow{catalase}$$
$$CH_3CHO + 2H_2O \qquad \text{(13-3)}$$

The hydrogen peroxide may be generated from either hypoxanthine or NADPH as follows:

$$\text{Hypoxanthine} + H_2O + O_2 \xrightarrow{xanthine\ oxidase}$$
$$\text{xanthine} + H_2O_2 \qquad \text{(13-4)}$$

or

$$NADPH + H^+ + O_2 \xrightarrow{NADPH\ oxidase}$$
$$NADP^+ + H_2O_2 \qquad \text{(13-5)}$$

Following the oxidation of alcohol by one of these routes, the acetaldehyde is oxidized to acetate by **aldehyde dehydrogenase** in the following reaction:

$$CH_3CHO + NAD^+ + H_2O$$
$$\xrightarrow{aldehyde\ dehydrogenase} CH_3COOH$$
$$+ NADH + H^+ \qquad \text{(13-6)}$$

Acetaldehyde oxidation occurs in the liver and in other tissues containing aldehyde dehydrogenase. Alcohol thus contributes to the body pool of acetyl-CoA. In the process of

converting 1 g of ethanol to carbon dioxide and water, the body obtains 7.1 kcal. It also is important to note that there is an increase in the NADH/NAD ratio. The overall reaction is

$$C_2H_5OH + 3O_2 \longrightarrow$$
$$2CO_2 + 3H_2O + 18\ ATP \qquad \text{(13-7)}$$

The relative importance of these three pathways is the subject of some debate. The weight of opinion is that alcohol dehydrogenase is responsible for the oxidation of most alcohol. The importance of the involvement of the MEOS is controversial. Overall, the evidence suggests that ADH is the only active enzyme at low ethanol concentration, but at higher concentrations (those above 10 mmol/L) ADH accounts for 60% and MEOS for 40%.[3] This seems to leave no role for catalase. However, it has been suggested that catalase may be involved in pathologic conditions, when there is increased purine breakdown and formation of H_2O_2.[7] The role of catalase in alcohol metabolism in pathologic conditions requires further investigation.

The major pathway for alcohol oxidation, then, provides us with acetaldehyde and hydrogen to consider when we examine the next steps in the metabolism of alcohol. First, we will consider the hydrogen (Figure 13-3).

The main pathway for the hydrogen metabolism requires transfer of hydrogen into the mitochondria where it is oxidized for energy production, supplanting fat. Ethanol oxidation in the liver is obligatory — that is, it takes precedence. The lipids, which would otherwise be oxidized, accumulate, producing a fatty liver. The excess hydrogen can also be used for the synthesis of fatty acids and alpha-glycerophosphate with subsequent formation of triglyceride, also contributing to the fatty liver. Pyruvate obtained in the process of gluconeogenesis is reduced to lactate instead of being used for glucose synthesis. In the alcoholic who has not been eating, liver glycogen reserves, which are important for maintaining normal blood glu-

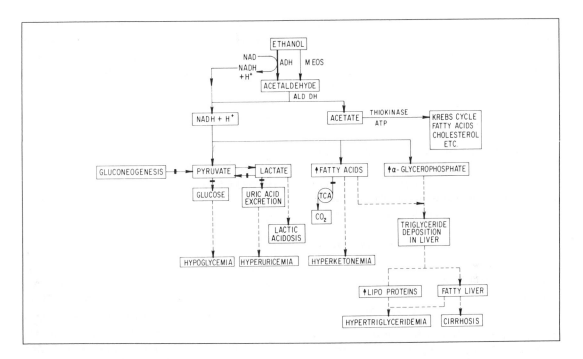

Figure 13-3. *Effects of ethanol on metabolism.*
ADH = alcohol dehydrogenase; MEOS =
microsomal ethanol oxidizing system;
ALD DH = aldehyde dehydrogenase.

cose concentrations, will also be depleted and hypoglycemia then can develop (see Chapter 11). The increased lactic acid can interfere with uric acid excretion, precipitating an attack of gout in susceptible individuals.

The liver must now dispose of the lipid, if possible. The lipid is "packaged" into lipoproteins (see Chapter 10). This process is facilitated by proliferation of the smooth endoplasmic reticulum and increased activity of the necessary enzymes. This reaction is the basis for the recommendation for abstinence in hyperlipoproteinemia. In addition, the conversion of excess fat to ketone bodies is used to dispose of lipid. In some patients, this can result in a condition similar to diabetic ketoacidosis.

Acetaldehyde, the other product of alcohol dehydrogenase activity, is converted into acetate and then to acetyl-CoA. This occurs primarily in the liver mitochondria, although

a small amount of acetaldehyde escapes into the blood and is metabolized in other tissues. Acetaldehyde may be central in the process of liver damage because it decreases mitochondrial functions.[8] It is reported to interfere with protein synthesis in the heart and has effects on the brain. It has been suggested that acetaldehyde may be the substance primarily involved in the predisposition to alcoholism and in the development of alcohol dependence.[8] Some individuals develop a limited tolerance to alcohol — that is, it requires a slightly larger dose to achieve a given pharmacologic effect on the CNS. The basis for this may be the induction of the MEOS so that ingested alcohol is metabolized faster and more must be drunk to achieve a given blood alcohol level.

Mechanism of Injury

The precise mechanism of hepatocyte injury is not always known. The following have been suggested as the primary alterations:

1. *Altered redox state:* The oxidation of ethanol transfers hydrogen to NAD and thus

increases the NADH:NAD ratio. The consequences of this change can include hyperlacticacidemia, increase in α-glycerophosphate, and decreases in gluconeogenesis, overall metabolic activity, or protein synthesis.

2. *Increased acetaldehyde* is produced in ethanol metabolism: Secondary effects may be inhibition of oxidative phosphorylation, decreased fatty acid oxidation in mitochondria, decreased glutathione levels predisposing to membrane damage from peroxide activity, and neurologic damage.

3. *Induction of the mitochondrial ethanol-oxidizing system* (MEOS) aggravates the other effects listed.

Nutritional Status of the Alcoholic

Alcoholism is a major cause of malnutrition. The reasons are threefold. First, alcohol interferes with central mechanisms that regulate food intake, and food intake decreases. Second, toxic effects and adaptive responses to ethanol interfere with the absorption, metabolism, or storage of nutrients. Various organs, primarily the liver and brain, can be damaged in this process; the cardiovascular, endocrine, immune, and hematopoietic systems also can be damaged. Third, the nutrient content of the diet often is depressed, even if total energy intake is adequate. The nonalcohol calories in the diet of the chronic alcoholic equal 70% or less of their caloric need. In addition, their energy intake often is in the form of pure carbohydrate and few other nutrients are provided. Excessive alcohol intake may provide less energy than an equicaloric amount of carbohydrate. As the MEOS is induced, it produces heat rather than ATP.

Food Intake and Alcoholism

Hunger and appetite are somewhat dependent on the amount of alcohol ingested. Light alcohol intake stimulates appetite, whereas excessive alcohol intake tends to cause anorexia, leading eventually to malnutrition. Other influences on food intake include socioeconomic factors and the user's psychological state. Funds to buy alcoholic beverages can be a major consideration, since alcoholics with limited incomes are known to buy alcohol in place of food.

Effects of Alcohol on Digestion and Absorption

Heavy alcohol intake has a detrimental effect on the gastrointestinal tract, liver, and pancreas, and malabsorption can occur even in the absence of liver disease. Large amounts of ethanol have a dose-dependent and direct toxic effect on the gastrointestinal mucosa, with resultant disaccharidase deficiency and disordered mucosal transport, as well as malabsorption of folate, thiamine, vitamin B_{12}, fat-soluble vitamins, calcium, magnesium, long-chain fatty acids, and amino acids.[9-15] Secretion of hydrochloric acid rises, and the incidence of peptic ulcer disease increases.

Effects of Chronic Alcoholism on Nutrient Metabolism

Dietary deficiencies are seen frequently in alcoholics. In addition, alcohol may affect nutrient metabolism because of its injurious effects on the liver and its influence on other organs and pathways. For example, it decreases protein synthesis, especially in the pancreas,[16] and glucose uptake and glycogen formation in muscle. The incidence of pancreatitis increases with resulting depression of enzyme secretion leading to steatorrhea.

Some changes in mineral metabolism are seen. Magnesium has been of particular interest, since the symptoms of magnesium deficiency and acute alcohol withdrawal (delirium tremens) are similar. A precise role for magnesium deficiency in delirium tremens has not been established, but the existence of a relationship is generally accepted.[17]

Various metabolic alterations, including abnormal pancreatic function, lead to changes in vitamin absorption and utilization. Thiamine deficiency is common. Supplementation is ineffective because alcohol interferes with thiamine metabolism. The most severe form of thiamine deficiency is **Wernicke's encephalopathy**, characterized by visual disorders, ataxia, confusion, and coma. This condition is thought to be a thiamine dependency syndrome in which vigorous treatment with thiamine and general nutritional support is required in conjunction with alcohol withdrawal. Despite treatment, some patients progress to a chronic degenerative condition known as **Korsakoff's psychosis** characterized by poor memory for recent events. The sequence sometimes is called **Wernicke-Korsakoff syndrome**. Other neurologic deficits associated with nutritional deficiency in alcoholics include **peripheral neuropathy** (thiamine and vitamin B_6 deficiency) and **pellagrous psychosis** (niacin deficiency).

Folate deficiency also occurs frequently in chronic alcoholics and presents important hematologic problems. Alcohol interferes with folate absorption, storage, and conversion to its active form.[18] Ethanol interferes with vitamin B_6 metabolism, too, and decreases intestinal absorption of fat-soluble vitamins. Vitamin A absorption and metabolism are altered.

Chronic alcohol intake also may cause immune suppression, cardiac myopathies, and respiratory disorders. Nutritional care is discussed in Chapters 6, 10, and 16.

Acute Adverse Effects of Alcohol Intoxication

Intoxication is defined as a blood alcohol level of 0.1% in an adult of average body composition of lean and fat tissue, 60% of which is water. Nondrinkers and children become intoxicated at lower blood alcohol concentrations. The acute neurologic effects of alcohol intoxication are dose-related, progressing from euphoria, relief from anxiety, and removal of inhibitions to ataxia, impaired vision, lack of muscle coordination, impaired reaction time, faulty judgment, and uninhibited behavior. If alcohol intake continues, it can progress from an anesthetic dose to lethal levels very quickly, but the anesthetic effect usually prevents intake of a lethal dose. It is important to remember that ethanol is a depressant, not a stimulant. The specific mechanisms by which ethanol produces these effects are unknown.

The causes of hangover also are incompletely understood. Effects usually are worse following the intake of alcoholic beverages containing many **congeners** (pharmacologically active molecules other than ethanol, including higher alcohols and benzene). Bourbon, whisky, rum, and brandy are high in congeners, whereas vodka is low. Hangover severity has also been related to the amount of metabolic acidosis and the degree of dehydration. These effects will occur in the novice drinker as well as in the chronic alcoholic.

Alcoholic Liver Disease

Alcoholic liver disease occurs in three forms — steatosis (fatty liver), alcoholic hepatitis, and cirrhosis.

Steatosis

Steatosis is seen in more than 80% of chronic alcoholics. This process of fatty metamorphosis was described in Chapter 1. Symptoms include malaise, anorexia, vomiting, weakness, and tenderness of an enlarged liver. More severely affected patients may show evidence of portal hypertension, fluid retention, and bleeding varices. Usual laboratory results include increased BSP retention and elevated serum globulin and transaminases. Serum albumin is depressed.

Fatty liver can often be treated by bed rest, abstinence from alcohol, and an adequate diet. With such treatment, fatty infiltration and abnormal serum bilirubin and enzyme levels disappear in four to six weeks. Abnormal BSP retention and serum albumin concentrations that persist may indicate residual liver impairment, but this condition is not known to lead to cirrhosis.

Alcoholic Hepatitis

Alcoholic hepatitis is less common than steatosis, occurring in approximately 30% of chronic alcoholics, but it is not necessarily a sequel to the fatty liver. It frequently is precipitated after a bout of heavy drinking. Symptoms include fatigue, weakness, anorexia, fever, and hepatomegaly. Laboratory results show elevated transaminases and glutamate dehydrogenase and decreased prothrombin time. The hepatocytes are necrotic, with an inflammatory reaction and hyaline degeneration (see Chapter 1). Some patients proceed to liver failure and encephalopathy. Alcoholic hepatitis can be fatal or can lead to chronic liver disease and cirrhosis.

Nutritional care may be similar to that provided for fatty liver. Some patients, especially those with vomiting and fever, require fluid and electrolyte therapy (see Chapter 2).

Alcoholic Cirrhosis

Alcoholic cirrhosis (**Laennec's cirrhosis**) develops in approximately 10% of chronic alcoholics who have a daily intake of 160 g of ethanol for ten years. It is described in detail in the section "Cirrhosis" in this chapter. **Hepatoma** (primary liver cancer) develops in 5% or more of the patients with Laennec's cirrhosis.

Nutritional Care of Alcoholics

Over the long term, alcoholics, whether they are abstinent or not, should have a diet adequate in all nutrients. Meals often are more acceptable if they are small and more frequent. Energy content of the diet should be individualized to maintain normal weight. Protein, fat, carbohydrate, and sodium are given as tolerated by the condition of the liver. Vitamin and mineral supplements are necessary if laboratory values indicate a deficiency, but there is no need for excessive nutrient medication.

During withdrawal, a chronic alcoholic may need parenteral support to correct fluid and electrolyte imbalance and hypoglycemia. Oral feeding should begin as soon as possible. Milk may be avoided if intestinal damage has resulted in lactose intolerance.

Several nutrition-related problems may arise in newly abstinent alcoholics. Hypoglycemic episodes, for example, may recur for several years. Some patients find it helpful to eat large breakfasts. Others reported to develop a craving for sweets. It has been suggested that this may be a substitute for alcohol. When alcohol intake stops, secretion of antidiuretic hormone increases, leading to overhydration; therefore, fluid restriction may be necessary.

Some patients are treated with disulfiram to decrease their dependency on alcohol. Disulfiram interferes with the metabolism of acetaldehyde to acetate, and alcohol intake then causes unpleasant symptoms (see Chapter 4). In addition to avoiding alcoholic beverages, it is important for the patient to avoid inadvertent alcohol intake in food. Some foods to be avoided are wine vinegar and apple cider. Foods cooked in wine and flamed desserts may also be avoided as a precaution because not all alcohol may evaporate during preparation.

The chronic alcoholic who continues to drink must understand that good nutrition will not prevent tissue damage from the alcohol, although it may moderate the severity of the damage if part of it was caused by malnutrition. Food-alcohol incompatibilities are summarized in Table 4-14.

Fetal Alcohol Syndrome

Serious effects on the infant are observed as a consequence of alcohol intake by the pregnant woman. This syndrome is described in Chapter 19.

CIRRHOSIS

Cirrhosis is a generic term rather than a single specific disease. It is the end stage of severe chronic liver diseases that result in hepatocyte destruction, regardless of cause. Causes include excess alcohol intake; chronic autoimmune or viral hepatitis; metabolic disorders such as alpha-1-antitrypsin deficiency, Wilson's disease, and idiopathic hemochromatosis; biliary disorders such as primary biliary cirrhosis and sclerosing cholangitis; obstruction of biliary drainage by tumors, gallstones, or postoperative strictures; vascular disorders such as hepatic vein occlusion or heart failure; or chronic use of hepatotoxic drugs such as isoniazid and Aldomet. As a result of these insults, which may be broadly categorized as physical destruction, ischemia, or infection, there is destruction of functioning hepatocytes. This, in turn, evokes the mechanisms of disorderly regeneration and repair described in Chapter 1.

As a consequence of hepatocyte destruction, attempts at regeneration occur. The hepatocyte is a stable cell — that is, it retains the ability to multiply — and the liver has remarkable powers of regeneration. Resections of 80–90% of the liver are replaced by enlarged and new cells in a very short time, although the factors that control this process are not understood very well. However, in the fibrotic liver, nonnecrotic hepatocytes attempt to regenerate the liver but cannot reinstate the normal architecture because the fibrotic bands of scar tissue get in the way. Instead, the hepatocytes multiply and form **nodules** of hepatocytes. These do not have a normal relationship to the vascular system and cannot perform normally. Thus there is **disorderly regeneration**, as described in Chapter 1.

The nodules derive their blood supply from the hepatic artery and are very sensitive to decreases in its blood flow. The hepatic artery, in turn, is sensitive to sympathetic vasoconstriction consequent to dehydration, shock, sepsis, or general anesthesia. Sudden deterioration in hepatic function can, therefore, result from these conditions.

Classification

There is no ideal classification of cirrhotic diseases. They often are grouped by etiology. An alternative classification is by morphological appearance. In the latter system, the liver may be **micronodular** with nodules less than 3 mm in diameter, separated by fine fibrous bands, or **macronodular** with larger nodules, or it may have **mixed nodules** of varying size.

Clinical Manifestations

Fibrosis and the presence of nodules throughout the liver are required for diagnosis of cirrhosis.[19] The liver has a large reserve capacity, and there is often a long period in the progress of the disease when the patient is asymptomatic. Common presenting symptoms are malaise and lethargy, dyspepsia, bloating, nausea, vomiting, and anorexia. The clinical manifestations vary somewhat with the etiology but merge as the disease progresses. Advanced cirrhosis is dominated by metabolic disorders, portal hypertension, ascites, edema, variceal bleeding, hemorrhages, secondary infections, and hepatic encephalopathy.[19] Additional complications of cirrhosis may be hepatocellular carcinoma and renal failure. Complications with nutritional significance will be described later.

In some patients, a progressive renal failure known as **hepatorenal syndrome** may follow gastrointestinal bleeding, infections, or excessive diuresis. The cause of this complication is unknown, but mortality is very high. Death occurs in uremia, in hepatic coma, or from gastrointestinal hemorrhage.

Portal Hypertension and Ascites

The fibrosis and nodules of regenerating hepatocytes together form a resistance to blood flow through the liver. The pressure in the portal vein rises as a consequence. When it exceeds 10 mm Hg, a collateral circulation develops between it and nearby veins so that blood can be diverted into the systemic veins. The veins with which the portal vein forms the collateral circulation are in the submucosa of the esophagus, stomach, and rectum, in the anterior abdominal wall, and the left renal vein, all of which drain into the vena cava. The collateral circulation develops by enlargement and proliferation of existing small blood vessels connecting these organs.

Portal hypertension can cause **ascites** (accumulation of fluid in the peritoneal cavity). Increased hydrostatic pressure in the portal vein in excess of the colloid osmotic pressure results in a transudation of fluid. Also, a block in the venous outflow from the liver causes an increased intrahepatic pressure with increased formation of hepatic lymph. When the capacity for lymph drainage is exceeded, the excess lymph exudes from the surface of the liver. Thus the abdominal cavity becomes distended with high-protein fluid.

The loss of protein from the blood lowers the colloid osmotic pressure, aggravating the problem. The pressure of this fluid accumulation can become so severe that it causes hernias and intestinal obstruction. Sometimes the hernia ruptures.

For the ascitic fluid to accumulate, renal excretion must be decreased. There are two mechanisms by which this may happen. In one, because of the loss of ascitic fluid from the circulation, the blood volume is decreased and renal perfusion declines. The renin-angiotensin-aldosterone system is activated (see Chapter 10), and the kidneys retain sodium. Thus sodium retention would be secondary to ascites formation.[20] An alternative or accompanying mechanism involves renal retention of sodium as the primary abnormality.[21] Overflow of fluid then occurs when other conditions, such as portal hypertension, make it possible. The mechanism for increased sodium retention is not clear but probably is multifactorial. The liver

may have a reduced capacity to inactivate aldosterone. Prostaglandins, natriuretic factors, the kallikrein-kinin system, and the sympathetic nervous system also may be involved.[22]

Varices and Hemorrhage in the Digestive System

The development of the collateral circulation is the cause of a number of added clinical manifestations. The high portal pressure is transferred to the systemic veins. In the esophagus, stomach, and intestine, the increased pressure causes **varices** (enlarged and tortuous veins such as those seen on the legs of some persons). Varices in the rectum result in hemorrhoids. Bleeding from tears of the esophagus, from gastritis, or from duodenal ulcers is also common. Complications that may result include adult respiratory distress syndrome (see Chapter 16) and acute renal failure. Bleeding in the esophagus or stomach contributes protein to the intestinal tract and exacerbates the tendency to hepatic encephalopathy, which will be described subsequently.

Alterations in Protein and Nitrogen Metabolism

Changes in protein metabolism have important consequences in the patient with liver disease. These changes involve protein synthesis, amino acid metabolism, and the metabolism of urea and ammonia.

Protein Synthesis. In hepatic failure, depressed synthesis of plasma protein leads to **hypoproteinemia**. This condition can be exacerbated by increased plasma protein catabolism, internal bleeding, and increased urinary excretion of amino acids.

Urea and Ammonia Metabolism. Urea synthesis may be depressed as much as 90% in liver disease, since the activities of the necessary enzymes that occur in the liver are decreased. At the same time, the blood ammonia level rises. There are five principal mechanisms by which this process can occur:

1. Amino acids in the intestine, from dietary protein, sloughed cells, or internal bleeding, are deaminated by intestinal bacteria, producing ammonia.
2. Urine output falls in some liver disease (**hepatorenal syndrome**), and retained blood urea nitrogen diffuses into the intestine. Urease from bacteria then converts it to ammonia.
3. Ammonia is produced from glutamine by the action of renal glutaminase and is shunted into the circulation.
4. At the same time, removal of ammonia for urea synthesis is reduced as a result of decreased hepatic function.
5. In the patient with portal hypertension, the blood in the venous anastomoses, which develop between the portal vein and systemic veins (portasystemic shunts), bypasses the liver. Sometimes, to reduce the danger of variceal hemorrhage, a portacaval shunt is created surgically, connecting the portal vein and the inferior vena cava. In either case, ammonia is not removed by the liver for detoxification.[23]
6. Hypokalemic acidosis causes production of ammonia from ammonium ion.

Amino Acid Metabolism. The liver also affects the concentration and metabolism of amino acids from the blood. As amino acids come to it in the portal and hepatic blood, the liver takes them up to a varying extent. The branched-chain amino acids (BCAAs)—valine, leucine, and isoleucine—are not absorbed by the liver normally but pass through to the systemic circulation. In sudden severe liver failure, the liver is unable to remove many of the amino acids from the plasma, and all amino acids except the BCAAs are increased in concentration. In chronic liver failure, there usually is an increase in the plasma concentrations of aromatic amino acids (AAAs)—phenylalanine and tyrosine—and also free (not total) tryptophan, whereas BCAA concentrations are decreased. The normal ratio of BCAAs to AAAs in plasma is 3 or 4; in hepatic disease, it may be 1.0 or less.[24-26] It is not entirely clear why this decrease occurs. Hyperinsulinema may suppress muscle output of BCAAs, or there may be an increase in their oxidation outside the liver.[27] It also is possible that they are used by the kidney to form glucose in an attempt to compensate for loss of hepatic gluconeogenesis to maintain the blood glucose at normal levels.

Fetor hepaticus is a musty odor of the breath and urine in coma patients and in patients with extensive collateral shunting. The odor is believed to be caused by **mercaptans**, metabolites of methionine.

Protein Metabolism and Hepatic Encephalopathy. In patients with hepatic failure (**hepatic decompensation**), neuropsychiatric disturbances (**hepatic encephalopathy**) can occur. The clinical manifestations indicate that there are alterations in the transmission of impulses in the central nervous system (CNS). Hepatic encephalopathy is characterized by acute and temporary or chronic and sustained disturbances in consciousness and electroencephalographic (EEG) changes. These disturbances progress from mild personality changes, forgetfulness, day-night reversal of sleep, and deterioration in personal care to intellectual deterioration and confusion, stupor, and eventually to deep coma. Many patients have **asterixis**, a flapping tremor in the precoma stage, but it is not invariable and is seen in other diseases as well.

There are several circumstances in which hepatic encephalopathy occurs. They differ somewhat in their manifestations, so it is possible that there are differences in their etiology. If liver failure is sudden, such as in **acute fulminant hepatitis**, the patient develops **acute encephalopathy** and progresses through the symptoms within a very short period, sometimes in a few hours. The clinical manifestations are severe and often resemble psychiatric disorders. The causes generally are reversible, and, if he or she survives, the patient may again become neurologically normal. However, if coma develops, the prognosis is grave.

Chronic encephalopathy occurs in some patients with chronic liver disease. The patient has intermittent attacks without apparent cause, or an attack can be precipitated by identifiable factors. These include, in order of frequency, increased dietary protein and azotemia, delivering more nitrogenous compounds to the liver, excessive sedation, use of tranquilizers, gastrointestinal hemorrhage, hypokalemia, and alkalosis. Hypokalemic alkalosis precipitates encephalopathy by converting ammonium ion (NH_4) to ammonia (NH_3), thereby facilitating its diffusion across the blood-brain barrier. In some patients, the cause is excessive use of diuretics. Infection increases the sensitivity of the brain to ammonia and other nitrogenous compounds.

The specific metabolic processes in the brain by which the neurologic symptoms are produced are not understood entirely, but the pathogeneses of hepatic coma in various conditions usually have some features in common. First, portal blood may be shunted around the liver either through spontaneously occurring shunts (**portasystemic**) or shunts that are created surgically (**portacaval**). Second, diminishing hepatic function usually contributes, but there are exceptions. Finally, the etiologic agent responsible for producing the clinical manifestations originate in the gut; gut bacteria have some role in the syndrome, and the etiologic agent or agents may be nitrogenous.

The identity of the etiologic agent is not known with certainty and is the subject of some very intriguing current research. To understand the theories of the specific causes of hepatic encephalopathy, some understanding of neurotransmitters is necessary.

Nerve impulses are transmitted from one neuron to another at **synapses** or from nerve to muscle at the **neuromuscular junction (motor end-plate)**. The end of the nerve

fiber contains vesicles enclosing minute amounts of a **neurotransmitter**. When the nerve impulse (**depolarization wave**) reaches the end of the fiber at the synapse, the vesicles fuse with the cell membrane and release their contents into the gap or synaptic cleft between it and the next nerve fiber or muscle fiber. The transmitter combines with the membrane of the affected neuron or muscle and makes it more permeable to particular ions. If permeability to sodium ion is increased, a wave of depolarization is triggered in the affected cell. At some synapses, the flow of potassium or chlorine ion, which have an inhibitory effect, is increased.

There are a number of neurotransmitters, most of which are either monoamines or peptides and therefore usually are products of amino acid metabolism. **Tyrosine** is oxidized in the adrenal medulla or nervous tissue to **3,4-dihydroxyphenylalanine** (DOPA). DOPA then is decarboxylated to **dopamine (dihydroxyphenylethylamine)** which is used as a transmitter in some neurons of the brain. Dopamine can be oxidized to produce **norepinephrine**, the transmitter in most sympathetic nerves. Norepinephrine is important in the CNS. Dopamine may also be methylated in the adrenal medulla to form **epinephrine**, using **methionine** as the methyl donor. Dopamine, epinephrine, and norepinephrine together are called **catecholamines**.

Adrenergic nerve fibers (those activated by epinephrine) have two different types of receptors, designated **alpha** and **beta**. Stimulation of these receptors may have opposite, and sometimes synergistic, effects. Norepinephrine has marked alpha-adrenergic receptor action and weaker beta-adrenergic receptor response. Epinephrine acts on both alpha-adrenergic and beta-adrenergic receptors. Adrenergic chemicals were studied first in the peripheral nervous system but also have demonstrated central effects in the brain.

Serotonin (5-hydroxytryptamine), synthesized from **tryptophan**, occurs primarily outside the nervous system (see Chapter 8) but acts as a neurotransmitter in some neurons in the CNS. It cannot cross the blood-brain barrier and therefore must be synthesized within the brain. **Acetylcholine**, a common transmitter between neurons that synapse outside the CNS, is formed from choline and acetylcoenzyme A (**acetyl-CoA**). Another transmitter is **4-aminobutyrate** or **gamma-amino-butyric acid** (GABA), which is formed from L-glutamate by transamination and increases chloride ion passage when released, producing an inhibitory effect. **Glycine** is an inhibitory transmitter. **Glutamate** and **aspartate** are excitatory.

With this knowledge of neurotransmitters we now can explore the relationship of protein metabolism and hepatic encephalopathy. In hepatic encephalopathy (HE), there is an abnormality in central neurotransmission. For many years, it was believed to be the result of toxic effects of ammonia on the brain even though the blood ammonia concentration and depth of coma are poorly correlated. Because of this poor correlation, it was suggested by some investigators that ammonia was not important in the etiology or was not the primary cause. However, it now is agreed that ammonia is a toxic substance. Normally, about 4 g of ammonia are absorbed daily. Sources are bacterial metabolism of urea in the gut, deamidation of glutamine in the renal tubules, and carbonic anhydrase inhibitors given as medication (e.g., Diamox). In addition, some foods contain preformed ammonia.

In hepatic disease, there apparently are changes in the blood-brain barrier or the brain itself that make the brain more sensitive to ammonia. In addition, HE can be produced experimentally in cirrhotic patients and others with portacaval shunts by giving ammonium compounds.[28,29] Other researchers have suggested that coma results from the effect on the brain of other substances such as methionine metabolites[30] or fatty acids.[31] Mercaptans and methanethiols, formed from methionine, have been impli-

cated.[32] Use of antibiotics prevents encephalopathy from these compounds,[33] suggesting that it is the bacterial metabolites, not the parent compounds, which are at fault. It has been suggested that the metabolites act by an interaction with ammonia.[34,35]

In addition, amino acids themselves, as well as amino acid metabolites, may be among the toxic materials. Normally these substances would be taken up by the liver, but in patients with portasystemic shunts, they bypass the liver and reach the brain, increasing the production of false neurotransmitters and possibly resulting in encephalopathy.[36]

Phenylalanine and tyrosine, it should be remembered, are precursors of catecholamines, and tryptophan is a precursor of serotonin. Products of microbial metabolism of tyrosine and tryptophan in the intestine include amines, indoles, and other substances that are weak or **false neurotransmitters**. Among these are **tyramine** and **octopamine**. Octopamine, produced from phenylalanine, tyrosine, or tyramine, has been studied in some depth and shown to be increased in the blood at levels that correlate well with the severity of the coma. **Phenylethanolamine**, another false neurotransmitter from phenylalanine, also increases. It is proposed that these substances are taken up by the nervous system, compete with true neurotransmitters, and create a widespread disturbance in neurotransmission.

The specific mechanisms by which alterations in amino acid concentrations alter neurotransmission is not entirely clear. Obviously, a theory is needed that accounts for all the facts, including provision for a role for ammonia and the derangements in plasma amino acid concentrations. Current proposals are summarized here, but these are very controversial.

Using information largely from research by Fischer,[37] we begin with the supposition that ammonia in the blood is increased and there is an apparent change in the blood-brain barrier by which its penetrability is altered, leading to an increase in ammonia levels in the brain. This ammonia is detoxified by astrocytes (the stroma cells in the brain) by forming glutamine from glutamic acid:

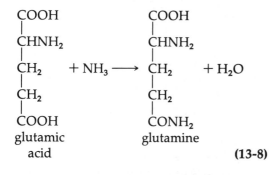

$$\begin{array}{ccc}
\text{COOH} & & \text{COOH} \\
| & & | \\
\text{CHNH}_2 & & \text{CHNH}_2 \\
| & & | \\
\text{CH}_2 & + \text{NH}_3 \longrightarrow & \text{CH}_2 \quad + \text{H}_2\text{O} \\
| & & | \\
\text{CH}_2 & & \text{CH}_2 \\
| & & | \\
\text{COOH} & & \text{CONH}_2 \\
\text{glutamic} & & \text{glutamine} \\
\text{acid} & &
\end{array}$$

$\hfill$ (13-8)

When glutamine leaves the cells and returns to the circulation (the theory continues), it exchanges with tyrosine, tryptophan, and methionine at the cell membrane so that they increase in concentration in the brain. Thus ammonia contributes indirectly to the accumulation of these amino acids in the brain, which in turn alters the neurotransmitter balance in the brain. Tyrosine is the main precursor of norepinephrine, but in hepatic failure, excess tyrosine or phenylalanine appears to cause an accumulation of octopamine rather than increased synthesis of norepinephrine.[36,38] There is a depletion of norepinephrine during hepatic coma. In hepatic failure, there also is a disturbance in serotonin metabolism. Glutamate, an excitatory transmitter, is decreased, presumably having been used to detoxify the ammonia. Tryptophan, present in the brain in increased quantities, is metabolized to serotonin. The increased serotonin, which is inhibitory, may be taken up in place of norepinephrine or dopamine. Gamma-aminobutyric acid, also inhibitory, has been shown to be increased in the blood plasma in patients in hepatic coma but has not yet been studied in the brain.

Branched-chain amino acids are neutral amino acids that are capable of competing with AAAs at the blood-brain barrier. Presumably, they could reduce the entrance of AAAs and thus cause disturbances in neurotransmission.

If these proposals are correct, they would, as pointed out by their authors,[39] account for the role of ammonia and the altered amino acid ratios, since both would affect neurotransmission. They would also explain why reduction of serum ammonia and restoration of normal amino acid ratios are effective in treating hepatic coma.

The effects of administering ornithine salts of the keto acid analogues of the BCAAs were compared with the effects of the BCAAs themselves in patients with portasystemic encephalopathy. Patients receiving the ornithine salts had the more significant improvement.[40] The reason is not known, and further investigation of the metabolic processes in the CNS obviously is needed.

There are those who disagree with the theory that the changes in amino acid pattern cause encephalopathy; they argue that the changes in plasma amino acid concentrations can occur along with encephalopathy but are not necessarily its cause.[41] Nevertheless, changes in amino acid concentrations are the basis for some of the newer nutritional care procedures discussed later in this chapter (see pp. 543–545).

Alterations in Carbohydrate Metabolism

Carbohydrate intolerance is seen in 70% or more of cirrhotic patients, and about half of these are diabetics.[42-46] Most of these are non-insulin-dependent.[47]

Portal-systemic shunting, impaired degradation, increased concentrations of ammonia, and amino acids stimulate glucagon secretion.[48,49] Insulin levels are increased, but the effect is mitigated by an elevation in peripheral insulin resistance.[27,50] Epinephrine and cortisol are also elevated.[51] Hepatic and muscle carbohydrate stores are depleted by an acceleration in glycogenolysis and impaired glucogenesis.

Hypoglycemia occurs in fulminant disease or far-advanced chronic disease. It is assumed to result from a failure of gluconeo-genesis but may be a consequence of reduced glycogenolysis.

Alterations in Lipid Metabolism

Very-low-density lipoproteins, high-density lipoproteins, and lecithin-cholesterol-acyl-transferase are synthesized in the liver. An alteration in any step in the process of lipid metabolism provides a potential mechanism for fat accumulation in the liver.[24] Possible alterations are listed here, and examples are given in parentheses:

1. Increased influx of fatty acids (diabetic ketosis; lipid mobilization from alcohol or corticosteroid intake).
2. Increased fatty acid synthesis (alcoholism; obesity).
3. Decreased fatty acid oxidation (alcoholism; obesity).
4. Increased availability of alpha-glycero-phosphate for triglyceride esterification (alcoholism; obesity).
5. Decreased apolipoprotein synthesis necessary for lipoprotein formation (effects of selected toxic chemicals).
6. Impaired lipoprotein synthesis from available lipid and apolipoprotein (alcoholism).
7. Impaired lipoprotein release from the liver (alcoholism).

Liver injury may lead to decreased serum cholesterol as a consequence of decreased cholesterol or apolipoprotein synthesis or both. In biliary tract obstruction, serum cholesterol levels often increase. The effects of reduction of bile salts in the intestine as a consequence of obstruction are described in Chapter 8.

Effects on Vitamin Metabolism

Low levels of folate,[52] thiamine, riboflavin, niacin, pyridoxine, vitamin B_{12}, and biotin[53] are commonly seen in patients with chronic hepatic failure. Folate is the most frequently deficient vitamin. Deficiencies of fat-soluble vitamins also are found frequently.[54] Poor diet, malabsorption, and metabolic aberrations are contributing causes.[52-55]

Other mechanisms that may explain production of deficiencies include

1. Alteration of metabolism of precursors (e.g., 5-methylhydrofolic acid → folic acid).
2. Increased demand for or loss of vitamins (B_6 and B_{12}).
3. Reduced absorption and storage of vitamins (fat soluble).

The expected clinical consequences of vitamin deficiency are seen in these patients. These include bleeding tendencies (vitamin K), night blindness (vitamin A), bone disorders (vitamin D), peripheral neuropathy (thiamine), glossitis and cheilosis (riboflavin), pellagra and Wernicke's encephalopathy (thiamine and niacin), and megaloblastic anemia (folate and vitamin B_{12}).[52-55]

Effects on Fluid, Electrolyte, and Acid-Base Balance

Sodium retention, hypokalemia, and reduced bicarbonate excretion occur frequently, resulting in hypokalemic metabolic alkalosis. Mild hypoxemia is also usual. The paO_2 may be 65–85 torr. This may be the consequence of ascites, with elevated diaphragms and abnormal distribution of blood flow consequent to distribution of vascular shunts. Mild hyperventilation is common ($paCO_2 = 30-35$ torr), resulting in respiratory alkalosis. The cause is uncertain; it does not appear to be related to the hypoxemia.

Other Effects

In addition to the effects already discussed, liver disease may result in alterations in concentrations of trace elements. **Anemia** is a common finding.

The liver synthesizes most of the proteins involved in coagulation of the blood. In severe liver disease, defects in coagulation may be the result of the decreased synthesis of factor V, and the vitamin K–dependent factors (II, VII, IX, and X). Cholestasis and malabsorption also seem to contribute to depressed synthesis of vitamin-K-dependent coagulant proteins. There are also abnormalities in fibrinogen structure. As a consequence, patients may have prolonged partial thromboplastin time and prothrombin time with a tendency to severe **bleeding tendencies**.

Malabsorption is a common finding in patients with liver disease. Suggested causes include abnormal intestinal flora, increased pressure in the portal vein and lymphatics, and pancreatic insufficiency, but the specific mechanisms have not been determined.

In patients with cirrhosis, **renal failure** may occur. The oliguria is usually caused by prerenal azotemia, acute tubular necrosis, or hepatorenal syndrome. The most common cause is ATN. It may be the result of treatments such as excess diuresis leading to prolonged volume depletion, the use of nephrotoxic antibiotics, and sepsis related to indwelling catheters. Many patients respond to volume replacement. Hepatorenal syndrome tends to follow volume depletion, paracentesis, or gastrointestinal bleeding. There is oliguria in which the urine is highly concentrated but almost free of sodium. These patients usually die in a short time.

Care of the Cirrhotic Patient

Specific treatment of cirrhosis is aimed at removing the etiologic agent, maximizing hepatic function, and minimizing the effects of complications such as ascites and encephalopathy. The nutritional care must be integrated with other aspects of treatment. Abstinence from alcohol is necessary in alcoholic cirrhosis. If the cause of cirrhosis is drug toxicity, use of the drug must be discontinued immediately. Hemochromatosis and Wilson's disease require the elimination of iron and copper, respectively. Some other etiologic agents respond to drug therapy.

General Nutritional Support

Nutritional care in cirrhosis is important because the use of drugs is limited by the reduced ability of the liver to metabolize them. Nutritional care is planned to support healing and regeneration of the damaged liver and to prevent or manage life-threatening complications. General nutritional support of the patient *without* impending encephalopathy consists of a high-calorie diet, 40 to 50 kcal per kg of dry body weight per day or BEE × 1.50 to 1.75, to minimize endogenous protein catabolism. If the patient has ascites, the calorie and protein content must be based on an estimate of body weight from which the weight of the ascites fluid has been subtracted.

Fat may be provided at 25–40% of total kilocalories. If there is evidence of fat malabsorption, part of the fat may be given as MCT. This is a reasonable procedure for patients with biliary cirrhosis. Fat may be restricted if there is evidence of jaundice.

The amount of protein is based on dry body weight, protein tolerance, and degree of malnutrition. A patient who has not shown hepatic encephalopathy may be given 1.5 g protein per kg dry weight.

The form in which the protein is given may be important. There is some evidence that cirrhotic patients tolerate the protein from dairy products and vegetable protein better than that from other sources.[56] The basis for this difference may lie in the amino acid patterns of the various proteins.[56] Vegetable proteins contain less methionine and fewer AAAs than do other proteins. They also may change the bacterial flora of the gut.[57] Given the proposed role of ammonia in the pathogenesis of hepatic encephalopathy, foods that contain preformed ammonia are omitted. Among these are various cheeses, salami, bacon, ham, ground beef, and gelatin. Analysis of ammonia in a number of foods has been provided by Rudman et al.[57]

The diet should contain 300 to 400 g of carbohydrate to spare protein. A patient weighing 60 kg, for example, might be given a diet containing 400 g of carbohydrate, 60 g of protein, 90 g of fat, and 2,650 kcal. Because the patient often is anorexic or nauseated, the foods might be offered in four to six smaller meals, or the patient might be given liquid supplements. To encourage food intake, the patient's preferences should be considered, and the patient should be consulted and encouraged frequently by the nutritional care specialist.

All patients need vitamin and mineral supplements. Vitamin B complex, vitamin A, zinc, magnesium, and phosphorus are needed. The dose depends on serum levels. Potassium should be monitored carefully because it enters new tissues as they are formed, and serum levels may be inadequate.

In addition to these general procedures, other modifications may be indicated by complications of the particular disease.

Esophageal and Gastric Varices

In a patient with esophageal and gastric varices, additional modifications are indicated. A diet reduced in roughage may be used to avoid damage to the mucosa and resultant gastrointestinal bleeding. At the same time, the patient must avoid constipation, since straining at the stool may cause hemorrhage. For this purpose, fluid intake should be maintained, and potassium intake should be generous, with ample intake of fruit or fruit juice. A soft, low-fiber diet is used. Lactulose, employed in the prevention of encephalopathy, is helpful. Meals should be small and frequent, and patients are advised to eat slowly and to chew their food well.

If the patient has an esophageal hemorrhage, bleeding may often be controlled with medication. Ranitidine reduces acid output and is used to control bleeding from duodenal ulcers. Unlike cimetidine, it does not affect drug metabolism in the liver. Usually surgery is unnecessary. If the bleeding is from gastritis, gastrectomy or a portacaval shunt may be necessary. There is a high mortality with these procedures.

In the patient who bleeds from varices, vasopressin may be used to constrict splanchnic blood flow and reduce blood pressure in the portal vein. Alternatively, the bleeding can sometimes be stopped in an emergency by inserting into the esophagus an appliance called a Sengstaken-Blackemore tube. It is a balloonlike device that can be inflated to stop the bleeding by pressure on the blood vessels. This procedure is known as **balloon tamponade**. Complications may include aspiration pneumonia, airway obstruction, or esophageal rupture.

A popular current method of controlling the bleeding is **endoscopic sclerotherapy**. In this method, a hardening agent is injected into or adjacent to the varices. Morrhuate sodium, the fatty acids of cod liver oil, is often used. The method is as effective as balloon tamponade plus vasopressin, but it may have complications including pain, ulcerations, esophageal strictures, aortic rupture, and adult respiratory distress syndrome (see Chapter 16). If these methods do not stop the bleeding, surgical creation of a portacaval shunt may be done. It has the same mortality rate as sclerotherapy.

Supportive treatment includes parenteral fluids and electrolytes, blood transfusions, and cleansing enemas to remove blood from the intestinal tract, thus preventing ammonia intoxication.[58]

Resumption of oral feeding, when it is possible, should be approached cautiously. Clear liquids, tea, water, and broth may first be given hourly or every two hours. All liquid should be at room temperature or cooler. The diet may be progressed from a full liquid diet to a nonroughage soft diet to a general nonroughage diet as tolerated. Small frequent meals may be helpful. Other modifications mandated by damage to the liver must be continued.

Ascites and Edema

Minimal fluid retention may disappear with bed rest alone; ascites disappears if the causes are removed. Therefore, the primary objective in the treatment of patients with ascites and edema is to improve liver function. Increased energy (1.5 × BEE) and protein (1.25–1.75 g/kg dry weight) are provided. Albumin replacements also improve osmotic pressure.

The diet is also sodium-restricted, sometimes to 10 or 20 mEq/day, sometimes with a fluid restriction to 1,000–1,500 ml. The sodium restriction is more severe than that used in renal and cardiovascular disease because diuretic drugs can be used only with caution in the cirrhotic patient. If any diuretic is used, it should be a potassium-sparing one like spironolactone, either alone or in combination with furosemide.

There is controversy concerning fluid restriction. It may be restricted to a volume equivalent to urine output the previous day. The objective is a weight loss of 0.5 to 1.0 kg/day. Others suggest unrestricted fluid intake as long as sodium intake is restricted and there is no evidence of further fluid retention. Potassium should be monitored if diuretics are used (see Chapter 9). If the patient does not respond to sodium restriction, sodium-containing antacids and intravenous antibiotics are discontinued, as are drugs that interfere with renal sodium excretion, such as anti-inflammatory drugs and beta blockers. Other approaches to control of fluid accumulation are paracentesis or creation of a peritoneovenous shunt.

Hepatic Encephalopathy

Encephalopathy varies in severity and, for convenience, is graded as follows:

Stage I: Euphoria or depression, subtle alterations in personality, mild confusion, slurred speech, difficulties in calculation, sloppy personal habits, difficulty in writing legibly.

Stage II: Lethargy, moderate confusion, asterixis, abnormal sleep, short attention span, inappropriate behavior, abnormal EEG.

Stage III: Marked confusion, incoherent speech, asterixis, short attention span, loss of fine motor control, sleeps much of time, grossly abnormal EEG.

Stage IV: Coma, may respond to noxious stimuli, no asterixis, depressed deep tendon reflexes, grossly abnormal EEG.[59]

There are no specific laboratory tests. Serum ammonia and cerebrospinal fluid glutamine levels are usually elevated, but not always. Diagnosis must rule out subdural hematoma or cerebral edema from head injury.

As the number of functioning hepatocytes declines, the established treatment is to restrict protein intake to 40 g/day, or less if necessary, to avoid encephalopathy. The protein must be distributed throughout the day. Maintenance of nitrogen balance is difficult if not impossible. The patient's anorexia is a complicating problem.

Precipitating factors must be removed or corrected. Standard therapy has centered on the gut, to reduce its protein content, alter the intestinal flora, or affect the rate of absorption of amino acids or their metabolites. **Neomycin** interferes with conversion of urea to ammonia by colonic bacteria. It reduces intestinal bacteria so that more protein, needed for liver regeneration, can be included in the diet. However, neomycin contributes to malabsorption.

Lactulose is a nonabsorbable disaccharide that is metabolized by colonic bacteria to organic acids, producing an acidic diarrhea, reducing bacterial action, and perhaps trapping some ammonia in the gut. It may also depress absorption of aromatic amino acids.[38] If there is gastrointestinal bleeding, it must be stopped.

Other precipitating factors include the use of sedatives or narcotics, acid-base disturbances, as described earlier, and infections to which cirrhosis patients are very prone. As necessary, sedatives and narcotics are discontinued and infections are treated with antibiotics.

Correction of the acid-base balance is very important because it affects movement of ammonia across cell membranes. Some gaseous un-ionized ammonia is found in the blood and diffuses freely with the concentration gradient across cell membranes. These membranes are not equally permeable to ammonium ion, which accumulates on the side of a membrane where there is a higher hydrogen ion concentration. Normal blood pH of 7.4 and cerebrospinal fluid (CSF) pH of 6.95 result in a pH gradient favoring movement of ammonia into the brain. In the systemic alkalosis seen in hepatic failure, this movement is enhanced by the increased gradient.

The hypokalemia also lowers the intracellular pH because of the exchange of hydrogen for potassium in the cells. As a result, there is even greater movement of ammonia into the brain.

If the patient has a history of encephalopathy, an amount of protein slightly less than that previously tolerated may be used in the diet. Powdered branched-chain amino acids to provide the remainder of the protein requirement is sometimes recommended to increase the total protein.[60] Others do not believe the use of BCAA is justified.[61] This method is clearly controversial and is very expensive.

In impending encephalopathy, the protein in the diet is reduced as necessary to 20 g or even none. When mental function improves, protein can be reintroduced at 0.25 g/kg and increased 0.25 g/kg every two or three days until reaching 1.5–2.0 g/kg. C:N ratio should be 400–800 kcal/g to conserve protein.

Carbohydrate is given as starch. Fat may be given as a mixture of MCT and LCT. For the patient being fed parenterally, fat emulsions apparently may be used safely. They are hydrolyzed by lipoprotein lipase in capillaries, and fatty acids are oxidized by the liver.[62] Excess carbohydrate, however, must be converted to fat and exported as lipoprotein by the liver. Thus large amounts of carbohydrates may cause a fatty liver, and partial substitution of fat for some carbohydrate will reduce the amount of fat that actually remains in the liver. A high carbohydrate content also presents a problem to patients with carbohydrate intolerance.

For patients with impending encephalopathy or those who have recovered, other products are available. Though 40 g of protein may not be sufficient to maintain nitrogen balance, greater amounts cannot be used. For these patients, liquid supplements containing increased amounts of branched-chain amino acids and reduced AAAs may be helpful. Two such products, **Hepatic-Aid** and **Travasorb Hepatic** are available (see Appendix G). Hepatic-Aid comes in a pudding form, also. Nothing is known yet of the effects of these products on long-term survival.

Feeding Techniques

Decisions about feeding methods to be used require consideration of the degree of organ failure, gastrointestinal function, and electrolyte and fluid tolerance, nutritional status, and the ability of the patient to eat conventional foods. The consumption of conventional foods can be limited by anorexia and encephalopathy.[53,63] In addition, the restriction of protein, sodium, fluid, and food consistency may make the diet unpalatable. Nonetheless, a great amount of food is necessary to provide adequate energy.

If the patient's intake remains insufficient, parenteral or enteral feeding may be necessary. Indications for parenteral feeding include

- Nonfunctional gastrointestinal tract
- Intolerance to enteral feeding methods
- High risk of aspiration (e.g., hepatic encephalopathy)

The content of the TPN must be adjusted to the patient's tolerance of the formula. Carbohydrate tolerance is demonstrated by maintenance of a blood glucose level < 200 mg/dl. Otherwise, insulin may be given. Intolerance to lipid at 25–40% of total kilocalories, demonstrated by hypertriglyceridemia or decreased clearance of the IV lipid, may be approached by limiting lipid to twice weekly doses.

Protein content of the TPN formula must be established with care. The amount and amino acid profile may depend on

- Adequacy of protein nutrition
- Severity of hepatic encephalopathy
- Aminogram including BCAA/AAA ratio

In the case of grade II or more severe hepatic encephalopathy, some institutions use Hepatamine (see Table 13-2) to correct a BCAA/AAA of 2 or less. Once hepatic encephalopathy is corrected, a standard amino acid solution may be substituted. The total amino acid amount must be adjusted to meet the adequacy of the protein nutrition. In addition, the formula should be given cautiously, possibly 0.5–0.75 g amino acid per kg dry body weight per day at first and increased slowly (0.25 g/day) to 1.5 g/kg/day.

Vitamins, electrolytes, and trace elements in the formula are established individually, with particular attention to the need to make up for deficiencies. The patient may need restriction of sodium and repletion of mag-

Table 13-2. Parenteral Amino Acid Formulas for Hepatic Failure

Content	Hepatamine[a] (Kendall McGaw)	Veinamine 8% (Cutter)	Aminosyn 8.5% (Abbott)
Osmolarity (mOsm/L)	785	950	850
Amino acid concentrations (%)	8	8	8.5
Amino acids, essential (mg/dl)			
Isoleucine[b]	900	493	620
Leucine[b]	1,100	347	810
Lysine	610	667	624
Methionine	100	427	340
Phenylalanine	100	400	380
Threonine	450	160	460
Tryptophan	66	80	150
Valine[b]	840	253	680
Amino acids, nonessential (mg/dl)			
Alanine	770		1,100
Arginine	600	749	850
Histidine	240	237	260
Proline	800	107	750
Serine	500		370
Tyrosine			44
Glycine	900	3,387	1,100
Cysteine	<20		
Glutamic acid		426	
Aspartic acid		400	
Electrolytes (mEq/L)			
Sodium	10	40	
Potassium		30	5.4
Magnesium		6	
Chloride	<3	50	35
Acetate	62	50	90
Phosphate (mM/L)	10		
Nitrogen (g/dl)	1.2	1.33	1.34

[a] Branched-chain-amino-acid–enriched formula for hepatic failure.
[b] Branched-chain amino acids.

nesium, phosphorus, zinc, folate, thiamine, and vitamin B$_{12}$.

Patients may be fed by tube if they have a functional gastrointestinal tract but their intake is insufficient. Esophageal varices are no longer a contraindication to tube feeding. A No. 8 French silastic tube is well tolerated. Patients needing fluid restriction may be given a calorie-dense formula. Formula should be given slowly in dilute form and advanced as tolerated. Patients need to be monitored carefully for formula tolerance.[62] Available prepared formulas listed in Appendix G for general use contain too much sodium and water and sometimes too much protein for many patients with hepatic disease. Instead, **modular formulas**, those tailor-made to the tolerance of the individual patient, may be used.[64]

The formulas high in BCAAs, Hepatic-Aid and Travasorb Hepatic (see Appendix G), are also usable for tube feeding. They differ in some important ways. Travasorb Hepatic contains 10.6% protein, the nitrogen of which is approximately 50% BCAA. It also contains vitamins and minerals to provide 100% of the recommended dietary allowances if 2,300 kcal are given. It contains 1.1 kcal/ml at the recommended dilution, and its osmolarity is 650 mOsm/L. The caloric density may be inadequate for patients whose fluid must be restricted. The inclusion of minerals reduces the potential for modifying the formula. Hepatic-Aid, on the other hand, provides 10.3% protein with 36% of the nitrogen as BCAA. It is essentially free of vitamins and minerals, so these must be added if the formula is used for a long period. Its osmolarity is 950 mOsm/L at the recommended dilution, requiring slow administration. The caloric density, 1.6 kcal/ml, may be an advantage for use with patients who require fluid restriction.

Abnormal hepatic function may reduce the ability to synthesize tyrosine from phenylalanine and cystine from methionine.[65] Travasorb Hepatic and Hepatic-Aid are free of both cystine and tyrosine, so these amino acids may have to be supplemented for some patients.[66]

Specific Forms of Cirrhosis

Laennec's Cirrhosis

Laennec's cirrhosis is also known as **alcoholic**, **fatty**, or **portal cirrhosis**, although the disease does not always resemble these descriptive terms exactly.

Etiology. Many studies have linked chronic alcoholism with Laennec's cirrhosis, but the amount of alcohol intake, in terms of quantity or duration, that will cause this disease is unknown. A pint of whisky or several quarts of wine daily for five to ten years is typical in these patients.

At one time, it was thought that the condition was caused by the malnutrition common to alcoholics. However, investigations have shown that Laennec's cirrhosis can develop in the presence of adequate nutrition.[67] Nevertheless, since many alcoholics are malnourished, the currently held view is that **malnutrition** is a contributory factor to the liver cell damage.

Only 10–20% of chronic alcoholics develop cirrhosis. As a consequence, it has been suggested that some patients have a **genetic predisposition** to its development.

Clinical Manifestations. Laennec's cirrhosis is a progressive disease, but if the patient strictly avoids alcohol and is treated properly, it can often be arrested and some repair may take place. Then, the five-year survival rate is approximately 60%. If alcohol intake continues, the survival rate is 40% in five years.

At first, the liver is enlarged with much fatty infiltration. The fat disappears with therapy unless the patient continues alcohol intake. As the disease progresses, nodules form as previously described. A decrease in fatty infiltration and reduction in the liver cell mass causes the liver to become shrunken and hard as the disease progresses. If the disease is not arrested, the number of liver cells dwindles until the disease progresses to irreversible **end-stage cirrhosis**.

Presenting symptoms are insidious in onset and may consist of fatigue, weakness, anorexia, jaundice, edema, and ascites. If alcohol intake continues, the disease progresses with fever, nausea, and vomiting. Jaundice deepens, ascites becomes more severe, and neurologic symptoms occur, progressing to weakness, portal hypertension, and a general worsening of other symptoms. Many patients die in hepatic coma, often precipitated by hemorrhage of esophageal varices or by infection.

Laboratory findings include increased BSP retention and elevated transaminases and alkaline phosphatase in serum. Serum albumin is depressed, as are clotting factors. White and red blood cells are decreased in number, possibly from a direct effect of alcohol on the bone marrow. Serum ammonia is elevated, and serum electrolytes are deranged in patients with ascites.

Nutritional Care. General nutritional care of patients with Laennec's cirrhosis is as described previously for cirrhotic patients in general. In addition, since the patient is likely to be an alcoholic and therefore may be malnourished, nutritional care must include abstinence from alcohol, if possible, and correction or prevention of malnutrition. The direct toxic effects of alcohol on digestion, absorption, and metabolism of nutrients must be considered. Nutritional care in malabsorption disorders is described in Chapter 8.

Postnecrotic Cirrhosis

The cause of postnecrotic cirrhosis is unknown, but it is preceded by hepatitis in many individuals. In some cases, it follows infections or exposure to industrial chemicals or other toxic materials. In other cases, evidence indicates that nutritional factors are involved in the cirrhotic process.[68]

Clinical manifestations are variable but can include symptoms similar to hepatitis or can consist of abdominal pain, ascites, jaundice, portal hypertension, and variceal hemorrhage. Laboratory tests show hyperbilirubinemia, BSP retention, elevated transaminases and alkaline phosphatase in serum, and elevated gamma globulin, but depressed albumin. Deficiencies of clotting factors are common, as is anemia.

Nutritional care requires avoidance of excess protein and control of ascites. Other aspects of care are rest and avoidance of drugs, except in some cases that respond to corticosteroids. Infections must be treated promptly, and portal hypertension may be treated surgically if there is variceal hemorrhage.

Biliary Cirrhosis

Biliary cirrhosis is a disorder in which there is excessive copper storage in the liver, kidneys, and spleen, impaired bile excretion, progressive destruction of the small bile ducts, and parenchymal destruction centered on the bile ducts. The disease is classified as primary or secondary. The cause of **primary biliary cirrhosis** is unknown but may be an autoimmune or endocrine disorder. It occurs almost exclusively in middle-aged women. **Secondary biliary cirrhosis** occurs as a consequence of the obstruction of the bile duct.

Clinical manifestations of biliary cirrhosis include severe pruritis (itching), prolonged progressive jaundice, hepatomegaly, and portal hypertension. Because bile flow is compromised, patients have steatorrhea and diarrhea by the mechanism described in Chapter 8. The patients also develop xanthomas and xanthelasma (see Chapter 10). Laboratory tests show elevated serum levels of cholesterol, other lipids, bilirubin, and alkaline phosphatase. There is a chronic inflammation of hepatocytes around the portal ducts and the interlobular ducts. The disease progresses for months or years, and cirrhosis is a late phase.

In the secondary disease, treatment consists of correction of the obstruction. The primary disease is incurable and progressive. Patients succumb, on the average, six to seven years following the onset of symptoms.

In addition to those items previously described in relation to cirrhotic disease in general, nutritional care includes the following features:

1. A high-calorie diet limited in cholesterol and saturated fat.
2. Reduction of dietary fat to 30 to 40 g/day, especially if the patient has steatorrhea.
3. Limitation of foods containing copper.
4. Water-miscible fat-soluble vitamins, given parenterally.
5. Calcium supplements if patient is osteopenic.

Patients may have edema, ascites, and esophageal varices. If so, their diets should be modified accordingly. Patients with severe jaundice may be given cholestyramine to chelate bile salts and reduce itching. Cholestyramine can cause severe constipation.

Wilson's Disease

Wilson's disease or **hepatolenticular degeneration** is an inherited metabolic disorder. Principal signs are cirrhosis of the liver, softening of the basal ganglia of the brain, and greenish brown rings, known as Kayser-Fleischer rings, around the cornea. Clinical disease usually presents between six and twenty years of age, rarely prior to age four.

It is believed to be the consequence of the genetic absence of an enzyme to synthesize ceruloplasmin, a copper-binding protein. Copper then accumulates in body tissues.

Treatment consists of penicillamine, a copper-chelating agent, given before meals. Its side effects may include skin rash, leukopenia, aplastic anemia, nephrotic syndrome, hemolytic anemia, and a lupus-like syndrome. If penicillamine alone is insufficient, a low-copper diet may be used. The diet limits copper intake to 1 mg/day. It is necessary to exclude organ meats, shellfish, nuts, dried legumes, broccoli, whole wheat, chocolate, cocoa, and tea. Tap water should also be assayed for copper content. Demineralized water should be used if the tap water contains more than 100 μg of copper per liter.[69]

NUTRITION SUPPORT IN HEPATIC FAILURE

If the patient is unable to meet nutritional requirements with conventional foods but has a functional gastrointestinal tract, tube feeding may be necessary. For some patients, formulas containing standard proteins or amino acid mixtures may be used. The formula should be calorically dense and lactose-free. The patient who has encephalopathy grade 2 or higher may be given a modified amino acid mixture (Hepatic Aid II or Travasorb Hepatic). The same products are also used if the plasma BCAA : AAA ratio is 2 or less. The ratio is calculated with the following equation in which amino acids are given in molar concentrations:

$$\text{Molar ratio} = \frac{(\text{leucine}) + (\text{isoleucine}) + (\text{valine})}{(\text{phenylalanine}) + (\text{tyrosine})} \quad \text{(13-9)}$$

The tube feeding should be given at $\frac{1}{4}$ to $\frac{1}{2}$ strength and administered very slowly (20–40 ml/hr). A silastic tube size of No. 8 French or less is tolerated reasonably well even if the patient has esophageal varices.[70]

Parenteral nutrition may be necessary if the gastrointestinal tract is not functioning or if encephalopathy has increased the risk of aspiration. The infusion may use Hepatamine for patients who do not tolerate a standard amino acid mixture. Carbohydrate and fat proportions must be adjusted to the patient's tolerance for carbohydrate and fat. Sodium may need to be restricted. Repletion should be provided for other minerals and for vitamins.[70]

Recommendations for monitoring the nutrition support patient include the following. Each observation should be made initially and then repeated at the intervals given:

Daily: Calorie count, body weight, fluid intake and output.

Daily until stable: Na^+, K^+, Cl^-, HCO_3^-, glucose (then repeat every three days).

Twice a week: Mg^{++}, PO_4^-, Zn^{++}, Ca^{++}, liver function test.

Weekly: Triglyceride, nitrogen balance, transferrin, leukocytes, hemoglobin, hematocrit.

Monthly: Albumin.

As needed: Plasma amino acids.[70]

NUTRITIONAL ASSESSMENT

With an understanding of the clinical manifestations of liver failure and available methods of care, approaches to nutritional assessment may be discussed.

The most common anthropometric measurements may be of limited use. Body weight, skinfold measurements, MAC, and MAMC are often inaccurate, secondary to fluid imbalance and edema. They may, however, be used to follow changes over a relatively long period.

Some information obtainable from the patient's medical record is of particular use. This includes weight change, possibly related to edema and to anorexia. The existence of steatorrhea and diarrhea and the use of lactulose are important considerations. Patient complaints of muscle cramps might be related to magnesium deficiency, and decreased taste sensation, to zinc deficiency.

Biochemical indices of malnutrition are of varying value. Serum albumin and transferrin do not accurately reflect the influence of diet on visceral protein status because hepatic synthesis is reduced as a consequence of the disease. Calculation of nitrogen balance must be based on total urinary nitrogen, rather than urinary urea nitrogen, because hepatic urea nitrogen formation is reduced. The calculation is inaccurate in the patient with ascites, oliguria, and lactulose therapy. In hyperammonemic patients or those whose renal function is affected, nitrogen is retained. In evaluation of nitrogen balance,

these patients then appear less catabolic than is actually the case.

Dietary analysis must include information on the quantity, pattern, and duration of alcohol intake. This information, however, is often particularly difficult to extract. It may be obtained from the patient or from a family member or friend. Since the information is often unreliable, it is useful to check 24-hour recall against a food frequency questionnaire. A specific alcohol intake questionnaire[69] is used in some institutions. The energy yield of the alcohol intake should be calculated in the diet evaluation along with the energy content of materials used for mixing. Since alcoholic patients tend to deny their drinking problems, it may be more accurate to double any self-reported intake.

Certain dietary risk factors are commonly associated with chronic liver disease and pancreatic disease. The diet evaluation should provide special attention to these factors:

1. High fat intake increases risk of pancreatitis in the alcoholic.[71]

2. High salt intake is associated with higher incidence of hypertension in the alcoholic.[71]

3. In view of the frequent incidence of vitamin and mineral deficiencies in alcoholic patients, the diet evaluation should consider those nutrients. Special consideration should be given to nutrients commonly associated with alcohol abuse: folate, thiamine, pyridoxine, riboflavin, niacin, vitamin A, and zinc.

4. The patient should be questioned about use of nutrient supplements, and also about the use of drugs that influence nutrient absorption or metabolism (see Chapter 4).

The adequacy of the diet may be evaluated, in addition to usual methods, by observations of muscle wasting and loss of body fat. Tolerance of dietary protein is assessed by monitoring the symptoms of encephalopathy (see p. 535). These observations may be used to judge the need to alter dietary protein and to evaluate methods of nutritional support. Water and sodium needs may be assessed by monitoring the peripheral edema and ascites. Clinical manifestations of vitamin and mineral deficiencies are not unusual. Particular attention may be directed to specific signs of deficiency of zinc, magnesium, phosphorus, vitamin A, and vitamin B complex.

LIVER TRANSPLANT

Orthoptic (in its normal place) liver transplant for patients with end-stage liver disease is a relatively new treatment that has had increasing success. One-year survival rates are 50% in adults and 70% in children. Liver transplant is considered for patients with progressive irreversible liver disease with failure of conventional treatments. Diagnoses in candidates for transplant commonly include primary biliary cirrhosis, sclerosing cholangitis, chronic active hepatitis with cirrhosis, α-1-antitrypsin deficiency, Wilson's disease, and chronic Budd-Chiari syndrome. Common diagnoses in children are biliary atresia or inborn errors of metabolism. On the other hand, patients with alcoholic cirrhosis, duct cell carcinoma, or other hepatic tumors are often not considered candidates for transplant because of a high rate of recidivism. Contraindications include sepsis, advanced pulmonary or renal disease, and multiple previous abdominal surgeries.

Aggressive nutritional support may help to lessen the risk of surgery. Therefore, the nutritional care specialist has an important role in pretransplant nutritional assessment and intervention for optimum nutritional support. In addition to the nutritional care previously described, the patient is given antibiotics to reduce gastrointestinal fungi and gram-negative bacteria. Also, a low-bacteria diet is recommended in the pretransplant period.[69] The essentials of such a diet are as follows:

1. Avoid all cheese and yogurt products, raw vegetables including salads and garnish, and raw fruits that are not peeled.
2. Do not use foods that are stored at room temperature or kept heated for long periods.
3. Defrost frozen foods in refrigerator or microwave.
4. Serve foods quickly following preparation.
5. Cover and freeze leftovers quickly.
6. Use refrigerated leftovers within two days.

This diet begins in the pretransplant period and continues posttransplant.

The patient receives clear and full liquids postoperatively. TPN or tube feedings may be necessary.

Case Study: Alcoholic Cirrhosis

Mr. K., a 39-year-old man, was brought to the hospital emergency room when he began vomiting blood in a nearby bar. The immediate need was, of course, to stop the bleeding. The patient was admitted to the hospital as a bed patient.

The admission examination found the patient to be approximately 8 kg under desirable weight, slightly dehydrated, and jaundiced. The abdomen was distended, and the liver was firm and enlarged. There was a moderate pedal edema. The following values were obtained in laboratory tests:

Serum alkaline phosphatase	12 Bodansky units
SGOT	208 units/ml
SGPT	172 units/ml
Serum albumin	2.8 g/dl
Serum bilirubin, total	8.7 mg/dl
Serum sodium	145 mEq/L
Serum magnesium	1.3 mEq/L
Serum potassium	3.2 mEq/L

The patient admitted to heavy alcohol use for the last ten years. He said he had experienced abdominal pain, loss of appetite, and chronic fatigue for the last month. Mr. K. was given a soft diet containing 70 g of protein, 1,000 mg of sodium, 3,000 kcal, and 1,000 ml of fluid per day in six equal feedings. Multivitamin supplements and a potassium-sparing diuretic were prescribed.

Three days later, the patient became lethargic and mentally confused. He had EEG changes and a flapping tremor. Treatment included neomycin and magnesium citrate. The diuretic was discontinued, and all protein in his diet was eliminated. At this time, laboratory results were as follows:

Serum potassium	3.2 mEq/L
Serum sodium	154 mEq/L
Blood urea nitrogen	6 mg/dl

In another three days, Mr. K. was mentally alert, and his diet prescription was changed to 10 g of protein, 500 mg of sodium, 500 ml of fluid, and 2,000 kcal. Protein was increased at a rate of 5 g every other day up to 50 g; with increases above this level, blood ammonia began to rise, and so the diet was maintained at 50 g of protein.

On discharge from the hospital, the patient was referred to the mental health counselor and the alcohol abuse clinic.

Exercises

1. Compare each of the laboratory values with normal values.
2. What abnormalities of liver function are indicated by each of the following: serum albumin, transaminases, alkaline phosphatase, serum bilirubin, serum sodium?
3. If the patient drank 750 ml of 80-proof whisky daily, how much alcohol would he get? How many kilocalories would he get from this source?
4. Why were vitamin supplements given to this patient?
5. Explain the pathogenesis of the patient's encephalopathy, jaundice, and fluid retention.
6. Give the rationale for each diet modification.
7. What diet do you think was recommended to this patient when he was discharged from the hospital?

References

1. Khatra, B.S., Chawla, R.K., Sewell, L.W., and Rudman, D. Distribution of branched-chain and keto acid dehydrogenase in primate tissue. *J. Clin. Invest.* 59:558, 1977.
2. Wright, R., Millward-Sadler, G.H., Alberti, K.G.M.M., and Karran, S., Eds. *Liver and Biliary Disease*, 2nd ed. London: W.B. Saunders, 1985.
3. Badaway, A.A.-B. The metabolism of alcohol. *Clin. Endocrinol. Metab.* 7:247, 1978.
4. Orme-Johnson, W.H., and Ziegler, D.M. Alcohol mixed function oxidase activity of mammalian liver microsomes. *Biochem. Biophys. Res. Commun.* 21:78, 1965.
5. Loomis, T. The pharmacology of alcohol. In N. J. Estes and M.E. Heinemann, Eds., *Alcoholism*, 2nd ed. St. Louis: C. V. Mosby, 1982.
6. Keilin, D., and Hartree, E.F. Properties of catalase. Catalysis of coupled oxidation of alcohols. *Biochem. J.* 39:293, 1945.
7. Lundquist, F. Enzymatic pathways of ethanol metabolism. In J. Tremolieres, Ed., *International Encyclopedia of Pharmacology and Therapeutics.* Sec. 20, *Alcohol and Alcoholism*, vol. 1. Oxford: Pergamon Press, 1970.
8. Lieber, D.S. The metabolism of alcohol. *Scientific American* 234:25, 1976.
9. Roe, D.A. *Alcohol and the Diet.* Westport, Conn.: AVI, 1979.
10. Shanbour, L.L. Effects of ethanol on the de-
terminants of intestinal transport. *Alcohol. Clin. Exp. Res.* 3:142, 1979.
11. Kuo, Y.-J., and Shanbour, L.L. Effects of ethanol on sodium, 3-O-methyl glucose and L-alanine transport in the jejunum. *Am. J. Dig. Dis.* 23:51, 1978.
12. Perlow, W., Baraona, E., and Lieber, D.S. Symptomatic intestinal disaccharidase deficiency in alcoholics. *Gastroenterology* 72:680, 1977.
13. Halsted, C.G., Robles, E.A., and Mezey, E. Decreased jejunal uptake of labeled folic acid (^{3}H-PGA) in alcoholic patients. Roles of alcohol and nutrition. *N. Engl. J. Med.* 285:701, 1971.
14. Thomson, A.L., Baker, H., and Leevey, C.M. Patterns of ^{35}S-thiamine hydrochloride absorption in the malnourished alcoholic patient. *J. Lab. Clin. Med.* 76:34, 1970.
15. Worthington-Roberts, B. Alcoholism and malnutrition. In N.J. Estes and M.E. Heinemann, Eds., *Alcoholism*, 2nd ed. St. Louis: C.V. Mosby, 1982.
16. Israel, Y., Valenzuela, J.E., Salazar, I., and Ugarte, G. Alcohol and amino acid transport in the human small intestine. *J. Nutr.* 98:222, 1969.
17. Sinclair, H.M. Nutritional aspects of alcoholism. *Proc. Nutr. Soc.* 31:117, 1972.
18. Flink, E.B., Shane, S.R., Jacob, W.H., and Jovans, J.E. Some aspects of magnesium deficiency and chronic alcoholism. In V.M. Sar-

desai, Ed., *Biochemical and Clinical Aspects of Alcohol Metabolism.* Springfield, Ill.: Charles C Thomas, 1969.

19. Hellman, R.S., and Steinberg, S.E. The effects of alcohol on folate metabolism. *Annu. Rev. Med.* 33:345, 1982.

20. Millward-Sadler, G.H., and Wright, R. Cirrhosis. An Appraisal. In R. Wright, G.H. Millward-Sadler, K.G.M.M. Alberti, and S. Karran, Eds., *Liver and Biliary Disease,* 2nd ed. London: W.B. Saunders, 1985.

21. Wilkinson, S.P., and Williams, R. Ascites, electrolyte disorders and renal failure. In R. Wright, G.H. Millward-Sadler, K.G.M.M. Alberti, and S. Karran, Eds., *Liver and Biliary Disease,* 2nd ed. London: W.B. Saunders, 1985.

22. Leiberman, F.L., Denison, E.K., and Reynolds, T.B. The relationship of plasma volume, portal hypertension, ascites, and renal sodium retention in cirrhosis. The overflow theory of ascites formation. *Ann. N.Y. Acad. Sci.* 170:202, 1970.

23. Carithers, R.L., and Fairman, R.P. Critical care of patients with severe liver disease. In W.C. Shoemaker, S. Ayres, A. Grenvik, P.R. Holbrook, and W.L. Thompson, Eds., *Textbook of Critical Care,* 2nd ed. Philadelphia: W.B. Saunders, 1989.

24. Alpers, D.H., and Isselbacher, K.V. Derangements of hepatic metabolism. In R.E. Petersdorf et al., Eds., *Harrison's Principles of Internal Medicine,* 8th ed. New York: McGraw-Hill, 1977.

25. Wu, C.V., Gollman, G., and Butt, H.R. Changes in free amino acids in the plasma during hepatic coma. *J. Clin. Invest.* 34:845, 1955.

26. Fischer, J.E., Yoshimura, N., James, J.H., et al. Plasma amino acids in patients with hepatic encephalopathy. Effects of amino acid infusions. *Am. J. Surg.* 127:40, 1974.

27. Soeters, P.B. and Fischer, J.E. Insulin, glucagon and amino acid imbalance and hepatic encephalopathy. *Lancet* 2:880, 1976.

28. Rosen, H.M., Yoshimura, N., Hodgman, J.M., and Fischer, J.E. Plasma amino acid patterns in hepatic encephalopathy of differing etiology. *Gastroenterology* 72:483, 1977.

29. Gabuzda, G.J., Jr., Phillips, G.B., and Davidson, C.S. Reversible toxic manifestations in patients with cirrhosis of the liver given cation-exchange resins. *N. Engl. J. Med.* 246:124, 1952.

30. McDermott, W.V., Jr., and Adams, R.D. Episodic stupor associated with an Eck fistula in the human with particular reference to the metabolism of ammonia. *J. Clin. Invest.* 33:1, 1954.

31. Muto, Y. Clinical study of the relationship of short chain fatty acids and hepatic encephalopathy. *Japan. J. Gastroenterol.* 63:19, 1966.

32. Chen, S., Zieve, L., and Mahadevan, V. Mercaptans and dimethyl sulfide in the breath of patients with cirrhosis of the liver. Effect of feeding methionine. *J. Lab. Clin. Med.* 75:628, 1970.

33. Phear, E.A., Ruebner, B., Sherlock, S., et al. Methionine toxicity in liver disease and its prevention by chlortetracycline. *Clin. Sci.* 15:93, 1956.

34. Zieve, L., Doizaki, W.M., and Zieve, F.J. Synergist between mercaptans and ammonia or fatty acids in the production of coma. A possible roll for mercaptans in the pathogenesis of hepatic coma. *J. Lab. Clin. Med.* 83:16, 1974.

35. Zieve, F.J., Doizaki, W.M., Zieve, L., and Gilsdorf, R.B. Synergism between ammonia and fatty acids in production of coma. Implications for hepatic coma. *J. Pharmacol. Exp. Ther.* 191:10, 1974.

36. Fischer, J.E., Rosen, H.M., and Ebeid, A.M. The effect of normalization of plasma amino acids on hepatic encephalopathy in man. *Surgery* 80:77, 1976.

37. Fischer, J.E., and Bower, R.H. Nutritional support in liver disease. *Surg. Clin. North Am.* 61:653, 1981.

38. Fischer, J.E. Portasystemic encephalopathy. In R. Wright, G.H. Millward-Sadler, K.G.M.M. Alberti, and S. Karran, Eds., *Liver and Biliary Disease,* 2nd ed. London: W.B. Saunders, 1985.

39. Bernardini, P., and Fischer, J.E. Amino acid imbalance and hepatic encephalopathy. *Annu. Rev. Nutr.* 2:419, 1982.

40. Herlong, H.F., Maddrey, W.C., and Walser, M. The use of ornithine salts of branched chain keto acids in portal systemic encephalopathy. *Ann. Intern. Med.* 93:945, 1980.

41. Morgan, M., and Sherlock, S. Presented in discussion at the Conference on Fulminant Hepatic Failure, Washington, D.C., Feb. 7–8, 1977.

42. DeMoura, M.C., and Cruz, A.G. Carbohydrate metabolism studies in cirrhosis of the liver. *Am. J. Dig. Dis.* 13:891, 1968.

43. Rehfeld, J.R., Juhl, E., and Hilden, M. Carbohydrate metabolism in alcohol-induced fatty liver. Evidence for an abnormal insulin response to glucagon in alcoholic liver disease. *Gastroenterology* 64:445, 1973.

44. Berkowitz, D. Glucose tolerance, free fatty acid and serum insulin responses in patients with cirrhosis. *Am. J. Dig. Dis.* 14:691, 1969.

45. Megyesi, L., Samols, E., and Marks, V. Glucose tolerance and diabetes in chronic liver disease. *Lancet* 2:1051, 1967.

46. Conn, H.O., Schreiber, W., Elkington, S.G., and Johnson, T.R. Cirrhosis and diabetes. I. Increased incidence of diabetes in patients with Laennec's cirrhosis. *Am. J. Dig. Dis.* 14:837, 1969.

47. Jacques, W.E. The incidence of portal cirrhosis and fatty metamorphosis in patients dying with diabetes mellitus. *N. Engl. J. Med.* 249:442, 1953.

48. Sherwin, R., Joshi, P., Hendler, R., et al. Hyperglucagonemia in Laennec's cirrhosis. *N. Engl. J. Med.* 290:239, 1979.

49. Strombeck, D.R., Rogers, Q., and Stern, J.S. Effects of intravenous ammonia infusion on plasma levels of amino acids, glucagon and insulin in dogs. *Gastroenterology* 74:1165, 1978.

50. Soeters, P.B., Weir, G.C., Ebeid, E.M., et al. Insulin, glucagon, portal systemic shunting and hepatic failure in the dog. *J. Surg. Res.* 23:183, 1977.

51. Eigler, N., Sacca, L., and Sherwin, R.S. Synergistic interactions of physiologic infusion of glucagon, epinephrine and cortisol in the dog. A model for stress-induced hypoglycemia. *J. Clin. Invest.* 63:114, 1979.

52. Halsted, C.H., Robles, E.A., and Mezey, E. Intestinal malabsorption in folate-deficient alcoholics. *Gastroenterology* 64:526, 1973.

53. Leevy, C.M., Baker, H., and Tenhorne, W. B-complex vitamins in liver disease of the alcoholic. *Am. J. Clin. Nutr.* 16:339, 1965.

54. Morgan, A.G., Kellcher, V., Walker, B.E., and Losowsky, M.S. Nutrition in cryptogenic cirrhosis and chronic aggressive hepatitis. *Gut.* 17:113, 1976.

55. Mezey, E. Liver disease and nutrition. *Gastroenterology* 74:770, 1978.

56. Greenberger, N.J., Carley, J., Schenker, S., et al. Effect of vegetable and animal protein diets in chronic hepatic encephalopathy. *Am. J. Dig. Dis.* 22:845, 1977.

57. Rudman, D., Smith, R.B., Salam, A., et al. Ammonia content of food. *Am. J. Clin. Nutr.* 26:487, 1970.

58. Conn, H.O. Cirrhosis. In L. Schiff and E.R. Schiff, Eds. *Diseases of the Liver,* 5th ed. Philadelphia: J.B. Lippincott, 1982.

59. Lamont, J.T., Koff, R.S., and Isselbacher, K.L. Cirrhosis. In R.E. Petersdorf et al., Eds., *Harrison's Principles of Internal Medicine,* 10th ed. New York: McGraw-Hill, 1983.

60. Shronts, E.P., Teasley, K.M., Thoele, S.L., and Cerra, F.B. Nutrition support of the adult liver transplant candidate. *J. Am. Diet. Assoc.* 87:441, 1987.

61. Krevsky, B., and Godley, J. Nutritional support in advanced liver disease. *Nutr. Supp. Serv.* 5:8, 1985.

62. Wretlind, A. Current states of Intralipid and other fat emulsions. In H.C. Meng and D.W. Wilmore, Eds., *Fat Emulsion in Parenteral Nutrition.* Chicago: American Medical Association, 1976.

63. Hurlow, A. Diet in the treatment of liver disease. *J. Hum. Nutr.* 31:105, 1977.

64. Smith, J., Horowitz, J., Henderson, J.M., and Heymsfield, S. Enteral hyperalimentation in undernourished patients with cirrhosis and ascites. *Am. J. Clin. Nutr.* 35:56, 1982.

65. Rudman, D., Kutner, M., Ansley, J., et al. Hypotyrosinemia, hypocystinemia, and failure to retain nitrogen during total parenteral nutrition of cirrhotic patients. *Gastroenterology* 81:1025, 1981.

66. Wade, J.E., Echenique, M., and Blackburn, G.L. Enteral feeding in liver failure. In I.D. Johnston, Ed., *Second Bermuda Symposium on Clinical Nutrition.* Lancaster, England: MTP Press, 1983.

67. Leiber, D.S., and Salaspuro, M.P. Alcoholic liver disease. In R. Wright, G.H. Millward-Sadler, K.G.M.M. Alberti, and S. Karran, Eds., *Liver and Biliary Disease.* London: W.B. Saunders, 1985.

68. Cossa, J.P., and Teti, S.P. Nutritional support of the patient in hepatic failure. *Nutr. Supp. Serv.* 1:39, 1981.

69. Zeman, F.J., and Ney, D.M. *Applications of Clinical Nutrition.* Englewood Cliffs, N.J.: Prentice-Hall, 1988, p. 313.

70. Shronts, E.P. and Fish, J. Nutrition support in hepatic failure. In E.P. Shronts, Ed., Nutrition Support Dietetics Care Curriculum 1989, Silver Spring, Md.: Amer. Soc. Parenteral and Enteral Nutr., 1989.

71. Durbec, J.P., and Sarles, H. Multicenter survey on the etiology of pancreatic disease. *Digestion* 18:337, 1978.

72. Pemberton, C.C., Moxness, K.E., German, M.J., Nelson, J.K., and Gastineau, C.F. *Mayo Clinic Diet Manual,* 6th ed. Toronto: Decker, 1988.

Bibliography

Davidson, C.S., Ed. *Problems in Liver Diseases.* New York: Stratton Intercontinental Medical Book Co., 1979.

Estes, N.J., and Heinemann, M.E., Eds. *Alcoholism,* 3rd ed. St. Louis: C.V. Mosby, 1986.

Goldstein, D.B. *Pharmacology of Alcohol.* New York: Oxford Press, 1983.

Kruk, Z.L., and Pycock, C.J. *Neurotransmitters and Drugs,* 2nd ed. London: Croom Helm, 1983.

Leiber, C.S., Ed. *Metabolic Aspects of Alcoholism.* Lancaster, England: MTP Press, 1977.

Roe, D.A. *Alcohol and the Diet.* Westport, Conn.: AVI, 1979.

Schiff, L., and Schiff, E.R., Eds. *Diseases of the Liver,* 6th ed. Philadelphia: J.B. Lippincott, 1987.

Wright, R., Millward-Sadler, G.H., Alberti, K.G.M.M., and Karran, S., Eds. *Liver and Biliary Disease,* 2nd ed. London: W.B. Saunders, 1985.

Zeman, F.J., and Ney, D.M. *Applications of Clinical Nutrition.* Englewood Cliffs, N.J.: Prentice-Hall, 1988.

Sources of Current Information

Alcoholism: Clinical and Experimental Research
Gastroenterology
Hepato-Gastroenterology
Hepatology

14. Nutrition in Hypermetabolic Conditions

Bruce M. Wolfe, M.D.

I. The Hypermetabolic Response
   A. Metabolic effects of starvation
      1. Early starvation
      2. Prolonged starvation
   B. Metabolic effects of injury or sepsis

II. Nutrient Requirements in Hypermetabolic Illness
   A. Energy
   B. Protein
   C. Protein-energy ratio
   D. Micronutrients

III. Sepsis
   A. Agents that produce infection or inflammation
   B. Specific infectious diseases

IV. The Patient Undergoing Major Surgery
   A. Preoperative nutrition
   B. Postoperative nutrition

V. The Burn Patient
   A. Estimation of the extent of injury
   B. Pathophysiology of burn injury
      1. Effects on the skin
      2. Effects on blood cells and the vascular system
      3. Hemodynamic and metabolic effects
   C. Management of the burn patient

Malnutrition or, more precisely, undernutrition not only follows reduced food intake but also may occur if the patient has increased need even in the presence of an amount of food intake that is adequate under normal circumstances. Many of the earlier chapters in this text described conditions in which the patient becomes malnourished as a result of anorexia or inability to ingest, digest, or absorb nutrients. In this chapter, we will consider conditions in which malnutrition may be caused by increased, unmet needs for nutrients. Particular emphasis will be placed on conditions classified as **hypermetabolic** or **hypercatabolic**, such as major surgery, major traumatic injuries, or **sepsis** (the presence of pathogenic organisms or their toxic metabolites). These conditions have a common effect in that they impose stress on the body. The consequences and factors unique to each of these stresses will be described. Cancer and pulmonary disease are also hypermetabolic illnesses, but because a number of unique aspects of nutritional care are associated with them, they are considered in the ensuing chapters.

THE HYPERMETABOLIC RESPONSE

Metabolic Effects of Starvation

The metabolic response to deficient nutrient intake is described here, since studies of metabolism in starvation are helpful in understanding metabolism in hypermetabolic conditions as well as in conditions in which the food intake of patients is decreased. Energy expenditure continues in starvation despite the lack of energy intake. It measures approximately 1,800 kcal/day in a normal human, and this energy must be mobilized from body stores. As shown in Figure 14-1, certain tissues—most notably the nervous system, red blood cells, bone marrow, phagocytes, fibroblasts, and the renal medulla—require glucose as their source of energy. Approximately 180 g of glucose must be supplied to these tissues. Under normal circumstances, the brain metabolizes 100 to 150 g of glucose to carbon dioxide and water each day,[1] and the other tissues metabolize 30 to 40 g of glucose to lactate and pyruvate.[2,3] The lactate is recycled to glucose using energy, and the pyruvate can be a substrate for gluconeogenesis or for formation of ATP. During normal nutrition, the skeletal muscle, heart, and renal cortex primarily use glucose. The liver derives much energy from the oxidation of free fatty acids to ketones.

Early Starvation

In early starvation, the glycogen reserves are depleted quickly. Body fat, though, contains large energy stores in most patients. It would be ideal if all of the energy needs in starvation could be met from stored carbohydrate and fat, but studies have shown that in starvation this is not the case. Once the liver glycogen reserves are exhausted, the body adjusts by hydrolyzing skeletal muscle pro-

Figure 14-1. Approximate daily flow of fuels in a fasting human, emphasizing amino acid release from muscle as a source of glucogenic substrate for liver. ~ P = energy; RBC = red blood cells; WBC = white blood cells. (From Cahill, G.F., Jr., Physiology of insulin in man. Diabetes 20:787, 1971. Reproduced with permission from the American Diabetes Association, Inc.)

tein and using the amino acids as sources of glucose (see Figure 14-1).

Gluconeogenesis occurs mainly in the liver and kidney.[4] In the liver, the main substrate is alanine, which comes to the liver from the muscle by means of the glucose-alanine cycle.[5] In the muscle, the branched-chain amino acids, leucine, isoleucine, and valine, are transaminated to provide most of the nitrogen for synthesis of alanine from pyruvate.[6] The alanine circulates to the liver,[7] where it is used for gluconeogenesis;[6] urea is the main by-product. In the kidney, the main substrate for gluconeogenesis is glutamine,[8] but other amino acids can be converted to glutamine by transamination, with ammonia as the main by-product. Approximately half of the total glucose is derived from the kidney as starvation continues.[4] The primary source of glucose in early starvation is the increased rate of gluconeogenesis.

In early starvation, and persisting for five to seven days, the urinary nitrogen excretion is approximately 12 g/day, of which 80–90% is urea. This loss represents a deficit of approximately 75 g of protein or 360 g of

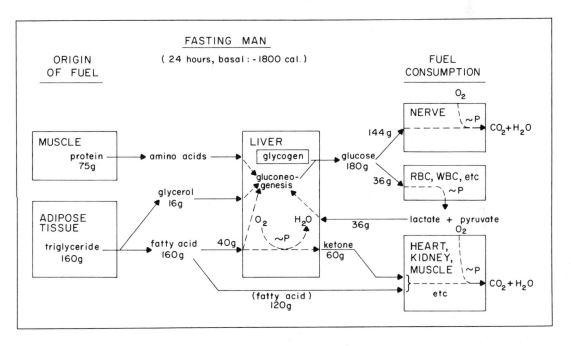

lean wet tissue per day. During seven days of starvation, as much as 500 g of protein or 5% of the total body intracellular protein may be lost. Important metabolic proteins are lost, such as those in the plasma and liver and the digestive enzymes.[9,10] Extracellular protein in bone matrix, tendons, and other supporting structures turns over slowly and so generally is preserved.

For each 1,800 kcal, 160 g of adipose tissue are metabolized.[2] Lipolysis releases free fatty acids and glycerol. The glycerol may provide approximately 18 g of glucose per day.[2] The free fatty acids serve as an energy source by direct oxidation to carbon dioxide or partial oxidation to ketone bodies in the

Figure 14-2. Substrate metabolism in a human after a prolonged period of fasting (five to six weeks). ~ P = energy; RBC = red blood cells; WBC = white blood cells. (From Cahill, G.F., Jr., Starvation in man. Reprinted with permission of the New England Journal of Medicine *282:669, 1970.)*

liver. The ketones are then released from the liver and may replace a portion of the glucose requirement of the central nervous system and other tissues.

Prolonged Starvation

In prolonged starvation (Figure 14-2), adaptive mechanisms conserve protein by enabling a greater portion of the energy needs to be met by fat metabolism, with a decreased requirement for glucose. The production of ketone bodies from fatty acids is accelerated, and the brain gets a significant proportion of its energy from these ketones. Muscle protein continues to be catabolized but at a decreased rate, thus prolonging survival. During prolonged starvation, protein catabolism falls to 20 g/day, and the efficiency of amino acid reuse increases so that urea nitrogen excretion decreases. The principal energy substrate is adipose tissue, with 60% of calories derived from the metabolism of fat to carbon

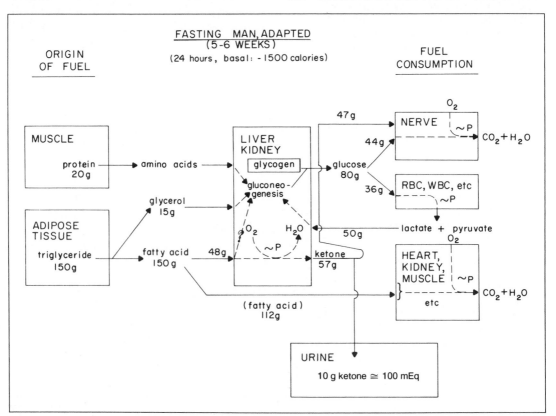

dioxide, 10% from the metabolism of free fatty acids to ketone bodies, and 25% from the metabolism of ketone bodies.

Metabolic rate and total energy expenditure decrease and are manifested by decreased activity, increased sleep, and decreased body temperature. If starvation continues, the body loses most of the intercostal muscles necessary for respiration. It becomes impossible to clear pulmonary secretions, and the patient may die of pneumonia and respiratory failure.[11]

Metabolic Effects of Injury or Sepsis

The metabolic response to injury or sepsis resembles the response to starvation in some

respects but differs in others (Figure 14-3). The metabolic rate is increased and tissue **catabolism** (breakdown into simpler compounds) predominates over **anabolism** (synthesis), resulting in a net destruction of tissue called the **catabolic response**.

Continued catabolism, particularly of protein, impairs the capacity to recover from injury or illness, since many aspects of recovery are dependent on active protein synthesis. For example, healing of traumatic or surgical wounds, tissue repair, replacement of red blood cells and lost plasma protein (as in hemorrhage), and immune response to infection are all processes of synthesis of new protein.

The metabolic consequence of this response to trauma and sepsis are reasonably well defined, although not all of the mechanisms have been established. The response was characterized by Cuthbertson[12] using nitrogen balance studies in subjects with fractures. Excretion of as much as 40 g of nitrogen in the urine per day, equivalent to approximately 1 kg of muscle, is not unusual

Figure 14-3. Estimation of daily fuel flux in a severely traumatized human. $\sim P$ = energy; RBC = red blood cells; WBC = white blood cells. (Reprinted with permission from Cahill, G. Carbohydrates. In Symposium on Total Parenteral Nutrition. Nashville, Tenn., 1/17–19, 1972. *Chicago: American Medical Association, 1972, pp. 50–51.)*

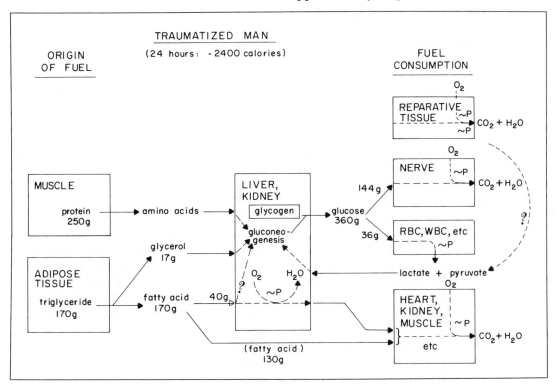

in traumatized adults,[13] and depletion of lean body mass occurs rapidly. As much as 20% of body protein may be lost in two weeks following a major injury. This is an amount much in excess of the amount of tissue injured. Other pathways of loss are transudates, exudates, wound drainage, intestinal losses, and hemorrhage in which 30.4 g of nitrogen are lost per liter of blood. Focus on the factors involved in the accelerated protein loss is therefore appropriate.

As in starvation, energy requirements must be met from endogenous sources if not available from exogenous intake. Deficiencies of energy supply relative to expenditure therefore accelerate the use of amino acids as energy sources. The increased energy expenditure seen in hypermetabolic conditions is thus one component of the negative nitrogen balance (protein catabolic state) seen in injured or septic patients.

In the presence of a hypermetabolic condition with inadequate nutritional support, protein-calorie malnutrition may develop rapidly as marasmus, kwashiorkor, or marasmic kwashiorkor. Methods of identifying these conditions during nutritional assessment have been described in Chapter 3.

The mechanisms by which stressful stimuli cause an increase in the metabolic rate are not understood completely. Afferent stimuli to the central nervous system through nervous pathways or circulating mediators ultimately lead to hypothalamus stimulation and release of catecholamines.[14] Prostaglandin synthesis and release appear to be involved in the mediation of hypermetabolism, including the release of catecholamines and the development of fever.[15] Mediators such as substances released from white blood cells (interleukin) also generate both the systemic responses of hypermetabolism and the stimulation of the **acute-phase proteins** crucial to the body's response to the stress. The functions of many of these proteins in the body's defense mechanisms are not understood completely, but some possibilities include amplification of the immune response, aid in tissue repair, removal of he-

moglobin from lysed red cells, and the minimizing of further tissue damage from phagocytosis.[16,17] Protein also is required for tissue repair. Both of these categories of anabolic processes are superimposed on the normal needs for homeostasis.

The rate of anabolism is, however, slower than the rate of catabolism, resulting in a net protein loss. Skeletal muscle makes the major contribution to both anabolic activity and gluconeogenesis, with lesser contributions from the skin and lower intestine.

In the body's response to trauma, hypermetabolism is associated with negative nitrogen balance and increased oxygen consumption, whereas in chronic starvation, the metabolic rate decreases in response to diminished nutrient intake. This constitutes a major difference between the response to trauma and the response to starvation. With an increased metabolic rate, there may be impairment of the usual metabolic pathways for use of energy sources.

Alterations in endocrine function play a major role in mediating the response to trauma. Several hormones are involved. **Catecholamine** secretion is particularly increased by stress and persists as long as the stress continues.[18] The consequences of the action of the increased catecholamines include an elevation in the metabolic rate and the production of hyperglycemia. Catecholamines also stimulate **glucagon** release. Increased circulating levels of glucagon are found consistently in stressed patients, whereas serum insulin may be depressed.[19] These changes, too, contribute to the production of hyperglycemia.

The catecholamine and glucagon responses are immediate. An acutely injured patient may have **hypovolemia** (diminished blood volume), and so blood flow to the central nervous system may be decreased. Consequently, a higher concentration of nutrients in the blood is necessary so that the brain can extract sufficient nutrients from the limited flow. The development of hyperglycemia, then, appears to be protective in cases of acute injury.

Catecholamines also stimulate adrenocorticotropic hormone (ACTH) release, resulting in increased glucocorticoid levels,[18] which may be two to five times normal and may last seven to ten days in minimal injury or for months in prolonged stress.[20-22] These corticoids increase lipolysis, amino acid mobilization, and glucagon release and inhibit protein synthesis and insulin secretion.[23-25] **Growth hormone** levels also are increased. The effects of glucocorticoid and growth hormone are not felt as quickly as the catecholamine and glucagon responses, but both contribute to the hyperglycemia.

When blood glucose levels are high, the normal physiologic response is an increase in insulin release and inhibition of glucagon. In the traumatized patient, however, hyperglucagonemia persists despite the presence of hyperglycemia. The glucagon stimulates gluconeogenesis in the liver. Cortisol is synergistic with glucagon in the stimulation of gluconeogenesis, so that their combined actions significantly increase urea formation and nitrogen loss.

The traumatized patient has an increased rate of glucose uptake by peripheral tissue and an increased release of lactate which is circulated to the liver and resynthesized into glucose via the Cori cycle. Thus glucose metabolism may be limited to anaerobic glycolysis, an inefficient means of metabolizing glucose for energy. The mechanisms of this altered metabolism are currently being investigated and may involve a failure of entry of carbon fragments into the tricarboxylic acid cycle.

The metabolism of fatty acids and the resulting acetyl-CoA is even less well understood than the altered glucose metabolism. Based on the observation that glucose supports nitrogen balance as well as, if not better than, fat emulsion during acute stress, it is believed that defects in fatty acid metabolism do occur in cases of injury or sepsis.

All of these metabolic events combine in accelerating the rate of development of malnutrition. If the patient has insufficient nutrient intake, these metabolic effects of stress are added to the metabolic effects of starvation. The simultaneous occurrence of diminished intake and hypermetabolic conditions is common in hospitalized patients.

NUTRITIONAL REQUIREMENTS IN HYPERMETABOLIC ILLNESS

The formulation of a nutritional support plan for patients with a hypermetabolic illness requires the assessment of the patient's nutritional status and the severity of the stress, an estimate of the likely duration of the stress, and consideration of the patient's age. The techniques for nutritional assessment described in Chapter 3, are applicable to hypermetabolic patients; however, the need for nutritional support is obvious in patients whose critical illness is coupled with a lack of food intake. Detailed assessment procedures rarely are necessary in these circumstances to establish the nutritional status. However, nutritional assessment is useful in such patients to monitor the efficacy of nutritional therapy.

To formulate a nutritional care plan, an estimate must be made of the patient's nutrient requirements. These requirements must take into consideration normal maintenance needs, the increased needs related to the hypermetabolic conditions, and the needs for repair and repletion.

Energy

Formulas and procedures that are useful in estimating the basal metabolic rate (BMR) in a normal healthy subject have limitations when applied to hospitalized patients. Patients are affected by a number of variables that increase or decrease the metabolic rate. The most influential factors in determining energy expenditures are the injuries or disease processes themselves and the activity of the patient. Recent food intake may raise the BMR by 5% to 15%. Conversely, fasting or nutritional depletion may decrease the BMR by as much as 30%. This presumably is the result of diminished thyroid stimulation and decreased sympathetic activity that occur during fasting. Loss of active metabolic tissue also may play a role. Fever can be most influential, with a 10–13% increase in heat production for each degree centigrade that the body temperature rises. Finally, pain, fear, and anxiety may contribute to additional energy expenditure.

In practice, the resting energy expenditure (REE) of a normally nourished hospitalized patient is estimated to be at least 10% greater than the estimated BMR of the patient when he or she is not ill. The minimally elevated expenditure can be attributed to eating and to some limited physical activity (see Chapter 3). The REE can be elevated, sometimes spectacularly, by the effects of illness or injury.

A number of tables and charts predicting the effects of injury or illness on energy expenditure have been published. One of these is provided in Table 14-1. As might be expected, the values given in different tables are variable and should be used as general guidelines only.

These tables and charts theoretically include only minimal physical activity. If phys-

ical activity is above minimal, an additional factor must be included. These **activity energy expenditures** increase the energy expenditure by approximately 20% in patients who are largely confined to bed and 30% for the more ambulatory patients.[26] Thus the equations for energy expenditure given in Chapter 3 must be adapted to include corrections for activity and for injury or illness:

Energy expenditure for men =
$(66 + 13.7W + 5H - 6.8A) \times$ activity
    factor $\times$ injury factor   **(14-1)**

Energy expenditure for women =
$(655 + 9.6W + 1.7H - 4.7A) \times$ activity
    factor $\times$ injury factor   **(14-2)**

where W = weight in kilograms; H = height in centimeters; A = age in years.

The activity factor is 1.2 if a patient is confined to bed or 1.3 if the patient is allowed to be out of bed. The injury factors are as follows: minor operation, 1.2; skeletal trauma, 1.35; major sepsis, 1.6; or severe thermal burn, 2.1.

These formulas may be made more precise by substituting specific values from other tables for the injury factor, but it is more important to remember that these equations are, at best, only broad guidelines. The nutritional care specialist must be alert for signs of caloric excess or deficiency in patients and must adjust the regimens accordingly.

In addition to the ongoing increased expenditure in hypermetabolic patients, the dimensions of any existing deficits must also be considered. Both protein and energy must be supplied in amounts in excess of expenditure if lost tissue is to be restored. There are no firm criteria established to determine the amount in excess of current expenditure that should be provided to depleted patients. In general, patients who are not energy deficient are given 20% more than the expenditure for current needs, whereas patients exhibiting substantial energy deficits are provided with up to 40% more energy than the current level of expenditure. Occasion-

Table 14-1. Increase in Energy Expenditure and Nitrogen Excretion Following Injury or Illness

Type of Injury or Illness	Percentage Increase above BEE[a]	Urinary Nitrogen (g/kg/day)[b]
Elective surgery	24	0.214
Skeletal trauma	32	0.317
Blunt trauma	37	0.332
Head trauma and steroids	61	0.338
Sepsis	79	0.368
Burns	132	0.360

Reprinted with permission from Long, C.L., Schaffel, N., Geiger, J.W., et al., Metabolic response to injury and illness. Estimation of energy and protein needs from indirect calorimetry and nitrogen balance. *JPEN* 3:452, 1979. ©1979, American Society of Parenteral and Enteral Nutrition.

[a] BEE = basal energy expenditure.
[b] Normal urinary nitrogen measures 0.085 g/kg/day.

ally, 60% excess is recommended[27] but this amount rarely is given.

Protein

The requirement for protein is poorly defined in patients with hypermetabolic conditions. Protein intake usually is increased above the minimum requirements for healthy adults, provided the patient has normal cardiac, renal, and hepatic function. Intakes of from 1 to 2 g of protein per kilogram of body weight per day are commonly used. For the great majority of patients, 1.2 to 1.5 g/kg/day is sufficient. Higher intakes are used for children. Efficacy of treatment with regard to the protein response can be estimated in the clinical setting by nitrogen balance studies, but the clinical importance of such studies is not established.

Requirements for specific amino acids have been studied in a variety of clinical conditions. Essentially all formulations of tube feeding and intravenous feeding products provide adequate amounts of essential amino acids. Increased feeding of specific amino acids such as the branched-chain amino acids and glutamine have been proposed. Their role in clinical practice is discussed in Chapters 6 and 13.

Protein-Energy Ratio

Since energy is needed to support anabolism, the nitrogen-calorie ratio must be considered. Healthy people with a relatively high energy expenditure due to activity require increased energy intake, although their protein requirement is not known to be increased. An adequate diet in such subjects may have a nitrogen-energy ratio of 1 : 300 (1 g of nitrogen per 300 kcal) or more.

In contrast, hospitalized patients are thought to have higher protein requirements despite their relative inactivity. The nitrogen-energy ratio that supports optimal use of amino acids for protein synthesis in these patients has been estimated to be from 1 : 100 to 1 : 180.[28] The ratio of nitrogen to energy supplied must be raised in patients with dis-

orders of nitrogen metabolism or disposal, as in hepatic or renal disease. A daily weight increase of 0.5 to 1 lb. is the maximum possible increase in lean tissue. Weight gain in excess of this amount represents water or fat.

Micronutrients

Little is known about the requirements for vitamins in hypermetabolic diseases. As a consequence, large increases to therapeutic doses of many vitamins have been recommended. There is, however, little evidence of a need for significantly increasing a patient's intake of ascorbic acid or the B vitamins. However, it is important to identify existing deficiencies in such vitamins as thiamine or folate that are common among chronic alcoholics. Therapeutic doses may be required for correction of such deficiencies.

In addition to provision of vitamins to maintain normal availability and function relative to the vitamin, pharmacologic effects may be attributed to additional supplementation. For example, pharmacologic doses of vitamin A have been shown to enhance wound healing and immune function and prevent gastrointestinal stress ulceration in animal models.[29]

Vitamin A is transported from the liver bound to retinol-binding protein (RBP). Protein deficiency decreases RBP and, thus, serum retinol levels. If large amounts of vitamin A are given to a patient deficient in RBP, there is a rise in plasma levels of vitamin A ester associated with lipoprotein. This is the form that apparently causes the symptoms of toxicity, even in the case of moderate elevation of intake.[30] The nutritional care specialist should be alert for signs of toxicity when large doses of vitamin A are prescribed. Appropriate dosage of vitamin A in the hypermetabolic patient is unknown and requires investigation.

Cellular destruction from trauma or the subsequent catabolic response is accompanied by losses of potassium, phosphate, magnesium, sulfur, zinc, creatine, creatinine, and uric acid.[31] After surgery or trauma, patients will often be dehydrated and have decreased blood volume. Immobilization of a large part of the body affects calcium and phosphorus turnover as well as nitrogen metabolism. After fractures, there is a great calcium loss, but the negative calcium balance is not corrected by administration of calcium. Fluid and electrolyte disorders and requirements have been discussed in Chapter 2. Monitoring of serum concentrations of potassium, phosphorus, and magnesium in particular is necessary in catabolic patients, since appropriate intake is difficult to predict.

SEPSIS

Sepsis (the presence of pathogenic microorganisms or their toxins in blood or tissue) from catheter contamination and many other infections is accompanied by fever and an increase in metabolic rate. **Fever** is defined as an increase in central body temperature. It occurs in response to infection, inflammation, or both. Heat stroke and increased intracranial pressure which cause **hyperthermia** (increased body temperature) are not classified as fevers. In these two conditions, body temperature rises because the "thermostat" that controls body temperature fails, and so temperature control is lost. In a fever, the normal setting of the thermostat is at a higher point as a result of the toxins released by an infectious or inflammatory process. Other factors that can alter body temperature are drugs, some hormones, and ionic changes in the posterior hypothalamus.

The **preoptic area** of the hypothalamus in the brain contains sites that detect changes in body temperature, integrating responses from the thermal receptors of the body. The preoptic area stimulates the anterior or posterior hypothalamus to increase and prevent heat loss. The hypothalamus, then, serves as the thermostat. It normally is set at approximately 37°C (98.6°F). Under normal conditions, when the body temperature rises, the

body's heat-losing mechanisms are activated. These include vasodilation and sweating. Conversely, when the body temperature drops, heat-producing responses such as shivering and vasoconstriction are initiated.

In a fever, the thermostat in the hypothalamus is set at a higher temperature. Mechanisms for heat production and heat conservation are activated, and body temperature rises until the new setting is reached. At that time, the balance is maintained at the new higher setting.

Agents That Produce Infection or Inflammation

Any agent that produces an infection or inflammation or both is a **pyrogen**. Pyrogens may be endogenous or exogenous. **Exogenous pyrogens**, which produce a fever when introduced into the body, include bacteria, viruses, fungi, and other microorganisms. **Endogenous pyrogens** are produced within the body and may include damaged tissue, necrotic cells, and antigen-antibody reactions, including graft rejection.

The agent believed to be primarily responsible for fever in humans is interleukin 1 (IL-1). Tumor necrosis factor and IL-6 also contribute to the febrile effects.[32,33] When IL-1 is released, it circulates via the bloodstream. Interleukin-1 stimulates prostaglandin E_1 from the hypothalamus. Prostaglandin E_1 then stimulates the release of norepinephrine, which stimulates adenyl cyclase production. It is theorized that adenyl cyclase then catalyzes conversion of ATP to cAMP, which, in turn, alters the calcium-to-sodium ratio in the hypothalamus, thus altering its firing rate. This process resets the thermostat to a higher level and produces a fever.

Body heat is produced by an increase in the metabolic rate. This is accomplished by stimulation of the sympathetic nervous system, thyroid hormone secretion, and shivering.[34] The accelerated metabolic activity increases the demand for oxygen and nutrients. Metabolic waste products build up. Excess carbon dioxide stimulates respiration, removing carbon dioxide and water. Fluid loss may eventually cause dehydration, with dry skin, dry mucous membranes, sunken eyeballs, and a concentrated urine of small volume. Intracellular potassium is lost, and sodium and chloride move into the cell.

If the fever is prolonged, body proteins are catabolized, with decreased activity, malaise, weakness, muscle aching, and albuminuria. Anorexia, fat catabolism, ketosis, and acidosis also may occur, although sepsis may slow the development of ketosis; it is not known whether fever has any beneficial effects. It can be very debilitating but does not appear to destroy microorganisms. During the febrile period, the patient's nutritional status should be assessed at intervals. Fluids, electrolytes, proteins, and energy supplies must be adequate.

Specific Infectious Diseases

Some infectious diseases have unique characteristics that require consideration in nutritional care.

Typhoid fever is rare in the United States and Canada but does occur occasionally. It is caused by bacteria *Salmonella typhosa,* which enter the patient by way of the gastrointestinal tract. Common sources are water or food contaminated by feces from a carrier. The organism penetrates the intestinal wall and produces inflammation of the lymph nodes and spleen. It also may localize in the lungs, gallbladder, central nervous system, or kidneys. The principal locale is in the Peyer's patches of the small intestine, sometimes causing intestinal hemorrhage or perforation. The accompanying fever is very high.

Primary treatment is with antibiotics. The patient may need parenteral glucose solution to maintain fluid balance. A high-calorie, low-residue diet is recommended when oral intake is possible.

Poliomyelitis became rare once an effective vaccine was made available; however, it, too, does occur sometimes. It may be non-

paralytic or paralytic. Paralytic poliomyelitis may present special nutritional problems. One form is bulbar poliomyelitis in which cranial nerves are affected. Symptoms include dysphagia, difficulty in chewing, inability to swallow, loss of gag reflex, and loss of movement of palatal and pharyngeal muscles. Respiratory paralysis is the most life-threatening aspect, and patients may require a mechanical respirator. Complications of this disease include urinary tract infections and renal stones.

Nasogastric tube feeding may be necessary. To reduce renal stone formation, it often is recommended that the diet be low in calcium (0.5 mg/day or less) with no milk. Fluid intake should be generous.

Tuberculosis is a chronic disease caused by *Mycobacterium tuberculosis.* It usually occurs in the lungs but may also be found in bones, kidneys, or lymph nodes. Malnutrition, diabetes, measles, chronic cortiocosteroid therapy, and general debility are predisposing factors to progression of the disease.

The principal drug used in treatment of tuberculosis is isoniazid (INH) which interferes with DNA synthesis and intermediary metabolism of the bacillus. Isoniazid increases the urinary excretion of pyridoxine and can cause a vitamin deficiency. Supplementary doses of 25 to 50 mg of pyridoxine per day are given.

The usual recommended diet for the patient with tuberculosis contains kilocalories for maintenance of normal body weight with generous allowances of protein, minerals, and vitamins to promote healing. If patients are hospitalized for long periods, attention to their personal preferences is important.

THE PATIENT UNDERGOING MAJOR SURGERY

Nutritional care of the surgical patient can be divided into the preoperative and postoperative periods.

Preoperative Nutrition

Nutritional deficiencies should be corrected and reserves established if time permits prior to surgery. Obese patients should be reduced only if adequate protein intake and preservation of lean body mass can be assured.

Major controversy has arisen regarding the practice of delaying surgical procedures for the purpose of nutritional repletion. If definite malnutrition is present and the delay in accomplishment of surgical treatment does not appear detrimental, such nutritional intervention may reduce complications and improve overall outcome. At least ten days of feeding appears to be necessary to prove beneficial. The cost-effectiveness of such feeding is an important issue. Tube feeding or oral nutritional repletion as an outpatient or simultaneously with other necessary hospitalization is most cost-effective, whereas parenteral nutrition as the primary purpose for hospitalization is exceedingly expensive and requires individual justification.

In the immediate preoperative period, nothing is given by mouth for at least eight hours, since food in the stomach may interfere with the surgical procedure, lead to vomiting and aspiration, and increase gastric retention. If surgery is on the gastrointestinal tract itself, the patient may not be fed for several days preoperatively to remove all fecal matter. These patients may be given a chemically defined diet (see Appendix G) during this interval.

Postoperative Nutrition

A surgical patient commonly undergoes a brief postoperative period of starvation. This is well tolerated if the patient is well nourished before the surgery. In the immediate postoperative period, fluid, electrolytes, and some energy are provided intravenously. When the gastrointestinal tract begins to function, oral feeding can begin. In minor surgery, diet as tolerated is given as soon as the patient is fully reactive. In more extensive surgery, the patient may be given a clear liquid diet and then progress through full liquid and soft diets to the house diet, according to tolerance. The patient should be advanced to solid foods as rapidly as possible (see Chapter 5).

For patients who are malnourished prior to surgery or who have extensive periods of inadequate intake postoperatively, additional support can be provided with supplements and tube feeding (see Chapter 5) or with parenteral nutrition as previously described. Patients who are unable to resume oral feeding by the tenth postoperative day or patients requiring reoperation should be started on active nutritional support. Specific procedures for nutritional care are described elsewhere for patients undergoing surgery of the upper and lower digestive system (see Chapters 7 and 8) and for those with cancer (see Chapter 15).

THE BURN PATIENT

The nutritional care of burn patients requires special attention for a number of reasons. Nutritional requirements are higher among burn patients than in any other single group of hospitalized patients. At the same time, intake is decreased significantly. If these needs are not met, the time required for full recovery from extensive burns is so prolonged that the patient becomes seriously depleted. If vigorous nutritional support is not provided, healing is delayed and infection is more common. There also is considerable weight loss, decreased immunocompetence with increased susceptibility to infection, and inability to maintain the work of breathing, leading to multiple organ failure and increased mortality.

Estimation of the Extent of Injury

The severity of burns is determined by the depth of the burn wound and the percent of body surface area burned. A **superficial burn** (formerly referred to as first-degree) involves only the epidermis (the outermost, nonvascular layer of the skin). Superficial burns are characterized by erythema (redness), which may appear several hours after the injury. Sunburn is an example. Because the tissue damage is superficial, systemic manifestations are mild. Pain and some edema are the chief manifestations. These burns heal in five to ten days.

Partial-thickness (second-degree) burns involve all of the epidermis and a portion of the **dermis** or **corium** (the fibrous inner layer of the skin, containing blood vessels, nerves, glands, and hair roots). The dermis extends between the epidermis and subcutaneous fat. Preservation of epidermal appendages, including sweat glands and hair follicles, makes regeneration of epithelium possible unless infection supervenes. These wounds are characterized by blisters and accompanied by considerable subcutaneous edema. Less severe partial-thickness burns may heal uneventfully in 10 to 14 days, whereas deeper ones may require 25 to 35 days for healing. Thus skin grafting may be used on these wounds.

Full-thickness (third-degree) burns are wounds in which the entire dermis down to the subcutaneous fat is destroyed and thrombosis of small vessels in the underlying tissue occurs. Coagulation necrosis produces the **eschar**, a dry, leathery, inelastic slough composed of the former elements of the skin. As all of the elements of the skin are destroyed, the functions of the skin are lost entirely. These functions include retention of heat and moisture and formation of a barrier against invasive infection. Untreated third-degree burns routinely become infected. Third-degree burns have no epithelial elements remaining and require skin grafting for wound closure.

The extent of burn injury commonly is expressed as the percent of body surface area burned. Superficial burn areas generally are not included in this percent determination. Diagrams that map the percent of specific areas of body surface are available to facilitate accurate estimation of percent of body burned. The "rule of nines" may be used for a rough estimation of body surface area in adults. In this system, each of the upper extremities is considered to have 9% of the body surface, the lower extremities, 18% each, the anterior and posterior trunk, 18% each, the head, 9%, and the perineum, 1%. More precise formulas are available particularly for children. At the time of initial evaluation, the distinction between partial- and full-thickness burns may be difficult. Preservation of the sensation of touch and pain in a burn wound suggests preservation of at least a portion of the dermal elements and indicates a partial-thickness burn. The burn wound that is anesthetic or numb suggests destruction of all elements of the skin and is presumed initially to represent a full-thickness burn.

Minor burns include those partial-thickness burns of less than 10% of the body surface and full-thickness burns of less than 2% of the body surface. Hospitalization usually is not required, and nutritional intake is easily maintained. Small full-thickness burns about the face or hands, however, may require hospitalization for specialized treatment but generally do not cause sufficient systemic metabolic response to impair nutritional intake. Partial-thickness or full-thickness burns of 10–20% of the body surface area require hospitalization. Generally, sepsis can be avoided in these patients, and the nutritional consequences are not severe. Burns of greater than 20% of the body surface area severely alter the metabolic response and increase the challenge of accomplishing adequate nutritional care. Children, particularly infants, require hospitalization and aggressive nutritional therapy for smaller burn wounds than do adults. In general, the survival rate declines with increasing depth of burn, area of burn, and with advancing age.

Pathophysiology of Burn Injury

Effects on the Skin

The skin has important functions in preventing heat and water loss and preventing the invasion of pathogenic organisms. Both of these functions are lost when the body surface is burned. Great care must be taken to prevent infection in partial-thickness and full-thickness burns.

Effects on Blood Cells and the Vascular System

The effect of loss of blood volume in burn patients is the same as that which occurs in hemorrhagic shock. Ischemia of the kidneys may cause oliguria and acute tubular necrosis.

At the same time, red cell mass declines by approximately 10% in the first 24 hours after the occurrence of deep burns, as a result of damage or destruction of cells in the burn area and as a consequence of dehydration. Later, red cell production may be depressed. Total losses may reach 185% of normal over the course of the illness.

Hemodynamic and Metabolic Effects

Hemodynamic and metabolic changes in burn patients occur in three phases. For the first 48 hours, there is the **hypovolemic** or **shock phase**. This is followed by a **hypermetabolic phase** until the wound closes. An **anabolic phase** succeeds wound closure.

In the early shock phase, the patient has tachycardia, hypotension, and subnormal cardiac output. The changes in renal function are largely the effects of hypovolemia, renal vascular restriction, and adrenocortical hormone activity. Inadequate therapy may result in acute renal failure.

Hypermetabolism is common and is proportional to the size of the burn wound up to at least 50% of body surface area. Resting energy expenditure may be increased as much as 100–150% above basal resting expenditure. Increased metabolic requirements of the burn wound itself[35] and systemic hypermetabolism mediated by catecholamines[14] account for most of the increased energy expenditure in burn patients. Loss of heat occurs through increased surface water evaporation and increased radiation losses. Both mechanisms result from loss of the intact skin. Normal skin limits loss of water by evaporation of 700 to 1,000 ml per day in unstressed adults. This protection is lost in the burned area, and water losses through the burn wound are as high as 2.5 to 4.0 L of water per day. Evaporation of 1 ml of water requires 0.58 kcal of heat as the heat of vaporization of water. Apparently, a portion of this energy is derived from environmental heat such that measurement of heat loss by evaporation is difficult. Heat loss by evaporation is a contributing factor to hypermetabolism in burn patients.[36]

The evaporated water is essentially free of electrolytes. If fluid is not replaced, the patient may develop hypertonic dehydration. The burn injury also causes a significant increase in capillary permeability, mostly in and around the site of the injury but also in other areas. Fluid and protein rapidly escape from the circulatory system. Blood volume decreases and interstitial fluid volume increases to create edema. In addition, some fluid and protein are lost from the burn surface. In extensive third-degree burns, the fluid loss can approach 10% of the body weight, primarily in the first 24 hours. In 48 hours, resorption of edema fluid occurs.

This hypermetabolism is temperature-sensitive, particularly in patients with burns covering more than 50% of body surface area.[35] Prevention of shivering and reduction of loss of body heat by radiation can be accomplished by maintenance of an ambient temperature of 32°C as opposed to room temperature (20–23°C).

Endocrine effects are those already described for other forms of trauma (see p. 558) but are of greater magnitude and return to normal only when the wound is closed.[37] The summation of these effects and evaporative heat losses results in severe negative energy and nitrogen balances. Increases in caloric requirements of 4,000 kcal or more have been documented. Positive nitrogen balance is achieved only when the wound is closed.

Other factors that contribute to changes of nutritional status are

The occurrence of infection.

Surgical procedures, such as skin grafting.

Curling's ulcer (an acute gastric ulcer with bleeding), which possibly is the result of ischemia. Patients are given antacids to maintain gastric pH above 5. If hemorrhage occurs, vagotomy and partial gastrectomy may be necessary.

Adynamic ileus, which prevents oral feeding for a variable period. The increased catecholamine levels cause vasoconstriction in the splanchnic bed, slowing peristalsis.

Management of the Burn Patient

Early treatment of a patient with a major burn includes establishment of an airway with a tracheostomy if necessary, insertion of a urinary catheter, administration of analgesic drugs, antibiotics, and tetanus immunization, care of the wound, and fluid replacement. The type of fluids given vary with the circumstances, but several formulas are available as guidelines in estimating therapy. One formula, for example, estimates fluid and electrolytes as follows:

Volume of fluid to be administered in the first 24 hours = 4 ml Ringer's lactated solution $\times W \times$ %BSA burned   **(14-3)**

where BSA = body surface area; W = body weight in kilograms. According to this formula, a 70-kg man with a burn over 40% of his body would require 11.2 liters of fluid to replace his loss ($4 \times 70 \times 40$). The difficulties of treatment with this volume of fluid are obvious.

The goal in long-term therapy of burn patients is to accomplish healing of all the burn wounds. A variety of techniques are used, including prevention of infection and allowance for spontaneous healing of partial-thickness burns. Full-thickness burn management requires removal of the eschar and application of split-thickness skin grafts taken from an area of unburned skin elsewhere on the body. Excision of the eschar (**debridement**) and application of skin grafts may be done as early as a few hours following injury to as late as several weeks postinjury. Patients with burns of 50% of the body surface area can be expected to require many weeks for ultimate recovery, because skin graft donor sites may have to heal and serve a second time to provide sufficient skin for grafting and wound coverage.

Specific formulas for estimation of nutritional requirements in burn patients have been devised. These formulas consider the size of the burn wound, because the extent of burn wound correlates closely with the severity of the hypermetabolism. During the course of hospitalization, as burn wounds heal and the percent of body surface area unhealed decreases, the energy expenditures may be adjusted downward.

These formulas should consider the depth and area of the burn. An example of such a burn formula is the one used at the University of California, Davis, Medical Center:

Kilocalories required for 24 hours = 33 kcal $\times$ kg IBW + the sum of calculations for various burn injury depths: **(14-4)**

Superficial burns:

0.20 kcal $\times$ % BSA burned $\times$ kg IBW

Partial-thickness burns:

0.33 kcal $\times$ % BSA burned $\times$ kg IBW

Full-thickness burns:

0.45 kcal $\times$ % BSA burned $\times$ kg IBW

Using this formula, a 70-kg IBW patient with a 50% BSA burn (10% superficial, 15% partial-thickness, and 25% full-thickness burn) would be calculated to need:

33 kcal $\times$ 70 = 2,310 kcal

$$0.20 \text{ kcal} \times 10 \times 70 = 140 \text{ kcal}$$

$$0.33 \text{ kcal} \times 15 \times 70 = 346 \text{ kcal}$$

$$0.45 \text{ kcal} \times 25 \times 70 = \frac{787 \text{ kcal}}{3,583 \text{ kcal}}$$

Protein losses also are increased significantly. In addition to the loss of protein through muscle catabolism in stress, the burn patient can lose large amounts of protein through the burn wound. This loss may average 1 to 3 g or more for each percent of burn.[38,39]

Protein needs can be determined by first calculating ideal caloric intake and then establishing protein intake based on a kilocalorie-to-nitrogen ratio of 150 : 1. One gram of nitrogen equals 6.25 g of protein. Assuming 150 kcal per gram of nitrogen, our 70-kg patient then would receive the following:

$$3,583/150 = 23.9 \text{ g nitrogen per 24 hours}$$

and

$$23.9 \times 6.25 = 150 \text{ g protein per 24 hours}$$

Remember that any formula provides an estimate only. Patient progress must be monitored carefully.

The burned patient represents a challenge to the nutritional care specialist. The patient's energy and protein needs are considerable, and great encouragement is needed to increase food intake owing to the patient's discomfort and depression. The patient is not fed until the postinjury ileus resolves, usually in 36 to 48 hours. In addition, the many surgical procedures require that the patient fast in preparation for anesthesia. The missed meals can represent a substantial loss. Despite these problems, most burn patients are able to eat considerable amounts of food in a high-protein, high-calorie diet with frequent feedings and between-meal supplements. Attention must be paid to the patient's preferences to make the food as appealing as possible.

A patient with burns over more than 40% of his or her body seldom eats enough to meet the increased needs. Tube feeding may be used to supplement oral intake. The location of the tube depends on the location of the burn. A nasogastric tube cannot be used for a patient with burns about the head and neck. Patients who are eating reasonably well may receive tube feedings during sleep, whereas those who are eating poorly or not at all may be fed continuously.

Supplementation of nutrient intake by intravenous infusion may be employed in burn patients, but in some burn centers it is avoided if possible. The primary reasons for this policy are the danger of infection and the limitation of access sites in patients burned over a large area. Nutritional intake is a higher priority, however, so that if enteral feeding is unsuccessful, parenteral feeding is used.

References

1. Ferrendelli, J.A. Cerebral utilization of non-glucose substrates and their effect in hypoglycemia. In F. Plum, Ed., *Brain Dysfunction in Metabolic Disorders*. New York: Raven Press, 1974.
2. Cahill, G.F., Jr., Herrera, M.G., Morgan, A.P., et al. Hormone-fuel interrelationships during fasting. *J. Clin. Invest.* 45:1751, 1966.
3. Levine, R., and Haft, D.E. Carbohydrate homeostasis. *N. Engl. J. Med.* 282:175, 1970.
4. Owen, O.E., Felig, P., Morgan, A.P., et al. Liver and kidney metabolism in prolonged starvation. *J. Clin. Invest.* 48:574, 1969.
5. Saudek, C.D., and Felig, P. The metabolic events of starvation. *Am. J. Med.* 60:117, 1976.
6. Felig, P., Owen, O.E., Wahren, J., and Cahill, G.F., Jr. Amino acid metabolism during prolonged starvation. *J. Clin. Invest.* 48:548, 1969.
7. Mallette, L.E., Exton, J. H., and Park, C.R. Effects of glucagon on amino acid transport and utilization of the perfused rat liver. *J. Biol. Chem.* 244:5724, 1969.
8. Pitts, R. F. Renal production and excretion of ammonia. *Am. J. Med.* 36:720, 1964.
9. Whipple, G. H. *The Dynamic Equilibrium of Body Proteins.* Springfield, Ill.: Charles C Thomas, 1956.
10. Filkins, J. P. Lysosomes and hepatic regres-

sion during fasting. *Am. J. Physiol.* 219:923, 1970.

11. Shils, M.E., and Randall, H.T. Diet and nutrition in the care of the surgical patient. In R. S. Goodhart and M.E. Shils, Eds., *Modern Nutrition in Health and Disease,* 6th ed. Philadelphia: Lea & Febiger, 1980.

12. Cuthbertson, D.P. The disturbance of metabolism produced by bony and non-bony injury, with notes on certain abnormal conditions of bone. *Biochem. J.* 24:1244, 1930.

13. Cahill, G.F., Jr., Felig, P., and Marliss, E.B. Some physiological principles of parenteral nutrition. In C.L. Fox, Jr., and G. G. Nahas, Eds., *Body Fluid Replacement in the Surgical Patient,* part IV. New York: Grune and Stratton, 1970.

14. Wilmore, D.W., Long, J.M., Skreen, R.A., et al. Catecholamines. Mediator of the hypermetabolic response of thermal injury. *Ann. Surg.* 180:653, 1974.

15. Dinarelli, C.A. Interleukin-1. *Rev. Infect. Dis.* 6:51, 1984.

16. Wannemacher, R.W., Jr. Protein metabolism (applied biochemistry). In H. Ghadimi, Ed., *Total Parenteral Nutrition.* New York: John Wiley and Sons, 1975.

17. Powanda, M.C. Changes in body balance of nitrogen and other key nutrients. Description and underlying mechanisms. *Am. J. Clin. Nutr.* 30:1254, 1977.

18. Egdahl, R.J. Pituitary-adrenal response following trauma to the isolated leg. *Surgery* 46:9, 1959.

19. Iverson, J. Adrenergic receptors and the secretion of glucagon and insulin from the isolated perfused canine pancreas. *J. Clin. Invest.* 52:1202, 1973.

20. Hume, D.M. The neuro-endocrine response to injury. Present status of the problem. *Ann. Surg.* 138:548, 1953.

21. Moore, F.D., Steenburg, R.W., Ball, M.R., et al. Studies in surgical endocrinology. I. The urinary excretion of 17-hydroxycorticoids and associated metabolic changes, in cases of soft tissue trauma of varying severity and in bone trauma. *Ann. Surg.* 141:145, 1955.

22. Ross, H., Johnston, I.D.A., Welborn, T.A., and Wright, A.D. Effect of abdominal operation on glucose tolerance and serum levels of insulin, growth hormone and hydrocortisone. *Lancet* 2:563, 1966.

23. Clark, E. Effect of cortisone upon protein synthesis. *J. Biol. Chem.* 200:69, 1953.

24. Perley, M., and Kipnis, D.M. Effects of glucocorticoids on plasma insulin. *N. Engl. J. Med.* 274:1237, 1966.

25. Marco, J., Calle, C., Roman, D., et al. Hyper-glucagonemia induced by glucocorticoid treatment in man. *N. Engl. J. Med.* 288:128, 1973.

26. Killey, J.M. Energy requirements of the surgical patient. In W.F. Ballinger, J.A. Collins, J.A. Drucker, et al., Eds., *Manual of Surgical Nutrition.* Philadelphia: W.B. Saunders, 1973.

27. Dudrick, S.J., Jensen, T.G., and Rowlands, B.J. Nutritional support. Assessment and indications. In M. Dietel, Ed., *Nutrition in Clinical Surgery.* Baltimore: Williams and Wilkins, 1980.

28. Kinney, J.M. Energy requirements for parenteral nutrition. In J.E. Fischer, Ed., *Total Parenteral Nutrition.* Boston: Little, Brown, 1976.

29. Winsey, K., Simon, R.J., Levenson, S.M., et al. Effect of supplemental vitamin A on colon anastomatic healing in rats given preoperative irradiation. *Am. J. Surg.* 153:153, 1987.

30. Smith, F.R., and Goodman, D.S. Vitamin A transport in human vitamin A toxicity. *N. Engl. J. Med.* 294:805, 1976.

31. Moore, F.D. Homeostasis. Bodily changes in trauma and surgery. In D.C. Sabiston, Ed., *Davis-Christopher Textbook of Surgery,* 11th ed. Philadelphia: W.B. Saunders, 1977.

32. Wan, J.M.–F., Haw, M.F., and Blackburn, G.L. Nutrition, immune function, and inflammation: an overview. *Proc. Nutr. Soc.* 48:315, 1989.

33. Kluger, M.J. Body temperature changes during inflammation: Their mediation and nutritional significance. *Proc. Nutr. Soc.* 48:337, 1989.

34. Guyton, A.C. *Textbook of Medical Physiology,* 5th ed. Philadelphia: W.B. Saunders, 1976.

35. Aulick, L.H., Wilmore, D.W., Mason, A.D., Jr., and Pruitt, B.A., Jr. Influence of the burn wound on peripheral circulation in thermally injured patients. *Am. J. Physiol.* 233H:520, 1977.

36. Harrison, H.N., Moncrief, J.A., Duckett, J.W., Jr., and Mason, A.D., Jr. The relationship between energy metabolism and water loss from vaporization in severely burned patients. *Surgery* 56:203, 1964.

37. Wilmore, D.W. Nutrition and metabolism following thermal injury. *Clin. Plast. Surg.* 1:603,1974.

38. Nylen, B., and Wallenius, G. The protein loss via exudation from burns and granulating wound surfaces. *Acta Chir. Scand.* 122:97, 1961.

39. Soroff, H.S., Pearson, E., and Artz, C.P. An estimation of the nitrogen requirements for equilibrium in burned patients. *Surg. Gynecol. Obstet.* 112:159, 1961.

Bibliography

Berk, J.L., Sampliner, J.E., Artz, J.S., and Vinocur, B., Eds. *Handbook of Critical Care.* Boston: Little, Brown, 1976.

Cerra, F.B. Hypermetabolism, organ failure, and metabolic support. *Surgery* 101:1, 1987.

Deitel, M., Ed. *Nutrition in Clinical Surgery.* Baltimore: Williams and Wilkins, 1980.

Fischer, J.E., Ed. *Total Parenteral Nutrition.* Boston: Little, Brown, 1976.

Grant, J.P. *Handbook of Total Parenteral Nutrition.* Philadelphia: W.B. Saunders, 1980.

Wilson, J.L., Ed. *Handbook of Surgery,* 5th ed. Los Altos, Calif.: Lange Medical, 1973.

Sources of Current Information

Annals of Surgery
JPEN, Journal of Parenteral and Enteral Nutrition
Nutrition Support Services
Surgery

15. Nutrition and Cancer

I. Reproduction of the Normal Cell
II. Classification of Neoplasms
III. Natural History of Neoplastic Growth
IV. Pathogenesis of Cancer
V. Etiology of Cancer
  A. Nutrition and diet
  B. Hormone-nutrient interactions
  C. Stress
  D. Radiation
  E. Inflammation and infections
VI. Host Effects on Carcinogenesis
VII. Metabolic and Nutritional Alterations in Malignancy
  A. Systemic effects
    1. Decreased food intake
    2. Altered metabolism and competition for nutrients
    3. Interrelationships of nutritional status and systemic effects of cancer
  B. Effects on specific organ systems
  C. Nutritional consequences of cancer therapy
    1. Surgery
    2. Radiation therapy
    3. Chemotherapy
    4. Immunotherapy
VIII. Cause of Death from Cancer
IX. Nutritional Management of the Cancer Patient
  A. Nutritional assessment
  B. Nutritional care
X. Special Considerations in Leukemia
XI. Case Study

Cancer is the second most common cause of death in adults and children in the United States, preceded only by cardiovascular disease in adults and accidents in children. The medical specialty that is concerned with cancer is **oncology**.

A **neoplasm** or **tumor** is a relatively autonomous growth of tissue. It occurs only in multicellular organisms where its growth is uncontrolled by the mechanisms that govern normal growth. The growth may be by cell division or by synthesis of macromolecules and apparently is unrelated to the demands of the host.

REPRODUCTION OF THE NORMAL CELL

To understand the nature of neoplastic growth, we need to review normal cell division. The reproductive cycle in the cell is represented in Figure 15.1.

Mitosis (the M phase), or cell division, is divided into four steps known as **prophase**, **metaphase**, **anaphase**, and **telophase**. **Interphase** (the period between cell divisions) is divided into (1) the **first growth period** (G_1), in which the cell size increases after the previous division; (2) **synthesis** (S), in which chromosomes reproduce; and (3) the **second growth period** (G_2), in which cells rearrange for division.

This cycle applies only to continuously dividing (**labile**) cells such as those in the crypts of Lieberkühn in the intestines (see Chapter 1). A second group of cells are the **permanent** cells, which lose their ability to divide once they reach a certain stage in their development. Neurons are among these. There is also a third group, the **stable** cells, that enter a quiescent stage, the G_0 phase (see Figure 15-1), in which they do not divide but remain capable of doing so if stimulated. In the liver, for example, cells will divide after partial hepatectomy. Some of the reasons that have been given for prolonged resting phases include cell crowding, contact inhibition, undernutrition, hypoxia, and effects of accumulation of metabolites or other substances.

Neoplasms can arise only in cells that have the ability to proliferate—that is, labile and

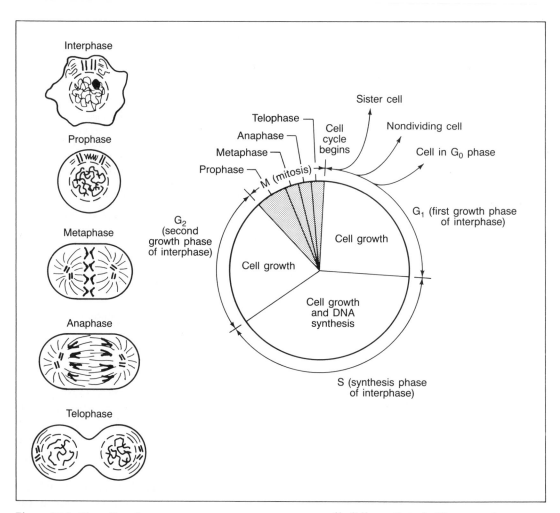

Figure 15-1. The cell cycle.

stable cells. Cancer cells apparently have the same components of the cell cycle but do not respond similarly to the control mechanisms. Undernutrition, for example, interferes with growth in a child, but a cancer continues to grow in an undernourished host.

CLASSIFICATION OF NEOPLASMS

Neoplastic diseases are believed to be a group of disorders rather than one disease and have been classified according to their behavior. **Benign tumors** are circumscribed, encapsulated growths of cells that usually

are well differentiated. They tend to grow slowly but may cause obstruction or atrophy of adjacent tissue as a result of pressure. They may be fatal when they occur at some sites, such as in the brain. They also sometimes become malignant. **Malignant tumors (or cancers)** often contain less-well-differentiated cells. They usually grow more rapidly and tend to invade surrounding tissue. In addition, malignant tumor cells may be released and be carried by the blood or lymph to distant sites where secondary tumors, known as **metastases**, appear.

Neoplasms also are named for the tissue from which they arise (Table 15-1). Some examples of benign tumors classified according to the tissue from which they arise are **fibroma** (from fibrous tissue), **chondroma** (from cartilage), and **adenoma** (from

Table 15-1. Examples of Neoplasms According to the Histogenetic Classification

Tissues of Origin	Benign	Malignant
Epithelial neoplasms		
Epidermis	Epidermal papilloma	Epidermal carcinoma
Stomach	Gastric polyp	Gastric carcinoma
Biliary tree	Cholangioma	Cholangiocarcinoma
Adrenal cortex	Adrenocortical adenoma	Adrenocortical carcinoma
Connective tissue neoplasms		
Fibrous tissue	Fibroma	Fibrosarcoma
Cartilage	Chondroma	Chondrosarcoma
Bone	Osteoma	Osteogenic sarcoma
Fat	Lipoma	Liposarcoma
Smooth muscle	Leiomyoma	Leiomyosarcoma
Skeletal muscle	Rhabdomyoma	Rhabdomyosarcoma
Blood or lymph vessel		Angiosarcoma
Neoplasms of the hemopoietic and immune systems		
Lymphoid tissue	Brill-Symmers disease	Lymphosarcoma (lymphoma)
		Lymphatic leukemia
		Reticulum cell sarcoma
		Hodgkin's disease
Thymus	Thymoma	Thymoma
Granulocytes		Myelocytic leukemia
Erythrocytes	Polycythemia vera	Erythroleukemia
Plasma cells		Multiple myeloma
Neoplasms of the nervous system		
Glia	Astrocytoma	Glioblastoma multiforme
	Oligodendroglioma	
Meninges	Meningioma	Meningeal sarcoma
Neurons	Ganglioneuroma	Neuroblastoma
Adrenal medulla	Pheochromocytoma	Pheochromocytoma
Brain, retina, pituitary, pineal		Glioma
Neoplasms of multiple histogenetic cellular origin		
Breast	Fibroadenoma	Cystosarcoma phylloides
Kidney		Wilms' tumor
Ovary, testis, etc.	Dermoid cyst (benign teratoma)	Malignant teratoma
Lung		Oat cell carcinoma or small cell carcinoma
Mesothelium		Mesothelioma
Miscellaneous neoplasms		
Melanocytes	Nevus	Melanoma
Placenta	Hydatidiform mole	Choriocarcinoma
Ovary	Granulosa cell tumor	Granulosa cell tumor
	Cystadenoma	Cystadenocarcinoma
Testis		Seminoma

Adapted with permission from Pitot, H.C., *Fundamentals of Oncology*, 3rd ed. New York: Marcel Dekker, 1986, p. 30. Also taken from Maillet, J.O., The cancer patient. In C.E. Lang, Ed., *Nutritional Support in Critical Care.* Rockville, Md.: Aspen, 1987.

glandular tissue). Tumors may be classified according to the histologic type (for example, **cystic** or **follicular**). They sometimes are named after their discoverer. Two of the best known of these are **Hodgkin's disease** in the lymph tissue and **Wilms' tumor** in the kidney, both malignant processes.

Another classification system refers to the embryonic origin. Malignant tissues from ec-

toderm and endoderm are called **carcinomas**, and those from mesoderm are **sarcomas**. If malignant cells appear very primitive and resemble embryonic tissue, the tumor is called a **blastoma**, as in **neuroblastoma**. Those tumors derived from two cell layers are **carcinosarcomas**, and those from all three cell layers are **teratomas**. Sometimes terms are combined to be more specific about a tumor's source: examples are **adeno-carcinoma**, **chondrosarcoma**, and **liposar-coma**. Obviously, the suffix **-oma** indicates a tumor. An exception to this is the **granu-loma**, a nonneoplastic growth that occurs in response to inflammation. **Leukemia** refers to malignant growth of white blood cells.

Cancers also are graded or "staged," using one of several available systems. One of the most commonly used is the **TNM system** (for "tumor, nodes, metastases"). It provides a description of the cancer according to the size of the primary tumor, the involvement of adjacent lymph nodes, and the number of metastases. The system varies somewhat with the identity of the primary tumor, but in general T_1 is a small, relatively circumscribed tumor, whereas T_4 indicates invasion of neighboring structures. Similarly, N_0 desig-nates no regional lymph node involvement. The other extreme of the scale, N_4, indicates involvement of multiple regional lymph nodes. Finally, M_0 indicates that no distant metastases are known, and M_1 designates their presence. Thus, $T_1N_0M_0$ indicates a small primary tumor with no regional lymph node involvement or known metastases, whereas $T_4N_4M_1$ indicates a large primary tumor, extensive lymph node involvement, and evidence of metastases.

NATURAL HISTORY OF NEOPLASTIC GROWTH

A sequence of change in the morphology of some cells has been observed in the genesis of cancer:

1. **Metaplasia** is replacement of one cell type with another. For example, in cases of irritation or inflammation of a mucosal sur-face, the underlying cells may differentiate into squamous cells instead of columnar cells. Frequently, this is a precancerous change. It may precede the development of a tumor by years.

2. **Dysplasia** or **anaplasia**, an alteration in adult cells with changes in their size, shape, or arrangement also is precancerous. It, too,

can precede tumor development by months or years.

3. **Hyperplasia** is an increase in the num-ber of cells. It occurs normally in fetal growth, wound healing, callus formation, and in the bone marrow, crypt cells of the intestine, and the basal layer of the skin. Ab-normal hyperplasia usually occurs in neo-plastic disease but is not required. Instead, the tissue may synthesize excess quantities of macromolecules.

4. **Neoplasia** — uncontrolled, progressive multiplication of cells — constitutes the fully developed disease.

Each primary tumor progresses indepen-dently, even in the same animal. In addition, characteristics of a particular tumor, such as growth rate, invasiveness, metastatic tend-ency, responsiveness to hormones, morphol-ogy, and **karyotype** (the arrangement of chromosomes) change independently.

When a tumor changes from benign to malignant or becomes more malignant, there is a change in morphology and activity. It is believed that, rather than a change in all cells, a few cells grow and metabolize faster and thus become predominant.

The mechanisms by which a tumor in-vades surrounding tissue is unknown. Fac-tors involved may include proteolysis, de-creased pH, differences in osmotic pressure, and others. Metastases tend to follow the routes of blood and lymph. Those carried in the blood usually are found first in the small capillaries at new sites.

PATHOGENESIS OF CANCER

Cancer cells are derived from normal cells. A current theory proposes that **carcinogenesis** (the process of cancer production) occurs in two stages, **initiation** and **promotion**. The initiation phase consists of a **mutation** (a transmissible alteration in a gene) in the cell, which then becomes neoplastic. Presum-ably, the mutation occurs in genes that regu-late cell production. Such a mutation could account for the irreversible nature of the neoplastic change, the tendency for the tumor cells to reproduce, and the great variety of tumors. However, a neoplastic cell can remain dormant for years. The dormant cell may later be activated in the promotion phase. Promoters are agents that alter gene expression, but the exact nature of promotion is not understood clearly.

Both initiators and promotors are believed to be environmental factors in almost all cases. If this is so, then the majority of cancers are preventable. The initiation phase of carcinogenesis is theorized to be irreversible, but the action of promoters is time-dependent and dose-dependent. The theory further states that if an environmental promoter is present in very low dose or is applied for only a short period, its effects may subside. An initiator or promotor that is widespread in the environment, present in larger quantities, and difficult to avoid would be a particular hazard. Some agents are thought to be both initiators and promoters and are called **complete carcinogens**.

ETIOLOGY OF CANCER

A wide variety of agents are thought to be initiators or promoters in carcinogenesis, including chemicals, microorganisms, and radiation. Although a large number of chemicals are known to be carcinogenic, they have no common structure or mode of action. Most carcinogenic agents contained in food are chemical agents.

Nutrition and Diet

Dietary and nutritional factors are thought to influence the incidence of cancer in animals, but their effects in humans are understood less clearly. Food items may provide a source of carcinogens or potentially carcinogenic substances. Some are naturally occurring, and others occur as the result of processing. Mutagens that are the result of processing include products of bacterial, fungal, or chemical action, products of cooking, additives, and contaminants such as pesticide residues, agricultural contaminants, and products of fuel combustion. Carcinogenic contaminants and additives that may be used in processing are assumed to be avoidable if they can be identified and eliminated from use. Mutagens from foods are believed to include **alkaloids** or **flavonoids** in edible plants and **aflatoxin B_1**, produced by *Aspergillus flavus*, a contaminant mold that may grow in grains and peanuts stored in warm, humid environments. Aflatoxin is a **hepatocarcinogen** (causes liver cancer) but is not a common problem in the United States. **Polycyclic hydrocarbons**, produced in cooking methods that result in charred or browned protein foods, also can be carcinogenic. Lastly, **nitrosamines** are **gastrocarcinogenic** (causing stomach cancer). These are formed from amines present in some foods plus nitrites added to some fish or meat as a preservative. Nitrites can also be produced by reduction of nitrates in vegetables.

Foods may also affect the occurrence of cancer by influencing the formation of carcinogens. Some nutritive factors are reported to be carcinogenic, and others, anticarcinogenic. Vitamin C inhibits the conversion of nitrates to nitrosamines, and thus is anticarcinogenic in nitrite-containing foods.[1] Derivatives of vitamin A, antioxidant food additives such as butylated hydroxytoluene (BHT), ethoxyquin, or coumarin, and some materials in the cabbage family (*Brassica*) are thought to be anticarcinogenic. However, the modes of action of these dietary factors are unknown. It has been suggested that they may alter the intestinal flora (fiber, meat), the mixed function oxidase system, other enzyme systems (meat, fat, indoles in vegetables, trace elements, and antioxidants), the endocrine or immune systems (fats, total energy), the availability of substrates for neoplastic growth, or the rate of activation of the carcinogen.

Caloric restriction in animals has been associated with a low incidence of most neoplasms,[2] although the incidence of hepatic tumors is increased. Mitosis during caloric restriction may be inhibited by energy deficit or hormonal changes. The effect of diminished energy intake in humans is unknown.

High-fat diets have been associated with intestinal cancer in both sexes and breast cancer in females in some studies, but other studies were negative.[3] In addition, there are still insufficient data to distinguish the effects of animal versus vegetable fats, saturated versus unsaturated fats, cis- versus trans-fatty acids, or the cholesterol content. It has also been suggested that the effect of fat intake is mediated by energy intake. It is obvious that more research is needed on the relationship between fat and malignancy. Some foods may modify the effects of carcinogens by affecting concentration in the bowel (fiber), exerting an effect on transport (fiber, alcohol), or inhibiting promotion (vitamin A, carotene). Increased intake of animal fat or protein has been associated with increased incidence of malignancies of the colon.[2,4-5] Increases in colon cancer have also been associated with low dietary fiber.[6-7] It is hypothesized that high-fiber foods pass through the gut quickly, allowing less time for the intestinal flora to produce carcinogens or for carcinogens to act on intestinal cells. Alternatively, colon cancer may arise following potentiation of carcinogens by increased amounts of bile acids, production of which is stimulated by dietary fat. Fiber may be anticarcinogenic by binding fecal bile acids.

Other relationships between diet and cancer have been reported. Pickled vegetables, potatoes, salted fish, and abrasive food grains have been associated with an increase in gastric cancers.[8] Alcohol appears to act as a promoter, associated with cancer of the liver, mouth, larynx, and esophagus, particularly in smokers.[9,10]

Risk factors in humans cannot be extrapolated from effects in animals. In general, dietary factors are believed to be promoters, not initiators. The observed relationships between diet and cancer do not identify the specific carcinogen involved, and mechanisms are unknown; however, the National Research Council has suggested the following guidelines as likely to reduce cancer risk:[11]

1. Decrease fat intake to 30% of kilocalories.
2. Increase intake of fruits, vegetables, and whole grains.
3. Minimize intake of cured, pickled, and smoked foods.
4. Minimize contamination of foods with carcinogens.
5. If alcoholic beverages are consumed, intake should be moderate.

Hormone-Nutrient Interactions

There is some evidence that hormones are involved in carcinogenesis and that nutrition may influence their action. Among the most common cancers are those of tissues whose growth is hormone-regulated—the breast, uterus, and prostate. It is not believed, however, that hormones are primary carcinogens. Instead, they might have an effect on the cells that render them susceptible to the primary agent.[12] The relationship of nutritional factors to hormone action are unclear, but it is known that obesity alters the metabolism of estrogen, a hormone associated with cancers of the vagina, uterus, breast, and liver.[13] Fat intake has also been associated with endometrial cancer.[14] Obese postmenopausal women convert a larger portion of androstenedione from the adrenal cortex to estrone than do thin women, and higher estrone levels indicate increased risk of endometrial cancer.[15] Increased dietary fat and increased kilocalorie intake have been associated with breast cancer,[16-18] and dietary fat, with prostate cancer.[19]

Stress

There may be a relationship between the incidence of cancer and stress. Possible mechanisms are stress damage to the thymus or other parts of the immune system or a hormonal effect involving the hypothalamus, pituitary gland, and adrenal cortex.

Radiation

Radiation may be carcinogenic under appropriate circumstances. It can cause chromosomal damage with abnormal repair. Sources of ionizing radiation in the environment include X-rays, radioactive materials used in diagnostic tests or in the work place, and exposure to atomic wastes. Ultraviolet light from sunlight is a nonionizing radiation which has been reported to be associated with an increased incidence of skin cancer. It is not known whether microwaves are carcinogenic. The predominant current opinion states that radiation is an initiator.

Inflammation and Infections

Chronic inflammation, some infectious agents (such as parasitic worms), and a number of **oncogenic** (tumor-causing) **viruses** also are carcinogenic. An oncogenic virus is a mass of chromosomes with six genes or less plus a protein coat. It adds to a cell new genetic material which may express itself as a malignancy. Oncogenic viruses have been identified in animals, but their importance in human cancer is unknown. One controversial theory states that chemical carcinogens act by activating an oncogenic virus.

HOST EFFECTS ON CARCINOGENESIS

In children, the cause of cancer may involve a genetic predisposition plus environmental influences in utero or during the neonatal period. The incidence of cancer increases with age, with a particular increase in later middle age and in old age. It is not known whether this occurs as a consequence of longer exposure to factors in the environment or is inherent in the aging process. Sex, too, is known to have an influence, since the type of cancer varies in men and women, even when genital system cancers are not included.

METABOLIC AND NUTRITIONAL ALTERATIONS IN MALIGNANCY

A malignancy can affect the patient's nutritional status in three ways. First, it may have a general systemic effect. Second, depending on its location, it may have local effects on specific organs. Finally, cancer therapy often affects nutritional status.

Systemic Effects

As malignancy progresses, cancer cells tend to become less differentiated. This does not mean, however, that the "dedifferentiated" cell is equivalent to the cells in the developing embryo. One of the important differences is that embryonic development is controlled very precisely, whereas malignancies do not respond to these controls. Cancer cells do tend to become less like their tissue of origin. As growth proceeds, different types of neoplasms become more alike, with many similarities in their metabolism. Thus we can describe some metabolic alterations that are seen commonly in patients with neoplastic disease, regardless of the specific tissue involved.

The major symptom complex common to many, but not all, neoplasms is **cachexia**,[20,27] characterized by anorexia, tissue wasting, weakness, impaired organ function, apathy, water and electrolyte imbalance, and decreased resistance to infection.[20] The patient becomes so emaciated that he or she appears to die of starvation. It has been estimated that the immediate cause of death in 20% to 40% of cancer patients is starvation. The severity of cachexia is not related entirely to the size of the neoplasm. Cachexia is common and severe, for example, in gastrointestinal neoplasms, but not in breast cancer. The etiology of the tissue catabolism in other patients is not entirely clear. Possibilities for consideration are, of course, decreased energy intake, increased energy expenditure, or both.

Decreased Food Intake

In some patients there are mechanical barriers to food intake, such as those that can occur in cancers of the head and neck, esophagus, gastrointestinal tract, or adjacent organs. Even when mechanical barriers are not present, the nutrient intake in most cancer patients tends to decrease, primarily as a result of anorexia.[22,23] In fact, anorexia sometimes appears so early that it is the warning symptom that leads to the original diagnosis.

The mechanisms for the production of anorexia are not understood entirely. Abnormalities of taste and smell occur in proportion to the tumor burden and probably contribute to decreased food intake.[24-27] The abnormalities frequently encountered include an increased threshold for sweet taste and a lower threshold for bitter taste. Thus patients must have sweeter food to taste the sweetness. The increased bitter taste causes early difficulty in eating protein foods, especially beef and pork. Fish and poultry are tolerated for a longer period, but patients also may find these unacceptable as the disease progresses.

The mechanisms producing these abnormalities still are under investigation. DeWys[22] has suggested that cell renewal in the taste buds is decreased in the patient with cancer, causing the elevated sweet threshold. Zinc deficiency may cause an increase in some thresholds, whereas altered plasma amino acids may lower the threshold for bitter taste.[25]

Patients also complain of a feeling of fullness, sometimes after only a few bites of food. Decreased gastrointestinal secretion, slowing digestion, and atrophy of the epithelium or muscle wall of the intestinal tract may be the mechanisms altering the sense of fullness.

Certain metabolites also are thought to affect food intake. Serotonin, synthesized from tryptophan, is known to stimulate the satiety center in the brain of rats and reduce their food intake. Krause et al.[28] postulate a mechanism that begins with a meal containing carbohydrate to induce plasma insulin release. As a result of this release, peripheral amino acid use is increased, and tryptophan in the blood is transferred across the blood-brain barrier, thereby competing with the branched-chain amino acids (BCAAs). When plasma BCAAs are reduced, tryptophan can be transported into the brain faster; this increases the brain serotonin level, presumably causing a reduction in food intake by stimulating the satiety center. This theory raises the possibility that food intake may be stimulated by administering BCAAs, but whether this is effective in humans is not yet known.

Other metabolites that possibly affect food intake are lactate, fatty acids, peptides, oligonucleotides, and imbalances of amino acids. These may act through an effect on neuroendocrine cells or on the hypothalamus and other central nervous system cells.[29] Hormonal changes, particularly insulin resistance, and psychological factors stimulating catecholamine release also may reduce appetite (see Chapter 12).

Altered Metabolism and Competition for Nutrients

Decreased food intake does not account entirely for the weight changes seen in cancer patients. Weight loss often is disproportionate to the decrease in nutrient intake and may occur even in the presence of seemingly normal intake. It may occur at a rate in excess of that seen in starvation,[30] suggesting either alterations in host metabolism, decreasing efficiency of nutrient use, or competition for nutrients between host and tumor in which the tumor prevails.

It is obvious that neoplastic tissue competes successfully for nutrients, since tumor growth commonly is seen even though the host is wasting.[31] The tumor has a high energy requirement to maintain sodium and potassium gradients,[32] to support protein synthesis, and to supply substrates for growth. This increased fuel consumption results in an increased resting metabolism in the tumor-host complex.[33,34] Increases of 35% to 74% have been reported,[35] but in many patients, the total tumor burden is not thought to be large enough to produce the observed amount of wasting.

Although reduced food intake and use of nutrients by the tumor contribute, a major cause of the observed inanition is alteration in the patient's metabolism (see Table 15-2). There is a systemic insulin resistance, with decreased peripheral glucose uptake and de-

Table 15-2. Metabolic Alterations in Malignancy

Metabolic Factor	Direction of Change
General effects	
Body weight	↓
Food intake	↓
Total energy expenditure	↑
Resting metabolic energy expenditure[a]	↑[b]
Thyroid hormone	↓
Glucose	
Lactate production	↑
Insulin sensitivity	↓
Glucose uptake	↑
Glucose utilization	↓
Gluconeogenesis	↑
Serum glucose	↓
Protein	
Whole body turnover	↑
Alanine and glutamine release from muscles	↑
3-methylhistidine excretion	↑
Hepatic protein synthesis	↑
Activity of cathepsin D, glucuronidase	↑
Activity of hexokinase, phosphofructokinase, lactate dehydrogenase, cytochrome *c* oxidase	↓
Urinary cortisone	↑
Lipids	
Serum triglyceride	↑
Lipolysis	↑
Serum glycerol	↑
Glycerol turnover	↑
Total body fat	↓
Deficiency or inactivation of bile salts and pancreatic lipase	↑
Other	
Extracellular fluid	↑
Total body sodium	↑
Intracellular fluid	↓
Total body potassium	↓

[a] Varies with tumor site.
[b] In advanced disease.

creased formation of glycogen. At the same time, gluconeogenesis is increased.[35–38]

Many tumors have a particularly accelerated rate of glycolysis and lactic acid production. The glycolysis of each mole of glucose provides 2 moles of ATP, but this ATP is used by the tumor. The lactic acid produced is returned to the liver and kidney, resynthesized to glucose through the Cori cycle, and recycled back to the tumor. This process requires the expenditure of 6 moles of ATP. There is increased or poorly regulated gluconeogenesis from the lactate in the liver, which may be the consequence of insulin resistance. The resulting increase in Cori cycle activity in cancer patients causes a total loss of 8 moles of ATP to the host.[38,39] Although it has been argued that this is not a significant loss,[41] it may also be argued that the oxidative metabolism of 1 mole of lactate could have yielded 30 moles of ATP that now are lost.

The patient's lipid metabolism may be abnormal as well. Serum free fatty acids are elevated, but clearance of lipid is increased.[42] At the same time, fat stores are depleted. The mechanism involved in the apparent increased mobilization of lipids is unknown, but some evidence suggests that tumors produce lipolytic substances.[43] The severe fat wasting may also be the result of the high energy expenditure. A shift from carbohydrate to lipid metabolism may be the result of alterations in insulin, glucagon, and catecholamine balance.[44]

Cancer patients have altered protein metabolism. There is decreased protein synthesis in the host, with a decrease in serum albumin[45] and many enzymes.[36] It is not known to what extent these are the consequence of substrate deficiency and decreased synthesis or of increased catabolism. The mechanisms for nitrogen conservation in starvation (see Chapter 14) appear to remain intact. Nevertheless, nitrogen loss in the host persists, even when amino acid and energy intakes are adequate.

Tumors have a great capacity to concentrate amino acids and have been called a "nitrogen trap."[34,46] The nitrogen turnover in a tumor is very low—that is, the amino acids are not recycled. Protein synthesis is increased, whereas amino acid breakdown, gluconeogenesis and urea cycle enzymes are depressed. Purine, pyrimidine, and DNA synthesis are increased, but degradation of purines and pyrimidine is diminished. As a consequence of these factors, patients with rapidly growing cancers may be in a positive nitrogen balance although they are losing weight.

Tumors not only retain exogenous proteins efficiently, but animal experiments have shown that they grow at the expense of the host. They draw some protein from host body tissue, largely from skeletal muscle.[47] The tumor thus contains even more nitrogen than was retained for positive nitrogen balance. Some tumors appear to have a special capacity to degrade selected essential amino acids, thereby producing an amino acid imbalance. Another possibility is that rapidly growing tumors have a heightened ability to concentrate amino acids or take up circulating proteins, such as albumin. Some protein is lost as the result of increased gluconeogenesis in the host.[48] The extent to which a tumor is a metabolic drain contributing to tissue wasting in the human host is unclear.

Additional effects on protein metabolism are indicated by the finding of novel proteins and peptides in the urine of patients with advanced cancer.[49,50] The activities of a number of enzymes of host tissue also are affected by the presence of neoplasms, even at distant sites. The mechanism by which this occurs is unknown.[50]

Fluid often is retained as neoplastic disease advances, masking tissue loss, although clinical edema may not be evident. In these circumstances, body weight is not useful as an indicator of nutritional status.

Overall, the metabolism of the cancer patient differs from that seen in starvation. Whereas healthy subjects show a decrease in basal metabolic rate (BMR) and decreased oxidative metabolism in starvation, BMR in cancer patients often increases, and oxygen consumption persists in the postabsorptive period. The patient thus may be hypermetabolic, and in many respects, metabolism resembles the acute phase response described in Chapter 6. Research is currently investigating the use of blockers of cytokine action in the treatment of cachexia.

Interrelationships of Nutritional Status and Systemic Effects of Cancer

It has been shown that improved nutrition accelerates tumor growth, but these experiments were done in animals with large transplanted tumors. In human patients with spontaneous tumors, no acceleration of tumor growth was observed following improved nutrition.[51] It has been suggested that inducing a deficiency of essential amino acids might impede tumor growth; however, this approach has not been successful because it also deprives normal tissue. Although the host and tumor are interdependent in some ways, they also are independent of each other to a great extent. A neoplasm, once it reaches a certain size, continues to grow regardless of the nutritional needs of the host. Therefore, nutritional deprivation harms the host more than it harms the tumor.

Effects on Specific Organ Systems

In addition to their systemic effects, cancers may have other effects that depend on their specific location, particularly in the digestive system.[52,53] Gastric carcinomas can cause losses of blood and other protein-rich fluids. Nausea and vomiting develop as a result of obstruction in the gastrointestinal tract and can lead to fluid, electrolyte, and protein losses. Intestinal damage can result in malabsorption with steatorrhea, diarrhea, lactase deficiency, and protein-losing enteropathy. Reduced intake may produce alterations in the intestinal mucosa known as **cancer enteropathy**. Pancreatic insufficiency caused by neoplastic growth can lead to impairment of nutritional status. (See Chapter 8 for nutritional care in these conditions.) Cancer of the liver may cause decreased albumin production with consequent hypoalbuminemia. Prothrombin deficiency also occurs in carcinoma of the liver, if the liver is unable to synthesize prothrombin or if decreased bile production interferes with vitamin K absorption.

Some malignancies affect nutrition by secreting one or more hormones in pharmacologic quantities. Some of these conditions, described in Chapters 7 and 8, include Zollinger-Ellison syndrome, pancreatic cholera, carcinoid syndrome, and villous adenoma. Medullary carcinoma of the thyroid secretes excess thyrocalcitonin that causes diarrhea by stimulating jejunal mucosal secretion of fluids and electrolytes. Bronchogenic and oat cell carcinomas cause fluid and electrolyte imbalances, as do carcinoma of the adrenal cortex and corticotropin-secreting tumors in the lung.

Neoplasms of the central nervous system have less specific effects. The mental symptoms may interfere with food intake in a variety of ways.

Cancers of the head and neck areas can result in severe malnutrition. There is a high rate of alcoholism and of tobacco use in these patients; thus many patients are at risk of malnutrition prior to the illness. In addition, food intake is adversely affected by fear, anxiety, and depression. In addition to the effects of site-specific malignancies themselves, the effects of the treatments also may vary with the site.

Nutritional Consequences of Cancer Therapy

The nutritional deprivation seen in the cancer patient is aggravated by therapy. The major approaches to anticancer therapy, all of which have nutritional significance, are **surgery**, **radiation**, and **chemotherapy**. Bone marrow transplant is a specialized surgical procedure discussed later in this chapter in connection with leukemia. **Immunotherapy** is a promising approach that will probably be used more frequently in the future with further development of techniques. Often, combinations of these methods are used.

Surgery

The systemic effects and nutritional implications of surgery in cancer patients are the same as those seen in other surgical patients (see Chapter 14). Patients sometimes develop complications among which are fistulas, obstruction, and sepsis. Other complications can arise, depending on the specific site of the resections.

In head and neck cancers, the surgery of the tongue, oral cavity, pharynx, and larynx can result in extensive alterations in the normal physiology. Loss of the cranial nerves involved in eating, for example, often affects chewing and swallowing (see Chapter 9).

There are 12 pairs of cranial nerves that branch from the brain and mainly innervate structures of the head and neck. Some are sensory nerves, some are motor nerves, and others are mixed sensory and motor nerves. A knowledge of their functions makes it possible to anticipate nutritional problems.

There are five pairs of these cranial nerves that are related to food intake:

1. The **trigeminal** (fifth cranial) **nerves** are a pair of mixed nerves which innervate muscles involved in chewing. Their three branches are the ophthalmic, maxillary (upper-jaw), and mandibular (lower-jaw) nerves. Paralysis of a trigeminal nerve causes the jaw to deviate toward the side of the lesion, resulting in difficulty in chewing.

2. The **facial** (seventh cranial) **nerves** innervate various structures of the face, head, and neck, including the skin and mucous membranes of the cheeks, gums, some of the teeth, and the anterior two-thirds of the tongue. Injury can cause paralysis resulting in facial droop and difficulty in lip closure on the affected side. It is then difficult to keep food in the mouth, with particular difficulty with liquids.

3. The **glossopharyngeal** (ninth cranial) **nerves** innervate the posterior third of the tongue and the pharynx. Damage causes absence of a gag reflex on the side of the lesion and loss of taste on the tongue in the affected areas.

4. The **hypoglossal** (twelfth cranial) **nerves** innervate the tongue. Damage causes the tongue to deviate toward the affected side. The patient has difficulty in pushing food to the side for chewing. A resection of the floor of the mouth or base of the tongue leaves the residual part of the tongue immobile. Removal of an acoustic neuroma can also destroy this nerve, resulting in a facial droop.

5. The **vagus** (tenth cranial) **nerves** are the only ones that extend beyond the head. Their motor fibers extend to the lungs, stomach, gallbladder, small intestine, and part of the large intestine. Some of the fibers control the release of gastric gland secretions and pancreatic secretions. The vagus supplies sensory fibers to the tongue, pharynx, and larynx, and motor fibers to the pharynx, larynx, and esophagus. Parasympathetic fibers and visceral fibers innervate thoracic and abdominal viscera. Damage to this nerve has many consequences. Lesions in the head and neck region can result in dysphagia and loss of a sense of taste. A **radical neck dissection** can involve loss of the ninth, tenth, and twelfth cranial nerves.

Another type of surgery that results in severe problems related to food intake is the **supraglottic laryngectomy** for cancers of the epiglottis and surrounding structures. The epiglottis is the structure that overhangs the larynx and prevents food and drink from entering the larynx and trachea. When it is removed, vocal cords are the only barrier to aspiration, and serious swallowing problems result.

In the esophagectomy patient, problems may arise with an increased tendency to regurgitation and with early satiety and ensuing reduction in food intake. An accompanying vagotomy can lead to gastric stasis, hypochlorhydria, steatorrhea, and diarrhea.

Nutritional care of patients with chewing and swallowing problems are described in Chapters 7 and 19.

Complications arising from the resections of the gastrointestinal tract are listed in Table 15-3. Some patients require total pancreatectomy, resulting in malabsorption and diabetes mellitus. Nutritional care in these conditions is described in Chapters 7, 8, and 11.

Radiation Therapy

Radiation disrupts the chemical bonds required in DNA reproduction and synthesis,[54] thus interfering with reproduction of dividing cells. It may be used in the form of X-rays or radioactive isotopes to produce **gamma rays** or atomic particles such as **electrons** (from **beta emitters**), **neutrons**, or **protons**. Radiation is used to treat tumors that respond to doses that are tolerable to normal tissues or those that can be targeted so that overlying tissue is not damaged. A typical protocol for treatment provides for radiation therapy five days a week for four to six weeks. The treatment has its greatest effect on cells in the G_2 or M phase of the cell cycle.

Table 15-3. Complications of Gastrointestinal Surgery in the Cancer Patient

Gastrectomy (total or high subtotal)
Dumping syndrome
Malabsorption
Hypoglycemia
Early satiety
Achlorhydria and intrinsic factor deficiency
Jejunectomy
Malabsorption of many nutrients
Ileal resection
Bile salt losses, fat malabsorption, steatorrhea, diarrhea
Fat-soluble vitamin malabsorption
Vitamin B_{12} malabsorption
Calcium and magnesium depletion
Hyperoxaluria and renal stones
Massive bowel resections
Malabsorption
Malnutrition
Dehydration
Metabolic acidosis
Blind loop syndromes
Ostomies: salt and water imbalance

Radiation is used for approximately half of all cancer patients, often in combination with chemotherapy or surgery or both. It can cause severe anorexia, nausea, and sometimes vomiting. Tumors of the central nervous system may cause increased intracranial pressure leading to nausea and vomiting. Cerebral edema may follow radiation therapy and exacerbate the symptoms.

When radiation is applied to the head or neck, an altered and unpleasant or decreased sense of taste and alterations in the sense of smell may be caused by damage to the taste buds and olfactory receptors.[55,56] In rats, radiation has been shown to cause the release of histamine, producing very strong learned taste aversions. These taste aversions can be blocked by administering an antihistamine to the animal prior to exposure to radiation. Levy et al.[57] proposed that the histamine production after radiation exposure represented the physiologic basis of radiation-induced taste aversions and noted that *humans treated with antihistamines immediately after radiation exposure showed a marked decline in incidence of nausea, vomiting, irritability, anorexia, and similar symptoms of radiation sickness.* Normal taste acuity returns one to two months after treatment.

Mucositis (inflammation of the mucosal lining of the mouth and pharynx) can cause severe pain and reduce food intake. Xerostomia can result from damage to the salivary glands, and that saliva which is produced may be particularly thick and viscous. The development of rampant caries, periodontal disease, and **osteoradionecrosis** (necrosis of the bone due to excessive radiation) often occurs. Some patients show **trismus**, a motor disturbance of the trigeminal nerve with difficulty in opening the jaw.

Radiation to the organs of the thorax, the esophagus, lungs, or mediastinum may cause esophagitis, dysphagia, nausea, stenosis, or fistulas. Fibrosis of the esophagus may result in esophageal strictures.

Low-dose radiation to the stomach is tolerated reasonably well and usually creates few problems, but high-dose radiation may cause ulceration with bleeding, vomiting, and weight loss.[58] The usual ulcer regimens are not effective, and partial gastrectomy may be necessary.[59] Radiation damage to the pancreas is rare.

Irradiation of the abdomen or pelvic region for gastrointestinal or genitourinary tract cancer tends to denude the mucosal lining and cause a loss of intestinal villi. There are changes in the vascular bed with intimal thickening, interfering with blood circulation. In addition to nausea, vomiting, and anorexia, steatorrhea and diarrhea are common. These conditions develop as early as two weeks after treatment begins. Other effects include strictures and obstructions, inflammation, ulcers, fistulas, thromboses, and acute or chronic enteritis or colitis. Whereas some of these effects are temporary, long-term injury also can result from radiation therapy. Ulceration, for example, can develop a month to a year after radiation is terminated.

Chemotherapy

Chemotherapy involves the use of antineoplastic drugs that disrupt the reproductive cycle of cells. These drugs affect cancer cells and normal cells in the same way. The mechanisms by which they do so include:

Interference with the synthesis of purines and pyrimidines for incorporation into the nucleic acids necessary for DNA synthesis.

Disruption of normal DNA structure or replication of RNA.

Prevention of normal cell division by causing spindle damage.

Creation of a hormone imbalance.

Making essential amino acids unavailable.

There are six general categories of antineoplastic agents, and each group functions a different way to interfere with cell reproduction. **Alkaloids**, obtained from plants, disorganize the chromosome spindles during mitosis. Examples of alkaloids are vincristine and vinblastine. **Alkylating agents**, such as nitrogen mustard and cyclophosphamide, bind with DNA, RNA, or some enzymes to interfere with cell division. **Antimetabolites** block reactions necessary to produce precursors to DNA synthesis. This category includes methotrexate, which reduces available folic acid, and 6-mercaptopurine, 5-fluorouracil, and cytosine arabinoside. Some **antibiotics**, such as mithramycin, bleomycin, and doxorubicin, interfere with the structure or function of DNA or other cell structures. The **antineoplastic enzyme** asparaginase interferes with the reactions necessary to produce a required amino acid. **Hormones** may affect the cell or otherwise interfere with cell metabolism by altering the hormone balance. These include estrogens, androgens, progestins, and prednisone. The sites of action of the major classes of chemotherapeutic drugs are shown in Figure 15-2.

The **log kill hypothesis** is used as a basis for chemotherapy. It assumes that a single dose kills a constant proportion, up to 99.9%, of the tumor cells. Repeated doses further reduce the number of neoplastic cells. A single surviving malignant cell, however, can multiply and eventually kill the host. Therefore, the maximum tolerable dose is used in a series that is repeated. In addition, it is common to use several antineoplastic agents for their synergistic effects. Since the treatment consists of repeated doses over a period of time, nutritional effects must be expected to occur for weeks or months.

The effectiveness of chemotherapeutic agents depends on their greater toxicity to cancer cells than to normal cells. Unfortunately, all existing agents are toxic to normal cells to some extent, and their use is limited by this toxicity. When an antineoplastic drugs interferes with cell reproduction, it follows that it affects cells that are reproducing (kinetic resistance), including reproducing normal cells. A major toxic effect is on the bone marrow, manifested by **leukopenia** (deficiency of leukocytes), **thrombocytopenia** (insufficient platelets), and **anemia**. These conditions limit the dose that may be used. When the red blood cell and platelet count is reduced severely, the therapy must be stopped until the cells multiply sufficiently. This is one of the major reasons that antineoplastic drugs are used in repeated series with intermittent recovery periods.

In addition to kinetic resistance, **genetic resistance** to anticancer drugs results from spontaneous mutations. These may result in resistance to a number of drugs. Drugs are often given in combination so that a single mutation will be unlikely to provide resistance to all.

If response to a single treatment is poor, combinations of chemotherapy with radiation or surgery, radiation with surgery, or all three methods may be used.

Antineoplastic drugs extensively affect the nutritional status of the patient. They have many effects on the gastrointestinal tract, since the lining is constantly renewed (Table 15-4). Toxic effects include oral ulcerations, glossitis, stomatitis, and mucositis, all of which cause severe pain during food intake. Nausea, vomiting, and diarrhea are seen commonly with all classes of antineoplastic drugs. They are believed to be the result of drug effects on a **chemoreceptor trigger zone** in the brain.[60,61] Anorexia with decreased food intake also usually occurs. Aversions to specific foods eaten before a treatment that caused gastrointestinal discomfort have been shown to develop. Some drugs cause altered taste sensations. Diarrhea occurs as a side effect of some drugs, and constipation is a side effect of others. Other nutrition-related side effects of chemotherapy include hepatotoxicity, electrolyte imbalances, and nephrotoxicity. Products of destroyed cancer cells and some of the drugs, especially alkylating agents, may be nephrotoxic.

In studies of the effects of nutritional status on a patient's response to antineoplastic drugs, it has been shown that cachectic patients respond poorly to chemotherapy, largely because they are unable to tolerate the usual doses. Hence, nutritional status both influences and is influenced by these agents.

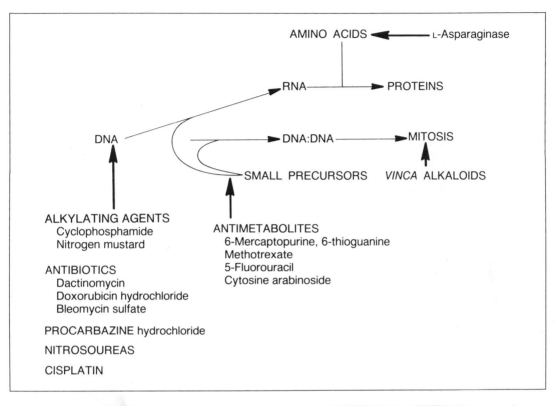

AMINO ACIDS ◄━━━━━ L-Asparaginase

RNA━━━━━► PROTEINS

DNA ━━► DNA:DNA ━━━━━► MITOSIS

SMALL PRECURSORS   *VINCA* ALKALOIDS

ALKYLATING AGENTS
  Cyclophosphamide
  Nitrogen mustard

ANTIBIOTICS
  Dactinomycin
  Doxorubicin hydrochloride
  Bleomycin sulfate

PROCARBAZINE hydrochloride

NITROSOUREAS

CISPLATIN

ANTIMETABOLITES
  6-Mercaptopurine, 6-thioguanine
  Methotrexate
  5-Fluorouracil
  Cytosine arabinoside

Figure 15-2. Site of action of chemotherapeutic agents. (Reprinted with permission from Cline, M.J., and Haskell, C.M. Cancer Chemotherapy, 3rd ed. Philadelphia: W.B. Saunders, 1980, p. 3.)

Immunotherapy

Treatment with interleukin-2 may result in fluid retention, azotemia, and hypotension. Nausea, anorexia, diarrhea, and dysgeusia with resultant weight loss may be the consequences of treatment with interferon.

CAUSE OF DEATH FROM CANCER

Although the effects of cancer are poorly understood, certain factors are recognized as being among the immediate causes of death in cancer victims. Cachexia is the primary cause of death in many, or perhaps most, cancer patients. Other causes are (1) organ failure, especially renal; (2) obstruction of a vital organ, airway, or blood vessel; (3) increased intracranial pressure; (4) circulatory

system effects such as hemorrhage, stroke, or embolus; and (5) infection.[62]

NUTRITIONAL MANAGEMENT OF THE CANCER PATIENT

In considering nutritional management in cancer, the question must be asked whether nutritional support to prevent or treat malnutrition makes any difference in the final analysis. Weight loss has been shown to be a good predictor of complications and death,[63,64] but it is unclear whether nutritional intervention increases the survival time or rate of cure. It *is* clear that nutritional support is well tolerated by the cancer patient and that it is possible to improve nutritional status in these patients.

Nutritional intervention can cause nitrogen retention and weight gain, although complete reversal of the tendency toward cachexia is rare. It decreases susceptibility to infection by supporting defense mecha-

Table 15-4. Nutrition-Related Side Effects of Chemotherapy

Chemotherapeutic Agent	Nausea	Vomiting	Anorexia	Diarrhea	Inflammation or Ulceration of Oral Cavity	Other
Amethopterin (methotrexate, MTX, Folex, Mexate)	X	X–	X	X	X	Gastrointestinal ulcerations; abdominal pain; hepatotoxicity; cirrhosis
Aminoglutethamide (Cytadren)	X	X				
L-Asparaginase (Elspar, L-ASP, crasnitin, amidohytrolate, colaspase)	X	X	X			Hepatic dysfunction; nephrotoxicity; pancreatitis; allergy
Bleomycin sulfate (Blenoxane, Bleo, BLM-2)	X	X–	X		X	Weight loss
Busulfan (Myleran, BUS, BSF, BAN)	X	X				
Carboplatin (Paraplatin)	X	X				Bone marrow depression
Carmustine (BCNU, BiCNU)	XX	XX	X			Hepatotoxicity; nephrotoxicity
Chlorambucil (Leukeran, CHL, CB-1348)	X	X–				
Cisplatin (cis-platinum, Platinol, DDP, CPDD, PDD, CPD, CACP)	XX	XX	X			Nephrotoxicity
Cyclophosphamide (Cytoxan, Endoxan, CYT, CTX, CYC, CPM)	XX	XX	X			Abdominal or epigastric pain
Cytosine arabinoside (cytarabine, ARA-C, Cytosar-U, CA)	XX	XX	X		X	Gastrointestinal ulcerations
Dacarbazine (DTIC-Dome, DIC, imidazole carboxamide)	XX	X				
Dactinomycin (ACT-D, ACT, DSCT, ACD, Cosmegen)	XX	XX	X	X	XX	Abdominal pain; dysphagia
Daunomycin hydrochloride (daunorubicin, DNR, rubidomycin, Cerubidine)	XX	X	X		X	Abdominal or epigastric pain
Doxorubicin hydrochloride (Adriamycin)	XX	X	X	XX	XX	
Estramustine (Emcyt)	X			XX		
Etoposide (VP 16, Ve-Pe-sid)	XX	XX	X	XX	XX	
Floxuridine (FUDR)	X	X			X	
5-Fluorouracil (5-FU, fluorouracil, Adrucil, Efudex, Fluoroplex)	X–	X–	X	XX	XX	
Flutamide (Eulexin)	X	X		X		Galactorrhea
Hydroxyurea (Hydrea, HYD, HU, HUR)	X	X–		X	X	Constipation
Ifosfamide (Ifex)	X	X				Bone marrow depression; lethargy; confusion, hallucinations
Interferon-Alfa 2A recombinant (Roferon)	X		X	X		Dysgeusia; weight loss
Interferon-Alfa 2B recombinant (Intron)	X		X	X		Dysgeusia; weight loss
Leuprolide acetate (Lupron)	X		X	X		Hepatotoxicity

Drug				Other effects
Lomustine (CCNU, CeeNU)	XX	XX		Constipation
Mechlorethamine hydrochloride (nitrogen mustard, Mustargen)	XX	XX	X	Jaundice; dysgeusia
Megestrol acetate (Megace)	X	X		Fluid retention
Melphalan (phenylalanine mustard, Alkeran, L-PAM)	X	X	X	Hypersensitivity
6-Mercaptopurine (Purinethol, 6-MP)	X–	X–	X	Hepatotoxicity
Mithramycin (Mithracin)	XX	XX	X	Hepatotoxicity
Mitomycin (Mutamycin, Mitomycin C, MTC, Ametysin)	X	X		
Mitotane (Lysodren)	X	X–	X	
Mitoxantrone (Novantrone)	X–	X–	X	
Plicamycin (Mithracin)	X	X	X	Hepatotoxicity; mental depression; fever; hypocalcemia; hypokalemia; hypophosphatemia
Procarbazine hydrochloride (methyl hydrazine, Matulane, Ibenzmethyzin, MIH)	XX	XX	X	Gastrointestinal ulceration; xerostomia; constipation
Streptozocin (Streptozotocin Zanosar)	XX	XX	X	Nephrotoxicity; may lead to diabetes
Tamoxifen (Nolvadex)	X	X		
6-Thioguanine (6-TG, Tabloid)	X–	X–		
Triethylenethiophosphoramide (Thiotepa, THIO, TESPA, TSPA)	X	X		
Vinblastine sulfate (Velban, VBL, Velbe, Vinkaleukoblastine sulfate)	X		X	Constipation; ileus
Vincristine sulfate (VCR, Oncovin, LCR, leucocristine sulfate)	X	X	X	Constipation; ileus; abdominal pain
Hormones				
Adrenocorticoids (prednisone, Medrol)	X			Weight gain; increased appetite; fluid retention; gastrointestinal ulcers
Androgens (Halotestin, Teslac, Depo-Testosterone, Deca-Durabolin, Methosarb)	X	X		Fluid retention; liver damage
Antiestrogens (tamoxifen citrate)	X	X		(Transient)
Estrogens (diethylstilbestrol [DES], TACE, Stilphostrol)	X	X		Fluid retention

Information compiled from Visconti, J.A., *Drug-Food Interactions*. Columbus, Ohio: Ross Laboratories, 1979; Wollard, J.J., Ed., *Nutritional Management of the Cancer Patient*. New York: Raven Press, 1979; Carter, S.K., Nutritional problems associated with cancer chemotherapy. In G.R. Newell and N.M. Ellison, Eds., *Nutrition and Cancer: Etiology and Treatment*. New York: Raven Press, 1981; See Lasley, K., and Ingnoffo, R.J., *Manual of Oncology Therapeutics*. St. Louis: C.V. Mosby, 1981; Donaldson, S.S., and Lenon, R.A., Alterations of nutritional status. Impact of chemotherapy and radiation therapy. *Cancer* 43:2036, 1979; U.S. Public Health Service, National Cancer Institute, *Chemotherapy and You*. NIH Publication No. 81 1136. Washington, D.C.: U.S. Department of Health and Human Services, 1980.

X = present; X– = minimal; XX = extreme.

587

nisms, including delayed hypersensitivity, cough, mucous protection of membranes, and ciliary function.[65,66] It also helps to minimize the symptoms of high-dose radiation and chemotherapy, making it possible to complete the course of treatment.[67-70] The advantages of nutritional intervention allow patients to be more active and have an increased feeling of well-being. As a consequence, nutritional support now is commonly used as an adjunct to other forms of therapy to at least improve the quality of life.

The role of the nutritional care specialist in the oncology unit is less firmly established than is the need for nutritional support. A recent survey indicated that, although physicians regarded the nutritional care specialist as the primary source of nutrition information, they believed that they, not the nutrition specialist, should relay the information to the patient.[71] Nutritional care specialists must be more assertive in demonstrating their value in direct care of the cancer patient.

Nutritional Assessment

All cancer patients should be considered to be at risk of malnutrition. Nutritional assessment should be done early and repeated at intervals. Patients who will be treated by surgery, radiation, or chemotherapy should receive preventive support. Oncology patients receiving the house diet should also be a concern of the nutritional care specialist. Although there may be no indication for restriction of specific foods, increased need and reduced intake may place them at risk. Risk factors to be considered during assessment include alcoholism, poor dentition, decreased appetite, nausea, vomiting, and diarrhea. In determining risk, plans for treatment must be taken into account even if the patient is not currently malnourished.

Initial screening should consider preillness and present body weight, and weights should be followed serially. In addition to weight, serum albumin and electrolytes are influenced by the presence of edema and ascites, hepatic or renal metastases, and drug

toxicities. These factors must be considered in interpretation. Serial weight changes and daily input and output are useful.

Patients who are found to be at risk in the initial screening should be assessed in depth, including a detailed diet history. Plans for nutritional support should be integrated with dental and mouth care. The financial resources of and facilities to provide an adequate diet for ambulatory patients must also be considered. Since the location of the tumor, size of the tumor burden, and nature of the treatment vary, the assessment and plans for support must be carefully individualized.

Nutritional Care

The procedures for nutritional care of each patient must be individualized, since needs vary from one patient to another, with the progress of the disease, and with the treatments used. It is not possible to establish a protocol that can be applied to all patients. Nevertheless, some guidelines can be provided.

Nutritional support is necessary to correct poor nutritional status, but in the cancer patient, it may also be used in anticipation of future problems. The nutritional care specialist should make every effort to prevent the weight loss typical of many cancer patients. In patients who are already depleted, repletion, although more difficult, should be attempted. For maintenance, 2,000 kcal/day often are sufficient, whereas repletion may require 3,000 to 4,000 kcal/day. Protein for maintenance may be 90 to 100 g/day, whereas repletion may require 100 to 200 g/day.

Oral feeding is recommended if the gastrointestinal tract is functional and oral intake is tolerated. Particular approaches to anorexia include the use of small frequent meals with foods of high nutrient density and individualization of the diet for the patient's needs and preferences. The patient needs personal attention and encouragement to eat.

Bloating sometimes occurs and may be

Table 15-5. Guidelines for Oral Feeding of Cancer Patients

Symptom	Suggested Remedies
Anorexia	Use small, frequent feedings
	Use high-calorie, calorically dense feedings
	Use favorite foods; avoid disliked foods
	Use small amount of alcohol before meals
	Provide foods with aroma, spiced to current likes
	Substitute eggs, cheese, yogurt for meats
	Use high-calorie liquids to take medications
	Eat most when appetite is best (usually mornings)
Taste and smell changes	Suck on sour candy or peppermint
	Avoid offensive odors
	Rinse mouth before eating
	Maintain good oral hygiene
	Serve food at room temperature
	Vary texture and temperature of a meal
	Use meals with odor and eye appeal
	Avoid greasy or fried foods
	Use acid foods to stimulate taste
Dry mouth	Use moist foods
	Use soft, pureed foods
	Add sauces, gravy, juices
	Serve liquid with meals
	Avoid spicy or acidic foods
	Use sugarless gum or candy to stimulate saliva
	Use artificial saliva
Sore mouth	Avoid acidic, salty, spicy, hard, or crunchy foods
	Use cold, soft, or pureed foods
	Use a straw when possible
Dysphagia	Use soft, moist foods
	Use butter, gravy, cream sauces, custards, puddings, milk shakes
	Avoid salty, spicy, coarse, or rough foods, and bread
	Cut foods in small pieces
	Have small, frequent meals
	Eat while seated upright
	Use high-calorie liquids and supplements
	Adjust food temperature to tolerance
	Avoid alcoholic beverages, smoking
Nausea and vomiting	Take antiemetic medications before usual meal times
	Eat dry, bland foods before meals
	Avoid offensive odors
	Eat bland, easy-to-digest meals several hours before treatment
	Eat and drink slowly in larger amounts when possible
	Try clear, cool beverages
	Avoid favorite foods at this time
	Choose foods that can be prepared quickly
	Use cool foods
	Keep head slightly elevated
	Perform frequent oral care
Early satiety	Use small, frequent, high-calorie foods
	Limit liquids taken with foods
	Limit fatty, greasy foods
Fatigue	Eat most nutritious meal in A.M.
	Use foods not requiring much chewing
	Plan rest periods
Mucositis and stomatitis	Use analgesic medications before meals
	Avoid very hot or cold, acidic, crisp, grainy, or raw foods
	Avoid milk and milk products
Bloating	Avoid greasy, fried foods
	Use small, frequent meals
	Eat slowly
	Avoid carbonated beverages, milk, gas-producing foods
Indigestion	Take antacid 1–2 hours before meals (a.c.) and h.s.
	Use small, frequent meals
	Avoid foods that are spicy or greasy
	Avoid milk and milk products
	Avoid alcoholic beverages and smoking

related to the type of food eaten. The elimination of fried, greasy, and fatty foods, gas-producing foods, milk, carbonated beverages, and chewing gum may help.

The patient's diet may be modified to reduce pain, avoiding very hot or cold foods, decreasing spices and acidic foods, and providing foods with a smooth texture. A rinse containing an analgesic sometimes is given before meals to reduce pain. Patients with a dry mouth may be given more liquid foods and provided with an artificial saliva. A summary of suggestions is given in Table 15-5. A decrease in sucrose in the diet is helpful in caries prevention.

If intake of usual foods cannot be maintained at a level sufficient to maintain normal weight, supplemental feedings often are used. Tube feedings may be used to replace or supplement oral intakes if these are inadequate. Nasogastric tubes, however, may be refused by the patient with oral inflammations. Some patients have gastrostomies or jejunostomies for feeding. If they cannot be fed in this way, intravenous hyperalimentation is used.

Low-fiber, high-fiber, or soft diets and other modifications may be indicated by a patient's specific symptoms. In patients receiving antineoplastic drugs, an increase in fluid intake is indicated to improve renal excretion of drugs and the products of cell breakdown, reduce the incidence of urinary infection, and replace losses from gastrointestinal disturbances, fevers, and infections. This may present particular problems in the patients with chewing and swallowing difficulties.

Head and neck cancer patients may need extensive rehabilitation. Sometimes, changes in food consistency are helpful. Others must use special devices such as feeding syringes, which place food at the back of the tongue. An occupational therapist is useful in providing exercises to restore muscle function. Some patients need nasogastric feeding tubes or a feeding gastrostomy. If the swallowing problem is sufficiently severe and recalcitrant to treatment, a laryngectomy may be performed with a physical separation of the alimentary and respiratory tracts, but this procedure results in loss of voice.

Care of renal disease may also be needed. Patients receiving cyclophosphamide should receive 2 to 3 liters of fluid per day. Nutritional management of the patient who has radiation injury to the liver is the same as for hepatitis (see Chapter 13). The terminal cancer patient should be provided with any food requested and any food that makes the patient comfortable.

Because nutritional care of the cancer patient must be individualized to meet the needs of the specific patient, the nutritional care specialist must have extensive skill and knowledge. Many of the techniques used in the management of gastrointestinal symptoms were described in Chapters 7 and 8, and so they are not repeated here. Procedures for nutritional support with supplements, tube feedings, and total parenteral nutrition are included in Chapter 5.

SPECIAL CONSIDERATIONS IN LEUKEMIA

Leukemia is a general term referring to a neoplastic disease of the blood-forming tissues. It is characterized by a significant increase in the numbers of leukocytes or their precursors. The lymphocytes do not function normally. In addition, the lymphoid tissues of the spleen, liver, lymph nodes, and bone marrow enlarge and proliferate. Clinical manifestations include anemia, thrombocytopenia, tendency to bleed from the nose, gums, joints, and other internal organs, increased incidence of skin infections and pneumonia, heat intolerance, and exhaustion.

Leukemias are broadly classified as **acute** or **chronic** according to the duration and rate of progression of the disease and also according to the type of cell involved. **Lymphocytic leukemia** involves lymphocytes and lymphoblasts, whereas **myelocytic leu-**

kemia involves the granulocytes. The features of these main types of leukemia are described in Table 15-6.

The cause of leukemia is unknown, but contributing factors are largely those seen in other forms of cancer: ionizing radiation, exposure to carcinogenic chemicals, or viruses. Heredity is thought to be a factor, since there is an increased incidence in the siblings of leukemia patients. An increased incidence accompanying Down syndrome (see Chapter 19) also indicates genetic involvement.

The aim of leukemia treatment usually is remission. **Remission** is defined as relief of symptoms, normal red blood cell and platelet counts, and the maintenance of competent white blood cells with as low a count of leukemic cells as possible.

Since the leukemic cells are spread throughout the body, surgical excision is not possible. The most frequently used form of treatment is chemotherapy. The drugs used have the various side effects previously described (see Table 15-4), and nutritional care must be based on the side effects. In addition, since many leukemia patients are children, the diet must be adjusted for age.

If chemotherapy is ineffective, bone marrow transplantation (BMT) may be used. It consists of several steps. First, the patient has four to eight days of an antileukemic and immunosuppressive "conditioning" regimen consisting of total body irradiation (TBI) and chemotherapy with cyclophosphamide, sometimes combined with busulfan, to kill leukemia cells. These treatments will eradicate the tumor cells, decrease the risk of graft rejection, and create physical space for the graft. Nutrition-related complications of TBI include infections, nausea, vomiting, diarrhea, and mucositis.[72] Side effects of the chemotherapy can include nausea, vomiting, stomatitis, and hepatic abnormalities.[73] These acute effects subside in 24–48 hours. More delayed effects include changes in taste and salivation, esophagitis, and damage to the intestinal epithelium. Liver failure may be mild to fatal, and infections are common.

Transplants may be in one of three categories:

1. *Autologous:* The patient's own stem cells in 250–750 ml of marrow are removed prior to chemotherapy, frozen, and reinfused intravenously after chemotherapy is finished. The malignancy must be one which does not affect the bone marrow, such as in solid tumors and lymphomas. This treatment allows doses in treatment during "conditioning" that would otherwise be lethal from aplasia of the marrow.
2. *Allogeneic:* The diseased bone marrow is destroyed and replaced intravenously with marrow cells "harvested" by aspiration from marrow at the iliac crest of a normal donor. This treatment is used in leukemia, and also in severe combined immune deficiency disease, aplastic anemia, and Wiskott-Aldrich syndrome.
3. *Syngeic:* Replacement cells are from an identical twin.

Nutritional needs of the BMT patients are estimated to be as follows:

Energy	BEE × 1.7 in the posttransplant period[74,75] or 45–65 kcal/kg/day in children less than ten years and 30–50 kcal/kg/day for adolescents and adults[76]
Protein	1.5 g/kg ideal body weight for adults
	1.8 g/kg ideal body weight at age 15–18 years
	2.0 g/kg ideal body weight at age 11–14
	2.4 g/kg ideal body weight at age 7–10
	2.5–3.0 g/kg ideal body weight at age 4–6
	3.0 g/kg ideal body weight at age 1–3

Patients generally cannot eat enough food to meet these needs in the immediate posttransplant period. Until adequate oral intake

Table 15-6. *Characteristics of the Main Types of Leukemia*

Type	Age and Sex Incidence	Onset of Symptoms	Treatment	Prognosis
Acute lymphocytic leukemia	Most commonly 3 to 4 years old; rare after age 15. Slightly increased among men	Sudden onset; symptoms rarely present more than six weeks prior to diagnosis	Very responsive to chemo-therapy	Five-year survival: 50%. Some indefinite disease-free survivors; slightly poorer prognosis in adults
Chronic lymphocytic leukemia	Most commonly 50 to 70 years old; rare before age 35; increased incidence with age. Greatly increased among men	Symptoms may not interfere with life of patient for years	Not very responsive to chemotherapy; main treat-ment is to fight infections	Variable; median survival is 7 years
Acute myelogenous leukemia	Most commonly young adults, but nearly equal frequency among all age groups. Slightly increased among men	Onset of symptoms may be abrupt, but usually a prodromal period of one to six months	Similar to acute lymphocytic leukemia, but needs increased chemotherapy (more resistant to treatment)	Untreated, median survival: 2 months. Treated, median survival: 13 months
Chronic myelogenous leukemia	Most commonly 30 to 50 years old; uncommon be-fore age 20. Slightly increased among men	Usually gradual	Chemotherapy, splenectomy (for splenic enlargement)	Median survival: 3 to 5 years, but eventually all reach blastic crisis

Reprinted with permission from Saunders, B., Nutritional management of the leukemia patient. In J.J. Woollard, Ed., *Nutritional Management of the Cancer Patient.* New York: Raven Press, 1979, p. 121.

is achieved, TPN is recommended. The recommended formula contains 70–75% of nonprotein calories from glucose and 25–30% from lipid. The TPN feeding is, of course, sterile.

In the case of an allogeneic graft, a unique complication is graft-versus-host disease (GVHD) (see Chapter 6). The transplanted cells attack the host, which the cells see as "foreign." It particularly tends to affect the skin, gastrointestinal tract, and liver. It may be acute, that is, occurring within 100 days of transplant, or chronic, occurring after 100 days.

The skin in acute GVHD develops a rash and may desquamate. Gastrointestinal symptoms include anorexia, nausea, vomiting, and watery diarrhea. There may be ileus and severe abdominal pain.[72–74,77] Liver function is depressed.[72] The condition is treated with immunosuppressants such as antithymocyte globulin, prednisone, and cyclosporin. Hypertension and severe magnesium wasting may be a consequence of the nephrotoxicity of the cyclosporin.[73,74] Chronic GVHD affects the upper gastrointestinal tract but not the small intestine.[77] It is treated with corticosteroids.

In GVHD, a diet regimen based on experience with a large number of patients has been suggested.[78] These recommendations are summarized in Table 15-7. Patients receive total parenteral nutrition through a central line, sometimes for an extended period (see Table 15-7). This support is continued while oral intake increases from liquid formulas to a low-fat, low-lactose, low-fiber, low-acid diet. The diet is liberalized as tolerated.

Most patients are receiving steroid medications that can induce osteoporosis. They should ingest 1,200 to 1,500 mg of calcium and 400 IU of vitamin D daily. High-potassium food may be needed to provide 3,000 mg/day to patients with diarrhea. Supplements may be needed in addition.

Another complication of BMT is **veno-occlusive disease** (VOD) of the liver. The treatments given in the "conditioning" phase cause fibrosis of the liver, obstructing the small veins. There is an increase in serum bilirubin, abnormal liver function tests, abdominal pain, ascites, and enlarged liver. The condition may progress to hepatic encephalopathy.[72–74]

There is no treatment for VOD other than resting the liver and supporting the patient. In nutritional support, the patient is given a sodium restricted diet, and fluid is restricted. If the patient is encephalopathic, protein is reduced as necessary, to possibly 0.5 g per kg body weight. In the TPN-fed patient, this would of course be given as amino acids.

Caloric support must also be provided. This presents some difficulties in view of the fluid restriction. Solutions for TPN must be very concentrated, and hemofiltration (see Chapter 9) may be necessary.

In addition, BMT patients are very prone to infections because they are immunosuppressed. Opportunistic bacterial infections in the early posttransplant period are often from *Pseudomonas*, *Klebsiella*, *Staphylococcus*, and *Candida*. During the acute period to 100 days, viral infections become more common. Interstitial pneumonia, resulting from cytomegalovirus, is frequent. After 100 days, in the chronic phase, varicella zoster infections occur often.

When TPN is discontinued, the immunosuppressed patient must be protected from infections carried in the food. Methods used vary widely. Some patients have simple isolation and regular diet. At the other extreme is the patient in a laminar air flow (LAF) room, given nonabsorbable antibiotics into the gut, and either a **sterile diet** or a **low-microbial diet**.

The sterile diet consists of foods sterilized by irradiation, autoclaving, canning, or prolonged baking. Trays are assembled in an LAF hood with aseptic technique. The procedure is labor-intensive and thus expensive. In addition, food quality suffers.

The low-microbial diet is less expensive, and many items are more acceptable. Only cooked foods are used, but they are those produced routinely. Raw fruits and vegeta-

Table 15-7. Sample Diet Progression in Graft-Versus-Host Disease

Approximate Days Following Onset	Intravenous Feeding[a]	Oral Feeding
0–16[b]	Kcal/day: 1.8 × BEE Protein, as crystalline amino acids: 2 g/kg IBW for adults; 2.5–3.0 g/kg IBW for children Fat emulsion: 500 ml/day for adults; 250 ml/day or a maximum of 4 g/kg IBW for children	None
17–25[b]	Continue as above	60 ml every 2 to 3 hours of iso-osmotic low-residue beverages.
26–34[b]	Continue as above	Add one solid food every 3 to 4 hours. Foods must be low in fiber, low in acid, low in fat, free of gastric irritants, and contain minimal amounts of lactose. Fat should not exceed 20 to 40 g/day. Include pectin-containing foods.
35–80[b]	As necessary to meet nutritional needs	Low fiber, low acid, no gastric irritants, minimal amounts of lactose; less than 40 g of fat per day if fat is malabsorbed.
81 or later[b]	Discontinue when nutritional needs are met by oral intake	Add foods containing fiber, lactose,[c] or acids one at a time. Add only one food per day, in order of patient's preference. If patient has no steatorrhea, liberalize fat content.

[a] BEE = basal energy expenditure; IBW = ideal body weight.
[b] Or as tolerated.
[c] Add lactase (LactAid [SugarLo Co.]) to reduce lactose concentration in dairy products.

bles are eliminated as are foods naturally containing large numbers of microorganisms, such as some cheeses, yogurt, and sweet acidophilus milk. Single-serving items are used whenever possible, and these patients are served first from any bulk containers. The relative safety of the sterile and low-microbial diets for BMT patients is not known.

Case Study: Leukemia and Chemotherapy

(Adapted from a case study provided by Mary Ellen Collins, R.D., of Brigham and Women's Hospital, Boston, Mass.)
Mrs. R. is a 32-year-old woman who was admitted with a recent diagnosis of acute myelogenous leukemia and fever. She is to be started on chemotherapy. The patient complains of vomiting, loss of appetite, mucositis, and oral lesions, but denies feeling nauseous. Her chart includes the following information:

Procedures: Multiple bone marrow aspirates
Medications
  Serax
  ARA-C
  Daunorubicin
  Trilafon
  Nembutal
  Lomotil
  Neutra-Phos
  K-Lor
  Tobramycin sulfate
  Ticarcillin disodium
  Amphotericin B
  Mycostatin
  Xylocaine 2% Viscous Solution
  Mylanta

Laboratory values
Admission:

Red blood cell count	$3.12 \times 10^6/mm^3$
Hemoglobin	9.0 g/dl
Hematocrit	27.3%
White blood cell count	$2.3 \times 10^3/mm^3$
Blood urea nitrogen	2 mg/dl

Serum cholesterol	103 mg/dl
Others	Within normal limits

Three weeks later:

Serum albumin	2.8 g/dl
Serum calcium	8.2 mg/dl
Serum phosphate	1.8 units/dl
Serum creatinine	0.4 mg/dl
Others	Unchanged

Height: 5 ft. 3 in.
Weight

Usual	47.7–50 kg
At admission	46.4 kg
At three weeks	44.3 kg

Without dentures: Secondary lesions
Social history: Married; lives with husband and 15-year-old son. Works as a hairdresser.
Food dislikes: "Thick foods," gravies, mayonnaise, fish, spicy foods.

Exercises

1. How does each laboratory value compare to normal values?
2. Give the purpose of each medication.
3. What nutrition problems would you anticipate as a result of chemotherapy?
4. Using the information given, how would you assess the patient's nutritional status?
5. What diet would you recommend?
6. What are the advantages of preventing weight loss?

References

1. Rawson, R.W. The role of nutrition in the etiology and prevention of cancer. *Nutr. Cancer* 2:17, 1980.
2. Colman, K.C. Nutrition and cancer. In J.R. Richards and J.M. Kinney, Eds., *Nutritional Aspects of Care of the Critically Ill.* Edinburgh: Churchill Livingstone, 1977.
3. Vogel, V.G., and McPherson, R.S. Dietary epidemiology of colon cancer. *Hemat./Oncol. Clin. North Am.* 3:35, 1989.
4. Carroll, K.K., and Khor, H.T. Dietary fat in relation to tumorigenesis. *Prog. Biochem. Pharmacol.* 10:308, 1970.
5. Wynder, E.L., and Reddy, B.S. Metabolic epidemiology of colorectal cancer. *Cancer* 34:801, 1974.
6. Burkitt, D.P. Epidemiology of cancer of the colon and rectum. *Cancer* 28:3, 1971.
7. Burkitt, D.P. Benign and malignant tumors of the large bowel. In D.P. Burkitt and H.C. Trowell, Eds., *Refined Carbohydrate Foods and Disease.* London: Academic, 1975.
8. Weisburger, J.H., Reddy, B., Hill, P., et al. Nutrition and cancer—on the mechanisms bearing on causes of cancer of the colon, breast, prostate, and stomach. *Bull. N.Y. Acad. Med.* 56:673, 1980.
9. Wynder, E.L., Covey, L.S., Mabucki, K., and Mushinski, M. Environmental factors in cancer of the larynx. *Cancer* 38:1591, 1976.
10. Chronic effects of alcohol. *Br. Med. J.* 2:381, 1978.
11. Committee on Diet, Nutrition and Cancer. *Diet, Nutrition and Cancer.* Washington, D.C.: National Academy of Sciences, 1982.
12. Berenblum, I. Established principles and unresolved problems in carcinogenesis. *J. Natl. Cancer Inst.* 60:723, 1978.
13. Lipsett, M.B. Interaction of drugs, hormones and nutrition in the causes of cancer. *Cancer* 43:1967, 1979.
14. Armstrong, B., and Doll, R. Environmental factors and cancer incidence and mortality incidence in different countries with special reference to dietary practices. *Int. J. Cancer* 15:617, 1975.
15. MacDonald, P.C., Edman, C.D., Hemsell, D.L., et al. Effect of obesity on conversion of plasma androstenedione to estrone in postmenopausal women with and without endometrial cancer. *Am. J. Obstet. Gynecol.* 130:448, 1978.
16. Carroll, K.K., Gammel, E.B., and Plunkett, E.R. Dietary fat and mammary cancer. *Can. Med. Assoc. J.* 98:590, 1968.
17. Drasar, B.S., and Irving, D. Environmental factors and cancer of the colon and breast. *Br. J. Cancer* 27:167, 1973.
18. Hems, G. Epidemiological characteristics of breast cancer in middle and late age. *Br. J. Cancer* 24:226, 1970.
19. Jackson, M.A., Ahluwalia, B.S., Herson, J., et al. Characterization of prostatic carcinoma among blacks: A continuation report. *Cancer Treat. Rep.* 61:167, 1977.
20. Theologides, A. Nutritional management of the patient with advanced cancer. *Postgrad. Med.* 61:97, 1977.
21. Costa, G., and Donaldson, S.S. Effects of cancer and cancer treatment on the nutrition of the host. *N. Engl. J. Med.* 300:1471, 1979.
22. DeWys, W.D. Anorexia in cancer patients. *Cancer Res.* 37:2354, 1977.

23. DeWys, W.D. Anorexia as a general effect of cancer. *Cancer* 43:2013, 1979.

24. DeWys, W.D. Taste and feeding behavior in patients with cancer. In M. Winick, Ed., *Nutrition in Cancer.* Current Concepts in Nutrition, vol. 5. New York: John Wiley and Sons, 1977.

25. DeWys, W.D., and Walters, K. Abnormalities of taste sensation in cancer patients. *Cancer* 36:1888, 1975.

26. DeWys, W.D. Changes in taste sensation and feeding behavior in cancer patients. A review. *J. Hum. Nutr.* 32:447, 1978.

27. Nielsen, S.S., Theologides, A., and Vickers, A.M. Influence of food odors on food aversions and preferences in patients with cancer. *Am. J. Clin. Nutr.* 33:2253, 1980.

28. Krause, R., James, H., Humphrey, C., et al. Cancer anorexia. A plasma amino acid–mediated phenomenon. Presented at the First European Congress on Parenteral and Enteral Nutrition, Stockholm, September 1979.

29. Theologides, A. Anorexia-producing intermediary metabolites. *Am. J. Clin. Nutr.* 29:552, 1976.

30. Douglas, H.O. Hyperalimentation in gastrointestinal cancer. *Contemp. Surg.* 13:35, 1978.

31. Munro, H.N. Tumor-host competition for nutrients in the cancer patient. *J. Am. Diet. Assoc.* 71:380, 1977.

32. Levinson, C., and Hemping, H.G. The role of ion transport in the regulation of respiration in Ehrlich mouse ascites—tumor cells. *Biochim. Biophys. Acta* 135:306.

33. Warnold, I., Lundholm, K., and Schersten, T. Energy balance and body composition in cancer patients. *Cancer Res.* 38:1801, 1978.

34. Waterhouse, C. How tumors affect host metabolism. *Ann. N.Y. Acad. Sci.* 230:86, 1974.

35. Kisner, D.L., and DeWys, W.D. Anorexia and cachexia in malignant disease. In G.R. Newell and N.M. Ellison, Eds., *Nutrition and Cancer: Etiology and Treatment.* Progress in Cancer Research and Therapy, vol. 17. New York: Raven Press, 1981.

36. Kisner, D., Hamosh, M., Blecker, M., et al. Malignant cachexia. Insulin resistance and insulin receptors. *Proc. Am. Assoc. Cancer Res.* 19:199, 1978.

37. Heber, D., Byerly, L., and Chlebowski, R. Metabolic abnormalities in the cancer patient. *Cancer* 55:225, 1985.

38. Holroyde, C.P., Gabuzda, T.G., Putnam, R.C., et al. Altered glucose metabolism in metastatic carcinoma. *Cancer Res.* 35:3710, 1975.

39. Waterhouse, C. Lactate metabolism in patients with cancer. *Cancer* 33:66, 1974.

40. Brennan, M., and Ekman, L. Metabolic consequences of nutritional support of the cancer patient. *Cancer* 54:2627, 1984.

41. Young, V.R. Energy metabolism and requirements in the cancer patient. *Cancer Res.* 37:2336, 1977.

42. Wright, C.J., Duff, J.H., McLean, A.P.H., and MacLean, L.D. Regional capillary blood flow and oxygen uptake in severe sepsis. *Surg. Gynecol. Obstet.* 132:637, 1971.

43. Liebelt, R.A., Liebelt, A.G., and Johnstone, H.M. Lipid mobilization and food intake in experimentally obese mice bearing transplanted tumors. *Proc. Soc. Exp. Biol. Med.* 138:482, 1971.

44. Stein, T.P. Cachexia, gluconeogenesis and progressive weight loss in cancer patients. *J. Theor. Biol.* 73:51, 1978.

45. Steinfield, J.L. I^{131}-albumin degradation in patients with neoplastic disease. *Cancer* 13:974, 1960.

46. Mider, G.B., Tesluk, J., and Morton, J.J. Effects of Walker Carcinoma 256 on food intake, body weight and nitrogen metabolism of growing rats. *Acta Unio Int. Contra Cancrum* 6:409, 1948.

47. Buzby, G.P., Mullen, J.L., Stein, T.P., et al. Host-tumor interaction and nutrient supply. *Cancer* 45:2940, 1980.

48. Gold, J. Cancer cachexia and gluconeogenesis. *Ann. N.Y. Acad. Sci.* 230:103, 1974.

49. Rodman, D., Del Rio, A., Akgun, S., and Frumin, F. Novel proteins and peptides in the urine of patients with advanced cancer disease. *Am. J. Med.* 46:174, 1969.

50. Theologides, A. Cancer cachexia. *Cancer* 43:2004, 1979.

51. Mullen, J.L., Buzby, G.P., Gertner, M.H., et al. Protein synthesis dynamics in human gastrointestinal malignancies. *Surgery* 87:331, 1980.

52. Lawrence, W. Effects of cancer on nutrition. Impaired organ system effects. *Cancer* 43:2020, 1979.

53. Leffall, L.D. Summary of the informal discussion of impaired organ system effects of cancer on nutrition. *Cancer Res.* 37:2379, 1977.

54. Welch, D. Nutritional consequences of carcinogenesis and radiation therapy. *J. Am. Diet. Assoc.* 78:467, 1981.

55. Conger, A.D. Loss and recovery of taste acuity in patients irradiated to the oral cavity. *Radiat. Res.* 53:338, 1973.

56. Cooper, G.P. Receptor origin of the olfactory bulb response to ionizing radiation. *Am. J. Physiol.* 215:803, 1968.

57. Levy, C.J., Carroll, M.E., Smith, J.C., and Hofer, K.G. Antihistamines block radiation-

induced taste aversions. *Science* 186:1044, 1974.

58. Roswit, B. Complications of radiation therapy. The alimentary tract. *Semin. Roentgenol.* 9:51, 1974.
59. Bowers, R.F., and Brick, I.B. Surgery in radiation injury of the stomach. *Surgery* 22:20, 1947.
60. Borison, H.L. Area postrema. Chemoreceptor trigger zone for vomiting—Is that all? *Life Sci.* 14:1807, 1974.
61. Cockel, P. Anti-emetics. *Practitioner* 206:56, 1971.
62. Warren, S. The immediate cause of death in cancer. *Am. J. Med. Sci.* 184:610, 1932.
63. Costa, G., and Donaldson, S. The nutritional effects of cancer and its therapy. *Nutr. Cancer* 2:22, 1980.
64. Buzby, G.P., Mullen, J.L., Matthews, D.C., et al. Prognostic nutritional index in gastrointestinal surgery. *Am. J. Surg.* 139:160, 1979.
65. Copeland, E. M., MacFadyen, B.V., and Dudrick, S.J. Effect of intravenous hyperalimentation on established delayed hypersensitivity in the cancer patient. *Ann. Surg.* 184:60, 1976.
66. Newhouse, M., Sanchis, J., and Bienenstock, J. Lung defense mechanisms. *N. Engl. J. Med.* 295:990, 1976.
67. Copeland, E.M., MacFadyen, B.V., MacComb, W.S., et al. Intravenous hyperalimentation in patients with head and neck cancer. *Cancer* 35:606, 1975.
68. Copeland, E.M., Suchon, E.A., MacFadyen, B.V., et al. Intravenous hyperalimentation as an adjunct to radiation therapy. *Cancer* 39:609, 1977.
69. Filler, R.M., Jaffe, N., Cassady, J.R., et al. Parenteral nutritional support in children with cancer. *Cancer* 39:2665, 1977.
70. Copeland, E.M., Daly, J.M., and Dudrick, S.J. Nutrition as an adjunct to cancer treatment in the adult. *Cancer Res.* 37:2451, 1977.
71. Cooper-Stephenson, C., and Theologides, A. Nutrition in cancer. Physicians' knowledge, opinions and educational needs. *J. Am. Diet. Assoc.* 78:472, 1981.
72. Ford, R., and Ballard, B. Acute complications after bone marrow transplantation. *Semin. Oncol. Nurs.* 4:15, 1988.
73. Rosenfield, C.S., Mangan, K.F., and Shadduck, R.K. Bone marrow transplantation. In W.C. Shoemaker, S. Ayres, A. Grenvik, P.R. Holbrook, and W.L. Thompson, Eds., *Textbook of Critical Care*, 2nd ed. Philadelphia: W.B. Saunders, 1989.
74. Lenssen, P., and Aker, S.N. *Nutritional Assessment and Management during Marrow Transplantation: A Resource Manual.* Seattle:

Fred Hutchinson Cancer Research Center, 1985.
75. Cunningham, B.A., Lenssen, P., Aker, S.N., Gitterre, K.M., Cheney, C.L., and Hutchinson, M.N. Nutritional considerations during marrow transplantation. *Nurs. Clin. North Am.* 18:585, 1983.
76. Szeluga, D.J., Stuart, R.K., Brookmeyer, R., Utermohlen, V., and Santos, G.W. Energy requirements of parenterally fed bone marrow transplant recipients. *JPEN* 9:139, 1985.
77. Leff, R.S., and Messerschmidt, G.L. Critical care aspects of autologous and allogeneic bone marrow transplantation. In W.C. Shoemaker, S. Ayres, A. Grenvik, P.R. Holbrook, and W.L. Thompson, Eds., *Textbook of Critical Care*, 2nd ed. Philadelphia: W.B. Saunders, 1989.
78. Gauvreau, J.M., Lenssen, P., Cheney, C.L., et al. Nutritional management of patients with intestinal graft-versus-host disease. *J. Am. Diet. Assoc.* 79:673, 1981.

Bibliography

Aker, S.N., and Cheney, C.L. The use of sterile and low microbial diets in ultraisolation environments. *JPEN* 7:390, 1983.

Boisaubin, E.V. Ethical issues in the nutritional support of the terminal patient. *J. Am. Diet. Assoc.* 84:529, 1984.

Buzby, G.P., Mullen, J.L., Stein, T.P., et al. Host-tumor interaction and nutrient supply. *Cancer* 45:2940, 1980.

Carson, J.A.S., and Gormican, A. Taste acuity and food attitudes of selected patients with cancer. *J. Am. Diet. Assoc.* 70:361, 1977.

Greenwald, P., Ershow, A.G., Novelli, W.D., and Benton, C.M. *Cancer, Diet, and Nutrition: A Comprehensive Sourcebook.* Chicago: Marquis, 1985.

Hegedus, S., and Pelham, M. Dietetics in a cancer hospital. *J. Am. Diet. Assoc.* 67:238, 1975.

Munro, H.N. Tumor-host competition for nutrients in the cancer patient. *J. Am. Diet Assoc.* 71:380, 1977.

Newell, G.R., and Ellison, N.M., Eds., *Nutrition and Cancer: Etiology and Treatment. Progress in Cancer Research and Therapy*, vol. 17. New York: Raven Press, 1981.

Oram-Smith, J.C., Stein, T.P., Wallace, H.W., and Mullen, J.L. Intravenous nutrition and tumor-host protein metabolism. *J. Surg. Res.* 22:499, 1977.

Pitot, H.C. *Fundamentals of Oncology*, 2nd ed. New York: Marcel Dekker, 1981.

Shamberger, R.J. *Nutrition and Cancer.* New York: Plenum Press, 1984.

Suen, J.Y., and Myers, E.N., Eds., *Cancer of the Head and Neck.* New York: Churchill Livingstone, 1981.

Theologides, A. Pathogenesis of cachexia in cancer. *Cancer* 29:484, 1972.

Theologides, A. Anorexia-producing intermediary metabolites. *Am. J. Clin. Nutr.* 29:552, 1976.

vanEys, J., Seelig, M.S., and Nichols, B.L., Jr. *Nutrition and Cancer.* New York: SP Medical and Scientific Books, 1979.

Wollard, J.J., Ed. *Nutritional Management of the Cancer Patient.* New York: Raven Press, 1979.

Sources of Current Information

British Journal of Cancer
Cancer
Cancer Research
International Journal of Cancer
Journal of the National Cancer Institute
JPEN Journal of Parenteral and Enteral Nutrition
Nutrition and Cancer
Radiation Research

16. Nutrition in Pulmonary Diseases

I. Anatomy of the Respiratory System
   A. Structure of the airways
   B. Lungs
   C. The pump

II. Physiology of the Respiratory System
   A. Respiration
      1. Mechanics of inspiration
      2. Elasticity of the lungs
      3. Airways resistance
      4. Work of breathing
   B. Ventilation
   C. Other functions

III. Diagnosis of Pulmonary Disease

IV. Effect of Malnutrition on Respiration

V. Chronic Obstructive Pulmonary Disease
   A. Etiology and pathogenesis
   B. Nutritional assessment
   C. Management of COPD

VI. Respiratory Failure
   A. Nutritional assessment
   B. Nutritional care
   C. Monitoring response to therapy

VII. Bronchopulmonary Dysplasia
   A. Pathology
   B. Prevention
   C. Nutritional assessment
   D. Nutritional care

VIII. Case Study

Nutrition is an important component in a number of pulmonary diseases in both adults and children. For an understanding of these disorders, a knowledge of the anatomy and function of the respiratory system is useful.

ANATOMY OF THE RESPIRATORY SYSTEM

The anatomy of the respiratory system includes neural tissue in the brainstem that is sensitive to oxygen and carbon dioxide and drives the whole system; the gas exchange system, which can be divided into the airways and the lung proper; and the surrounding rib cage and muscles that serve as a pump.

Structure of the Airways

The **trachea**, leading from the external source of air toward the lung, is made of horseshoe-shaped cartilage. The posterior wall is flaccid, making it possible to cough. The trachea is lined with ciliated epithelium and includes some goblet cells.

The trachea divides first into two main **bronchi**, one for each side of the chest. The left bronchus is longer and comes off at an abrupt angle, allowing space for the heart. The right bronchus comes off at an angle that is almost in a direct line with the trachea. Therefore, inhaled material goes into the right lung more readily.

The bronchi, which are not lined by capillaries, divide further into **lobar** and then **segmented bronchi**. All are composed of cartilage (see Figure 16-1). This tracheobronchial tree not only serves as a conduit for gas exchange, but also serves as a barrier for infections and toxic agents. The epithelial surface serves as a mechanical barrier. The ciliated surface moves particles up and out. The mucus traps particles for removal by the cilia or by coughing.

When these divisions no longer contain cartilage, they are **bronchioles**. From the bifurcation of the trachea to the terminal bronchioles, there may be nine to 32 divisions. Some of the final generation of the bronchioles are called **terminal**, and others are **respiratory bronchioles**. These latter have a few alveoli arising directly from their walls. Mostly they give off **alveolar ducts** that lead to rounded **alveolar sacs**. The alveolar ducts

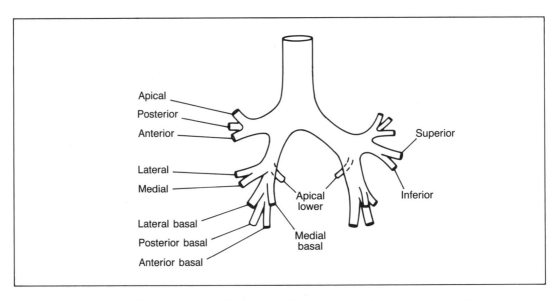

Figure 16-1. Structure and nomenclature of the bronchi.

have small outpocketings known as alveoli. These are thin-walled air sacs in a mesh of capillaries. Oxygen and carbon dioxide diffuse through the alveolar epithelium and capillary endothelium for oxygenation of the blood. There is a potential space between these two tissues, but the space is visible only in disease. The alveoli also have minute openings that make it possible for air to pass from one alveolus to those adjacent. The **pores of Kohn** provide communication between lobule parts supplied by different bronchioles, making collateral ventilation possible.

Lungs

The right lung consists of three lobes, and the left lung has two lobes. The lobes are separated by invaginations of pleural space. A bronchus goes to each lobe. The lobe is divided by fibrous septa that separate the lung into bronchopulmonary segments, each of which is supplied by a segmental bronchus. Smaller septa separate these segments into **lobules** supplied by a bronchiole. A lobule contains about four acini, each of which is supplied by a terminal bronchiole. These divide into respiratory bronchioles, which

branch into alveolar ducts leading to the alveolar sacs.

An alveolus is lined with two types of cells:

1. **Type I pneumocytes** have extensive flattened areas that cover most of the internal surfaces of the alveoli.
2. **Type II pneumocytes** are fewer in number and are more globular in shape. They contain **lamellar bodies** that are the source of **surfactant**. Surfactant reduces surface tension, about which more will be said later.

The acini also contain phagocytic macrophages, described in Chapter 6.

The outer surface of the lungs and inner surface of the chest wall are lined by the pleura, a serous membrane; therefore, the thoracic cavity is also called the **pleural cavity**. The thoracic cavity is divided into the right and left sides by the **mediastinum**, a partition containing all major organs except the lungs—for example, the heart and esophagus. The **diaphragm** below separates the pleural cavity from the abdominal cavity (see Figure 16-2).

The Pump

Breathing is initiated in the respiratory centers of the pons and medulla. The rate is

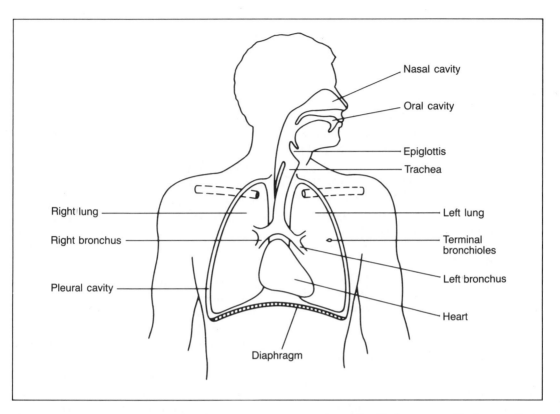

Figure 16-2. Anatomical relationship of the major airways and the lungs to the other organs of the thoracic cavity.

controlled by arterial partial pressures of carbon dioxide (pCO_2) and oxygen (pO_2) and pH. The diaphragm responds to the pons and medulla to act like a bellows to move air.

PHYSIOLOGY OF THE RESPIRATORY SYSTEM

Respiration

Mechanics of Inspiration

The process of respiration is based on Boyle's law, which states that, given a closed space and constant temperature, gas pressure varies inversely with its volume. The thoracic cavity is a closed space at constant body temperature. The available volume is altered by movement of the surrounding muscles:

1. The **diaphragm** contracts and moves down to increase the volume of the tho-

racic cavity. It also causes the lower ribs to rise and move outward.
2. The **external intercostal** muscles contract to pull ribs upward and forward.
3. The **scalene** muscles elevate the first and second ribs.
4. The **sternocleidomastoid** muscles elevate the sternum.

As a consequence, the size of the thoracic cavity increases; however, the last two function only at high levels of ventilation or in the presence of inflow obstruction.

As the chest enlarges, thoracic cavity pressure falls, and air rushes in until the pressure equals atmospheric pressure. Expiration normally is a passive process. The muscles relax and the lungs recoil with expulsion of the air.

Elasticity of the Lungs

Normally, the lung is easily distended within the normal range of pressures (-2 to -10 cm H_2O), a property commonly called

compliance. Factors commonly affecting compliance are given in Table 16-1.

Another property affecting the lung is surface tension, the force across a liquid-gas surface whereby the liquid surface tends to become as small as possible. The inner surfaces of alveoli are covered by surfactant, which reduces surface tension and allows the lung to expand more easily, that is, become more compliant.

Surfactant also promotes the stability of the alveoli. Ordinarily, in a foam, small bubbles have a higher pressure than larger bubbles. As a consequence, they tend to empty into larger bubbles whose total surface area is lower. Alveoli are basically a collection of small bubbles. Surfactant decreases surface tension and reduces the tendency in the lungs to form one large bubble with less surface area for gas exchange.

In addition, surface tension tends to suck fluid from capillaries. Surfactant reduces this effect and keeps alveoli dry. These actions stabilize the alveoli and decrease the tendency to **atelectasis** (partial collapse).

Airways Resistance

The flow of air through the airways resembles that seen in the flow of liquids or gases through a tube. There are three types of rate and patterns of flow:

1. **Laminar flow** (streamlined flow parallel to the sides of the tube) occurs at low pressure.
2. Local **eddies**, especially at branches, develop with increased flow.
3. **Turbulence** occurs at high flow rate.

Table 16-1. Factors Commonly Affecting Compliance

Decrease	Increase
Increased pulmonary venous pressure: Lung becomes engorged with blood	Age
Alveolar edema	Emphysema
Diseases causing lung fibrosis	

Resistance to laminar flow (R) is directly proportional to the viscosity of the gas (n) and length of the tube (l) and inversely proportional to the fourth power of the tube radius (r):

$$R = \frac{n \cdot l}{r^4} \qquad (16\text{-}1)$$

Therefore, tube radius is critical. If the radius is divided in half, resistance increases 16 times. On the other hand, if tube length increases by two, resistance increases by two.

In the bronchial tree, there are many branches with changes in caliber (r) and irregular wall surfaces. Laminar flow is believed to occur in very small airways, and turbulence occurs in the trachea. The major resistance arises in medium-sized bronchi. Very small bronchioles show little resistance because the total r is large. As a consequence, considerable disease to these small airways can occur before unusual resistance is detected.

The contraction of bronchial smooth muscle narrows airways and increases the airways' resistance. This contraction can occur as a result of stimulation of receptors in the trachea and bronchi by irritants (e.g., cigarette smoke) and parasympathetic stimulation by drugs (e.g., acetylcholine). On the other hand, bronchodilation can be caused by sympathetic stimulation by drugs (e.g., isoproterenol, norepinephrine).

Work of Breathing

Energy is required to move the lung and chest wall. Therefore, with progressive respiratory failure from any cause, the muscles must work harder. They need more oxygen and substrates to provide energy. Conversely, malnutrition can contribute to respiratory failure.

Ventilation

In studying lung function, one must consider not only the static volumes of gas contained in the lung, but also the amount of air flow in a given time.

The amount of ventilation is also influenced by nutrients metabolized. The ratio of CO_2 exhaled to O_2 inhaled is the respiratory quotient:

$$RQ = \frac{CO_2}{O_2} \qquad (16\text{-}2)$$

Examples of RQ values related to nutrients metabolized are as follows:[1]

Glucose oxidation:

$$C_6H_{12}O_6 + 6\,O_2 \longrightarrow 6\,CO_2 \\ + 6\,H_2O \qquad (16\text{-}3)$$

Therefore, $6\,CO_2 \div 6\,O_2 = 1.0$

Protein (amino acid) oxidation:

$$1 \text{ amino acid} + 5.1\,O_2 \longrightarrow 4.1\,CO_2 \\ + 28\,H_2O + 0.7 \text{ urea} \qquad (16\text{-}4)$$

Therefore, $4.1\,CO_2 \div 5.1\,O_2 = 0.8$

Triglyceride (e.g., tripalmitin) oxidation:

$$2\,C_{51}H_{98}O_6 + 145\,O_2 \longrightarrow 102\,CO_2 \\ + 98\,H_2O \qquad (16\text{-}5)$$

Therefore, $102\,CO_2 \div 145\,O_2 = 0.7$

Triglyceride synthesis from glucose:

$$26\,C_6H_{12}O_6 + 3.5\,O_2 \longrightarrow 2\,C_{54}H_{101}O_6 \\ + 48\,CO_2 + 55\,H_2O \qquad (16\text{-}6)$$

Therefore, $48\,CO_2 \div 3.5\,O_2 = 13.71$

Thus it is clear that an excess of kilocalories in the form of carbohydrate produces a large excess of carbon dioxide and thereby increases the respiratory load. An $RQ > 1.0$ is undesirable, indicating accumulating carbon dioxide and leading to acidosis (see Chapter 2).

Other Functions

In addition to gas exchange, the lung performs a number of other functions. These are listed in Table 16-2.

Table 16-2. Functions of the Lungs

Gas exchange
Synthesis of surfactant, mucopolysaccharides and immunoglobulins (in bronchial mucus), collagen, and elastin
Conversion of angiotensin I to angiotensin II
Inactivation of bradykinin, serotonin, prostaglandins
Storage of megakaryocytes, mast cells

DIAGNOSIS OF PULMONARY DISEASE

A number of methods useful in diagnosis and monitoring of pulmonary disease must be understood by the nutritional care specialist. Some of the items are necessary to nutritional assessment, and others must be understood in order to be able to read the patient's medical record. These methods are summarized in the following paragraphs:

1. Take the patient's history carefully. Factors to be considered include the following:

   Is the patient dyspneic? Duration? On exertion? When resting? Related to position? At night?

   Is there chest pain? Location? Type? On exertion? When resting?

   Is there coughing? Nonproductive? Duration? Productive? Duration? Amount, color, consistency, odor of sputum? Presence of blood?

   Is occupation related to disease? Duration and level of exposure? Material involved?

   Family history of cardiopulmonary disease? Members affected? Degree of illness?

   History of smoking: Duration? Cigarette, cigar, or pipe? Amount? If quit, how long?

2. Observations of the patient should be made to ascertain the following:

   Position? Leaning forward, on furniture or other positions suggesting respiratory distress?

   Color? Pallor? Cyanosis? Flushing?

   Respiratory rate? (Twelve to 16 breaths

per minute is normal in an adult.) Tachypnea (increased)? Bradypnea (decreased)?

Abnormal breathing pattern?

Apnea (absence of breathing)?

Apneustic (prolonged inhalation)?

Obstructive (prolonged exhalation)?

Biot's (irregular — periods of apnea and gasping ventilation)?

Cheyne-Stokes (increased, then decreased ventilation, then variable apnea)?

Kussmaul's (increased rate and depth of ventilation)?

Chest movement? Symmetrical? Normal up and out in respiration?

Chest shape? (Normal transverse diameter is 2:1 to anterior-posterior [A-P] diameter.) "Pigeon chest"? "Barrel chest"? "Funnel chest"?

Spinal abnormalities? Kyphosis (forward curving when viewed laterally)? Scoliosis (lateral curvature viewed from back)?

Figure 16-3. Subdivisions of pulmonary capacity. TLC = total lung capacity; IRV = inspiratory reserve volume; TV = tidal volume (normal breathing); ERV = expiratory reserve volume; RV = residual volume (never expired); VC = vital capacity; IC = inspiratory capacity (IRV + TV); FRC = full residual capacity (ERV + RV).

Digital clubbing? (Fingernail has $>180°$ angle to finger although normal is $<160°$. Cause unknown.)

Neck vein distention?

Peripheral edema?

3. Does palpation reveal tenderness? Masses? Emphysema? Location? Amount of involvement?

4. Type of sound produced by percussion (striking chest with fingers) may be of diagnostic value.

5. Auscultation (listening for breath sounds, usually with a stethoscope) may reveal the following abnormal sounds:

Rales — crackling sounds, usually on inspiration. Do not usually clear on coughing.

Ronche — gurgling sounds of air through secretions. May clear after coughing.

Wheezes — continuous; may be musical.

Pleural friction rubs — caused by rubbing of pleurae.

6. Arterial blood gas analysis is very important in pulmonary disease (see Chapter 2).

7. Pulmonary function may be assessed with a spirometer. The various subdivisions that must be understood are as follows (see also Figure 16-3):

TLC   *Total lung capacity:* Amount of air in lungs following maximum inspiration.

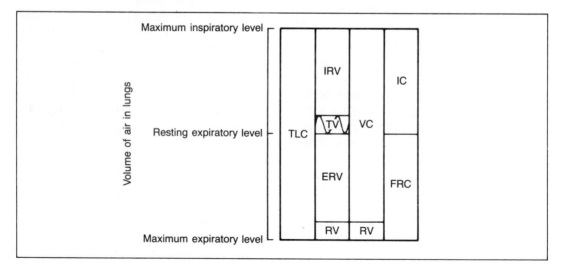

TV   *Tidal volume:* Amount of air inhaled and exhaled during rest.

IRV   *Inspiratory reserve volume:* Amount of air maximally inhaled from resting inspiration.

ERV   *Expiratory reserve volume:* Amount of air maximally exhaled from resting expiration. Also known as functional residual volume (FRV).

RV   *Residual volume:* Amount of air in lungs after maximum expiration.

VC   *Vital capacity:* Amount of air in maximal expiration following maximal inspiration. Also known as forced vital capacity (FVC).

FEV_1 *Forced expiratory volume in 1 second:* The volume forcefully expired in 1 second after maximal inspiration.

8. Other methods include **bronchoscopy**, in which a bronchofiberscope allows direct visualization. It is particularly useful in suspected neoplasms. **Needle biopsies** are used for obtaining lung tissue for study, useful in a number of situations.

EFFECT OF MALNUTRITION ON RESPIRATION

Malnutrition increases the risk, morbidity, and mortality of respiratory failure.[2] It has been associated with decreased function of the parenchyma of the lungs, wasting of respiratory muscles, and reduced ventilatory drive.[3] The incidence of pulmonary infection is often increased also. Animal studies have demc   .rated loss of pulmonary connective tissue, decreased lung weight, and enlarged terminal air spaces.[4-6] In addition to these morphological changes, malnutrition has been shown in young animals to result in reduced surfactant production, impaired antioxidant protective mechanisms, and reduced immune responses. Data on the extent to which these changes apply to human young or in adult pulmonary disease is very limited. However, kwashiorkor and marasmus have been shown to have these effects.

An increase in the work of breathing can lead to protein depletion, including depletion of the diaphragm mass. This will, in turn, contribute to decreased pulmonary function, to altered immune function, and possibly to a higher incidence of respiratory infection.

Some other effects of specific nutrient deficiencies include the following:

Phosphate depletion depresses the ventilatory response to hypoxia.

Magnesium depletion leads to respiratory muscle fatigue.

Sodium depletion also occurs in patients given diuretics. Marked depletion leads to appetite depression and then slowing of the ventilatory drive.

Iron deficiency occurs consequent to low food intake, frequent venipuncture, and related acute illnesses.

Vitamin A deficiency can suppress mucus secretion and loss of cilia, reducing defense against infection.

Vitamin C deficiency also suppresses mucus secretion.

Vitamin E deficiency effects are uncertain.

CHRONIC OBSTRUCTIVE PULMONARY DISEASE

Chronic obstructive pulmonary disease (COPD) is also known as chronic obstructive lung disease (COLD), chronic airflow obstruction (CAO), or chronic airflow limitation. It is a major public health problem, with 50,000 deaths per year in the United States. From 10% to 25% of adults have some degree of chronic bronchitis, with chronic symptoms or permanent disability. However, a large majority of cases are preventable by cessation of smoking.

Limited air flow and pulmonary insufficiency are characteristic of COPD. There is interference with the inflow of oxygen and with elimination of carbon dioxide. As a consequence, blood gases are abnormal. The acronym COPD refers to a combination of chronic bronchitis and emphysema that may be present in variable proportions. The terms have been defined as follows:

Chronic bronchitis consists of excessive mucus secretion in the bronchial tree manifested by a chronic or recurring productive cough. Infection and bronchospasm are common.

Emphysema is an anatomic alteration of the lung characterized by dilation and destruction of airspaces distal to terminal bronchioles with overinflation, collapse of airways, and dyspnea. This has a poorer prognosis than does chronic bronchitis.

The presence of either of these in pure form with clear distinctions is rare. Nevertheless, two forms are commonly described:

In **type A** ("pink puffer"), airways obstruction is severe, but ventilatory drive is preserved. Dyspnea is intense, with pursed-lip breathing. The patient is thin and often elderly. Blood gas volume is near normal until the disease is far advanced. Lung capacity is increased. There may be radiological evidence of emphysema. The patient rarely develops edema or overt heart failure.

In **type B** ("blue bloater"), obese patients have poor respiratory drive (reason unknown), their weight is stable or above normal, and they easily drift into congestive heart failure. There is usually fairly normal lung capacity with only moderate airways obstruction. Patients tend to have abnormal blood gases with elevated plasma HCO_3^-. Another complication is **cor pulmonale**, heart disease caused by respiratory disorders, often resulting in right ventricular hypertrophy.

Other causes of ventilatory failure are as follows:

1. Some cases of chronic severe asthma.
2. Central failure of respiratory drive. Those who are severely obese are "Pickwickian syndrome" patients.
3. Nonobese patients with central failure may have bronchiectasis (dilation of the bronchioles) or narrowing of small airways.
4. Restriction of chest wall movement from, for example, kyphoscoliosis, ankylosing spondylitis, or severe muscular weakness.

Etiology and Pathogenesis

Smoking is considered a major etiological factor. Other factors include urban air pollutants, industrial pollutants, increasing age, genetic predisposition, and infection. In addition, there is a rare inborn error of metabolism producing an $alpha_1$ antitrypsin deficiency. Normally, proteases digest inflammatory debris in the lung, and $alpha_1$ antitrypsin prevents these proteases from attacking normal tissue. In $alpha_1$ antitrypsin deficiency, the lung is attacked by proteases that degrade the lung tissue. There are varying degrees of severity of this condition, the more severe of which result in COPD.

Nutritional Assessment

Weight loss is common in COPD and is associated with a poor prognosis.[7,8] Therefore, regular monitoring of body weight is mandatory. It has been suggested that weight loss results at least partially from decreased intake, although this conclusion is controversial, but the decrease, if it does exist, may be secondary to shortness of breath during preparation of meals and eating, peptic ulcers, bronchodilator medications that are gastric irritants, nausea and vomiting with the use of theophylline medications, and chronic sputum production. Determination of the cause of decreased food intake will indicate appropriate approaches to correction.

An alternative, or additional, cause of weight loss is increased energy expenditure. The causes may include the increased work of breathing and the effects of infection. The patient may be in a hypermetabolic state, as described in Chapter 14.

Anthropometric measures of triceps skinfold and midarm muscle circumference are needed to relate changes in body weight to changes in body composition. These will indicate whether changes in weight are the result of alterations in body fat stores, muscle mass, or edema.

Catabolism of muscle mass in malnutrition will include catabolism of both inspiratory and expiratory muscles. Malnutrition also decreases the ability of the diaphragm to contract. Therefore, loss of muscle mass must be detected.

Other parameters, frequently abnormal in COPD patients, include serum albumin, serum transferrin, creatinine-height index, total iron-binding capacity, serum zinc, and immune function. Tests of respiratory function are useful in monitoring the respiratory muscle response to nutritional support.[9]

Management of COPD

Patients should be strongly encouraged to stop smoking. They may be given steroid (15 mg prednisone q.d.) to determine whether there is an allergic component. Other medications commonly used include

- Broad spectrum antibiotic, e.g., amoxycillin 250 mg t.i.d. or tetracycline 250 mg q.i.d.
- Bronchodilator, e.g., theophylline.
- Mucolytic, e.g., bromhexine 16 mg q.i.d.
- Influenza vaccine.

If the patient becomes severely ill and is admitted to the hospital, management often includes antibiotics, bronchodilators, encouragement to expectorate, and management of respiratory failure with artificial ventilation. Other aspects of management that may be necessary include IV for rehydration, percussion, and postural drainage.

The goals of nutritional care are as follows:

1. To provide adequate nutrition so that the patient is more resistant to stresses, such as infection, that worsen the disease manifestations.
2. To provide a nutrient mix that benefits the patient's pulmonary function by reducing

production of carbon dioxide and maintaining respiratory muscle function.

The respiratory quotients (see Equations 16-3 to 16-6) demonstrate that the least carbon dioxide per unit of oxygen consumed is produced in the metabolism of fat, and the most is produced in the metabolism of carbohydrate, when considering the three sources of energy. The quotients also indicate that a very large amount of carbon dioxide is produced when carbohydrate in excess of maintenance needs is being converted to fat. Therefore, there is a theory that increased fat and decreased carbohydrate may be indicated, and that carbohydrate should not be given in amounts that would promote lipogenesis.

Nutritional status tends to decline as COPD progresses, and malnutrition and infection tend to exacerbate each other. In addition to promotion of wasting of respiratory muscles with a decrease in their strength and leading to declining vital capacity and oxygen utilization, other effects of COPD plus infection include

- Declining serum albumin and resulting oncotic pressure → possible pulmonary edema.
- Declining surfactant production → decreased compliance leading to pulmonary collapse.

The respiratory muscles may require four to ten times normal oxygen. Eating requires energy, and one-third or more of total kilocalories may be expended in respiration. To reduce dyspnea, the patient should rest for a half hour before eating and avoid exercise, therapy, or treatment for one hour after eating. Oxygen may be needed while eating. If the patient uses oxygen routinely, he or she should continue its use and eat slowly.

Thus caloric intake must be increased to meet need. At the same time, excess intake must be avoided. Energy needs are best determined by indirect calorimetry, but can be estimated with the Harris-Benedict equation.

Protein intake should be adequate, neither deficient or excessive. Protein deficiency, as well as administration of steroids, causes muscle wasting. It can also decrease theophylline elimination, possibly causing toxicity.

High-protein diets, on the other hand, stimulate the ventilatory drive. It has been suggested that the effect is a function of the amino acid profile. Increased levels of branched-chain amino acids may stimulate ventilation by altering neurotransmitter synthesis in the brain.[10] If the patient has no alveolar reserves, the work of breathing and the resulting dyspnea can then increase.[11]

In COPD patients, positive nitrogen balance has been achieved when energy intake is about twice REE and the calorie-nitrogen ratio is about 150:1.[12]

To reduce gastric distention, bloating, and the oxygen needed for chewing and digestion:

- Give six small meals per day.
- Take fluids between meals to prevent excess stomach distention and pressure on diaphragm.
- Restrict fluids for volume-sensitive patients (those with cor pulmonale and congestive heart failure).
- Give 2–3 liters fluid/day to non-volume-sensitive patients (for hydration, preventing constipation, thinning mucus).

RESPIRATORY FAILURE

Respiratory failure may be acute or chronic. Among the symptoms are malaise, difficulty in sleeping, headaches, weakness, palpitations, breathlessness, cough, tachycardia, arrhythmias, ascites, and edema. Arterial blood gases and pH must be measured for diagnosis. The causes are given in Table 16-3.

Respiratory failure occurs when the lungs are unable to provide enough oxygen to the tissues or remove carbon dioxide adequately

Table 16-3. Causes of Respiratory Insufficiency

Intrinsic lung diseases:
COPD
Infections
Interstitial lung diseases
Tracheal blockage
Drowning
Status asthmaticus
Toxic gas inhalation
Chest trauma
Extensive pneumonia
Respiratory distress syndrome (infant and adult)
Neuromuscular:
Chest trauma
Selected drugs
Thoracic surgery
High abdominal surgery
Kyphoscoliosis
Cervical spinal cord injuries
Neuromuscular diseases
   Myasthenia gravis
   Amyotrophic lateral sclerosis
   Myotonic dystrophy
   Guillain-Barré syndrome
   Botulism
   Tetanus
   Poliomyelitis
Central ventilatory drive:
Pickwickian syndrome (massive obesity)
Myxedema
Stroke
Brain trauma
Shock
Drug overdose
Others:
Asthma
Pulmonary embolism
Acute heart failure
Pulmonary edema
Carbon monoxide inhalation

from the blood. It is defined as paO_2 between 50 and 70 torr (normal = 80–100) and $paCO_2 > 50$ (normal = 35–45). The low oxygen levels are potentially lethal, but elevated CO_2 levels are intoxicating though not normally lethal.

Hypoxemia is treated with oxygen and respiratory acidosis with increased alveolar ventilation. Sometimes bicarbonate is given. The patient may need endotracheal intubation and mechanical ventilation.

Nutritional Assessment

Body weight and most anthropometrics are useful in the usual fashion (see Chapter 3) unless the patient is fluid-overloaded. Usual biochemical parameters are also useful. History and physical examination should look for drugs or concurrent illness causing fluid overload. For patients on ventilatory support, indirect calorimetry is most useful to determine their RME.

Nutritional Care

A diet that minimizes the production of carbon dioxide while maintaining good nutrition is indicated, as is the case for the COPD patient who is not in failure. In addition, the patient in respiratory failure may require the assistance of a ventilator to correct abnormal blood gases.

In early respiratory failure, if intake does not meet requirements, the use of calorically dense supplementary feedings may be useful. If these do not meet nutritional needs, tube feeding is indicated.

Common recommendations for stressed pulmonary patients are

25–35 kcal/kg/day for maintenance.
45 kcal/kg/day for anabolism.
0.2 g nitrogen (1.5 g amino acid) per kg per day.
2–4 g carbohydrate per kg per day for obligatory needs for brain and blood cell metabolism (about 200 g/day).
50–60% kcal as lipid.[13]

The tube feedings may begin at 30–50 ml/hr. and are increased by 25 ml/hr. each day until the 150 ml/hr. rate is reached. Details of the procedure are given in Chapter 5.

Tube feedings that are relatively rich in fat and somewhat lower in carbohydrate may be chosen from the following:

Compleat B	Must use large bore tubes. Milk-based—do not use if lactase deficient.
Nutri-1000	46.7% lipid; low residue; lactose-free; usable in very fine bore tubes.
Isocal	37% lipid.
Magnacal	36% lipid.
Ensure	31.5% lipid.
Vipep	22% lipid. Low residue; lactose-free; fine bore tubes; elemental diet.
Precision Isotonic	28.1% lipid.
Pulmocare	Designed especially for pulmonary disease.
Modular formulas	For patients with special needs.

Some special considerations in the pulmonary patients are the following:

1. Special precautions against aspiration are needed. Using a tube that extends beyond the pylorus is helpful.
2. Reduce aspiration by elevating the head of the bed.
3. Add blue food coloring to the formula so that aspiration is easily detected if it occurs.
4. It is recommended that formulas that are blenderized diets (low tonicity) or defined formulas (neutral pH and free of large particles) are best to use. Either of these may reduce lung damage.

For patients with ileus, fistulas, or pancreatitis, or if the patient cannot swallow because of the presence of an endotracheal tube, TPN may be used. Peripheral support (PPN) has fewer risks than CPN. This method, however, is limited by the following factors:

1. The large volume of fluid needed to contain sufficient calories.
2. The limitation in total energy which can be provided.
3. The limited length of time that the method is usable (see Chapter 5).

For extended support, CPN can be more useful, but it too has its limitations:

1. High glucose concentrations can lead to excess carbon dioxide production. If problems of carbon dioxide retention persist, the use of fat in the formula may be necessary.
2. Fat administration and resultant lipemia can decrease the diffusing capacity of oxygen. Alternatively, it has been suggested that intravenous fat emulsions may have a therapeutic effect on pulmonary function through an increase in prostaglandin synthesis.[10] Serum triglycerides and arterial blood gases must be monitored.
3. Since phosphate depletion reduces respiratory drive, phosphate supplementation may be necessary.

An estimate of total energy expenditure is 25–35 kcal/kg/day for maintenance and 45 kcal/kg/day for anabolism. Since patients are often admitted as trauma emergencies, they may not be undernourished. It is often recommended that 1.0–1.2 × daily kcal for maintenance and 1.4–1.6 × daily kcal for anabolism be given these patients.

Fat frequently is provided in one 500 ml bottle of 10% or 20% fat emulsion per day. Too much lipid should not be given to very catabolic patients. It has been suggested that triglyceridemia with prolonged clearing can be the consequences of (1) deficiencies of muscle carnitine to transport long-chain fatty acids across the mitochondrial membrane and (2) depressed tissue lipoprotein lipase activity. As a result, fat in excess, as well as excess carbohydrate, may delay weaning from the ventilator.

Protein can be given as 1.25 g amino acid per kg per day (0.2 g nitrogen per kg per day).

Patients who are starved have depressed metabolic rate and depressed minute ventilation. For these patients, a 3.5% amino acid solution may increase both minute ventilation and metabolic rate to normal by increasing the neurogenic ventilatory drive. On the other hand, those with very high protein intakes may become dyspneic because of the tendency to increase respiratory effort.

Therefore, amino acid administration concentrations must be moderate.

Patients on a ventilator frequently need nutritional support. They may be given tube feedings if they have a tracheostomy. Those with endotracheal tubes must be fed with TPN. In formulating either feeding, increased calories are required, but glucose should not be given in excess of energy requirement, or the RQ will be more than 1.00, and more CO_2 will be produced. In order to excrete this excess CO_2, increased tidal volume or minute volume would be necessary. Since the patient's respiratory failure makes these impossible, the patient's dependence on mechanical ventilation increases.

Nutritional support should begin immediately if long-term mechanical ventilation is likely.

Two other problems may arise as a result of mechanical ventilation. First, the patient may retain salt and water. Therefore, there is a need to monitor fluid volume status to prevent left ventricular failure. Second, acid-base imbalance may arise. Carbon dioxide retention results in respiratory acidosis. If mechanical ventilation is excessive, respiratory alkalosis may be produced (see Chapter 2). Thus the physician must stabilize the fluid, electrolyte, and acid-base balance.

Another problem arises when it is desirable to wean the patient from the ventilator. Usually, when the patient is clinically stable, ventilation is gradually decreased. The ability of a patient with a carbohydrate-excess diet to breathe on his or her own is compromised, and the weaning process is difficult and sometimes impossible.

Monitoring Response to Therapy

If the patient is not retaining fluid, body weight is useful, as are anthropometric values, but significant changes are not expected in less than monthly intervals. Biochemical parameters are not reliable in patients with fluid overload. Indirect calorimetry is helpful in monitoring the effects of changes in feeding formulas.

The nutritional care specialist must monitor the transition from parenteral to tube feeding to conventional feeding (see Chapter 5).

BRONCHOPULMONARY DYSPLASIA

Bronchopulmonary dysplasia (BPD) affects primarily low-birth-weight infants. Nutritional problems are a combination of increased requirements related to respiration and functional limitations of the gastrointestinal tract to meet those needs.

Infants who are born prematurely or at low birth weight may have immature lungs in which their ability to synthesize surfactant is undeveloped. As a result, they are unable to inflate the lungs for adequate ventilation. This condition is known as **hyaline membrane disease** or **infantile respiratory distress syndrome** (IRDS). Frequently, BPD is a complication of the treatment of IRDS with positive pressure ventilation and oxygen administration, that is, a hyperoxic environment. Other risk factors include pneumonia, meconium aspiration, tracheoesophageal fistula, and congenital heart disease.

Pathology

The patient can have failure-to-thrive (FTT), including slower growth of the lung tissue. The slower growth in these children can result from prolonged hypoxia, increased oxygen dependency, hypercapnia, and prolonged emotional deprivation from long hospitalization. Other signs and symptoms include tachypnea, dyspnea, and a characteristic radiographic appearance. Some of the complications of BPD include pulmonary edema and cor pulmonale.

The pathogenesis of BPD and of its complications are poorly understood. High partial pressures of oxygen are toxic to plants and mammals. In mammals, if this oxygen is at high pressure (hyperbaric hyperoxia), tissue injury occurs first in the central nervous system, producing convulsions. If pressure is normal (normobaric hyperoxia), injury occurs first in the lung. This damage occurs after a period of about 24 hours. This delay suggests there must be a period in which toxic materials accumulate or defense materials are depleted.[14]

In oxygen toxicity, the toxic materials are apparently free radicals of oxygen.[14] A free radical is any molecule with unpaired electrons. In the case of free radicals of oxygen, there is superoxide (O_2^-), hydrogen peroxide, and the hydroxyl radical ($OH\cdot$) produced by the following reactions:

$$Fe^{+3} + O_2^- \longrightarrow Fe^{+2} + O_2$$

$$Fe^{+2} + H_2O_2 \longrightarrow Fe^{+3} + OH\cdot + OH\cdot$$

These free radicals can be formed by a variety of normal cellular and enzymatic reactions, by exposure to a hyperoxic environment, and by exposure to ionizing radiation, environmental gases and particles, antibiotics, antineoplastic drugs, and various chemicals.

This exposure to oxidizing agents has been shown to damage the endothelial cells of the lung early. It may also alter connective tissue, producing more chronic abnormalities.[14]

Prevention

Nutritional management must consider protective agents and factors in treatment. Protective agents in the lung, acting as antioxidants, may include the enzymes superoxide dismutase, catalase, and glutathiones. Others may be vitamins E and C, beta carotene, unsaturated fatty acids, and uric acid.[15-17] Many of these may protect against pulmonary oxygen toxicity by binding and detoxifying some reactive forms of oxygen.

It has been shown in animals that survival is improved in a hyperoxic environment if the animals are well nourished. Infants fed human milk or commercial formulas are unlikely to be deficient in the protective nutrients. Those fed by TPN may be at risk unless they receive supplements of these nutrients.[16]

Nutritional Assessment

A number of factors must be considered in nutritional assessment of the BPD patient. These items can be categorized as follows:

Gestational history: Gestational age at birth? Prenatal history, including medications? Perinatal history?

Growth and feeding: Growth pattern? Age of achievement of feeding milestones? Composition, volume, frequency of formula and food intake? Feeding behavior? Emesis?

Physical exam: Visual and auditory development? Urine and stool production? Work of breathing? Laboratory values— hematocrit, hemoglobin, transcutaneous oxygen, serum urea nitrogen, serum electrolytes, urine specific gravity?

Social and environmental: Home facilities? Bonding? Community and economic resources?

Drug treatment: What drugs is the child taking? Bronchodilators? Diuretics? Corticosteroids? Antibiotics? Cardiac medications?

Nutritional Care

Caring for the infant or child with BPD presents several problems. A major consideration is the provision of adequate energy to support growth despite limited gastrointestinal function.

The BPD patient has an increased basal metabolic rate compared with term infants or very-low-birth-weight (VLBW) infants without BPD. To a large extent, this increased BMR is the consequence of persistent tachypnea, using 50–70% of basal metabolism, while normal breathing accounts for less than 5% of the BMR. In addition, BPD infants are irritable compared to VLBW infants, further increasing the metabolic rate.

BPD may be considered to occur in three phases that influence feeding methods to meet these caloric needs:

1. In the **acute phase**, the infant is acutely ill, and oral feeding is difficult. The caloric needs are estimated to be 50–70 kcal/kg/day, usually provided parenterally. There may be some difficulty in meeting the total need, since the low-birth-weight infant has limited ability to handle a large fluid load. When these infants retain fluid, there is increased risk of necrotizing enterocolitis in the intestine[18] and of patent ductus arteriosus in the heart (PDA).[19,20] Excess fluid prevents the PDA from closing normally postnatally. These infants often also have a reduced sensitivity to insulin and a consequent increased risk of hyperglycemia.

2. In the **intermediate phase**, there is clinical improvement. Total energy needs are 95–120 kcal/kg/day. Oral intake can be gradually introduced. Fluid overload can be partly avoided by providing high-caloric-density infusates and infant formulas. Energy requirement may be controlled by avoiding thermal losses. Intravenous fat emulsions in the parenteral infusions are also helpful.

3. In the **convalescent phase**, the infant is being fed orally exclusively. Caloric needs are 120–130 kcal/kg/day, similar to the needs of patients without BPD. A formula providing 24 kcal/oz. meets this need without fluid overload. This caloric density can be achieved by mixing a 13-oz. can of formula concentrate with 9 ounces of water (instead of 13 oz. of water) or 3 unpacked level scoops of a powdered formula with 5 ounces of water.

Case Study: Respiratory Failure

William E., age 54 years, was admitted to the hospital with pneumococcal pneumonia. The patient had a history of 38 years of smoking. He also had a history of COPD treated in the clinic.

On the present admission, he developed respiratory failure. The Nutrition Support Service was asked to evaluate the patient. Nutritional assessment indicated moderate malnutrition. Food intake was less than need.

A nasoduodenal feeding tube was placed for

continuous feeding by pump. The head of the bed was elevated.

After four days, the patient developed an acute abdomen. After surgery, the assessment indicated severe protein malnutrition. Bowel sounds were absent. A central venous catheter was placed for continuous feeding by pump. A high-carbohydrate formula with phosphate supplementation was prescribed.

The patient also developed respiratory failure and was placed on ventilatory support.

Exercises

1. Describe the morphological changes which occur in COPD.

2. How can COPD lead to malnutrition?
3. Describe the diet modifications used for COPD patients and their rationale.
4. Describe methods that may be used to test for aspiration.
5. Compare the advantages of central and peripheral parenteral nutrition.
6. What is the purpose of the supplementary phosphate in the TPN formula?
7. What effect on RQ would you expect from the high-carbohydrate feeding? Why?
8. Describe the effect of this feeding on weaning from a ventilator.
9. What action might be taken to resolve this problem?

References

1. Heymsfield, S.B. Influence of formula composition and caloric infusion rate on respiratory and cardiovascular function. *Dietetic Currents* 12:7, 1985.
2. Selivanov, V., Sheldon, G.F., and Fantini, G. Nutrition's role in averting respiratory failure. *J. Respir. Dis.* 4(9):29, 1983.
3. Bell, L.P., and Shronts, E.P. Nutritional support in respiratory failure. In C.E. Lang, Ed., *Nutritional Support in Critical Care.* Rockville, Md.: Aspen, 1987.
4. Sahebjami, H., and Macgee, J. Changes in connective tissue composition of the lungs in starvation and refeeding. *Am. Rev. Respir. Dis.* 128:644, 1983.
5. Sahebjami, H., and Vassalo, C.L. Effects of starvation and refeeding on lung mechanics and morphometry. *Am. Rev. Respir. Dis.* 119:443, 1979.
6. Doekel, R.C., Zwielich, C.W., Scoggin, C.H., et al. Clinical semistarvation. Depression of hypoxic ventilatory response. *N. Engl. J. Med.* 295:358, 1976.
7. Vandenberg, E., van de Woestijne, K.P., et al., Weight changes in the terminal stages of chronic obstructive pulmonary disease. *Am. Rev. Respir. Dis.* 95:556, 1967.
8. Vandenberg, E., van de Woestijne, K.P., and Gyselin, A. Weight changes in the terminal stages of chronic obstructive pulmonary disease. Relation of respiratory function and prognosis. *Am. Rev. Respir. Dis.* 95:1556, 1967.
9. Hunter, A.M.B., Carey, M.A., and Larsh, H.W. The nutritional status of patients with chronic obstructive pulmonary disease. *Am. Rev. Respir. Dis.* 124:376, 1981.
10. Askanazi, J., Goldstein, S., Kvetan, V., and Kinney, J.M. Respiratory diseases. In *Nutrition and Metabolism in Patient Care*, eds. J.M.

Kinney, K.N. Jeejeebhoy, G.L. Hill, and O.E. Owen. Philadelphia: W.B. Saunders, 1988.
11. Askanazi, J., Weissman, C., La Sala, P.A., et al. Effect of protein intake on ventilatory drive. *Anesthesiology* 60:106, 1984.
12. Goldstein, S.A., Askanazi, J., Weissman, C., et al. N balance during nutritional support in malnourished COPD patients. *JPEN* 10:165, 1986.
13. Rothkopf, M.M., Stanislaus, G., Haverstick, L., Kvetan, V. and Askenazi, J. Nutritional support in respiratory failure. *Nutr. Clin. Prac.* 4:166, 1989.
14. Fanburg, B.L., Deneke, S.M., Lee, S.-L., and Hill, N.S. Mediators of lung injury in oxygen toxicity. *Report of the Ninetieth Ross Conference on Pediatric Research*, p. 16. Columbus, Ohio: Ross Laboratories, 1986.
15. Roberts, R.J. Antioxidant systems of the developing lung. *Report of the Ninetieth Ross Conference on Pediatric Research*, p. 24. Columbus, Ohio: Ross Laboratories, 1986.
16. Bell, E.F. Prevention of bronchopulmonary dysplasia. Vitamin E and other antioxidants. *Report of the Ninetieth Ross Conference on Pediatric Research*, p. 77. Columbus, Ohio: Ross Laboratories, 1986.
17. Zachman, R.D. Vitamin A. *Report of the Ninetieth Ross Conference on Pediatric Research*, p. 86. Columbus, Ohio: Ross Laboratories, 1986.
18. Bell, E.F., Warburton, D., Stonestreet, B.S., and Oh, W. High volume fluid intake predisposes premature infants to necrotizing enterocolitis. *Lancet* 2:90, 1979.
19. Stevenson, J.G. Fluid administration in the association of patent ductus arteriosus complicating respiratory distress syndrome. *J. Pediatr.* 90:257, 1977.
20. Bell, E.F., Warburton, D., Stonestreet, B.S., and Oh, W. Effect of fluid administration on the development of symptomatic patent

ductus arteriosus and congestive heart failure in premature infants. *N. Engl. J. Med.* 302:598, 1980.

Bibliography

Bernard, M.A., Jacobs, D.O., and Rombeau, J.L. *Nutritional and Metabolic Support of Hospitalized Patients.* Philadelphia: W.B. Saunders, 1986.

Miller, L.G., and Kazemi, H. *Manual of Clinical Pulmonary Medicine.* New York: McGraw-Hill, 1985.

Mitchell, R.S., and Petty, T.L. *Synopsis of Clinical Pulmonary Disease,* 3rd ed. St. Louis: C.V. Mosby, 1982.

Noller, C., and Mobarhan, S. Enteral feeding in patients with advanced chronic obstructive pulmonary disease. *Nutr. Supp. Services* 6(2A):37, 1986.

Scarpelli, E.M., Ed. *Pulmonary Physiology: Fetus, Newborn, Child and Adolescent,* 2nd. ed. Philadelphia: Lea & Febiger, 1990.

Weinberger, S.E. *Principles of Pulmonary Medicine.* Philadelphia: W.B. Saunders, 1986.

17. Inborn Errors of Metabolism

I. Fundamentals of Genetics
A. Transmission of the genetic code
B. Expression of the genetic code
   1. Genotype and phenotype
   2. Sex-linked traits
   3. Mutations
   4. Chromosomal abnormalities
II. Introduction to Inborn Errors of Metabolism
A. Pathophysiology
   1. Abnormal enzyme function in major metabolic pathways
      a. accumulation of a precursor to toxic levels
      b. deficiency of end product
      c. production of toxic by-products from a normally minor pathway
      d. overproduction of intermediate products through loss of feedback control
   2. Defective plasma membrane transport
   3. Reduced coenzyme production or binding
   4. Deficiency or abnormality of circulating proteins
   5. Abnormality of structural protein
   6. Abnormalities of enzymes that regulate drug metabolism

B. Clinical manifestations
C. Diagnosis
D. Management
   1. General principles of prevention and management
   2. Principles of nutritional management
III. Disorders of Amino Acid Metabolism
A. The hyperphenylalaninemias
   1. Classic phenylketonuria
      a. metabolic abnormalities
      b. clinical manifestations
      c. heredity and incidence
      d. diagnosis and monitoring
      e. nutritional management
      f. follow-up
      g. duration of the diet
      h. maternal phenylketonuria
   2. Variant forms of phenylketonuria
B. Disorders of tyrosine metabolism
   1. Variant forms
   2. Diagnosis and monitoring
   3. Nutritional management
C. Branched-chain ketoaciduria
   1. Biochemical abnormalities
   2. Diagnosis and monitoring
   3. Nutritional care
   4. Variant forms
   5. Duration of diet

D. Isovaleric acidemia
   1. Metabolic abnormalities
   2. Clinical manifestations
   3. Diagnosis and monitoring
   4. Treatment
E. The homocystinurias
   1. Biochemical and clinical abnormalities
   2. Diagnosis and monitoring
   3. Nutritional management
F. Urea cycle disorders
   1. Metabolic defects and clinical manifestations
   2. Diagnosis
   3. Treatment
   4. Monitoring treatment effects
G. Other disorders of amino acid metabolism
IV. Disorders of Carbohydrate Metabolism
A. Disorders of galactose metabolism
   1. Biochemical abnormalities
   2. Screening and diagnosis
   3. Clinical manifestations
   4. Nutritional management
   5. Nutritional assessment and monitoring
B. Disorders of fructose metabolism
   1. Essential fructosuria
   2. Hereditary fructose intolerance
      a. biochemical abnormalities

This chapter, originally coauthored by Sushma Palmer, has been adapted from chapter 10 in the first edition.

   b. clinical
      manifestations
   c. diagnosis
   d. nutritional
      management
   3. Hereditary fruc-
      tose-1, 6-bisphos-
      phatase deficiency
C. Glycogen storage
   diseases
   1. Biochemical
      abnormalities
   2. Diagnosis and
      nutritional
      management

V. Disorders of Lipid
   Transport
   A. Refsum's disease
VI. Disorders of Purine and
    Pyrimidine Metabolism
    A. Gout
       1. Biochemical
          abnormalities
       2. Clinical features
       3. Treatment
    B. Hereditary xanthin-
       uria
VII. Vitamin Dependency
     Disorders
     A. Folate dependency

   B. Vitamin B_{12} depen-
      dency
   C. Pyridoxine depen-
      dency
   D. Vitamin D–
      dependent rickets
   E. Familial vitamin
      D–resistant rickets
VIII. Disorders of Mineral
      Metabolism
      A. Wilson's disease
      B. Acrodermatitis
         enteropathica
IX. Case Study

The diseases discussed in this chapter are known as **inborn errors of metabolism**, sometimes called **congenital metabolic disorders**. They are primarily those disorders in which a mutation of a single gene or a small number of related genes causes a metabolic abnormality. There are a large number of these conditions, but we will discuss here only those for which nutritional care is an essential component of management, with an emphasis on those which occur most often. Table 17-1 provides a list of inborn errors in which modifications of nutrient intake are indicated.

Because genetic aberration is the basis for inborn errors of metabolism, the fundamental concepts of genetics that are necessary for an understanding of these diseases will be explained first. Some general principles of pathophysiology and nutritional care applied to the inborn errors will then be described, followed by a description of specific disorders and their nutritional management.

FUNDAMENTALS OF GENETICS

The hereditary information in each cell is contained in its nucleus. It is necessary to understand, first, how this information is transmitted to new cells during growth in an individual.

Transmission of the Genetic Code

The hereditary information in the nucleus is contained in **chromosomes**. These consist of strands of **DNA**, the basic genetic material of all cells. DNA is a generic term that refers to many specific compounds, just as the word **protein** encompasses many compounds formed from amino acids. It now is well established that DNA molecules consist of chains of nucleotides, usually found in pairs, that are twisted around each other to form a coiled double helix. The two strands are held together by hydrogen bonds between pairs of nitrogenous bases, one on each strand, arranged so that the base, adenine, always is bonded to thymine or a similar analogue and guanine always is bonded to cytosine or a similar analogue. Thus the nitrogenous base on one strand can serve to identify the nitrogenous base on the other. If the strands are separated, each serves as a template for the structure of the other, and two double helixes, exactly like the first, can be made from the two separated strands. This process of replication underlies the function of DNA as the hereditary material.

In the nonreplicating cell, the strands of DNA are not visible but, in preparation for cell duplication, the double helix unwinds and duplicates itself as just described. At the beginning of cell replication (called **mitosis**), the two strands become visible under the microscope. The formations seen at the begin-

Table 17-1. Inborn Errors of Metabolism Requiring Nutrient Intake Modification

Protein or amino acid modifications	*Vitamin modifications*
Alcaptonuria	Biotinidase deficiency
Argininemia	Chediak-Higashi syndrome
Argininosuccinic aciduria	Cystathioninuria
β-methyl-crotonylglycinuria	Ehlers-Danlos syndrome
Branched-chain α ketoaciduria	Folic acid reductase deficiency
Carbamylphosphate synthetase deficiency	Folic acid transport defect
Citrullinemia	Hartnup disease
Dibasic aminoaciduria	Homocystinuria
Glutamate aspartase transport defect	Cystathionine β-synthase deficiency
Glutaric acidemia	N^5–N^{10}–methylenetetrahydrofolate deficiency
Hyperbeta-alaninemia	CH_3-cobalamine deficiency
Isovaleric acidemia	Hydroxykynurenenuria
Lysine intolerance	Methylmalonic aciduria
Methionine malabsorption	Defective reductase or transport
Nonketotic hyperglycinemia	Impaired synthesis
Ornithine transcarbamylase deficiency	Mutase deficiency
Phenylketonuria	Racemase deficiency
Propionic acidemia	Multiple carboxylase deficiency
Tyrosinemia, type I	Oxalosis
Tyrosinemia, type II	B_6-dependency with seizures
Valinemia	Pyruvate dehydrogenase deficiency
	Tryptophanuria with dwarfism
Carbohydrate modifications	Vitamin A defect
Fructose intolerance	Vitamin B_{12} defect
Fructose-1,6-diphosphatase deficiency	Vitamin D–dependent rickets
Galactokinase deficiency	Vitamin K–dependent coagulation defect
Galactosemia	Xanthurenic aciduria
Glucose-galactose malabsorption	
Glucose-6-phosphate dehydrogenase deficiency	*Mineral modifications*
Glycogen storage disease	Acrodermatitis enteropathica
Glucose-6-phosphatase deficiency	Chloride diarrhea
Amylo-6-glucosidase deficiency	Cystinosis
Phosphorylase deficiency	Hyperphosphatemia
Phosphorylase kinase deficiency	Periodic paralysis
Lactose intolerance	
Porphyria	*Other modifications*
Sucrose-isomaltose malabsorption	Cystic fibrosis
	Diabetes insipidus
Lipid modifications	Diabetes mellitus
Abetalipoproteinemias	Gout
β-sitosterolemia	Ketoacidosis of infancy
Combined hyperlipidemia	Lactic acidosis, intermittent
Hypercholesterolemia	Orotic aciduria
Hyperlipoproteinemia I	Refsum's disease
Dihydropteridine reductase deficiency	Renal tubular acidosis
Biopterine biosynthetic blocks	Xanthinuria
Hypertriglyceridemia	

ning of mitosis, the chromosomes, contain the DNA strands. Following duplication of the DNA, each chromosome will consist of two identical strands (**chromatids**) joined at a point called the **centromere**. When the cell replicates, the centromere divides so that one chromatid becomes a new chromosome in each of the daughter cell nuclei, leaving each cell with the same genetic code as the original nucleus.

Every organism has a number of chromosomes characteristic of its species. There are 46 chromosomes in humans. Humans, along with other higher plants and animals, are **diploid** — that is, they inherit a complete set of 23 chromosomes from each parent. The human chromosomes, therefore, occur in pairs, known as **homologous pairs**.

Every living organism must be able to synthesize its own characteristic proteins. The instructions for the structure of these proteins are carried in the DNA molecules. This is the information transmitted as inherited traits. In specifying the sequence of amino acids that make up a protein, a sequence of either two or three contiguous nucleotides function as a code word or **codon** that identifies a specific amino acid. When amino acids, such as glycine, that are identified by only two nucleotides form part of the sequence, the identity of the third nucleotide becomes irrelevant. However, a third nucleotide is always present to maintain the sequence of triplets. There are also codons that specify the beginning and end of a sequence of amino acids.

The genetic code also must be transmitted from one generation to the next. In the germ cells or **gametes** (**ovum** and **sperm**), the cells divide by a special process called **meiosis** in such a way that the germ cell contains 23 chromosomes. It is called **haploid** because it has half the usual number of chromosomes. The process by which this is accomplished distinguishes meiosis from mitosis. In the first phase of meiosis, the original chromosomes replicate to create two chromatids that are joined at the centromere in the same fashion as in mitosis. However, the homologous pairs then become attached at their centromeres to form a **tetrad**. At this point, an interchange (**crossover**) can occur between the segments of one chromosome and the corresponding segments of the homologous chromosomes, resulting in new combinations so that the two chromatids of each chromosome are no longer identical. The chromatids of the homologous chromosomes are assorted randomly as these new chromosomes separate to form two new nuclei. This separation is the first meiotic division.

The time of the second meiotic division differs in the sperm and ovum. In the sperm, the sister chromatids separate, each forming two more nuclei with only half as many chromosomes. Since the chromatids are not identical, there are now four sperm cells, each with unique chromosomes. This process occurs prior to the fertilization of the ovum. The ovum, still containing 46 chromosomes, is fertilized after the first meiotic division by a sperm containing 23 chromosomes. The second meiotic division of the ovum occurs after fertilization and provides the 23 maternal chromosomes constituting the genetic inheritance of the new infant.

The units of heredity within the chromosomes are the **genes**, the part of the total DNA molecule that specifies the code for a given function (a structural protein or enzyme, for example). The position of a gene for a given trait is known as the **locus**. The genes for many traits exist in variant forms (**alleles**) that account for variation in a trait. Some traits have only one allele, but others have many. A simple example would be alleles for brown eyes and blue eyes. As described in Chapter 9, there are many alleles for histocompatibility. Although the general population may have many alleles for some traits, a given individual can have a maximum of two for any one trait, one from each parent.

The function of many genes, as described for DNA, is to specify the structure of a polypeptide. Genes sometimes work as a group. An **operon** is a group of structural genes that operate somewhat as a single unit and code for enzymes or other proteins. They usually lie adjacent to each other and are controlled as a unit. All cells of the body have the same genetic information. Therefore, following differentiation, much of the DNA code is silenced — that is, made nonfunctional — so that the cells can perform different functions. Thus, adjacent to the operon is an **operator gene**, which serves as an on-off switch for the operon, and a **regulator gene**, which may bind to the operator to turn it off.

Expression of the Genetic Code

Genotype and Phenotype

Each individual normally possesses two genes for each trait. If both genes for a given trait are identical, the person is **homozygous** for that trait but, if the alleles are different, the person is **heterozygous** for that trait. The genetic makeup of an individual is termed the **genotype**, and its visible expression is the **phenotype**. For example, if a person with brown eyes has one allele for brown eyes and one allele for blue eyes, these two alleles constitute the genotype, and the phenotype includes brown eyes. If a trait is expressed when it is present on only one of a pair of chromosomes, it is a **dominant** trait. If it is expressed only when present on both of the chromosomes (homozygous), it is a **recessive** trait. In the brown-eyed example used previously, there is a dominant gene for brown eyes and a recessive gene for blue eyes. Sometimes, the gene expression is intermediate between the forms of the traits specified by the allele (**incomplete dominance**), or two dominant alleles are fully expressed (**codominant**).

The relationship between genotype and phenotype is variable. Some genes have **incomplete penetrance** — that is, the allele is expressed in some individuals but not others, as in diabetes mellitus. Incomplete penetrance often is accompanied by **variable expressivity**, in which the trait may be expressed in somewhat different ways.

Some genes are **pleiotropic**; they affect several apparently unrelated aspects of the phenotype. In many cases, however, the affected aspects may indeed be related and may share some similar steps in their metabolism.

A single feature may be controlled by more than one gene pair and may also be influenced by the environment. For example, genetic effects on height sometimes are modified by diet. The expression of some genes is affected by the internal environment so that the trait is not expressed at birth but appears postnatally.

Sex-Linked Traits

An additional concept that must be understood is that of **sex-linked traits**. There are 22 homologous pairs of chromosomes known as **autosomes** present in both males and females. The 23rd pair (**sex chromosomes**) differ in males and females. Females have two X chromosomes, and males have one X chromosome and a much smaller Y chromosome. Females receive one X chromosome from each parent and provide an X chromosome to each offspring. Males receive an X chromosome from their mothers and a Y chromosome from their fathers. They provide an X chromosome to their daughters and a Y chromosome to their sons. Thus it is the father who determines the sex of the child.

The Y chromosome has no genes related to traits other than those involved in sex determination, but the X chromosome carries genes affecting other functions. The expression of these genes, called **sex-linked** or **X-linked** traits, may be different in the two sexes. Thus, there are four basic modes of inheriting single gene mutations in humans: **autosomal recessive, autosomal dominant, X-linked recessive,** and **X-linked dominant**.

Males are always **hemizygous** for the genes on the X chromosome, since they have only one X chromosome. A sex-linked allele that is recessive in the female will be expressed in the male, since there is no alternative allele. Also, a male can receive and transmit to his daughters a sex-linked trait that he received from his mother, but he cannot transmit it to his sons because the sons will not receive an X chromosome from him. However, he can pass X-linked traits to his grandsons through his daughters.

Since females have two X chromosomes, they may be homozygous or heterozygous for sex-linked traits. If they are heterozygous for a sex-linked recessive trait, they become **carriers** who do not exhibit the trait but can transmit it to half their offspring of either sex. Daughters express sex-linked recessive traits if a male who expresses the trait (their father) mates with a female homozygote (their mother). They may or may not express the trait if the mother is a carrier (heterozygote).

Mutations

Genes usually are very stable, but they can undergo **mutation**, an inheritable change in structure, so that a different allele is formed. We do not know all the causes of mutations, nor can we generally identify the cause of a specific mutation. We do know that X-radiation, ionizing radiation, and some chemicals are among their causes.

Mutations causing disorders of interest to nutritionists may be subdivided into two categories: chromosomal aberrations and point mutations. **Point mutations** involve only a small number of nucleotide pairs in the DNA molecule. The change may consist of insertion, deletion, or substitution of a base pair. Since the code for the amino acid structure of a polypeptide consists of sets of nucleotides, these shifts sometimes lead to the production of a new polypeptide. If the code for an amino acid is identified by the first two nucleotides, there is no effect of a mutational change in the third. This is known as a **silent mutation**. Many mutations are this type.

Approximately one-fourth of all mutations involving a substitution do cause changes in amino acid sequence (**missense mutations**). The severity of the effect depends on the function of the polypeptide whose structure has been altered. Initially, it was believed that one gene contained the code for one enzyme. Subsequently, it was found that this belief is not precisely accurate. Therefore, the concept has been changed to "**one gene, one polypeptide**." If an enzyme contains more than one chain, each of which is specified by a different gene, mutations of any of these genes have the potential to alter the activity of that enzyme. On the other hand, if a single chain has more than one active site and catalyzes more than one metabolic reaction, a single mutation would affect more than one enzyme action. Missense mutations may thus have effects of varying severity. The conditions discussed in this chapter are, in many cases, the consequences of this type of mutation, but are less severe than those that cause prenatal death.

In other cases, known as **no-sense mutations**, the codon for an amino acid might be mutated to a "stop" signal. Under these circumstances, the synthesis is stopped before the chain is completed, usually resulting in the complete absence of a trait (or enzyme). Deletion or insertion of a base also will cause a no-sense mutation because it will cause a shift in the whole sequence of triplets. No-sense mutations are, however, relatively rare.

Some conditions occur with a frequency that suggests they are the result of a combination of multiple gene mutations and environmental effects. Diabetes mellitus (Chapter 11) and cleft palate (Chapter 19) have been included in this category.

It is important to know the frequency with which a point mutation will be expressed in succeeding generations. This is particularly important when the mutation results in an adverse effect such as an inborn error of metabolism. When each parent carries an autosomal recessive trait, the probability that the trait will be expressed is the same for *each* pregnancy. Let us assume, as an example, that the mode of inheritance of an inborn error of metabolism from a given pair of parents carries the probability that there will be one affected child (homozygote), two carriers (heterozygotes), and one child who does not carry the trait. The probability that the child from the first pregnancy will have the disease is one in four. If the first child is a homozygote—that is, has the disease—there is no guarantee that the next three offspring from successive pregnancies will include one normal child and two carriers. Rather, in the second pregnancy (and all others), the probability that the child will be a homozygote is still one in four.

Chromosomal Abnormalities

Chromosomal abnormalities can have many effects because they affect many genes. They are of two general types: variations in the normal number of chromosomes or gross structural abnormalities of individual chromosomes. A fragment of a chromosome can become attached to another chromosome and thus become **translocated**. Sometimes a piece of a chromosome is **deleted**. Some deletion syndromes result in conditions described elsewhere in this book. They include cleft palate, low birth weight, seizures, failure-to-thrive, and congenital heart disease. A third type of chromosomal abnormality is an **inversion** in which two breaks occur in the structure of a chromosome. The free piece then is realigned after a 180-degree reversal of its orientation. Chromosomal abnormalities may lead to fetal death, various congenital malformations (most of which are associated with mental retardation), and, in some cases, to neoplasia.[1]

INTRODUCTION TO INBORN ERRORS OF METABOLISM

The concept that an abnormal gene could impair metabolism and produce a pathologic condition called an **inborn error of metabolism** was first introduced by Garrod[2] in 1908. These inborn errors of metabolism now are known to cause defects of structural proteins, transport proteins, functioning proteins, and proteins that regulate gene expression or gene repair.

In most of the conditions described in this chapter, there is a block in a metabolic pathway caused by a mutation in a single gene. Because one gene is supposed to control the synthesis of one polypeptide, a change in the gene structure could result in a change in the structure of that polypeptide and a consequent change in the activity of the protein product. The protein product may be an enzyme, and the condition is classified as an **enzyme defect**. More recently, **defects in transport** have also been recognized as a form of inborn error.

Pathophysiology

The pathophysiologic consequences of the product of a mutant gene depend on the normal metabolic role of the affected pathway.

In general, the causes of pathophysiologic effects are categorized as follows.[1]

Abnormal Enzyme Function in Major Metabolic Pathways

The generalized diagram of a metabolic pathway in Figure 17-1 illustrates the means by which a disorder may be produced. If we assume that the mutant gene product is an abnormal enzyme with reduced or absent activity resulting in a metabolic block in the major pathway, the consequences of such a metabolic block may include accumulation of a precursor to toxic levels, deficiency of an end product, production of toxic products from a normally minor pathway, and overproduction of intermediate products through loss of feedback control.

Accumulation of a Precursor to Toxic Levels. The most commonly described inborn error of metabolism is the accumulation of a precursor to toxic levels. If we assume, in Figure 17-1, that enzyme cd is missing and there is a block in the metabolic step from product C to product D, the immediate precursor, product C, or more remote precursors, A or B, might increase in concentration in body tissues. The means by which the toxic effects are produced frequently are unclear. If a substance that accumulates is relatively insoluble and difficult to excrete, it may be stored, producing one of the inborn errors known as **storage diseases**.

Deficiency of End Product. Sometimes a pathologic condition occurs because an essential end product is reduced in concentration. In our model (Figure 17-1), if product D is essential and there is no alternative pathway, a block at enzyme ab, bc, or cd would result in a deficiency of product D.

Production of Toxic By-products from a Normally Minor Pathway. In some disorders, the precursor in the major pathway is not the immediate cause of the disease. Instead, a minor pathway may become more

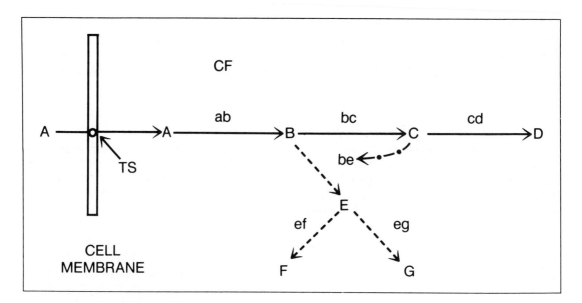

Figure 17-1. A model metabolic pathway. Substrates and metabolic products are indicated in capital letters. Enzymes are represented by lowercase letters corresponding to the substrate and product at their site of action. Solid arrows indicate the major pathway; broken lines, the minor pathways; and the line of dots and dashes, an example of feedback control. CF = cofactor; TS = transport system.

active, as a consequence of precursor accumulation, and produce large quantities of a material normally present in minute quantities. In Figure 17-1, let us assume that there is a block at bc or cd and product B accumulates. The pathways B→E→F, B→E→G, or both, might then become more active and possibly produce pathologic consequences.

Overproduction of Intermediate Products Through Loss of Feedback Control. A pathologic condition may result from a loss of feedback regulation when an essential end product is missing. For example, in our model, if product D in Figure 17-1 controls the production of product E, the absence of feedback control from product D might cause overproduction of product E, F, or G, with consequent pathologic effects.

Defective Plasma Membrane Transport

The transport of essential substances from outside to inside the cell is compromised in some inborn errors. There is some evidence, primarily in microbes, of the existence of permeases. Errors in permease activity might result in transport defects. In humans, most transport defects have been identified in the kidney tubules or intestinal absorptive cells, leading to decreased intestinal absorption, increased renal excretion, or both. Malfunction of the transport system (see Figure 17-1) could lead to a deficiency of any of the products, A, B, C, or D.

Reduced Coenzyme Production or Binding

Disorders related to reduced coenzyme production or binding have been called **vitamin-dependent inborn errors** or **vitamin dependency syndromes**. Theoretically, a very large number of disorders is possible. However, very few are understood completely. It has been suggested that defects in production or binding of cofactors might result from (1) failure to transport the vitamin into certain cells, (2) failure to produce the coenzyme from the vitamin, or (3) failure to bind the cofactor to the apoenzyme to form the active enzyme.[1] In some cases, vitamins or coenzymes in larger than normal quantities may stabilize and increase the activity or concentrations of affected enzymes and prevent the adverse effects which would otherwise result from a metabolic block. Because cofactors function with many apoenzymes, their defects affect many reactions and thereby alter many functions.

Deficiency or Abnormality of Circulating Proteins

A variety of protein materials that circulate in blood cause disease when their concentration or structure and function are altered. Very few of these diseases are amenable to dietary manipulation.

Abnormality of Structural Protein

Genetic abnormalities of collagen-related protein have been associated with metabolic disease. Most abnormalities of this type are not amenable to specific dietary treatment; however, some cause organ dysfunction that requires nutritional care. One such abnormality of collagen-related material causes kidney failure.

Abnormalities of Enzymes That Regulate Drug Metabolism

Abnormalities of enzymes that regulate drug metabolism are expressed only if a patient is exposed to the drug in question. Generally, such disorders are not treated with diet, although a large dose of vitamin B_6 is useful in some patients receiving isoniazid.

Clinical Manifestations

Some inborn errors of metabolism are lethal, whereas others cause varying degrees of incapacitation, and still others are benign. In general, if an infant shows unexplained failure-to-thrive (see Chapter 19), vomiting, feeding difficulties, lethargy, coma, acidosis, jaundice, hepatomegaly, irritability, or hy-

peractivity, inborn errors must be considered in the differential diagnosis.

The more specific consequences of an inborn error will vary not only with the type of defect, but also with the degree of impairment. Some patients have variants of the classic disease, and the consequences of these variants differ in severity from those of the classic disease. The consequences of a metabolic disorder can sometimes be moderated by appropriate treatment, especially if the disease is diagnosed early. It is important to begin treatment early in most types of treatable inborn errors of metabolism. The central nervous system of the newborn infant is very vulnerable to damage, and many inborn errors, if untreated, can result in mental retardation. The consequences of individual disorders will be described later in this chapter. In some disorders, there is no known method of treatment.

Diagnosis

Most inborn errors of metabolism are not accompanied by pathognomonic symptoms, and thus a variety of diagnostic procedures are necessary to identify specific errors. Genetic screening (the search in the population for certain genotypes) can be used to detect certain inborn errors. In most developed countries, for example, it is common practice to screen all neonates for phenylketonuria. Other conditions are so rare or their consequences so mild that mass screening is not considered to be cost-effective. In others, adequate screening methods are lacking.

The general types of diagnostic tests used include biochemical analysis of blood, urine, other body fluids, or tissue samples obtained by biopsy. Concentrations of normal substrates, metabolites, or products may be identified as being abnormally high or abnormally low, or the presence of unusual substrates may be detected. In other assays, enzyme activity is determined. Variants of normal proteins sometimes are identified by electrophoresis, enzyme kinetics, or alterations in such properties as response to heat, pH, substrates, inhibitors, or cofactors. Other recent methods include tissue cultures of fibroblasts, blood cells, and cells in the amniotic fluid.

These methods as well as others sometimes are used to identify heterozygote carriers. Many inborn errors are autosomal recessive traits, and the trait can be detected by diagnostic tests. If carriers can be identified, the incidence of the disease can sometimes be reduced by genetic counseling. In addition, if heterozygote carrier parents can be identified, the disease can sometimes be diagnosed before the child is born. **Amniocentesis** (sampling of cells from amniotic fluid) is used for prenatal detection of some inborn errors. This procedure carries some risk but may be necessary in families in which the trait is known to exist. The risk is especially justified in diseases in which early diagnosis and treatment can prevent severe physiologic consequences, impaired growth, and mental retardation.

Management

General Principles of Prevention and Management

The types of treatment available for inborn errors of metabolism depend to some extent on our knowledge of the pathologic processes involved. In some diseases, little is known about these processes, and management must be limited to rehabilitation or to genetic counseling to reduce incidence.

When the impaired metabolic pathway is known, other possibilities exist. It is for this group of patients that nutritional care often is important. The general types of procedures might include the following:

1. For accumulation of precursor to toxic levels: restrict source of the precursor.
2. For deficiency of end product: provide replacement.
3. For production of toxic by-product: restrict source of its precursor.
4. For diseases involving sensitivity to environmental factors (e.g., drugs): avoid exposure.

5. For deficient coenzymes: give increased quantities of the vitamin involved.

In some disorders, the specific product of a defective gene, whether an enzyme, a structural protein or a regulator, is known and influences possible treatment. For instance, if an enzyme is deficient, it might be replaced. One such disorder is cystic fibrosis of the pancreas (see Chapter 8), for which replacement of pancreatic enzymes is a common method of treatment. The number of disorders that can be treated in this way is very limited, however. If the defective gene affects regulation, replacement of the missing repressor, inducer, or inhibitor is a theoretical approach to treatment; currently, though, this is seldom possible and is the subject of ongoing research. The production of abnormal structural proteins can sometimes be prevented, or its consequences can be treated with drugs.

Another area of ongoing research involves genetic engineering to "repair" a defective gene. This approach could be applied only if the specific mutation is known. In some disorders, organ transplants are useful.

Principles of Nutritional Management

Inborn errors that respond to alterations in diet, although relatively few in number, are of particular interest to the nutritional care specialist and provide an opportunity to perform an important service. Proper nutritional management of some of these disorders is sometimes lifesaving and sometimes prevents profound mental retardation.

From the foregoing discussion, it is clear that approaches to nutritional management include (1) restriction of sources of accumulated products, or their precursors or by-products, (2) replacement of end products, or (3) increased vitamin dosage.

In some inborn errors, it is necessary to restrict severely the intake of certain nutrients. If the adverse effect is the result of accumulation of a nonessential nutrient, such as galactose or fructose, the offending material might be eliminated from the diet. If the nutrient occurs widely in food, the patient or family will need counseling on sources of that nutrient, substitute foods, and menu planning to assure nutritional adequacy.

On the other hand, if the disease requires the restriction of an essential nutrient, the process consists of restriction of that nutrient to the level of minimum requirements and becomes more hazardous and complex. Disorders of amino acid metabolism are good examples of this type of problem. The amino acid must be provided in amounts necessary for normal growth and development and the maintenance of essential metabolic processes, but an excess must be avoided. In addition, essential end products, if deficient as a result of the metabolic block, must be provided. Thus the patient is walking a fine line between excess and deficiency.

There are two general methods by which adequate but not excessive administration of amino acids can be achieved. In some disorders, total protein intake can be reduced to minimal levels with an increase in nonprotein energy sources. Alternatively, if natural proteins contain an excess of the offending amino acid, a semisynthetic formula with reduced amounts of the offending substrate may be used. These formulas are either protein hydrolysates from which the amino acid in question has been removed or mixtures of pure amino acids. Most of them contain added carbohydrate, fat, vitamins, and minerals to provide adequate nutrition.

The length of time that a child may need a restricted diet varies. If the primary adverse consequence is impaired myelination of the brain, the diet may be liberalized or may become unnecessary once myelination is complete. In other disorders, the diet is needed for a lifetime.

The tolerance of the patient for an offending amino acid can vary with the circumstances. In diseases in which products of amino acid metabolism tend to accumulate, the patient will have the greatest tolerance for natural protein during periods of rapid growth and when the nutritional status is optimum. In these circumstances, much protein is being used for synthesis, preventing accumulation of toxic metabolites. If, on the other hand, the use of the offending amino acid for growth is impaired by illness or lack of other essential nutrients, the load on the affected degradative pathway is increased, and a toxic metabolite is more likely to accumulate. Therefore, the maintenance of optimum nutrition is highly desirable.

The daily requirements for various nutrients in infancy and childhood are given in Table 17-2. The nutritional care specialist must be familiar with these requirements that serve as guidelines in assessing nutritional adequacy and planning diets for patients with inborn errors to assure normal growth and physical and mental development.

DISORDERS OF AMINO ACID METABOLISM

Of the inborn errors of metabolism that are amenable to nutritional management, errors of amino acid metabolism, particularly those involving essential amino acids, are among those that occur most commonly. Nutritional management requires careful continuing cooperation of the nutritional care specialist and the patient, his or her family members (especially parents), teachers, and others. In many disorders of amino acid metabolism, failure of nutritional management can have devastating consequences.

The Hyperphenylalaninemias

Phenylalanine is essential for growth, and in children 50% to 60% of dietary phenylalanine is used in formation of new tissue. This amount decreases with age to about 10% in adults.[3,4] The remainder of the dietary phenylalanine is the subject of concern in these conditions because it is the accumulation of this material that leads to the disease manifestations.

The **hyperphenylalaninemias** are a group of disorders that manifest themselves by abnormally high blood levels of phenylalanine. One of these, **phenylketonuria**

Table 17-2. Approximate Daily Requirements for Various Nutrients at Different Ages in Infancy and Childhood

Nutrient	Unit of Measure	0–2 Months	2–5 Months	6–12 Months	1–2 Years	2–3 Years	3–4 Years	4–6 Years	6–8 Years	8–10 Years
Calories[a]	kcal	120/kg	110/kg	100/kg	1,100	1,250	1,400	1,600	2,000	2,200
Volume (H$_2$O)	ml	100/kg	110/kg	100/kg	1,100	1,250	1,400	1,600	2,000	2,200
Carbohydrate[b]	g					Total kilocalories × 0.50 ÷ 4				
Protein[c]										
Infants	g/kg	1.8–2.2	1.8–2.0	1.8						
Children	g/day				25	25	30	30	35	40
Fat	g					Total kilocalories × 0.35 ÷ 9				
Sodium	mEq/kg	3	3	3	3	3	3	3	3	3
Potassium	mEq/kg	3	3	3	3	3	3	3	3	3
Calcium	mg	400	500	600	700	800	800	800	800	800
Phosphorus	mg	200	400	500	700	800	800	800	900	1,000
Magnesium	mg	40	60	70	100	150	200	200	250	250
Iron	mg	6	10	15	15	15	10	10	10	10
Iodine	μg	25	40	45	55	60	70	80	100	110
Phenylalanine										
Infants	mg/kg	47–90	47–90	25–47						
Children[d]	mg/day				200–500	200–500	200–500	200–500	200–500	200–500
Histidine	mg/kg	16–34	16–34	16–34						
Leucine										
Infants	mg/kg	76–150	76–150	76–150						
Children	mg/day				750–1,000	750–1,000	750–1,000	750–1,000	750–1,000	750–1,000
Isoleucine										
Infants	mg/kg	79–110	79–110	50–75						
Children	mg/day				500–750	500–750	500–750	500–750	500–750	500–750
Valine										
Infants	mg/kg	65–105	65–105	50–80						
Children	mg/day				400–600	400–600	400–600	400–600	400–600	400–600
Methionine[e]										
Infants	mg/kg	20–45	20–45	20–45						
Children	mg/day				400–800	400–800	400–800	400–800	400–800	400–800
Cyst(e)ine[f]										
Infants	mg/kg	15–50	15–50	15–50						
Children	mg/day				400–800	400–800	400–800	400–800	400–800	400–800

Nutrient	Units									
Lysine										
Infants	mg/kg	90–120	90–120	90–120						
Children	mg/day				1,200–1,600	1,200–1,600	1,200–1,600	1,200–1,600	1,200–1,600	1,200–1,600
Threonine										
Infants	mg/kg	45–87	45–87	45–87						
Children	mg/day				800–1,000	800–1,000	800–1,000	800–1,000	800–1,000	800–1,000
Tryptophan										
Infants	mg/kg	13–22	13–22	13–22						
Children	mg/day				60–120	60–120	60–120	60–120	60–120	60–120
Vitamin B_1 (thiamine)	μg	200	400	500	600	600	700	800	1,000	1,100
Vitamin B_2 (riboflavin)	μg	400	500	600	600	700	800	900	1,100	1,200
Vitamin B_6 (pyridoxine)	μg	200	300	400	500	600	700	900	1,100	1,200
Vitamin B_{12}	μg	1.0	1.5	2.0	2.0	2.5	3.0	4.0	4.0	5.0
Folic acid	μg	50	50	100	100	200	200	200	200	300
Niacin	mg	5	7	8	8	8	9	11	13	15
Vitamin C	mg	35	35	35	40	40	40	40	40	40
Vitamin A	IU	1,500	1,500	1,500	2,000	2,000	2,500	2,500	3,500	3,500
Vitamin D	IU	400	400	400	400	400	400	400	400	400
Vitamin E	IU	5	5	5	10	10	10	15	15	15

Reprinted with permission from the American Academy of Pediatrics Committee on Nutrition, Special diets for infants with inborn errors of amino acid metabolism. *Pediatrics* 57:786, 1976. Copyright the American Academy of Pediatrics, 1976.

a The caloric requirement is increased when protein is provided as a mixture of the corresponding free L-amino acids.

b Minimum fraction is 50% of total calories; optimum value is given.

c Minimum fraction is 4% of total calories; optimum value is given.

d More phenylalanine (>800 mg) is required in the absence of tyrosine.

e More methionine is required in the absence of cyst(e)ine.

f More cyst(e)ine is required in the presence of a blocked transsulfuration outflow pathway for methionine metabolism.

Note: These data are compiled from National Academy of Sciences/National Research Council data on Recommended Dietary Allowances (RDA) and from amino acid data of Holt and Snyderman (Holt, L.E., and Snyderman, S.E.: The amino acid requirements of infants. *J.A.M.A.* 175:100, 1961; and The amino acid requirements of children. In W.L. Nyhan, Ed., *Amino Acid Metabolism and Genetic Variation.* New York: McGraw-Hill, 1967). These dietary RDA have the limitations of any statement of dietary requirement because of the individual variations a physician will encounter in working with a patient. This limitation is particularly true with amino acid requirements for which amounts in excess of the requirement are toxic. There is limited information on amino acid requirements of infants and children at different ages; the figures given here are in excess of the minimum requirements. Consequently, this table should be used only as a guide and should not be regarded as an authoritative statement to which individual patients must conform.

(PKU), was discovered by Folling,[5] who found phenylpyruvic acid in the urine of two mentally retarded children. A number of variant forms of PKU have also been identified. Each of these forms involves a defect in the conversion of phenylalanine to tyrosine.

Classic Phenylketonuria

Metabolic Abnormalities. The biochemical defect in classic PKU, or **type I hyper-**

phenylalaninemia, is a deficit of liver **phenylalanine hydroxylase**, the enzyme that catalyzes the conversion of phenylalanine to tyrosine (Figure 17-2). Oxygen, tetrahydrobiopterin reductase, and NADH + H$^+$ also participate in this pathway.

In classic PKU, the enzyme activity is less than 2% of normal.[3] Normal levels are <2 mg/dl (120 μmol/L), but levels may rise to 20 mg/dl (1,200 μmol/L) in classic PKU. As a consequence, there is an accumulation of phenylalanine in body fluids.

As the blood phenylalanine concentration rises, the activity of alternative pathways increases (see Figure 17-2). The increased concentration of the substrate induces the action of phenylalanine transaminase and increases phenylpyruvic acid production.

Figure 17-2. Sites of metabolic blocks in phenylalanine and tyrosine metabolism. **A.** *Phenylketonuria.* **B.** *Dihydropteridine reductase deficiency.* **C.** *Tyrosinemia, type 2.* **D.** *Neonatal tyrosinemia and hereditary (type 1) tyrosinemia.* **E.** *Alkaptonuria.* **F.** *Tyrosinemia.*

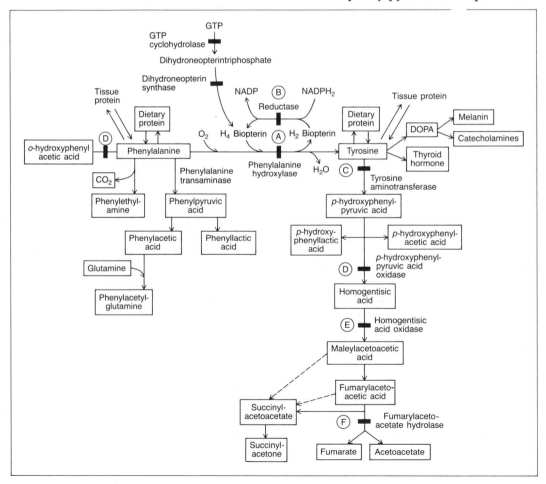

The phenylpyruvic acid then is converted to phenyllactic and phenylacetic acids and phenylacetylglutamine. These are found in increased quantities in the urine. Thus PKU is an example of a disorder in which precursors accumulate and in which there is enhanced activity in minor metabolic pathways.

Excess phenylalanine also affects the metabolism of other amino acids. The absorption of tryptophan from the intestine is inhibited by phenylalanine. Bacterial action on the tryptophan in the intestine increases production of indoleacetic and indolelactic acids from tryptophan. These are absorbed and excreted in increased quantities in the urine. The concentration of blood serotonin, a metabolite of tryptophan, is decreased, and the excretion of 5-hydroxyindoleacetic acid, the metabolite of serotonin, is decreased secondarily.

Tyrosine becomes an essential amino acid for PKU patients, because they cannot form tyrosine from phenylalanine. In addition, tyrosine metabolism is inhibited by the presence of excess phenylalanine. The production of tyrosine metabolites, such as melanin, epinephrine, and thyroxin, thus are reduced.

Clinical Manifestations. The phenylketonuric infant generally is considered to be mentally normal at birth, since appropriate postnatal treatment results in normal mental development. However, some effects may occur before birth. A study of a group of infants with PKU showed lower birth weights, increased numbers of premature births, and perinatal difficulties.[1] Therefore, the prenatal effects deserve further study.

The postnatal consequences of PKU have deservedly received much more attention, since the untreated disease has a devastating effect on the central nervous system. The most severe consequence is impaired mental development, and it has been estimated that an untreated phenylketonuric infant can lose 50 IQ points in its first year. Most untreated patients eventually have an IQ of about 20,

and only a few have an IQ higher than 60 (on a scale in which normal is approximately 100). Many require institutionalization.

The effect on the brain in an untreated phenylketonuric infant becomes particularly noticeable at four to six months of age. Some behavioral and neurologic manifestations such as hyperactivity, feeding difficulties, and vomiting occur within the first three months but may be mistaken for other disorders. The condition progresses to listlessness and apathy, or it may include psychotic behavior and hyperactivity. Patients may have muscle tremors and later develop an abnormal gait and posture. Approximately one in four patients has convulsions.

The cause of mental retardation in PKU is not completely understood. The brain is smaller, and myelination is deficient. It has been suggested that the brain damage could be the consequence of lack of the phenylalanine or tyrosine needed for protein synthesis, the action of phenylalanine catabolites, the lack of tyrosine by-products, or a combination of these.[6,7]

The reduced production of melanin and the consequent deficiency of melanin pigment in the skin, hair, and eyes causes the child to be fairer in coloration than the rest of the family. Many phenylketonuric patients have a mousy or musty odor that has been attributed to phenylacetic acid in the urine and perspiration. Some patients have eczema of unknown origin. Other manifestations of classic PKU include **microcephaly** (a small head in proportion to body size) and reduced life expectancy, possibly related to institutionalization.

The consequences of PKU can be considerably moderated and, in some cases, entirely avoided if treatment is begun in the early postnatal period, ideally in the first two weeks. If this is done, the patient should grow and develop normally both mentally and physically. Failure to institute treatment in the first few weeks postnatally is likely to lead to brain damage and mental retardation. The brain damage is irreversible, but other biochemical and clinical manifestations subside to some degree if the child is treated later.

Heredity and Incidence. Phenylketonuria is inherited as an autosomal recessive trait, and classic PKU occurs in homozygotes for the trait. Therefore, the parents are assumed to be heterozygous carriers. The incidence of hyperphenylalaninemia varies. It is highest in Germany, Belgium, Scotland, Ireland, Czechoslovakia, and Poland and lowest in Finland and Japan. Incidence in the United States is intermediate, approximately 1 in 11,000 live births, and similar to that seen in Australia, Austria, Denmark, and England.

Diagnosis and Monitoring. Because the consequences of untreated PKU are so serious, most states now require testing of neonatal infants to detect PKU. The normal infant has a serum phenylalanine level of less than 2 mg/dl. A test result of 4 mg/dl or higher must be investigated further. If serum phenylalanine is 20 mg/dl or more and serum tyrosine is normal (1 to 4 mg/dl), treatment is begun immediately.

Several types of diagnostic tests have been used. For years, a commonly used test consisted of the reaction between ferric chloride and phenylpyruvic acid in the infant's urine to form a green color. Ferric chloride (in the form of Phenistix) or 2,4-dinitrophenylhydrazine (DPNH) may be used at home to detect phenylpyruvic acid and is useful for monitoring identified cases. These tests give a general guide to the effectiveness of treatment. However, they have serious disadvantages for use in initial diagnosis, because they are not specific for phenylpyruvic acid but will react with other compounds, and some metabolites interfere with the reaction. Also, they are not sufficiently sensitive, and appreciable brain damage may occur if treatment is delayed owing to false-negative results in these tests.

More recently developed methods for measuring serum phenylalanine are preferable for diagnosis. The **Guthrie bacterial in-**hibition assay uses a drop of blood obtained by heel prick and can detect phenylalanine levels greater than 4 mg/dl of whole blood. The blood on the filter paper is applied to the surface of agar containing the organism *Bacillus subtilis* and **beta-2-thienylalanine**, a phenylalanine antagonist. High levels of phenylalanine will overwhelm the action of the antagonist, allowing the organism to grow at a rate proportionate to the phenylalanine concentration. Alternatively, the blood sample can be eluted from the filter paper and the phenylalanine level measured by a photofluorometric assay.

Newborn infants with blood phenylalanine concentrations of 4 to 8 mg/dl must be retested immediately. With earlier discharges of infants from the nursery after birth, phenylalanine concentrations of 2 to 4 mg/dl are often considered positive. These infants should also be retested.

When the screening test indicates phenylalanine above 8 mg/dl, quantitative determinations of serum phenylalanine and its metabolites and of tyrosine (<50 μmol/dl) should be done promptly. High levels of plasma phenylalanine, low levels of plasma tyrosine, and the presence of *o*-hydroxyphenylacetic acid in the urine are pathognomonic for PKU.

The blood phenylalanine concentration rises postnatally as the infant is fed protein containing excess phenylalanine. Thus it is important that the test not be done too early. It is estimated that 5% of cases are missed because of inadequate protein feeding prior to the test.

The general criteria for diagnosing classic PKU are (1) two measurements, 24 hours apart, of phenylalanine greater than 20 mg/dl when dietary intake of phenylalanine is normal; (2) tyrosine <5 mg/dl and failure of plasma tyrosine to rise after loading with phenylalanine; and (3) presence of metabolic excretion products of phenylalanine in the urine.[8]

Nutritional Management. Experience in recent years has demonstrated normal mental and physical development in patients with classic PKU if they are managed properly with low-phenylalanine diets. Although there is some disagreement as to the length of time that the diet is required and a few untreated phenylketonuric individuals have normal intelligence, a large body of evidence now supports the use of the phenylalanine-restricted diet indefinitely.[8]

Excess phenylalanine must be avoided, but the minimum requirement must be provided in carefully measured quantities since it is an essential amino acid. Care must also be taken to assure intake of enough phenylalanine and other nutrients to avoid tissue catabolism. If the patient is undernourished and tissue is catabolized, phenylalanine is released, with possible subsequent brain damage.[9,10] Therefore, the objectives of nutritional management of PKU patients are

1. To supply an adequate diet to support normal growth rate.
2. To supply sufficient phenylalanine for protein synthesis.
3. To avoid excessive phenylalanine that would lead to elevated concentrations in the blood.

Blood levels should be maintained as close to normal (50 μmol) as possible.

When the diagnosis is made, the blood phenylalanine level should be lowered rapidly, but with care to avoid phenylalanine deficiency, by feeding a low phenylalanine or phenylalanine-free formula. This is done more rapidly, often in three days, if the infant is hospitalized so that the patient can be monitored frequently. In nonhospitalized patients, the approach must be more cautious and may take up to ten days. The blood phenylalanine concentrations should be under control by three weeks of age.[4]

For long-term care, guidelines for approximate daily intakes of phenylalanine, tyrosine, protein, and energy are given in Table 17-3. In infants, the larger amounts in the range given are used earlier in the age range during the time that growth is more rapid.

Infants with PKU usually are bottle-fed, but they may be breast-fed if great care is taken. They must be given tyrosine as a supplement, since tyrosine is an essential amino acid in PKU. Some tyrosine will be present in the food the patient eats. An additional 20–35 mg/kg/day is needed to provide a total of 120–150 mg/kg/day.

Natural foods offer variety but also are sources of phenylalanine. Thus their use is limited by the need to limit phenylalanine intake. As a consequence, a formula free of or low in phenylalanine is used to help meet the child's nutritional requirements. If too much or too little phenylalanine is present, protein metabolism may be inefficient and may interfere with normal growth and development.

Steps in planning a phenylalanine-restricted diet. Steps in planning a phenylalanine-re-

Table 17-3. *Approximate Recommended Daily Intakes of Phenylalanine, Tyrosine, Protein, and Energy in Phenylketonuria*

Age (years)	Phenylalanine (mg/kg/day)	Tyrosine (mg/kg/day)	Protein (g/kg/day)	Energy (kcal/kg/day)
0.0–0.5	70–20	80–60	2.2–2.5	120–110
0.5–1	50–15	60–40	2.0–2.5	120–100
1–3	40–15	60–30	1.8–2.0	100–90
4–6	35–15	50–25	1.5–1.8	90–80
7–10	30–15	40–20	1.2–1.5	85–80
11–14	30–15	30–15	1.0–1.2	70–60
15–18	30–10	30–10	0.8–1.0	60–40

Based on data from Berry, H.K., Hyperphenylalaninemias and tyrosinemias. *Clin. Perinatal.* 3:15, 1976; Elsas, L.J., II, and Acosta, P.B., Nutritional support of inherited metabolic disease. In M.E. Shils and V.R. Young, *Modern Nutrition in Health and Disease,* 7th ed. Philadelphia: Lea & Febiger, 1988; and Acosta, P.B. et al. *Microcomputers in Nutrition Support of Genetic Disease.* Tallahassee: Florida State University, 1984.

Table 17-4. Composition of Phenylalanine-Low and -Free Formula Products (per 100 g of product)

Nutrients	Analog XP[a]	Lofenalac[b]	Maxamaid XP[a]	Maxamum XP[a]	Phenyl-Free[b]	PKU 1[c]	PKU 2[c]	PKU 3[c]
Energy (kcal)	475	460	350	340	406	278	298	286
Carbohydrate (g)	59.0[d]	60.0[e]	62.0[f]	45.0[f]	66.0[e,f]	19.3[f]	7.6[f]	3.4[f]
Fat (g)	20.9	18.0[g]	0	0	6.8[h]	0	0	0
Protein equivalent (g)	13.00[i]	15.0[i]	25.0[i]	39.0[i]	20.3[i]	50.3[i]	66.8[i]	68.0[i]
Alanine (g)	0.58	0.68	1.03	1.60	0	2.40	3.10	3.10
Arginine (g)	1.03	0.56	2.21	3.02	0.69	2.00	2.70	2.70
Aspartic acid (g)	0.96	1.40	1.85	2.81	5.30	5.70	7.60	7.60
Carnitine (g)	0.095	Added	0	0.02	0	0	0	0
Cystine (g)	0.38	0.06	0.71	1.11	0.35	1.40	1.80	1.80
Glutamic acid (g)	1.17	4.00	2.40	4.56	6.70	12.00	16.00	16.00
Glutamine (g)	0.11	?	0.22	0.34	0	0	0	0
Glycine (g)	0.90	0.38	1.77	2.82	3.30	1.40	1.80	1.80
Histidine (g)	0.59	0.49	1.27	1.71	0.47	1.40	1.80	1.80
Isoleucine (g)	0.90	0.87	1.70	2.66	1.10	3.40	4.50	4.50
Leucine (g)	1.55	1.70	2.91	4.56	1.71	5.70	7.60	7.60
Lysine (g)	1.05	1.66	2.22	3.49	1.87	4.00	5.40	5.40
Methionine (g)	0.25	0.55	0.48	0.73	0.63	1.40	1.80	1.80
Phenylalanine (g)	0	0.075	0	0	20	0	0	0
Proline (g)	1.10	1.42	2.05	3.23	0	5.40	7.10	7.10
Serine (g)	0.67	0.94	1.26	1.99	0	3.00	4.00	4.00
Taurine (g)	0.19	0.027	0	0.13	0	0	0	0
Threonine (g)	0.76	0.79	1.42	2.23	0.93	2.70	3.60	3.60
Tryptophan (g)	0.30	0.20	0.57	0.89	0.28	1.00	1.40	1.40
Tyrosine (g)	1.37	0.80	2.56	4.03	0.93	3.40	4.50	6.00
Valine (g)	0.99	1.38	1.85	2.92	1.26	4.00	5.40	5.40
Minerals								
Calcium (mg)	325	434	810	670	508	2,400	1,312	1,312
Chloride (mEq)	8.0	9.2	12.9	16.0	26.7	47.1	28.2	28.2
Chromium (µg)	15	?	0	50	0	0	0	0
Copper (mg)	0.4	0.4	2.0	1.4	0.6	6.7	2.0	3.6
Iodine (µg)	47	32	134	107	45	234	120	143
Iron (mg)	7.0	8.7	12.0	23.5	12.2	34.0	15.0	21.0

Nutrient							
Magnesium (mg)	34	50	200	285	152	521	156	536
Manganese (mg)	0.6	0.14	1.30	1.7	1.02	2.40	0.70	4.8
Molybdenum (μg)	35.00	?	60.0	110	0	107.00	32.00	476
Phosphorus (mg)	230	324	810	670	508	1,860	1,014	1,014
Potassium (mEq)	10.8	12.1	21.5	17.9	35.1	59.8	34.1	34.1
Selenium (μg)	15	?	0	50	6.1	0	0	0
Sodium (mEq)	5.3	9.4	25.2	24.3	17.7	46.4	27.8	27.8
Zinc (mg)	5.0	3.6	13.0	13.6	7.1	26.0	7.8	23.8
Vitamins								
Vitamin A (μg)	530	432	300	705	366	2,800	1,560	1,190
D (μg)	8.5	7.2	12.0	8.0	3.8	25.0	33.0	12.0
E (mg)	4.9	14.4	6.5	7.8	9.2	34	18.0	12.0
K (μg)	21	72	0	70	102	167	167	167
Ascorbic acid (mg)	40	37	135	90	53	234	80	100
Biotin (mg)	0.026	0.036	0.12	0.140	0.030	0.100	0.300	0.179
B_6 (mg)	0.52	0.29	1.00	2.1	0.9	2.20	1.50	3.2
B_{12} (μg)	1.25	1.4	4.0	4.0	2.5	7.9	3.0	5.0
Choline (mg)	50	61	110	320	85	434	261	261
Folate (μg)	38	72	150	500	127	340	400	952
Inositol (mg)	100	22	56	86	30	500	300	300
Niacin, preformed (mg)	4.5	5.8	12.0	13.6	8.1	54.0	24.0	18.0
Pantothenic acid (mg)	2.65	2.2	3.7	5.0	3.0	25.0	11.0	8.3
Riboflavin (mg)	0.60	0.3	1.20	1.4	1.0	4.00	2.00	1.8
Thiamine (mg)	0.50	0.36	1.08	1.4	0.6	2.70	1.40	1.8

Compiled from Elsas, L.J., II, and Acosta, P.B., Nutrition support of inherited metabolic diseases. In M.E. Shils and V.R. Young, Eds., *Modern Nutrition in Health and Disease*, 7th ed. Philadelphia: Lea & Febiger, 1988; Committee on Nutrition, American Academy of Pediatrics, Special diets for infants with inborn errors of amino acid metabolism. *Pediatrics* 57:583, 1976; and Acosta, P.B. et al., *Microcomputers in Nutritional Support of Genetic Disease*. Tallahassee: Florida State University, 1984.

[a] Ross Laboratories.
[b] Mead Johnson.
[c] Milupa.
[d] Maltodextrins + galactose.
[e] Corn syrup solids + tapioca starch.
[f] Sucrose.
[g] Corn oil.
[h] Corn oil + coconut oil.
[i] Free L-amino acids.
[j] Casein hydrolysate + free L-amino acids.

stricted diet are described in detail and will serve as a model for planning nutritional management of other inborn errors described later in this chapter.[11]

Step 1: Use Table 17-3 to *compute the daily requirement for protein, phenylalanine, and energy.* For example, let us assume the patient is a six-month-old infant weighing 7 kg, with a good control of serum phenylalanine and normal growth and development, with 30 mg of phenylalanine, 2.5 g of protein, and 110 kcal/kg body weight in the diet. The total daily requirements would then be

Phenylalanine requirement: 30 mg/kg × 7 kg = 210 mg

Protein requirement: 2.5 mg/kg × 7 kg = 17.5 g

Energy requirement: 110 kcal × 7 kg = 770 kcal

Adjustments in these values must be made frequently, sometimes weekly, as the child grows.

Step 2: Calculate the amount of low-phenylalanine powdered formula required to meet 80–90% of the daily protein requirement. Most of the protein must be derived from this source, since natural foods, which may serve as protein sources, contain too much phenylalanine. Compositions of low-phenylalanine formulas generally available in the United States are given in Table 17-4. The ages for which each is designed are given in Table 17-5. However, the following differences must be considered:
1. Lofenalac and PKU 1 are intended for in-

fants. Lofenalac is a "complete" formula, but a fat source and extra carbohydrate must be added to PKU 1.
2. For children, Phenyl-Free is a "complete" formula (without phenylalanine). It may be used to adulthood. PKU 2 is intended for use from 1 year of age to adolescence, and PKU 3, from adolescence to adulthood. A fat source must be added and extra carbohydrate may be needed. Maxamaid XP is intended for ages 2 to 8 years. A fat source must be added. Carbohydrate and vitamin K may be needed. It is orange-flavored. Maxamum XP is intended for use from age 8 to adulthood. A fat source must be added. Extra carbohydrate may be needed. It is available plain or orange-flavored.
3. For pregnancy, PKU 3 and Maxamum XP are available. Vitamin and mineral supplements may be necessary.

In the example of the calculation, Lofenalac will be used because it was the first to be available and thus has "seniority." The general procedure in calculation is the same if the other products are used.

The calculation should be as follows: Protein to be derived from Lofenalac:

80% of 17.5 = 14 g

Thus the amount of Lofenalac needed is 14.0 g of protein divided by 1.4 g/Tbsp. or 10.0 Tbsp. (10 "measures"). A measuring device is included in the container and holds 1 Tbsp. or 10 g.

Step 3: Calculate the amount of evapo-

Table 17-5. Reduced Phenylalanine Formulas for Varying Patient Ages

Patient Age	Manufacturer		
	Ross	Mead Johnson	Milupa
Infant	Analog XP	Lofenalac	PKU 1
Child, age 2–8	Maxamaid XP	Phenyl-Free	PKU 2
Child, 8 years to adolescence	Maxamum XP	Phenyl-Free	PKU 2
Adolescent	Maxamum XP		PKU 3
Pregnancy	Maxamum XP		PKU 3

rated milk to be added to provide enough phenylalanine for growth. The relevant nutritive values for evaporated milk or alternatives are given in Table 17-6.

Again using our example of a six-month-old, 7-kg infant, the amount of evaporated milk may be calculated as follows:

Phenylalanine in Lofenalac = 10 Tbsp. × 7.5 mg/Tbsp. = 75 mg
Phenylalanine to be provided from milk or other sources = 210 mg − 75 mg = 135 mg
Therefore, add 1 oz. evaporated milk × 104 mg/oz. = 104 mg

The calculated amount of milk is mixed with Lofenalac so that the child does not develop a taste for milk.

The remaining amount of phenylalanine will be provided by solid foods (see Step 5).

Step 4: Calculate the amount of fluid needed including that mixed with the Lofenalac powder. The amount varies with age and preference.

Let us assume that the fluid requirement of our hypothetical infant is 100 ml/kg.

Thirty ml equals approximately 1 oz. Then:

$$100 \times 7 \text{ kg} = 700 \text{ ml}$$

$$\frac{700 \text{ ml}}{30 \text{ ml/oz.}} = 23.3 \text{ oz. of fluid, which may be rounded to 24 oz.}$$

The Lofenalac and evaporated milk are diluted, and the mixture can be made up to a total volume of 24 oz. The number of formula feedings and the size appropriate for various ages are given in Appendix K. For the

Table 17-6. Phenylalanine, Tyrosine, Protein, and Energy Content of Selected Food Groups

Food Group	Phenylalanine (mg)	Tyrosine (mg)	Protein (g)	Energy (kcal)
Evaporated milk, 1 oz.	104		2.1	42
Breast milk, 1 oz.	12.3		0.27	21
Similac 20, 1 oz.	22		0.45	20
Similac 24, 1 oz.	32		0.66	24
Enfamil 20, 1 oz.	17		0.40	20
Enfamil-Pre, 1 oz.	23		0.72	24
SMA 20, 1 oz.	24		0.24	20
SMA 24, 1 oz.	29		0.54	24
Isomil-20, 1 oz.	29		0.54	20
Prosobee 20, 1 oz.	29		0.6	20
Vegetables (variable serving)[a]				
Strained and junior	15	10	0.5	20
Table	15	10	0.5	10
Fruits (variable serving)[a]				
Strained and junior	15	10	0.5	Var.
Table and juices (unsweetened)	15	10	0.5	60–70
Breads, crackers, cereals[a]	30	20	0.6	30
Miscellaneous (mostly potatoes and pastas)	30		0.6	32
Soups, canned, condensed[a]	15			
Fats[a]	5	4	0.1	60
Free foods (candies, carbonated beverages, sugars, starch, nondairy creams)	0		0	Var.

[a] For lists of specific foods and serving sizes, see Acosta, P.B., and Wenz, E., *Diet Management of PKU for Infants and Preschool Children*, D.H.E.W. Publication No. (HSA) 78–5209. Washington, D.C.: U.S. Department of Health, Education, and Welfare, 1978; The Waisman Center, *The Low Protein Food List*. Madison: University of Wisconsin Press, 1981; Acosta, P.B. et al., *Microcomputers in Nutritional Support of Genetic Disease*. Tallahassee: Florida State University, 1984.

infant in our example, four bottles of 6 oz. each might be appropriate.

Older children with PKU generally will demand more fluids than do nonphenylketonuric children. The extra fluid reduces the solute load excreted by the kidneys and assists in the elimination of by-products of phenylalanine metabolism.

Step 5: Calculate the amounts of solid foods to be included in the diet. Solid foods should be introduced at the same age as for the nonphenylketonuric child. Appropriate ages at which various solid foods are given to the normal child are shown in Appendix K. Examples of the phenylalanine content of groups of foods are contained in Table 17-6. These groups may be used in a manner similar to the way the exchange lists are used for diabetic diets (see Chapter 11).

For PKU, 15 mg of phenylalanine is often considered an exchange, and serving sizes are adjusted to provide this amount. Breads and cereals are usually given in serving sizes equal to two exchanges. Detailed lists of the contents of each solid food group with exchange lists are available in diet manuals supplied by hospitals and formula companies, and in various educational materials for patients. The phenylalanine, protein, and energy content are listed for individual foods within each list. Serving sizes vary within each list. For example, 5 Tbsp. of strained carrots contain 0.5 g of protein and 19 kcal, and 2 Tbsp. of strained green beans contain 0.3 g of protein and 7 kcal: Despite the difference in serving size, both will provide 15 mg of phenylalanine. Serving sizes generally are small, often expressed in tablespoons, since the patient is very young. On the average, phenylalanine makes up 5% of the protein in breads, cereals, and fat, 3.3% of the protein in vegetables, and 2.6% of the protein in fruit. Meat, fish, and poultry are excluded, since they are too high in phenylalanine content. The parent is instructed in menu planning using the exchanges. Phenylalanine should be distributed evenly in planning meals. In addition, phenylalanine from natural foods must be offered within an hour of the time that the formula is given to ensure that all the amino acids necessary for protein synthesis are available simultaneously.

Step 6: Provide additional energy sources if needed. For example, corn syrup, honey, or sugar can be added to the formula if the formula and solid foods do not provide sufficient energy. For example, assume the kilocalorie requirement is 770 and the following energy is supplied:

Energy Source	Kilocalories
10 Tbsp. Lofenalac	430
1 oz. evaporated milk	42
1 serving fruit puree	150
1 serving vegetable puree	20
Total	642

The deficit is 128 kcal (770 − 642). This amount could be provided in 2 Tbsp. of corn syrup to be added to the Lofenalac.

Sometimes, a mother prefers to continue to breast-feed. A procedure for partial breast feeding of PKU infants is available for use in this situation.[12] Human milk has 0.8 to 0.9 g/dl of protein compared to 3.3 g/dl in cow's milk. It is lower in phenylalanine and higher in nonprotein nitrogen. A mean value of 41 mg of phenylalanine per deciliter of breast milk is used for purposes of calculation. The diet is calculated to allow for a combination of breast feeding and Lofenalac feeding. The amount of breast milk ingested is determined by weighing the baby before and after feeding. The amount of breast milk the infant takes can be controlled by limiting the time allowed for breast feeding.

Making dietary adjustments for age. As the child grows older, adjustments must be made to meet increased need for nutrients for growth and development. Some general guidelines follow.

The addition of solid foods and self-feeding should begin on a normal schedule. One such schedule is as follows:

Feed the formula powder partly as a paste beginning at 3 to 4 months. It may be mixed with fruit or honey.

Add fruit puree at 2 to 3 months, and vegetable puree and strained cereals at 3 to 4 months.

Low-phenylalanine breads may be given at 5 to 8 months.

Add coarsely chopped foods and begin cup feeding at approximately 9 months.

Begin finger and spoon self-feeding at 10 to 12 months.

Raw foods can be given at 15 to 18 months.

Other formulas, containing less phenylalanine, are substituted as the child gets older to allow greater use of solid foods. "Free" foods—that is, foods that are phenylalanine-free—may be added to provide adequate energy. These foods are forms of pure carbohydrates and fats. Excess use should be avoided to assure that other foods are not refused. In addition, a multiple vitamin and iron supplement may be needed.

Feeding problems. Feeding problems may arise as they do in nonphenylketonuric children, but are likely to be the source of great anxiety to the parents of a child with PKU. The nutritional care specialist can be very helpful in counseling such parents. Koch et al.[13] have suggested some reasons for certain common problems:

If a child is **unduly hungry**, the prescribed diet may be inadequate, or the child may be refusing the formula, and solid foods do not satisfy the appetite. Possibly, the prescribed foods are being refused in order to obtain sweet foods.

Loss of appetite may occur if the child is ill or if there are too many sweet foods in the diet. Overprescription of formula may lead to reduced appetite for other foods, or there may be a phenylalanine deficiency.

Refusal of formula can result temporarily from a normal fluctuation of appetite, or there may be failure to offer the formula consistently. Other causes of refusal may be the inclusion of calorie-containing beverages, or too much water added to the formula, making the volume excessive. Also, the formula may be too thick and unpalatable, or the child may be manipulating the parents.

Refusal of solid foods can result from a normal fluctuation of appetite or the refusal

of prescribed food to obtain sweet free foods. Possibly, the formula has been overprescribed. Alternatively, the child may be manipulating the parents.

Follow-up. Frequent measurements of blood phenylalanine levels and urinary metabolites are used as guidelines to determine the effectiveness of dietary control in PKU patients. A generally used schedule for determination of blood phenylalanine levels includes twice-per-week assays until the age of three months, followed by assays once a week for infants to one year of age, once every two or three weeks for toddlers, and once monthly thereafter. A record of food ingested prior to blood sampling should be kept to aid in interpretation of the test results.

A blood phenylalanine concentration greater than 4 mg/dl (250 μmol) is an indication for a decrease in the phenylalanine prescription and more frequent blood tests until blood phenylalanine is between 50 and 150 μmol.[4]

The diet must be continually monitored and adjustments made when control is lost. Loss of dietary control with increased blood phenylalanine may be the result of (1) prescription of more protein and phenylalanine than is needed; (2) failure to follow the diet; or (3) infection, undernutrition, or trauma that causes tissue catabolism with release of its phenylalanine content; and (4) inadequate energy or protein intake reducing tissue synthesis and allowing accumulation in the blood of phenylalanine that would otherwise be used for growth. If serum phenylalanine rises beyond the acceptable level, corrective measures must be taken promptly.

The diet prescription should be recalculated as necessary. In some circumstances, however, the primary need is more careful adherence to the prescribed diet, and nutritional counseling can be very important. The parents must understand the importance of the diet and the procedures for following the diet and for record keeping. They must make every effort to assure that siblings, grandparents, neighbors, and others do not feed the child foods that are not allowed. These procedures are relatively simple when the patient is fed only a bottled formula. However, the formula is fairly expensive, and many parents react unfavorably to its odor and taste. When solid foods are added, the process becomes more complicated. Planning meals and record keeping are difficult, and so parents must be instructed very thoroughly. In addition, the child's condition can place stress not only on parents but on siblings, who may resent the attention provided to the affected child.

When a child becomes ill and tissue catabolism causes a rise in serum phenylalanine, a diet lower in phenylalanine may be needed. Sometimes a phenylalanine-free diet is needed.

Problems may also arise from amino acid deficiency. A deficiency can occur as a consequence of lack of understanding of the diet by the parents; food refusal; vomiting or malabsorption, which reduces the amount of amino acid available; or inadequate intake due to an excess volume of formula or other food. A deficiency also can arise when the prescribed amount of phenylalanine is inadequate. This can occur, for example, following an illness when the amino acid requirement is increased to provide for healing or if energy intake is inadequate.

The first symptoms of a deficiency of phenylalanine are feeding difficulties, reduced rate of weight gain, and skin rash. These occur when plasma phenylalanine is less than 1 mg/dl (60 μmol/L). If the deficiency continues, gastrointestinal upsets, edema, lethargy, anemia, and bone changes ensue. The condition may progress to mental retardation, convulsions, and death. In addition, periodic measurements of physical growth, nutritional adequacy of the diet, and psychological and neurologic evaluations are necessary to monitor the patient's progress.

Duration of the Diet. It had formerly been suggested that the diet can be safely discontinued when the patient is four to 12 years old.[14-16] However, investigation of intelligence and performance has shown deterioration as phenylalanine concentration rises in both children[17,18] and adults.[19] Elevated phenylalanine may be concentrated into the neurones by the blood-brain barrier and depress synthesis of L-DOPA and serotonin by competing for tyrosine and tryptophan hydroxylases. As a consequence, in the United States, there is a trend toward later discontinuation. Current practice varies greatly, but recent studies suggest that the diet should be continued at least through adolescence if not indefinitely.

Maternal Phenylketonuria. Some children with PKU who received proper early treatment have grown to adulthood and reproductive age. As a result, an additional complication, maternal PKU, has appeared in recent years.[20,21]

A high blood phenylalanine level in the mother is toxic to the fetus, resulting in intrauterine growth retardation (40%), congenital heart disease (12%), mental retardation (92%), and microcephaly (73%) when the fetus was exposed to high phenylalanine levels in utero.[22] Abnormal myelin, abnormal cell migration, and abnormal protein synthesis have been described in these patients.[23] It is important that the adult woman who has PKU and who is contemplating pregnancy be given genetic counseling so that she understands the high risks involved.

Normal infants have been produced by women who restrict phenylalanine intake prior to conception and during pregnancy. While the subject is still under investigation, current objectives are to maintain maternal phenylalanine levels at 2 to 6 or 8 mg/dl. At the same time, care must be taken to avoid restriction of phenylalanine in the diet during pregnancy to the extent that microcephaly and intrauterine growth retardation would ensue. Although more than 90% of children of women with PKU who were untreated during pregnancy (serum phenylalanine >20 mg/dl) were mentally retarded, women with milder elevations of phenylalanine (3–10 mg/dl) were at lower risk. Maternal phenylalanine levels of 4 to 8 mg/dl are not detrimental to the fetus.[8]

Recommended formulas for use in pregnancy are Phenyl-Free, PKU 3, or Maxamum XP. Phenylalanine must be provided, usually with 5–10 mg/kg in the first trimester and subsequent increases as indicated by monitoring procedures. Blood phenylalanine must be monitored weekly and the diet adjusted as needed. Tyrosine supplements may also be needed. Products designed for treating infants with PKU are not recommended for use in pregnancy. When used in amounts necessary to fulfill protein requirements of pregnancy, they provide excess amounts of fat-soluble vitamins.

Variant Forms of Phenylketonuria

It is apparent that persistent elevation in phenylalanine levels postnatally is not suffi-

cient evidence by itself for diagnosis of classic PKU. There are a number of variants of PKU (Table 17-7) that appear to have a substantially lower incidence than classic PKU. From the biochemical standpoint, as Table 17-7 shows, it is important to distinguish classic PKU from **atypical** and **transient** forms in which the enzymatic defect is similar but the effects are not as severe as in the classic disease. In these cases, plasma phenylalanine levels can be maintained within the normal range by moderate or temporary restriction of phenylalanine in the diet.

Another group of patients, approximately one-fourth of all patients with hyperphenylalaninemia, have a mild or benign disease without the clinical manifestations of classic PKU. The postnatal rise in plasma phenylalanine in these patients is slow, seldom reaching 20 mg/dl. Phenylpyruvate deriva-

Table 17-7. Differential Diagnosis of Hyperphenylalaninemia

Disorder	Enzyme Affected	Mode of Inheritance	Biochemical Findings
Classic phenylketonuria	Phenylalanine hydroxylase	Autosomal recessive	Plasma phenylalanine >16 mg/dl; diet therapy with 250–500 mg phenylalanine per day needed to normalize plasma levels
Atypical phenylketonuria	Phenylalanine hydroxylase	Probably autosomal recessive	Plasma phenylalanine >16 mg/dl; responds to diet with >500 mg phenylalanine per day
Transient phenylketonuria	Phenylalanine hydroxylase	Autosomal recessive	Transient plasma phenylalanine levels >16 mg/dl; condition becomes benign or normal several months or years after birth
Benign hyper-phenylalaninemia	Phenylalanine hydroxylase	Autosomal recessive	Plasma phenylalanine >16 mg/dl; clinically benign; no diet therapy needed
Phenylketonuria (dihydropteridine reductase deficiency)	Dihydropteridine reductase	Probably autosomal recessive	Resembles classic phenylketonuria but no central nervous system response to low-phenylalanine diet

Based on Rosenberg, L.E., and Scriver, C.R., Disorders of amino acid metabolism. In P.K. Bondy and L.E. Rosenberg, Eds., *Metabolic Control and Disease*, 8th ed. Philadelphia: W.B. Saunders, 1980.

tives usually are not produced in significant amounts. Measurements of phenylalanine hydroxylase activity and oral loading tests with L-phenylalanine are used to distinguish this form of hyperphenylalaninemia from classic PKU. The need for dietary restriction varies, and surveys show that intellectual development usually is normal in untreated patients with mild hyperphenylalaninemia.[24]

In contrast, biochemical findings in **dihydropteridine reductase deficiency** are similar to those of classic PKU in the newborn period, but dietary restriction of phenylalanine is not sufficient to control the neurologic symptoms.[25] The patient has normal phenylalanine hydroxylase activity but may have a defect in metabolism of biopterin (see Figure 17-2), which acts as a hydrogen ion donor. It also acts as a coenzyme for tyrosine hydroxylase and tryptophan hydroxylase.[26] Tyrosine and tryptophan are involved in the synthesis of neurotransmitters (L-DOPA and serotonin). In the absence of this action, neurological disease progresses. Tetrahydrobiopterin, the hydrogen donor, L-DOPA, and serotonin must be replaced.[26]

Disorders of Tyrosine Metabolism

Variant Forms

Several disorders of tyrosine metabolism are responsive to nutritional management.

Transient or **neonatal tyrosinemia** occurs in approximately 0.5% of full-term infants, and there is a greater incidence in premature infants. The condition subsides quickly in most infants but may persist in a few. In these, it generally disappears by three months of age, even without treatment.

The condition is exacerbated by a high-protein diet, including many infant formulas made with cow's milk, which is high in tyrosine. As a consequence, a low intake of phenylalanine and tyrosine has been suggested for management. This may be accomplished temporarily by restricting the total protein content of the diet. Ascorbic acid is required for normal p-HPPA oxidase, and doses of 50 to 100 mg of ascorbic acid per day sometimes will correct the metabolic

consequences. There is some controversy regarding the necessity for treatment because the condition generally is benign. However, retardation has been reported in some affected infants.

Hereditary tyrosinemia or **tyrosinemia type 1**, also known as **inborn hepatorenal dysfunction**, is a more serious condition. It is an autosomal recessive trait that occurs in 1 in 50,000 to 100,000 births, and is characterized by severe impairment of liver and renal tubule function. Clinical manifestations in the **chronic form** include failure to thrive, cataracts, hypoglycemia, hypotonia, rickets, and hyperpigmentation. Mental retardation may occur but is not invariable.[27] Hereditary tyrosinemia may be fatal if untreated.

Originally, it was thought that the condition was a deficit in activity of p-HPPA oxidase. More recently, it has been suggested that it may be secondary to a primary defect in hepatic fumarylacetoacetate hydrolase resulting in the production of succinylacetoacetate and succinylacetone (see Figure 17-2).[28] Succinylacetone accumulation is associated with impaired transport and alterations in p-hydroxyphenylpyruvic acid oxidase (p-HPPA oxidase) function and delta-aminolevulinic acid (ALA) dehydratase.[29] The pathway for action of ALA dehydratase is shown in Figure 17-3. In this pathway, ALA accumulates and is neurotoxic. With decreased heme production, PBG also accumulates.[30-32]

The diet must be tyrosine-restricted and phenylalanine-restricted because phenylalanine is a source of tyrosine. Two other disorders of tyrosine metabolism, possibly related to tyrosine aminotransferase dysfunction, have been described. One, referred to as **tyrosinosis (Medes type)**, is known to have occurred in one case only. It may be similar to type 1.

The second disorder has been called **tyrosinemia type 2, hypertyrosinemia**, or **tyrosinosis (Oregon variety)**.[33] It is thought to represent a deficit of the soluble form of tyrosine aminotransferase that occurs in the cytosol of the liver cells, as opposed to a less soluble form that exists in the mitochondria.

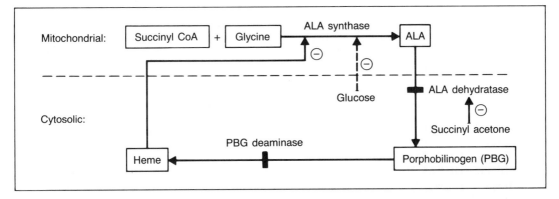

Figure 17-3. Suggested metabolic abnormality in tyrosinemia type I. Succinylacetone is formed as a result of a defect in hepatic fumarylacetoacetate hydrolase. Succinylacetone impairs delta-amino-levulinic acid (ALA) dehydratase. Minus signs indicate points of negative feedback. Black bars show points of metabolic blocks.

The patients have elevated serum tyrosine, increased excretion of the phenolic acids (*o*-hydroxyphenylpyruvic, *o*-hydroxyphenyl-lactic, and *o*-hydroxyphenylacetic acids [see Figure 17-2]), erythematous palmar and plantar lesions, mental retardation, and corneal ulcers. Some of the lesions respond to dietary manipulation. A diet restricted in phenylalanine and tyrosine is recommended.[34,35]

Last, a disorder of tyrosine metabolism that is due to a deficit of **homogentisic acid oxidase** leads to **alkaptonuria**, one of the four conditions originally described by Garrod.[2] Biochemical manifestations include lifelong homogentisic aciduria. The condition seems benign at first, but the homogentisic acid forms a dark compound of unknown composition, possibly a polymer, which accumulates in connective tissue and gives it a black color. This condition, known as *ochronosis*, is accompanied by a crippling arthritis.

Once they are established, there is no treatment for the ochronosis and the arthritis, but the use of a phenylalanine-restricted and tyrosine-restricted diet has been suggested as a possible approach to prevention. Since the diet is relatively unpalatable and alkaptonuria appears benign at first, this approach has not been tried for a sufficiently protracted period to be evaluated.

Diagnosis and Monitoring

In a newborn screening program, blood tyrosine above 4 mg/dl, or sometimes 8 mg/dl, indicates the need for further investigation. Other methods can involve assays for plasma amino acids and urinary organic acids by gas chromatography and mass spectroscopy, evaluation of renal and hepatic function, and urine tests for *p*-hydroxyphenyl acids and succinylacetone.

Type 1 tyrosinemia has been diagnosed prenatally by measurement in amniotic cells

Table 17-8. Guidelines for Daily Intake of Phenylalanine, Tyrosine, Protein, and Energy in Tyrosinemias

Age (years)	Phenylalanine (mg/kg)	Tyrosine (mg/kg)	Protein (g)	Energy (kcal)
0–0.5	70–20	80–60	2.5/kg BW	145–95/kg BW
0.5–1	50–15	60–40	2.2/kg BW	135–80/kg BW
1–3	40–15	60–30	25/day	1,300/day
4–8	35–15	50–25	30/day	1,700/day
9–10	30–15	45–20	35/day	2,400/day
11–14	30–15	30–15	45–50/day	2,200–2,700/day
15–19	30–10	30–10	45–55/day	2,100–1,800/day

Table 17-9. Composition of Tyrosine-Low or -Free Formula Products (per 100 g of product)

Nutrients	Analog X PHEN, TYR [a]	Analog X PHEN, TYR, MET [a]	Low-Phe/Tyr Diet Powder [b]	Maxamaid X PHEN, TYR [a]	Maxamaid X PHEN, TYR, MET [a]	TYR 1 [c]	TYR 2 [c]
Energy (kcal)	475	475	460	350	350	280	300
Carbohydrate (g)	59.0[d]	59.0[d]	60.0[e]	62.0[f]	62.0[f]	22.7[f]	12.1[f]
Fat (g)	20.9	20.9	18.0[g]	0	0	0	0
Protein equivalent (g)	13.0[h]	13.0[h]	15.0[i]	25.0[h]	25.0[h]	47.4[h]	63.0[h]
Alanine (g)	0.64	0.65	0.68	1.25	1.28	2.40	3.10
Arginine (g)	1.12	1.14	0.56	2.21	2.23	2.00	2.70
Aspartic acid (g)	0.94	0.95	1.40	1.84	1.86	5.70	7.60
Carnitine (g)	0.01	0.01	added	0	0	0	0
Cystine (g)	0.42	0.43	0.06	0.82	0.83	1.40	1.80
Glutamic acid (g)	1.26	1.28	4.00	2.46	2.50	12.00	16.00
Glutamine (g)	0.11	0.11	?	0.24	0.25	0	0
Glycine (g)	1.00	1.02	0.38	1.96	1.99	1.40	1.80
Histidine (g)	0.64	0.65	0.46	1.26	1.27	1.40	1.80
Isoleucine (g)	1.00	1.02	0.88	1.96	1.99	3.40	4.50
Leucine (g)	1.72	1.75	1.70	3.36	3.42	5.70	7.60
Lysine (g)	1.17	1.19	1.66	2.28	2.32	4.00	5.40
Methionine (g)	0.27	0	0.55	0.54	0	1.40	1.80
Phenylalanine (g)	0	0	0.075	0	0	0	0
Proline (g)	1.22	1.24	1.42	2.38	2.42	5.40	7.10
Serine (g)	0.75	0.77	0.94	1.46	1.49	3.00	4.00
Taurine (g)	0.02	0.02	0.027	0	0	0	0
Threonine (g)	0.84	0.86	0.79	1.64	1.68	2.70	3.60
Tryptophan (g)	0.34	0.34	0.20	0.66	0.67	1.00	1.40
Tyrosine (g)	0	0	0.038	0	0	0	0
Valine (g)	1.10	1.12	1.38	2.14	2.18	4.00	5.40
Minerals							
Calcium (mg)	325	325	431	810	810	2,400	1,312
Chloride (mEq)	8.3	8.3	9.3	12.9	12.9	47.1	28.2
Chromium (µg)	15	15	?	0	0	0	0
Copper (mg)	0.45	0.45	0.4	2.0	2.0	6.7	2.0
Iodine (µg)	47	47	32	134	134	234	120

Iron (mg)	7.0	7.0	8.6	12.0	12.0	34.0	15.0
Magnesium (mg)	34	34	50	200	200	521	156
Manganese (mg)	0.6	0.6	0.7	1.30	1.30	2.40	0.70
Molybdenum (µg)	35	35	?	60.0	60.0	107.00	32.00
Phosphorus (mg)	230	230	324	810	810	1,860	1,014
Potassium (mEq)	10.8	10.8	12.0	21.5	21.5	59.8	34.1
Selenium (µg)	15	15	?	0	0	0	0
Sodium (mEq)	5.2	5.2	9.4	25.2	25.2	46.4	27.8
Zinc (mg)	5.0	5.0	2.9	13.0	13.0	26.0	7.8
Vitamins							
Vitamin A (µg)	530	530	345	300	300	2,800	1,560
D (µg)	8.5	8.5	7.2	12.0	12.0	25.0	33.0
E (mg)	4.9	4.9	14.4	6.5	6.5	34.0	18.0
K (µg)	21	21	72	0	0	167	167
Ascorbic acid (mg)	40	40	37	135	135	234	80
Biotin (mg)	0.026	0.026	0.036	0.12	0.12	0.100	0.300
B6 (mg)	0.52	0.52	0.3	1.00	1.00	2.20	1.50
B12 (µg)	1.25	1.25	1.4	4.0	4.0	7.9	3.0
Choline (mg)	50	50	61	110	110	434	261
Folate (µg)	38	38	72	150	150	340	400
Inositol (mg)	100	100	22	56	56	500	300
Niacin, preformed (mg)	4.5	4.5	5.8	12.0	12.0	54.0	24.0
Pantothenic acid (mg)	2.65	2.65	2.2	3.7	3.7	25.0	11.0
Riboflavin (mg)	0.60	0.60	0.43	1.20	1.20	4.00	2.00
Thiamine (mg)	0.50	0.50	0.36	1.1	1.1	2.70	1.40

Compiled from Elsas, L.J., II, and Acosta, P.B., Nutrition support of inherited metabolic diseases. In M.E. Shils and V.R. Young, Eds., *Modern Nutrition in Health and Disease*, 7th ed. Philadelphia: Lea & Febiger, 1988; Committee on Nutrition, American Academy of Pediatrics, Special diets for infants with inborn errors of amino acid metabolism. *Pediatrics* 57:583, 1976; and Acosta, P.B. et al., *Microcomputers in Nutritional Support of Genetic Disease*. Tallahassee: Florida State University, 1984.

a Ross Laboratories.
b Mead Johnson.
c Milupa.
d Maltodextrins + galactose.
e Corn syrup solids + tapioca starch.
f Sucrose.
g Corn oil.
h L-amino acids.
i Casein hydrolysate + free amino acids.

for succinylacetone and fumarylacetoacetate hydrolase. Accurate differential diagnosis is essential both prenatally and postnatally for appropriate treatment.

A recommended program for monitoring includes plasma tyrosine determinations three times a week for two weeks after diagnosis and weekly thereafter until stabilization.[11] Plasma tyrosine and phenylalanine then are determined monthly. A three-day diet record should precede blood sampling to aid in interpretation of results. Growth, development, liver function, and renal tubular function should also be evaluated at intervals.

Nutritional Management

The restriction of phenylalanine and tyrosine in diets for tyrosinemias is intended to maintain plasma tyrosine between 50 and 150 μmol and plasma phenylalanine between 40 and 80 μmol. The diet is calculated by a procedure very similar to that used for PKU. The recommended intakes of tyrosine, phenylalanine, protein, and energy need to be estimated. Some currently used guidelines are contained in Table 17-8. Restrictions are less severe in type 2 than in type 1.

Formula products useful for these patients are described in Table 17-9. Additional water to meet the fluid requirement is provided separately if necessary. As the child gets older, vegetables, fruit, and breads and cereals are calculated into the diet using exchange lists and the procedures described previously. The average content of phenyl-

alanine and tyrosine in the food groups in the exchange lists is given in Table 17-10.

It is not known whether some patients have less ability to metabolize methionine or whether increased methionine concentrations (> 40 μmol) are the result of liver damage. Some physicians also restrict methionine. Supplementation of L-cysteine may then be necessary.

In type 1, to control attacks of porphyria, high-carbohydrate diets may be used to decrease Δ-ALA synthase activity. The patient may also need replacement of renal tubule losses.

Branched-Chain Ketoaciduria

Branched-chain ketoaciduria (BCK) is known also as **maple syrup urine disease** (MSUD). In addition to the classic form of the disease, there are several genetic variants — **intermittent, intermediate,** and **thiamine-responsive.**[25]

Classic BCK is an autosomal recessive disorder. The infant appears normal at birth. However, after ingesting a feeding containing protein, the infant may develop apnea and convulsions. There is a progressive neurologic dysfunction, a peculiar maple syrup – like odor, feeding difficulties, and a constant shrill cry. These are soon followed by neurologic symptoms, which include a loss of **tendon reflexes** and **Moro's reflex** (see Chapter 19). Alternating periods of hyperactivity and flaccidity commonly are seen along with opisthotonos (a spasm with head and feet back and body bowed forward) and seizures.

Table 17-10. Average Phenylalanine, Tyrosine, Protein, and Energy Content of Food Groups for Use in Phenylalanine- and Tyrosine-Restricted Diets

Food Groups	Phenylalanine (mg)	Tyrosine (mg)	Protein (g)	Energy (kcal)
Milk				
Whole, 100 ml	185	163	3.5	67
Evaporated, 100 ml	336	357	7.0	137
Vegetables[a]	15	10	0.5	10
Fruits[a]	15	10	0.5	60
Breads and cereals[a]	30	20	0.6	30
Fats[a]	5	4	0.1	60

[a] Serving size varies. See exchange lists for phenylalanine-restricted and tyrosine-restricted diets.

There is poor sucking and irregular respiration. The patient may die during the first few weeks or months.[3] Brain damage and mental retardation commonly occur in untreated survivors in the classic disease. Its incidence is estimated to be 1 in 216,000 live births.

Biochemical Abnormalities

The metabolic defect in classic BCK consists of a deficiency of **branched-chain keto acid decarboxylase**, the enzyme complex that is necessary for oxidative decarboxylation of

Figure 17-4. Biochemical block in branched-chain ketoaciduria. The deficiency or absence of branched-chain decarboxylase prevents oxidative decarboxylation of leucine, isoleucine, and valine, thereby preventing the formation of acetyl-CoA, acetoacetate, and succinic acid. (Adapted from Scribanu, N., and Palmer, S., Maple syrup urine disease. In S. Palmer and S. Ekvall, Eds., Pediatric Nutrition in Developmental Disorders. Springfield: Charles C Thomas.)

the branched-chain amino acids (BCAAs) leucine, isoleucine, and valine[36] (see Figure 17-4). The affected amino acids and their keto derivatives accumulate in the plasma and urine. Keto derivatives accumulate and clinical symptoms appear when the amino acid levels exceed 1 mmol in the plasma.[37] Leucine accumulates to the greatest extent, although the block affects all three amino acids.

The accumulation of the amino acids themselves, rather than their metabolites, is believed to be responsible for the mental retardation. The mechanism responsible for retardation appears to be defective myelination in the brain.[38] Specifically, there are thought to be effects on enzymes involved in myelination and inhibited amino acid transport and oxidative phosphorylation.[36]

Diagnosis and Monitoring

Homozygous BCK patients can often be identified because of the characteristic odor

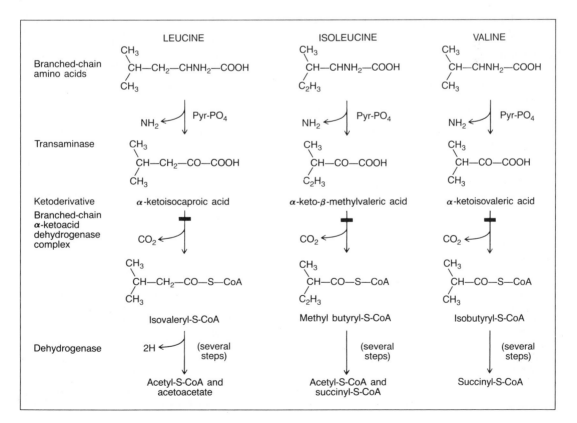

of the urine that usually appears in the first week of life. A mass screening technique uses a bacterial inhibition assay for blood leucine. Concentrations of >4 mg/dl in the screening test should be evaluated further. Diagnosis is confirmed by quantitative determination of the plasma levels of BCAAs and of alloisoleucine, which is a metabolite of the accumulated isoleucine, and urine levels of branched-chain alpha-keto acids.

Plasma amino acids and urine ketoacids should be determined twice monthly on samples obtained immediately before the midday feeding. After discharge from the hospital, parents test the patient's urine for ketoacids using dinitrophenylhydrazine (DNPH). A written diet record is useful in interpreting a positive test. A positive test can be the result of underrestriction of BCAA, overrestriction of BCAA that depresses tissue synthesis, or an intercurrent infection. The Guthrie test is also used weekly. Heterozygotes can be detected by the presence of alloisoleucine in fasting blood samples, by tolerance tests for the BCAAs, or by a test for the ability of leukocytes or dermal fibroblasts to metabolize leucine keto derivatives.

Table 17-11. Composition of Branched-Chain-Amino-Acid-Free Formula Products (per 100 g of product)

Nutrient	Analog MSUD[a]	Maxamaid MSUD[a]	MSUD Diet Powder[b]	MSUD 1[c]	MSUD 2[c]
Energy (kcal)	475	350	466	286	307
Carbohydrate (g)	59.0[d]	62.0[e]	63.3[f]	30.5[e]	22.5[e]
Fat (g)	20.9	0	20.0[g]	0	0
Protein equivalent (g)	13.0[h]	25.0[h]	8.2[h]	40.9[h]	54.3[h]
Alanine (g)	0.76	1.48	0.44	2.40	3.10
Arginine (g)	1.33	2.60	0.49	2.00	2.70
Aspartic acid (g)	1.11	2.17	1.14	5.70	7.60
Carnitine (g)	0.01	0	0.008	0	0
Cystine (g)	0.49	0.96	0.25	1.40	1.80
Glutamic acid (g)	1.49	2.90	2.10	12.00	16.00
Glutamine (g)	0.11	0.28	0	0	0
Glycine (g)	1.19	2.31	0.60	1.40	1.80
Histidine (g)	0.76	1.49	0.25	1.40	1.80
Isoleucine (g)	0	0	0	0	0
Leucine (g)	0	0	0	0	0
Lysine (g)	1.38	2.69	0.51	4.00	5.40
Methionine (g)	0.32	0.63	0.25	1.40	1.80
Phenylalanine (g)	0.90	1.75	0.55	2.40	3.20
Proline (g)	1.44	2.81	0.89	5.40	7.10
Serine (g)	0.89	1.73	0.60	3.00	4.00
Taurine (g)	0.02	0	0.028	0	0
Threonine (g)	1.00	1.94	0.55	2.70	3.60
Tryptophan (g)	0.40	0.77	0.20	1.00	1.40
Tyrosine (g)	0.90	1.75	0.65	2.90	3.90
Valine (g)	0	0	0	0	0
Minerals					
Calcium (mg)	325	810	491	2,400	1,312
Chloride (mEq)	8.3	12.9	10.5	47.1	28.2
Chromium (μg)	15	0	0	0	0
Copper (mg)	0.45	2.0	0.44	6.7	2.0
Iodine (μg)	47	134	33	234	120
Iron (mg)	7.0	12.0	9.0	34.0	15.0
Magnesium (mg)	34	200	52	521	156
Manganese (mg)	0.6	1.30	0.15	2.40	0.70

(continued)

Variant forms of BCK are differentiated from the classic disease on the basis of the same tests. In addition, clinical features vary somewhat. Comparison of the level of keto acid decarboxylase activity to normal controls can be useful in diagnosis. Some variants have enzyme levels of 5% to 15% of normal. The enzyme activity should be determined.

Nutritional Care

If diagnosis is prompt in the newborn, that is, within eight to ten days, the child may be given a feeding free of branched-chain amino acids (see Table 17-11). If necessary, gastrostomy feeding or parenteral nutrition, free of BCAAs, may be provided. The objective of early feeding is to promote anabolism. Approximately 75% of BCAAs are used for anabolism, thus lowering their plasma concentrations. For variant forms, if the patient has enzyme activity at 15% of normal, a protein intake of 1.5 g/kg/day may be safely used.

Chronic treatment is based on alterations in the diet, on the same principles as seen in PKU. Plasma concentrations of the BCAAs should be controlled to be within the follow-

Table 17-11. (Continued)

Nutrient	Analog MSUD[a]	Maxamaid MSUD[a]	MSUD Diet Powder[b]	MSUD 1[c]	MSUD 2[c]
Molybdenum (μg)	35.00	60.0	0	107.00	32.00
Phosphorus (mg)	230	810	268	1,860	1,014
Potassium (mEq)	10.8	21.5	12.5	59.8	34.1
Selenium (μg)	15	0	0	0	0
Sodium (mEq)	5.2	25.2	8.0	46.4	27.8
Zinc (mg)	5.0	13.0	3.7	26.0	7.8
Vitamins					
Vitamin A (μg)	530	300	444	2,800	1,560
D (μg)	8.5	12.0	7.4	25.0	33.0
E (mg)	4.9	6.5	14.8	34.0	18.0
K (μg)	21	0	74	167	167
Ascorbic acid (mg)	41	135	39	234	80
Biotin (mg)	0.026	0.12	0.040	0.100	0.300
B_6 (mg)	0.52	1.00	0.30	2.20	1.50
B_{12} (μg)	1.25	4.0	1.50	7.9	3.0
Choline (mg)	50	110	63	434	261
Folate (μg)	38	150	74	340	400
Inositol (mg)	100	56	22	500	300
Niacin, preformed (mg)	4.5	12.0	5.9	54.0	24.0
Pantothenic acid (mg)	2.65	3.7	2.2	25.0	11.0
Riboflavin (mg)	0.60	1.20	0.45	4.00	2.00
Thiamine (mg)	0.50	1.1	0.37	2.70	1.40

Compiled from Elsas, L.J., II, and Acosta, P.B., Nutrition support of inherited metabolic diseases. In M.E. Shils and V.R. Young, Eds., *Modern Nutrition in Health and Disease,* 7th ed. Philadelphia: Lea & Febiger, 1988; Committee on Nutrition, American Academy of Pediatrics, Special diets for infants with inborn errors of amino acid metabolism. *Pediatrics* 57:583, 1976; and Acosta, P.B. et al., *Microcomputers in Nutritional Support of Genetic Disease.* Tallahassee: Florida State University, 1984.

[a] Ross Laboratories.
[b] Mead Johnson.
[c] Milupa.
[d] Maltodextrins + galactose.
[e] Sucrose.
[f] Corn syrup solids and modified tapioca starch.
[g] Corn oil.
[h] Free L-amino acids.

ing ranges to allow maximum development of intelligence:

Isoleucine 40–90 μmol
Leucine   80–200 μmol
Valine   200–425 μmol

Plasma leucine in excess of 600 μmol is associated with ketoacidemia and ataxia. Protein (25–30 g/kg) and energy (140–170 kcal/kg) must be supplied in sufficient quantity to prevent protein catabolism and to promote normal growth. The plasma concentrations of all three BCAAs usually are not reduced simultaneously. Once each is normalized, supplements of that amino acid must be given in physiologic amounts or provided as natural foods to prevent deficiency. Leucine often falls most slowly and may require eight to ten days to reach normal levels.

Once the concentration of all three BCAAs in the serum is normalized, a more complete diet can be calculated. The recommended amounts of BCAAs, protein, and energy to be given to patients with classic MSUD are shown in Table 17-12. However, the individual prescription may need to be adjusted daily for several weeks and twice weekly for

six months. The need for the BCAAs declines during this period as growth rate decreases, and care must be taken to avoid their excess intake and accumulation.

The procedures for calculating the diet for the patient with BCK are very similar to those used for PKU patients:

1. Calculate the requirements for protein, energy, isoleucine, leucine, and valine (Table 17-12).
2. Calculate the amount of milk or other foods required to provide BCAAs for normal growth (see Table 17-13). Many clinicians specifically prescribe only the leucine, which is controlled within narrow limits of 1–2%. Isoleucine and valine may vary 10–30% but should be monitored also.
3. Calculate the amount of formula required to supply *at least* the protein requirement (Table 17-11).
4. Calculate the amount of fats and carbohydrates necessary to supply the required energy, and the necessary minerals must be added separately.
5. Add water to meet fluid needs.
6. Provide vitamin supplements as required.

Table 17-12. Guidelines for Daily Intake of Protein, Isoleucine, Leucine, Valine, and Energy for Children with Branched-Chain Ketoaciduria

Age (years)	Isoleucine (mg/kg)	Leucine (mg/kg)	Valine (mg/kg)	Pure Amino Acids (g)	Energy (kcal)
0–0.5	60–30	100–40	90–40	2.5/kg	95–145/kg
0.5–1	70–30	75–40	60–30	2.2–5.0/kg	80–135/kg
1–3	85–20	70–40	80–30	25/day	900–1,800/day
4–6	80–20	65–35	70–30	35/day	1,300–2,300/day
7–10	30–20	60–30	30–25	40/day	1,600–3,300/day
11–15					
Female	30–20	50–30	30–20	55/day	1,500–3,000/day
Male	30–20	50–30	30–20	50/day	2,000–3,700/day
15–19					
Female	30–10	40–15	30–15	55/day	1,200–3,000/day
Male	30–10	40–15	30–15	65/day	2,100–3,900/day
>19					
Female	30–10	40–15	30–15	50/day	1,400–2,500/day
Male	30–10	40–15	30–15	65/day	2,000–3,300/day

Compiled from Elsas, L.J., II, and Acosta, P.B., Nutrition support of inherited metabolic diseases. In M.E. Shils and V.R. Young, Eds., *Modern Nutrition in Health and Disease*, 7th ed. Philadelphia: Lea & Febiger, 1988; and Elsas, L.J., II, and Naglak, M., Nutrition support of maple syrup urine disease. *Metabolic Currents* 1(3):15, 1989.

Table 17-13. Nutrient Composition of Foods for Children with Branched-Chain Ketoaciduria

Food and Serving Size	Protein (g)	Isoleucine (mg)	Leucine (mg)	Valine (mg)	Energy (kcal)
Whole milk, 100 ml	3.5	223	344	240	67
Vegetables[a]	0.6	22	30	24	15
Fruits[a]	0.6	17	25	22	90
Breads and cereals[a]	0.5	18	35	25	30
Fats[a]	0.1	7	10	7	75

[a] Serving size varies. See exchange lists for isoleucine-restricted, leucine-restricted, and valine-restricted diets.

Solid foods should be added at normal times during growth and development. Normal ages for addition of solid foods to the infant's diet are given in Appendix K. See Table 17-13 for categories of acceptable foods and their nutritional values. These foods are grouped into four lists: vegetables, fruits, breads and cereals, and fats. Detailed exchange lists stating serving sizes that vary within the lists are given to parents. Foods within a list can be exchanged in a manner similar to that used in planning a low-phenylalanine diet. Additional energy, if needed, can be provided with fats and pure carbohydrates.

If therapy is begun in the immediate postnatal period with a synthetic diet restricted in the amounts of BCAAs, the following results can be expected:

Mental development may be normal.

The typical odor fades as chemical control is achieved.

Hypertonicity becomes less noticeable and disappears.

Normal tendon reflexes reappear with improvement in the sucking and swallowing reflexes.

The seizures cease, followed by a return of the electroencephalogram to normal.

Leucine levels greater than 10 mg/dl are associated with the appearance of **ataxia** (failure of muscle coordination). A recommended schedule suggests monitoring until normal levels are reached, and then monitoring weekly until one year of age, twice monthly up to three years of age, and monthly thereafter. A three-day diet record should be kept prior to obtaining each blood sample and submitted with the sample to assist in interpretation.

Possibly as a result of a defect in gluconeogenesis, hypoglycemia is a common complication in untreated BCK patients.[39] Another frequent complication is the onset of infections. Because they lead to a rapid breakdown of body protein and to amino acid imbalance in the plasma, they are potentially life-threatening. Several patients have died at age ten years or later from infections or from severe acidosis, which is also a common occurrence.

As is the case with PKU, the duration of diet therapy is still a matter of much debate. Because the chief anatomic lesion in this disease is defective myelination, the necessity for dietary control may be assumed to be reduced after myelination is complete. In older, untreated patients, the degree of developmental delay appears to be less severe. Whether this represents a less severe form of the disease or some form of compensation is not clear.

Variant Forms

The **intermittent** form of BCK consists of attacks that are similar to classic BCK, but the biochemical findings disappear periodically. Onset may be as late as at eight years of age and often is precipitated by an infection. An attack may be fatal. Peritoneal dialysis may be necessary during acute episodes, followed by a low-protein diet as a precaution between episodes. Mental retardation may result, but some patients are reported to have normal intelligence.

A few patients have an **intermediate** or **mild** type of the disease. Branched-chain amino acids and keto acids accumulate, but their concentrations are lower than those seen in the classic form of the disease. Mental retardation has been present in most patients described, and protein restriction was not helpful.[3]

Some patients respond to the administration of thiamine. It has been suggested that thiamine may stabilize the deficient enzymes. In **thiamine-responsive BCK**, the Committee for Improvement of Hereditary Disease Management[40] recommends the administration of approximately 10 mg of thiamine per day and a moderately-low-protein diet (2 g/kg/day).

Duration of Diet

In classic MSUD, the diet must be followed throughout life. This necessity may also apply to patients with the variants. It is believed that the accumulated alpha-keto acids are neurotoxic, interfering with oxygen consumption and ATP production in the brain.[36]

Isovaleric Acidemia

Isovaleric acidemia is known as "sweaty feet syndrome" as a result of the characteristic odor of the patient.

Metabolic Abnormalities

This disease is characterized by a deficiency of **isovaleryl-CoA dehydrogenase**. This results in a block in leucine metabolism in the step after the location of the block causing MSUD (see Figure 17-5). As a result, isovaleric acid (IVA), 3-OH-isovaleric acid (3-hydroxy IVA), and isovalerylglycine (IVG) accumulate in the blood and other body fluids. The IVA is the cause of the sweaty-feet odor. The IVG is consistently found in the urine, but 3-hydroxy IVA is only seen during ketotic attacks.

Clinical Manifestations

The disease has two forms. **Acute IVA** patients develop, a few days postnatally, poor feeding, vomiting, diarrhea, tachypnea, the characteristic odor, tremors, and lethargy. Some patients do not respond to treatment and die of unknown causes. Others survive and develop a chronic intermittent disease.

Chronic IVA develops between two weeks of age and late infancy. Signs and symptoms include vomiting, acidosis, coma, and the characteristic odor. It may follow an infection, administration of aspirin, or a high protein intake.

Diagnosis and Monitoring

Diagnosis may be made by measurement of urinary IVG. Affected patients excrete 40 to 250 mg of IVG per day. Normal is 2 mg/day or less. The diagnosis may be confirmed by tissue culture demonstrating decreased ability of affected patient's cells to metabolize leucine.

Treatment

The main features of dietary treatment are high calorie intake and glycine. During attacks of ketosis, parenteral therapy and correction of acidosis are appropriate. Over the long term, protein intake may be reduced moderately, but reductions in protein intake cannot be sufficient without creating deficiencies of isoleucine and valine. Supplementation with glycine (50–150 mg/kg) is used to remove IVA through an alternate pathway.

The Homocystinurias

Several different forms of **homocystinuria** are recognized. From the nutritional standpoint, the homocystinurias are important because of their relatively high frequency, which is estimated to be 1 in 35,000 to 1 in 350,000 live births for the classic form.[41] Except for PKU, they may be the most common

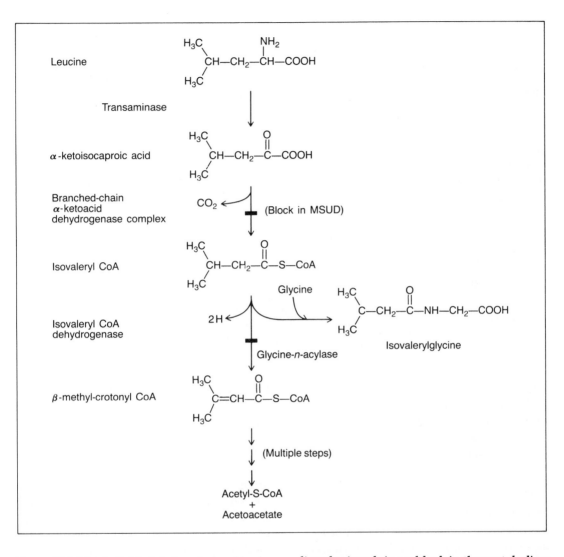

Figure 17-5. Metabolic block in isovaleric acidemia. Black bar shows point of block.

treatable inherited disorder of amino acid metabolism.

Biochemical and Clinical Abnormalities

The biochemical and clinical features of three forms of homocystinuria are summarized in Table 17-14.

Cystathionine beta-synthetase deficiency homocystinuria, the most common form, is inherited as an autosomal recessive disorder involving a block in the metabolism of homocysteine to cystathionine (Figure 17-6). In addition to the clinical features shown in Table 17-14, patients with this type of homocystinuria commonly have a light complexion and growth failure, but these features are not present in all cases. Homocystinurics frequently have significant skeletal abnormalities. Arterial and venous thromboses may be fatal in early adulthood. Mental retardation affects about half the patients. Others may be normal or above in intelligence.

Homocystinuria is characterized by severe elevation of methionine (approximately 30

Table 17-14. Comparison of Clinical and Biochemical Features in Three Forms of Homocystinuria

Feature	Cystathionine Beta-Synthetase Deficiency	Defective Cobalamin Coenzyme Synthesis	$N^{5,10}$-Methylene-tetrahydrofolate Reductase Deficiency
Mental retardation	50% affected	Common	Common
Growth retardation	Absent	Common	Absent
Dislocated optic lenses	Almost always	Absent	Absent
Thromboembolic disease	Common	Absent	Rare
Skeletal changes	Osteoporosis		
Homocystine in blood and urine	Increased	Increased	Increased
Cystathionine in blood and urine	Decreased	Normal or increased	Normal or increased
Methylmalonate in blood and urine	Normal	Increased	Increased
Serum cobalamin	Normal	Normal	Normal
Serum folate	Normal or decreased	Normal or increased	Normal or decreased
Response to vitamin	Pyridoxine	Cobalamin (vitamin B_{12})	Folate
Dietary methionine restriction	Helpful	Harmful	Harmful

Compiled from Rosenberg, L.E., and Scriver, C.R., Disorders of amino acid metabolism. In P.K. Bondy and L.E. Rosenberg, Eds., *Metabolic Control and Disease*, 8th ed. Philadelphia: W.B. Saunders, 1980; Elsas L.J., II, and Acosta, P.B., Nutrition support of inherited metabolic diseases. In M.E. Shils and V.R. Young, Eds., *Modern Nutrition in Health and Disease*, 7th ed. Philadelphia: Lea & Febiger, 1988; and Acosta, P.B., et al., *Microcomputers in Nutritional Support of Genetic Disease.* Tallahassee: Florida State University, 1984.

mg/dl, as compared with slightly more than 0.45 mg/dl normally) and homocysteine (5 mg/dl, as compared with normally undetectable levels) in the plasma and excessive excretion of homocystine in the urine (270 mg/L as compared with normally undetectable levels).

As shown in Table 17-14, there are two other genetic defects that result in less common forms of homocystinuria. Homocystinuria accompanies any condition in which the rate of homocysteine methylation catalyzed by N^5 – methyltetrahydrofolate–homocysteine methyltransferase is reduced significantly (see Figure 17-6). This reduction can occur from failure to form N^5 – methyltetrahydrofolate, as a consequence of a reductase deficiency, thereby resulting in a decreased rate of transfer, or in failure to form methyl-B_{12}, a cofactor required by N^5 – methyltetrahydrofolate – homocysteine methyltransferase. This may occur in cases of vitamin B_{12} deficiency or through impaired cellular uptake or metabolism of vitamin B_{12}.

Diagnosis and Monitoring

For preliminary screening, the urine is tested with nitroprusside, which produces a red color if there are excess levels of homocysteine and cysteine. A positive test is confirmed with a bacterial inhibition test. The concentration of methionine must be measured to determine the exact enzyme involved. An elevated methionine level indicates a deficiency of cystathionine beta-synthetase, whereas a normal or reduced methionine level suggests that another enzyme is involved. Assays for specific enzymes will assist in identifying the metabolic block (see Figure 17-6). After diagnosis, plasma methionine and cysteine are determined twice weekly for three months, weekly to age six months, and twice monthly thereafter. A three-day diet record should accompany blood samples. Laboratory results should show little or no homocysteine and $15 - 30\,\mu$mol of methionine.[4] In addition, patients should be routinely evaluated for normal growth and development.

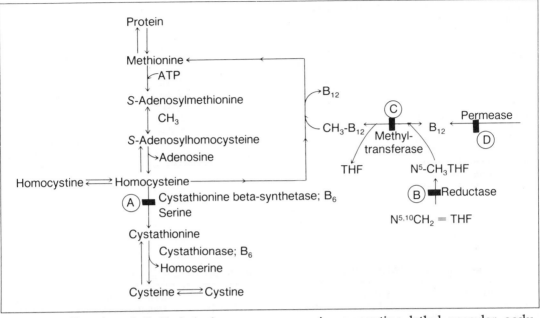

Figure 17-6. Sites of metabolic blocks in the homocystinurias, shown by solid bars. **A.** *Classic disease due to impaired cystathionine beta-synthetase.* **B.** *Reductase deficiency with failure to form N^5-methyltetrahydrofolate.* **C.** *Methyltransferase deficiency with failure to form methyl-B_{12}.* **D.** *Impaired cellular uptake of vitamin B_{12}.*

Nutritional Management

The major objectives in the nutritional management of the form of homocystinuria due to synthetase deficiency are to reduce the intake of the precursors of homocysteine and yet to supply the dietary elements necessary for growth and development. Patients diagnosed at birth and treated since early infancy have been reported to grow normally, both physically and mentally.[41] The methionine requirement per kilogram of body weight needs to be reduced and adjusted as the child grows. General guidelines to determine the approximate amounts of methionine, protein, and energy needed are contained in Table 17-15. In older, untreated cases, dietary restriction is unable to reverse dislocated lenses, mental retardation, or other clinical features; however, it may be of assist-

ance in preventing lethal vascular occlusions.

In newly diagnosed patients, increased doses of some vitamins can be tried first to differentiate between the types of homocystinuria. Some homocystinuric patients have been successfully treated with 250 to 750 mg of pyridoxine, suggesting that their form of homocystinuria is vitamin B_6-responsive.[41,42] The biochemical basis for vitamin B_6 responsiveness is not clear,[3] but vitamin B_6 is a coenzyme for cystathionine synthetase and may act by stabilizing the subunits of the mutant enzyme.

Patients with the transferase deficiency produced by cobalamin malabsorption or a defect in vitamin B_{12} metabolism are reported to respond to parenteral cobalamin administration, whereas one case with decreased N^5-methylenetetrahydrofolate reductase deficiency showed dramatic psychological improvement with folate supplements. These forms of homocystinuria do not respond to methionine restriction.[3]

A low-protein, low-methionine diet has been used successfully by some to treat patients who are identified early but who do not respond to vitamin therapy.[41] In addi-

Table 17-15. Guidelines for Daily Intake of Methionine, Cystine, Protein, and Energy in Homocystinuria Due to Synthetase Deficiency

Age (years)	Methionine (mg/kg BW)	Cystine (mg/kg BW)	Protein (g)	Energy (kcal)
0–0.5	50–20	300	2.5/kg BW	145–95/kg BW
0.5–1	40–15	200	2.2/kg BW	135–80/kg BW
1–3	30–10	150	25/day	1,300/day
4–6	20–10	100	30/day	1,700/day
7–10	20–10	100	35/day	2,400/day
11–15	20–10	100	45–50/day	2,200–2,700/day
15–19	5–10	100	45–55/day	2,100–1,800/day

BW = body weight.

Table 17-16. Composition of Methionine-Low or -Free Products (per 100 g of product)

Nutrient	Analog X MET[a]	HOM 1[b]	HOM 2[b]	Low Methionine Diet Powder[c]	Maxamaid X MET[a]
Energy (kcal)	475	277	296	518	350
Carbohydrate (g)	59.0[d]	17.7[e]	5.2[e]	51.0[f]	62.0[d]
Fat (g)	20.9	0	0	28.0[g]	0
Protein equivalent (g)	13.0[h]	51.6[h]	68.8[h]	15.5[i]	25.0[h]
Alanine (g)	0.59	2.40	3.10	0.79	1.1
Arginine (g)	1.04	2.00	2.70	0.88	2.04
Aspartic acid (g)	0.87	5.70	7.60	1.76	1.70
Carnitine (g)	0.01	0	0	added	0
Cystine (g)	0.39	2.50	3.40	0.14	0.75
Glutamic acid (g)	1.16	12.00	16.00	5.10	2.27
Glutamine (g)	0.11	0	0	?	0.22
Glycine (g)	0.93	1.40	1.80	0.53	1.81
Histidine (g)	0.59	1.40	1.80	0.36	1.16
Isoleucine (g)	0.93	3.40	4.50	0.73	1.81
Leucine (g)	1.59	5.70	7.60	1.20	3.10
Lysine (g)	1.08	4.00	5.40	0.95	2.10
Methionine (g)	0	0	0	0.16	0
Phenylalanine (g)	0.70	2.40	3.20	0.77	1.37
Proline (g)	1.13	5.40	7.10	2.40	2.19
Serine (g)	0.69	3.00	4.00	1.36	1.35
Taurine (g)	0.02	0	0	0.03	0
Threonine (g)	0.78	2.70	3.60	0.51	1.52
Tryptophan (g)	0.31	1.00	1.40	0.19	0.61
Tyrosine (g)	0.70	2.90	3.90	0.54	1.37
Valine (g)	1.01	4.00	5.40	0.73	1.97
Minerals					
Calcium (mg)	325	2,400	1,312	480	810
Chloride (mEq)	8.0	47.1	28.2	12.0	12.8
Chromium (μg)	15	0	0	?	0
Copper (mg)	0.45	6.7	2.0	0.48	2.0
Iodine (μg)	47	234	120	52	134
Iron (mg)	5.5	34.0	15.0	9.7	12.0
Magnesium (mg)	34	521	156	56	200
Manganese (mg)	0.31	2.40	0.70	0.16	1.30
Molybdenum (μg)	25.00	107.00	32.00	?	60.0

(continued)

tion, supplements of cystine are necessary. The mutation prevents the production of cysteine from methionine, and cysteine (or cystine) becomes an essential amino acid. In addition, foods low in methionine are also low in cystine.

The formulas that may be used are described in Table 17-16. The procedure used for calculation of the formula is similar to that used for PKU and BCK. Methionine is provided to infants through addition of milk to the formula. Calcium cystinate is also added to the formula (Table 17-15). Exchange lists are available for vegetables, fruits, breads and cereals, and fats. The me-

thionine requirement is small; therefore, amounts of foods that can be given also are small. Items from a list of selected foods are used to increase the energy content of the diet. Mean values for these food groups are given in Table 17-17. Specific lists of the foods contained in each exchange list are available in some hospital and clinic diet manuals and in instruction materials for patients. These lists must be supplied to patients or parents.

Although dietary restriction may be difficult to maintain in older patients, there is no indication that the diet can be discontinued without considerable risk of clinical mani-

Table 17-16. (Continued)

Nutrient	Analog X MET[a]	HOM 1[b]	HOM 2[b]	Low Methionine Diet Powder[c]	Maxamaid X MET[a]
Phosphorus (mg)	226	1,860	1,014	380	810
Potassium (mEq)	10.2	59.8	34.1	15.4	21.5
Selenium (μg)	15	0	0	?	0
Sodium (mEq)	5.3	46.4	27.8	9.6	25.2
Zinc (mg)	3.9	26.0	7.8	4	13.0
Vitamins					
Vitamin A (μg)	530	2,800	1,560	387	300
D (μg)	8.5	25.0	33.0	8	12.0
E (mg)	4.9	34.0	18.0	8	6.5
K (μg)	21	167	167	80	0
Ascorbic acid (mg)	40	234	80	42	135
Biotin (mg)	0.026	0.100	0.300	0.04	0.12
B_6 (mg)	0.52	2.20	1.50	0.32	1.00
B_{12} (μg)	1.25	7.9	3.0	1.61	4.0
Choline (mg)	50	434	261	40	110
Folate (μg)	38	340	400	80	150
Inositol (mg)	100	500	300	24	56
Niacin, preformed (mg)	4.5	54.0	24.0	6.4	12.0
Pantothenic acid (mg)	2.65	25.0	11.0	2.4	3.7
Riboflavin (mg)	0.60	4.00	2.00	0.48	1.20
Thiamine (mg)	0.50	2.70	1.40	0.4	1.08

Compiled from Elsas, L.J., II, and Acosta, P.B., Nutrition support of inherited metabolic diseases. In M.E. Shils and V.R. Young, Eds., *Modern Nutrition in Health and Disease,* 7th ed. Philadelphia: Lea & Febiger, 1988; Committee on Nutrition, American Academy of Pediatrics, Special diets for infants with inborn errors of amino acid metabolism. *Pediatrics* 57:583, 1976; and Acosta, P.B. et al., *Microcomputers in Nutritional Support of Genetic Disease.* Tallahassee: Florida State University, 1984.

[a] Ross Laboratories.
[b] Milupa.
[c] Mead Johnson.
[d] Maltodextrins + galactose.
[e] Sucrose.
[f] Corn syrup solids.
[g] Corn oil and coconut oil.
[h] L-amino acids.
[i] Soy protein isolate.

Table 17-17. Nutrient Content of Foods Used in a Methionine-Restricted Diet

Food	Total Protein (g)	Methionine (mg)	Energy (kcal)
Milk, whole, 100 ml	3.5	85	67
Vegetables[a]			
Group 1	0.7	10	10
Group 2	1.5	10	35
Fruits[a]	0.8	5	75
Breads and cereals[a]	1.5	20	55
Fats[a]	0.1	2	65
Free foods[a]	0	0	Variable

Modified with permission from Acosta, P.B., and Elsas, L.J., II, *Dietary Management of Inherited Metabolic Disease.* Atlanta: ACELMU Publishers, 1976, p. 56.

[a] Serving size varies. See exchange lists for methionine-restricted diets.

festations, particularly thromboembolisms and lens dislocation. Patients with low or normal levels of plasma methionine should not be treated with a low-methionine diet.

Urea Cycle Disorders

The urea cycle disorders are a group of defects in fixation of ammonia and formation of urea.

Metabolic Defects and Clinical Manifestations

There is a urea cycle disorder (UCD) for each missing enzyme (see Figure 17-7). Each is characterized by hyperammonemia and accumulation of intermediaries in the cycle, as shown in Table 17-18. When protein is fed, there is development of hyperammonia leading to poor feeding, vomiting, irritability, respiratory distress, lethargy, and hypotonia or spasticity, convulsion, and coma.[43] These clinical signs are common to all the disorders. Some patients die, and survivors are mentally retarded. It may be possible to prevent nervous system effects if high blood ammonia levels can be prevented in the newborn. Older patients often suffer from cyclic vomiting and migraine headaches.

In addition, some clinical manifestations specific to the defect of an individual enzyme also occur.[43-46] In AL deficiency, the hair is dry, brittle, and sparse (**trichorrhexis nodosa**). Males with OTC deficiencies have less than 5% enzyme activity and usually die in the neonatal period. However, a variant form with 25% activity allows survival. There may be more than one gene for some enzymes (AS, ARG), and thus other variants are possible. This problem is under study.

Diagnosis

Screening methods are available, but routine screening of newborns is not done in most states. Diagnosis is based on the presence of high concentrations of ammonia in the blood and assays for the specific metabolite that tends to accumulate. Excess ammonia occurs also in liver disease, Reye's syndrome, various organic acidurias, and a number of other conditions. Thus differential diagnosis is important.

Heterozygotes are sometimes identified by milder symptoms. These include mild protein intolerance leading to migraine in adults and cyclic vomiting in children.[47]

Treatment

In the acute stage, when plasma ammonia levels are high, the patient may become comatose. It is important to reduce ammonium levels. Peritoneal dialysis is sometimes used for this purpose.[48]

A more conservative approach is the use of a gavage feeding (orogastric) with a high-energy formula (150 kcal/kg) day to which arginine (350–500 mg/kg/day) is added. Alternatively, parenteral nutrition may be used with 10–20% glucose plus Intralipid (2–4 g/kg).[4]

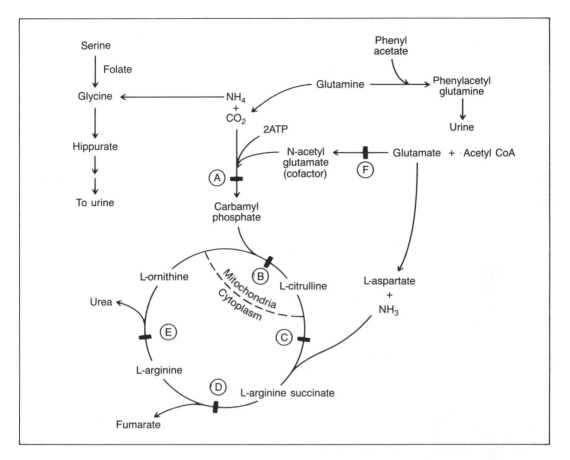

Figure 17-7. The urea cycle. **A.** *Carbamyl phosphate synthase I (CPS).* **B.** *Ornithine transcarbamylase (OTC).* **C.** *Argininosuccinate (AS).* **D.** *Argininosuccinate lyase (AL).* **E.** *Arginase (ARG).* **F.** *N-acetylglutamate synthetase (NAG). Reactions of the cycle may be summarized as follows:*

1. $NH_4^+ + HCO_3^- + 2ATP \xrightarrow[Mg^{2+}]{NAG}$
   carbamyl phosphate $+ 2 ADP^{3-} + HPO_4^{2-}$

2. *Glutamate* $+$ *Acetyl-CoA* $\xrightarrow{Arginine}$
   N-acetylglutamate $+$ *CoA*

3. *Carbamyl Phosphate* $+$ *Ornithine* $\longrightarrow$
   Citrulline $+ HPO_4^{2-} + H^+$

4. *Citrulline* $+$ *Aspartate* $+$ *Mg-ATP* $\rightleftharpoons$
   Argininosuccinate $+$ *AMP* $+$ *Mg-pyrophosphate* $+ 2H^+$

5. *Argininosuccinate* $\underset{\xrightarrow{Argininosuccinate/lyase}}{\rightleftharpoons}$
   Arginine $+$ *Fumarate*

6. *Arginine* $\xrightarrow{Mn^{2+}}$ *Ornithine* $+$ *Urea*

Some medications are also useful in lowering blood ammonium levels. **Sodium benzoate** is sometimes used to remove ammonium by forming hippuric acid, which is excreted. **Phenylacetate** combines with glutamine to form phenylacetylglutamine, also excreted (see Figure 17-7).[4] As ammonium levels fall, protein feeding may begin cautiously with 1.0–1.5 g protein per kg per day. The protein-free feeding should not be extended so that the patient becomes catabolic.

The objectives of chronic therapy for the survivors are to control ammonium levels to less than 50 μmol and to supply amino acids for optimum growth and development. To reduce ammonium levels, intake of precursors is limited with a diet containing only essential amino acids, and catabolism of tissue protein is minimized with a generous energy supply. The amount of protein and energy recommended are given in Table 17-19.

Table 17-18. Characteristics of Urea Cycle Disorders

Defective Enzyme	Genetics	Effect	Site of Action
Carbamyl phosphate synthase I	Autosomal recessive	Decreased plasma citrulline	Mitochondria
N-acetyl glutamate synthase	Autosomal recessive	As above—cofactor for CPS-I	Mitochondria
Ornithine transcarbamylase	X-linked dominant, usually lethal in males	Orotic aciduria	Mitochondria
Argininosuccinate synthetase	Autosomal recessive	Increased plasma and urine citrulline (citrullinuria) and orotic aciduria	Cytoplasm
Argininosuccinate lyase	Autosomal recessive	Increased plasma and urine argininosuccinate	Cytoplasm
Arginase	Autosomal recessive	Increased plasma and urine arginine	Cytoplasm

Formula products useful for these patients are described in Table 17-20. Nitrogen-free products useful to lower ammonium levels and provide carbon skeletons for synthesis of nonessential amino acids in UCD include Moducal and Polycose (see Appendix G). These products are also useful in diseases previously discussed where supplementation of energy intake is desirable.

When ammonium concentrations are within normal limits, other foods may be added at appropriate ages. Average values for the various food groups are given in Table 17-21. The diet is calculated using the same principles as diets for PKU.

Arginine supplementation for all except those who have an arginase defect is required. Sodium benzoate and phenylacetate may be given to increase nitrogen excretion, as described previously. Folate is supplemented to enhance synthesis of glycine from serine and avoid glycine depletion. Pyridoxine is supplemented to support transamination. Carnitine supplementation may be needed, and the addition of methionine and cysteine may be needed to synthesize taurine and sulfur amino acids.[4]

Monitoring Treatment Effects

The specific therapy will depend on the laboratory results in the monitoring procedures. A recommended protocol is as follows:

0–6 months	Weekly: Height, weight; blood NH_3; daily diet record Monthly: Plasma arginine, ornithine, ASA enzyme, complete blood count; routine developmental and neurological exam
6–12 months	Bimonthly: Blood NH_3 and diet records Monthly: Plasma amino acids; height, weight; developmental and neurological exam
1 year and up	Monthly: Blood NH_3 and diet records Every 2–3 months: Plasma amino acids; height, weight; developmental and neurological exam

Table 17-19. Guidelines for Daily Intake of Protein, Energy, and Arginine in Urea Cycle Disorders

Age (years)	Protein (g/kg)	Arginine (mg/kg)	Energy (kcal/kg)
0–0.25	1.6–1.2	250–500	145–125
0.25–0.5	1.3–1.0	250–500	145–125
0.5–0.75	1.3–1.0	250–500	125–120
0.75–1	1.2–0.9	250–500	135–115
1–4	1.0–0.7	200–450	120–110
4–7	0.8–0.6	150–400	110–100
7–11	0.7–0.5	100–350	90–80
11–18	0.6–0.4	50–300	65–55
19+	0.5–0.3	50–30	50–35

Other Disorders of Amino Acid Metabolism

Table 17-22 summarizes the major clinical and biochemical manifestations, principles of diagnosis, and dietary management in other inborn errors of amino acid metabolism.[49-78] Although most of these are known to be transmitted as autosomal recessive disorders and most of them are rare, it should be noted that ornithine transcarbamylase deficiency is thought to be an X-linked disorder, and that histidinemia, Hartnup disease, and cystinuria occur fairly frequently. The incidence of each is estimated to be in the general range of 1 in 10,000 to 1 in 30,000 live births.

DISORDERS OF CARBOHYDRATE METABOLISM

In this section, we review the role of nutrition in the diagnosis and management of inborn

Table 17-21. *Protein and Energy Composition of Foods for Patients with Urea Cycle Disorders*

Food	Protein (g)	Energy (kcal)
Breads and cereals	0.6	30
Fruits	0.5	60
Vegetables	0.5	15
Fats	0.1	60

Table 17-20. *Composition of Products for Urea Cycle Disorders (per 100 g of product)*

Nutrient	UCD 1[a]	UCD 2[a]	Nutrient	UCD 1[a]	UCD 2[a]
Energy (kcal)	258	290	Chromium (μg)	0	0
Carbohydrate (g)	8.00[b]	5.8[b]	Copper (mg)	8.0	2.0
Fat (g)	0	0	Iodine (μg)	274	120
Protein equivalent (g)	56.4[c]	66.7[c]	Iron (mg)	40.0	15.0
Alanine (g)	0	0	Magnesium (mg)	0	0
Arginine (g)	0	0	Manganese (mg)	2.8	0.7
Aspartic acid (g)	0	0	Molybdenum (μg)	128	32
Carnitine (g)	0	0	Phosphorus (mg)	2,195	1,014
Cystine (g)	3.10	0	Potassium (mEq)	70.6	34.1
Glutamic acid (g)	0	0	Selenium (μg)	0	0
Glutamine (g)	0	0	Sodium (mEq)	54.6	27.8
Glycine (g)	0	0	Zinc (mg)	31.0	7.8
Histidine (g)	3.10	3.60	Vitamins (%)	2.1	1.0
Isoleucine (g)	7.60	8.90	Vitamin A (μg)	3,360	1,560
Leucine (g)	12.80	15.00	D (μg)	30	33
Lysine (g)	9.00	10.70	E (mg)	41	18
Methionine (g)	3.10	7.10	K (μg)	200	167
Phenylalanine (g)	5.30	14.10	Ascorbic acid (mg)	280	80
Proline (g)	0	0	Biotin (mg)	0.12	0.30
Serine (g)	0	0	B_6 (mg)	2.6	1.5
Taurine (g)	0	0	B_{12} (μg)	8	3
Threonine (g)	6.00	7.10	Choline (mg)	512	261
Tryptophan (g)	2.20	2.80	Folate (μg)	400	400
Tyrosine (g)	6.50	0	Inositol (mg)	590	300
Valine (g)	9.00	10.70	Niacin (mg)	65	24
Minerals (%)	18.1	8.7	Pantothenic acid (mg)	30	11
Calcium (mg)	2,832	1,312	Riboflavin (mg)	4.8	2.0
Chloride (mEq)	55.5	28.2	Thiamine (mg)	3.2	1.4
			Water (%)	4.1	3.7

Compiled from Elsas, L.J., II, and Acosta, P.B., Nutrition support of inherited metabolic diseases. In M.E. Shils and V.R. Young, Eds., *Modern Nutrition in Health and Disease*, 7th ed. Philadelphia: Lea & Febiger, 1988; Committee on Nutrition, American Academy of Pediatrics, Special diets for infants with inborn errors of amino acid metabolism. *Pediatrics* 57:783, 1976; and Acosta, P.B. et al., *Microcomputers in Nutritional Support of Genetic Disease*. Tallahassee: Florida State University, 1984.

[a] Milupa.
[b] Sucrose.
[c] L-amino acids.

Table 17-22. Diagnosis and Dietary Treatment of Selected Disorders of Amino Acid Metabolism

Disorder, Inheritance, and Incidence	Enzymatic Defect	Clinical and Biochemical Findings	Diagnosis	Dietary Management
Disorders of branched-chain amino acids				
Hypervalinemia (Wada et al.[49] Wada[50]); autosomal recessive	Valine aminotransferase? Possible defect in transamination or decarboxylation	Vomiting, lethargy, failure to thrive, mental retardation, delayed motor development, increased plasma and urinary valine	Hypervalinemia and hypervalinuria, concentration of other branched-chain acids normal	Provide nutrient intake sufficient to maintain growth[51,52] and maintain plasma valine in normal range. MSUD Diet Powder plus leucine and isoleucine. When plasma valine approaches normal (2.6 mg/dl), add milk to provide approximately 65–105 mg of valine per kilogram of body weight for maintenance of normal plasma valine in infants. Replace milk with solid foods as appropriate for age[53]
Methylmalonic acidemias (Oberholzer et al.[54]); autosomal recessive in most cases	Two disorders: methylmalonyl-CoA mutase deficiency or defect of cobalaminocoenzyme synthesis; possible methylmalonyl-CoA racemase defect	Poor feeding, dehydration, hypotonia, intermittent apnea, persistent vomiting,[53] elevated urinary and plasma methylmalonic acid, severe ketoacidosis and hyperglycinemia in early infancy, hyperammonemia, absence of megaloblastic anemia in some. May be fatal. In milder cases, methylmalonic acid in urine up to 5 g/day (compared to <5 mg) and up to 34 mg/dl in plasma (normally undetectable)[25]	Diagnosis of unexplained ketoacidosis, elevated methylmalonic acid in urine, elimination of B_{12} deficiency (in cobalamin-responsive cases), homocystinuria, hypermethioninemia, assay of methylmalonyl-CoA mutase activity in fibroblasts to differentiate the two forms[55]	Rosenberg and Scriver[25] suggest 1,000-μg/day vitamin B_{12} injection to test for B_{12}-responsive trait. In B_{12}-responsive cases, cobalamin injection of up to 200 μg/day, starting with lower doses. Low-protein diet (0.5–1.0 g/kg/day) in non-B_{12}-responsive form[56,57] low-methylmalonate precursor formulas also useful. Reduce valine, isoleucine, methionine, threonine. Product 80056 with the required amino acids added[53]
Propionic acidemia (ketotic hyperglycinemia (Childs et al.[58]); autosomal recessive	Propionyl-CoA carboxylase	Recurrent attacks of ketoacidosis, vomiting, seizures, electroencephalographic changes, hyperammonemia, neu-	Propionic acid in plasma or urine; propionicacidemia more reliable feature than hyperglycinemia since it does not occur in	Provide calories from carbohydrate; add vitamins and minerals. May use Product 80056.[53] Limit protein to control

Disorder	Enzyme defect	Clinical features	Diagnosis	Treatment
		tropenia aggravated by infection or high-protein diet; symptoms vary in severity, and death may occur in early infancy; branched-chain amino acids induce hyperglycinemia and propionate formation	nonketotic hyperglycinemia,[59] confirmation by enzyme assay in leukocytes or fibroblasts[60]	propionic acidemia and infections. Limit odd carbon chain fatty acids and cholesterol,[61] some patients respond to biotin[62]—5 mg biotin twice daily until plasma propionate is normal. Give S-14 (Wyeth) at 0.5 g of protein per kilogram and increase until ketones are positive; then decrease to prior protein intake. Limit isoleucine, leucine, methionine, threonine, valine, which precipitate propionate; add even-carbon-chain fatty acids and cholesterol[53]
Histidinemia (Auerbach et al.[63]); autosomal recessive; 1:15,000	Histidase (L-histidine alpha-deaminase)	Accumulation of histidine and its derivatives in blood, urine, other tissues; impaired formation of urocanic acid; impaired speech, mental retardation in 40%; excessive imidazole pyruvic acid in urine	Excessive histidine in plasma or urine by chromatography or other method; may be confused with PKU; direct or indirect evidence of histidase deficiency for confirmation	Low-histidine diet may control biochemical and potential clinical consequences (controversial)[64,65]

Disorders of amino acid metabolism

Disorder	Enzyme defect	Clinical features	Diagnosis	Treatment
Hyperprolinemia, types I and II (Scriver)[66]; autosomal recessive	Type I: proline oxidase; type II: pyrroline-5-carboxylic acid dehydrogenase	Block in proline metabolism; clinical symptoms not well defined. *Type I:* probably benign; elevated plasma proline (<2 mmol). *Type II:* probably benign; may affect brain development; hyperprolinemia usually more severe than in type I (>1.5 mmol)	Plasma proline >0.45 mmol considered abnormal; partition paper chromatography or more precise chemical method to detect proline in urine and plasma	Low-protein diet (approximately 6 mg/kg/day compared to normal intake of 125–300 mg/kg/day) may lower plasma proline.[67,68] Need for diet therapy questionable if condition is benign
Hyperhydroxyprolinemia (Efron et al.[69]); autosomal recessive	4-Oxoproline reductase	Probably benign; elevated plasma hydroxyproline (normal, 0.01 mmol); other amino acids normal; urinary hydroxypyroline elevated; may have	Partition paper chromatography of serum, plasma, or whole blood to detect hydroxyproline; elevated urine levels alone not definitive diagnosis	Low-hydroxyproline diet not effective in lowering hydroxyproline in body fluids.[70] Need for therapy questionable

(continued)

Table 17-22. (Continued)

Disorder, Inheritance, and Incidence	Enzymatic Defect	Clinical and Biochemical Findings	Diagnosis	Dietary Management
		hyperactivity and mental retardation, but not proved		
Disorders of tryptophan metabolism				
Xanthurenic aciduria, pyridoxine-responsive (Knapp[71]); possibly X-linked	Kynureninase	Kynureninase requires pyridoxal phosphate as a coenzyme; the mutation may reduce affinity for the latter. Significant xanthurenic aciduria, sometimes with mental retardation	Significant reduction in kynureninase activity in liver biopsy in absence of pyridoxal phosphate; abnormal tryptophan loading test[72]	Favorable response to pyridoxine supplements[72]
Disorders of amino acid transport				
Hartnup disease (Baron et al.[73]) autosomal recessive; 1 : 26,000	Defect in intestinal absorption and renal transport of tryptophan; increased absorption of indole derivatives from gut	Pellagra-like skin rash, attacks of transient cerebellar ataxia, constant aminoaciduria; symptoms may be absent in infancy. *During attacks*: unsteady gait, change in mental state; may be delirium. Elevation of indole derivatives in plasma and urine, decreased niacinamide synthesis because of reduced tryptophan absorption, mental retardation in some cases	Reduced plasma tryptophan (30% of normal), characteristic aminoaciduria, and increased fetal excretion of threonine, tyrosine, phenylalanine, histidine, and tryptophan only. On tryptophan loading: increased urinary output of indican, indoleacetic acid, and its glutamine derivatives[25]	Variable clinical picture makes evaluation of therapeutic regimens difficult. Significant improvement of skin rash with niacinamide supplements (40–250 mg/day).[25,74] High-protein diet
Cystinuria (Garrod,[2] Wollaston,[75] Scriver and Rosenberg[3]) most common IEM (with possible exception of PKU); autosomal recessive; 1 : 20,000 or higher	Defect in intestinal and renal transport for dibasic amino acids and cystine[76]	Aminoaciduria characterized by great excess of cystine, lysine, arginine, and ornithine; cystine excess predisposes to renal, bladder, and ureteral calculi, possibly growth retardation, and impaired cerebral function	Hexagonal flat cystine crystals in concentrated urine; detection of cystine with cyanide-nitroprusside test; confirmation by characteristic aminoaciduria; need to distinguish from homocystinuria and cystinosis	Object is to reduce urinary cystine excretion and prevent cystine calculi formation; increasing urine volume and alkalinity helpful.[77] Low methionine, low-protein diet may lower urinary cystine excretion[78]

PKU = phenylketonuria; CSF = cerebrospinal fluid; IEM = inborn error of metabolism.

errors of galactose, fructose, and glycogen metabolism. These disorders range in effect from benign to lethal. Other inherited conditions related to carbohydrate metabolism, described in other chapters, include errors of carbohydrate digestion and absorption (Chapter 8) and diabetes mellitus (Chapter 11).

Disorders of Galactose Metabolism

The term **galactosemia** encompasses three autosomal recessive disorders characterized by impaired galactose metabolism.[79] They represent defects in two different enzymes that participate in the metabolism of galactose to glucose.

Figure 17-8. Pathways of galactose metabolism. Black bars show sites of blocks. **A.** *Site of metabolic block in galactokinase deficiency.* **B.** *Site of metabolic block in transferase deficiency.* **C.** *Site of metabolic block in epimerase deficiency.*

Biochemical Abnormalities

The normal pathways of galactose metabolism are summarized in Figure 17-8, which also indicates the metabolic blocks in galactosemia. The first type is the result of a **galactokinase deficiency** that blocks the formation of galactose-1-phosphate from galactose, the first step of galactose metabolism. This metabolic error results in the accumulation of galactose in the body tissues. The increase in the concentration of galactose in the lens of the eye enhances the activity of the alternative pathway for the formation of galactitol (see Figure 17-8). Galactitol is nondiffusible. It accumulates in the lens and causes cataracts.[80] In addition, galactose and galactitol are excreted in the urine.

The second type, "classical" galactosemia, is more severe. It results from the absence of or decrease in activity of **galactose-1-phos-**

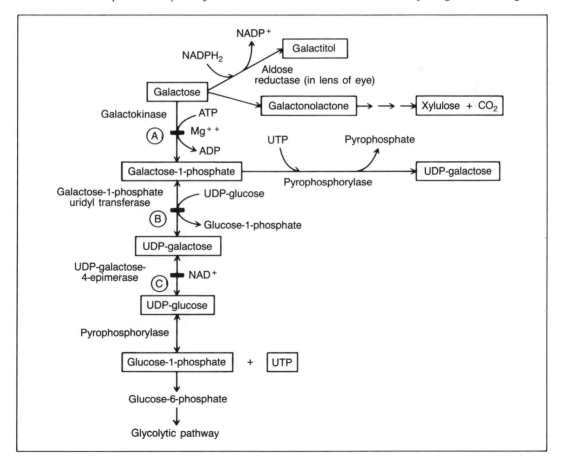

phate uridyl transferase. This enzyme normally catalyzes the second step of galactose metabolism in which UDP-galactose is formed from galactose-1-phosphate and UDP-glucose (see Figure 17-8). Inactivity of this transferase leads to the accumulation of both galactose and galactose-1-phosphate in erythrocytes, liver, spleen, lens of the eye, kidney, heart, muscle, cerebral cortex, and other tissues.[81] Galactose accumulates because the excessive galactose-1-phosphate inhibits the previous step, the conversion of galactose to galactose-1-phosphate. Galactose and galactitol are excreted in the urine in transferase, as well as kinase, deficiency.

There also are secondary metabolic blocks. Excessive galactose-1-phosphate inhibits conversion of glucose-1-phosphate to glucose-6-phosphate, which functions in the release of glucose from liver glycogen. Glucose release is inhibited secondarily.

In addition to galactitol formation, there are two proposed alternative pathways. First, the reaction involving the oxidation of galactose to galactonic acid and xylulose operates in some patients.[82] Second, the activity of pyrophosphorylase for conversion of galactose-1-phosphate to UDP-galactose (see Figure 17-8) is believed to be minimal and does not increase in galactosemia. Therefore, it does not provide an effective alternative pathway for galactose metabolism.

The reaction involving UDP-galactose-4-epimerase activity is reversible. As a consequence, UDP-glucose can be converted to UDP-galactose. The body thus is able to provide endogenous galactose for the formation of brain cerebrosides and complex polysaccharides. As a consequence, dietary galactose is not an essential nutrient. The epimerase has been found to be deficient in a few cases only and deficient only in erythrocytes, and the condition is symptom-free.

Screening and Diagnosis

Transferase deficiency has been estimated to occur in 1 in 50,000 persons, or it may be as frequent as 1 in 18,000. The most common screening test is the Beutler fluorescent test, which uses a small blood sample on filter paper and determines the ability to produce NADPH, which is fluorescent in UV light.[4] An alternative uses *E. coli* in a bacterial test.

If either test is positive, all lactose should be removed from the infant's diet at once while further tests are made. A definitive diagnosis is obtained by measurement for galactose-1-P-transferase in red blood cells. Homozygotes for the "classic" disease have no activity, and heterozygotes have 50% of normal activity. There are variants based on amount of activity and isoenzyme patterns. Galactose should be restricted for any mutant form in which galactose-1-P is greater than 2 mg/dl. If the presence of galactosemia is suspected based on family history, amniotic fluid cells can be tested for galactose-1-P, and amniotic fluid, for galactitol.[83]

Clinical Manifestations

Galactokinase deficiency, as previously described, is associated with cataract development in the first few weeks of life, but cataracts may develop in utero. There are no other clinical symptoms. Mental retardation usually is not a feature of galactokinase deficiency.

Transferase deficiency, on the other hand, is characterized by vomiting, anorexia, diarrhea, hypoglycemic attacks, jaundice, cirrhosis of the liver (see Chapter 13), ovarian failure, and hepatomegaly (enlarged liver), as well as cataracts. The presence of renal damage is indicated by albuminuria and aminoaciduria. Mental retardation occurs in severe cases. The disease has varying degrees of severity and may express itself as no more than gastrointestinal hyperirritability in mild cases. The symptoms may appear at birth unless a galactose-free diet was used during pregnancy. In that case, the symptoms develop rapidly after milk feeding is begun, usually within three to five days. The high lactose content of milk, 7% in human milk and 5% in cow's milk, contributes significantly to the galactose load in infancy.

The mechanisms by which the toxic effects are produced in transferase deficiency are not understood completely. The secondary block of the pathway to glycolysis may be responsible for the liver cell damage. The inhibition of glucose-6-phosphatase interferes with glucose release from liver glycogen and results in hypoglycemia. Since liver and kidney damage are not seen in galactokinase deficiency, it is likely that these effects are associated with the accumulation of galactose-1-phosphate.

Mental retardation in transferase deficiency also is thought to be related to the failure to metabolize galactose-1-phosphate. Normally, the brain does not use galactose readily but does so when blood galactose levels are high. Large quantities of galactose-1-phosphate in the neurons may inhibit normal neuronal metabolism and cause brain damage.

Nutritional Management

The biochemical and clinical manifestations of both transferase deficiency and galactokinase deficiency can be well controlled by elimination of the sources of galactose from the diet.[84]

Treatment has to be started within the first month of life to avoid or at least arrest cataract formation. Because cataracts can form in utero, restriction of galactose during pregnancy is necessary if maternal galactosemia is suspected.[85]

Because milk and milk products contain lactose, they are omitted from the galactose-free diet in infancy. Lactose yields approximately 50% galactose when metabolized. Several commercial milk substitutes — Nutramigen, Pregestimil, ProSobee, and Isomil — that are essentially free of lactose and galactose can be used. Their composition is given in Appendix G. Requirements for protein, calcium, and riboflavin, for which milk is an important dietary source, can be met adequately by using these milk substitutes. If the infant does not accept any of these products, a meat-based formula is an acceptable alternative. Recently developed milk analogues are devoid of cow's milk products and use soy protein and sodium caseinate as the source of protein. However, these products need to be supplemented with calcium or protein in the diet. Soybeans contain oligosaccharides of which galactose is a constituent. Although it is assumed that these substances are not metabolized to free galactose, soy products should be used with caution unless the patient can be monitored carefully.

Examples of other foods that must be restricted are fruits and vegetables that are processed with lactose. Peas, lima beans, and sugar beets also are sources of galactose and must be eliminated. Organ meats such as liver, pancreas (sweetbreads), and brain contain galactose. Meat products containing fillers must be avoided unless it is certain that they contain no milk products. Creamed dishes need to be eliminated, and breads, cereals, and margarines must be milk-free. The labels on margarines must be read carefully to assure that the product is usable. Pure oils, lard, and hydrogenated shortening are devoid of milk, lactose, and galactose and are safe to use.[11] Desserts such as cakes, pastries, cookies, puddings, and frozen desserts also must be avoided unless they are lactose-free. Some artificial sweeteners contain lactose as an extender. Some drugs contain lactose and must be replaced by a "sugar-free" equivalent if they are needed.

The parents, and later the child, should be carefully instructed in avoidance of milk, milk products, and any foods, drugs, or toiletries containing lactose or galactose. The nutritional care specialist must provide information on foods to avoid, instruction on reading and interpreting labels, recipes for acceptable milk-free substitutes for common foods, and information on menu planning for normal nutrition.

Nutritional Assessment and Monitoring

The objectives of the diet are to reduce erythrocyte galactose-1-phosphate to less than 3 mg/dl and urinary galactose to less than 10 mg/dl. The newly diagnosed patient is monitored weekly until normal levels are reached, then monthly throughout infancy, and four to six times per year thereafter. The nutritional care specialist should assess the diet periodically. It also is essential to monitor the progress of children on galactose-restricted diets by means of physical examination, including palpation of the liver, anthropometric measurements, and urine tests for hexitol. In addition, they should undergo wrist roentgenography for bone age, psychological evaluation, and slit-lamp examination for cataracts annually and an electroencephalogram every two years.[86]

Dietary control instituted early in infancy usually can prevent the development of cataracts and hypoglycemia and permit normal liver function and normal physical growth. If cataracts are present at birth, the diet may prevent their further development but may not cause them to regress. Mental development may be impaired if dietary control is inadequate. Mental deficiency, once established, is not reversed by galactose restriction. Severe restriction of galactose is necessary during the first year of life; however, opinions differ about the required duration of dietary restriction thereafter.[87] Segal[88] contends that there is no good evidence to suggest that a relaxation of the restricted diet is warranted. However, older patients may have psychological problems associated with stringent galactose restriction, and the use of some snacks may have to be considered.

Disorders of Fructose Metabolism

Pathways of fructose metabolism and the primary metabolic blocks in fructose metabolism are shown in Figure 17-9.

Essential Fructosuria

Essential fructosuria is an autosomal recessive trait characterized by a deficiency of **hepatic fructokinase**. Fructose accumulates and blood fructose levels rise. Fructose is excreted in the urine when it reaches the renal threshold of 10 to 20 mg/dl. The condition is asymptomatic and does not require treatment.[89] Therefore, it will not be discussed further.

Hereditary Fructose Intolerance

Hereditary fructose intolerance has much more serious effects. It is a rare autosomal recessive trait characterized by a defect in **fructose-1-phosphate aldolase** (aldolase B).[90] It occurs once in 20,000 to 30,000 live births in Europe but much less often in North America.[90]

Biochemical Abnormalities. The enzymatic defect results in the accumulation of fructose-1-phosphate, and there is a secondary inhibition of fructokinase leading to fructosemia and fructosuria. Apparently a secondary inhibition of the metabolism of fructose-1,6-bisphosphate also occurs. The accumulation of fructose-1-phosphate and fructose-1,6-bisphosphate appears to inhibit phosphorylase in the liver, thereby reducing the release of glucose from glycogen. Gluconeogenesis also is blocked at the step involving the mutant aldolase.

The formation of fructose-1-phosphate binds and sequesters phosphate, causing hypophosphatemia. The availability of ATP apparently is decreased. The inhibition of phosphorylase, hypophosphatemia, and inhibition of gluconeogenesis all are believed to contribute to the hypoglycemia seen in this condition.[89]

Clinical Manifestations. The clinical manifestations of hereditary fructose intolerance vary with the age of the patient and the severity of the disease. The condition is manifested in infants at a later age than is galactosemia, since sources of fructose normally are fed later. When fructose is fed, some consequences are immediate and short-lived, whereas others become chronic. Aldolase B occurs only in the liver, kidney, and intes-

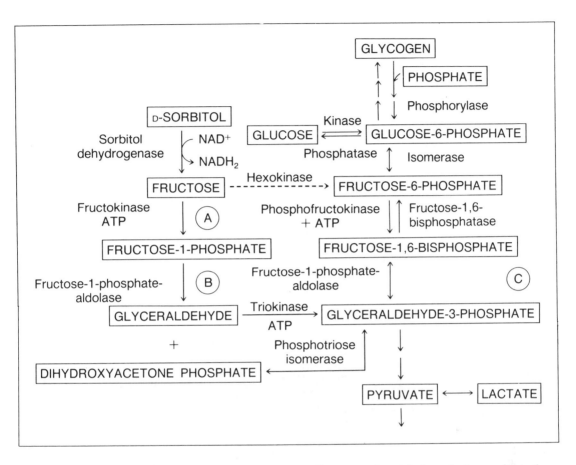

Figure 17-9. Pathways of fructose metabolism, and sites of blocks in errors of fructose metabolism.
A. *Essential fructosuria.* **B.** *Hereditary fructose intolerance.* **C.** *Fructose-1,6-bisphosphatase deficiency.*

tines. Signs and symptoms of the disorder involve only these tissues.

Major manifestations can be related to the effects of accumulation of fructose-1-phosphate, which is osmotically active and toxic to tissue and which sequesters phosphate.[90] The osmotic activity results in nausea, vomiting, and intestinal pain and bloating.

Tissue toxicity occurs in the liver and kidneys. Hepatomegaly, jaundice, hyperbilirubinemia, increased serum levels of hepatic enzymes, and hepatic failure are related to hepatic toxicity. Renal dysfunction also occurs, demonstrated by inability to acidify the urine, albuminuria, and aminoaciduria.[90]

Sequestration of phosphate results in hypophosphatemia, hypoglycemia, and elevations in blood levels of lactic acid and uric acid. Signs of hypoglycemia include sweating, trembling, and disturbances of consciousness, including coma. A deficit of phosphate for ATP formation may contribute to the liver damage.

There are additional signs and symptoms that differ in severity with the variation in the severity of the disease. General malaise is common. Dehydration, edema, ascites, seizures, failure-to-thrive, and growth failure have been observed in some cases. Death may occur from cachexia if the condition is not treated.

Later, affected children and adults develop a strong aversion to fruit and sweets. The effects on the liver and kidneys apparently are reversible. Patients generally have no dental caries. The disease does not appear to cause brain damage, and intelligence is normal. Symptoms tend to decrease with age.

Diagnosis. An intravenous fructose tolerance test is used for diagnosis. Affected persons will respond with a fall in plasma glucose and inorganic phosphorus. The diagnosis can be confirmed by liver biopsy and measurement of aldolase activity.

Nutritional Management. The patient must be given a diet free of fructose. Since sucrose and sorbitol are sources of fructose, the diet must also be free of these substances. The diet requires the elimination of all infant formulas containing fructose or sucrose, all fruits and fruit juices, most vegetables, and all products to which fructose, sucrose, or sorbitol has been added. These include many breads and cereals, meat products that are sugar-cured or breaded, and milk drinks that are sweetened. Desserts containing sugar, honey, fruit, or fruit juice must be eliminated. (Honey contains fructose.) Desserts labeled *dietetic* may be used if they do not contain sugar, fructose, or sorbitol.

Unfortunately, data on sucrose and fructose content of foods are scarce and sometimes contradictory. A summary of the available data,[90] however, lists the foods given in Table 17-23. Using these lists, the following recommendations have been made:[90]

1. Fructose should be rigidly restricted during infancy.
   a. Naturally sweet foods or products with added sugar should not be used.
   b. Animal foods without added sugar are allowed.
   c. Introduction of solid foods should not be delayed and should begin with strained meat.
   d. Allowed foods of vegetable origin (see Table 17-24) should be introduced only after the age of two or three years with frequent assessment of weight, height, and liver size.
   e. Foods of vegetable origin should contain less than 1.0 g fructose per day or occasionally 1.5 g/day. They should include no more than two servings of allowed vegetables and no more than five servings of allowed cereal products per day.
2. Fructose intake may be liberalized after infancy. The amount of fructose that may be allowed and the age at which it may safely be given have not been established. Therefore, fructose increase must be approached with caution, and patients must be monitored at frequent intervals.
3. Fructose-free sweeteners may eventually be introduced with caution.
4. Patients should be given routinely an ascorbic acid supplement. The supplement must be free of fructose, as should any other medication.
5. Patients and parents should receive continuing nutritional counseling.

Hereditary Fructose-1,6-Bisphophatase Deficiency

Hereditary fructose-1,6-bisphosphatase deficiency is a rare disorder that is associated with hypoglycemia and lactic acidosis. The symptoms resemble those of tyrosinosis. The clinical manifestations often are precipitated by an infection, and the mortality is high. As a consequence, nutritional management is not a common approach.

Glycogen Storage Diseases

A group of disorders known as the **glycogen storage diseases** are associated with abnormalities in glycogen metabolism. These disorders, shown in Table 17-24, are associated with the absence or reduction in activity of different enzymes involved in glycogen metabolism. The glycogen storage diseases are rare, but the exact incidence of each has not been determined yet. Not all are amenable to nutritional management but all are shown in the table to demonstrate their interrelationship.

Table 17-23. Food Lists for Hereditary Fructose Intolerance

Foods Allowed	Foods Not Allowed	Foods Allowed	Foods Not Allowed
Milk and milk products		*Group B* (0.1 – 0.2 g per serving; limit to one or two servings a week):	
Infant formulas without sucrose or fructose	Infant formulas containing sucrose or fructose (Isomil, Prosobee, Nursoy, Nutramigen, RCF)	Whole wheat flour	Legume products:
Milk		Wheat bran, 2 Tbsp.	Carob powder
Milk products without added sugar		Brown rice	Soy sauce
		Shredded wheat	Tofu
Fruits		Cream of Wheat	Miso
Rhubarb, unsweetened	All others	Cream of Rice	Nuts; peanut butter
Avocado	Commercial infant fruits	Crackers and breads made from white flour without added sugar	Seeds
Lemon juice, unsweetened			
Vegetables		*Meats and meat substitutes*	
Group A (< 0.2 g per 50-g serving; limit to two servings a day):		Meat, muscle	Meats, fish, or poultry processed with sugar or breaded
Endive	All others	Meat, organ	
Escarole	Commercial infant vegetables	Poultry, plain	
Celery		Fish, plain	
Lettuce		Egg	
Potato, white (mature, freshly harvested)		*Fats and oils*	
Spinach		Fats without added sugar	
Swiss chard		*Sweetening agents*	
Group B (0.2 – 0.5 g per 50-g serving; limit to one or two servings a week):		Glucose	Fructose (levulose)
Broccoli		Glucose polymer	Invert sugar
Brussels sprouts		Galactose	Sucrose, table:
Cauliflower		Lactose	Sugar, beet
Cucumber		Maltose	Sugar, cane
Green pepper		Aspartame	Sugar, fruit
Radish		Saccharin	Sugar, confectioner's sugar
Summer squash			Maple syrup
Cereals, seeds, grains, legumes (limit to five servings a day)			Molasses
			Honey
			Corn syrup
Group A (< 0.1 g per serving):		*Miscellaneous*	
White wheat flour	Commercial baby food	Gelatin	Vanilla
White bread, 1 slice	Cereals containing germ or added sugar	Vinegar	
Rye flour		Tea	
Degermed cornmeal	Wheat germ	Coffee	
White rice	Cookies, cakes	*Use sparingly* (lack of information)	
Puffed wheat, 25 g	Candy	Mustard	
Puffed rice, 25 g	Carbonated beverages, sweetened	Herbs	
	Legumes	Spices	
		Cocoa	

Compiled from information contained in Bell, L., and Sherwood, W.G., Current practices and improved recommendations for treating hereditary fructose intolerance. *J. Am. Diet. Assoc.* 87:771, 1989.

Biochemical Abnormalities

The major pathways of glycogen metabolism and the enzymatic effects associated with various glycogen storage diseases are shown in Figure 17-10. The predominant biochemical defect due to the enzymatic disturbance in the pathway of glycogen synthesis or degradation is the storage of excessive amounts or an abnormal form of glycogen in various body tissues, mainly in the liver. The usual human content of glycogen is less than 5 g per 100 g of wet weight of liver and less than 2 g per 100 g of wet weight of muscle.

The diseases of glycogen storage affect primarily either the liver or the skeletal muscle and myocardium, although other organs sometimes are involved. In the diseases with

Table 17-24. Major Clinical Symptoms, Diagnosis, and Management of Glycogen Storage Diseases

Disease Type and Enzyme Defect	Clinical Manifestations	Diagnosis	Nutritional Management
Type I (von Gierke's disease; hepatorenal glycogen storage disease); glucose-6-phosphatase	Anorexia, weight loss, vomiting, enlargement of liver and kidney, failure to thrive, stunted growth, severe hypoglycemia in infancy, acidosis hyperlacticacidemia, hyperlipemia, hyperuricemia, and gout	Increased glycogen storage (normal structure), glucose-6-phosphatase absent in fresh liver biopsy, subnormal response to glucagon or epinephrine	Treatment is symptomatic: surgical construction of portacaval anastomosis; feeding medium-chain triglycerides, and frequent small feedings (six to eight per day) of normal diet with high-glucose feedings between meals; nocturnal glucose infusions and feeding cornstarch q6h useful.
Type II (Pompe's disease); α-1,4-glucosidase	Hepatomegaly, hypotonia, cardiomegaly, maybe cardiorespiratory failure and death	Muscle biopsy analysis for α-1,4-glucosidase; can be detected in utero	No known effective treatment; low-carbohydrate, high-protein, high-fat diet attempted but not generally effective
Type III (Cori's disease); amylo-1,6-glucosidase (debranching enzyme)	Similar to type I but milder; lipids, glucose, and electrocardiogram normal; muscle wasting and weakness	Liver biopsy or leukocytes for enzyme assay; excessive storage of abnormal glycogen	Similar to type I, but a diet high in protein is recommended; give night feeding to avoid hypoglycemia
Type IV; Brancher enzyme deficiency amylo-1,4→1,6-transglucosylase (branching enzyme)	Hepatosplenomegaly, cirrhosis, ascites, liver failure, accumulation of abnormal glycogen; muscle hypotension	Absence of amylo-1,4→1,6 transglucosylase activity in leukocytes, excessive storage of abnormal glycogen	No known effective treatment; death usually before age five

(continued)

the hepatic enzymatic effect, the liver is greatly enlarged. Other symptoms are severe hypoglycemia, hypertriglyceridemia, hypercholesterolemia, and increased blood urate and lactate levels. Death in childhood is uncommon. If the disease affects the muscle primarily, it causes cramps, muscular weakness and atrophy, massive glycogen infiltration into the muscles, reduced muscular function and, in some cases, myocardial failure and death.

Diagnosis and Nutritional Management

In the glycogen storage diseases, the most reliable diagnostic test is the demonstration of the absence of or reduction in the activity of the specific enzyme. As shown in Table 17-24, differential diagnosis is necessary to distinguish between the different types of glycogen storage diseases.

The management and prognosis of these diseases varies considerably. In some instances—for example, type I—severe metabolic abnormalities eventually may lead to death, whereas in other types, such as type V, there is minimal disability. Dietary modification usually is not effective in controlling the outcome of most glycogen storage diseases, although some of the symptoms (e.g., hypoglycemia) can be relieved by specific intervention.[91] Techniques for nutritional management are summarized in Table 17-24.

Table 17-24. (Continued)

Disease Type and Enzyme Defect	Clinical Manifestations	Diagnosis	Nutritional Management
Type V (McArdle's disease); muscle phosphorylase	Weakness, cramping of muscles on exercise in young adults, failure of blood lactate to rise	Absence of phosphorylase and increased glycogen on muscle biopsy	Intravenous glucose infusions to relieve muscular pain
Type VI (Hers' disease); liver phosphorylase(?)	Hepatomegaly, normal spleen; absence of hypoglycemia, lipemia, and acidosis; mild clinical course	Depressed liver enzyme activity, normal glucose-6-phosphatase and amylo-1,6-glucosidase, and increased liver glycogen	A high-protein diet and frequent small feedings
Type VII: Tarui's disease muscle phosphofructokinase	Weakness and cramping of skeletal muscle on exercise; similar to type V	Decrease in muscle phosphofructokinase on biopsy	No dietary treatment known
Type VIII; liver phosphorylase b kinase	Hepatomegaly, cerebral degeneration	Reduction in liver phosphorylase activity	No dietary treatment known
Type IX; liver phosphorylase b kinase deficiency	Hepatomegaly; no splenomegaly; mild hypoglycemia	Deficient WBC or hepatic liver phosphorylase b kinase	No dietary treatment known
Type X, XI, XII	Very rare—one case only		
Type O; UDPG transferase deficiency	Hypoglycemic seizures; mental retardation	Absence or reduction in activity of glycogen synthase	Frequent small feedings with high sugar content, high-protein feedings in between

Compiled from Palmer, S., Glycogen storage diseases. In S. Palmer and S. Ekvall, Eds., *Pediatric Nutrition in Developmental Disorders.* Springfield, Ill.: Charles C Thomas, 1978; Bondy, P.K., and Rosenberg, L.E., Eds., *Metabolic Control and Disease,* 8th ed. Philadelphia: W.B. Saunders, 1980; Howell, S.R., and Williams, J.C., The glycogen storage diseases. In J.B. Stanbury, J.B. Wyngaarden, D.S. Frederickson, et al., *Metabolic Basis of Inherited Disease,* 5th ed. Philadelphia: W.B. Saunders, 1983; and Sidbury, J.B., The glycogenoses. In A.M. Rudolph and J.I.E. Hoffman, *Pediatrics,* 19th ed. Norwalk, Conn.: Appleton-Century-Crofts, 1982.

DISORDERS OF LIPID TRANSPORT

The disorders of lipid transport resulting from single gene mutations that are closely related to cardiovascular disease were discussed in Chapter 10. Another disorder in this category, abetalipoproteinemia, is described in Chapter 8. This section contains another example of lipid transport disorders, Refsum's disease.

Refsum's Disease

Refsum's disease is known also as **phytanic acid storage disease**. Phytanic acid is a twenty-carbon branched chain acid that is found in some foods. The biochemical lesion

consists of a failure to convert phytanic acid to alpha-hydroxyphytanic acid, the initial step in its conversion to pristanic acid (Figure 17-11).[92] The activity of the enzyme phytanic acid alpha-hydroxylase, which catalyzes this step, is absent. Subsequent steps in the metabolism of pristanic acid by beta-oxidation are not affected.

Refsum's disease is a rare autosomal recessive disorder.[93,94] It is characterized by peripheral neuropathy, ataxia, **retinitis pigmentosa** (a progressive sclerosis, pigmentation, and atrophy of the retina leading to blindness), and disorders of the skin and bones.[92] These symptoms result from the accumulation of phytanic acid in tissues, particularly the liver and kidneys.[93] Normal

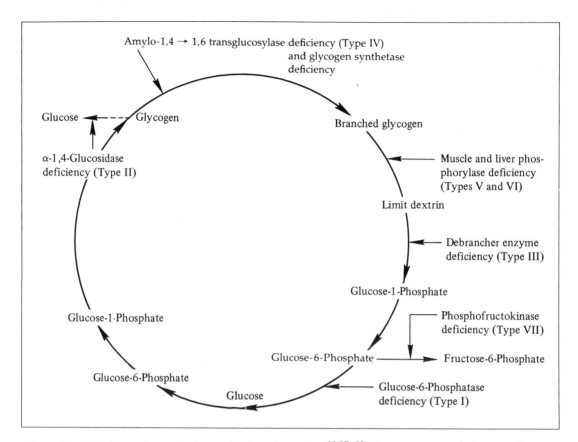

Figure 17-10. Major pathways in the synthesis and degradation of glycogen in glycogen storage diseases.

human plasma contains only traces (0.3 mg/dl) of phytanic acid, but in patients with this disease, 5–30% of total fatty acids are phytanic acid.

The sources of phytanic acid probably are exclusively dietary. The major dietary sources have been identified as dairy products,[95] with traces in some vegetables (e.g., squash and tomatoes) and fish oils.[96] Phytol, a component of chlorophyll that is ubiquitous in green leafy vegetables, is also a precursor of phytanic acid. However, it is present in the bound form in the chlorophyll molecule in green vegetables and, in its bound form, is not thought to be an important dietary source of phytanic acid.[97]

Several investigators have reported success in treating Refsum's disease by restricting the phytanic acid content of the diet.[92,97–99] The response of plasma phytanate to dietary treatment is associated with improvement or even regression of peripheral neuropathy.[97,98] Reducing the intake of phytanic acid from its estimated level of approximately 60 mg/day can lower plasma phytanic acid levels, but a drastic reduction to approximately 3 mg of phytanate daily is reported to be necessary for normalizing plasma phytanic acid levels.[97] Severe restriction of total caloric intake may be necessary. Therefore, careful monitoring of the diet and follow-up of patients is recommended. Therapeutic benefits are reported to be maximized if the diet therapy is initiated early.[92]

DISORDERS OF PURINE AND PYRIMIDINE METABOLISM

A number of hereditary syndromes are associated with abnormalities in purine and pyrimidine metabolism. Here we will briefly

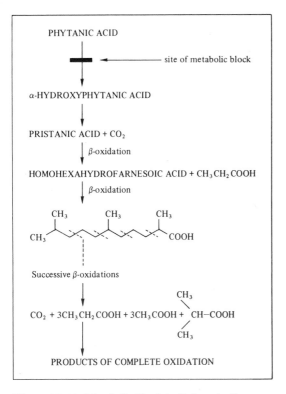

PHYTANIC ACID

site of metabolic block

α-HYDROXYPHYTANIC ACID

PRISTANIC ACID + CO_2

β-oxidation

HOMOHEXAHYDROFARNESOIC ACID + CH_3CH_2COOH

β-oxidation

Successive β-oxidations

CO_2 + 3CH_3CH_2COOH + 3CH_3COOH + CH–COOH

PRODUCTS OF COMPLETE OXIDATION

Figure 17-11. Metabolic block in Refsum's disease.

describe two such syndromes, gout and hereditary xanthinuria.

Gout

The term **gout** is used to describe a cluster of clinical symptoms associated with hyperuricemia (increased levels of uric acid in the blood). It is a form of arthritis found in a variety of hereditary disorders and in some disorders related to environmental factors. Gout is a common ailment, accounting for 4–5% of all patients with arthritis in major clinics in the United States, and with an overall incidence of 0.3%. It occurs much more frequently in men than women.

Biochemical Abnormalities

The hyperuricemia of gout results most commonly from a genetic defect that leads to excessive synthesis of the purine precursors of uric acid or, in other cases, from normal purine synthesis but diminished uric acid excretion.

A variety of enzymatic defects may result in excessive purine synthesis. The ones leading to hyperuricemia and gout are (1) deficiency of glucose-6-phosphatase (glycogen storage disease type I), (2) hypoxanthine-guanine phosphoribosyl transferase (HPRT) deficiency in patients with the Lesch-Nyhan syndrome, and (3) increased activity of phosphoribosylpyrophosphate synthetase. Hyperuricemia and gout also may appear in association with a number of other hereditary disorders.

Clinical Features

Clinically, gout is characterized by recurrent, paroxysmal, acute attacks due to severe inflammation in peripheral joints, followed by complete transient remission. Gradually, these episodes become more frequent and lead to chronic disability and joint destruction. The incidence of renal calculi and renal and vascular damage is exceedingly high. The clinical features are the result of urate deposits in tissues because of the limited solubility of uric acid and its salts in biologic fluids. At the low pH of the urinary tract, free acid forms calculi in the kidney and bladder, and at the high pH of the plasma, crystals of monosodium urate monohydrate are precipitated in and around the joints, tendons, **subchondral** (beneath cartilage) bones, and kidney parenchyma. Only a small percentage of hyperuricemic patients develop gouty arthritis.

Treatment

Acute attacks of gouty arthritis respond well to therapy with a variety of **antiinflammatory drugs**, and **antihyperuricemic** drugs are used for lowering plasma uric acid levels.[100] **Diet therapy** now is used only as an adjunct to drugs, although it was used more extensively before the advent of effective drugs.

Dietary restriction of foods high in purine can lower serum urate concentration, but the response to even a purine-free diet has been reported as moderate at best.[101] Nevertheless, a purine-restricted diet (in essence, a restriction of high-protein foods) containing 200 g of meat, poultry, or fish twice weekly and low in dried beans, lentils, bran, and wheat germ frequently is recommended as adjunctive therapy. Organ meats are exceedingly high in purine and may have to be eliminated.[102] High-fat diets, consumption of alcohol, and very-low-calorie diets tend to increase serum urate concentration and may provoke acute attacks of gout.[103,104] Increased consumption of fluids and maintenance of an alkaline pH in the urine also assist in the treatment of gout.[100]

Hereditary Xanthinuria

Hereditary xanthinuria results from a deficiency of xanthine oxidase and leads to excessive secretion of hypoxanthine and xanthine, the precursors of uric acid. The enzyme deficiency results in reduced formation of uric acid and consequent hypouricemia and sometimes is accompanied by hypercalciuria.

In most patients with xanthinuria, the disease has a benign course and requires no treatment. However, in patients with recurrent renal calculi, a high-fluid diet, maintenance of an alkaline pH in the urine, and dietary restriction of purine-containing foods may be beneficial in delaying recurrences.[99]

VITAMIN DEPENDENCY DISORDERS

There is increasing awareness that some inborn errors of metabolism are associated with an increase in the requirement for certain vitamins that function as coenzymes at different steps in metabolic pathways. This heterogeneous group of disorders, often referred to as **vitamin dependency syndromes**, is poorly understood. Interest in these disorders has focused chiefly on conditions involving folate, vitamin B_{12} (cobala-

min), pyridoxine, and vitamin D. Hartnup disease might be considered a vitamin dependency syndrome with a transport defect or a disorder of amino acid metabolism. For convenience, it was included in Table 17-22. The vitamin dependency disorders will be described briefly, since the primary treatment is administration of vitamins.

Folate Dependency

A number of inborn errors of folate metabolism have been described recently. For example, increased folate requirement is known to occur in homocystinuria owing to $N^{5,10}$-methylenetetrahydrofolate reductase deficiency, and in inborn errors of vitamin B_{12} metabolism,[105] Lesch-Nyhan syndrome,[106] sickle cell disease (see Chapter 18), and **psoriasis** (a chronic skin disease).[107]

Vitamin B_{12} Dependency

Vitamin B_{12} (cobalamin) has been associated with several inborn errors of metabolism. It acts as a coenzyme in several reactions, particularly those involving transfer of single-carbon atoms.

The reactions of two enzymes in mammalian cells are known to require cobalamin coenzymes. One of these enzymes is **methyl-cobalamin-dependent homocysteine-N^5-methyltetrahydrofolate methyltransferase**, the metabolic function of which is illustrated in Figure 17-6 in relation to homocystinuria. The second enzyme is **adenosylcobalamin-dependent methylmalonyl–CoA mutase**. This enzyme catalyzes a step in the metabolism of propionyl-CoA to methylmalonyl-CoA and then to succinyl-CoA. Propionate is an intermediate product in the metabolism of isoleucine, valine, methionine, threonine, odd-chain fatty acids, and cholesterol. A variety of inherited defects in this metabolic pathway lead to one form or another of **methylmalonic acidemia** (MMA). Some types of MMA are not vitamin-dependent, whereas other defects involve steps in cobalamin metabolism and lead to impaired methylmalonyl-CoA mutase activity and thus to methylmalonic acidemia. These conditions respond to pharmacologic doses of cyanocobalamin. Additional abnormalities in cobalamin metabolism have also been identified and are accompanied by homocystinuria, cystathioninuria, and hypomethioninemia.[105]

Pyridoxine Dependency

Pyridoxine or **vitamin B$_6$** is a cofactor in approximately 50 decarboxylase and transaminase enzymes. Hunt et al.[108] were the first to report a case of intractable seizures in an infant on an apparently pyridoxine-sufficient diet. The seizures were unresponsive to anticonvulsant drugs and physiologic doses of pyridoxine; however, a massive dose of pyridoxine (10 mg) relieved the symptoms. The seizures were thought to be due to a deficiency of the neurotransmitter gamma-aminobutyric acid, the synthesis of which requires glutamic acid decarboxylase and pyridoxal phosphate as a cofactor.[109] Additional types of vitamin B$_6$ dependency involve an increased requirement of the coenzyme in disorders of cystathionine synthetase (homocystinuria) and kynureninase (hyperxanthurenic aciduria).[110] Laboratory experiments also suggest that impaired vitamin B$_6$ function may contribute to the pathogenesis of PKU.[111] Other inborn errors that are reported to respond to high doses of pyridoxine are glycinuria, cystathioninuria, and Hartnup disease.[112]

Hereditary pyridoxine dependency usually occurs soon after birth, although some symptoms may develop only later. Dietary deficiency of vitamin B$_6$ must be ruled out in diagnosing this condition.

Pyridoxine dependency states respond promptly; however, an oral dose of up to 50 mg of pyridoxine daily may be required to achieve control.

Vitamin D – Dependent Rickets

Vitamin D – dependent rickets is an autosomal recessive trait that is responsive to large doses of vitamin D. The affected enzyme, 1-alpha-hydroxylase in the renal tubular cells, catalyzes the conversion of 25-(OH)-vitamin D$_3$ to 1,25-(OH)$_2$D$_3$. Vitamin D–dependent rickets is thought to arise from a defect in this enzyme, but this theory has not been confirmed.[113]

The condition responds dramatically to supplements with vitamin D and phosphate. A well-balanced diet is an adjunct to therapy,[114] and the nutritional care specialist should work with parents or patients on planning for adequate nutrition.

Familial Vitamin D – Resistant Rickets

Familial vitamin D – resistant rickets (FVDRR), in contrast to vitamin D–dependent rickets, is an X-linked dominant trait with an estimated incidence of 1 in 25,000 live births. The condition is characterized by rickets in children and osteomalacia in adults. Stature may or may not be affected. The cardinal biochemical sign in FVDRR is hypophosphatemia associated with decreased tubular resorption of inorganic phosphate and a consequent increase in urinary phosphate.

The exact mechanism for the hypophosphatemia is poorly understood. The abnormality usually is attributed to a defect in renal tubular phosphate reabsorption. It is possible that there is decreased conversion of vitamin D to the biologically active form, 25-hydroxycholecalciferol. There is increased fecal excretion of vitamin D in plasma and urine. The primary biochemical abnormalities mentioned could be responsible for decreased intestinal absorption of calcium. The reduced calcium absorption might then lead to rickets in children, osteomalacia in adults, or secondary hyperparathyroidism with attendant hypophosphatemia and phosphaturia.

Alternatively, Albright's group[115,116] has proposed that decreased calcium absorption is the primary, not a secondary, defect in FVDRR, and that hyperparathyroidism is the secondary effect. So far, no theory has explained the disorder completely. Since the condition affects transport, it is included in those disorders classified as transport defects.

The objectives of treatment are to control the bone disease and promote growth. Current treatment consists of oral supplements of inorganic phosphate and large doses of vitamin D,[114] but the treatment is not always completely effective, especially in males.[113] The effective vitamin dose sometimes is in the toxic range, with a potential for renal damage. The nutritional care specialist should observe the patient for signs of vitamin toxicity and monitor the diet for nutritional adequacy.

DISORDERS OF MINERAL METABOLISM

Considerable attention has been directed to the etiology and treatment of **Wilson's disease**, a metabolic disease known to be due to an inherited abnormality of copper metabolism, and to **acrodermatitis enteropathica**, a disorder of zinc metabolism.

Wilson's Disease

Wilson's disease, also known as **hepatolenticular degeneration**, is an autosomal recessive disorder, although it appears to be slightly more common in males than in females. The incidence of Wilson's disease is unknown.

It is characterized by degenerative changes in the brain, cirrhosis of the liver, and **Kayser-Fleischer rings** (greenish brown pigmented rings at the outer margin of the cornea).[117] Hepatic and renal impairment, especially progressive failure in the renal tubular transfer of amino acids and other substrates, are common. Clinical symptoms rarely occur in early childhood.

The exact enzymatic defect has not been identified, but the abnormal gene product causes impaired incorporation of copper into ceruloplasmin (the blue copper-containing protein) and results in the excretion of copper in the bile. Excess copper is deposited in various tissues, particularly the liver, brain, cornea, and kidney. Serum copper and ceruloplasmin usually are decreased in Wilson's disease.[117] Urinary copper excretion is increased, and serum phosphate and urate levels are decreased.

The diagnosis of Wilson's disease is based on the presence of Kayser-Fleischer rings, neurologic features, and liver disease. Positive diagnostic tests include measurement of decreased serum ceruloplasmin and copper levels and increased liver stores of copper.

The objective of treatment is to relieve the tissues of copper and prevent its reaccumulation. Wilson's disease is treated with penicillamine, a copper-chelating agent. The disease can be controlled effectively but is invariably fatal if untreated. Treatment must be continued indefinitely.

Nutritional management is an adjunct to penicillamine therapy. The patient is advised to avoid liver, nuts, mushrooms, cocoa, chocolate, and shellfish, which are high in copper content. Follow-up is essential to ensure a well-balanced diet. Oral administration of potassium sulfide to precipitate copper in the bowel in the form of insoluble copper sulfide also is helpful in preventing the reaccumulation of copper. Pyridoxine supplements are needed to prevent pyridoxine deficiency that could result from prolonged penicillamine therapy.

Acrodermatitis Enteropathica

The primary biochemical abnormality in acrodermatitis enteropathica has not been identified, although a defect in some factor responsible for the absorption or gastrointestinal transport of zinc has been hypothesized.[118] Acrodermatitis enteropathica is characterized by severe diarrhea, dermatitis of the oral, anal, and genital areas, and **alopecia** (hair loss) in early infancy, often following the change from breast milk to cow's milk. Chronic diarrhea, malabsorption, steatorrhea, and lactose intolerance are common. Ophthalmic manifestations include blepharitis, conjunctivitis, photophobia, and corneal opacities. Tremor, irritability, and occasional cerebellar ataxia occur, infections are common, and retarded growth and hypogonadism are characteristic.[118] If untreated, the condition is fatal in most cases.

Acrodermatitis enteropathica is diagnosed by the clinical picture, especially the dermatitis and gastrointestinal manifestations in younger children. In addition, the biochemical parameters of zinc deficiency—low plasma and urinary zinc levels and reduced serum alkaline phosphatase and erythrocyte zinc levels—have been reported in many patients. Another consistent biochemical finding is aberrant fatty acid metabolism with some impairment in the elongation-saturation system of fatty acid metabolism.[119]

Small daily supplements (35 mg) of zinc sulfate bring about complete relief of symptoms. The use of approximately 150 mg of oral zinc sulfate daily in divided doses is recommended to guard against intercurrent infections and to promote adequate growth during adolescence.[120-123] A diet high in zinc may be helpful as adjunctive therapy.[123]

Case Study: Phenylketonuria

Jennifer C. was ten days old when her parents were told that the screening test for PKU was positive. Further tests showed a serum phenylalanine concentration of 35 mg/dl. The parents were instructed by the nutritionist on the use of a low-phenylalanine formula. Mrs. C. was very careful to follow the directions of the nutritionist at the clinic, and Jennifer's serum phenylalanine fell to 6 mg/dl. Jennifer liked her formula and grew at a normal rate. She also seemed to be developing normally mentally.

As Jennifer developed, solid foods were added to her diet at the usual times for normal children. On one occasion, Jennifer had an upper respiratory infection and refused to drink all her formula. When her serum phenylalanine was determined, it had risen to 15 mg/dl. The nutritionist examined carefully the three-day food intake record that Mrs. C. had brought to the clinic.

Exercises

1. What is the normal serum phenylalanine level in the newborn infant?
2. Why does serum phenylalanine increase in classic PKU?
3. What other metabolic alterations occur?
4. Calculate a Lofenalac formula to be given to Jennifer when she weighs 10 kg.
5. Later, Jennifer's diet prescription was altered to contain 340 mg of phenylalanine, with 120 mg of it from Lofenalac, 16 g of protein, and 800 kcal. Jennifer is capable of eating strained fruits and vegetables and infant cereals. Plan a diet for Jennifer, assuming she eats six times a day.
6. Why did Jennifer's serum phenylalanine level rise when she had an infection? What advice would you give Jennifer's mother concerning Jennifer's diet during such a period?
7. Assuming Jennifer is one year old and weighs 10 kg, calculate a diet for her if she has the following: (a) branched-chain ketoaciduria; (b) tyrosinemia, type 2; and (c) synthetase deficiency homocystinuria.

References

1. Elsas, L.J., II, and Priest, J.H. Medical genetics. In W.A. Sodeman, Jr., and T.M. Sodeman, Eds., *Sodeman's Pathologic Physiology,* 6th ed. Philadelphia: W.B. Saunders, 1979.
2. Garrod, A.E. The Croonian lectures on inborn errors of metabolism. *Lancet* 2:1, 73, 142, 214, 1908.
3. Scriver, C.R., and Rosenberg, L.E. *Amino Acid Metabolism and Its Disorders.* Philadelphia: W.B. Saunders, 1973.
4. Elsas, L.J., II, and Acosta, P.B. Nutrition support of inherited metabolic diseases. In M.E. Shils and V.R. Young, Eds., *Modern Nutrition in Health and Disease,* 7th ed. Philadelphia: Lea & Febiger, 1988.
5. Fölling, A. Uber Ausscheidung von Phenylbrenztraubensaure in den Harn als Stoff-

weschselanomalie in Verbindung mit Imbezillitat. *Hoppe-Seylers Z. Physiol. Chem.* 227:169, 1934.

6. Woolley, D.W., and van de Hoeven, T. Serotonin deficiency in infancy as one cause of a mental defect in phenylketonuria. *Science* 144:883, 1964.

7. Udenfriend, S. The primary enzymatic defect in phenylketonuria and how it may influence the central nervous system. In J.A. Anderson and K.F. Swaiman, Eds., *Proceedings of a Conference on Phenylketonuria and Allied Metabolic Diseases.* Washington, D.C.: U.S. Government Printing Office, 1979.

8. Koch, R., and Wenz, E. Phenylketonuria. *Annu. Rev. Nutr.* 7:117, 1987.

9. Bickel, H., Gerrard, J., and Hickmans, E.M. Influence of phenylalanine intake on phenylketonuria. *Lancet* 2:812, 1953.

10. Koch, R., Blaskovics, M., Wenz, E., Fishler, K., and Schaeffler, G. Phenylalaninemia and phenylketonuria. In W.L. Nyhan, Ed., *Heritable Disorders of Amino Acid Metabolism.* New York: John Wiley and Sons, 1974.

11. Acosta, P.B., and Elsas, L.J., II. *Dietary Management of Inherited Metabolic Disease: Phenylketonuria, Galactosemia, Tyrosinemia, Homocystinuria, Maple Syrup Urine Disease.* Atlanta: ACELMU Publishers, 1975.

12. Ernest, A.E., McCabe, E.R.B., Neifer, M.R., and O'Flynn, M.E. *Guide to Breast Feeding the Infant with PKU.* Washington, D.C.: U.S. Government Printing Office, 1979.

13. Koch, R., Wenz, E., and Steinber, M.S. *PKU —Guide to Management.* Los Angeles: Children's Hospital of Los Angeles and California State Department of Health, 1977.

14. Holtzman, N.A., Welcher, D.W., and Mellits, E.D. Termination of restricted diet in children with phenylketonuria. A randomized controlled study. *N. Engl. J. Med.* 293:1121, 1975.

15. Hudson, F.P. Termination of dietary treatment of phenylketonuria. *Arch. Dis. Child.* 42:198, 1967.

16. Horner, F.A., Streamer, C.W., Alejandrino, L., Reed, L.H., and Ibbott, F. Termination of dietary treatment of phenylketonuria. *N. Engl. J. Med.* 266:79, 1962.

17. Seashore, M.R., Friedman, E., Novelly, R.A., and Bapat, F. Loss of intellectual function in children with phenylketonuria after relaxation of phenylalanine restriction. *Pediatrics* 75:226, 1985.

18. Holtzman, N.A., Kronmal, R.A., van Doorninck, W., Azen, C., and Koch, R. Effect of age at loss of dietary control on intellectual performance and behavior of children with

phenylketonuria. *N. Engl. J. Med.* 314:593, 1986.

19. Krause, W., Epstein, C., Averbrook, A., Dembure, P., and Elsas, L. Phenylalanine alters the mean power frequency of electroencephalograms and plasma L-dopa in treated patients with phenylketonuria. *Pediatr. Res.* 20:1112, 1986.

20. Mabry, C.C., Nelson, I.L., and Denniston, J.C. Newly appreciated cause of mental retardation. Observation on two phenylketonuric mothers and their children. *J. Pediatr.* 63:877, 1963.

21. Lenke, R.R., and Levy, H.L. Maternal phenylketonuria and hyperphenylalaninemia. An international survey of the outcome of untreated and treated pregnancies. *N. Engl. J. Med.* 303:1202, 1980.

22. Lenke, R.R., and Levy, H.L. Maternal phenylketonuria and hyperphenylalaninemia. *N. Engl. J. Med.* 303:1202, 1980.

23. Okano, Y., Chow, I.Z., Isshiki, G., Inoue, A., and Oura, T. Effects of phenylalanine loading on protein synthesis in the fetal heart and brain of rat. An experimental approach to maternal phenylketonuria. *J. Inherited Metab. Dis.* 9:15, 1986.

24. Levy, H.L., Shih, V.S., Karolkewicz, V., et al. Persistent mild hyperphenylalaninemia in the untreated state. A prospective study. *N. Engl. J. Med.* 285:424, 1971.

25. Rosenberg, L.E., and Scriver, C.R. Disorders of amino acid metabolism. In P.K. Bondy and L.E. Rosenberg, Eds., *Metabolic Control and Disease,* 8th ed. Philadelphia: W.B. Saunders, 1980.

26. Kaufman, S. Raine memorial lecture. *J. Inherited Metab. Dis.* 8 (Suppl. 1):20, 1985.

27. Halvorsen, S., and Gjessing, L.R. Tyrosinosis. In H. Bickel, F.P. Hudson, and L.E. Woolf, Eds., *Phenylketonuria and Some Other Inborn Errors of Metabolism.* Stuttgart: Georg Thieme, 1971.

28. Lindblad, B., Lindstedt, S., and Steen, G. On the enzymic defects in hereditary tyrosinemia. *Proc. Natl. Acad. Sci.* 74:4641, 1971.

29. Sassa, S., and Kappas, A. Hereditary tyrosinemia and the heme biosynthetic pathway. *J. Clin. Invest.* 71:625, 1983.

30. Christensen, E., Jacobsen, B.B., Gregersen, N., Hjeds, H., Pedersen, J.B., Brandt, N.J., and Baekmark, U.B. Urinary excretion of succinylacetone and α-aminolevulinic acid in patients with hereditary tyrosinemia. *Clin. Chim. Acta* 116:331, 1981.

31. Kvittengen, E.A., Halvorsen, S., and Jellum, E. Deficient fumarylacetoacetate fumaryl hydrolase activity in lymphocytes and fibro-

blasts from patients with hereditary tyrosinemia. *Pediatr. Res.* 14:541, 1983.

32. Furukawa, N., Kinugasa, A., Sea, T., Ishi, T., Ota, T., Machida, Y., et al. Enzyme defect in a case of tyrosinemia, type I, acute form. *Pediatr. Res.* 18:463, 1984.

33. Kennaway, N.G., and Buist, N.R. Metabolic studies in a patient with hepatic cytosol tyrosine aminotransferase deficiency. *Pediatr. Res.* 5:287, 1971.

34. Buist, N.R., Kennaway, N.G., and Fellman, J.H. Disorders of tyrosine metabolism. In W.L. Nyhan, Ed., *Heritable Disorders of Amino Acid Metabolism.* New York: John Wiley and Sons, 1974.

35. Llenado, M., and Ekvall, S. Tyrosinosis. In S. Palmer and S. Ekvall, Eds., *Pediatric Nutrition in Developmental Disorders.* Springfield, Ill.: Charles C. Thomas, 1978.

36. Danner, D.J., and Elsas, L.J., II. Disorders of branched chain amino acid metabolism. In C.R. Scriver et al., Eds., *The Metabolic Basis of Inherited Disease,* 6th ed. New York: McGraw-Hill, 1989.

37. Lancaster, G., Mamer, O.A., and Scriver, C.R. Branched-chain alpha-ketoacids isolated as oxime derivatives. Relationship to the corresponding hydroxyacids and amino acids in maple syrup urine disease. *Metabolism* 23:257, 1974.

38. Bowden, J.A., Brestel, E.P., Cape, W.T., et al. α-Keto-isocaproic acid inhibition of pyruvate and α-ketoglutarate oxidative decarboxylation in rat liver slices. *Biochem. Med.* 4:69, 1970.

39. Haymond, M.M., Karl, I.W., Feign, R.D., et al. Hypoglycemia in maple syrup urine disease. Defective gluconeogenesis. *Pediatr. Res.* 7:500, 1973.

40. Committee for Improvement of Hereditary Disease Management. Management of maple syrup urine disease in Canada. *Can. Med. Assoc. J.* 115:1005, 1975.

41. Mudd, S.H., Levy, H.L., and Skovby, F. Disorders of transsulfuration. In C.R. Scriver et al., Eds., *The Metabolic Basis of Inherited Disease,* 6th ed. New York: McGraw-Hill, 1989.

42. Abel, E., Michell, M., and Ekvall, S. Homocystinuria. In S. Palmer and S. Ekvall, Eds., *Pediatric Nutrition in Developmental Disorders.* Springfield, Ill.: Charles C. Thomas, 1978.

43. Levin, B., Abraham, J.M., Oberholzer, V.G., and Burgess, E.A. Hyperammonaemia. A deficiency of liver ornithine transcarbamylase occurrence in mother and child. *Arch. Dis. Child.* 44:152, 1969.

44. Cederbaum, S.D., Shaw, K.N.F., and Valente, M. Hyperargininemia. *J. Pediatr.* 90:569, 1975.

45. Kennaway, N.G., Harward, P.J., Ramberg, D.A., Koler, R.D., and Buist, N.R.M. Citrullinemia. Enzymatic evidence of genetic heterogeneity. *Pediatr. Res.* 9:554, 1975.

46. Glick, N.R., Snodgrass, P.J., and Schafer, I.A. Neonatal arginosuccinic aciduria with normal brain and kidney but absent liver arginosuccinate lyase activity. *Am. J. Hum. Genet.* 28:22, 1976.

47. Russell, A. The implications of hyperammonemia in rare and common disorders, including migraine. *Mt. Sinai J. Med.* 40:723, 1973.

48. Batshaw, M.L., and Brusilow, S. Acute management of hyperammonemic coma in congenital urea cycle enzymopathies (UCE). Peritoneal dialysis (PD) vs. exchange transfusion (ET). *Pediatr. Res.* 13:472, 1979.

49. Wada, Y., Tada, K., Minagawa, A., et al. Idiopathic hypervalinemia. *Tohoku J. Exp. Med.* 81:46, 1963.

50. Wada, Y. Idiopathic hypervalinemia. Valine and alpha ketoacids in blood following an oral dose of valine. *Tohoku J. Exp. Med.* 87:322, 1965.

51. Holt, L.E., Jr., Gyorgy, P., Pratt, E.L., et al. *Protein and Amino Acid Requirements in Early Life.* New York: University Press, 1960.

52. Brooks, E. Hypervalinemia. In S. Palmer and S. Ekvall, Eds., *Pediatric Nutrition in Developmental Disorders.* Springfield, Ill.: Charles C. Thomas, 1978.

53. Crump, I. Inborn Errors of Metabolism. Dietary Therapy. In San Diego Pediatric Nutrition Group, *Pediatric Nutrition Manual.* San Diego: University of California Medical Center, 1981.

54. Oberholzer, V.G., Levin, B., Burgess, E.A., and Young, W.F. Methylmalonic aciduria, an inborn error of metabolism leading to chronic metabolic acidosis. *Arch. Dis. Child.* 42:492, 1967.

55. Willard, H.F., and Rosenberg, L.E. Inborn errors of cobalamin metabolism. Effect of cobalamin supplementation in culture on methylmalonyl CoA mutase activity in normal and mutant human fibroblasts. *Biochem. Genet.* 17:57, 1979.

56. Palmer, S., Ekvall, S., and Umali, M. Methylmalonic aciduria. In S. Palmer and S. Ekvall, Eds., *Pediatric Nutrition in Developmental Disorders.* Springfield, Ill.: Charles C. Thomas, 1978.

57. Nyhan, W.L., Fawcett, N., Ando, T., et al. Response to dietary therapy in B_{12} unre-

sponsive methylmalonic acidemia. *Pediatrics* 51:539, 1973.

58. Childs, B., Nyhan, W.L., Borden, M., et al. Idiopathic hyperglycinemia and hyperglycinuria. A new disorder of amino acid metabolism. *Pediatrics* 27:522, 1961.

59. Ando, T., Rasmussen, K., Nyhan, W.L., et al. Propionic acidemia in patients with ketotic hyperglycinemia. *J. Pediatr.* 78:827, 1971.

60. Hsia, Y.E., Scully, K.J., and Rosenberg, L.E. Inherited propionyl-CoA carboxylase deficiency in ketotic hyperglycinemia. *J. Clin. Invest.* 50:127, 1971.

61. Brandt, I.K., Hsia, Y.E., Clement, D.H., et al. Propionicacidemia (ketotic hyperglycinemia). Dietary treatment resulting in normal growth and development. *Pediatrics* 53:391, 1974.

62. Barnes, N.D., Hull, D., Balbogin, L., et al. Biotin-responsive propionicacidaemia. *Lancet* 2:244, 1970.

63. Auerbach, V.H., DiGeorge, A.M., Baldridge, R.C., et al. Histidinemia. A deficiency in histidase resulting in the urinary excretion of histidine and of imidazolepyruvic acid. *J. Pediatr.* 60:487, 1962.

64. Gatfield, P.D., Knights, R.M., Devereaux, M., et al. Histidinemia. Report of four new cases in one family and the effect of low histidine diets. *Can. Med. Assoc. J.* 101:465, 1969.

65. Stevens, F., and Ekvall, S. Histidinemia. Histidine alpha-deaminase deficiency. In S. Palmer and S. Ekvall, Eds., *Pediatric Nutrition in Developmental Disorders.* Springfield, Ill.: Charles C Thomas, 1978.

66. Scriver, C.R., Smith, R.J., and Phang, J.M. Disorders of proline and hydroxyproline metabolism. In J.B. Stanbury, J.B. Wyngaarden, D.S. Fredrickson, et al., Eds., *The Metabolic Basis of Inherited Disease*, 5th ed. New York: McGraw-Hill, 1983.

67. Harries, J.T., Piesowics, A.T., Seakins, J.W.T., et al. Low proline diet in type-I hyperprolinaemia. *Arch. Dis. Child.* 46:72, 1971.

68. Simila, S. Dietary treatment in hyperprolinemia type II. *Acta Paediatr. Scand.* 63:249, 1974.

69. Efron, M.L., Bixby, E.M., Palattao, L.G., et al. Hydroxyprolinemia associated with mental deficiency. *N. Engl. J. Med.* 267:1193, 1962.

70. Efron, M.L. Treatment of hydroxyprolinemia and hyperprolinemia. *Am J. Dis. Child.* 113:166, 1967.

71. Knapp, A. Über eine neue, hereditäre, von

Vitamin-B_6 abhängige Störung im Tryptophan-Stoffwechsel. *Clin. Chim. Acta* 5:6, 1960.

72. Tada, K., Yokoyama, Y., Nakagawa, H., et al. Vitamin B_6-dependent xanthurenic aciduria. (The second report.) *Tohoku J. Exp. Med.* 95:107, 1968.

73. Baron, D.N., Dent, C.E., Harris, H., et al. Hereditary pellagra-like skin rash with temporary cerebellar ataxia, constant renal aminoaciduria, and other bizarre biochemical features. *Lancet* 2:421, 1956.

74. Llenado, M., and Ekvall, S. Hartnup disease. In S. Palmer and S. Ekvall, Eds., *Pediatric Nutrition in Developmental Disorders.* Springfield, Ill.: Charles C Thomas, 1978.

75. Wollaston, W.H. On cystic oxide, a new species of urinary calculus. *Philos. Trans. R. Soc. Lond. [Biol.]* 100:223, 1910.

76. Milne, M.D., Asatoor, A.M., Edwards, K.D.G., et al. The intestinal absorption defect in cystinuria. *Gut* 2:323, 1961.

77. Dent, C.E., Friedmann, W., Green, H., et al. Treatment of cystinuria. *Br. Med. J.* 1:403, 1965.

78. Kolb, R.O., Earll, J.M., and Harper, H.A. 'Disappearance' of cystinuria in a patient treated with prolonged low methionine diet. *Metabolism* 16:378, 1967.

79. Mason, H.H., and Turner, M.E. Chronic galactosemia. *Am. J. Dis. Child.* 50:359, 1935.

80. Gabbay, K.H. The sorbitol pathway and the complication of diabetes. *N. Engl. J. Med.* 288:831, 1973.

81. Quan-Ma, R., Wells, H.J., Wells, W.W., et al. Galactitol in the tissues of a galactosemic child. *Am. J. Dis. Child.* 112:477, 1966.

82. Segal, S., and Cuatrecasas, P. The oxidation of C^{14} galactose by patients with congenital galactosemia. Evidence for a direct oxidative pathway. *Am. J. Med.* 44:340, 1968.

83. Jakobs, C., Warner, T.G., Sweetman, L., and Nyhan, W.L. Stable isotope dilution analysis of galactitol in amniotic fluid. An accurate approach to prenatal diagnosis of galactosemia. *Pediatr. Res.* 18:714, 1984.

84. Kromrower, G.M., and Lee, D.H. Long-term follow-up of galactosaemia. *Arch. Dis. Child.* 45:367, 1970.

85. Schapira, F., Gregori, C., Boue, J., et al. Prenatal diagnosis of galactosemia. *Biomedicine Express* 29(4):136, 1978.

86. Wenz, E., and Michel, M. Galactosemia. In S. Palmer and S. Ekvall, Eds., *Pediatric Nutrition in Developmental Disorders.* Springfield, Ill.: Charles C. Thomas, 1978.

87. Donnell, G.N., and Bergren, W.R. The ga-

lactosemias. In D.N. Raine, Ed., *The Treatment of Inherited Metabolic Disease.* New York: Elsevier, 1974.

88. Segal, S.D. Disorders of galactose metabolism. In J.B. Stanbury, J.B. Wyngaarden, and D.S. Fredrickson, Eds., *The Metabolic Basis of Inherited Disease,* 4th ed. New York: McGraw-Hill, 1978.

89. Gitzelman, R., Steinmann, B., and van den Berghe, G. Disorders of fructose metabolism. In C.R. Scriver et al., Eds., *The Metabolic Basis of Inherited Disease,* 6th ed. New York: McGraw-Hill, 1989.

90. Bell, L., and Sherwood, W.G. Current practices and improved recommendations for treating hereditary fructose intolerance. *J. Am. Diet. Assoc.* 87:721, 1987.

91. Chen, Y.T., Cornblath, M., and Sidbury, J. Cornstarch therapy in type I glycogen storage disease. *N. Engl. J. Med.* 310:171, 1984.

92. Steinberg, D. Phytanic acid storage disease (Refsum's disease). In J.B. Stanbury, J.B. Wyngaarden, D.S. Fredrickson, et al., Eds., *The Metabolic Basis of Inherited Disease,* 5th ed. New York: McGraw-Hill, 1983.

93. Refsum, S. Heredopathia atactica polyneuritiformis. *Acta Psychiatr. Scand. [Suppl.]* 38:9, 1946.

94. Refsum, S. Heredopathía atáctica polyneuritiformis reconsideración. *World Neurol.* 1:334, 1960.

95. Ackman, R.G., and Hooper, S.N. Isoprenoid fatty acids in the human diet. Distinctive geographical features in butterfats and importance in margarines based on marine oils. *Can. Inst. Food Sci. Technol. J.* 6:159, 1973.

96. Sen Gupta, A.K., and Peters, H. Isolation and structure determination of polybranched-chain fatty acids from fish oil. *Fette Seifen, Anstrichmittel* 68:349, 1966.

97. Steinberg, D., Mize, C.E., Herndon, J.H.K., Jr., et al. Phytanic acid in patients with Refsum's syndrome and response to dietary treatment. *Arch. Intern. Med.* 125:75, 1970.

98. Lundberg, A., Lilja, L.G., Lundberg, P.O., et al. Heredopathia atactica polyneuritiformis (Refsum's disease). Experiences of dietary treatment and plasmapheresis. *Eur. Neurol.* 8:309, 1972.

99. Stokke, O., and Eldjarn, L. Biochemical and dietary aspects of Refsum's disease. In P.J. Dyck, P.K. Thomas, and E.H. Lambert, Eds., *Peripheral Neuropathy,* vol. 2. Philadelphia: W.B. Saunders, 1975.

100. Seegmiller, J.E. Diseases of purine and pyrimidine metabolism. In P.K. Bondy and L.E. Rosenberg, Eds., *Metabolic Control and Disease,* 8th ed. Philadelphia: W.B. Saunders, 1980.

101. Seegmiller, J.E., Laster, L., and Howell, R.R. Biochemistry of uric acid and its relations to gout. *N. Engl. J. Med.* 168:712, 764, 821, 1963.

102. Hine, J. Hyperuricemia (Lesch-Nyhan syndrome). In S. Palmer and S. Ekvall, Eds., *Pediatric Nutrition in Developmental Disorders.* Springfield, Ill.: Charles C. Thomas, 1978.

103. Ogryzlo, M.A. Hyperuricemia induced by high fat diets and starvation. *Arthritis Rheum.* 8:799, 1965.

104. Maclachlan, M.J., and Rodnan, G.P. Effects of food, fast and alcohol on serum uric acid and acute attacks of gout. *Am. J. Med.* 42:38, 1967.

105. Maloney, M.J., and Rosenberg, L.E. Inherited defects of B_{12} metabolism. *Am. J. Med.* 48:584, 1970.

106. Felix, J.S., and Demars, R. Purine requirement of cells cultured from humans affected with Lesch-Nyhan syndrome (hypoxanthine-guanine phosphoribosyltransferase deficiency). *Proc. Natl. Acad. Sci. U.S.A.* 62:536, 1969.

107. Baer, M.T. Folic acid deficiency. In S. Palmer and S. Ekvall, Eds., *Pediatric Nutrition in Developmental Disorders.* Springfield, Ill.: Charles C Thomas, 1978.

108. Hunt, A.D., Jr., Stokes, J., Jr., McCrory, W.W., et al. Pyridoxine dependency. Report of a case of intractable convulsions in an infant controlled by pyridoxine. *Pediatrics* 13:140, 1954.

109. Scriver, C.R., and Whelan, D.T. Glutamic acid decarboxylase in mammalian tissue outside the central nervous system and the possible relevance to vitamin B_6 dependency with seizures. *Ann. N.Y. Acad. Sci.* 166:83, 1969.

110. Kappas, A., Sassa, S., Galbraith, R.A., and Nordmann, Y. The porphyrias. In C.R. Scriver et al., Eds., *The Metabolic Basis of Inherited Disease,* 6th ed. New York: McGraw-Hill, 1989.

111. Loo, Y.H., and Ritman, P. Phenylketonuria and vitamin B_6 function. *Nature* 213:914, 1967.

112. Berry, H.K. Inborn errors of metabolism. *J. Am. Diet. Assoc.* 49:44, 1966.

113. Rasmussen, H., and Tenenhouse, H.S. Hypophosphatemias. In C.R. Scriver, et al., Eds., *The Metabolic Basis of Inherited Disease,* 6th ed. New York: McGraw-Hill, 1989.

114. Palmer, S. Familial vitamin D–resistant rickets. In S. Palmer and S. Ekvall, Eds., *Pediatric Nutrition in Developmental Disorders.* Springfield, Ill.: Charles C. Thomas, 1978.
115. Albright, F., Butler, A.M., and Bloomberg, E. Rickets resistant to vitamin D therapy. *Am. J. Dis. Child.* 54:529, 1937.
116. Albright, F., and Sulkowitch, H.W. The effect of vitamin D on calcium and phosphorus metabolism. Studies on four patients. *J. Clin. Invest.* 17:305, 1938.
117. Danks, D.M. Disorders of copper transport. In C.R. Scriver, et al., Eds., *The Metabolic Basis of Inherited Disease,* 6th ed. New York: McGraw-Hill, 1989.
118. National Academy of Sciences. *Zinc.* Subcommittee on Zinc, Committee on Medical and Biologic Effects of Environmental Pollutants. Division of Medical Sciences, Assembly of Life Sciences, National Research Council. Baltimore: University Park Press, 1978.
119. Nelder, K.H., Hagler, L., Wise, W.R., et al. Acrodermatitis enteropathica. A clinical and biochemical survey. *Arch. Dermatol.* 110:711, 1974.
120. Moynahan, E.J. Acrodermatitis enteropathica. A lethal inherited human zinc-deficiency disorder. *Lancet* 2:399, 1974.
121. Nelder, K.H., and Hambidge, K.M. Zinc therapy of acrodermatitis enteropathica. *N. Engl. J. Med.* 292:879, 1975.
122. Michaelson, G. Zinc therapy in acrodermatitis enteropathica. *Acta Derm. Venereol.* (Stockh.) 54:377, 1974.
123. Palmer, S. Human zinc deficiency. In S. Palmer and S. Ekvall, Eds., *Pediatric Nutri-* tion in Developmental Disorders. Springfield, Ill.: Charles C Thomas, 1978.

Bibliography

Bondy, P.K., and Rosenberg, L.E., Eds. *Metabolic Control and Disease,* 8th ed. Philadelphia: W.B. Saunders, 1980.
Nyhan, W.L., *Abnormalities in Amino Acid Metabolism in Clinical Medicine.* Norwalk, Conn.: Appleton-Century-Crofts, 1984.
Nyhan, W.L., Ed. *Heritable Disorders of Amino Acid Metabolism.* New York: John Wiley and Sons, 1974.
Palmer, S., and Ekvall, S., Eds. *Pediatric Nutrition in Developmental Disorders.* Springfield, Ill.: Charles C Thomas, 1978.
Raine, D.N., Ed. *The Treatment of Inherited Metabolic Disease.* New York: Elsevier, 1974.
Schuett, V.E. *Low Protein Cookery for PKU,* 2nd ed. Madison: University of Wisconsin Press, 1988.
Scriver, C.R., et al., Eds. *The Metabolic Basis of Inherited Disease,* 6th ed. New York: McGraw-Hill, 1989.

Sources of Current Information

American Journal of Diseases of Children
Archives of Disease in Childhood
Journal of Inherited Metabolic Disease
Journal of Mental Deficiency Research
Journal of Pediatrics
New England Journal of Medicine
Pediatric Research
Pediatrics

18. Nutritional Anemias

Robert B. Rucker, Ph.D.

I. Erythropoiesis and Hemoglobin Synthesis
  A. Sites and developmental stages of red blood cell formation
  B. Red blood cell maturation
    1. Role of erythropoietin
    2. Role of hemoglobin
    3. Steps in the maturation process
  C. Hemoglobin synthesis and degradation
  D. Important nutrients involved in erythropoiesis
    1. Iron
    2. Folic acid and vitamin B_{12}
    3. Other nutrients
II. The Anemias
  A. Normocytic anemias
  B. Megaloblastic anemias
  C. Microcytic anemia
  D. Sickle cell anemia and other hemoglobinopathies
  E. Hemolytic anemia
III. Concluding Comments
  A. Anemia and athletic performance

Anemia most often implies a reduction in the quantity of **hemoglobin** or in the number of **red cells (erythrocytes)** in blood. Its major pathophysiologic effect is a reduction in the oxygen-carrying capacity of blood that can lead to tissue **hypoxia** (low oxygen content). Signs of anemia are common to many diseases and disorders; therefore, anemia is a symptom of disease rather than a disease itself.

Almost all forms of anemia involve nutrition in their treatment. In this chapter, some of the major types of anemias will be described and the roles of various nutrients in **erythropoiesis** (production of red blood cells) and hemoglobin synthesis will be discussed. Normal values are given in Appendix C. Nutrients such as iron, folic acid, vitamin B_{12}, protein, and ascorbic acid are very important to normal red blood cell and hemoglobin formation; defective erythropoiesis may result from defects in the metabolism of copper, vitamin A, vitamin E, niacin, pyridoxine, riboflavin, and thiamine. Fortunately, the understanding of how this diverse array of nutrients may alter normal erythropoiesis or hemoglobin synthesis is facilitated by the knowledge that many nutrients act through related mechanisms. Steps involved in the development of erythrocytes and the synthesis of hemoglobin are described in the following sections. It is important to understand the key features of these steps to understand the mechanisms that underlie nutrition's role in the treatment of anemias.

ERYTHROPOIESIS AND HEMOGLOBIN SYNTHESIS

Sites and Developmental Stages of Red Blood Cell Formation

The first signs of vascular system development occur during the third week of embryogenesis. As described in Chapter 1, the cells associated with the development of the vascular system are **mesenchymal** (mesodermal) in origin. The mesenchymal cells destined to become hemoglobin-synthesizing cells (**erythroblasts**) first form unique clusters of cells called **blood islands**. In the fetus, the blood islands are initially confined to the yolk sac, spleen, and liver. However, by the fourth month of development, erythropoiesis also occurs in bone.[1,2] Throughout fetal development, erythropoiesis is both **medullary** (in the bone marrow) and **extramedullary** (in tissues other than bone).[2] After birth, the bone marrow progressively takes over the function of erythropoiesis. In young children and adults, significant extramedullary erythropoiesis usually is observed only under abnormal circumstances. Figure 18-1 illustrates the expansion and regression of hematopoietic or erythropoietic tissue during fetal and adult life. With time, hematopoietic function from medullary sources is progressively reduced, as only replacement of red blood cells is needed by the time that adolescent growth is completed. In bone marrow, the major types of blood cells are derived from progenitor or **stem cells**, as described in Chapter 6.

Major factors that influence red blood cell development and formation are (1) the con-

centration of hemoglobin within the cell, (2) **erythropoietic stimulating factor**, also referred to as **erythropoietin**, and (3) the supply of essential nutrients (Figure 18-1).

Red Blood Cell Maturation

Role of Erythropoietin

Erythropoietin causes an acceleration in the maturation of erythroid-committed cells to form erythroblasts.[3,4] When tissue oxygen tension is low, the kidney releases an enzyme that activates an inactive erythropoietin precursor found in plasma. Once activated, erythropoietin stimulates erythrocyte maturation. Erythropoietin also influences hemoglobin synthesis by stimulating the synthesis of messenger RNA (mRNA) for hemoglobin. Figure 18-2 depicts the role of

Figure 18-1. Relative contribution of different hematopoietic tissues to and time course of red blood cell production during fetal and adult life.

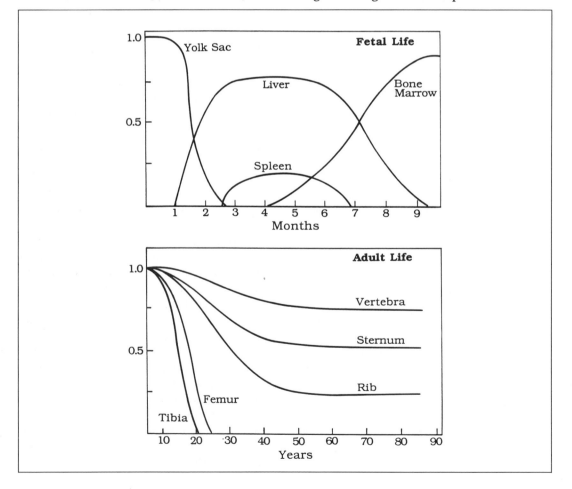

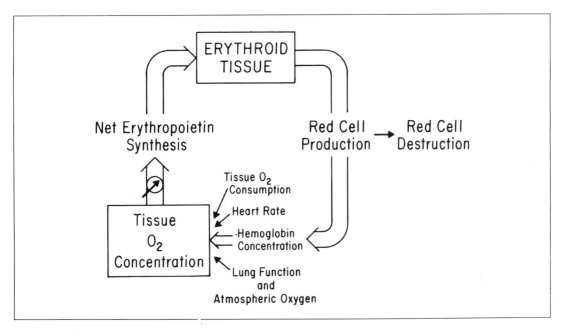

Figure 18-2. Regulation of erythroid cell maturation by erythropoietin. The body tissue concentration of oxygen (O₂) is influenced by numerous factors, such as O₂ consumption by tissues, heart rate, hemoglobin concentration, and lung function. When the tissue concentration of O₂ is lowered, erythropoietin precursors in circulation are activated to stimulate formation of new red blood cells.

erythropoietin in the erythroid cell cycle. It is based on observations that a loss of red blood cells and increased hypoxia cause an increase in net erythropoietin production.

Role of Hemoglobin

The concentration of hemoglobin and by-products of hemoglobin synthesis also are important in the regulation of erythropoiesis.[4] High concentrations of hemoglobin cause relatively fewer cell divisions to take place before an erythroblast is transformed into a reticulocyte. Further, the concentration of hemoglobin acts as an internal negative feedback control on hemoglobin synthesis. Thus both hemoglobin concentration and erythropoietin can influence considerably the steps in red blood cell maturation.

Steps in the Maturation Process

Figure 18-3 depicts the red blood cell maturation process and highlights important steps in red blood cell formation. First, there is differentiation of totipotent stem cells to **burst-forming units** (BFU) and then to **colony-forming units** (CFU). These are the steps that are particularly responsive to erythropoietin. The CFU next transform by rapid cell division into erythroblasts. Erythroblasts have mitochondria and function to synthesize abundant quantities of messenger RNA for hemoglobin synthesis. With increased hemoglobin accumulation, however, there is a gradual reduction in nuclear size. Eventually, the nucleus of the erythroblast is actually extruded, giving rise to cells called **reticulocytes**. These cells are characterized by netlike fibers in their cytoplasm. Reticulocytes are young red blood cells that are still capable of synthesizing hemoglobin, because they contain mRNA and the machinery for protein synthesis, but no nucleus and little or no DNA.[1]

Reticulocytes are capable of penetrating the sinusoidal wall that separates marrow from blood. Therefore, the reticulocyte is the most immature red blood cell that normally

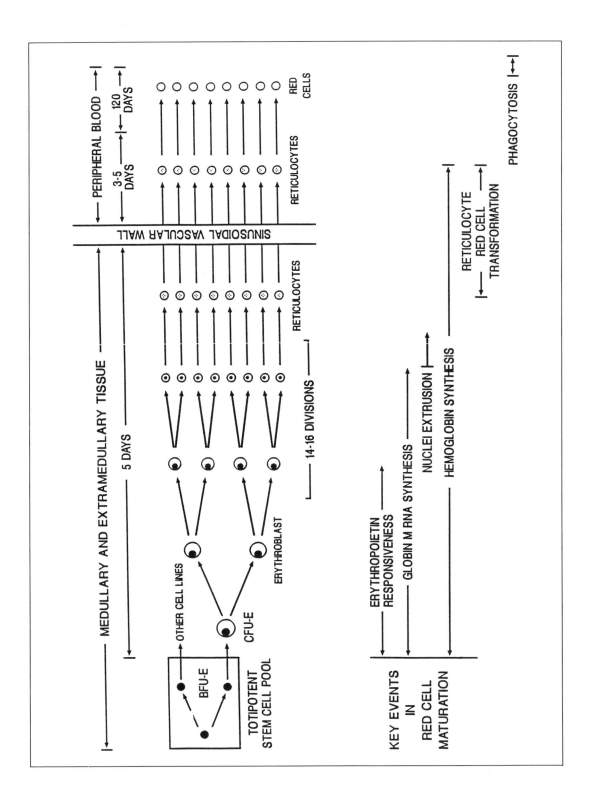

appears in circulating blood. These cells soon lose their potential for hemoglobin synthesis as they transform into mature red blood cells, that is, erythrocytes. Soon after the reticulocyte enters into the circulation, it takes on the shape of a red blood cell, a biconcave disk, and loses its protein synthetic activity. Its metabolic activity now is governed largely by the initial content of nutrients, which gradually are depleted as the cell ages.

Erythrocytes remain in the circulation for approximately 120 days before they are destroyed by phagocytic processes. With shape changes due to denaturation and the abnormal packing of hemoglobin, aged red blood cells become vulnerable to phagocytic action of macrophages in organs such as the spleen and liver. The steps in this final process are depicted in Figure 18-4.

Hemoglobin Synthesis and Degradation

Since erythroid cell maturation is controlled in part by hemoglobin concentration, it is important to appreciate some of the steps in hemoglobin biosynthesis.[5] Hemoglobin is composed of four protein subunits. The oxygen-binding capacity of hemoglobin depends on the appropriate association of two identical subunits and two other subunits that may or may not be identical. For exam-

Figure 18-3. Stepwise maturation of erythroid cells. From the stem cell pool, the totipotent stem cells may differentiate into a number of different cell lines. The earliest identifiable cell in the erythropoietic (E) series is a highly nucleated cell referred to as a burst-forming unit (BFU-E). These BFU-E differentiate into smaller colony-forming units (CFU-E), which quickly divide to form erythroblasts. After 14 to 16 cell divisions, the nucleus of the erythroblast is extruded, and there is transformation to reticulocytes. Next, reticulocytes are released into peripheral blood and transform into mature red blood cells. Approximate times for some of these transformations are given, as well as some key events in the various steps of red blood cell maturation.

ple, in normal adults, 95% of the hemoglobin is composed of two identical subunits designated as alpha chains and two identical subunits designated as beta chains. Other nonalpha chains predominate in hemoglobin during fetal development and in certain diseases, such as thalassemia. The chemical characteristics of the protein or **globin** subunits are different enough so that it is possible to distinguish fetal blood from adult blood by a variety of clinical procedures.[1,2,5]

Before these subunits are converted to active hemoglobin, there is need for the attachment of **heme**. Heme consists of a porphyrin ring structure that contains **iron**. The synthesis of heme occurs in the mitochondria of pronormoblasts. Nutritional deficiencies, such as iron or pyridoxine deficiency, often cause decreased heme biosynthesis. The importance of heme lies in its ability to bind oxygen. Thus factors that influence heme synthesis can ultimately influence systemic oxygen concentration.

When red blood cells are fragmented, the hemoglobin that is released from the red cell is degraded by lysosomal proteinases. The heme portion undergoes several modifications that give rise to products which are excreted by way of bile. As shown in Figure 18-5, heme is first degraded to biliverdin and eventually to bilirubin. When heme is degraded in nonhepatic tissue, bilirubin is released into circulation and binds to albumin. Following its transport to the liver, it mixes with the liver pool of bilirubin and normally is excreted via the bile. Note that abnormally elevated blood plasma levels of bilirubin often serve as a clinical marker for liver damage and biliary obstruction.[6,7]

Important Nutrients Involved in Erythropoiesis

Many nutrients influence the rate of red blood cell formation and hemoglobin synthesis. The body's need for iron,[6] folic acid, vitamin B_{12}, and other vitamins[7] is closely related to synthesis of new red blood cells and hemoglobin.

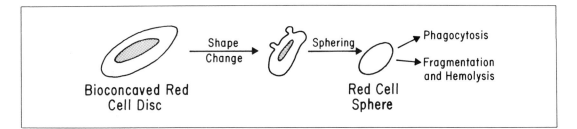

Figure 18-4. Steps in the destruction of the red blood cell. The aged red blood cell transforms from a biconcave disk into a sphere. The spheres are trapped in the fenestrated vasculature of organs such as the spleen. The trapping is then followed by phagocytosis. Some red blood cells also are fragmented as they penetrate small capillaries and are lost owing to hemolytic processes.

Iron

The iron required for synthesis of a normal concentration of hemoglobin to replace 1% of the red blood cell mass (the amount lost each day) is approximately 25 mg. Most of this iron comes from internal storage or is released from degraded hemoglobin. The released iron usually is stored in liver, spleen, and muscle, bound to the intracellular protein complexes **ferritin** or **hemosiderin**. The term **hemosiderin** is used for poorly defined iron-protein complexes in cells. The presence of hemosiderin in high amounts in liver or the release of ferritin into circulation often indicates excessive or optimal iron storage.[1,5,8,9]

An important feature of iron regulation is the consistent reuse of internal stores of iron. Iron is not readily excreted from the body, and the major losses of iron occur only when red blood cells or epithelial cells are lost. Entry of iron from intestinal mucosal cells, however, is rapid when the body stores of iron are low. To a degree, intestinal cells appear to be able to sense when the body stores of iron are low or elevated, and they regulate iron absorption accordingly. In part, intestinal absorption is controlled by the amount of iron that is bound to transferrin. The intestinal absorption of iron is increased when the amount of iron bound to transferrin is low. For the internal circulation of iron,

plasma contains enough transferrin to bind 300 to 400 μg of iron per deciliter of blood. However, in normal individuals, only 30% or so of this capacity is reached. A level of 30% saturation provides for a continual entry of iron into the body from the intestine. Transferrin saturation that is lower than 30% causes increased entry of iron.

With respect to the sites in the body where iron is utilized, those cells with high iron requirements have specific receptors for transferrin. For example, erythroblasts have numerous receptors for plasma transferrin. Once associated with these receptors, iron is taken up by the erythroblast and transported to mitochondria for eventual use in heme synthesis.[8]

Approximately 70% of the body's iron ultimately is delivered for hemoglobin synthesis, and the other 30% is directed toward the synthesis of other iron-containing proteins such as myoglobin and various oxidases. When iron is needed for erythropoiesis or by other iron-requiring cells, the removal of iron from transferrin is very efficient. For example, erythroid marrow receives only 5% of the cardiac output but extracts 85% of the circulating iron. When a cell is saturated with enough iron, it no longer takes up iron efficiently or stores it as ferritin for future use. With a deficiency of dietary iron, there is first a reduction in the saturation of transferrin, which is followed by a reduction in the iron associated with cellular ferritin. These losses subsequently lead to reduced net heme synthesis and, in turn, reduced hemoglobin synthesis.

For the nutritional assessment of iron status, anemia with a low plasma or serum iron or with abnormal plasma total iron-binding capacity may indicate a significant

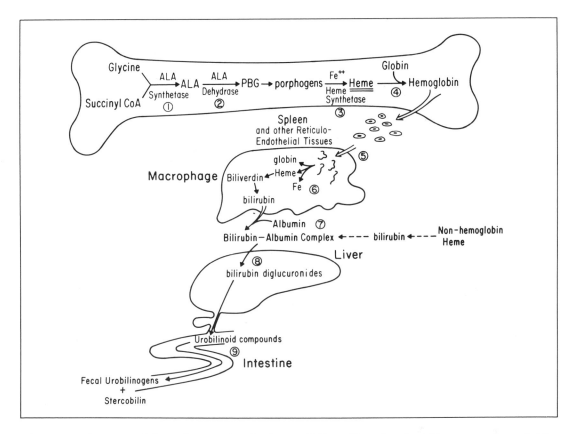

Figure 18-5. Summary of the major steps involved in heme synthesis and degradation. The initial steps (1 and 2) take place in the mitochondria of erythroid cells and require first the synthesis of alpha-aminolevulinic acid (ALA) and porphobilinogen (PBG). The third step comes at the end of the pathway and represents the site where iron is inserted into heme. Heme then combines with each of the four globin chains of hemoglobin in the red blood cell. After the red blood cell has served its function (step 4), it is degraded (step 5). Iron is released, globin is degraded, and heme first is converted to biliverdin (step 6) and then is transported to the liver (step 7) for eventual conjugation to glucuronide and elimination (steps 8 and 9) in the form of urobilinogens and stercobilin. CoA = coenzyme A.

loss of iron over an extended period, whereas normal hematological values with a low plasma or serum iron may indicate a loss of iron over a recent and shorter period of time.[9]

Another dimension of iron absorption and metabolism is the variability of iron utilization or availability from differing food sources.[10] The relative absorption or avail- ability of iron is related in part to the solubility of iron complexes derived from digestion of food. Iron complexes from foods of animal origin often are more soluble and available than iron complexes from foods of plant origin (Table 18-1).

Folic Acid and Vitamin B_{12}

Folic acid and vitamin B_{12} are important factors in erythropoiesis.[11] These vitamins are involved in purine synthesis, thymidine synthesis, and ultimately, DNA and RNA synthesis (Figure 18-6). With deficiencies of either folic acid or vitamin B_{12}, the pronormoblast cannot divide normally, and its rate of maturation is decreased.

A variety of metabolic and nutritional conditions can promote deficiencies of either vitamin B_{12} or folic acid. Some of these conditions are listed in Table 18-2. They include the impaired synthesis of **intrinsic factor**, a protein derived from the gastric mucosa that is essential for B_{12} absorption, and impaired

Table 18-1. Estimation of Absorbable Iron from Different Types of 3000 kilo Joule (720 kcal) Meals[a]

Type of Meal	Composition	Total Iron (mg)	Heme Iron (mg)	Estimated Upper Limit of Iron Absorption[a] (mg)
Low availability[b] containing 25 mg of ascorbic acid	30 g protein from vegetables and legumes	2.0–2.5	0	0.06–0.075
	Yogurt	0.1–0.2	0	0.003–0.006
	Brown rice, 1 cup	1.0–1.5	0	0.02–0.045
	Small apple or ripe banana	0.5–1.0	0	0.015–0.03
		3.6–5.2		0.098–0.156
Medium availability[c] containing 50 mg of ascorbic acid	30 g protein from vegetables and legumes	2.0–2.5	0	0.1–0.13
	Yogurt	0.1–0.2	0	0.005–0.01
	Brown rice, 1 cup	1.0–1.5	0	0.05–0.075
	Large orange juice	0.1	0	0.005
		3.2–4.3		0.16–0.21
Medium availability[c] containing 25 mg of ascorbic acid	30 g protein from meat	2.8	0.7	0.11+(0.14)
	Assorted vegetables	0.6–0.8	0	0.03–0.04
	Milk, 1 cup	0.1–0.2	0	0.005–0.01
	Cake (50–60 g) and legumes	0.3–0.4	0	0.015–0.02
		3.8–4.2		0.30–0.32
High availability[d] containing 50 mg of ascorbic acid	30 g protein from beef (>90 g raw)	3.0	1.4	0.13+(0.32)
	Assorted vegetables	0.5–0.6	0	0.04–0.05
	Bread	0.5–0.6	0	0.04–0.04
	Fruit cocktail	0.5–0.6	0	0.04–0.05
		4.5–4.8		0.57–0.60

[a] Absorbable iron is estimated by assuming that on the average 23% of heme iron is absorbed, whereas only 3 to 8% of non-heme iron is absorbed. The four examples were chosen to reflect that both the ascorbic acid content and 1 protein source influences iron availability.[10]

[b] Three percent × the iron content is used to estimate absorbable iron from a low-availability meal, which is defined as a meal containing <30 g as meat, poultry, or fish and 25 mg or less ascorbic acid.

[c] Five percent is used as the factor for a medium-availability meal, which is defined as a meal containing 30–90 g of raw meat, poultry, or fish, or alternatively a vegetable-based meal that contains about 50 mg ascorbic acid.

[d] Eight percent is used for a high-availability meal, which is defined as > 90 g of meat, poultry, or fish and ingestion of 50 or more mg of ascorbic acid.

folic acid absorption. Folic acid is found in many foods as polyglutamyl folic acid or "conjugated" folate. Factors that inhibit activity of intestinal conjugase, an enzyme responsible for the cleavage of glutamyl residues from polyglutamyl folate, interfere with folic acid absorption. These points will be emphasized again in the section "Megaloblastic Anemias" (p. 693).

Other Nutrients

In addition to iron, folic acid, and vitamin B_{12}, many other nutrients are involved in erythropoiesis and hematopoiesis. **Pyridoxine** is a cofactor for the enzyme alpha-aminolevulinic acid synthetase (see Figure 18-5). A deficiency of pyridoxine can result

in decreased heme synthesis and, eventually, anemia. Impaired red blood cell formation may also be observed in severe vitamin C, niacin, and thiamine deficiencies.[12]

The dietary intake of **vitamins E** and **A** may also influence erythropoiesis and red blood cell integrity. Vitamin A toxicity can cause changes in red blood cell membranes which, in some instances, result in anemia because of increased red cell destruction. On the other hand, vitamin A deficiency appears to cause an increased accumulation of iron in storage tissues so that iron is not readily released for hematopoiesis.[13] Vitamin E protects red blood cell membranes from oxidative damage. Red blood cell membranes tend to rupture more easily in the presence of oxidants when the vitamin E concentration in

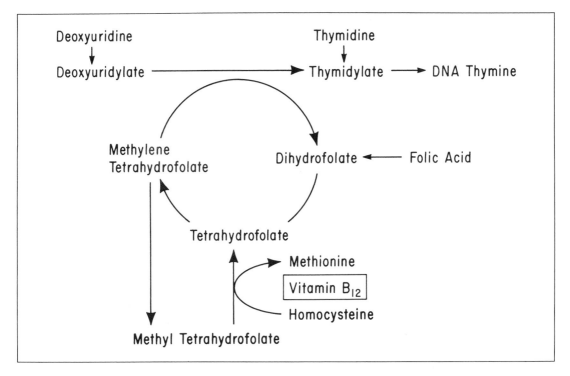

Figure 18-6. Interrelationship between folic acid and vitamin B_{12}. Elevated plasma methyltetrahydrofolate levels are observed in patients with vitamin B_{12} deficiency because of the inability to convert methyl tetrahydrofolate to tetrahydrofolate or other active forms of folic acid. Because of this lack of active intracellular folates, there is reduced conversion of deoxyuridylate to thymidylate. Unused folate is "trapped" as methyltetrahydrofolate. Note that the tetrahydrofolate form of the vitamin is the active form. The dihydrofolate form of the vitamin must first be reduced to tetrahydrofolate.

the red cell membrane is reduced. There also are reports from experimental animal studies that suggest that decreased activity of alpha-aminolevulinic acid synthetase is associated with vitamin E deficiency. This role, however, is secondary to the more important one of protection of the lipid-rich membranes of red blood cells from oxidative damage.[14]

Decreased protein synthesis due to severe protein deficiency can also result in impaired red blood cell formation. This fact is one of the bases for the use of hemoglobin concentration in nutritional assessment, as described in Chapter 3. Finally, **essential fatty acid** deficiency has also been reported

to cause alterations in red blood cell membrane composition and structural integrity. Lists of some of the anemias and presumed mechanisms involving deficiency of selected nutrients are given in Tables 18-3 and 18-4.

THE ANEMIAS

A classification of anemias is given in Table 18-3. It is emphasized that the general term **anemia** is defined relative to standards that are derived from studies on large populations; therefore, there is no definitive separation between anemic and nonanemic patients. Further, anemia most often is the secondary manifestation of a disease. Although the underlying cause of an anemia may not be nutritional in origin, usually some type of nutritional management is important in the treatment of the anemia.

Normocytic Anemias

The term **normocytic anemia** is used to describe the condition in which cell size, cell hemoglobin concentration, and reticulocyte

Table 18-2. Typical Reasons for Vitamin B$_{12}$ and Folic Acid Deficiency

Category	Etiologic Mechanisms
Vitamin B$_{12}$ deficiency	
Decreased absorption	Poor diet
	Intrinsic factor deficiency
	Pernicious anemia
	Gastrectomy (total or partial)
	Destruction of gastric mucosa by caustics
	Anti–intrinsic factor antibody in gastric juice
	Abnormal intrinsic factor molecules
	Intrinsic intestinal disease and selective malabsorption syndromes
	Ileal resection, ileitis (ileum is site for B$_{12}$ absorption)
	Sprue, celiac disease
	Infiltrative intestinal disease (lymphoma, scleroderma, etc.)
	Drug-induced malabsorption
	Competitive parasites
	Fish tapeworm infestation
	Bacteria in diverticula of bowel, blind loops (bacteria compete for B$_{12}$)
	Chronic pancreatic disease
Increased requirement	Pregnancy
	Neoplastic disease
	Hyperthyroidism
Folic acid deficiency	
Decreased absorption	Poor diet
	Alcoholism
	Infancy
	Hemodialysis
	Intestinal short circuits
	Steatorrhea
	Sprue, celiac disease
Decreased requirement	Intrinsic intestinal disease
	Anticonvulsants, oral contraceptives
Increased requirement	Pregnancy
	Infancy
	Hyperactive hematopoiesis
	Neoplastic disease
	Skin disease
Blocked activation	Folic acid and B$_{12}$ antagonists (various chemotherapy drugs)
	Metabolic inhibitors
	Purine synthesis: 6-mercaptopurine, 6-thioguanine
	Pyrimidine synthesis: 6-azauridine
	Thymidylate synthesis: 5-fluorouracil
	Deoxyribonucleotide synthesis: hydroxyurea, cytosine arabinoside
	Inborn errors
	Lesch-Nyhan syndrome
	Hereditary orotic aciduria
	Deficiency of formiminotransferase methyltransferase, and the like
	Unexplained disorders
	Pyridoxine-responsive megaloblastic anemia
	Thiamine-responsive megaloblastic anemia
	Erythremic myelosis (Di Guglielmo syndrome)

count are within normal limits, but the **hematocrit** (packed cell volume or proportion of cells in blood) is low. Normocytic anemias usually are the result of a decreased proliferation of red blood cells from bone marrow. This is **bone marrow failure** in the sense that red blood cells are not released at a normal rate, so there are fewer cells, but the cells that are released have a normal appearance.[1]

Normocytic anemias are the least well understood of all of the hematologic disorders. One form of normocytic anemia is **aplastic anemia**. It is an anemia in which the bone marrow appears to be morphologically

Table 18-3. The Anemias

Anemias due to decreased red blood cell production
Normocytic anemias
  From primary bone marrow failure
    Aplastic anemia
    Myelopathic (e.g., leukemia-related) anemias
  From secondary causes
    Chronic inflammation
    Uremia
    Hepatic disease
    Endocrine disorders
Megaloblastic (macrocytic) anemias
  From primary nutritional deficiencies
    Vitamin B_{12}
    Folic acid
    Thiamine and pyridoxine (rare)
  From secondary causes
    Drugs acting as B_{12} and folate antagonist
    Orotic aciduria
    Erythroleukemias
    Pernicious anemias
Microcytic anemias
  From primary nutritional deficiencies
    Iron
    Pyridoxine (sideroblastic anemia)
    Ascorbic acid and vitamin A deficiency
  From other causes
    Hemorrhage
    Forms of thalassemia
    Drugs and heavy metal intoxication (e.g., lead, cadmium)
Anemias due to increased destruction of red blood cells
Hemoglobinopathies
  Sickle cell anemia
  Thalassemia
Hemolytic anemias
  From primary nutritional deficiencies: vitamin E
  From secondary causes
    Favism
    Glucose-6-phosphate dehydrogenase deficiency
    Drugs
    Mechanical damage
    Infection (e.g., malaria)
    Immunologic disorders

---

and functionally hypoplastic—that is, the amount of functional marrow is decreased. Aplastic anemias often are unresponsive to medicinal iron. They may be caused by ionizing radiation or by drugs and chemical agents such as benzidine, chloramphenicol, selected antimicrobial drugs, and drugs used as anticonvulsants. In rare instances, the use of aspirin or even chemicals in hair dyes have been known to cause aplastic anemia. When aplastic-like anemias are seen in childhood, they usually are genetic in origin. When they are seen in adults, they sometimes are associated with renal failure and thymomas (a relatively rare form of thymic tissue cancer). In patients with chronic renal disease, the red blood cell life span often is shortened, and, as noted previously, there may be decreased net erythropoietin production.[14]

The treatment of anemias associated with diseases such as chronic renal failure usually is directed at treatment of the primary disease. Often, normocytic anemia associated with the diseases given in Table 18-3 is mild. If the anemia is severe, **blood transfusions** are used to correct the anemia. The transfusions generally are performed to "buy time" until remission occurs. Diets modified to provide additional nutrients usually are not helpful. The blood transfusion itself can supply iron and other nutrients. Thus the potential always exists for iron toxicity with repeated transfusions, since the body has no way to eliminate excess iron. One pint of blood contains approximately 250 mg of iron, so fifteen transfusions or more can double the total body iron content of 3.5 g. Medicinal iron therapy is not needed in these circumstances. Therefore, apart from supplementing the diet with B vitamins such as folic acid and vitamin B_{12}, any diet therapy for the patient with normocytic anemia is not directed at the anemia but at the primary disease or condition underlying the anemia. However, the patient may profit from a diet reduced in dietary iron.

Megaloblastic Anemias

Megaloblastic (large primitive cell, or macrocytic) **anemias** usually are the result of a deficiency of vitamin B_{12} or folic acid or are caused by drugs or conditions that interfere with folic acid and vitamin B_{12} metabolism.[15] For example, megaloblastic anemias may be secondary to enteropathies, such as tropical sprue or gluten sensitivity, or to drug-induced disorders of DNA synthesis, particularly drugs such as methotrexate that act as folic acid antagonists. As described earlier, there is retarded development of the erythroblasts in megaloblastic anemia, which causes a decrease in the rate of erythroblast maturation to reticulocytes and erythrocytes.

Table 18-4. Mechanisms by Which Common Nutrition-Related Anemias Are Promoted

Anemia	Causative Nutrient or Food Component Deficiency	Mechanism
Macrocytic	Vitamin B_{12} and folic acid	Decrease DNA synthesis that retards or inhibits cell division
	Thiamine and pyridoxine	Presumed to be related to decreased DNA synthesis owing to impaired purine synthesis
Microcytic	Iron	Reduced heme synthesis and, subsequently, hemoglobin synthesis
	Ascorbic acid	Presumed to be related to decreased iron utilization
	Vitamin A	Presumed to be related to increased iron storage so that iron is not available for heme synthesis
	Vitamin E	Presumed to be related to decreased heme synthesis
	Pyridoxine	Reduced heme synthesis
	Lead	Reduced heme synthesis
	Copper	Reduced iron use and release for heme synthesis
	Cadmium	Reduced iron and copper use
Hemolytic	Vitamin E	Impaired integrity of red blood cell membrane, which leads to increased susceptibility to damage by oxidants

Megaloblastic cells are easily detected because of their larger size and nuclear contents. Abnormal megaloblasts also are often packed with hemoglobin but contain fragmented remnants of nuclear material. The term **megaloblast** also denotes any myeloid cell in the leukocyte series that is in transition before mitosis.

The classic form of megaloblastic anemia is **pernicious anemia**, which is caused most often by the inability to produce sufficient intrinsic factor. The current thought is that pernicious anemia is an autoimmune disorder caused by the presence of the high amounts of anti–intrinsic factor antibodies in serum and gastric juice. There are also very rare forms of juvenile pernicious anemia in which there is failure of intrinsic factor secretion or the production of biologically inert intrinsic factor.

Vitamin B_{12} is efficiently stored, and several years may pass before clear signs of macrocytic anemia due specifically to vitamin B_{12} deficiency are observed. Only in very strict vegetarians, however, should a simple deficiency of vitamin B_{12} be observed, since foods of plant origin do not contain vitamin B_{12} unless contaminated by soil and bacteria. Most often, diet-related macrocytic anemias are due to folic acid deficiency. In contrast to vitamin B_{12}, folic acid may be depleted from the body in two to four months. Moreover,

the absorption and metabolism of folic acid appear to be influenced by a broader spectrum of enteropathies and drug-related problems (particularly those associated with alcohol).

Before initiating nutritional therapy, it is important that the cause of the megaloblastic anemia be determined. For example, administration of only folic acid in the presence of a primary vitamin B_{12} deficiency may correct, in part, the megaloblastic anemia, but it will not correct other signs of vitamin B_{12} deficiency, such as progressive nervous tissue degeneration.[16]

Symptoms of megaloblastic anemia common to both vitamin B_{12} and folic acid deficiency are weakness, dyspnea, and intestinal disorders characterized by either diarrhea or constipation. Other common signs of water-soluble vitamin deficiencies, as well as the clinical signs of macrocytic anemia, may be present. If vitamin B_{12} deficiency is the underlying cause of the anemia, the peripheral and central nerve degeneration may first appear as numbness and tingling in the extremities, diminution of vibratory or postural sense, poor muscle control, or poor memory.

When there is no underlying genetic or systemic cause of megaloblastic anemia, usually a normal diet with increased amounts of protein, iron, vitamin B_{12}, and folic acid is all that is required to correct the condition. With a simple deficiency of vitamin B_{12} or folic acid, recovery is rapid.

Microcytic Anemia

Microcytic (small cell) **anemia** usually is the result of decreased hemoglobin biosynthesis. Red blood cells that are not fully packed with hemoglobin are fairly small. Also, they sometimes do not have the dark red color of normal red blood cells; thus the term **hypochromic microcytic** is used to describe their appearance. **Hypochromic** connotes less color or pigmentation.[1,2]

Iron deficiency is a major cause of microcytic anemia. For an adult consuming 2,500 calories/day, 10 to 20 mg of iron usually is adequate, assuming that at least 10% of the total ingested iron is absorbed. Excessive blood loss, pregnancy, and menstrual losses of iron increase demands for iron. For example, during pregnancy there is expansion of the mother's hemoglobin mass that requires approximately 0.5 to 1.5 mg of absorbed iron per day in addition to the normal requirement. The formation of the placenta, cord, and fetus requires another 400 mg of total iron over the course of pregnancy. The loss of blood at delivery (usually 500 to 600 ml) requires an additional 300 to 350 mg of total iron. Thus the total iron costs of pregnancy in excess of the normal basal requirements of 1 to 2 mg of absorbed iron per day is equal to approximately 4 mg/day.

In the early stages of iron deficiency, ferritin stores are depleted and iron absorption increases. Typical of all true anemic states, weakness and dyspnea may occur. A severe iron deficiency also may cause structural and functional changes in epithelial tissues.

Although iron is best absorbed when little food is given, excessive amounts of elemental iron or iron salts without food can cause gastric irritation; therefore, it is best to administer iron supplements at or following a meal. The gastrointestinal side effects of iron supplements may also be minimized by increasing the supplement slowly over a few days until the required amount is reached.[8,9]

The amounts of iron that are given often amount to 1 to 2 mg/kg of body weight (100 to 200 mg/day). With a simple iron deficiency, this amount usually causes a rapid stimulation of heme synthesis and hemoglobin synthesis. Parenteral administration of iron or injection with iron dextran may be necessary for patients who are unable to take iron orally.

It should be appreciated that in high doses, iron can be very toxic, particularly in children. Doses of 3 to 10 g/day are known to be fatal. High amounts of iron can cause metabolic acidosis and **cirrhosis**—that is, damage to the parenchymal cells in a number of tissues because of the inability of these tissues to store excessive amounts of iron.

It has also become clear that iron plays important roles in the body's general **host defense mechanisms** against infection.[17,18] With sustained low levels of iron intake, defective cell-mediated immunity and polymorphonuclear leukocyte dysfunction are often observed. A severe anemia due to iron deficiency may coincide with increased susceptibility to infection. In experimental animal models of infection, acute and severe lack of dietary iron during pregnancy results in offspring with impaired resistance. In part, this appears to be due to a compromise in the activity of myeloperoxidase, an important iron-containing enzyme that is found in high concentrations in phagocytic cells. Myeloperoxidase is an essential component in the degradative processing of bacterial components, also referred to as opsonic activity (see Table 18-5).

On the other hand, it is documented that a number of bacterial organisms are highly responsive and proliferate in an iron-enriched environment. For example, *Salmonella* and *Mycobacterium tuberculosis* proliferate very rapidly when iron is made available, either in the intestine or in lung fluids.[18] In response to infections that result in fever, the concentration of iron in liver, spleen, and other storage tissues often increases, and the amounts of circulating iron decrease. This phenomenon is thought to be a host defense mecha-

Table 18-5. Iron and Susceptibility to Infectious Disease

Iron status[a]	Immunoglobulin Levels[b]	Cutaneous Sensitivity[c]	Opsonic Activity of Plasma[d]	Myeloperoxidase Activity[e]	Bacterial Growth[f] Without Iron	With Iron
Hemoglobin <5 g/dl	↓	↓	↓	↓	↓	↓↑
Hemoglobin 5–10 g/dl	↑↓	↑↓	↓	↓	↓	↓↑
Hemoglobin >10 g/dl	↑↓	↑↓	↑↓	↑↓	↑↓	↑↓

Decreased, ↓; sometimes decreased, ↓; sometimes increased, ↑; increased, ↑; variable or no change, ↓↑.
[a] Hemoglobin values were chosen to correspond to an acute and severe iron deficiency, a moderately severe iron deficiency, or a relatively normal iron intake.
[b] Typical direction of change in immunoglobulin levels.
[c] Potential for positive reactions to Candida, Trychophyton, streptokinase-streptodornase, or mumps.
[d] Relative measure of bacterial particles ingested by plasma phagocytic cells.
[e] Myeloperoxidase activity in eosinophils, macrophages, and neutrophils.
[f] Growth of tubercle bacilli in human serum with or without the addition of iron.

nism against infection (see Table 18–5). As a consequence of the decrease in circulating iron, anemia may result from chronic infection. Some clinicians now believe that aggressive iron supplementation should be approached cautiously, particularly if the iron supplementation is recommended for only a mild anemia and there are signs of bacterial infection.

In addition to iron deprivation, hypochromic microcytic anemia may also arise from severe protein deficiency such as that seen in kwashiorkor, from intoxication with heavy metals such as lead, and in deficiencies of vitamin A, vitamin E, copper, or pyridoxine. Copper deficiency causes iron to accumulate in storage tissues so that the delivery of iron to bone marrow is impaired.[1,12] Likewise, pyridoxine deficiency can cause anemia even in the presence of a high level of iron in serum and tissue. Pyridoxine-dependent anemia is distinctive because of the accumulation of iron in erythroblasts. With a decrease in heme synthesis (see Figure 18-5), iron remains in the mitochondria of erythroblasts and forms inorganic iron complexes. Erythroblasts that contain an excess of iron are called **sideroblasts**. These cells are identified in the laboratory by staining for iron. Sideroblastic anemia can also be a result of inherited defects in the formation of alpha-aminolevulinic acid or defects in other

steps in the heme pathway. It should be appreciated, however, that neither copper nor pyridoxine deficiency occurs frequently in humans.

The mechanisms by which many heavy metals or deficiencies of vitamins A or E cause microcytic anemia appear to involve decreased heme synthesis or impaired release of iron from storage tissues. (See Table 18-4, which contains suggestions for mechanisms related to common forms of anemia. Note that most of the nutrition-related microcytic anemias involve defects in either iron release from storage tissue or heme biosynthesis.)

Sickle Cell Anemia and Other Hemoglobinopathies

There are many variants in hemoglobin that result from substitutions of only a single amino acid in one or more of the hemoglobin chains. More than 220 human **hemoglobin variants** are known. Most were discovered during the course of population survey studies and are not the cause of clinical syndromes; however, several hemoglobin variants cause serious anemias.[1,19,20] One such variant causes **sickle cell anemia**, which occurs predominantly in blacks. In this form of anemia, the red blood cell takes on a peculiar elongated or sickled shape. With inappropriate amino acid substitutions in hemoglobin, there is abnormal packaging of hemoglobin in red blood cells, and the red cell takes on a bizarre shape at low oxygen tension. As the cells sickle, they become ridged and can obstruct capillary blood flow. The cells also are ruptured easily so that there is damage to various organs and tissues. Any organ or system may be involved. Approximately 8% of blacks in the United States are **heterozygous** for this variant. The **genetic** or **gene frequency** is as high as 30% in parts of Central Africa.

The most important feature of nutritional therapy in sickle cell anemia is to assure that there is not excessive iron storage. The diet should be normally low in iron. Iron-rich foods such as liver and iron-fortified cereals should be excluded from the diet. In addition, the diet should be low in fat (less than 30% of the total calories), particularly if liver and gallbladder disease accompany the anemia.

Requirements for water-soluble vitamins, however, are often high, because of the need to continually synthesize large numbers of new red blood cells. It has been suggested that zinc supplementation may be helpful. A considerable quantity of zinc is found in erythrocytes, bound to the enzyme carbonic anhydrase. This zinc is lost as the cells are lysed. In contrast to iron, zinc is more readily excreted from the body. Also, the sickle cell patient may suffer from ulcerative lesions; supplements of zinc (20 to 30 mg/day) may help to promote normal wound healing.

Thalassemias are another group of disorders that result in anemia.[20] In the thalassemia syndromes, there usually is an absence of or diminished synthesis of one of the globin chains of hemoglobin. For example, in **alpha-thalassemia**, the alpha chain of hemoglobin is absent or reduced in content in the red blood cell. In beta-thalassemia, the beta chain of hemoglobin is absent or reduced in content.

Of the two forms, beta-thalassemia occurs most often and frequently is seen in people of Mediterranean origin. Similar to the sickled red cell, red blood cells in beta-thalassemia take on abnormal shapes. These red blood cells are fragile and rupture easily. Untreated children with beta-thalassemia usually die at an early age. With blood transfusions, however, many children can survive to their early twenties. The nutritional care in this condition is directed toward provision of a well-balanced diet rich in water-soluble vitamins and, if transfusions are a part of the treatment, low in iron.

Hemolytic Anemia

There are always red blood cells of varying age in circulation and, since the red blood cell has a finite life span, there are always red blood cells undergoing destruction. An increased rate of destruction of red blood cells can occur because of mechanical damage (e.g., that which is a result of an artificial heart valve), the effects of various autoimmune disorders, or alterations in red cell shape. Red blood cell membrane defects also may cause rupture of red cells. Increased lysis may occur owing to defects in certain metabolic pathways within the red blood cell that protect against oxidative damage. When red blood cell lysis or **hemolysis** is increased because of one of these processes, **hemolytic anemia** may occur.[11,21]

Vitamin E deficiency can result in hemolysis of red blood cells. Hemolysis of red cells is, in fact, one of the few deficiency signs that has been observed consistently in vitamin E–deficient humans. When hemolysis is observed in young infants, vitamin E deficiency may be an underlying cause, since infants are born with low stores of vitamin E. In some instances, this condition appears to result in red blood cell membranes that are more susceptible to oxidative damage and hemolysis. Red cell membranes are composed in part of polyunsaturated lipids. Since unsaturated fats are easily oxidized, the potential for oxidative damage of the red blood cell membrane is high. Hydrogen peroxide and lipid peroxides form when oxygen tension is high. Thus it is very important for

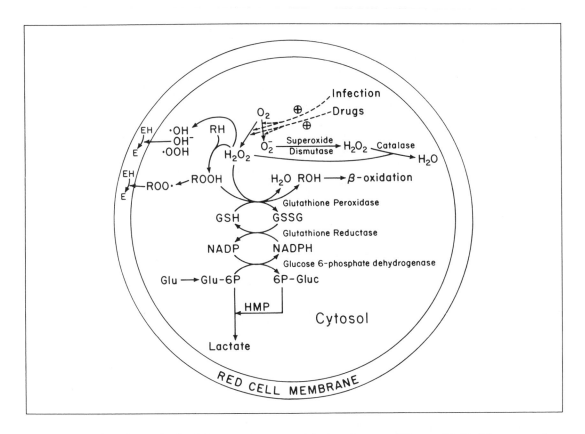

Figure 18-7. Selected steps in the defense against oxidants that alter red blood cell metabolism and membrane integrity. Infections, certain drugs, and some dietary components appear to increase production of peroxides by red blood cells. Superoxide (O_2^-), hydrogen peroxide (H_2O_2), organic and lipid-derived peroxides (ROOH), hydroxyl anions and radicals (OH^-, $\cdot OH$), or hydrogen peroxide radicals ($\cdot OOH$) in high concentration can alter hemoglobin structure and cellular membrane lipids so that hemolysis of the cell may result. Vitamin E (EH) acts within the membrane to protect against the destructive action of oxidants. In the cytosol, superoxide dismutase, glutathione peroxidase (catalyzes the oxidation of glutathione [2GSH → GSSG]), and catalase act to reduce the levels of superoxide and hydrogen peroxides. Essential to these steps is a high cellular concentration of NADPH derived from NADP following the oxidation of glucose-6-phosphate (Glu-6P) to 6-phosphoglucuronic acid (GP-Gluc). These compounds are then metabolized further in the hexose monophosphate shunt pathway.

the red blood cell to control the level of peroxide-containing compounds.

Vitamin E works directly within the membrane to protect against oxidative and perox-

idative damage (Figure 18-7). There are also a number of enzymes that act in the cytosol of red blood cells to control the levels of damaging oxidants. One form of oxygen that is particularly damaging to red blood cells is the **superoxide radical**. The enzyme **superoxide dismutase** functions to limit this form of oxygen to low concentrations. The enzymes **catalase** and **glutathione peroxidase** function to keep cytosol concentrations of hydrogen peroxide low.

Glutathione peroxidase is particularly important in that it reduces both the levels of hydrogen peroxide and lipid peroxides in red blood cells. That glutathione peroxidase is coupled to other enzymes in the red blood cell is also important. An NADPH-synthesizing system is required. NADPH is derived from the production of 6-phosphogluconate from 6-phosphoglucose. The NADPH is used by glutathione reductase to maintain a high level of glutathione, which serves as a cofactor for glutathione peroxidase.

Inherited deficiencies of selected enzymes

that result in low levels of NADPH, such as **glucose-6-phosphate dehydrogenase deficiency**, can give rise to increased concentrations of hydrogen peroxide or peroxide-containing compounds within the red blood cell, because of the reduction of NADPH and, subsequently, of glutathione and glutathione peroxidase activity.[21]

The effects of low vitamin E, low NADPH, or low glutathione peroxidase levels, however, usually are not observed until there is stress on the red cell because of increased hydrogen peroxide or superoxide radical formation. Infections and the metabolism of many drugs often generate hydrogen peroxide and other oxidants as end products. Antimalarial drugs, sulfonamides, nitrofurans, and, occasionally, aspirin can precipitate hemolysis in individuals who have a red blood cell deficiency of glucose-6-phosphate dehydrogenase. In patients receiving these drugs, vitamin E has been suggested to be therapeutically helpful in lessening hemolysis.

Other diet-derived factors can also precipitate a hemolytic crisis in susceptible individuals. Signs of acute hemolytic anemia have been observed in individuals (usually of Mediterranean descent) when **fava beans** are consumed as part of the diet. In this case, components of the fava bean exacerbate peroxidative damage to the red blood cell.

CONCLUDING COMMENTS

There are a number of nutritional variables to consider when anemia is observed as a secondary response to disease. For each case, good clinical information is needed to determine the anemia classification and the appropriate therapy. The role of the nutritional care specialist is made easier when a good history of the patient is available, since chronic infection, pregnancy, hemorrhage, or large menstrual losses are common underlying causes of anemia. In most instances, the approach to dietary treatment is to establish a well-balanced diet with appropriate supplements. In special instances, however,

reduction of intake of selected nutrients such as iron may be indicated.

Anemia and Athletic Performance

Anemia is sometimes observed in well-trained athletes such as endurance athletes and cross-country runners. This form of anemia, so-called sports anemia, is usually transient, with a decrease in hematocrit to 85–90% of normal values during the intense training phase, followed by gradual normalization. The mechanisms for sports anemia, however, are complex, and may be due to multiple factors. Obviously, iron-deficiency anemia can bring about a decrease in hemoglobin and hematocrit; however, the conscious effort by many athletes to optimize performance usually encourages them to direct special attention to nutrition. Such attention often translates into overzealous use of nutritional supplements; thus simple deficiencies of iron or vitamins are not likely to be common in athletes. Other causes of sports anemia are increased erythrocyte destruction, gastrointestinal loss, expansion of the normal blood volume, or loss of blood from constant abrasions. A daily loss of 1 to 2 ml of blood can result in a 0.5–1.0-mg loss of iron per day, which can result in a 20–40-mg loss of iron over a four-week period. Such losses may promote microcytic anemia. Alternatively, erythrocyte destruction has been demonstrated in a number of studies.[22] The evidence for erythrocyte destruction is based on higher than normal reticulocyte counts, decreased hemoglobin, and increased levels of free erythrocyte porphyrin. Consequently, whether or not nutritional intervention is appropriate when anemia is observed depends upon so many factors that it is difficult to make clear assessments. If the athlete is training intensely, and only the hematocrit is depressed (i.e., low normal values), then the anemia is possibly the result of an expanded plasma volume. An elevated free porphyrin level, however, could indicate that the intensity of the training has promoted red cell destruction, and other information—for example, serum iron or transferrin saturation — is needed before a clear evaluation may be made.

References

1. Williams, W.J., Beutler, E., Ersley, A.J., and Lichtman, M.A., Eds. *Hematology,* 3rd ed. New York: McGraw-Hill, 1983.
2. Hillman, R.S., and Finch, C.A. *Red Cell Manual,* 5th ed. Philadelphia: F.A. Davis Company, 1985, pp. 1–32.
3. Ogawa, M., Porter, P.N., and Nakahata, T. Renewal and commitment to differentiation of hemopoietic stem cells. An interpretive review. *Blood* 61:823, 1983.
4. Finch, C.A. Erythropoiesis, erythropoietin and iron. *Blood* 60:1241, 1982.
5. Bunn, H.F., and Forget, B.G. *Hemoglobin: Molecular, Genetic and Clinical Aspects.* Philadelphia: W.B. Saunders, 1984.
6. Bunn, H.F. Erythrocyte destruction and hemoglobin metabolism. *Sem. Hematol.* 9:317, 1972.
7. Berlin, N., and Berk, P.D. Quantitative aspects of bilirubin metabolism for hematologists. *Blood* 57:983, 1981.
8. Finch, C.A., and Huebers, H. Perspectives in iron metabolism. *N. Engl. J. Med.* 306:1520, 1982.
9. Cook, J.D. Clinical evaluation of iron deficiency. *Sem. Hematol.* 19:6, 1982.
10. Monsen, E.R., Hallberg, L., Layrisse, M., Hegsted, D.M., Cook, J.D., Mertz, W., and Finch, C.A. Estimation of available dietary iron. *Am. J. Clin. Nutr.* 31:134, 1978.
11. Shane, B., and Stokstad, E.L.R. Vitamin B_{12} – folate interrelationships. *Annu. Rev. Nutr.* 5:115, 1985.
12. Lindenbaum, J., Ed. *Nutrition in Hematology.* New York: Churchill Livingstone, 1983.
13. Hodges, R.E., Sauberlich, H.E., Canham, J.E., Wallace, D.L., Rucker, R.B., Mejia, L.A., and Mohanram, M. Hematopoietic studies in vitamin A deficiency. *Am. J. Clin. Nutr.* 31:876, 1978.
14. Basu, T.K., and Stein, R.M. Erythropoiesis associated with chronic renal disease. *Arch. Intern. Med.* 133:442, 1974.
15. Herbert, V., and Das, K.C. The role of B_{12} and folic acid in hemato- and other cell poiesis. *Vitam. Horm.* 34:1, 1976.
16. Reynolds, E.H. Neurological aspects of folate and vitamin B_{12} metabolism. *Clin. Haematol.* 6:661, 1976.
17. Weinberg, E.D. Iron and susceptibility to infectious disease. *Science* 184:952, 1974.
18. Strauss, R.G. Iron deficiency, infections and immune function. A reassessment. *Am. J. Clin. Nutr.* 31:660, 1978.
19. Wood, W.G., and Weatherall, D.J. Developmental genetics of human haemoglobins. A review. *Biochem. J.* 215:1, 1983.
20. Weatherall, D.J., and Clegg, J.B. *Thalassemia Syndromes,* 3rd ed. Oxford: Blackwell Scientific, 1981.
21. Valentine, W.N. Hemolytic anemia and inborn errors of metabolism. *Blood* 54:549, 1979.
22. McDonald, R., and Keen, C.L. Iron, zinc and magnesium nutrition and athletic performance. *Sports Med.* 5:171, 1988.

19. Nutritional Care in Neurological, Muscular, and Skeletal Disorders

I. Cleft Lip and Cleft Palate
  A. Prenatal development
  B. Nutritional care of the affected infant
  C. Nutritional care and surgical repair
II. Neuromuscular and Nervous System Disorders
  A. Developmental disabilities
    1. Anatomy and physiology of food intake
    2. Nutritional care in developmentally delayed patients
      a. feeding skills and food intake problems
        (1) total body reflexes
        (2) oropharyngeal reflexes
        (3) arm and hand control and eye-hand coordination
        (4) learned eating skills
        (5) self-feeding skills
      b. assessing feeding skills
      c. diet texture
      d. nutritional assessment of the developmentally disabled child
      e. behavioral problems
      f. nutritional needs and problems
        (1) growth retardation
        (2) overweight
        (3) underweight
        (4) constipation
        (5) fluid intake
        (6) drug-related problems
    3. Some specific conditions associated with developmental disabilities
      a. cerebral palsy
      b. Down syndrome
      c. fetal alcohol syndrome
      d. Prader-Willi syndrome
      e. spina bifida
      f. failure to thrive
      g. other feeding problems
  B. Neurological and neuromuscular problems in the older child or adult
    1. Epilepsy and other seizure disorders
      a. diagnosis
      b. treatment
    2. Brain and spinal cord injuries
      a. brain injury
        (1) nutritional assessment
        (2) nutritional support
        (3) food intake in early rehabilitation
      b. spinal cord injury
    3. Progressive neurological disorders
      a. Parkinson's disease
      b. Guillain-Barré syndrome
      c. amyotrophic lateral sclerosis
      d. dementia
      e. Huntington's chorea
      f. multiple sclerosis
      g. myasthenia gravis
    4. Muscular dystrophy
      a. pathogenesis
      b. nutritional assessment
      c. management
  C. Psychosis
  D. Schizophrenia
  E. Mood Disorders
  F. Drug Addiction
III. Diseases of the Musculoskeletal System
  A. Osteoarthritis
  B. Rheumatoid arthritis
  C. Juvenile rheumatoid arthritis
    1. Nutritional assessment
    2. Nutritional care
IV. Comment

A number of conditions involving the nervous system, muscles, skeleton, or a combination of these tissues affect nutritional status. Since many of these disorders lead to permanent disabilities with features in common and since many require similar nutritional care, they are included in this one chapter. For convenience, other conditions involving the neuromuscular and musculoskeletal systems also are described in this chapter.

CLEFT LIP AND PALATE

Prenatal Development

In normal prenatal development, at approximately four to six weeks' gestation, the upper lip is formed from a central flap and two side flaps that grow toward each other and fuse. If the fusion fails to take place, the child is born with a **cleft lip**, which may be unilateral or bilateral, complete (extending up into the nostril) or incomplete (sometimes only a slight notch on the upper lip). At the same time, the infant may have a **cleft palate**. Normally, the palate develops as tissue grows in from the sides and joins in the middle at seven to eight weeks' gestation. It consists of the **hard palate**, a bony shelf immediately behind the front teeth, and the **soft palate**, which extends toward the back of the mouth and divides the oral pharynx from the nasal cavity. If the normal fusion during gestation does not occur, an opening exists between the mouth and nose. The cleft may be in the soft palate alone or in both soft and hard palate. Hard palate clefts may be partial or total. The width of the cleft also varies. Cleft lip and cleft palate may occur separately or together, but bilateral cleft palate is usually accompanied by a cleft lip.[1]

The incidence of cleft lip and palate (CL/P) is about one in every 700 to 800 live births.[2] The cause is thought to be a combination of genetics and environment. The condition tends to recur in families. In addition, use of alcohol, tobacco, or heroin in the first trimester tends to increase the incidence.[1] In animals, maternal deficiencies of vitamin A, riboflavin, or folate or high doses of vitamin A have been associated with CL/P.[3] However, the application to human subjects is unknown.

Nutritional Care of the Affected Infant

Cleft lip and palate cause feeding and respiratory problems. The infant is also prone to ear infections, which may lead to hearing problems and then to difficulties in speech development.[4] It is important to provide good nutrition for these infants in preparation for their surgery and to promote resistance to ear infections.

The infant with CL/P cannot create an airtight seal necessary for the production of negative pressure and therefore has difficulty in sucking. Subnormal growth has been related to the resulting feeding problems,[5] but also to the type of cleft.[6] Infants with unilateral clefts of lip and palate or of the palate alone were significantly shorter than those with bilateral clefts of lip and palate or clefts of the lip alone.[6]

The infant who has a cleft of the lip, whether unilateral or bilateral, or a cleft of the soft palate can be breast-fed, but must be held upright to prevent the feeding from entering the nose.[7] It is not always possible to breast feed the infant with a cleft of both the hard and soft palate, but breast milk may instead be expressed and fed in a bottle.

Because of the lack of suction in cleft of both the hard and soft palate, special equipment for bottle feeding is necessary. Two types are available. The **Breck feeder** consists of a bulb-type syringe with a rubber or plastic tube. The **Beniflex feeder** is a soft bag with a cross-cut nipple. It is used for soft palate or partial hard palate clefts.

In place of sucking, the child learns to squeeze or chew the nipple. While this technique is being learned, feeding may be slow and tiring for some infants. The feeding period then must be lengthened and may need to be more frequent, sometimes every two hours. If necessary to increase nutritive value, a formula may be concentrated to 24 kcal/oz. instead of the usual 20 kcal/oz.

Another problem is excessive air intake. Feeding in an upright position with frequent burping is necessary. If there is choking and gagging, several techniques may be suggested to parents during counseling:

1. Feed in a more upright position.
2. Feed more slowly.
3. Use a smaller nipple opening.
4. Reduce pressure if using a soft container.
5. Direct flow toward the cheek.

As the infant learns to suck, swallow, and breathe in normal rhythm, the nipple may be changed to one that is firmer and has a smaller opening. The increased effort necessary to feed helps to develop facial musculature for chewing and speech.

Other problems include dental decay or malocclusion that interfere with sufficient food intake. The child may need supplements of vitamins C and D and fluoride.

Nutritional Care and Surgical Repair

A cleft lip is repaired when the infant has achieved a weight gain of 10 lb. or at ten weeks of age. Postoperatively, the infant may again be breast-fed, or a Breck feeder may be used with care not to press on the suture line. Clear liquids are given for two days, after which breast or formula feeding may begin. Each of these feedings is followed by some water to prevent contamination of the suture line. The Breck feeder may be abandoned in one to one and a half months.

Prior to palate repair, an **obturator** may be used. It is an acrylic plate that is molded to the infant's mouth to cover the cleft and to hold the dental arches. It may be worn all day or only during feeding, as tolerated by the infant.

Solid foods should be added at the usual ages. Acidic and spicy foods should be avoided, since they tend to cause irritation of the mouth and nose. Other foods to avoid for some children are round pieces of food such as sliced carrots, foods that are sticky and can form a plug, and those that are difficult to chew. Nuts, peanut butter, leafy vegetables, peelings of raw fruit, grapes, wieners, jelly beans, hard candies, popcorn, chewing gum, biscuits, cookies, and creamed dishes are reported to get caught in the cleft and may then slip into the trachea and block the airway.

Repair of a cleft palate is done later than lip repair, but before speech patterns are established, usually at 12 to 14 months. The child is weaned from the feeder at the age of four to six months and accustomed to the use of a cup and spoon for feeding. Solid foods are added at this time. Prior to surgery, clear liquids are given occasionally so the infant becomes accustomed to them. In addition, the child should also become accustomed preoperatively to arm restraints that prevent the child's putting the hands in the mouth. Postoperatively, the child is fed from a cup only, not with a spoon or through a straw, to avoid injuring the repair site. No foreign materials (silverware, straws, nipples, pacifiers, or toothbrushes) are allowed in the mouth.

A common protocol for postoperative feeding consists of clear liquids for five days, then full liquids for ten days, followed by progression for ten to 20 days to a soft, finely pureed, or mashed diet. The normal diet for age may then be resumed, except that very hard foods such as crackers and zwieback should be avoided for up to two months.

NEUROMUSCULAR AND NERVOUS SYSTEM DISORDERS

Neuromuscular and nervous system disorders accompanied by nutritional problems occur in both children and adults. Disabilities are seen in individuals of various ages who become senile or who have other conditions affecting the neuromuscular, nervous, or skeletal systems. Accompanying eating problems vary in nature and severity. Enlarged tonsils and throat infections may cause minor problems that require correction. Other individuals have disorders that are very serious.

Developmental Disabilities

Approximately 3% of the population in the United States are mentally retarded or have other developmental problems. Nearly half of these are children or adolescents, many of whom survive to adulthood. Many have multiple handicaps. These conditions, collectively known as **developmental disability** or **developmental delay**, are described as "significant physical, mental, or sensory impairment often accompanied by associated disabilities found in various combinations of a visual-perceptual-motor, language, or behavioral nature that can affect major life activities."[8]

Many factors may cause brain damage during the course of development. Some genetic abnormalities, such as phenylketonuria, may lead to hereditary metabolic disorders with effects on the brain (see Chapter 17). Chromosomal abnormalities cause conditions such as Down syndrome, described later in this chapter. Later in pregnancy, maternal drug addiction, toxemia, and conditions causing fetal malnutrition may cause brain damage. In the perinatal period, prematurity, trauma during the birth process, hypoglycemia, and hyperbilirubinemia contribute to brain damage, and in childhood, infections, tumors, and trauma may damage the brain. In a child who is normal at birth, disability may be the result of environmental deprivation, including children who have had multiple hospitalizations and perhaps have not eaten orally for a long period. Abused or depressed children, those with failure to thrive (discussed later in this chapter), and just picky, fussy, slow eaters are also at risk of feeding-skill delay. Children who survive drowning accidents or other incidents causing anoxia sometimes are permanently brain-damaged. At the same time, it is important to remember that, although many brain-damaged children are mentally retarded, this is not invariably the case. Some children have motor dysfunction without a decrease in intelligence. In either case, problems associated with feeding often provide the first clue to the existence of central nervous system deficit.

Anatomy and Physiology of Food Intake

As in other parts of the body, the bones provide the foundation, and the muscles, controlled by the nerves, provide power for movement involved in food intake. The **skeletal structure** involved in eating consists of three bones. The **mandible** (lower jaw bone) is important in eating, since it is the only bone in the face that is free to move. The muscles attached to the mandible are under voluntary control and, when normally coordinated, make it possible for a person to elevate and lower the mandible to close and open the mouth. The muscles also make it possible to protrude and retract the mandible, to move it laterally, and to maintain it in a position so that the mouth is closed at rest. The **maxillae** are actually two bones that form the upper jaw and hard palate. They are stationary, and so the mandible must rise to meet the upper jaw for chewing. The **hyoid bone** is suspended from the temporal bone by ligaments but is not attached to any other bone. Some muscles of the tongue and floor of the mouth are attached to the hyoid bone, which moves up involuntarily during swallowing to aid in sealing off the epiglottis.

Using the bones as levers, the **muscles** contract to cause movement if stimulated by the nerves. Muscles can only pull by **contracting** (shortening). They return to their original length by relaxing, but there is no mechanism by which a muscle can push. A muscle's potential for work is related to its **tone** or **tension** (degree of firmness). In general, three possible categories of tone are described: **hypotonic, flaccid,** or **floppy** and **atonic** muscles are soft and flabby; **hypertonic, spastic,** or **stiff** muscles are rigid and hard in a continuous contraction or convulsion; and muscles with **normal tone** have some resilience when at rest. The muscle must have sufficient tone to perform its function but not so much that further contraction is difficult.

The amount of muscle tension is influenced by the number of muscle fibers stimulated by the **nerves.** When there is a disturbance in the impulses from the central nervous system, there will be a disturbance in the related muscles. Depending on the nature of the disorder in the nervous system, the muscle may be hypertonic, weak, or paralyzed, or they may have alternating tone. If the nerve supply to the muscle is severed, the fibers of the muscle atrophy so that the muscle will be much smaller than its normal size. The degenerated fibers are replaced by fibrous tissue. Therefore, it is important that the muscles used in eating not be allowed to atrophy from disuse. Loss of function from disuse is difficult, sometimes impossible, to correct. An equally important consideration is that many muscles for eating are used also for speech. If these muscles are allowed to atrophy, speech will be affected.

The brain and many nerves are involved in the eating process. When the nervous system malfunctions, either in the brain itself or in peripheral nerves, a variety of problems is possible. In addition to the problems related to the muscles, nerve disorders can cause loss of sensation in the face, mouth, or soft palate, thereby causing loss of taste perception and inability to locate, and thus control, food in the mouth. Nerve disorders can affect salivary gland function as well.

There are a number of reflexes that are important functional components of the eating process. Eating disorders may involve hyperactive, hypoactive, absent, or abnormal reflexes. Sometimes, a normal reflex may persist beyond the age at which it usually comes under voluntary control. In other cases, feeding difficulties arise because of lack of control of total body posture.

Nutritional Care in Developmentally Delayed Patients

Nutritional problems in developmentally delayed children may be classified as those related to (1) feeding skills, (2) nutrient intake and function, and (3) behavior.

Feeding Skills and Food Intake Problems. The normal infant develops feeding skills in a specific sequence. In a developmentally delayed child, this same sequence often is followed, but the rate at which progress occurs may be slowed. Also, reflexes that normally disappear during development may persist past the time when they are useful. In other cases, these developmental landmarks are abnormal. Thus it is important to be familiar with normal development and to be able to relate these to nutritional needs in handicapped children.

A child exhibits typical patterns of posture and movement as he or she develops. In motor development, reflex contraction is followed by voluntary contraction and muscle control develops **cephalocaudally** (from the head downward). Large muscle movement precedes fine motions.

The infant begins with certain simple reflexes which are modified and inhibited (controlled) as he or she develops. Although these reflexes are significant in their relation to each other, they are described separately for clarity.

Total body reflexes. The total body reflexes are present in the normal infant for a few months and then fade, but they can interfere with development of eating if they persist beyond the age at which they normally are brought under control.[9] Children with **persistent flexor reflexes** are hard to position for feeding. They tend to be bent in a fetal position, making feeding or eating difficult. Poor equilibrium and poor head control make chewing and swallowing difficult.

Tongue control and hand-to-mouth coordination are poor.

Extensor thrusting (extension reflexes) can be initiated in some brain-damaged patients by stimulation or pressure in the occipital area of the skull or on the balls of the feet. The arms and legs become extended with a stiff trunk and with the head and neck thrown back. Hand-to-mouth movements or movements across the midline of the body are inhibited.

Moro's reflex is elicited if the head drops back suddenly. There is a rapid extension and then flexion of the limbs as if embracing something. It occurs normally in an infant to the age of approximately four months. If it persists beyond that age, it interferes with sitting balance and hand-to-mouth movement.

The **asymmetric tonic neck reflex** occurs normally in infants from birth to four to seven months of age.[10-13] When the face is turned to one side, the arm and leg on that side will become extended and the opposite side will become flexed. This sometimes is referred to as the "fencing position." The normal infant can move away from this position and bring a hand to his or her mouth to suck on the fingers. The developmentally disabled infant who has a dominant asymmetric tonic neck reflex cannot bring food to his or her mouth while looking at the food. The reflex interferes with head and trunk control and with normal arm and head movements in feeding.

A strong **tonic labyrinthine reflex** can force a child into an extensor position, holding his or her head and neck in extension. This posture makes swallowing difficult.[9]

Normal muscle tone makes possible the sitting position, arm and head movement, and mouth movements for eating. An infant with increased muscle tone may be unable to bend at the hips in order to sit or to control the head and neck to stay in a sitting position. Increased tonus sometimes prevents movement of the lips, tongue, and jaw for chewing. The hypotonic infant may have diffi-

culty in maintaining a sitting posture and in maintaining lip closure or jaw movement.

Suckling infants are fed in a semirecumbent, flexed position, allowing the baby to swallow easily. Normally, at approximately six months of age, a child may be placed in a high chair for eating. At approximately 18 to 24 months, the normal child is sufficiently coordinated that a baby high chair is no longer needed.

If the child has no head and trunk control, support must be provided with the trunk and head flexed forward. If the head is extended, the child will gag. His or her head, trunk, and feet should be supported in an upright symmetric position for feeding.

Oropharyngeal reflexes. Other reflexes, classified as oropharyngeal reflexes, are involved in eating. These will be described individually for the sake of clarity, but it is important to remember that the sequence of action is crucial.

The **rooting reflex** is present at birth or appears soon after birth except when urinating and for two hours or so after eating. It fades at approximately three months of age. It is a food-seeking behavior in which the infant will turn its head toward the stimulus if the cheek or corner of the mouth is touched with a nipple or a finger. If rooting movement continues after the food source is located, it may interfere with the development of sucking.

There is a difference between suckling and sucking. From birth to approximately five months, **suckling** can be seen. At first, it can be elicited by stimulating almost any body part but, within a few days, only the lips, cheeks, and inside of the mouth are responsive. Suckling is a continuous process in which the passage from the nose is open so that nose breathing and swallowing occur simultaneously. It occurs with the body in a flexed position and will not take place when the infant's body is extended.

Sucking follows the more primitive suckling. It is a discontinuous process in which liquid accumulates in the mouth. Before swallowing, there must be a pause in breathing. The sucking-swallowing reflex begins soon after birth, but becomes a voluntary activity by six months of age. The reflex consists of opening the mouth to accept a nipple followed by sucking whenever the corners or center of the upper lip are touched.

Some premature or retarded infants do not have the ability to suck and must be assisted. They must be able to create a seal with the lips and closure of the soft palate to create a negative pressure. The posterior tongue provides the pumping action.

In the **sucking reflex**, when the mouth has moved to the stimulus, the tongue retracts and the lips close. The movement of the hyoid bone shows that swallowing occurs. The sucking-swallowing reflex is replaced after approximately one year with a mature swallowing pattern.

The **bite reflex** is present at birth and normally comes under voluntary control in three to six months. It consists of a sudden, snapping viselike closure of the mandible elicited by touching the lips, teeth, gums, or tongue.[6] If it persists past five to six months of age or if it is oversensitive, it interferes with other developmental activities such as taking food from a cup or spoon, chewing, and speaking. In addition, it can cause damage to the lips, tongue, or cheeks. The patient may need help in overcoming this reflex.

Drooling, although not a reflex, begins in the normal infant at approximately three months and subsides before 12 months. The child with poor lip closure and weak swallowing almost always drools excessively. It is associated with wet clothing, unpleasant odors, and social stigma. Development of strong lip closure controls drooling.

The **gag reflex** normally is present at birth and is located at the tip of the tongue. It moves to the back of the mouth in the ensuing six to eight months. It is not a normal part of taking food but is a protective mechanism. It consists of contraction of the constrictor muscles of the pharynx[12] and is elicited by pressure at the middle of the tongue and

areas back to the **uvula** (the fleshy mass that descends from the back of the soft palate above the root of the tongue). Its decrease is associated with the development of chewing, but it never disappears completely, even in the adult.

A **hypoactive gag reflex** is a serious problem because the child is unable to sense choking. It is seen in Down syndrome and also is present in floppy infant syndrome and pseudobulbar palsy, conditions in which hypotonia is prominent.

The **hyperactive gag reflex** is elicited by stimulation of other areas of the mouth. It interferes with eating and can make the swallowing of solid food difficult or impossible. In swallowing, it may be helpful to have the head tilted back slightly. This causes the tongue to drop down and back, reducing its stimulation. Parents may be counseled to feed the child from straight ahead to avoid triggering abnormal reflexes.

Arm and hand control and eye-hand coordination. The normal child also develops controlled arm and hand movements and eye-hand coordination at appropriate ages. The newborn infant usually can bring its hand to its mouth for sucking. The ability to reach and grasp large objects usually develops at three to four months, and a pincer movement to pick up tiny objects develops at approximately six months. In central nervous system dysfunction, the hand-to-mouth movement may be abnormal.[13] Persistent asymmetric tonic neck reflex causes the head to turn away as the hand comes to the mouth. A persistent primitive grasp interferes with handling of utensils. The child's grasp and movement to the mouth may need to be guided at first. Adaptive equipment may be necessary.

In evaluation of arm and hand movement for self-feeding, factors that should be observed include finger grasp, palmar grasp, wrist and elbow flexion, wrist rotation, hand and arm steadiness, and coordination of hand-to-mouth movement. A normal infant has a reflexive **palmar grasp** at one to two days of age which persists for approximately three months.[14] If it persists beyond the time when the child is ready for independent use of his or her hands, as for finger feeding, the child will not be able to voluntarily grasp or release objects.[15]

The normal infant regards the feeding bottle and may touch it at approximately five months. He or she can hold or stabilize it with a palmar grasp at seven months or so.[16] This visual coordination is a necessary development in normal feeding.

The **palm-chin reflex** is present in premature and some newborn infants but disappears by three to four months.[12] As a result of this reflex, the jaw is open as long as any pressure is applied to the **thenar eminence** (the bulge on the palm at the base of the thumb). If the reflex persists, a child cannot hold food in his or her mouth when the palms are stimulated.

Learned eating skills. To progress in eating skills, the child must develop jaw stability and tongue and lip control. He or she also must know how to chew and swallow. These are learned eating skills, not reflexes. Swallowing is a reflex only after the bolus of food reaches a critical point.

Jaw stability is indicated by the position of the lower jaw. Normally, when a child is at rest, the mandible is elevated or closed. Need for treatment is indicated if the mandible is (1) open or depressed, (2) protracted or jutting outward, (3) retracted or drawn inward, or (4) closed and cannot be voluntarily opened.

Some patients require treatment to achieve adequate **lip closure** and control of the lips when they are at rest or while eating.

Tongue control is important in eating and is a prerequisite for speech. It positions food for both chewing and swallowing. Normally, at six months, the child is capable of elevation, depression, lateralization, retraction, and protraction of the tongue. The protraction or forward thrust is the most common action of the tongue.

Some children have abnormal **tongue thrust** in which the tongue extends forward or laterally between or against the teeth. It can be the result of tonsillitis, early thumb sucking, or early loss of primary incisors. Often the child has a hypersensitive mouth, and tongue movement occurs on stimulation of the lips, tongue, or palate. If the child has a minor problem, it may correct itself in time, but correction without treatment is unlikely if the condition persists after the age of ten years.[17] Tongue thrust prevents getting food in the mouth or keeping it there. It also interferes with swallowing. The objective of treatment, then, is for the tongue to remain in an appropriate position in the mouth.

If **chewing** is to develop, the diet must be progressed appropriately from liquid to pureed to chopped foods as the child matures. Normally, all food is liquid for three months, with soft pureed food used in the next two months. Chopped foods are introduced at approximately seven months.

Rotary chewing, a process distinct from biting, begins at nine months or slightly later. At that time, usual table foods may be used, adjusted for the eruption of the molars for grinding. At first, chewing occurs in an up-and-down motion, but gradually, the side-to-side motion develops.

The incisors erupt at six to nine months to provide for biting. Molars erupt between 12 and 24 months, at which time lateral jaw movements for chewing occur. The first permanent molars erupt at six years.[18] Tongue movements must be coordinated and controlled to keep food between the molars for chewing, and the lips must remain closed.

To develop the normal **mature swallowing pattern**, the child must have jaw stability, contracted masseter muscles but relaxed muscles in the floor of the mouth, and tongue control. It is a complex combination of voluntary and involuntary actions involving 22 muscles and is learned over a period of time. In the handicapped child, jaw closure, tongue placement, and lip closure may have to be taught separately and then coordinated.

Self-feeding skills. Self-feeding skills are important objectives in correcting eating handicaps. The techniques progress from bottle or breast feeding to assisted spoon feeding and finger self-feeding and, finally, to the use of utensils.

The first of these skills is drinking from a cup or glass. The normal infant can sip liquids from a cup or glass at the age of eight to ten months, drink with help at 12 to 14 months, and drink with little help at approximately 18 months. For developmentally disabled children, teaching this technique may begin with the use of thin liquids, advancing to thicker liquids as ability increases. Some children, however, have greatest difficulty with thin liquids and so teaching must begin with thicker mixtures.

Finger self-feeding is the next step. A child may begin self-feeding with his or her fingers as soon as he or she can pick up objects and put the hands to the mouth. Foods that are suitable for this purpose include pieces of fruit or vegetables, crackers, cheese, or dry cereals. A child with an eating handicap may need help in learning to finger-feed, a skill that must precede self-feeding with a spoon. The piece of food may be placed in the child's hand and guided to his or her mouth at first. As skill develops, self-feeding as much as possible should be encouraged.

Self-feeding with a spoon should then be encouraged. When a child can pick up food with his or her fingers and bring it to the mouth, he or she can begin to practice with a spoon. The child should begin with a **pronated grasp** (with the palm down). The normal child learns to hold the spoon with the hand in the **supinated** (palm upward) position at 18 to 24 months. At the same age, a normal child will begin to stab with a fork, but this maneuver is not well established until approximately four years of age. A normal child of eight can cut with a knife.[15,19,20]

Sometimes special equipment for eating is helpful. Depending on specific need, special utensils may be provided with padded, extended, or bent handles or with a ring or cuff on the handle to facilitate holding. The plate on which the food is placed may be anchored and have sides so the food can be "trapped."

At first, food that tends to stick to the spoon should be used. Very liquid or slippery foods should be avoided until the child has developed some skill in the use of utensils.

In simplified form, the five basic feeding skills may be summarized as follows:

Birth to four months	suck/swallow reflex
Four to six months	Elevation tongue movement
Five to six months	Up-and-down chewing
Eight to ten months	Lateral tongue movement
Ten to 12 months	Rotary chewing

Table 19-1 summarizes in more detail the normal developmental landmarks related to feeding.

Assessing Feeding Skills. Assessment of feeding skills must take into account the age of the child. The nutritional care specialist can do an initial screening as follows:[21]

For infants up to eight months, use baby food and infant formula during assessment. Older infants can be given a soft cracker. The infant often chews with the mouth open, making observation easy.

In the **suck-swallow** action, the tongue lies on the bottom of the mouth and thrusts out to massage the nipple. Look for the position of the tongue.

To see **tongue elevation**, watch to see the tip of the tongue move to the roof of the mouth, rather than thrusting out.

Up-and-down chewing can be felt by cupping the hand under the child's jaw. There should be no grinding motion.

To see **lateral tongue movement**, look for the tip of the tongue to move to the side. Food will then shift to the side between the jaws.

Rotary chewing can also be felt by cupping the hand under the child's jaw. It feels like a circular or side-to-side motion.

Table 19-1. Normal Development of Reflexes and Feeding Skills

Approximate Age[a]	Reflexes and Skills	Approximate Age[a]	Reflexes and Skills
Newborn	Lack of head and trunk control; must have total support Rooting reflex; sucking-swallowing primarily through up-and-down jaw movement Palm-chin reflex Extrusion reflex (pushes out solid food placed on tongue)	6–8 months	Sits well in high chair Holds bottle alone Reaches for dish, spoon Begins up-and-down chewing if given chewable foods Transfers objects between hands Can grasp large pieces of food Chews easily dissolved foods Finger-feeds
1–2 months	Palm-chin reflex diminished Begins head control but still requires support Some hand-to-mouth skill Protraction-retraction tongue movement Solid foods involuntarily ejected		Uses fingers in grasping
		8–9 months	Sits independently Bite reflex disappears Tongue lateralization begins Finger-feeds bite-size pieces of food Can grasp small pieces Lips close when swallowing
2½–3 months	Mature sucking Reflexive palmar grasp disappears at approximately 12 weeks	9–11 months	Good eye-hand-mouth coordination Can pick up small pieces of food
4–5 months	Asymmetric tonic neck reflex disappears at 4–7 months Extrusion reflex disappears at approximately 4 months Head and upper trunk control—may sit in infant seat or high chair Frequently puts hands to mouth Elevation tongue movement; negative pressure sucking		Finger-feeds easily Bites off correct amount Lateral tongue movement Rotary chewing begins at approximately 10 months
		12–18 months	Finger-feeds much of meal, but messy Uses spoon at approximately 15 months; may rotate spoon near mouth Drinks from cup with moderate spillage
5 months	Sits in high chair with support Up-and-down chewing movement Can drink from cup if it is held by others	18 months	Drinks from glass or cup with little spillage Uses spoon without rotation
		24 months	Good rotary chewing Competent spoon feeding
6 months	Good head control Some independent sitting Bites on soft food; chews Can hold bottle, hold and eat biscuit Can reach for and grasp objects	30 months	Straw sucking complete Chews well
		36 months	Uses utensils Feeds self well

[a] The range of normal variability is wide and the ages given are merely approximations.

Diet Texture. Many of the problems of nutrient intake in developmentally delayed patients are avoidable if guidance is provided to parents or other caretakers on food texture changes and appropriate expectations of feeding skills.

Once the infant's most advanced skills are identified, the most appropriate texture can be chosen. The texture of the diet must be varied as eating skill advances. If the texture is not appropriate, there is risk of choking or gagging, or of aspirating food into the lungs. If appropriately textured foods are not provided at the time that the patient is developmentally ready to advance to the next stage, his or her development may be further delayed and may be irreparably damaged. Table 19-2 lists various feeding skills and the feeding procedures indicated. If delays are detected, the child should be referred for further evaluation and rehabilitation by a team that includes speech, physical, and occupational therapists.

Nutritional Assessment of the Developmentally Disabled Child. The assessment of the developmentally delayed child must include both nutritional assessment and evaluation of feeding skills. It sometimes requires the effort of a health care team composed of individuals from many areas of ex-

Table 19-2. Guide for Choice of Textures in Development of Feeding Behaviors

Skill Developed	Recommended Texture	Example
Sucking	Use fluids	Milk
Elevation of tongue moves food to back of mouth	Continue using liquids	Milk
Elevation tongue movement	Pureed	Iron-fortified infant cereals Pureed or strained fruits and vegetables Mashed potatoes Applesauce
Up-and-down chewing plus beginning lateral tongue movement	Mashed	Iron-fortified infant cereals Mashed fruits and vegetables Lumpy mashed bananas Mashed tofu Mashed egg yolk Pureed meats and poultry
Up-and-down chewing and complete lateral tongue movement	Ground and finely chopped	Iron-fortified infant cereals Rice, crackers Cooked macaroni Soft cooked vegetable pieces Banana slices Chopped soft fruit Soft cheeses Tofu cubes Pureed meats and poultry
Complete lateral tongue movement plus rotary chewing	Chopped	Iron-fortified adult cereals Crackers, biscuits, toast strips, tortillas Pastas Cooked vegetables; finely chopped coleslaw Tofu cubes Chopped ground beef Finely chopped meats and poultry Casseroles
Reaches for and grasps objects; brings hands to mouth	Begin finger feeding with large pieces	Crackers; teething biscuits; oven-dried toast; cheese sticks
Voluntary release	Finger feeding with small pieces	Dry cereals Small pieces of meat Cottage cheese
Puts lips on cup rim	Begin cup feeding	
Reaches for spoon; ulnar deviation of wrist	Self-feeding	Foods that adhere to spoon Cooked cereal Mashed potato Applesauce Cottage cheese
Increased rotary movement of jaw	Increase texture and variety	Chopped meats Raw vegetables and fruits

pertise. The nutritional care specialist on the team can provide a large part of the nutritional assessment. Since many of the same structures and functions are involved in both eating and speaking, the participation of a speech therapist is important in some cases. Table 19-3 provides a list of nutrition-related factors that may be observed.

Alterations in the standard procedures for anthropometric measurements given in Chapter 3 may be necessary. For those incapable of standing upright, **recumbent length** may be substituted for height. If a child's legs are deformed, **sitting height** is used as an alternative to total height. **Crown-rump length** is the equivalent measure in infants. In some cases, measurement of **arm span** or **tibia length** is used for estimation of total length.[22] **Serial head circumferences** sometimes are recorded also. **Fat fold measurements** are used to estimate the percentage of body fat. **Midarm circumference** and **triceps skinfold** are useful for this purpose.

Table 19-3. Possible Considerations in Feeding Assessment in Neurological Patients

Medical History
Diagnosis
Primitive or abnormal reflexes
Physical handicaps and motor abnormalities
Abnormalities of spin
Respiration
Ambulation
Allergy
Special diet
Medications: type? dosage? when given?
Past feeding history
Current feeding therapy
   Techniques and goals
Obstetric history
Bowel function: normal? constipation? diarrhea?
Vision
Communication and speech skills
Nutritional Assessment
Anthropometry
Clinical findings
Laboratory findings
Usual food intake (one- to three-day recall or diaries)
Appetite
Total fluid intake
Feeding Assessment Observations

Skeletal maturity is not always related to height in handicapped children. For these individuals, estimates of bone age may be obtained from roentgenograms. This procedure requires a pediatrician or radiologist with skill in interpretation. Similarly, **dental roentgenograms** can be used as an index of development, requiring the services of a dentist. Scoring methods for deciduous teeth have not been developed; therefore, this procedure is not useful for very young children.

The nutrition of developmentally delayed children should be assessed at frequent intervals and followed closely. After infancy, the child should be evaluated at six-month intervals. If nutritional problems develop, assessment should occur more frequently to evaluate progress under treatment. If delays are detected, the child should be referred for further evaluation and rehabilitation by a team that includes speech, physical, and occupational therapists.

Behavioral Problems. Some feeding problems are primarily behavioral in nature. They may occur in developmentally delayed children and in children who are able to eat but who are considered problem eaters. There are several types of behavioral problems.

In some cases, eating is associated with unpleasant consequences. This can occur in patients for whom food intake must be frequent, is time-consuming, or is associated with discomfort. Additional incentives must be offered to offset these negative factors.

Some patients use the feeding situation to manipulate the environment, including the parents, and parents often profit from counseling to regain control in such cases. Sometimes, however, it is the parent who institutes the inappropriate feeding programs. Some stressed families need professional family counseling to help them to cope with these situations.

Nutritional Needs and Problems. The developmentally disabled child needs the same nutrients as the normal child. In some cases, however, the quantities required are different. There are several problems that are seen frequently.

Growth retardation. Many brain-damaged children are retarded in growth. The reason for this is often unknown, but since eating handicaps are common, it is important to assure that malnutrition does not contribute to the growth deficit. When a child is shorter than normal, age should not be used as a basis for estimation of energy need, or the child will become overweight. The kilocalorie ration to maintain normal body weight should be provided in proportion to the child's height and activity.

Overweight. Handicapped patients whose capacity for activity is limited often are obese. The therapist should not reward progress in the obese handicapped child with food. Exercise should be increased if possible.

Underweight. Patients with eating and swallowing problems or who fall asleep during meals may be underweight. Some patients have increased muscle tone, increasing their caloric need at the same time that food intake is decreased. In addition to the development of self-feeding skills, an increase in the number of meals per day and the use of liquid supplements and foods of high caloric density are helpful. Some patients apparently are unable to sense hunger and are anorexic. They, too, may be given a high-density diet.

Constipation. Constipation is a commonly occurring problem, particularly in patients receiving soft low-fiber foods or inadequate fluid and in those whose activity is limited. Some developmentally delayed patients may have decreased muscle tone in the intestinal tract. Suggestions for diet modifications for chronic constipation are provided in Chapter 8. These must be altered as necessary for age and the nature of the handicap. In general, increased fluid and fiber are helpful. If the patient is unable to chew raw fruits and vegetables, prunes and soaked bran in the diet may be beneficial.

Fluid intake. Fluid intake must be carefully monitored in the patient who cannot respond to thirst or who is unable to express a desire for fluid.

Drug-related problems. A number of drugs useful in the management of patients with developmental disabilities or behavioral problems have effects that have nutritional implications. **Amphetamine** causes alterations in taste, extreme drowsiness, and depressed appetite. Steroids, on the other hand, increase appetite and can cause obesity.

Many developmentally disabled children are seizure-prone and receive medications for this reason. The effects of these drugs on nutrition will be described later in this chapter.

Some Specific Conditions Associated with Developmental Disabilities

Several of the more common conditions associated with developmental disability will be described in some detail here to illustrate a number of the problems previously described.

Cerebral Palsy. Cerebral palsy, occurring in 1 or 2 in 1,000 live births, is a group of nonprogressive disorders caused by damage to the brain centers for motor control from anoxia, trauma, or infection. The damage occurs in the prenatal or perinatal period or occasionally in the early years. Approximately 50% of these patients have subnormal intelligence, but others have normal intelligence, and some may be gifted. Sometimes sight, hearing, or speech is impaired. Approximately one-third experience seizures. The physical handicaps may be mild or severe. There are several different forms of the condition:

1. In **spasticity**, which occurs in 60% of cases, the patient has hyperactive stretch reflexes, increased muscle tone, and muscle weakness. Movement is blocked by antagonist muscles, and freedom of movement is limited. It may affect the arm and leg on one side only (**hemiparesis**), all four extremities

(tetraparesis), the legs more than the arms (spastic diplegia), or both legs but not the arms (paraparesis). Spasticity occurs in 70% of cerebral palsy patients.

2. **Dyskinesia** is indicated by many involuntary, uncontrolled, and purposeless movements, which disappear during sleep. The most common form (15% of patients) is **athetosis**, in which the patient has slow writhing movements, usually involving the face, neck, trunk, and all four extremities.

3. **Ataxia** produces incoordination and balance problems. The patient has difficulty in turning and falls frequently. This form is the least common. It occurs in combination with other types.

4. **Flaccidity** is demonstrated by decreased muscle tone.

5. **Mixed types** have elements of more than one of the others. For example, athetosis and spasticity can occur in the same patient.

Therapy in cerebral palsy is most effective if there is team treatment. Depending on the specific dysfunctions, team members may include physicians in neurology, orthopedics, pediatrics, psychiatry, and rehabilitation along with nurses and physical, occupational, and speech therapists, as well as nutritionists.

The use of energy in cerebral palsy is inefficient, and varies with the type of disease. Spastics have low activity and may require as little as 1,200 kcal/day. On the other hand, the constant movement of athetoids may increase their need to as much as 6,000 kcal/day.[23,24] If these needs are not met, general growth retardation may occur.[25-27] Other problems include delayed bone maturation, microcephaly, hormone dysfunction, and general malnutrition. A number of reasons have been suggested for growth retardation and malnutrition:

1. Feeding problems associated with incoordination of muscles involved in chewing and swallowing.
2. Slow development consequent to action of hypothalamic centers.

3. Caries and other dental problems.
4. Poor dietary habits.
5. Mineral depletion related to anticonvulsant drug use or lack of exercise.[8]

Energy requirements are estimated on the basis of height. If the subject is nonambulatory, 11.1 kcal/cm will be needed, while ambulatory subjects may be given 13.9 kcal/cm.[28] Exercise should be encouraged if it is possible.

Feeding problems commonly seen include almost all those previously described. Muscle incoordination in the lips, tongue, and palate can lead to difficulties in sucking and swallowing and persistent drooling. Persistent bite reflex and asymmetric tonic neck reflex, tongue thrust, and hyperactive gag also are seen. A high-arched palate, small lower jaw, and lack of lateral jaw movement cause chewing problems. Hand-to-mouth coordination often is delayed. Infants may need to have oral tissues desensitized and be fed with special nipples and other devices. Older children must be encouraged to eat meat, fruit, and vegetables, rather than an excess of milk. Gastroesophageal reflux occurs in about 25% of severely affected children.

Dental problems, contributing to difficulties in self-feeding include caries, gingivitis, malocclusion, and tooth loss. Good dental hygiene is essential, including the use of fluoridated water.

Medications frequently used include anticonvulsants, discussed later in the chapter in relation to epilepsy. Others are laxatives, (see Chapter 8) and muscle relaxants such as diazepam (see Chapter 4). Effects of these drugs must be considered in providing nutritional care.

Tube feeding, sometimes through a gastrostomy, may be necessary. TPN is occasionally required but is less common. When non-oral feedings are used before oral intake is firmly established in an infant, strong resistance to oral feeding develops. While oral feeding is being reinstated, a combination of oral and non-oral feeding may be required to meet nutritional needs.

Down Syndrome. A patient with Down syndrome (mongolism) has either an extra chromosome 21, a condition known as trisomy 21, or a chromosomal translocation. It occurs in approximately 1 in 660 live births. Trisomy 21 occurs primarily when mothers are 42 years old or more at conception, but translocation may occur at any maternal age.

Since individuals with Down syndrome have limited mental abilities, an understanding of terminology is helpful to those working with these patients. When a person functions at the very lowest end of the normal range of intellectual function, the level of ability is referred to as **borderline** function. Functions below borderline are called **mental retardation**. The degrees of retardation are graded as **mild, moderate, severe,** and **profound**. The majority of Down syndrome children are in the mild to moderate retardation range.

These patients are growth-retarded. Hypotonicity may lead to obesity and constipation, and frequently causes a protruding tongue. The tongue thrust reflex often persists. The patients have narrow nasal passages and tend to be mouth breathers. Development of oral reflexes is delayed, and swallowing is poor. A narrow palate interferes with a proper seal when sucking. Tooth eruption is delayed and chewing difficulties are common. Other dental problems include periodontal disease, malocclusion, hypocalcification, and caries. These add to the chewing problems. There is a high incidence of tracheoesophageal fistulas, pyloric stenosis, malabsorption, and heart defects. Biochemical defects in protein, fat, carbohydrate, vitamin, and mineral metabolism are seen.

Nutritional care involves development of feeding skills, prevention of obesity, and prevention of nutritional deficiency. Training must be provided to help the patient control the tongue and keep the mouth closed when eating. As the child becomes older, fiber and fluid in the diet may be increased to avoid constipation. To reduce dental problems, foods high in sucrose, including sweet, sticky snacks, should be eliminated. A soft diet may be necessary because of malocclusion and tooth loss, but intake of fresh fruits and vegetables should be increased if possible.

Energy content of the diet should be provided in proportion to the patient's height and activity, approximately 16.1 kcal/cm for male patients and 14.3 kcal/cm for females at five to 11 years of age. In the teen years, the intake is often reduced because the adolescent growth spurt in these children is depressed and is sometimes absent.[29] Growth must be monitored on special charts for Down syndrome patients. The NCHS charts are not appropriate for this group.[29]

Eventually, many patients make a transition to community groups or independent living. These individuals will need help in food selection and preparation for maintaining good nutritional status.

Fetal Alcohol Syndrome. Fetal alcohol syndrome (FAS) has been generally recognized only recently. Alcohol crosses the placenta and enters the fetal circulation very rapidly. It reaches the fetus within 30 minutes. The fetal blood alcohol level becomes equal to the amount in the maternal blood but is cleared more slowly. Alcohol persists in the amniotic fluid.

Fetal alcohol syndrome apparently can vary in severity. The major features of the condition consist of brain injury, growth deficiency, delayed development, and alterations in the structure of the face. The facial characteristics are most easily observed. The head is small, the bridge of the nose is flat, and the eyes have epicanthic folds which obscure the inner corners. The philtrum (the groove between the upper lip and nose) is indistinct, and the upper lip is thin and reddish. The severely affected infant may have a significant reduction in height and weight. Mental retardation and irritability also are seen. The condition is permanent, and older children may be hyperactive and have poor coordination.

An important unanswered question is whether there is a safe level of alcohol intake for the pregnant woman. It has been suggested that low levels of intake, in which all absorbed alcohol is detoxified by the liver and does not flow into the general circulation, may be safe. However, the safe level has not been specified. Even very moderate social drinking may cause some abnormalities. Pending further information, the most prudent course for pregnant women is to avoid any alcohol intake.

Maternal alcohol intake can damage the fetus, but the mechanisms are not understood. Alcohol may act directly, possibly by its dehydrating effect on fetal cells. It may affect protein synthesis or formation of neurotransmitters. Acetaldehyde is very toxic and crosses the placenta. This, therefore, may be the toxic agent. Alternatively, increased ethanol-metabolizing enzymes may have a role in the production of anomalies.[30]

The incidence of hypoglycemia and malnutrition, including amino acid, vitamin, and trace element deficiencies, is increased in alcoholics. However, the evidence does not suggest that malnutrition is the sole cause of FAS. Smoking, increased caffeine intake, and drug abuse occur with greater frequency in those who are heavy drinkers. The relative effects of these factors on the incidence of FAS is unknown.

Prader-Willi Syndrome. Prader-Willi syndrome is a congenital disorder, the cause of which is unknown. It occurs in one in 10,000 to 25,000 live births. A disturbance in brain development may account for all the symptoms. The clinical manifestations include hypotonic musculature, hypogonadism, failure-to-thrive, and, later, obesity, behavioral abnormalities, and mental dysfunction.[31]

About 40% of these individuals have IQs in the normal or borderline range. Others have functions described as learning disabilities. Many patients have craniofacial and limb abnormalities. The hypotonia of infancy includes poor sucking ability. Linear growth is low. In order to support adequate growth, the infant formula may be concentrated to 25 to 30 kcal/oz. and given in short, frequent feedings.[32]

Of great interest to nutritional care specialists is the tendency to excessive weight gain. Patients between the ages of two and four years develop a severe food-seeking behavior and tend to gorge themselves with any available food. This behavior is apparently of hypothalamic origin, since they do not sense satiety.[31] In addition, they have a decreased energy requirement,[33] and may consume as many as 5,600 kcals per day. The resulting obesity can be so severe as to result in early death.

Anorectic drugs are ineffective. It appears that the best treatment of the obesity is careful control of food intake. Weight maintenance has been reported at 10 to 11 kcal/cm, and weight loss, at 8 to 9 kcal/cm.[32] Control of food intake may require locks on refrigerators, food cupboards, and even garbage cans. If these are provided and food intake is controlled with weighed portions of food, weight control is possible. Exercise is also helpful.[31]

Spina Bifida. **Spina bifida** is a group of congenital disorders also referred to as **myelodysplasia**, **myelomeningocele**, and **meningomyelocele**. The term **neural tube defect** includes spina bifida and any other malformation resulting from defective or delayed closure of the neural tube in the embryo.

In spina bifida, there is a defect in the bone encasement of the spinal cord through which the cord herniates. A sac filled with cerebrospinal fluid protrudes from the midline of the back. It is covered with a membrane to which nerve roots adhere. Many patients have decreased intelligence, and a large proportion are hydrocephalic.

An **Arnold-Chiara malformation** of the brain (in which the cerebellum and medulla protrude down into the cervical spine) is often associated with spina bifida. In severe form, this condition causes weakness and atrophy of muscles in the neck and arm, hydrocephalus, and mental retardation. In some patients, paralysis in the laryngopharyngeal area of the neck, often called **bulbar palsy**, causes failure-to-thrive, aspiration, pneumonia, apnea, and cardiac arrest.[34] There may be poor gag and swallow reflexes and gastroesophageal reflex. Tube feeding may be necessary. Epilepsy occurs in 10–30% of these patients.

The patient has bladder and bowel incontinence and variable weakness or flaccid paralysis in the lower body below the defect. The **neurogenic bladder** (abnormal nervous system control of the bladder) causes an incomplete bladder emptying and a high incidence of **urinary tract infection** (UTI), which may, in turn, lead to renal disease. Some patients are given large doses of ascorbic acid to acidify the urine to a pH below 6 to prevent the infection.[34] Others may be given an acid-ash diet, which is low in fruits and vegetables, and high in meats, meat substitutes, fat, and cereals. However, this diet is contrary to recommendations for obesity control.

Constipation is an additional problem. Contributing factors are **neurogenic bowel**, inactivity, and anticholinergic medications used to treat neurogenic bladder. The patient needs to be counseled to assure adequate fluid and fiber intake for prevention and treatment of constipation.

Several nutrients have been associated with the etiology of spina bifida. These include folate,[35] zinc,[36] and copper.[37] Other studies have shown that the use of multivitamin supplements at the time around conception is associated with decreased incidence of neural tube defects.[38]

Spina bifida patients undergo multiple surgical procedures for hydrocephalus, orthopedic problems, removal of the original lesion, and prevention of renal damage. They may have depressed ascorbic acid saturation, possibly resulting from an inborn error of tyrosine metabolism,[39] and often have spontaneous fractures similar to those seen in scurvy. Vitamin supplementation may often be indicated for pregnant women as a preventive or for affected children, but the nutrient-disease relationship is as yet unclear.

Obesity is common. Muscle structure is decreased in the denervated area, and the proportion of fat is increased. Some patients are in a wheelchair, and the energy need may be as low as 50% of normal, frequently 7 to 10 kcal/cm, and should be provided in proportion to height to maintain normal weight.

Another problem is in the care of the skin. Those in a wheelchair are at high risk for developing **pressure sores**. A sore in the lower body where a patient has no feeling can become very deep, to the bone, and result in bone infection. Obesity increases the risk of developing pressure sores. Nutritional care for this problem is discussed later in this chapter.

Nutritional assessment of these patients presents some difficulties. Height and weight should be monitored regularly, but an accurate measure of height may be difficult to obtain. Recumbent length can be measured in young children and those unable to stand alone. If the person has **scoliosis** (lateral curvature from the straight vertical line of the spine) or **contractures of the legs**, arm span may be substituted for height on the NCHS growth charts. Arm span is the distance between the tips of the middle fingers when arms are outstretched as far as possible to each side. The ratio of arm span to height must sometimes be adjusted for loss of leg muscle in spina bifida:[34] For high lumbar and thoracic level defects (no leg muscle mass):

$$\text{Height} = \text{arm span} \times 0.9 \qquad \textbf{(19-1)}$$

For middle and lower lumbar level defects (partial loss of leg muscle mass):

$$\text{Height} = \text{arm span} \times 0.95 \qquad \textbf{(19-2)}$$

For sacral level defects (minimal or no loss of leg muscle mass):

$$\text{Height} = \text{arm span} \times 1.0 \qquad \textbf{(19-3)}$$

Body weight may be obtained with a chair scale or bed scale. If these are not available, an indication of changes in body fatness may be obtained by monitoring subscapular or triceps skinfold thickness.

Other factors that should be monitored in nutritional assessment are

- Fluid and fiber, related to bowel function
- Feeding skills and behaviors
- Drug-nutrient interactions
- Iron status

Failure to Thrive. Failure to thrive (FTT) has been defined in various ways. It usually applies to children less than three years old who are not gaining weight in proportion to height, who have a sudden decrease in rate of weight gain, or who have height or weight below the 3rd percentile, subcutaneous fat at the 5th percentile or less, or some combination of these.

Formerly, FTT cases were divided into organic and inorganic categories. Organic causes include congenital anomalies, post-neonatal medical illness, major illness, and organ system failure, while inorganic causes of FTT included parents who are described as isolated, overwhelmed, or emotionally or physically unavailable; social environments of loss, stress, or poverty; impoverished interactions in nonfeeding situations; and disorganized feeding situations resulting in inadequate energy supply.[40] Usually, several of these causes interact.

Because of the complexity of the etiology of FTT, evaluation is usually done by a team that may include a social worker, nurse, pediatrician, and nutritionist. The nutritional assessment includes height, weight, head circumference, and skinfolds.

If the child was premature, the standard growth grid is corrected until the age of two years. For example, a child who was two months premature would, at the age of eight months, be considered six months old for purposes of using the grid. Using the corrected grid, an ideal weight-for-height age is calculated, and FTT is then evaluated as follows:[40]

Mild FTT = <90% ideal weight-for-height age.
Moderate FTT = <80% ideal weight-for-height age.

Severe FTT = <70% ideal weight-for-height age.

Appropriate factors in the diet history may include

- Three-day food record or 24-hour recall
- Formula preparation: methods, content, amount
- Solid foods: amount, type, meal pattern
- Feeding abilities
- Number of meals, snacks
- Time used in feeding
- With whom does the child eat?
- Do others provide meals, e.g., daycare?
- Diet restrictions related to finances, religion, other?
- Resources available for food
- Medications
- Supplements used
- Mobility and activity
- Laboratory tests, in addition to usual assessment procedures (see Chapter 3): ova and parasites; sweat chloride, alkaline phosphatase

Once the causes have been determined, intervention may be provided by the same team. Families may receive counseling for psychosocial problems, be referred to specialty clinics such as neurology or endocrinology, or be referred to community resources for support.

In order for catchup growth to occur, protein and energy must be provided in excess. The amount needed may be calculated as follows:[41]

Step one: Plot the height and weight of the child on an NCHS growth chart.
Step two: Find the age at which the present weight would be at the 50th percentile. This is the "weight age."
Step three: Find the recommended calories for this weight age from the table of recommended dietary allowances (see Appendix A).
Step four: Find the weight at the 50th percentile for the child's present age.

Step five: Multiply values in steps three and four.

Step six: Divide the value obtained in step five by actual weight to obtain kcal/kg/day to be fed.

Protein can be calculated similarly.

Methods used to increase food intake must be adjusted for the age of the child. For the infant, the usual caloric density of the formula is 20 kcal/oz. This can be increased gradually, that is by 2 kcal/oz. steps, to 24 kcal/oz. by increasing the concentration of the formula. If higher caloric density is still needed, vegetable oil, MCT, or more carbohydrate may be added. This should also be done gradually in 2 kcal/oz. steps.[41]

When solid foods are added, those that are higher in energy content may be chosen. For example, choose sweet potatoes, peas and bananas in place of spinach, green beans and applesauce. In addition, infant cereals, dry milk powder, vegetable oil, and carbohydrate additives can be added to strained foods.[41]

Beverages containing 25–30 kcal/oz may be given to toddlers. Caloric density can be increased in 5 kcal/oz steps with dry milk or instant breakfast powders. Solid food energy content can be increased with procedures similar to those used for infants. Toddlers may also be given high energy snacks such as peanut butter and crackers.[41]

Nutritional counseling can include advice on preparation of more calorie-dense formulas and solid foods, development of feeding skills, and methods of handling behavior problems. Growth should be monitored weekly at first in infants, less often later or in older children. Repeated food records may be helpful.

Other Feeding Problems. Obstructive lesions or psychological factors may lead to feeding problems even though the child is neurologically normal. Other cases of feeding difficulties are the result of **mismanagement of behavior**, resulting in multiple food dislikes, bizarre food habits, and mealtime tantrums. Provision of information to the parents on normal feeding behavior may be helpful in avoiding the development of such problems. Behavioral problems, once they do develop, may become the responsibility of psychologists, although nutritional care specialists may have a cooperative role.

Neurological and Neuromuscular Problems in the Older Child or Adult

In addition to the developmentally disabled child who becomes an adult, some normal children and adults develop neurological disorders. There are a variety of reasons for this, including progressive neurologic diseases, cerebrovascular accidents, and surgery for tumors.

Epilepsy and Other Seizure Disorders

Epilepsy is a chronic nervous disorder with periodic excessive neuronal discharges in the brain during which the patient may have loss of consciousness with convulsions. Seizures may follow brain infection, drug abuse, or alcohol abuse and can occur, as described previously, in cerebral palsy, spina bifida, and other conditions. Epilepsy may also occur spontaneously in some families. It can occur at any age beginning in infancy, but 75% of patients have their first seizure before age 18. There are reported to be 100,000 new cases each year affecting 2 to 4 million people a year in the United States.

There are several types of seizures, which vary in their nature and severity:

1. **Tonic-clonic** or **grand-mal** seizures are characterized by a sudden loss of consciousness with the hazard of a fall leading to a head injury. The body becomes stiff (tonic phase) followed by thrashing (clonic phase). The patient may then fall into a deep sleep.
2. **Petit mal** or **absence** seizures are characterized by "blank spells" in which the patient, commonly a child, seems to be daydreaming. The seizures may be very frequent, sometimes hundreds per day, and interfere with learning so the child may be thought to be retarded.

Table 19-4. Nutritional Effects of Drugs for Patients with Neurological Conditions

Drug (Proprietary Name)	Reported Nutrition-Related Side Effects and Changes in Laboratory Values
Steroid	
Dexamethasone	Decreased water, sodium retention
	Abnormal glucose tolerance; increased serum glucose
	Increased protein catabolism; decreased serum protein
	Increased appetite
	Potassium loss; decreased serum potassium
	Decreased calcium absorption; decreased serum calcium
Anticonvulsants	
Phenobarbital (Luminal)	Increased appetite *or* anorexia
	Nausea, vomiting
	Increased vitamin D and K catabolism
	Decreased bone density
	Decreased serum calcium, vitamin B_6, B_{12}, folate
	Sedation
Phenytoin (Dilantin)	Nausea, vomiting, constipation
	Decreased taste sensitivity
	Increased vitamin D and K catabolism
	Increased serum glucose; glucose intolerance
	Decreased serum calcium, vitamins B_6 and B_{12}, folate
	Decreased serum vitamin D, magnesium, alkaline phosphatase
	Gum hyperplasia
Carbamazepine (Tegretol)	Nausea, vomiting, diarrhea
	Xerostomia
	Abdominal pain
	Glossitis, stomatitis
	Increased serum glucose
	Increased blood urea nitrogen
	Bone marrow suppression
	Drowsiness
	Blood dyscrasias
	Ataxia
Valproic acid (Depakene, Depakote)	Nausea, vomiting, indigestion
	Diarrhea, abdominal pain
	Constipation
	Anorexia and weight loss *or* increased appetite and weight gain
	Hepatic failure (in children less than two years old)

(continued)

3. **Complex-partial** seizures consist of automatic or odd behavior lasting a few minutes. Sometimes the person seems hostile or aggressive but later may be confused and have no recollection of the incident.

4. **Simple-partial** seizures consist of spasms on one side of the body (**Jacksonian seizures**) beginning in the fingers or toes, or there may be a distortion of sensations.

5. **Atonic seizures** are characterized by sudden loss of all muscle tone. The patient falls and may have a head injury.

A given patient may have more than one type of seizure. In addition, the number of seizures may vary greatly, for example, from one monthly to hundreds per day.

Status epilepticus consists of recurrent seizures. Between episodes, the patient does not completely regain consciousness. The condition may result in permanent brain damage.

Diagnosis. The undiagnosed patient who has had a seizure is given a thorough physical examination, and medical and family histories are obtained. The erratic electrical impulses in the brain are monitored with an **electroencephalograph** (EEG). Different

Table 19-4. (Continued)

Drug (Proprietary Name)	Reported Nutrition-Related Side Effects and Changes in Laboratory Values
Diazepam (Valium)	Nausea, constipation Increased appetite
Ethosuximide (Zarontin)	Gastrointestinal upset, nausea, vomiting, anorexia Weight loss Kidney dysfunction
Trimethadione (Tridione)	Gastrointestinal upset Weight loss
Primidone (Mysoline)	Gastrointestinal upset Weight loss
Clonazepam (Clonopin)	Hyperactivity Short attention span and impulsive behavior Drowsiness Ataxia, vertigo, dizziness Confusion Drooling Weight gain
Diuretics Mannitol	Nausea, vomiting Thirst Fluid and electrolyte imbalance
Furosemide (Lasix)	Nausea, vomiting, constipation, diarrhea Anorexia Stomatitis Abdominal cramps Thirst Fluid and electrolyte imbalance Increased BUN, serum glucose, urate, zinc, potassium, calcium, magnesium Decreased serum magnesium, chloride Increased urinary potassium, sodium, chloride, magnesium, calcium, glucose, thiamine, vitamin B_6

EEG patterns, interpreted by a neurologist, and the patient's symptoms are used to distinguish among different types of epilepsy. Other diagnostic procedures include the following:

1. Brain scan (CT or PET) to identify tumors or scars.
2. Brain X-ray.
3. Lumbar puncture to sample cerebrospinal fluid.
4. Blood tests for biochemical abnormalities.
5. Psychological tests.

Treatment. The most common treatment of epilepsy and other seizure disorders is one of the anticonvulsant drugs. There are several of these from which the neurologist may choose, depending on the type and severity of seizures, the age of the patient, and drug sensitivities (see Table 19-4). Many of these drugs have nutritional implications.

The use of phenytoin, phenobarbital, valproic acid, or primidone results in low serum folate and may cause megaloblastic anemia if the patient becomes very deficient, since anticonvulsants alter folate metabolism.[42] On the other hand, folate supplements may precipitate a seizure and should be provided cautiously.[43,44]

Anticonvulsants also increase the need for vitamin D,[45,46] possibly by inducing vitamin D–degrading enzymes. Serum calcium, phosphorus, and alkaline phosphatase should be monitored in these patients. Other effects of anticonvulsant therapy include neonatal coagulation defects, gingival hyperplasia, effects on pituitary, insulin, thyroid and adrenal hormones, congenital malformations in infants of mothers taking these drugs, and possibly deficiencies of copper, zinc, and pyridoxine. Patients receiving anticonvulsants are given routine vitamin-mineral supplements.

Anorexia may be approached with small, frequent feedings and vitamin B complex supplements. Patients receiving primidone may be in most need of this modification. Sometimes, the patient is given a ketogenic diet that results in the production of ketosis. The diet contains a fat-to-carbohydrate ratio of $3:1$ or $4:1$. Ketosis is reputed to control convulsions, but the diet is often considered unpalatable. An alternative is a formula of one part skim milk and two parts MCT Oil with vitamin and mineral supplements. Status epilepticus is treated with anticonvulsants and with intravenous fluids to avoid dehydration.

Brain and Spinal Cord Injuries

A number of disorders of the brain and spinal cord lead to disabilities. Nutrition can be important in helping these patients during rehabilitation.

Brain Injury. The brain can be injured in a variety of ways with direct destruction of neuronal cells or by interference with delivery of oxygen or glucose by the blood to the brain. Blunt or penetrating traumatic injuries from automobile and motorcycle accidents, industrial accidents, sports injuries, knife wounds, gunshot wounds, fights, and explosions are prominent among the causes of traumatic brain injury (TBI). Many involve the use of alcohol.

Another cause of brain injury is a **ruptured cerebral aneurysm**. An aneurysm is a weakness in a blood vessel wall. If it ruptures, the consequences of the bleeding depends on the location of the bleed. Some patients have an **arteriovenous malforma-**

tion (AVM), a congenital defect with a mass of tortuous, dilated arteries and veins with no intervening capillaries. Perfusion of the surrounding brain tissue is reduced. If the AVM ruptures, symptoms are similar to those in ruptured cerebral aneurysms.

In other cases, a **hematoma** (a localized collection of extravasated blood) may develop. Hematomas may be **intracerebral** (within the brain tissue), **epidural** (between the skull and the **dura** or covering of the brain), or **subdural** (between the dura and the brain). Any of these have the potential for damage to the brain.

Head injuries are often categorized as **open** or **closed**. In the open injury, there is a break in the skin, skull, or dura covering the brain. A closed head injury has no break in this covering and may be more serious.

Injury of the brain may have acute metabolic consequences as well as chronic sequelae that affect both feeding ability and nutritional status. The metabolic response to severe brain injury has been compared to that seen in severe burns over 20% of the body surface area (see Chapter 14). The brain-injured patient is hypermetabolic and hypercatabolic, a response that peaks in three to five days. Serum and urine levels of cortisol, epinephrine, and norepinephrine are elevated; oxygen consumption and urinary nitrogen excretion are increased. Fluid and electrolyte imbalances are common with **SIADH** (syndrome of inappropriate ADH secretion). Hyponatremia, excess fluid retention, and increased serum ADH result. Some patients have **diabetes insipidus** (insufficient ADH) with increased urine output, hypernatremia, dehydration, and hypotension. In addition, serum zinc and iron are depressed, and copper, ceruloplasmin, C-reactive protein, and other acute phase proteins are elevated.[47]

Studies indicate that patients receiving nutritional support had a more favorable outcome.[48-50] The effect of TPN was more favorable than enteral (tube) feeding, possibly because of a higher amount of protein and energy provided.[51,52]

Increased intracranial pressure (ICP) is seen with most brain injuries involving hypoxemia (as in near-drowning), intracranial bleeding, or cerebral edema. It occurs in traumatic injuries and other conditions such as brain tumors, abscesses, hemorrhages, and hydrocephalus. In addition, strokes, cerebral contusions, and meningitis are often accompanied by cerebral edema and increased pressure. If untreated, elevated ICP can result in herniation through openings in the skull and subsequent death.

One of the first goals of treatment is the control of the posttraumatic swelling of the brain. Patients are often given steroids (dexamethasone) and diuretics (mannitol or furosemide) to reduce cerebral edema. Phenobarbital, phenytoin, carbamazepine, and diazepam are used as anticonvulsants, as they are in the seizure disorders described earlier in this chapter. A combination of phenobarbital and phenytoin is often used.

Management also includes limitation of fluid intake sufficient to produce mild dehydration and mechanical ventilation to reduce carbon dioxide pressure to 25–30 torr. When fluid is restricted to reduce cerebral edema, hypertonicity must be avoided. If unrecognized, it may lead to coma and death. The use of tube feedings of high-nitrogen or high-calorie content (e.g., 2 kcal/ml) could contribute to the problem. Conversely, the extracellular fluid is hypotonic in some patients as a result of inappropriate secretion of antidiuretic hormone or cerebral salt wasting. In these circumstances, the use of calorie-dense feedings and fluid restriction is helpful.

Coma is an impairment of consciousness or profound stupor that may result from deranged cerebral or brainstem function. Possible causes are listed in Table 19-5. The discussion in this chapter will refer particularly to traumatic injuries. Coma in metabolic disorders, such as hepatic failure and renal failure, is discussed in other chapters.

The level of consciousness is commonly evaluated on the Glasgow Coma Scale (GCS), shown in Table 19-6. The GCS is

Table 19-5. Causes of Coma

Intracranial lesions
Tumor
Trauma: contusion; subdural, epidural, or intracerebral hematoma; brain edema
Infection: abscess, meningitis, encephalitis
Cerebrovascular disease:
   Hemorrhage
   Thrombosis affecting brainstem
   Cerebral embolism
   Subarachnoid hemorrhage (aneurysm; arteriovenous malformation)
   Disease of small vessels (systemic lupus erythematosus; fat embolism; disseminated intravascular coagulation; subacute bacterial endocarditis)
Toxins
Barbiturates; cyanide, ethyl alcohol; ethylene glycol; heavy metals; methyl alcohol; narcotics; organic phosphates; salicylates; tranquilizers
Metabolic disorders
Encephalopathy: uremic, hepatic, pulmonary (hypoxic, hypercapnic), Wernicke's (thiamine deficiency)
Diabetes mellitus: (hypoglycemia; ketoacidotic coma; nonketotic hyperosmolar coma)
Adrenal insufficiency
Thyroid: myxedema coma; thyroid storm
Hypernatremia or hyponatremia (inappropriate ADH)
Hypercalcemia
Reye's syndrome

based on eye opening and on motor and verbal response. Interpretation is given at the bottom of the table. Patients in an irreversible coma are said to be in a **persistent vegetative state**.

Nutritional assessment. Assessment of nutritional status can present a number of difficulties. For patients admitted as emergencies, height, weight, and information on diet may not be available. Visceral protein levels may be affected by fluid status. They cannot be compared with published standards but can be useful in monitoring the patient's progress. Total lymphocyte counts are not reliable if the patient is given steroids.

Nutritional support. In estimating the patient's energy requirements, steroid medications, infections, severity of injury, and length of time after injury are added to the usual considerations (see Chapter 3). On the other hand, sedatives may serve to decrease the REE. Overfeeding may lead to hyperglycemia and increased carbon dioxide produc-

Table 19-6. Glasgow Coma Scale

Parameter	Response	Score
Eyes	Open spontaneously	4
	To verbal command	3
	To pain	2
	No response	1
Best motor response	To verbal command: obeys	6
	To painful stimulus:	
	Localizes pain	5
	Flexion-withdrawal	4
	Decorticate (flex)	3
	Decerebrate (extend)	2
	No response	1
Best verbal response	Oriented, converses	5
	Disoriented, converses	4
	Inappropriate responses	3
	Incomprehensible sounds	2
	No response	1
Interpretation	Total range	3–15
	Mild head injury	13–15
	Moderate head injury	9–12
	Severe head injury	3–8

tion. Hyperglycemia tends to worsen the effects of ischemia, while carbon dioxide exacerbates high ICP. Energy needs may be as high as 50 kcal/kg with up to 2.5 g protein per kg.

An important objective of nutritional support is the prevention of **decubitus ulcers** or **pressure sores**. A decubitus ulcer is a localized area of tissue necrosis caused by pressure over bony sites of the body. Sites over the sacrum, coccyx, hips, and heels are particularly susceptible to ulcer formation. Other sites are the tips of shoulders, crests of the pelvis, greater trochanters of the thighs, inner and outer surfaces of ankles, and the outer sides of the feet, shoulder blades, and elbows. They occur in a number of conditions, particularly those in which patients are bedridden, wheelchair bound, or otherwise immobilized. Coma patients are among those at high risk.

Factors that tend to contribute to ulcer formation are heat, moisture, pressure, shearing forces, and malnutrition. Decubiti are painful, can become infected, and can lead to death. They can begin in a matter of hours, but can take months to heal. Therefore, prevention is very important, and *any patient*

with decubiti is considered to be at risk and in need of nutritional support.

Nutritional care must assure adequate intake of calories, protein, vitamins, minerals, and fluid. Supplemental feedings, tube feedings, or TPN may be necessary.

Prevention of decubiti requires both good nutritional care and good nursing procedures. Patients at risk—that is, those who are immobilized from paralysis, coma, heavy sedation, or spinal cord injuries and those in traction—should be turned frequently, often every two hours. The skin must be kept clean and dry. Physical activity should be encouraged if the patient's condition permits, and massage helps increase local circulation. Patients in a wheelchair are instructed to do push-ups with the arms to relieve pressure on the buttocks. Other patients at risk are the aged and those who are depressed or in pain.

Severity of these ulcers is staged as follows:

Stage I	Redness of skin that is not relieved by relief of pressure or by massage.
Stage II	Blistering, abrasions, or skin breaks with damage to superficial tissue and blood vessels.
Stage III	Loss of outer skin with drainage of blood fluid.
Stage IV	Involvement of deeper tissue; may include muscle and bone.

A tissue over a bony prominence is compressed, the blood vessels are compressed, and lack of oxygen damages the tissue. In addition, poor drainage leads to tissue breakdown. Shearing force at the sacrum when the patient slides down in a bed at an angle greater than 30 degrees also contributes to decubiti. Other contributors include moisture, heat, irritation from wrinkled sheets or foreign materials in the bed, and friction during turning.

Nutritional support of the neurological patient must not only provide nutritional requirements, but often must be provided by tube or TPN if the patient is in a coma or has dysphagia. Placement of a feeding tube may be hazardous in patients who have fractures of bones in the face and base of the skull; in these patients the feeding tube may go into the cranium. The location of the tube depends largely on the risk of aspiration and anticipated duration of tube feeding. Patients who are alert and have the required reflexes for swallowing and protection of the airway have a low risk of aspiration. A nasogastric tube is then a reasonable choice for the short term. For a longer term, weeks or even years, a gastrostomy tube is often inserted so the feeding can be supplied directly into the stomach.

The patient who cannot protect his airway because of a decreased level of consciousness, weakness, or impaired reflexes is at risk of aspiration. For these patients, a nasojejunal tube may be used. Another choice is a gastrostomy-jejunal (Rombeau) tube that provides feeding directly into the jejunum.

The choice of feeding formulas is discussed in Chapter 5. If the patient has persistent ileus or reduced gastrointestinal absorption, TPN may be necessary.

Swallowing problems may be seen when coma subsides, cognitive function returns, and attempts are made to return the patient to oral feeding. An evaluation of the patient's swallowing ability must first be conducted with videofluoroscopy. Many patients with neurological conditions have impaired ability to swallow, resulting from a lesion in the cerebral cortex or from cranial nerves from the brainstem. Table 19-7 shows the cranial nerves involved in swallowing. Other patients have mechanical problems as

Table 19-7. Cranial Nerves

Nerve Number	Nerve Name	Type	Function
I	Olfactory	Sensory	Sense of smell
II	Optic	Sensory	Sight
III	Oculomotor	Mixed	Control of muscles of eyelid, constriction of pupil, muscle sense in movement of eye, accommodation of eye
IV	Trochlear	Mixed	Movement of superior oblique muscle of eyeball, muscle sense
V	Trigeminal:		
	Ophthalmic	Sensory	Some of tongue and jaw muscles, from skin of upper eyelid, side of nose, and anterior half of scalp
	Maxillary	Sensory	From nose, skin of cheek, side of forehead, upper lip and upper teeth of forehead, upper lip and upper teeth
	Mandibular	Mixed	*Sensory:* from side of head, chin, mucous membrane of mouth, lower teeth and anterior $\frac{2}{3}$ of tongue *Motor:* to several muscles for chewing
VI	Abducens	Motor	Some muscles of eyeball
VII	Facial	Mixed	*Sensory:* sense of taste in forward $\frac{2}{3}$ of tongue, to salivary glands for secretion *Motor:* facial muscles for facial expression
VIII	Vestibulocochlear	Sensory	Serves vestibule of ear and semicircular canals; carries impulses for equilibrium and hearing
IX	Glossopharyngeal	Mixed	*Motor:* muscles of pharynx; soft palate and posterior $\frac{1}{3}$ of tongue *Sensory:* to taste buds on posterior $\frac{1}{3}$ of tongue; affects taste (posterior tongue)
X	Vagus	Mixed	*Sensory:* fibers to mucous membranes of larynx, trachea, bronchi, lungs, arch of aorta, esophagus, stomach *Motor:* swallowing, speech, peristalsis, secretions from stomach and pancreas; contractions of trachea, bronchi, bronchioles
XI	Accessory	Motor	To palate, pharynx, larynx
XII	Hypoglossal	Motor	Tongue muscles

a result of trauma, cancer, obstruction, or other damage to the organs of swallowing. Clinical manifestations of a swallowing problem include drooling, retention of food in the mouth, feeling a "lump in the throat," coughing or choking on attempts to swallow, and a "gurgly" voice. There may be pain on chewing and swallowing, and a decrease in sensitivity to taste and smell. A therapy team is necessary to help the patient overcome this problem. It is a slow process, and tube feeding must be continued until the patient's oral intake is equal to his needs.

In general, the "dysphagia diet" consists of groups of foods of varying consistencies, which the patient learns to swallow:

1. Pureed or blenderized smooth, moist foods; no liquids.
2. Mechanically soft foods, pureed or minced, soft; no liquids.
3. Thick liquids, e.g., farina, thickened cream soup, yogurt.
4. Medium liquids, e.g., milk shakes, regular cream soups.
5. Thin liquids, e.g., milk, clear liquids. Milk is not recommended until late in the patient's progress because it tends to cause production of mucus.

As a general rule of thumb, thick, smooth foods are easier to manage than those with pieces, and thicker liquids are easier to manage than thin liquids. Very hot and cold foods decrease oral sensations, but temperatures slightly above or below body temperature are helpful.

The patient should be seated upright with head slightly forward. The foods used must be individualized. When solid foods are given, they should be given in pieces that are sufficiently small that they will not obstruct the airway.

The patient must be monitored for adequacy of food intake. Some useful procedures to increase food intake are these:

• Give small, frequent meals.

• Provide high-kilocalorie, high-protein supplements of appropriate consistency.
• Feed orally insofar as possible.
• Supplement with tube feeding if necessary.

Several thickening agents are available to make foods more easily swallowed and retained. These materials are useful for patients with acquired neurological disorders as well as for children with developmental disabilities. Thickeners add to caloric intake and must be considered in nutritional assessment.[53] Foods that may be used as thickeners are listed in Table 19-8.[53]

Thickening agents are useful in swallowing problems and also in gastroesophageal reflux (GER). In some forms of neurological impairment, the esophageal sphincter does not close properly, or there is abnormal peristalsis and delayed stomach emptying. These children may benefit from thickened foods in smaller, more frequent feedings. Upright positions, at a 30- to 45-degree angle during and after feeding, are helpful.

Food intake in early rehabilitation. Additional problems arise if there are deficits in the patient's cognitive functions. The patient may need supervision at meals because of mental

Table 19-8. *Thickening Products for Use in Foods*

Product	Caloric Content per Tbsp.
Commercial products	
Diafoods Thick-it	16–18
Diafoods Thick-it 2	16–18
Crescent Frutex	52
Common foods to thicken liquids	
Pureed fruits	5–11
Pureed vegetables	5–11
Dried infant cereals	14
Yogurt	8–16
Soft tofu	10
Puddings	Variable
Common foods to thicken solid foods	
Dried infant cereals	14
Potato flakes	11
Wheat germ	27
Bread or cracker crumbs	22

lethargy or agitation, a short attention span, deficit of short-term memory, and poor judgment.[54]

Spinal Cord Injury. A great many patients with spinal cord injuries (SCI) are young with injuries related to automobiles and motorcycles (47%), falls and jumps (21%), diving accidents and other sports injuries (14%), gunshot wounds and other violence (15%), and other causes (3%). Most commonly, SCI from traumatic injuries occurs between 16 and 30 years of age, and 82% of the patients are male. Other cord injuries can be the result of tumors or congenital defects.

The long-term effects of spinal cord injury in which there may be loss of sensation and voluntary motor function are strongly influenced by the location of the injury and the degree of disruption. The greatest loss occurs when there is complete transection of the cord high in the spinal column.

The vertebrae are numbered from top to bottom as indicated in Table 19-9. The functions related to associated nerves suggest the types of loss that could be expected. As indicated in the table, an injury from C-3 to T-1 will result in **quadriplegia** (paralysis of all four limbs), and an injury below T-1 results in **paraplegia** (paralysis of legs and lower body).

Preexisting medical conditions are rare, but accidental injuries may include trauma to other parts of the body. Malnutrition may occur in more than two-thirds of rehabilitation patients. Possible causes of malnutrition include these:

1. Altered nutritional requirements as a result of the acute trauma, medical complications, and treatment.
2. Nausea, anorexia, dysphagia, and malabsorption.
3. Poverty.

Table 19-9. Effects of Spinal Cord Transections at Various Locations

Vertebrae	Results of Cord Transection	Functions of Nerves
Cervical		
1 and 2	Required ventilatory support; quadriplegia	Head control
3 and 4	Quadriplegia; may not require ventilatory support	Inspiration
5 and 6		Flexion of shoulder and elbows; have use of biceps
6 and 7		Wrist movement
7 and 8		Extension of elbows and fingers
Thoracic		
1		Spreading and closing of fingers; client has normal hands
2–6		Forced inspiration, expiration
6–12		Sitting up; assist inspiration, expiration; may ambulate with long braces on legs
Lumbar		
1–3	Paraplegia; loss of bladder and bowel function	Hip movement
3–4		Knee extension
4–5		Hip extension; standing; movement of feet; may ambulate with short leg braces
Sacral		
1		Hip extension; standing; movement of feet
2–4		
Coccygeal		
1		Motion and sensation

4. Social isolation; depression; altered mental states; disturbed relationships with family or other caretakers.
5. Alcoholism; drug abuse; effects of drug treatment.
6. Motor disabilities and dysphagia.

Many SCI patients lose weight in the acute phase. In addition to the items listed, muscle mass is lost. However, activity is decreased. When the hypercatabolic phase ends, BMR and energy needs are depressed, and there is a tendency to gain weight. Complications affecting other organ systems are listed in Table 19-10.

When patients are immobilized, the excretion of calcium in the urine becomes very high. It exceeds normal excretion in about a month and may remain elevated for 12 to 18 months. It may result in calcium oxalate kidney stones. Other signs and symptoms of hypercalciuria include anorexia, nausea,

Table 19-10. Possible Complications after Spinal Cord Injury

Organ System	Complication
Respiratory	Increased incidence of infections
	Lung collapse
	Pulmonary embolism
Gastrointestinal	Constipation
	Fecal impaction
	Peptic ulcer
	Superior mesenteric artery syndrome
	Amyloidosis
	Diverticulosis
	Hiatal hernia
	Gastroesophageal reflux
	Reduced vitamin K formation and absorption
Skeletal	Loss of bone mass; hypercalciuria
	Fractures of long bones
Urinary tract	Pyelonephritis
	Renal calculi
	Urethral fistula
	Infection of prostate gland
Circulatory	Sudden increases in blood pressure
	Profuse sweating and flushing
	Orthostatic hypotension
	Thrombophlebitis
Skin	Decubitus ulcers
Other	Mental depression

vomiting, abdominal pain, and cardiac irregularities.

Rehabilitation procedures are designed to prevent further disability and to restore function to the maximum extent possible. The nutritional care specialist has an important place in the rehabilitation of many patients in conjunction with the efforts of the physician, registered nurse, occupational, physical, and speech therapists, vocational counselor, orthotist, and social worker.

The patient's nutritional needs must, of course, be met. Energy content must be individually adjusted to avoid obesity, high enough to provide sufficient energy for physical therapy, but decreased for those patients whose activities are reduced. Because immobilized patients lose muscle, the estimations of energy needs are adjusted by reducing calculated desirable body weights by 4.5 kg for paraplegics and 9 kg for quadriplegics. For paraplegics, 28 kcal/kg/day and, for quadriplegics, 23 kcal/kg/day have been recommended.[55]

Protein intake should be at least 0.8 g protein per kilogram of body weight per day. If the patient has infections or decubitus ulcers, 1.0 to 1.5 g protein per kilogram may be required. The nitrogen : calorie ratio may vary from 1 : 150 to 1 : 100.

Adequate vitamins and minerals may be obtained from a standard supplement. Therapeutic doses may be desirable. Fluid intake of 2,500 to 3,000 ml is recommended in infection and for prevention of urinary calculi.

Bowel and bladder problems are frequent in patients with disabling injuries. A high-fiber diet with 2 to 3 liters of fluid per day is recommended for prevention of constipation or impaction if renal function is normal. Physical therapy providing for muscle tension and weight bearing may be helpful in reducing calcium loss from the skeletal system and in preventing decubitus ulcers.

Many patients need assistance in learning to manage the activities of daily living. For those with disabilities involving the upper body, arms, and hands, some of the same devices used to help the developmentally disabled child to self-feed may be useful. Tables, beds, or trays over wheelchairs may have to be adapted to provide a convenient place to eat. The adult patient also may need suggestions on methods for food preparation. Detailed information on equipment and techniques is available in *Mealtime Manual for the Aged and Handicapped.*[56] This volume is divided into sections for patients with only one hand, those with weakness in the upper extremities, those with incoordination, loss of sensation, and limited vision, those in wheelchairs, and those with other handicaps.

Patients often also have serious financial problems as a result of the medical cost of their injuries. They may need help in finding social programs to assist with the cost of food and special equipment.

Nutritional assessment of SCI patients uses the usual assessment procedures in general but must be individualized. A thorough, nutrition history should be obtained. If the patient's ability to communicate is impaired, family members may be necessary sources of information. Anthropometric data may include height and weight and comparison with desirable weight for height and weight prior to injury. It has been suggested that the Metropolitan Life Insurance Table recommended values be reduced by 5% to 10% for paraplegic patients and 10% to 15% for quadriplegics.[57] Triceps skinfold and mid-arm muscle circumference may be unreliable because of the muscle atrophy, decreased activity in these patients, and absence of reference standards. Patients with SCI have a high rate of elimination of serum albumin, which also may not be reliable for assessment.[57] Serum transferrin is believed to be more reliable for assessment.

Progressive Neurological Disorders

Parkinson's Disease. **Parkinson's disease** is a progressive neuromuscular disease of the elderly in which there is a progressive loss of dopaminergic neurons in the substantia nigra and a decreased concentration of do-pamine in the basal ganglia of the brain. It occurs in about 10% of the population over the age of 60 years.

Early clinical manifestations include tremors when at rest, rigidity, and abnormalities of gait. Some patients have bradykinesia (slow movement) while others show choreoathetoid movements and are in almost constant motion. Their energy expenditure is much increased. As the disease progresses, the tremor becomes more severe and the patient may become bedridden. The disease is treated with levodopa (L-DOPA), a precursor of dopamine, into which it is converted in the brain. A decarboxylase inhibitor is also given to prevent digestion of L-DOPA in the intestine, but tends to cause nausea and vomiting. Anticholinergic drugs are also used, with side effects of xerostomia and constipation.

Recently in Sweden, dopamine-rich neurons from eight- to nine-week-old aborted fetuses were grafted into the brains of patients with severe Parkinson's disease. Reports indicated that some symptoms subsided, but it is not clear whether the results are the effect of graft-induced dopaminergic transmission or whether there is a non-specific effect of the surgical procedures. Research is continuing.[58]

Parkinson's disease patients have a broad spectrum of feeding and nutrition problems.[59] Prominent among these are difficulties in chewing and swallowing. Swallowing problems stem from tongue tremor, difficulty in bolus formation in the mouth, hesitancy in initiating swallowing, and disturbances in pharyngeal motility. In addition, there is a tendency to aspiration. As facial muscles change, dentures may fit less well, contributing to chewing problems. Improper chewing leads to gastrointestinal distress, choking, and flatulence. Other factors leading to digestive discomfort are delayed gastric emptying, constipation, and alterations in appetite. The patient's energy requirement may be increased or decreased, depending on the type of movement that predominates. Because of the tremors and rigidity, patients experience difficulty in obtaining food, preparing food, and even transferring food from the plate to the mouth.

With these problems in mind, nutritional care is based on the following recommendations:[57]

1. Individualize energy intake to amount of involuntary muscle activity, limitation of movement, and exercise to achieve and maintain desirable body weight.
2. Neutral amino acids may compete with levodopa for carrier necessary for intestinal absorption and for crossing the blood-brain barrier. To optimize drug effects, a moderate amount of protein (e.g., 40 to 50 g/day) divided evenly into three or four meals is sometimes recommended. Alternatively, a low protein intake during the day and a larger intake in the evening has been suggested. The research basis for these diets is considered weak.
3. Provide adequate fiber and fluid to prevent constipation.
4. Provide special utensils and repair of dentures to facilitate eating.
5. Massage facial and neck muscles before eating.
6. Thicken liquids as necessary.
7. Avoid easily aspirated foods (e.g., nuts, peas).
8. In the presence of delayed gastric emptying, advise the patient to eat slowly, use small, frequent meals, and increase carbohydrate and decrease fat in the diet.
9. To avoid flatulence, chew food thoroughly and eat slowly.

Guillain-Barré Syndrome. **Guillain-Barré syndrome** is also known as **acute postinfectious polyneuritis** or **idiopathic polyneuritis**. It is an autoimmune reaction that often follows a viral infection and may follow an immunization. Myelin sheaths, and sometimes the axons, deteriorate. Nerve conduction is lost, resulting in partial or complete paralysis. Other clinical manifestations include muscular weakness, numbness, pain, and changes in blood pressure. The weakness of the legs progresses to arms, trunk, face, and head. There is a low-grade fever, respiratory failure, urinary tract infection, and personality changes. Nutrition-related symptoms include dysphagia if the seventh and ninth cranial nerves are involved, difficult mastication, anorexia, and weight loss.

During the acute phase, tube feeding or TPN may be required. Energy and protein content of these formulas may need to be increased. Fat is adjusted as necessary if the patient is on a ventilator (see Chapter 16). As the patient progresses and is ready to be fed orally, the consistency of the diet is adjusted to the swallowing ability. Nutrient content must be adjusted for weight loss and fever. When appropriate, the diet must be adjusted to promote weaning from the ventilator.

Amyotrophic Lateral Sclerosis. **Amyotrophic lateral sclerosis** (ALS) is also known as **Lou Gehrig's disease**, **progressive spinal muscular atrophy**, and **motor neuron disease**. It is a progressive, paralytic, terminal disease of unknown cause. It affects the anterior horn cells of the spinal cord, the corticospinal tract, and the motor nuclei of the cerebral cortex.

There are three forms of the disease: bulbar, upper motor neuron, and lower motor neuron. Bulbar ALS affects neurons in the brainstem that control breathing, swallowing, and speech. Upper motor neuron ALS affects neurons that extend from the brain through the spinal cord. It causes muscle weakness, exaggerated reflexes, and spasticity. Lower motor neuron ALS involves neurons originating in the spinal cord and results in muscle weakness, wasting of limbs, and loss of reflexes.

Early symptoms include muscle atrophy and weakness of the hands and arms, chewing and swallowing difficulties, and absent or delayed gag reflex. The disease advances with drooling and dysphagia, respiratory muscle weakness, and flaccid quadriplegia.

Weight loss of 10% of body weight is common, primarily from dysphagia. Other contributing factors include early satiety and increased risk of aspiration. Constipation results from soft food textures, low fiber intake, decreased physical activity and weakened muscles for defecation.[60]

The consistency of the diet must be adjusted to the swallowing ability with frequent, small meals. As the disease progresses, tube feedings through a percutaneous gastrostomy (PEG) or jejunostomy (PEJ) tube and then TPN may be needed. Caloric and protein intake should be high. Increased fiber and 2 to 3 liters of water per day counteract the constipation.[60]

Dementia. About half of all nursing home patients have **dementia**. As many as 21% of persons over 65 years of age may have mild or severe dementia. In those over age 80, incidence may be up to 36%. Therefore, dementia is a serious public health problem.[61]

The most common causes of dementia are Alzheimer's disease, multiple infarcts, and alcoholism. Other possible causes, occurring less often, are infections, brain tumors, hydrocephalus, drugs and toxins, and metabolic and endocrine disorders.[61]

In the diagnosis of dementia, a neuropsychiatric examination is followed by a thorough search for reversible causes of the condition.

Alzheimer's disease is a degenerative disease of the cerebral cortex that progresses slowly. There may be a genetic predisposition. There is an association with Down syndrome. Therefore, the gene for Alzheimer's disease may be on chromosome 21.

Loss of acetylcholine-containing neurons, particularly in the frontal lobe, results in deterioration of intellect, memory, and personality. Early clinical manifestations include memory loss, behavior changes, and poor judgment. As the condition progresses, the patient is severely demented, incontinent, and often bedridden. The condition may linger for three to twenty years before death, but usually six to ten years. The cause is unknown.

The brain of an Alzheimer's disease patient shows atrophy of the cerebral cortex,

Table 19-11. Progression of Alzheimer's Disease

Phase	General Symptoms	Nutrition-Related Effects
Phase I (early)	Patient complains of loss of memory Decrease in social and vocational skills Careless in work, housekeeping, financial management Easily lost Personality changes Recognizes faces Well oriented to time	Difficulty in shopping, cooking May forget to eat Changes in taste and smell Increased preference for sweets and salty foods Unusual food choices Degeneration of appetite regulation
Phase II (middle)	Inability to recall names Disorientation to time Delusions Depression Agitation Language problems	Increased energy requirement secondary to agitation May hoard food in mouth, forget to swallow, lose ability to use utensils, use spoon only, eat with hands
Phase III (final)	Complete disorientation Have forgotten their own names Do not recognize family No verbal skills Cannot do basic self care Urinary and fecal incontinence May be bedridden with spastic quadraplegia	May not recognize food May refuse to eat, or to open mouth for feeding Kluver-Bucy syndrome (eating non-food items) May require nasogastric feeding

Prepared from Gray, G.E. Nutrition and dementia. *J. Am. Diet. Assoc.* 89:1795, 1989.

loss of neurons, the presence of tangles of neurofilaments, and plaques of degenerating nerve terminals with an amyloid core. The number of plaques and the loss of neurons are correlated with the severity of the dementia.[61]

The progress of Alzheimer's disease has been divided into three phases. These phases and descriptions of functions are given in Table 19-11.

Nutrient requirements are not known to be altered by the disease process. Therefore, nutrients should be provided at levels appropriate for sex, age, and activity. Consistency of the diet should be modified to the swallowing ability for the dysphagic patient. Tube feedings may be necessary. Fluid and fiber should be adjusted as necessary to avoid constipation, but large quantities of fluid late in the day should not be given to incontinent patients.

Self-feeding at meal time should be encouraged, but it may be necessary to offer one course, or even one food, at a time to reduce confusion. Meal service and personal care should be routine in time and procedure.

There have been suggestions that the condition is related to aluminum toxicity. However, recent investigation suggests that aluminum toxicity is secondary to the disease.[61] There is some evidence that grafting nerve growth factor (NGF)-producing cells in the brain may be helpful.[62] However, little is known of the effects of this procedure, and some investigators suggest that it could actually be harmful.

Multi-infarct dementia results from multiple strokes. The onset is abrupt, in contrast to Alzheimer's disease, and the disease progresses as new infarcts occur. The course tends to fluctuate. Symptoms of motor and sensory disorders depends on the brain region in which the infarcts occurred. Mood changes are common. Risk factors are the same as for strokes in general, and diet for control of these risk factors is appropriate (see Chapter 10).

Nutritional requirements are apparently similar to those for healthy controls. The nu-

tritional care specialist's contribution in the care of these patients consists largely of management of feeding problems.

Alcohol dementia is sometimes difficult to differentiate from Alzheimer's disease. The total effects may be the sum of the effects of alcohol, nutritional deficiencies, and head trauma. Good nutrition and abstinence may result in improvement.

Huntington's Chorea. **Huntington's chorea** is an autosomal dominant genetic disease with cerebral degeneration. It is characterized by spasmodic irregular movements with onset at the age of 35 to 42 years. Behavioral changes begin about ten years prior to the movement disorder. The condition progresses for 15 to 30 years and ends in death.

During the course of the disease, the patient may become dysphagic, may lose the ability to self-feed, and may have problems with constipation. Nutritional care is similar to that in other neurological diseases with the same characteristics.

Multiple Sclerosis. **Multiple sclerosis** is a nervous system disease of unknown etiology. It occurs primarily in adults 20 to 50 years of age at onset. It runs a course of many years of exacerbations and remissions, during which the myelin sheaths in the central nervous system degenerate and are replaced by scar tissue. The cause of the disease is unknown, but it may be an autoimmune disease, a slow-acting virus, or a disease of fat metabolism. Clinical manifestations include fatigue; weakness; loss of position sense; impaired coordination; sensory impairment, including vision, touch, position, vibration, and pain; and respiratory, bowel, and urinary problems.

Serum lecithin and linoleate levels are subnormal, particularly when symptoms are severe. A linoleate supplement was reported to ameliorate the symptoms.[63] A low-fat diet containing 10 g of saturated fat, 40 to 50 g of polyunsaturated fat, and 1 tsp. of cod liver oil have also been suggested for treatment.[64,65] It was claimed that the diet retarded the progress of the disease, but its effectiveness is unproven. The effectiveness of vitamin and mineral supplementation is also not proven.

Nutritional care usually consists of an adequate diet in small frequent meals of a consistency appropriate to the degree of dysphagia and with attention to maintaining normal weight as activity decreases. Feeding aids are needed as the disease progresses. The diet may also be modified to avoid constipation. Sodium intake is reduced for those receiving steroid medication. Tube feeding may eventually be necessary.

Myasthenia Gravis. **Myasthenia gravis** is an autoimmune disease in which nerve impulses are not carried normally across the myoneural junction (from the nerve ending to the muscle), resulting from deactivation of acetylcholine receptor sites. As a consequence, muscle contraction is poor with easy fatigability, weakness, and paralysis. The disease commonly affects muscles innervated by the bulbar nuclei of the brain and therefore affects the eyes, face, lips, tongue and throat. It may, however, affect almost any muscle. The patient has difficulty in chewing and swallowing, and has a tendency to drool.

Strength decreases with increased muscle use; therefore, frequent rest is necessary. The main meal should be in the morning when muscles are rested. A half hour rest is provided prior to meals to reach maximum strength in affected muscles. Soft, easily chewed foods with high caloric density in small portions may be helpful to these patients. They eat slowly, so extra time for eating must be allowed and equipment provided to keep food warm. Supplementary feedings are given enterally. As the disease progresses, tube feedings may be required.

Muscular Dystrophy

Muscular dystrophy consists of a progressive degeneration of skeletal muscles with increasing weakness. There are several forms of this X-linked disease. They vary in genetic inheritance and severity. The most common and severe is Duchenne muscular dystrophy (DMD). The incidence of DMD in the United States is one in 3,000 boys.

When the child is two to five years of age, standing and walking become clumsy with many falls. The calf muscles appear to be enlarged. The muscles are infiltrated by fat and fibrous tissue, and muscle fibers degenerate. The heels are slightly off the ground and patients tend to walk on their toes. Lordosis increases gradually.

The patient gradually loses ambulation, usually between the ages of seven and thirteen years. The use of a wheelchair can sometimes be postponed by bracing and by orthopedic surgery.

Once a wheelchair is used, calf muscles shorten, stretch reflexes disappear, and contractures develop at ankles, knees and hips. With further progression of the disease, contractures also develop at the shoulders, elbows and wrist. Shoulders and arms weaken and become useless. Weakness of facial muscles reduces facial expression and gives the impression of mental dullness. Involvement of facial and neck muscles also cause lolling of the head, a slack mouth, and enlargement of the tongue.

The nervous system is not involved. Testing for intelligence indicates an I.Q. about 20 points below the mean, but the I.Q. does not deteriorate as the disease progresses. Sensation is normal.

Scoliosis develops and compromises the respiratory system. Respiratory infections become severe problems. Cardiomyopathy may also become severe. The immediate cause of death is most often from cardiac arrhythmia, pneumonia, or respiratory failure. Death usually occurs at 15 to 26 years of age.

Pathogenesis. Decreased protein synthesis is thought to be the immediate cause of the muscle wasting. One theory of the biochemical basis of the disease is that there is a defect in membrane permeability, possibly with movement of calcium into the muscle cells. The increase in intracellular calcium may then lead to the other biochemical alterations. Alternatively, there may be loss of intracellular substances from muscle cells.

Laboratory abnormalities include increased serum creatine kinase and creatine phosphokinase (CPK). Serum CPK is used for diagnosis and for evaluation of disease progression. An alteration in the cell membrane involving insulin receptors may be the basis for insulin resistance that is sometimes reported.

Nutritional Assessment. Usual methods of estimation of growth and body size and body composition are limited in usefulness. As fat accumulates and protein decreases, the amount of fat may be underestimated and protein overestimated.

Body weight of the very young DMD child is usually low. Later, the patient may be underweight or may be obese. Cachexia should be avoided, but moderate weight control may slow the progress of the disease and require less muscle strength for daily activity.

Obesity is often seen in patients in a wheel-chair. In addition to the basic disease process, the reduced activity and psychosocial problems contribute to the accumulation of fat.

Estimation of height is difficult in the DMD patient because of contractures. Crown-rump length or sitting height may be used if the legs are deformed. However, when the torso also becomes deformed, these methods are no longer useful. The knee height (see Chapter 3) may be useful but is quite variable in adolescent boys.

Weight alone is limited in usefulness. The contribution of fat, somatic protein, and visceral protein should be assessed. Triceps skinfold, midarm fat area, and midarm muscle area are helpful in younger patients but become more variable with disease progression. Therefore, results must be interpreted cautiously.

Management. There is no effective treatment, and the disease progresses inexorably.

In early stages, management is aimed toward maintaining ambulation. Stretching and braces are used to prevent contractures in the legs. Surgical incisions to release contractures may allow an additional two or three years of ambulation.

Once the patient is wheelchair bound, often at age 12 to 13, prevention of contractures and scoliosis is difficult. The scoliosis can lead to decreased pulmonary function. Spinal fusion is sometimes then recommended.

A number of drugs have been used in DMD with variable results. Because growth seems to be correlated with disease progression, the use of growth inhibitors has been investigated. Prednisone seems to slow the disease progression, possibly by stabilizing the cell membrane. No currently available drug offers a cure, although one promising product is currently under investigation. The nutritional care specialist needs to be aware of nutrition-related side effects of drugs in use and drugs now under development.

The major alteration in nutrient need in these patients is related to energy. Reduced activity and metabolic alterations reduce caloric need. The use of the wheelchair can decrease energy consumption by 25%.

The nutritional care specialist can contribute to the care of these patients in the following ways:

1. Counseling to reduce energy intake for maintenance of desirable body weight.
2. Counseling for adequate intake of other nutrients in a diet with reduced calories.
3. Advice to the primary caregiver to reduce stress.

Psychosis

Almost 20% of the hospital beds in the United States are occupied by patients with psychiatric illness. Many of these patients are malnourished, even though mental illness rarely increases nutrient requirements. There are many reasons for this high incidence of malnutrition. The diet of the patient may have been neglected during a period of emotional stress. Some patients are depressed, uninterested, forgetful, confused, and anxious, all of which can cause a decrease in food intake and lead to nutritional deficiency. Others are compulsive eaters and become obese.

Unfortunately, conditions in the hospital also may contribute to poor nutrition in the patient. Although, ideally, the hospital should provide a therapeutic environment, patients are "warehoused" in some institutions where funds are inadequate. A poor diet is provided in some hospitals, and patients with eating problems can be neglected because of a shortage of adequately trained personnel.

The objectives of nutritional care of the hospitalized mental patient are (1) prevention or correction of malnutrition, (2) correction of feeding problems, and (3) restoration of the patient's ability to eat with emotional satisfaction.

A variety of feeding problems are found in mental patients. For example, some patients refuse to eat from a fear of poisoning, a hallucination that they have no stomach, a feeling of guilt, or a desire for suicide. These patients may require tube feeding. Care must be taken to assure that suicidal patients are not provided with implements that can be used for self-destruction. Paper dishes and plastic implements may be needed. Other patients have bizarre, destructive, or disruptive behaviors related to food and may profit from eating in isolation. The anxious patient has difficulty in deciding where and what to eat. Those patients incapable of making a decision may need to be fed one food at a time and given one implement with which to eat. During retraining, cafeteria-style service is helpful to give practice in making choices.

Some patients are hyperactive and are unable to sit still long enough for normal food intake, yet their needs may be increased. These patients should be provided with supplemental foods that can be eaten during activity. Fluid intake of these patients should be monitored carefully.

It must also be remembered that food has symbolic meanings for everyone. In mental illness, these become exaggerated. Good food and a pleasant environment are important in therapy.

Large doses of vitamins have been suggested for treatment of mental illness, based on claims that some people need large quantities of some vitamins for optimal mental function. The procedure is known as **orthomolecular psychiatry**. The American Psychiatric Association does not advocate this treatment, stating that it is unsupported by scientific evidence and that results are not reproducible.[66] The matter remains somewhat controversial, since brain metabolism is not entirely understood. If the psychiatrist prescribes large doses of vitamins, the patient should be observed for signs of vitamin toxicity.

The mentally ill patient who is being treated as an outpatient or the former mentally ill patient who has been discharged from the hospital may have many problems. They often are inexperienced and poor, and have been abandoned by their families. There are many stigmas attached to mental illness by society, and patients have difficulty finding employment. Some of the patients live in halfway houses after discharge from the mental hospital. These facilities should employ a nutritional consultant to assure an adequate diet for residents, but a consultant is not always provided. Some day-care centers also exist to help mentally ill patients. A nutritional care specialist in this setting can teach skills in food shopping and preparation, cleanliness and safety, as well as social skills. Teaching of mentally ill patients requires careful planning, since the patients' attention spans often are short.

The following information on some specific mental illnesses may be helpful.

Schizophrenia

Schizophrenia affects 0.5% to 1.0% of the population. The onset is typically in patients aged 20 to 30 years. A family history of schizophrenia and a history of prenatal or perinatal complications are risk factors.

Symptoms include illogical or incoherent thinking, bizarre behavior, hallucinations, and delusions. The delusions can include the belief that the hospital food is poisoned or that certain foods have magical properties.

If the patient refuses food and drink, nasogastric feedings may be necessary. Schizophrenia is believed to be due to an increased number of dopamine receptors in the brain and is treated with dopamine-receptor blocking agents. Side effects of these medications are dry mouth, constipation, and weight gain.[67]

Many of these patients in the last 25 to 30 years have been released from psychiatric institutions. Some function adequately in home and family, but others need residential care and others become homeless.

Mood Disorders

Mood disorders are classified as **unipolar** (depression) or **dipolar** (mania with or without depression). Unipolar depression occurs in about 10% of women and 5% of men. It tends to recur, beginning in midlife. Dipolar disorder occurs in 0.5% to 1.0% of persons of either sex, beginning usually at age 20 to 30 years.

There is apparently a genetic basis for the disorders. The genes for bipolar illness are localized on chromosome 11 and on the X chromosome. Emotional stress also appears to contribute.[67]

Depression is treated with electroconvulsive therapy, psychotherapy, and antidepressive medications. Side effects of antidepressants include dry mouth, constipation, and either loss or gain of weight. Patients may find that food is tasteless and they may lose weight. Some depressed patients have delusions that interfere with food intake. Depending on the degree of malnutrition, the severity of the depression, and the effect of medication, the patients may need oral supplements, nasogastric feedings, or TPN.

Some patients gain weight during their depression. This occurs, for example, in those with **seasonal affective disorder**, that is, those who become depressed in the winter. They may eventually need counseling for weight loss.

The patient in the manic phase is hyperactive, irritable, and easily distracted. When symptoms are controlled with medication, they can be encouraged to eat and regain lost weight.

Manic episodes are treated with antipsychotics and also with lithium. Side effects of lithium may include nausea, vomiting, anorexia, abdominal pain, mild diarrhea, impaired glucose tolerance, polyuria, polydipsia, and weight gain. A sodium restriction can result in lithium retention and development of lithium toxicity. On the other hand, increased caffeine increases lithium excretion and may lead to a return of manic symptoms.[67]

Monoamine oxidase inhibitors are also used for their depressive effect. Their interactions with food are discussed in Chapter 4.

Drug Addiction

There is limited information on the nutritional status of and procedures for nutritional care of drug addicts. Nutritional assessment of those addicted to commonly abused narcotics (heroin, cocaine, or lysergic acid diethylamide [LSD]) showed that malnutrition is common; the addict develops a craving for sweets, and the diet generally is high in carbohydrate and may be low in vitamins A, B_{12}, and other B vitamins.[68] Fatty acid composition was altered. Consumption of alcohol was high, and hepatitis, hypertension, and infections were common.

The access of nutritional care specialists to drug addicts is limited until the addicts are associated with some form of residential institutional care or a clinic. Addicts or former addicts in clinics or halfway houses need nutritional counseling and assistance with psychosocial development. The nutritional care specialist skilled in interpersonal relationships could make an important contribution to the rehabilitation of the drug addict if the opportunity develops.

DISEASES OF THE MUSCULOSKELETAL SYSTEM

Musculoskeletal diseases are those that affect the bones, joints, and muscles. Some also affect the internal organs and skin. They may be classified into four broad categories:[69]

1. Diseases that usually affect only the joints (e.g., osteoarthritis).
2. Systemic diseases affecting primarily the musculoskeletal system but also affecting other tissues (e.g., rheumatoid arthritis).
3. Systemic diseases with pain in joints or muscles but without structural changes (e.g., polymyalgia rheumatica).
4. Diffuse connective tissue disease involving skin, internal organs, and the musculoskeletal system (e.g., systemic lupus erythematosus).

The term **arthritis** is used to designate the diseases in these categories in which there is inflammation of the joints. It occurs in more than 17 million people, and may be acute or chronic and primary or secondary to other diseases. The two most common forms are rheumatoid arthritis and osteoarthritis.

Osteoarthritis

Osteoarthritis is known also as **degenerative** or **hypertrophic arthritis**. It occurs almost universally in the elderly. The cause is not entirely clear, but it may develop from stress on the joints. As such, it occasionally develops in younger persons after athletic and other injuries.

The primary lesion is degeneration of the articular cartilage in the joints. It affects the thumb particularly, and also fingers, hips, knees, ankles, and spine. It begins with a feeling of stiffness, particularly in the morning or following a long period of immobilization. Soreness subsides after a warm-up. The disease usually involves only a few joints, but general involvement is possible. The severity of the degenerative lesion may vary from asymptomatic to widespread involvement and disability.

The primary feature of nutritional care is weight reduction if the patient is overweight. This is particularly important if arthritis is present in the spine or weight-bearing joints. Because arthritis tends to limit exercise, weight reduction may be very difficult.

Rheumatoid Arthritis

Rheumatoid (atrophic) arthritis is a progressive chronic debilitating disease of unknown etiology occurring in approximately 3% of the adult population. Average age at onset is 35 years, but the disease also occurs in children. The **synovium** (joint lining) is inflamed and painful. Fibroblasts, blood vessels, and inflammatory cells proliferate. The disease may affect any joint but is seen most often in the hands, knees, ankles, and feet. The patient is in negative nitrogen and calcium balance, with muscle atrophy and bone decalcification. The patient frequently is underweight and anemic. The anemia is hemolytic in origin and is not related to iron intake.

The patient may have fever, rash, and extreme fatigue. A **rheumatoid factor** is found in the blood and synovial fluid but is not specific for this disease; rheumatoid factor is found in other conditions as well. The disease occurs in a genetically susceptible individual after an infection that probably is viral. An immune mechanism is believed to perpetuate the joint inflammation.

There is no known cure, and treatment is not very successful. As a result, patients are prone, in desperation, to adopt unproved treatments, including fad diets. Among the so-called remedies suggested are the following:[70]

Take large doses of calcium, riboflavin, pantothenic acid, and vitamins D and E.
Eat only fresh fruit and honey for three days.
Eliminate potatoes, tomatoes, eggplant, and red or green peppers from the diet.
Eliminate dairy products, meat, fruit, egg yolk, vinegar, pepper, "hot spices," choco-

late, dry toasted nuts, alcoholic beverages, soft drinks, additives, preservatives, and "chemicals" from the diet.

Drink 1 cup of burdock root or burdock burr tea three times daily for $1\frac{1}{2}$ months and drink ginger tea while sitting in a ginger root or apple cider vinegar bath.

Eat watercress, cherries, raw liver, parsley, fish liver oil, or bone meal or drink alfalfa tea or lemon juice.

Drink 6 oz. of celery juice daily and eliminate bread.

Nutritional care actually is focused on:

Provision of an adequate diet. (Patients may have poor food intake, especially if hands and legs are affected.)

Achievement and maintenance of normal weight.

Help with problems of daily living, including preparation of meals.

Patients are given anti-inflammatory drugs such as aspirin or indomethacin. If these are ineffective, steroid drugs sometimes are used to reduce pain and stiffness. Among the agents that may be used are adrenocorticotropic hormone (ACTH), cortisone, prednisone, hydrocortisone, and dexamethasone. Medications should be taken after meals to reduce gastric irritation.

Juvenile Rheumatoid Arthritis

Juvenile rheumatoid arthritis (JRA) is considered to be distinct from adult rheumatoid arthritis. It is one of a large number of pediatric rheumatic diseases, having connective tissue inflammation in common. The most common of these are JRA, with an incidence of 14 per 100,000 children less than 16 years old, and systemic lupus erythematosus (SLE), with an incidence of 0.6 per 100,000. JRA is further subclassified as follows:

1. Pauciarticular: affects fewer than five joints, usually in lower extremities.
2. Polyarticular: affects more than four

joints, occurs in both upper and lower extremities; acute or insidious onset.
3. Systemic: has fever, rash, polyarthritis; involves heart, liver, spleen, and lymph nodes.

Patients sometimes cross over from one type to another.

Nutritional Assessment

Malnutrition has been documented in 26% of adult rheumatoid arthritis patients, but the incidence in children is not known.[71] Suggested tests for nutritional screening include the following:[71,72]

1. Anthropometric: weight, height, usual weight, percent weight change, triceps skinfold, midarm total and muscle circumference.
2. Biochemical: complete blood count, serum albumin. Tests for specific conditions; transferrin saturation; serum ferritin; reticulocyte counts and other evaluations as necessary for iron status.
3. Clinical: medications; disabilities.
4. Dietary: 24-hour or three-day diet history; feeding skills; modified diets in current or previous use; use of supplements.

Nutritional Care

There are no data that suggest that specific foods or diets cause or alleviate JRA, but nutritional care can be important in related problems such as malnutrition, growth retardation, weight loss, obesity, and nutritional anemia. In addition, diet modifications are sometimes indicated by nutrient-drug interactions. Some diet modifications that may be indicated for the JRA patient are given in Table 19-12.

COMMENT

Nutritional care specialists can make important contributions to the care of the han-

Table 19-12. Diet Modifications in Juvenile Rheumatoid Arthritis

Indication	Cause	Nutrition Modification
Decreased growth rate	Reduced appetite	Increase energy and intake Nutritional supplements
Weight gain; obesity	Decreased physical activity from pain and decreased joint movement Steroids	Reduced energy intake Advise increase in physical activity
Temporomandibular joint (TMJ) arthritis	Inability to open and close jaw	Soft diet Smaller portions Smaller pieces of food
Increased urinary ascorbic acid	Aspirin	Include good source of ascorbic acid in diet Multivitamin supplement
Increased urinary potassium	Furosemide Steroids	Include good source of potassium in diet Potassium supplement if necessary
Oral ulcers	Methotrexate	Rinse mouth with anesthetic Avoid acidic, salty, or spicy foods Avoid temperature extremes in food
Sodium retention	Steroids	Sodium-restricted diet (2 g Na)
Hyperglycemia and glycosuria	Steroids	Restrict carbohydrate
Increased serum cholesterol and triglycerides	Steroids	Cholesterol- and fat-restricted diet (30% of total kilocalories)

dicapped. Although they often are not involved in long-term direct training programs, they may take part in program planning, consultation on normal nutrition and feeding techniques, and direct evaluation, diagnosis, treatment, and rehabilitation of patients.[73]

References

1. Brooks, M.D. Nutrition overview of cleft lip and palate. *Top. Clin. Nutr.* 3(3):9, 1988.
2. Farnan, S. Nutrition and feeding of children with cleft lip/palate. *Nutrition News* 3(2):1, 1988.
3. Oka, S.W. Epidemiology and genetics of clefting. With implications for etiology. In H.K. Cooper, R.L. Harding, W.M. Krogman, et al., Eds., *Cleft Palate and Cleft Lip: A Team Approach to Clinical Management and Rehabilitation of the Patient.* Philadelphia: W.B. Saunders, 1979.
4. Starr, P., Pearman, W.A., and Peacock, J.L. *Cleft Lip and/or Palate.* Springfield, Ill.: Charles C Thomas, 1983.
5. Balluff, M.A., and Udin, R.D. Using a feeding appliance to aid the infant with a cleft palate. *Ear Nose Throat J.* 65:316, 1986.
6. Bowers, E.J., Mayro, R.F., Whitaker, L.A., et al. General body growth in children with clefts of the lip, palate, and craniofacial structure. *Scand. J. Plast. Reconstruct. Surg.* 21:7, 1987.
7. Grady, E. Breastfeeding the baby with a cleft of the soft palate. *Clin. Pediatr.* 16:978, 1977.
8. Denhoff, E., and Feldman, S.A. *Developmental Disabilities Management through Diet and Medication.* New York: Marcel Dekker, 1981.
9. Mueller, H.A. Facilitating feeding and prespeech. In P.H. Pearson and C.E. Williams, Eds., *Physical Therapy Services in Developmental Disabilities.* Springfield, Ill.: Charles C Thomas, 1972.
10. Fiorentino, M.R. *Reflex Testing Methods for Evaluating Central Nervous System Development.* Springfield, Ill.: Charles C Thomas, 1973.
11. Bobath, K., and Bobath, B. *The Motor Deficit in Patients with Cerebral Palsy.* London: Spastics Society Medical Education and Information Unit, in association with Heinemann Medical, 1966.
12. Peiper, A. *Cerebral Function in Infancy and Childhood.* New York: Consultants Bureau, 1963.
13. Paine, R.S., and Oppe, T.E. *Neurological Examination of Children.* London: Suffolk Lavenham Press, 1966.

14. Ingram, T.T.S. Clinical significance of the infantile feeding reflexes. *Dev. Med. Child. Neurol.* 4:159, 1962.

15. Twitchell, T.E. Normal motor development. *Phys. Ther.* 45:419, 1965.

16. Campbell, S.K. Facilitation of cognitive and motor development in infants with central nervous system dysfunction. *Phys. Ther.* 54:346, 1974.

17. Gallender, D. *Eating Handicaps. Illustrated Techniques for Feeding Disorders.* Springfield, Ill.: Charles C Thomas, 1979.

18. McDonald, R.E. *Dentistry for the Child and Adolescent.* St. Louis: C.V. Mosby, 1969.

19. Freud, A. *Normality and Pathology in Childhood.* New York: International Universities Press, 1966.

20. Illingworth, R.S. *The Development of the Infant and Young Child,* 5th ed. Baltimore: Williams and Wilkins, 1972.

21. Rice, S. Assessment of oral feeding skills. *WIC Currents* 12:23, 1986.

22. Pipes, P. *Nutrition in Infancy and Childhood.* St. Louis: Times Mirror/Mosby, 1985.

23. Phelps, W.M. Dietary requirements in cerebral palsy. *J. Am. Diet. Assoc.* 27:869, 1951.

24. Eddy, T.P., Nicholson, A.L., and Wheeler, E.F. Energy expenditures and dietary intakes in cerebral palsy. *Dev. Med. Child. Neurol.* 7:377, 1965.

25. Hammond, M.I., Lewis, M.N., and Johnson, E.W. A nutritional study of cerebral palsied children. *J. Am. Diet. Assoc.* 49:196, 1966.

26. Gourge, A.L., and Ekvall, S.W. Diets of handicapped children. Physical, psychological and socioeconomic correlations. *Am. J. Ment. Defic.* 80:149, 1975.

27. Pecks, S., and Lamb, M.W. Comments on the dietary practices of cerebral palsied children. *J. Am. Diet. Assoc.* 27:870, 1951.

28. Culley, W.J., and Middleton, T. Caloric requirement of mentally retarded children with and without motor dysfunction. *J. Pediatr.* 75:380, 1969.

29. Cronk, C., et al. Growth charts for children with Down syndrome 1 month to 18 years of age. *Pediatrics* 81:102, 1988.

30. Ouelette, E. The fetal alcohol syndrome. In J.J. Vitale and S.A. Broitman, Eds., *Advances in Human Clinical Nutrition.* Boston: John Wright–PSG, 1982.

31. Cassidy, S.B. Prader-Willi syndrome. *Curr. Prob. Pediatr.* 14:1, 1984.

32. McCamman, S., Rues, J., and Cannon, S. Prader-Willi syndrome. Intervention approaches based on differential phase characteristics. *Top. Clin. Nutr.* 3(3):1, 1988.

33. Bray, G.A., Dahms, R.S., Swerdloff, R.H.,

Fiser, R.H., Atkinson, R.L., and Carrel, R.E. The Prader-Willi syndrome. A study of 40 patients and a review of the literature. *Medicine* 62(2):59, 1983.

34. Brizee, L. Nutritional concerns associated with spina bifida. *Nutrition News* 3(4):1, 1988.

35. Laurence, K.M., James, N., and Campbell, H. Blood folate levels and quality of the maternal diet. *Brit. Med. J.* 285:216, 1980.

36. Bergmann, K.E., Makosch, G., and Tews, K.H. Abnormalities of hair zinc concentrations in mothers of newborn infants with spina bifida. *Am. J. Clin. Nutr.* 33:2145, 1980.

37. Nevin, N. Prevention of neural tube defects in an area of high incidence. In J. Dobbing, Ed., *Prevention of Spina Bifida and Other Neural Tube Defects.* New York: Academic Press, 1983.

38. Anonymous. Evidence for an association between periconceptual use of multivitamins and neural tube defects. *Nutr. Rev.* 48:15, 1990.

39. McKibben, B., Toseland, P.A., and Duckworth, T. Abnormalities in vitamin C in spina bifida. *Dev. Med. Child Neurol.* 15(suppl.):55, 1968.

40. Casey, S.C. Failure to thrive. A challenge that warrants teamwork. *Nutrition News* 4(1):1, 1989.

41. Rathbum, J.M., and Peterson, K.E. Nutrition in failure to thrive. In R.J. Grand, J.L. Sutphen, and W.H. Dietz, Jr., Eds. *Pediatric Nutrition: Theory and Practice.* Boston: Butterworths, 1987.

42. Norris, J.W., and Pratt, R.F. Folic acid deficiency and epilepsy. *Drugs* 8:366, 1974.

43. Reynolds, E.H. Folate metabolism and anticonvulsant therapy. *Proc. Roy. Soc. Med.* 67:6, 1974.

44. Chanarin, I. Effects of anticonvulsant drugs. In M.I. Botez and E.H. Reynolds, Eds., *Folic Acid in Neurology, Psychiatry and Internal Medicine.* New York: Raven Press, 1979.

45. Deluca, K., Masotti, R.E., and Partington, N.W. Altered calcium metabolism due to anticonvulsant drugs. *Dev. Med. Child Neurol.* 14:318, 1973.

46. Lifshitz, F., and Maclaren, N. Vitamin D–dependent rickets in institutionalized, mentally retarded children receiving long-term anticonvulsant therapy. I. A survey of 288 patients. *J. Pediatr.* 83:612, 1973.

47. Ott, L., Young, B., and McClain, C. The metabolic response to brain injury. *JPEN* 11:488, 1987.

48. Rapp, R.P., et al. The favorable effect of early

parenteral feeding on survival in head-injured patients. *J. Neurosurg.* 58:906, 1983.

49. Clifton, G.L., et al. The metabolic response to severe head injury. *J. Neurosurg.* 60:687, 1984.

50. Clifton, G.L., et al. Enteral hyperalimentation in head injury. *J. Neurosurg.* 60:687, 1984.

51. Young, B., Ott, L., Twyman, D., Norton, J., Rapp, J.R., Tibbs, P., Haack, D., Brivins, B., and Dempsey, R. The effect of nutritional support on outcome from severe head injury. *J. Neurosurg.* 67:668, 1987.

52. Twyman, D.L., Rapp, R.P., and Young, A.B. Parenteral vs. enteral feedings in severe head injury patients. A randomized study. *JPEN* 5:577, 1981.

53. Feucht, S. Guidelines for the use of thickening agents in foods and liquids. *Nutrition News* 3(6):1, 1988.

54. Stern, J. Nutritional rehabilitation in the closed head injury patients. *Diet. Crit. Care* 7(4):2, 1985.

55. Endersbe, L.A. Nutrition support in neurologic impairment. In E.P. Shronts, Ed., *Nutrition Support Dietetics: Core Curriculum 1989.* Silver Spring, Md.: American Society for Parenteral and Enteral Nutrition, 1989.

56. Institute of Rehabilitative Medicine, New York University Medical Center. *Mealtime Manual for the Aged and Handicapped.* New York: Essandess Special Edition, 1970.

57. Peiffer, S.C., Blust, P., and Leyson, J.F.J. Nutritional assessment of the spinal cord injured patient. *J. Am. Diet. Assoc.* 78:501, 1981.

58. Lindvall, O., Brundin, P., Widner, H., Rehncrona, S., et al. Grafts of fetal dopamine neurons survive and improve motor function in Parkinson's disease. *Science* 247:574, 1990.

59. Lieberman, D.A. Nutritional management of the patient with Parkinson's disease. *Top. Clin. Nutr.* 4(1):1, 1989.

60. Miller, C.A. Nutritional needs and care in amyotrophic lateral sclerosis. *Top. Clin. Nutr.* 4(1):15, 1989.

61. Gray, G.E. Nutrition and dementia. *J. Am. Diet. Assoc.* 89:1795, 1989.

62. Marx, J. NGF and Alzheimer's: Hopes and fears. *Science* 247:408, 1990.

63. Millar, J.H.D., Zilkha, K.J., Langman, M.J.S., et al. Double-blind trial of linoleate supplementation of the diet in multiple sclerosis. *Br. Med. J.* 1:765, 1973.

64. Swank, R.L., and Bourdillon, R.D. Multiple sclerosis. Assessment of treatment with a modified low fat diet. *J. Nerv. Ment. Dis.* 131:486, 1960.

65. Swank, R.L. Multiple sclerosis. Twenty years on a low fat diet. *Arch. Neurol.* 23:460, 1970.

66. American Psychiatric Association Task Force on Vitamin Therapy in Psychiatry. Megavitamin and orthomolecular therapy in psychiatry (excerpts from a report). *Nutr. Rev.* (Suppl.1)32:44, 1975.

67. Gray, G.E., and Gray, L.K. Nutritional aspects of psychiatric disorders. *J. Am. Diet. Assoc.* 89:1492, 1989.

68. Frankle, R.T., and Christakis, G. Some nutritional aspects of "hard" drug addiction. *Dietetic Currents* 2(3):1, 1975.

69. Houpt, J. Arthritic and Rheumatic Disorders. In A.G. Gornall, Ed., *Applied Biochemistry of Clinical Disorders.* Hagerstown, Md.: Harper and Row, 1980.

70. Meister, K.A. Can diet cure arthritis? *ACSH News and Views* 1:10, 1980.

71. Koenning, G.M. Nutritional management of the child with juvenile rheumatoid arthritis. *Top. Clin. Nutr.* 3(3):17, 1988.

72. Warady, B.D., McCamman, S.P., and Lindsley, C.B. Anthropometric assessment of patients with juvenile rheumatoid arthritis. *Top. Clin. Nutr.* 4(1):7, 1989.

73. Wallace, H.M. Nutrition and handicapped children. *J. Am. Diet. Assoc.* 61:127, 1972.

Bibliography

Acardo, P.J., Ed. *Failure to Thrive in Infancy and Early Childhood.* Baltimore: University Park Press, 1982.

Blackman, J.A., Ed. *Medical Aspects of Developmental Disabilities in Children Birth to Three.* Rockville, Md.: Aspen, 1990.

Diagnostic and Statistical Manual of Mental Disorders, 3rd ed., rev. Washington, D.C.: American Psychiatric Association, 1987.

Gines, D.J., Ed. *Nutrition Management in Rehabilitation.* Frederick, Md., Aspen, 1990.

Kaplan, H.I., and Sadock, B.J., Eds. *Comprehensive Textbook of Psychiatry/IV.* Baltimore: Williams and Wilkins, 1985.

Talbott, J.A., Hales, R.E., and Yudofsky, S.C., Eds. *The American Psychiatric Press Textbook of Psychiatry.* Washington, D.C.: American Psychiatric Press, 1988.

Sources of Current Information

American Journal of Clinical Nutrition
Developmental Medicine and Child Neurology
Journal of the American Dietetic Association
Journal of Pediatrics
Nutrition Focus (University of Washington)
Pediatric Research
Topics in Clinical Nutrition

III. Appendixes

Contents

A. Recommended Nutrient Intakes   746

B. Vocabulary and Abbreviations   751

C. Normal Laboratory Values   760

D. Conversion Factors   767

E. Osmolality and Specific Gravity   768

F. Caffeine   769

G. Formula-Feeding Products   771

H. Revised Daily Food Guide Food Groups   786

I. Age-Specific Lipid Values   790

J. Exchange Lists for Protein-, Sodium-, and Potassium-Restricted Diets   792

K. Appropriate Serving Sizes of Usual Foods for Infants and Children   805

L. Growth and Development Charts for Infants and Children   807

Appendix A. Recommended Nutrient Intakes

Table A-1. *Recommended Dietary Allowances,*[a] *Revised 1989,* Designed for the Maintenance of Good Nutrition of Practically All Healthy People in the United States

Category	Age (years) or Condition	Weight[b] (kg)	Weight[b] (lb.)	Height[b] (cm)	Height[b] (in.)	Protein (g)	Fat-Soluble Vitamins Vita-min A (μg RE)[c]	Vita-min D (μg)[d]	Vita-min E (mg α-TE)[e]	Vita-min K (μg)
Infants	0.0–0.5	6	13	60	24	13	375	7.5	3	5
	0.5–1.0	9	20	71	28	14	375	10	4	10
Children	1–3	13	29	90	35	16	400	10	6	15
	4–6	20	44	112	44	24	500	10	7	20
	7–10	28	62	132	52	28	700	10	7	30
Males	11–14	45	99	157	62	45	1,000	10	10	45
	15–18	66	145	176	69	59	1,000	10	10	65
	19–24	72	160	177	70	58	1,000	10	10	70
	25–50	79	174	176	70	63	1,000	5	10	80
	51+	77	170	173	68	63	1,000	5	10	80
Females	11–14	46	101	157	62	46	800	10	8	45
	15–18	55	120	163	64	44	800	10	8	55
	19–24	58	128	164	65	46	800	10	8	60
	25–50	63	138	163	64	50	800	5	8	65
	51+	65	143	160	63	50	800	5	8	65
Pregnant						60	800	10	10	65
Lactating	1st 6 months					65	1,300	10	12	65
	2nd 6 months					62	1,200	10	11	65

Reproduced with permission from *Recommended Dietary Allowances,* 10th edition, © 1990, by the National Academy of Sciences, National Academy Press, Washington, DC.

[a] The allowances, expressed as average daily intakes over time, are intended to provide for individual variations among most normal persons as they live in the United States under usual environmental stresses. Diets should be based on a variety of common foods in order to provide other nutrients for which human requirements have been less well defined. See text for detailed discussion of allowances and of nutrients not tabulated.

[b] Weights and heights of Reference Adults are actual medians for the U.S. population of the designated age, as reported by NHANES II. The median weights and heights of those under 19 years of age were taken from Hamill, P.V.V., Drizd, T.A., Johnson, C.L., Reed, R.B., Roche, A.F., and Moore, W.M. Physical growth: National Center for Health Statistics percentiles. *Am. J. Clin. Nutr.* 32:607, 1979. The use of these figures does not imply that the height-to-weight ratios are ideal.

[c] Retinol equivalents. 1 retinol equivalent = 1 μg retinol or 6 μg β-carotene.

[d] As cholecalciferol. 10 μg cholecalciferol = 400 IU of vitamin D.

[e] α-Tocopherol equivalents. 1 mg d-α tocopherol = 1 α-TE.

[f] 1 NE (niacin equivalent) is equal to 1 mg of niacin or 60 mg of dietary tryptophan.

Table A-1. (Continued)

	Water-Soluble Vitamins						Minerals						
Vitamin C (mg)	Thiamine (mg)	Riboflavin (mg)	Niacin (mg NE)[f]	Vitamin B₆ (mg)	Folate (µg)	Vitamin B₁₂ (µg)	Calcium (mg)	Phosphorus (mg)	Magnesium (mg)	Iron (mg)	Zinc (mg)	Iodine (µg)	Selenium (µg)
30	0.3	0.4	5	0.3	25	0.3	400	300	40	6	5	40	10
35	0.4	0.5	6	0.6	35	0.5	600	500	60	10	5	50	15
40	0.7	0.8	9	1.0	50	0.7	800	800	80	10	10	70	20
45	0.9	1.1	12	1.1	75	1.0	800	800	120	10	10	90	20
45	1.0	1.2	13	1.4	100	1.4	800	800	170	10	10	120	30
50	1.3	1.5	17	1.7	150	2.0	1,200	1,200	270	12	15	150	40
60	1.5	1.8	20	2.0	200	2.0	1,200	1,200	400	12	15	150	50
60	1.5	1.7	19	2.0	200	2.0	1,200	1,200	350	10	15	150	70
60	1.5	1.7	19	2.0	200	2.0	800	800	350	10	15	150	70
60	1.2	1.4	15	2.0	200	2.0	800	800	350	10	15	150	70
50	1.1	1.3	15	1.4	150	2.0	1,200	1,200	280	15	12	150	45
60	1.1	1.3	15	1.5	180	2.0	1,200	1,200	300	15	12	150	50
60	1.1	1.3	15	1.6	180	2.0	1,200	1,200	280	15	12	150	55
60	1.1	1.3	15	1.6	180	2.0	800	800	280	15	12	150	55
60	1.0	1.2	13	1.6	180	2.0	800	800	280	10	12	150	55
70	1.5	1.6	17	2.2	400	2.2	1,200	1,200	320	30	15	175	65
95	1.6	1.8	20	2.1	280	2.6	1,200	1,200	355	15	19	200	75
90	1.6	1.7	20	2.1	260	2.6	1,200	1,200	340	15	16	200	75

Table A-2. Median Heights and Weights and Recommended Energy Intake

Category	Age (years) or Condition	Weight (kg)	Weight (lb.)	Height (cm)	Height (in.)	REE (kcal/day)	Average Energy Allowance (kcal)[a] Multiples of REE	Average Energy Allowance (kcal)[a] Per kg	Average Energy Allowance (kcal)[a] Per Day[b]
Infants	0.0–0.5	6	13	60	24	320		108	650
	0.5–1.0	9	20	71	28	500		98	850
Children	1–3	13	29	90	35	740		102	1,300
	4–6	20	44	112	44	950		90	1,800
	7–10	28	62	132	52	1,130		70	2,000
Males	11–14	45	99	157	62	1,440	1.70	55	2,500
	15–18	66	145	176	69	1,760	1.67	45	3,000
	19–24	72	160	177	70	1,780	1.67	40	2,900
	25–50	79	174	176	70	1,800	1.60	37	2,900
	51+	77	170	173	68	1,530	1.50	30	2,300
Females	11–14	46	101	157	62	1,310	1.67	47	2,200
	15–18	55	120	163	64	1,370	1.60	40	2,200
	19–24	58	128	164	65	1,350	1.60	38	2,200
	25–50	63	138	163	64	1,380	1.55	36	2,200
	51+	65	143	160	63	1,280	1.50	30	1,900
Pregnant	1st trimester								+0
	2nd trimester								+300
	3rd trimester								+300
Lactating	1st 6 months								+500
	2nd 6 months								+500

Reproduced with permission from *Recommended Dietary Allowances*, 10th edition, © 1990, by the National Academy of Sciences, National Academy Press, Washington, DC.

[a] In the range of light to moderate activity, the coefficient of variation is ±20%.

[b] Figure is rounded.

Table A-3. Estimated Safe and Adequate Daily Dietary Intakes of Selected Vitamins and Minerals[a]

Category	Age (years)	Vitamins	
		Biotin (μg)	Pantothenic Acid (mg)
Infants	0–0.5	10	2
	0.5–1	15	3
Children and adolescents	1–3	20	3
	4–6	25	3–4
	7–10	30	4–5
	11+	30–100	4–7
Adults		30–100	4–7

Category	Age (years)	Trace Elements[b]				
		Copper (mg)	Manganese (mg)	Fluoride (mg)	Chromium (μg)	Molybdenum (μg)
Infants	0–0.5	0.4–0.6	0.3–0.6	0.1–0.5	10–40	15–30
	0.5–1	0.6–0.7	0.6–1.0	0.2–1.0	20–60	20–40
Children and adolescents	1–3	0.7–1.0	1.0–1.5	0.5–1.5	20–80	25–50
	4–6	1.0–1.5	1.5–2.0	1.0–2.5	30–120	30–75
	7–10	1.0–2.0	2.0–3.0	1.5–2.5	50–200	50–150
	11+	1.5–2.5	2.0–5.0	1.5–2.5	50–200	75–250
Adults		1.5–3.0	2.0–5.0	1.5–4.0	50–200	75–250

Reproduced with permission from *Recommended Dietary Allowances*, 10th edition, © 1990, by the National Academy of Sciences, National Academy Press, Washington, DC.

[a] Because there is less information on which to base allowances, these figures are not given in the main table of RDA and are provided here in the form of ranges of recommended intakes.

[b] Since the toxic levels for many trace elements may be only several times usual intakes, the upper levels for the trace elements given in this table should not be habitually exceeded.

Table A-4. Estimated Sodium, Chloride, and Potassium Minimum Requirements of Healthy Persons[a]

Age	Weight (kg)[a]	Sodium (mg)[a,b]	Chloride (mg)[a,b]	Potassium (mg)[c]
Months				
0–5	4.5	120	180	500
6–11	8.9	200	300	700
Years				
1	11.0	225	350	1,000
2–5	16.0	300	500	1,400
6–9	25.0	400	600	1,600
10–18	50.0	500	750	2,000
>18[d]	70.0	500	750	2,000

Reproduced with permission from *Recommended Dietary Allowances*, 10th edition, © 1990, by the National Academy of Sciences, National Academy Press, Washington, DC.

[a] No allowance has been included for large, prolonged losses from the skin through sweat.

[b] There is no evidence that higher intakes confer any health benefit.

[c] Desirable intakes of potassium may considerably exceed these values (~3,500 mg for adults).

[d] No allowance included for growth. Values for those below 18 years assume a growth rate at the 50th percentile reported by the National Center for Health Statistics (Hamill, P.V.V., Drizd, T.A., Johnson, C.L., Reed, R.B., Roche, A.F., and Moore, W.M. Physical growth: National Center for Health Statistics percentiles. *Am. J. Clin. Nutr.* 32:607, 1979).

Table A-5. Recommended Nutrient Intakes for Canadians[a]

Age	Sex	Weight (kg)	kcal/kg[b]	Protein (g/day)[c]	Fat-Soluble Vitamins			Water-Soluble Vitamins			Minerals				
					Vitamin A (RE/day)[d]	Vitamin D (μg/day)[e]	Vitamin E (mg/day)[f]	Vitamin C (mg/day)	Folacin (μg/day)[c,g]	Vitamin B$_{12}$ (μg/day)	Calcium (mg/day)	Magnesium (mg/day)[c]	Iron (mg/day)	Iodine (μg/day)	Zinc (mg/day)
Months															
0–2	Both	4.5	120–100	11[h]	400	10	3	20	50	0.3	350	30	0.4[i]	25	2[j]
3–5	Both	7.0	100–95	14[h]	400	10	3	20	50	0.3	350	40	5	35	3
6–8	Both	8.5	95–97	17[h]	400	10	3	20	50	0.3	400	50	7	40	3
9–11	Both	9.5	97–99	18	400	10	3	20	55	0.3	400	50	7	45	3
Years															
1	Both	11	101	19	400	10	3	20	65	0.3	500	55	6	55	4
2–3	Both	14	94	22	400	5	4	20	80	0.4	500	70	6	65	4
4–6	Both	18	100	26	500	5	5	25	90	0.5	600	90	6	85	5
7–9	M	25	88	30	700	2.5	7	35	125	0.8	700	110	7	110	6
	F	25	76	30	700	2.5	6	30	125	0.8	700	110	7	95	6
10–12	M	34	73	38	800	2.5	8	40	170	1.0	900	150	10	125	7
	F	36	61	40	800	2.5	7	40	180	1.0	1,000	160	10	110	7
13–15	M	50	57	50	900	2.5	9	50	150	1.5	1,100	210	12	160	9
	F	48	46	42	800	2.5	7	45	145	1.5	800	200	13	160	8
16–18	M	62	51	55	1,000	2.5	10	55	185	1.9	900	250	10	160	9
	F	53	40	43	800	2.5	7	45	160	1.9	700	215	14	160	8
19–24	M	71	42	58	1,000	2.5	10	60	210	2.0	800	240	8	160	9
	F	58	36	43	800	2.5	7	45	175	2.0	700	200	14	160	8
25–49	M	74	36	61	1,000	2.5	9	60	220	2.0	800	250	8	160	9
	F	59	32	44	800	2.5	6	45	175	2.0	700	200	14[k]	160	8
50–74	M	73	31	60	1,000	2.5	7	60	220	2.0	800	250	8	160	9
	F	63	29	47	800	2.5	6	45	190	2.0	800	210	7	160	8
75+	M	69	29	57	1,000	2.5	6	60	205	2.0	800	230	8	160	9
	F	64	23	47	800	2.5	5	45	190	2.0	800	220	7	160	8
Pregnancy (additional)															
1st trimester			100	15	100	2.5	2	0	305	1.0	500	15	6	25	0
2nd trimester			300	20	100	2.5	2	20	305	1.0	500	20	6	25	1
3rd trimester			300	25	100	2.5	2	20	305	1.0	500	25	6	25	2
Lactation (additional)			450	20	400	2.5	3	30	120	0.5	500	80	0	50	6

Adapted from *Recommended Nutrient Intakes for Canadians*. Ottawa: Canadian Government Publishing Centre, 1983. Reproduced with permission of the Minister of Supply and Services Canada.

[a] Recommended intakes during periods of growth are taken as appropriate for individuals representative of the midpoint in each age group. All recommended intakes are designed to cover individual variations in essentially all of a healthy population subsisting upon a variety of common foods available in Canada.

[b] Figures for energy are estimates of average requirements for expected patterns of activity. For nutrients not shown, the following amounts are recommended: thiamine, 0.4 mg/1,000 kcal (0.48 mg/5,000 kJ); riboflavin, 0.5 mg/1,000 kcal (0.6 mg/5,000 kJ); niacin, 7.2 NE/1,000 kcal (8.6 NE/5,000 kJ); vitamin B$_6$, 15 μg, as pyridoxine, per gram of protein; phosphorus, same as calcium.

[c] The primary units are expressed per kilogram of body weight. The figures shown here are only examples.

[d] One retinol equivalent (RE) corresponds to the biological activity of 1 μg of retinol, 6 μg of β-carotene, or 12 μg of other carotenes.

[e] Expressed as cholecalciferol or ergocalciferol.

[f] Expressed as d-α-tocopherol equivalents, relative to which β- and γ-tocopherol and α-tocotrienol have activities of 0.5, 0.1, and 0.3 respectively.

[g] Expressed as total folate.

[h] Assumption that the protein is from breast milk or is of the same biological value as that of breast milk and that between 3 and 9 months adjustment for the quality of the protein is made.

[i] It is assumed that breast milk is the source of iron up to 2 months of age.

[j] Based on the assumption that breast milk is the source of zinc for the first 2 months.

[k] After the menopause the recommended intake is 7 mg/day.

Appendix B. Vocabulary and Abbreviations

*Table B-1. Vocabulary**

Root Words

Adeno	Gland	Lith-	Stone
Andro-	Men	Lymph-	Waterlike
Ano-	Anus	Malac-	Softening
Arterio-	Artery	Mea-	Passage
Antr-	Cavity, cave	Meg-	Large, great, strong
Arthro-	Joint	Menin-	Membrane
-blast	Immature form, sprout, germ	Morph-	Form, shape
Broncho-	Bronchus	My-, myo-	Muscle
		Myelo-	Marrow
Canc-, carc-	Malignant tumor		
Cardi-, cardio-	Heart	Naso-	Nose
Chole-	Bile	Necro-	Dead
Cholecysto-	Gallbladder	Neph-, nephro-	Kidney
Choledocho-	Bile duct	Neuro-	Nerve
Chondro-	Cartilage		
Col-	Colon	Oligo-	Few, scant
Corp-	Body, mass	Oophor-	Ovary
Crani-, cranio-	Skull	Ophthalm-	Eye
Cyano-	Blue	Os-, oss-, ost-, osteo-	Bone
Cysto-	Bladder; any fluid-filled sac	-osis	Disease
Cyto-	Cell	Ot-	Ear
Derm-, dermato-	Skin	Ovar-	Ovary
Duodeno-	Duodenum		
		Pancreato-	Pancreas
Em-	Blood	Parieto-	Wall
Encephalo-	Brain, skull	Path-	Disease
Entero-	Intestine	Ped-	Child, feet
Erythro-	Red	Pneumo-, Pneumon-	Lung
Esophago-	Esophagus	Poly-	Many, much
Esthe-	Feeling, sensation	Proct-	Anus, rectum
Fis-	Cleavage, split	Pseud-	False
For-	Opening, aperture	Pulm-	Lung
Forn-	Arch, vault	Pyel-, pyelo-	Pelvis
		Py-, pyo-	Pus
Gastr-	Stomach	Pyr-	Fever, fire
Glosso-	Tongue		
Gynec-	Women (especially women's reproductive organs)	Recto-	Rectum
		Reni-, reno-	Kidney
		Retic-, reticulo-	Netlike
		Rhino-	Nose
Hem-, hemat-	Blood	Salping-	Tube
Hepato-	Liver	Sang-	Blood
Hist-	Tissue	Sclero-	Hard
Hydr-	Water	Seb-	Hard fat
Hyster-, hystero-	Uterus	Sept-	Thin wall
Idio-	Unknown, strange, peculiar	Septic-	Poison
Ileo-	Ileum	Sinu-	Curved, hollow
		Sta-	Stand
Jejuno-	Jejunum	Stomato-	Mouth
Laryngo-	Larynx	Tox-, toxic-	Poison
Leuc-, leuk-	White		
Lipo-	Fat		

(continued)

---

* The terms listed are divided into two sections. *Root words* usually refer to the part of the body or tissue, whereas prefixes and suffixes are *modifiers* that describe the variation from normal or the action on the root word.

Table B-1. (Continued)

Tracheo-	Trachea	Hyper-	Over, above, beyond, excessive
Uretero-	Ureter	Hypo-	Under, deficiency of
Urethro-	Urethra		
Utero-	Uterus	Im-, in-	In, into, not
Vari-	Bent, stretched	Infra-	Below, beneath
Veni-, veno-	Vein	Inter-	Between
Modifiers		Intra-	Within, during
		-itis	Inflammation of
A-	Without, from	Lev-, levo-	Left
Ab-, abs-	From	-lith	Stone
Ad-	To, toward, at	-lysis, -lytic	Destructive
-algia	Pain in	Mal-	Bad
Am-, ambi-, amphi-	Around	Meso-	Middle, between
-asis	Affected with, disease	-oid	Formed like
Ante-	Before, forward	-oma	Tumor
Anti-	Against, opposite	-osis	Disease
Brachy-	Short	Pan-	All, every
Brady-	Slow	Para-	Beside
-cele	Hernia of	-pathy	Disease
Circum-	Around	-penia	Without, lack of
-cleisis	Closure of	Peri-	Around
Con-	With	-phagia	To eat
-cyte	Cell	-phobia	Fear of
De-	Down, from, away	-pnea	Breathing air
Demi-	Half	-poiesis	To produce
Dextro-	Right	Poly-	Many
Dia-	Through	Post-	After
Dis-	Apart	Pre-, pro-	Before
-duct	Lead, guide	Privia-	Without, lack of
-dynia	Pain in	-ptosis	Falling of
Dys-	Difficult, painful	Quad-, quar-	Four
E-	From, out of, without	Re-	Again
Ec-	Out	Retro-	Backward
-ectasis	Deletion of	-rrhagia	Bursting from
Ecto-	Without, outside, external	-rrhaphy	Sewing of
-ectomy	Excision of	-rrhea	Flowing
-ectopy	Displacement of	-rrhexis	Rupture of
Ek-	From, out of, without	-scopy	Viewing of
Em-	In	Semi-	Half
-emesis	Vomiting	-spasm	Spasm of
-emia	In blood	-stenosis	Narrowing of
En-	In	-stomy	Making a mouth
Endo-, ento-	Within	Sub-	Under, below
Epi-	On, against	Super-	Over, above
-esthesia	Feeling, sensation	Supra-	Above
Eu-	Well, abundant, easy	Tachy-	Swift, fast
Ex-	From, out of, without	-tomy	Cutting of
Exo-	Outside, beyond	Trans-	Above, beyond, through, across
Extra-	Outside, beyond		
-genesis, -genic	Producing, forming	-trismus	Spasm of
Hemi-	Half	-trophy	Growth or mutation

Table B-2. Abbreviations Used in Medical Records

a	Before
A	Artery
A, Asmt	Assessment
AAA	Abdominal aortic aneurysm
A&B	Apnea and bradycardia
Ab	Antibody; abortion; antibiotic
Abd	Abdomen, abdominal
ABG	Arterial blood gases
a.c.	Before meals, ante cibum
ACTH	Adrenocorticotropic hormone
ad lib	As needed or desired
A.D.C. VAN DISSEL	Mnemonic for Admit, Diagnosis, Condition, Vitals, Activity, Nursing procedures, Diet, Ins and outs, Specific drugs, Symptomatic drugs, Extras, Labs
ADH	Antidiuretic hormone
ADL	Activities of daily living
AE	Above elbow
AEIOU TIPS	Mnemonic for Alcohol, Encephalopathy, Insulin, Opiates, Uremia, Trauma, Infection, Psychiatric, Syncope
AF	Afebrile, aortofemoral, or atrial fibrillation
AFB	Acid-fast bacilli
AFP	Alpha-fetoprotein
AI	Aortic insufficiency
A/G	Albumin/globulin ratio
AKA	Above knee amputation
Alb	Albumin
ALL	Acute lymphocytic leukemia
AML	Acute myelogenous leukemia
Amts	Amounts
Amb	Ambulate
AOB	Alcohol on breath
AODM	Adult-onset diabetes mellitus
AP	Angina pectoris; anterior-posterior; abdominal-perineal
ARF	Acute renal failure
AS	Aortic stenosis
ASCVD	Atherosclerotic cardiovascular disease
ASD	Atrial septal defect
ASAP	As soon as possible
ASHD	Arteriosclerotic heart disease
ASO	Antistreptolysin O
AV	Atrioventricular
A-V	Arteriovenous
a&w	Alive and well
B I&II	Billroth I and II
BBB	Bundle branch block
BCAA	Branched chain amino acids
BE	Barium enema
BEE	Basal energy expenditure
BF	Breast feeding
b.i.d., b.d.	Twice daily
BJ	Bone and joint
BK	Below knee
BKA	Below knee amputation
BM	Bone marrow; bowel movement
BMI	Body mass index
BMR	Basal metabolic rate
BOM	Bilateral otitis media
BP, b.p.	Blood pressure
BPM	Beats per minute
BRP	Bathroom privileges
B.S.	Bowel sounds; breath sounds
B.T.	Bedtime

(continued)

Table B-2. (Continued)

BUN	Blood urea nitrogen
Bx	Biopsy
c.	Cup
$\bar{c}$	With
ca.	Approximately
Ca, Ca^{++}	Calcium
CA	Cancer
CAA	Crystalline amino acids
CAD	Coronary artery disease
CAT, CT	Computerized (axial) tomography
CBC	Complete blood count
CC	Chief complaint
CCU	Coronary care unit; clean catch urine
CF	Cystic fibrosis
CHD	Coronary heart disease
CHF	Congestive heart failure
CHI	Creatinine-height index
chol.	Cholesterol
CHO	Complex carbohydrate
CI	Cardiac index
cm	Centimeter
CMI	Cell-mediated immunity
CML	Chronic myelogenous leukemia
CNS	Central nervous system
C/O	Complains of
CO	Cardiac output
COAD	Chronic obstructive airways disease
COLD	Chronic obstructive lung disease
COPD	Chronic obstructive pulmonary disease
CPK	Creatine phosphokinase
CRF	Chronic renal failure
CrCl	Creatinine clearance
CSF	Cerebralspinal fluid
c.v.	Cardiovascular
CVA	Cerebrovascular accident
CVP	Central venous pressure
CVR	Cardiovascular-renal
CVS	Cardiovascular system
CXR	Chest x-ray
DAT	Diet as tolerated
DBW	Desirable body weight
D/C	Discontinue; discharge
DCH	Delayed cutaneous hypersensitivity
decaf	Decaffeinated
def.	Deficiency
dex	Dexter (right)
DIC	Disseminated intravascular coagulation
dil	Dilate
DKA	Diabetic ketoacidosis
dl	Deciliter
DM	Diabetes mellitus
DOB	Date of birth
DOE	Dyspnea on exertion
DTR	Deep tendon reflexes
Dx	Diagnosis
D$_5$LR	5% dextrose in lactated Ringer's solution
D$_5$W	5% dextrose in water solution
ECG, EKG	Electrocardiogram
EAA	Essential amino acids
EEG	Electroencephalogram
ENT	Ear, nose, and throat

(continued)

Table B-2. (Continued)

EENT	Eye, ear, nose and throat
EFA(D)	Essential fatty acid (deficiency)
e.g.	For example
elec	Electrolytes
elim	Eliminate, elimination
esp	Especially
EtOH	Ethanol, ethyl alcohol
ESRD	End-stage renal disease
FBS	Fasting blood sugar
FFA	Free fatty acids
FH	Family history
fl.	Fluid
FMH	Family medical history
FTT	Failure to thrive
F/U	Follow-up
FUO	Fever of unknown origin
Fx	Fracture
g	Gram
G	Gravida
GA	General appearance
GB	Gallbladder
GC	Gonococcus; gonorrhea
GE	Gastroenteritis
gest	Gestation
GFR	Glomerular filtration rate
GI	Gastrointestinal
gluc	Glucose
Gt	A drop
gr	Grain
gtts	Drops
GTT	Glucose tolerance test
GU	Genitourinary
GYN	Gynecology
H&H	Hemoglobin & hematocrit
Hb, Hgb	Hemoglobin
HBP	High blood pressure
HBV	High biological value
H.C.	High calorie
HCG	Human chorionic gonadotropin
Hct	Hematocrit (See PCV)
HCVD	Hypertensive cardiovascular disease
HEENT	Head, eyes, ears, nose, and throat
H&N	Head and neck
HOB	Head of bed
H/O	History of
H&P	History and physical
Hp	Hemiplegia
HLP	Hyperlipidemia
HPI	History of present illness
HR	Heart rate
h.s.	At bedtime, hora somni
HTN, HPN	Hypertension
ht	Height
I	Infant
IBW	Ideal body weight
ICU	Intensive care unit
ID	Identification
IDDN	Insulin-dependent diabetes mellitus
i.e.	That is
IHD	Ischemic heart disease
IM, i.m.	Intramuscular

(continued)

Table B-2. (Continued)

IMP	Impression
I&O	Intake and output
IP	Intraperitoneal
IRDM	Insulin-resistant diabetes mellitus
IV, i.v.	Intravenous
IVC	Intravenous cholangiogram
IVP	Intravenous pyelogram
Jc.	Juice
JODM	Juvenile-onset diabetes mellitus
kg	Kilogram
KOR	Keep open rate
KUB	Kidney, ureter, bladder
KVO	Keep vein open
L	Liter, left
LBW	Low birth weight, low biological value
LDH	Lactic acid dehydrogenase
LE	Lupus erythematosus
LLE	Left lower extremity
LLL	Left lower lobe (lung)
LLQ	Left lower quadrant
LLSB	Left lower sternal border
LML	Left middle lobe (lung)
LMD	Local medical doctor
LMP	Last menstrual period
LOC	Loss of consciousness
LOM	Limitation of motion
LP	Lumbar puncture
LPN	Licensed practical nurse
LS	Lumbosacral; low salt
LSB	Left sternal border
LUE	Left upper extremity
L&W	Living and well
lytes	Electrolytes
MAC	Midarm circumference
MAFA	Midarm fat area
MAMA	Midarm muscle area
MAMC	Midarm muscle circumference
MBF	Meat-base formula
MCH	Mean cell hemoglobin
mEq	Milliequivalent
MH	Menstrual history
MI	Mitral insufficiency, myocardial infarction
ml	Milliliter
mm	Millimeter
mmol	Millimole
mo.	Months
mOsm	Milliosmole
MCH	Mean cell hemoglobin
MCHC	Mean cell hemoglobin concentration
MCL	Midclavicular line
MCT	Medium-chain triglyercide
MCV	Mean cell volume
meds	Medications
MP	Metatarsal-phalangeal
mg	Milligram
MS	Mitral stenosis; multiple sclerosis; morphine sulfate
MVI	Multivitamin injection
N, NML, Nl	Normal
NAD	No acute distress; no active disease
NCAT	Normocephalic atraumatic

(continued)

Table B-2. (Continued)

NCD	Normal childhood disease
NED	No evidence of disease
NERD	No evidence of return disease
ng	Nanogram
NG	Nasogastric
NIDDM	Non-insulin-dependent diabetes mellitus
NKA	No known allergies
NKDA	No known drug allergies
NPN	Nonprotein nitrogen
NPO	Nothing by mouth, non per os
NR	Not remarkable
NS	Normal saline; neurosurgery
NSR	Normal sinus rhythm
N&V	Nausea and vomiting
OB	Obstetrics
OBW	Optimal body weight
OC	Oral contraceptives
OCG	Oral cystogram
OD	Overdose; right eye
OK	Okay, suitable
OOB	Out of bed
O&P	Ova and parasites
OR	Operating room
OS	Left eye
OU	Both eyes
oz.	Ounce
$\bar{p}$	after
Para	Pregnancies; paraplegic
p.c.	After eating, post cibum
PC	Present complaint
PCM	Protein-calorie malnutrition
PCV	Packed cell volume (hematocrit)
PDA	Patent ductus arteriosus
PDR	Physician's Desk Reference
PE	Pulmonary embolus
pg	picogram
PG	Pregnant, pregnancy
PH	Past history
PI	Present illness; pulmonary insufficiency
PID	Pelvic inflammatory disease
PKU	Phenylketonuria
PMD	Private medical doctor
PMH	Past medical history
PMN	Polymorphonuclear leukocyte (neutrophil)
po	By mouth, given orally
P.O.	Postoperative
POD	Postoperative day
PP	Patient profile
pr	By rectum, given rectally
PR	Pulse rate
p.r.n.	Whenever necessary
prot.	Protein
Pt	Patient
PT	Physical therapy; prothrombin time
PTA	Prior to admission
PTH	Parathormone
PTT	Partial thromboplastin time or prothrombin time
PUFAs	Polyunsaturated fatty acids
PUD	Peptic ulcer disease
PVD	Peripheral vascular disease
PZI	Protamine zinc insulin

(continued)

Table B-2. (Continued)

q	Every
q.d.	Every day
qh	Every hour
q.i.d.	Four times daily
q.o.d.	Every other day
q2h, q3h	Every 2 hours, every 3 hours
quad	Quadriplegic
r.b.c.	Red blood cells
RBC	Red blood cell count
RCM	Right costal margin
RDAs	Recommended dietary allowances
RLE	Right lower extremity
RLL	Right lower lobe
RLQ	Right lower quadrant
RO, R/O	Rule out
ROM	Range of motion
ROS	Review of systems
RTA	Renal tubular acidosis
RTC	Return to clinic
RUE	Right upper extremity
RUL	Right upper lobe (lung)
RUQ	Right upper quadrant
rx	Take
Rx	Prescription, treatment
s̄	Without
SAA	Synthetic amino acids
S&A	Sugar and acetone
SBS	Short bowel syndrome
SCr	Serum creatinine
SG	Swan-Ganz (catheter)
SGA	Small for gestational age
SGOT	Serum glutamic oxaloacetic transaminase
SGPT	Serum glutamic pyruvic transaminase
SH	Social history
sig.	Label
SL	Sublingual
SLE	Systemic lupus erythematosus
SOAP	Mnemonic for Subjective, Objective, Assessment, Plan
SOB	Short of breath
SOBOE	Short of breath on exertion
sos	If necessary
S/P	Status postoperatively
SQ	Subcutaneous, given subcutaneously
S&S	Signs and symptoms
stat	At once
sub	Substitute
SUN	Serum urea nitrogen
Sx	Symptoms
T, Tbsp.	Tablespoon
t, tsp.	Teaspoon
T&A	Tonsillectomy and adenoidectomy
TB	Tuberculosis
TBLC	Term birth, living child
TDE	Total daily energy expenditure
temp	Temperature
TF	Tube feeding; transferrin
TG, trig.	Triglycerides
TIA	Transient ischemic attack
TIBC	Total iron-binding capacity
t.i.d.	Three times daily
TKO	To keep open

(continued)

Table B-2. (Continued)

TLC	Total lymphocyte count; tender loving care; total lung capacity
TPN	Total parenteral nutrition
TPR	Temperature, pulse, and respiration
TSF	Triceps skinfold
TSH	Thyroid stimulating hormone
TV	Tidal volume
Tx	Treatment
UA, U.A.	Urine analysis; uric acid
UBW	Usual body weight
UCD	Usual childhood diseases
UGI	Upper gastrointestinal
UNA	Urea nitrogen appearance
URI	Upper respiratory (tract) infection
US	Ultrasound
UTI	Urinary tract infection
UUN	Urinary urea nitrogen
Vag	Vaginal
VC	Vital capacity
V&P	Vagotomy and pyloroplasty
Vit.	Vitamin(s)
VMA	Vanillylmandelic acid
vs	Versus
VS	Vital signs
VSS	Vital signs stable
w.b.c.	White blood cells
WBC	White blood cell count
WDWN	Well developed, well nourished
WNL	Within normal limits
w/o	Without
W/U	Workup
w/v	Weight per volume
yr.	Years
y.o.	Years old
#	Pounds (lb.)
24°	24 hours
37°	37 degrees
↑	High, increased, elevated, more
↓	Low, decreased, depressed, less

Table B-3. Quantitative Symbols

=	Equal
≠	Unequal
>	Greater than
<	Less than
≥	Greater than or equal
≤	Less than or equal
↑	Increasing
↓	Decreasing
1°	Primary
2°	Secondary

Appendix C. Normal Laboratory Values

Table C-1. Whole Blood, Serum, and Plasma[a]

Test	Material	Normal Value
Acetone	Serum	0.3–2.0 mg/dl
Albumin	Serum	3.2–5.5 g/dl
Ammonia	Plasma	20–150 μg/dl
Amylase	Serum	50–200 Somogyi units/dl
Ascorbic acid (vitamin C)	Plasma	0.6–1.6 mg/dl
	Whole blood	0.7–2.0 mg/dl
Bicarbonate	Plasma	21–28 mEq/L
Bile acids	Serum	<1.0 mg/dl
Bilirubin	Serum	Up to 0.2 mg/dl (direct or conjugated)
		0.1–1.0 mg/dl (indirect or unconjugated)
		Total: 0.5–1.2 mg/dl
Blood gases	Whole blood	
Anion gap		8–16 mEq/L
pH		Arterial: 7.35–7.45
		Venous: 7.36–7.41
pCO_2		Arterial: 35–45 mm Hg
		Venous: 35–50 mm Hg
pO_2		Arterial: 50–100 mm Hg
BSP (Bromsulphalein) (5 mg/kg)	Serum	<5% retention after 45 min. or <4 mg/dl
Calcium	Serum	Total: 8.5–10.5 mg/dl
		4.3–5.5 mEq/L
		Ionized: 4.2–5.2 mg/dl
		2.1–2.6 mEq/L
Carbon dioxide	Whole blood	Arterial: 19–24 mEq/L
		Venous: 22–26 mEq/L
	Plasma	Arterial: 21–30 mEq/L
		Venous: 22–34 mEq/L
Carotene, beta	Serum	50–300 μg/dl
Chloride	Serum	95–108 mEq/L
Cholesterol, esters	Serum	68–76% of total cholesterol
Cholesterol, total	Serum	150–250 mg/dl (varies with age and diet)
Copper	Serum	110–160 μg/dl

(continued)

[a] The following works provide useful information on interpretation of tests: Bennington, J.L., Fouty, R.A., and Hougie, C., *Laboratory Diagnosis*. Toronto, Ont.: Macmillan, 1970; Byrne, C.J., Saxton, D.F., Pelikan, P.K., and Nugent, P.M., *Laboratory Tests. Implications for Nurses and Allied Health Professionals*. Menlo Park, Calif.: Addison-Wesley, 1981; Halsted, J.A., and Halsted, C.H., Eds., *The Laboratory in Clinical Medicine. Interpretation and Application*, 2nd ed. Philadelphia: W.B. Saunders, 1981; Ravel, R., *Clinical Laboratory Medicine*, 3rd ed. Chicago: Year Book Medical Publishers, 1978; Sabiston, D.C., Ed., *Textbook of Surgery*, 12th ed. Philadelphia: W.B. Saunders, 1981; Tilkian, S.M., and Conover, M.H., *Clinical Implications of Laboratory Tests*. St. Louis: C.V. Mosby, 1975; and Wallach, J., *Interpretation of Diagnostic Tests*, 2nd ed. Boston: Little, Brown, 1974.

Note: This is not exhaustive but contains those values most likely to be useful to nutritionists. The values were compiled from a number of sources that did not always agree; therefore, values given are representative.

Table C-1. (Continued)

Test	Material	Normal Value
Creatine	Serum or plasma	Men: 0.2–0.8 mg/dl Women: 0.6–1.0 mg/dl
Creatine phosphokinase (CPK)	Serum	Men: 5–35 units/ml Women: 5–25 units/ml
Creatinine	Serum or plasma	0.7–1.5 mg/dl
Creatinine clearance (endogenous)	Serum or plasma and urine	Men: 110–150 ml/min. Women: 105–132 ml/min.
Electrophoresis, lipoprotein	Serum	Alpha: 12–18%, 80–310 mg/dl Beta: 50–70%, 160–400 mg/dl Prebeta: 11–29%, 50–180 mg/dl Chylomicrons: 0–1%, 0–50 mg/dl
Electrophoresis, protein	Serum	Albumin: 53–68%, 3.5–5.5 g/dl Alpha-1: 2.0–5.0%, 0.1–0.4 g/dl Alpha-2: 8.0–13.0%, 0.4–1.0 g/dl Beta: 11.0–17.0%, 0.5–1.1 g/dl Gamma: 15.0–25.0%, 0.5–1.6 g/dl
Fatty acids, total	Serum	190–420 mg/dl
Folate	Serum	7–16 ng/ml (bioassay)
Gamma globulin	Serum	0.5–1.6 g/dl
Globulins, total	Serum	2.3–3.5 g/dl
Glucose, fasting	Blood Plasma or serum	60–100 mg/dl 70–115 mg/dl
Glucose-6-phosphate dehydrogenase (G6PD)	Erythrocytes	140–280 units/10^9 cells
Glutathione	Whole blood	24–37 mg/dl
Growth hormone	Serum	1–15 ng/ml
Hemoglobin	Serum or plasma Whole blood	0.5–5.0 mg/dl Women: 12.6–14.2 g/dl Men: 14.0–16.5 g/dl Pregnancy: >10.6 g/dl
α-Hydroxybutyric dehydrogenase	Serum	140–350 units/ml
Immunoglobulins	Serum, adults	
IgG		800–1,600 mg/dl, 80%
IgA		50–250 mg/dl, 15%
IgM		40–120 mg/dl, 0.5%
IgD		0.5–3.0 mg/dl, 0.2%
IgE		0.01–0.04 mg/100 dl, 0.0002%
Iron, total	Serum	60–200 μg/dl
Iron-binding capacity	Serum	250–410 μg/dl
Ketone bodies	Serum	Negative or 2–4 μg/dl
Lactic acid	Whole blood, venous Whole blood, arterial	5–20 mg/dl 3–7 mg/dl
Lactic dehydrogenase (LDH)	Serum	80–120 Wacker units 150–450 Wroblewski units 71–207 IU/L
Lactic dehydrogenase (heat stable)	Serum	30–60% of total LDH
Lactose tolerance	Serum	Serum glucose changes are similar to those seen in a glucose tolerance test
Lipase	Serum	0–1.5 Cherry-Crandall units/ml
Lipids, total	Serum	450–850 mg/dl
Cholesterol		120–260 mg/dl
Triglycerides		0–190 mg/dl
Phospholipids		150–380 mg/dl

(continued)

Table C-1. (Continued)

Test	Material	Normal Value
Fatty acids, free		25 mg/dl
Neutral fat		0–200 mg/dl
Macroglobulins, total	Serum	70–430 mg/dl
Magnesium	Serum	1.5–2.5 mEq/L (1.8–3.0 mg/dl)
Nonprotein nitrogen (NPN)	Serum	15–35 mg/dl
	Whole blood	25–50 mg/dl
Osmolality	Serum	285–295 mOsm/kg
Pantothenic acid	Whole blood	20–80 pg/ml
pH	Whole blood, arterial	7.35–7.45
Phenylalanine	Serum	Adults: <3.0 mg/dl
		Newborns (term): 1.2–3.5 mg/dl
Phosphatase, acid, total	Serum	0–1.1 units/ml (Bodansky)
		1–5 units/ml (King-Armstrong)
		0.13–0.63 units/ml (Bessey-Lowry)
		1.4–5.5 units/ml (Gutman-Gutman)
		0–0.56 units/ml (Roy)
		0–6.0 units/ml (Shinowara-Jones-Reinhart)
Phosphatase, alkaline, total	Serum	Adults:
		1.5–4.5 units/dl (Bodansky)
		4–13 units/dl (King-Armstrong)
		0.8–2.3 units/ml (Bessey-Lowry)
		15–35 units/ml (Shinowara-Jones-Reinhart)
		30–85 IU
		Children:
		5.0–14.0 units/dl (Bodansky)
		3.4–9.0 units/ml (Bessey-Lowry)
		15–30 units/dl (King-Armstrong)
Phosphate	Serum	Adults:
		1.8–2.6 mEq/L
		3.0–4.5 mg/dl
		Children:
		2.3–4.1 mEq/L
		4.0–7.0 mg/dl
Potassium	Plasma	3.5–5.0 mEq/L
Proteins, total	Serum	6.0–8.0 g/dl
Albumin		3.5–5.5 g/dl
Riboflavin	Whole blood	100–500 pg/ml
Sodium	Serum	136–145 mEq/L
Transaminase		
Glutamic oxaloacetic	Serum (SGOT)	8–40 units/ml
Glutamic pyruvic	Serum (SGPT)	5–35 units/ml
Triglycerides	Serum	0–150 mg/dl
Urea clearance	Serum and urine	Maximum clearance: 60–99 ml/min.
		Standard clearance: 41–65 ml/min. or more than 75% of normal clearance
Urea nitrogen	Blood (BUN)	10–20 mg/dl
	Serum (SUN)	11–23 mg/dl
Uric acid	Serum	Men: 2.5–8.0 mg/dl
		Women: 1.5–6.0 mg/dl

(continued)

Table C-1. (Continued)

Test	Material	Normal Value
Vitamin A	Serum	20–80 μg/dl
Vitamin B$_6$ (pyridoxine)	Plasma	30–80 ng/ml
Vitamin B$_{12}$	Serum	160–1,000 pg/ml
Vitamin E	Plasma	0.6 mg/dl
Zinc	Plasma	75–125 μg/dl

Table C-2. Urine

Test	Type of Specimen	Normal Value
Acetoacetic acid	Random	Negative
Acetone	Random	Negative
Albumin	Random	Negative
Aldosterone	24 hr.	2–26 μg/24 hr.
Alpha-amino acid nitrogen	24 hr.	100–290 mg/24 hr.
Ammonia nitrogen	24 hr.	500–1,200 mg/24 hr. 20–70 mEq/24 hr.
Amylase	24 hr.	80–5,000 Somogyi units/24 hr.
Ascorbic acid	Random 24 hr.	1–7 mg/dl >50 mg/24 hr.
Bence Jones protein	Random	Negative
Bilirubin	Random	Negative
Blood, occult	Random	Negative, 0.02 mg/dl
Chloride	24 hr.	110–250 mEq/24 hr.
Cortisol	24 hr.	<150 μg/24 hr.
Creatine	24 hr.	Men: 0–40 mg/24 hr. Women: 0–100 mg/24 hr. Higher in children and during pregnancy
Creatinine	24 hr.	Men: 15–26 mg/kg/24 hr. 1.0–2.0 g/24 hr. Women: 14–22 mg/kg/24 hr. 0.8–1.8 g/24 hr.
Glucose	Random 24 hr.	Negative 250 mg/24 hr.
Hemoglobin	Random	Negative
Homogentisic acid	Random	Negative
Homovanillic acid (HVA)	24 hr.	<15 mg/24 hr.
5-Hydroxyindoleacetic acid (5-HIAA)	Random 24 hr.	Negative <10 mg/24 hr.
Ketone bodies	Random	Negative
Lactose	24 hr.	12–40 mg/24 hr.
Magnesium	24 hr.	6.0–8.5 mEq/24 hr.
Osmolality	Random	38–1,400 mOsm/kg water

(continued)

Note: This list is not exhaustive but contains those values most likely to be useful to nutritionists. The values were compiled from a number of sources that did not always agree; therefore, values given are representative. Further information on interpretation of tests is available (see footnote a, Table C-1).

Table C-2. (Continued)

Test	Type of Specimen	Normal Value
Oxalic acid	24 hr.	10–55 mg/24 hr.
pH	Random	4.6–8.0
Phenolsulfonphthalein (PSP)	Urine, timed after 6 mg PSP IV	
	15 min.	28–50% dye excreted
	30 min.	16–24% dye excreted
Phenolsulfonphthalein (PSP)	60 min.	9–17% dye excreted
	120 min.	3–10% dye excreted
Phenylpyruvic acid	Random	Negative
Phosphorus	Random	0.9–1.3 g/24 hr.
		0.2–0.6 mEq/24 hr.
Potassium	24 hr.	25–100 mEq/24 hr.
Protein	24 hr.	10–150 mg/24 hr.
Reducing substances, total	24 hr.	0.5–1.5 mg/24 hr.
Sodium	24 hr.	40–260 mEq/24 hr.
Specific gravity	Random	1.016–1.022 (normal fluid intake)
		1.001–1.040 (range)
Sugars (excluding glucose)	Random	Negative
Titratable acidity	24 hr.	20–40 mEq/24 hr.
Urea nitrogen	24 hr.	6–17 g/24 hr.
Uric acid	24 hr.	250–750 mg/24 hr.
Urobilinogen	2 hr.	0.3–1.0 Ehrlich units
	24 hr.	0.05–2.5 mg/24 hr., or 0.5–4.0 Ehrlich units/24 hr.
Vanillylmandelic acid (VMA)	24 hr.	<8 mg/24 hr. (adults)
Volume, total	24 hr.	600–1,600 ml/24 hr.
Zinc	24 hr.	0.15–1.2 mg/24 hr.

Table C-3. Hematology

Red blood count	Men: $4.6–6.2 \times 10^6$/mm^3
	Women: $4.2–5.4 \times 10^6$/mm^3
	Pregnancy: $>3.6 \times 10^6$/mm^3
White blood cell count	5,000–10,000/ml
Differential white blood cell count	
Segmented neutrophils	54–62%, 3,000–5,800/ml
Bands	3–5%, 150–400/ml
Lymphocytes	25–33%, 1,500–3,000/ml
Monocytes	3–7%, 285–500/ml
Eosinophils	1–4%, 50–250/ml
Basophils	0.75%, 15–50/ml
Platelet count	150,000–400,000/ml
Hemoglobin	Men: 14.0–18.0 g/dl
	Women: 12.0–16.0 g/dl
	Pregnancy: >10.6 g/dl
Hemoglobin A_{1c}	3–5% of total

(continued)

Note: This is not exhaustive but contains those values most likely to be useful to nutritionists. The values were compiled from a number of sources that did not always agree; therefore, values given are representative. Further information on interpretation of tests is available (see footnote a, Table C-1).

Table C-3. (Continued)

Hematocrit (packed cell volume [PCV])	Men: 40–54% Women: 37–47% Pregnancy: >34%
Reticulocyte count	0.5–1.5%
Red blood cell indexes	
Mean corpuscular volume (MCV)	87–105 μ^3
Mean corpuscular hemoglobin (MCH)	27–35 pg
Mean corpuscular hemoglobin concentration (MCHC)	32–36%
Blood volume (7–8% of body weight in kilograms)	Men: 69 ml/kg Women: 65 ml/kg
Plasma volume	Men: 44 ml/kg Women: 40 ml/kg
Red blood cell volume	Men: 26 ml/kg Women: 21 ml/kg

Table C-4. Typical Test Panels

Test panels are the result of the development of automated analytical instruments. It is common for the physician to order an automated panel of tests, rather than ordering individual tests. The contents of some typical test panels are shown in this table.

Preliminary Screening (SMA 6)[a]
Bicarbonate (CO_2)
Sodium
Potassium
Chloride
Blood urea nitrogen (BUN)
Blood glucose
Reported in patient's chart thus:

Na	Cl	BUN
K	HCO₃	Glucose

For example:

142	102	10
4.0	28	102

Health Survey Screening
Albumin
Alkaline phosphatase
SGOT
Bilirubin (total)
Blood urea nitrogen (BUN)
Calcium
Cholesterol
Glucose
Lactic dehydrogenase (LDH)
Phosphorus
Protein, total
Uric acid

Routine Urinalysis
Color
Appearance
Specific gravity
pH
Albumin, qualitative
Glucose, qualitative
Ketone bodies, qualitative
Bilirubin, qualitative
Occult blood
Casts
Organisms
Mucus
Epithelial cells
Crystal
White blood cells
Red blood cells

Hemogram
Hemoglobin
Hematocrit
Red cells
White cells
Differential
    Neutrophils, segmented
    Neutrophils, nonsegmented
    Lymphocytes
    Monocytes
    Eosinophils
    Basophils
    Atypical lymphocytes
    Other
RBC morphology
Platelets:
    Morphology
    Count
Mean corpuscular volume (calculated)
Mean corpuscular hemoglobin (calculated)
Mean corpuscular hemoglobin
    concentration (calculated)

Some of these values are reported in patient's chart thus:

    Hgb Segs/Bands/Lymphs/Monos/
        Basos/Eos

(continued)

Table C-4. (Continued)

WBC —— MCV-MCH-MCHC
      Hct Platelet count

For example:

$$11,000 \ \frac{10.2}{30.4} \ \begin{array}{l} 40S, 20B, 30L, 6M, 1B, 3E \\ 80/27/32 \\ 286,000 \end{array}$$

A "complete blood count" (CBC) usually includes Hgb, Hct, RBC, WBC, MCV, MCH, MCHC.

Broad Spectrum Screening (SMA 20)[a]
Albumin
Alkaline phosphatase
Bicarbonate (CO_2)
Bilirubin, total
  Direct
  Indirect
Blood urea nitrogen (BUN)
BUN/creatinine ratio
Calcium
Ionized calcium (estimated)
Chloride
Cholesterol
Creatinine
Globulin
Glucose
Lactic dehydrogenase (LDH)
Inorganic phosphorus
Potassium
Serum glutamic oxaloacetic transaminase (SGOT)
Serum glutamic pyruvic transaminase (SGPT)
Sodium
Total protein
Triglycerides
Uric acid
Anion gap (calculated)

Lipid Panel
Cholesterol, total
Cholesterol, LDL
Cholesterol, HDL
Cholesterol, VLDL
LDH:HDL ratio
Triglycerides
VLDL: triglycerides ratio
Lipoprotein electrophoresis
Phospholipids
Total lipids
Glucose

Acute Heart Panel
Creatinine phosphokinase (CPK)
Hydroxybutyric dehydrogenase (HBD)
Lactate dehydrogenase (LDH)
LDH Isozymes
Potassium
SGOT

CHD Risk Profile
HDL
Cholesterol, total
Triglycerides
Glucose

Hypertension Panel
Renal panel
Blood gases:
  pH
  pCO_2
  Bicarbonate
Cholesterol
Glucose
LDH
Triglycerides

Liver Panel
Alkaline phosphatase
Bilirubin, total
  Direct
LDH
LDH isozymes
SGOT (AST)
SGPT (ALT)
Protein, total
Protein electrophoresis
Urine bile pigment
Albumin
Globulin

Pancreatic Panel
Serum amylase
Serum lipase
Urine amylase

Renal Panel
BUN
Creatinine
Creatinine clearance
Calcium
Chloride
Phosphorus
Potassium
Protein, total
Protein electrophoresis
Sodium
Urine specific gravity
Urine culture

Diabetes Mellitus Panel
Glucose
Glucose tolerance (if not contraindicated)
Serum ketones
Triglycerides
Urine glucose, 24 hour
Urine ketones

Diabetes Management Profile
Glucose
Hemoglobin A_{1c}

[a] SMA = sequential multiple analysis.

Appendix D. Conversion Factors

METRIC SYSTEM WEIGHTS

1 kilogram (kg) = 1,000 grams (g)
1 milligram (mg) = 0.001 gram (g)
1 microgram (μg) = 10^{-6} g or μ
1 nanogram (ng) = 10^{-9} g or mμ
1 picogram (pg) = 10^{-12} g or $\mu\mu$
1 femtogram (fg) = 10^{-15} g or m$\mu\mu$

METRIC AND AVOIRDUPOIS SYSTEMS OF VOLUME (FLUID)

1 liter (L) = 1,000 milliliters (ml)
1 milliliter (ml) = 1,000 microliters (μl)
1 deciliter (dl) = 100 milliliters

APPROXIMATE HOUSEHOLD EQUIVALENTS

1 teaspoon (tsp.) = 5 ml = 5 g
1 tablespoon (Tbsp.) = 15 ml = 15 g
1 cup (16 Tbsp.) = 237 ml (usually rounded to 240)
= 240 g

CONVERSION FACTORS

1 kilogram = 2.2046 pounds (usually rounded to 2.2)
1 pound = 0.4536 kg
1 ounce = 28.35 g (usually rounded to 30)
1 liter = 1.06 quarts
1 fluid ounce = 29.57 ml (usually rounded to 30)
1 inch = 2.54 centimeters
1 centimeter = 0.394 inch
Degrees Celsius = ($^\circ$F − 32) × $\frac{5}{9}$
Degrees Fahrenheit = ($^\circ$C × $\frac{9}{5}$) + 32

Parts per million (ppm) to percent:

1 ppm = 0.0001%
10 ppm = 0.001%
100 ppm = 0.01%
1,000 ppm = 0.1%

Milliequivalents (mEq) to milligrams:

mEq × atomic weight/valence = mg
Example: 30 mEq Na × 23/1 = 690 mg Na

Milligrams to milliequivalents:

(mg/atomic weight) × valence = mEq
Example: 1,482 mg K/39 × 1 = 38 mEq K

For other values, use the atomic weights shown in the following table:

		Atomic Weight	Valence
Calcium	Ca	40	2
Chlorine	Cl	35.4	1
Magnesium	Mg	24.3	2
Phosphorus	P	31	2
Potassium	K	39	1
Sodium	Na	23	1
Sulfate	SO$_4$	96	2
Sulfur	S	32	2
Zinc	Zn	65.37	2

STANDARD PREFIXES

Less Than 1			More Than 1		
atto	10^{-18}	a	deka	10^1	da
femto	10^{-15}	f	hecto	10^2	h
pico	10^{-12}	p	kilo	10^3	k
nano	10^{-9}	n	mega	10^6	M
micro	10^{-6}	μ	giga	10^9	G
milli	10^{-3}	m			
centi	10^{-2}	c			
deci	10^{-1}	d			

Appendix E. Osmolality and Specific Gravity

Osmosis is the movement of fluid across a semipermeable membrane from an area of lower concentration of solutes to an area of higher concentration. Osmotic pressure is the difference in the concentration of the number of particles of solutes. It is expressed in terms of **osmols** or **milliosmols** (mOsm). One millimole (mmol) of a substance that does not dissociate in solution equals 1 mOsm. If a substance dissociates, it contains milliosmoles equivalent to the number of particles produced. Sodium chloride dissociates into sodium ion (Na^+) and chloride ion (Cl^-), so 1 mmol equals 2 mOsm. One millimole of sodium phosphate (Na_2HPO_4) dissociates into two Na ions and one HPO_4 ion, making 3 mOsm.

Osmolality is measured in milliosmoles of solute per **kilogram** of solvent, whereas *osmolarity* is defined as milliosmoles of solute per liter of solution (solute plus solvent). When the solvent is water, as it is in most biologic systems, osmolarity is approximately 80% of osmolality.

Normal osmolality of serum is 280 to 295 mOsm/kg. It is determined mainly by the concentrations of sodium, urea, and glucose. Amino acids, small peptides, and other electrolytes also have an osmotic effect, whereas starch, whole protein, and long-chain fat have a low osmolality. Serum osmolality can be estimated using the formula

$$mOsm/kg = 2(Na^+ + K^+) + \frac{serum\ urea\ nitrogen}{2.8} + \frac{glucose}{18}$$

where Na^+ and K^+ (potassium ion) are given in milliequivalents per liter; serum urea nitrogen and glucose are given in milligrams per deciliter.

Specific gravity sometimes is used to measure urine concentrations. Specific gravity differs from osmolality in that it depends on the size and weight of dissolved particles in addition to the number of particles. Distilled water has a specific gravity of 1 g/ml. Normal range for urine is 1.001 to 1.025.

Appendix F. Caffeine*

RELATED COMPOUNDS

Compound	Formula	Source
Caffeine	1,3,7 trimethylxanthine	Coffee, tea, cocoa beans, kola nuts
Theobromine	3,7 dimethylxanthine	Cocoa
Theophylline	1,3 dimethylxanthine	Tea

ABSORPTION, METABOLISM, AND EXCRETION OF CAFFEINE

Absorbed rapidly

Distributed throughout body water within 1 hour

Readily transferred across placenta

Metabolic half-life $\cong$ 3 hours

Excreted in urine as methylxanthine derivatives, small amount of unchanged caffeine in urine; some fecal excretion; primary excretion product is 1-methyl uric acid

PHYSIOLOGIC EFFECTS OF CAFFEINE

Cardiac muscle stimulant

Smooth muscle relaxant

Central nervous system stimulant

Diuretic

Stimulates gastric acid secretion

Increases plasma glucose and free fatty acid concentrations

WITHDRAWAL SYMPTOMS

Nausea

Vomiting

Irritability

TOXICITY

Can cause vomiting and convulsions

Acute human fatal dose $\cong$ 170 mg/kg body weight

PHARMACOLOGIC USES OF METHYLXANTHINES

Caffeine: Cerebral stimulant; respiratory stimulant (in premature infants); chronic use does not decrease effect; pharmacologic dose for adult $\cong$ 200 mg

Theobromine: Diuresis

Theophylline: Coronary dilation

* The material in this appendix has been compiled from the following sources: Graham, D.M., Caffeine — Its identity, dietary sources, intake and biological effects. *Nutr. Rev.* 36:97, 1978; Coffee drinking and peptic ulcer disease. *Nutr. Rev.* 34:167, 1976; Stephenson, P., Physiologic and psychotropic effects on man. *J. Am. Diet. Assoc.* 7:240, 1977; Hospital Food Service, Clinical Dietetic Section, *Manual of Clinical Dietetics.* Los Angeles: University of California, 1977; Bunker, M.L., and McWilliams, M., Caffeine content of common beverages. *J. Am. Diet. Assoc.* 74:28, 1979; Nazy, M., Caffeine content of beverages and chocolate. *J.A.M.A.* 229:337, 1974; and American Dietetic Association, *Handbook of Clinical Dietetics.* New Haven, Conn.: Yale University Press, 1981.

METHYLXANTHINES IN FOOD AND DRINK

Food or Beverage	Caffeine (mg/6-oz. cup)	Theophylline (mg/6-oz. cup)	Theobromine (mg/6-oz. cup)
Roasted and ground coffee, brewed to varying strengths	60–150		
Instant coffee	60		
Nescafé	7		
Decaffeinated coffee	3		
Decaf	0.18		
Sanka	3.3		
Tea, brewed to varying strengths	34–65	2	1
Instant tea	55		2
Cocoa (mean, all types)	13		250
African			272
South American			232
Cola beverages			
Coca-Cola	64.7		
Diet Pepsi-Cola	36		
Diet-Rite Cola	31.7		
Dr. Pepper	60.9		
Diet Dr. Pepper	54.2		
Pepsi-Cola	43.1		
Royal Crown Cola	33.7		
Diet RC Cola	30.0		
Mountain Dew	54.7		

DRUG SOURCES OF CAFFEINE

Drug	Usual Purpose for Use	Caffeine Content (mg/tablet)
Anacin	Headache relief	32
A.P.C.	Analgesic	32
Bromoquinine	Cold tablet	15
Cope	Headache relief	32
Darvon	Prescription drug	32
Dristan	Allergy relief	30
Excedrin	Headache relief	32
Fiorinal	Prescription drug	40
Migral	Prescription drug	50
No Doz	Keep awake	100–200
Sinarest	Allergy relief	31
Vivarin	Keep awake	100–200

Appendix G. Formula-Feeding Products

Table G-1. Oral Supplementary Feedings

Product (ml to provide 100% RDA)	Composition (Source)			Caloric Density (kcal/ml)	Lactose	Residue	Notes
	Carbohydrate (g/100 kcal)	Protein (g/100 kcal)	Fat (g/100 kcal)				
Alterna[e] (powder)	13 (Corn syrup solids, sucrose)	2.7 (Whey powder, nonfat dry milk, caseinate)	4.0 (Soy oil)	0.36	Yes	Low	Indicated for patients with renal disease
Citrotein[a] (powder) (1180)	18.25 (Maltodextrins, sucrose)	6.25 (Egg albumin)	0.26 (Soy oil, monoglycerides, diglycerides)	0.66	No	Low	Protein and vitamin supplement to clear liquid diet. 263.4 g dry weight needed to give 1,000 kcal; 3.1 mEq Na/dl; 1.8 mEq K/dl Nonpro C:N ratio = 76:1. Gluten free; 496 mOsm/kg.
Delmark Eggnog[b]	13 (Nonfat dry milk, maltodextrins, sugar)	5.25 (Nonfat dry milk, egg white, egg yolk solids)	3.0 (Cottonseed oil, soy oil, egg yolk)	1.16	Yes		
Delmark Milkshake[b]	12.5 (Sugar, maltodextrins, ice cream mix)	3.8 (Egg, milk)	3.85 (Vegetable oil)	0.95	Yes		
Dietene[a]	15.75 (Nonfat milk, sucrose)	8.75 (Nonfat milk)	0.2	0.8	Yes		Add powder to milk.
dp High p.e.r. Protein[c]	2.0	20.6	1.0	2.58 kcal/g			Protein supplement; low electrolyte; 258 g dry weight to give 1,000 kcal.

(continued)

Table G-1. (Continued)

Product (ml to provide 100% RDA)	Composition (Source)			Caloric Density (kcal/ml)	Lactose	Residue	Notes
	Carbohydrate (g/100 kcal)	Protein (g/100 kcal)	Fat (g/100 kcal)				
Duocal[d]	15.5 (Maltodextrins)	0	4.7 (Vegetable: 34% MCT, 23% linoleate)	4.7	No	Low	Energy supplement; low electrolyte; 100 g = 28 mg Na, 3.5 mg K.
Forta Pudding[e]	13.6 (Sucrose, modified starch)	2.72 (Nonfat milk)	3.88 (Soy oil)	1.69	Yes	Low	Vanilla, chocolate, butterscotch, tapioca. 240 mg Na/serving; 330 mg K/serving.
Gevral[f]	6.68 (Lactose, sucrose)	17.1 (Ca Caseinate)	0.57 (Milk fat)	0.653	Yes	Low	Protein-calorie supplement; artificial flavors; 248.8 g dry weight to give 1,000 kcal.
Lolactene[a]	13 (Corn syrup solids, sucrose)	6.6 (Caseinate)	2.3 (Vegetable oil, mono and diglycerides)	0.8	Low	None	1,150 ml gives 1,000 kcal.
Lonalac[g]	30 (Lactose)	21 (Casein)	49 (Coconut oil)	0.67	High	Low	Low Na (4 mg/dl); high K, high protein; do not reconstitute with water high in Na.
MCT Duocal[d]	15.7 (Maltodextrins)	0	4.94 (82.5% MCT: 12.5% linoleate; 5% LCT vegetable oil)	4.7	No	Low	Energy supplement; 100 g contains 175 mg Na and 6 mg K.
Nutrex broth[h]	87 (Corn syrup solids)	13 (Caseinate)	0	1.39	No	Low	Clear soup: chicken, beef, vegetable. PER = 2.5; Nonpro C:N ratio = 175:1; mOsm/kg = 350.
Nutrex CLD[h]	12.9 (Sucrose)	11.4 (Egg white solids; gelatin)	0	0.95	No	Low	Clear gel; semisolid; mOsm/kg = 680.
Nutrex drink[h]	20 (Corn syrup solids; sucrose)	5.3 (Egg white solids)	0	0.71	No	Low	Clear liquid diet; six flavors.

Nutrex Protamin[h]	15 (Corn syrup solids; sucrose)	3.1 (Caseinate)	3 (Corn oil)	1.27	No	Low	Full liquid diet; three flavors; mOsm/kg = 450.
Nutricare[i] (1200)	11.8 (Maltodextrins; sucrose)	5.7 (Whey protein concentrate)	3.2 (Whey concentrate lecithin)	1.16	Yes		Mix with 8 oz. whole milk per serving.
Ross SLD[e] (840)	78 (Hydrolyzed cornstarch; sucrose)	21.4 (Egg white solids)	0.6	0.7	No	Low	Clear liquid; 3.6 mEq Na/dl and 2.1 mEq K/dl: Nonpro C:N ratio = 92:1; mOsm/kg = 545.
Sustacal Pudding[f]	53 (Nonfat milk; sucrose)	11 (Milk)	36 (Soy oil)	48/oz.	Yes		Vanilla, chocolate, butterscotch; 120 mg Na per serving; 46.2 mOsm per 5 oz. serving; Nonpro C:N ratio = 200:1.

a Sandoz
b Delmark
c General Mills
d Scientific Hospital Supplies
e Ross Laboratories
f Lederle Laboratories
g Mead Johnson Nutritionals
h Nutrex
i Advanced Healthcare

Note: The composition of these products is subject to change. Current product literature should be consulted before use. This table is not intended to be comprehensive.

Table G-2. Sources of Single Nutrients

Product (form)	Composition (source)			Caloric Density	Osmolality (mOsm/kg)	Lactose	Residue	Notes
	Carbohydrate (g/100 kcal)	Protein (g/100 kcal)	Lipid (g/100 kcal)					
Protein sources Casec[a] (powder)	0	23.78 (caseinate)	0.54	3.7/g		No	Low	Add to liquid or food; 270 g gives 1,000 kcal; low Na; no vitamins.
Dialume[b] (powder)	17.22	6.9	Trace	3.6/g	918 at 1:5 dilution	No		For oral or tube feeding; contains all essential amino acids, cystine, and histidine; gluten-free; orange flavor; tartrazine-free; 168 mg Na and 9.2 mg K/10 g.
Maxipro HBV[b] (powder)	Trace	22.56	1.02	3.09/g	165 at 1:5 dilution	Trace		For oral or tube feeding; 230 mg Na and 450 mg K/100 g; gluten-free.
Nutrisource Protein[c] (powder)	1.75	18.75 (delactosed lactalbumin; egg white solids)	2.1	4.02/g		No		Use only for modular tube feeding; 76 g protein/100 g.
Nutrisource Amino Acids[c] (powder)	0	24.87 (free amino acids)	0	3.9/g		No		Use only for modular tube feeding; 97 g protein/100 g.
Nutrisource Amino Acids–High Branched Chain[c] (powder)	0	24.87 (free amino acids)	0	3.9/g		No		Use only for modular tube feeding; 44% branched-chain amino acids.

ProMix[d] (powder)	1.39	20.85 (whey protein)	1.1	3.52/g	No		Add to liquids; no vitamins.
ProMod[e] (powder)	2.4	18.9 (whey protein)	2	4.3/g	0.4/5 g protein		Add to liquids; unflavored.
Pro-pac[f] (powder)	1.25	19.2 (whey protein)	20	4/g	Yes		Add to liquids; no vitamins.
Carbohydrate sources							
Cal-Power[c] (liquid)	27.2 (deionized corn syrup)	0.06	0	1.8/ml	No		For oral or tube feeding; 550 g gives 1,000 kcal; 30 mg Na and 3 mg K/8 fl. oz.; high osmolality.
Controlyte[g] (powder)	14.3 (cornstarch hydrolysate)	Trace	4.8 (soy oil)	2.0/ml 5.0/g	No	598	Low	For oral or tube feeding; add to liquid or food; high osmolality; 198 g gives 1,000 kcal; 60 mg Na and 16 mg K/14-oz. can.
Hy-Cal[h] (liquid)	24.41	0.01	0.01	2.5/ml	No	2,781	Low	Oral supplement; 16 mg Na and 0.7 mg K/4 oz.; 407 ml gives 1,000 kcal.

(continued)

[a] Mead Johnson Nutritional
[b] Scientific Hospital Supplies
[c] Sandoz
[d] Navaco Laboratories
[e] Ross Laboratories
[f] Sherwood Medical
[g] Kendall McGaw
[h] Beecham Laboratories
[i] O'Brien/KMI
[j] Wyeth

Note: The composition of these products changes frequently. Current product literature should be consulted before use. This table is not intended to be comprehensive.

Table G-2. (Continued)

Product (form)	Composition (source)			Caloric Density	Osmolality (mOsm/kg)	Lactose	Residue	Notes
	Carbohydrate (g/100 kcal)	Protein (g/100 kcal)	Lipid (g/100 kcal)					
L. C. Liquid Carbohydrate Supplement[d]	25 (glucose polymers)	0	0	2.5/ml				
Liquid Maxijul[b] (liquid)	26.7 (maltodextrins)	0	0	1.87/ml	400	No	Low	55% Maxijul powder in water; 23 mg Na and 0.42 mg K/dl.
Maxijul[b] (powder)	25.6 (maltodextrins)	0	0	3.75/g	525 in 40% solution	No	Low	Oral use; 46 mg Na and 3.9 mg K/100 g.
Maxijul LE[b] (powder)	25.6 (maltodextrins)	0	0	3.75/g	525 in 40% solution	No	Low	Oral use; 0.23 mg Na and 0.4 mg K/100 g.
Pure Carbohydrate Supplement[d] (powder)	25 (glucose polymers)	0	0	4/g	131 at usual dilution	No	Low	
Moducal[a] (liquid or powder)	25 (maltodextrins)	0	0	2/ml 3.8/g	725 (liquid) 206/60 g in 250 ml water	No	Low	
Nutrisource Carbohydrate[c] (liquid)	25 (deionized corn syrup solids)	0	0	3.2/ml		No	Low	For modular tube feeding only.
Pedialyte[e]	25	0	0	0.2/ml				Calorie and electrolyte source.
Polycose[e] (liquid or powder)	25 (hydrolyzed cornstarch)	0	0	2.8/ml 3.8/g	570	No	Low	100 g powder contains 380 kcal, 110 mg Na, and 10 mg K; 100 ml liquid contains 200 kcal, 70

Product								Comments
Sumacal[f] (liquid or powder)	25 (maltodextrins)	0	0	3.8/g	680	No	Low	150 mg Na and 40 mg K/12-oz. bottle.
Sumacal Plus[f] (powder)	3.2	0	0	2.5/g	890	No	Low	Low electrolyte.
Lipid sources Calogen[b] (liquid)	0	0	11.1 (Arachis oil)	4.5/ml		No	Low	Long-chain triglycerides; 77% linoleate; 20.7 mg Na and 19.6 mg K/100 ml.
High Fat Supplement[i] (powder)	6.5	0.75	7.7 (Partly hydrogenated corn oil)	6.12/g				
MCT Oil[a] (liquid)	0	0	12.05 (Coconut oil fraction)	8.3/ml	Negligible	No	Low	Oral supplement; 60% C_8 and 24% C_{10} fatty acids; 120.5 g gives 1,000 kcal; low electrolytes.
Microlipid[f] (liquid)	0	0	11.11 (Soy, corn, or safflower oil)	4.5/ml	80	No	Low	Oral supplement; P:S = 7.3:1; 73.7% linoleate; low electrolyte.
Nutrisource Lipid Long Chain Triglycerides[c] (liquid)	0	0	11.1 (Soy oil)	2.16/ml		No	Low	For modular tube feeding only; P:S = 2.4:1; 49% linoleate; electrolyte-free.
Nutrisource Lipid Medium Chain Triglycerides[c] (liquid)	0	0	11.9 (Coconut oil)	2.11/ml		No	Low	For modular tube feeding only; linoleate-free; electrolyte-free; 2 g LCT + 22 g MCT/100 ml.

(continued)

Table G-2. (Continued)

Product (form)	Composition (source)			Caloric Density	Osmolality (mOsm/kg)	Lactose	Residue	Notes
	Carbohydrate (g/100 kcal)	Protein (g/100 kcal)	Lipid (g/100 kcal)					
Electrolyte sources								
Lytren[a] (powder)	25.3	0	0	0.333/g	290	No	Low	Electrolyte source (mEq/L): Na, 30; K, 25; Ca, 4; Mg, 4; citrate, 36; SO$_4$, 4; Cl, 25; PO$_4$, 5.
Reosol[i]	25	0	24 g/dl		290	No	Low	Electrolyte source (mEq/L): Na, 50; K, 20; Cl, 50; Ca, 4; Mg, 4; citrate, 34.

Micronutrient sources (see manufacturer's literature for composition)

Product (form)	Notes
Nutrisource Vitamins[c]	Provides 100% of NRC-RDA for essential vitamins in each 10-g packet. For use in modular tube feeding.
Nutrisource Minerals for Protein Formulas[c]	Provides 100% of NRC-RDA for essential minerals in each 24-g packet if used with three packets of Nutrisource Protein; also provides safe levels of trace elements.
Nutrisource Minerals for Protein Formulas, Electrolyte Restricted[c]	Is essentially sodium-, potassium-, and chloride-free. Provides 100% of NRC-RDA of other minerals plus trace elements if used with three packets of Nutrisource Protein.
Nutrisource Minerals for Amino Acid Formulas[c]	Provides 100% of NRC-RDA for essential minerals in each 24-g packet plus trace elements if used with Nutrisource Amino Acids or Amino Acid–High Branched Chain packets.
Nutrisource Minerals for Amino Acid Formulas-Electrolyte Restricted[c]	Is essentially sodium-, potassium-, and chloride-free. Provides 100% of NRC-RDA of other minerals plus trace elements when used with Nutrisource Amino Acids or Amino Acids–High Branched Chain packets.

Other

Product (form)	Carbohydrate (g/100 kcal)	Protein (g/100 kcal)	Caloric Density	Residue	Notes
Fibrad[e] (powder)	(pea, oat, and sugar; beef fiber; xanthan gum)	0	0.56/g	0.78/g	Fiber supplement.

Table G-3. Complete Liquid Formula Diets

Product (form) (kcal to meet vitamin RDA)	Composition (source)			Electrolytes (mEq/dl at usual dilution)		Caloric Density (kcal/ml at usual dilution)	Osmolality (mOsm/kg) (flavors)	Lactose	Residue	Nonprotein kcal:N ratio	Renal solute load (mOsm)	Notes
	Carbohydrate (% of kcal)	Protein (% of kcal)	Lipid (% of kcal)	Na	K							
Hydrolyzed protein-based												
Accupep HPF[a] (powder) (1,600)	75.5 (Maltodextrin)	16 (Whey hydrolysate)	8.5 (MCT; corn oil)	3.0	2.9	1.0	490	0	Low	134:1		
Criticare HN[b] (liquid) (2,000)	83 (Maltodextrin; modified cornstarch)	14 (Hydrolyzed casein, 70% free amino acids; 30% small peptides)	3 (Safflower oil)	2.7	3.4	1.06	650	0	Low	148:1	23/100 kcal	Oral or tube
Elemental 028[c] (powder)	76.5 (Glucose polymer)	10 (Crystalline amino acids)	14.5 (Arachis oil)	2.61	2.39	0.5 at 1:5 dilution	450 at 1:5 dilution (Unflavored); 720 (Orange)	0	Low	220:1		
Isotein HN[d] (powder) (1,776)	52 (Maltodextrin; monosaccharides)	23 (Delactosed lactalbumin)	30 (Corn oil; MCT oil)	2.7	2.7	1.2	300	0		86:1		
Nutramigen[b] (powder)	52 (Sucrose; tapioca starch)	13 (Hydrolyzed casein)	35 (Corn oil)	1.38	1.76	0.68	479	0	Low		13/dl	Oral or tube; infant formula
Nutrex Aminex[e] (powder) (2,100)	82.2 (Maltodextrin; modified cornstarch)	15.3 (Amino acids)	2.5 (Safflower oil)	2.0	2.0	1.0	600 (Unflavored, also vanilla, chocolate, strawberry)	0		149:1		Oral or tube
Peptamer[f] (liquid) (2,000)	51 (Maltodextrins)	16 (Whey hydrolysate: 1% amino acids, 21% small peptides MW < 1000; 50% peptides MW < 5000)	33 (70% MCT; 30% LCT; lecithin and residual milk fat)	2.17	3.2	1.0	260	0	Low	131:1		Tube feeding

(continued)

a Sherwood Medical
b Mead Johnson Nutritional
c Scientific Hospital Supplies
d Sandoz
e Nutrex
f Clintec
g O'Brien/KMI
h Norwich-Eaton Pharmaceuticals
i Ross Laboratories
j Biosearch
k Kendall-McGaw

Note: Current product literature should be consulted before use. This table is not intended to be comprehensive.
C:N ratios are *nonprotein* calories to nitrogen.
MCT = medium-chain triglycerides; LCT = long-chain triglycerides.
BCAA = branched-chain amino acids; AAA = aromatic amino acids; EAA = essential amino acids.
MW = molecular weight.

Table G-3. (Continued)

Product (form) (kcal to meet vitamin RDA)	Composition (source)			Electrolytes (mEq/dl at usual dilution)		Caloric Density (kcal/ml at usual dilution)	Osmolality (mOsm/kg) (flavors)	Lactose	Residue	Nonprotein kcal:N ratio	Renal solute load (mOsm)	Notes
	Carbohydrate (% of kcal)	Protein (% of kcal)	Lipid (% of kcal)	Na	K							
Pepti-2000[a] (powder) (1,600)	75.5 (Maltodextrins)	16 (Hydrolyzed lactalbumin: 15% amino acids, 40% peptides MW < 1000, 30% peptides < 5000)	8.5 (MCT Oil; corn oil; mono- and diglyceride)	2.96	2.95	1.0	490	No	Low	130:1		
Pregestimil[b] (powder)	54 (Corn syrup solids; tapioca starch)	11 (Hydrolyzed casein; amino acids)	35 (Corn oil; MCT)	1.38	1.9	0.65 (infants); 1.5 (adults)	348	0	Low	13/day (infants at 20 kcal/ oz.)		
Reabilan[g] (liquid)	52.5 (Maltodextrins; tapioca)	12.5 (Whey and casein peptides: 8% amino acids, 56% peptides MW < 1000, 30% peptides MW < 5000)	35 (MCT; primrose oil; soy oil; mono- and di-glycerides; lecithin)	3.04	3.2	1.0	350	0	Low	175:1	27.5/dl	
Reabilan HN[g] (liquid)	47.5 (Maltodextrins; tapioca)	17.5 (Whey and casein peptides: 8% amino acids, 56% peptides MW < 1000, 30% peptides MW < 5000)	35 (MCT; primrose oil; soy oil; mono- and di-glycerides; lecithin)	4.34	4.23	1.33	490	0	Low	125:1		
Tolerex[k] (powder) (1,800)	92.4 (Glucose; oligo-saccharides)	8.2 (Crystalline l-amino acids)	1.3 (Safflower oil)	2.04	3.0	1.0	550 (Unflavored), 678 (Beef); 610 (Orange, grape, strawberry)	0	Low	284:1		Oral or tube
Travasorb STD[f] (powder) (2,000)	76 (Glucose; oligosaccharides)	12 (Hydrolyzed lactalbumin)	11 (7% MCT; 4% sunflower oil)	4.0	3.0	1.0	560	0	Low			
Travasorb HN[f] (powder) (2,000)	70 (Glucose oligosaccharide)	18 (Hydrolyzed lactalbumin; l- methionine)	11 (7% MCT; 4% sunflower oil)	4.0	3.0	1.0	560	0	Low			
Vital HN[j] (powder) (1,500)	75 (Hydrolyzed cornstarch)	17 (Partially hydrolyzed whey; meat soy; amino acids)	8 (5% safflower oil; 3% MCT)	1.67	2.98	1.0	460 (Various flavors)	0.8/dl	Low	125:1		
Vivonex HN[h] (powder) (3,000)	81.5 (Glucose oligosaccharide)	17.8 (Amino acids)	0.78 (Safflower oil)	2.3	3.0	1.0	810 (Unflavored); 920 (Beef); 850 (Orange, grape, strawberry)	0	Low	125:1		

Product (kcal)	Carbohydrate (g)	Protein (g)	Fat (g)				Osmolality (flavor)					Comments
Vivonex T.E.N.[h] (powder) (2,000)	82.2 (Maltodextrins; modified starch)	15.3 (Amino acids: 52% essential; 33% BCAA; 6% AAA)	2.5 (Safflower oil)	2.0	2.0	1.0	630 (Vanilla, strawberry, orange-pineapple, lemon-lime)	0	Low	139:1		
Isolates of intact protein												
Attain[a] (liquid) (1,060)	48 (Maltodextrins)	16 (Caseinate)	36 (Corn oil)	3.0	2.9	1.0	300	0	0	131:1		
Attain L.S.[a] (liquid) (1,600)	48 (Maltodextrins)	16 (Caseinate)	36 (Corn oil)	0.9	2.9	1.0	240	0	0	131:1		
Carnation Instant Breakfast[e] (+ 8 oz. milk) (powder) (1,124)	50.2 (Maltodextrins; sucrose; lactose)	22 (Milk; caseinate; whey)	26.3 (Milk fat)	4.3–5.4	5.4–7.91	1.06	671–715	9.51	Low	92:1		
Comply[a] (liquid) (1,500)	48 (Hydrolyzed cornstarch)	16 (Caseinate)	36 (Corn oil)	4.4	4.4	1.5	410/600	0	Low	134:1		
Enrich[i] (liquid) (1,530)	55 (Hydrolyzed cornstarch; sucrose; 13 g soy polysaccharide fiber/ 1,000 kcal)	14.5 (Caseinate; soy isolate)	30.5 (Corn oil)	3.7	4.0	1.1	480 (Vanilla)	0	High	148:1	344	
Ensure[i] (liquid) (2,000)	54.5 (Hydrolyzed cornstarch; sucrose)	14 (Caseinate; soy isolate)	31.5 (Corn oil)	3.5	3.8	1.06	450 (Flavor packets available)	0	Low	153:1		Oral or tube.
Ensure HN[i] (liquid) (1,400)	53.2 (Hydrolyzed cornstarch; sucrose)	16.7 (Caseinate; soy isolate)	30.1 (Corn oil)	3.83	3.8	1.06	470	0	Low	125:1		Oral or tube.
Ensure Plus[i] (liquid) (2,130)	53.3 (Hydrolyzed cornstarch; sucrose)	14.7 (Caseinate; soy isolate)	32 (Corn oil)	3.31	3.96	1.5	600	0	Low	146:1		Oral; tube feeding with caution only.
Ensure Plus HN[i] (liquid) (1,420)	53.3 (Hydrolyzed cornstarch; sucrose)	16.7 (Caseinate; soy isolate)	30 (Corn oil)	3.38	3.06	1.5	650	0	Low	125:1		Oral or tube.
Enteral[e] (liquid) (1,600)	55 (Maltodextrins; sucrose)	15 (Caseinate; soy isolate)	30 (Sunflower oil; MCT; mono- and diglycerides)	3.26		1.06	420	0	Low	140:1		Oral or tube.
Enteral 400[c] (liquid) (1,600)	57.6 (Glucose polymers)	11.6 (Whey isolate)	35.3 (Arachis oil; MCT)	2.7	2.99	1.00	330 at 1:4 dilution	Low		193:1		Oral or tube.
Entralife[e] (liquid) (1,250)	54.6 (Hydrolyzed cornstarch)	15 (Whey concentrate; soy protein)	31.4 (⅓ corn oil; ⅔ soy oil)	2.61	2.59	1.00	300	0		144:1		
Entralife HN[k] (liquid) (1,250)	52.9 (Maltodextrins)	16.7 (Caseinate)	30.4 (⅓ corn oil; ⅔ soy oil)	4.01	3.20	1.0	300 (Vanilla)	0	Low	125:1		
Entrition[l] (liquid) (2,000)	54.5 (Maltodextrins)	14 (Caseinate)	31.5 (Corn oil)	3.05	3.07	1.0	300	0	Low	154:1		Also available at ½ strength.
Entrition HN[l] (liquid) (1,300)	45.6 (Maltodextrins)	17.6 (Caseinate; soy isolate)	36.8 (Corn oil)	3.67	4.05	1.0	300	0	Low	117:1		
Introlite (powder) (1,321)	53.3 (Hydrolyzed cornstarch)	16.7 (Caseinates; soy isolate)	30 (MCT; corn oil; soy oil)	4.0	4.0	0.53		0	Low			
Isocal[b] (liquid) (2,000)	50 (Maltodextrins)	13 (Caseinate; soy isolate)	37 (Soy oil; MCT)	2.3	3.4	1.06	300	0	Low	167:1	210/ quart	

(continued)

Table G-3. (Continued)

Product (form) (kcal to meet vitamin RDA)	Composition (source) Carbohydrate (% of kcal)	Protein (% of kcal)	Lipid (% of kcal)	Electrolytes (mEq/dl at usual dilution) Na	K	Caloric Density (kcal/ml at usual dilution)	Osmolality (mOsm/kg) (flavors)	Lactose	Residue	Nonprotein kcal:N ratio	Renal solute load (mOsm)	Notes
Isocal HCN[b] (liquid) (2,000)	47 (Maltodextrins)	15 (Caseinate; soy isolate)	40 (28% soy oil, 12% MCT)	3.5	3.6	1.06	690	0	Low	125:1	383/ quart	
Isocal HN[b] (liquid) (1,250)	47 (Maltodextrins)	17 (Caseinate; soy isolate)	36 (Soy oil; MCT)	3.5	2.7	1.06	300	0	Low	125:1		
Isolife[a] (liquid) (2,000)	55 (Hydrolyzed cornstarch)	15 (Whey protein concentrate; soy protein)	30 (Corn oil; MCT)	3.13	2.56	1.0	300	0	Low	144:1		
Isosource[c] (liquid) (1,875)	56 (Maltodextrins)	14 (Caseinate)	30 (½ corn oil, ½ MCT)	0.78	4.3	1.25	300	0	Low	155:1		Tube or oral.
Isosource HN[c] (1,920)	53.3 (Maltodextrins)	17 (Caseinate)	30 (½ corn oil, ½ MCT)	0.78	4.3	1.28	300 (Vanilla)	0	Low	125:1		Tube or oral.
Isotein HN[c] (powder) (1,770)	52 (Maltodextrins; monosaccharides)	23 (Delactosed lactalbumin, casein)	25 (Soy oil, MCT)	2.7	2.74	1.2	300	0	Low	86:1		
Jevity[f] (liquid) (1,400)	53.3 (Hydrolyzed cornstarch; 13 g soy polysaccharide fiber/1,000 kcal)	16.7 (Caseinate)	30 (40% corn oil; 10% soy oil; 50% MCT)	4.05	4.02	1.06	310	0		125:1	374/L	Added fiber; use 10F tube or larger if gravity-fed.
Magnacal[a] (liquid) (2,000)	50 (Maltodextrins; sucrose)	14 (Caseinate)	36 (Soy oil)	4.3	3.2	2.0	590	0	Low	157:1		Oral or tube.
Meritene[c] (liquid) (1,200)	46 (Lactose; corn syrup solids; sucrose)	24 (Nonfat milk)	30 (Corn oil)	3.83	4.1	0.96	505 (Vanilla)	5.7	Low	79:1		Oral or tube.
Meritene[c] (powder) (1,100) (prepared with whole milk)	45 (Lactose; sucrose; corn syrup; sucrose)	26 (Casein)	29 (MCT/LCT 24/76; coconut oil, corn oil)	47.8	71.8	1.00	690 (Vanilla, also other flavors)			71:1		Oral or tube.
Newtrition 2.0[f] (liquid) (1,900)	52 (Maltodextrins; sucrose; glucose)	14 (Caseinate; soy isolate)	34 (Corn oil)	2.6	2.6	1.06	450	0		154:1		
Newtrition High Nitrogen[f] (liquid) (1,240)	52 (Maltodextrins)	19 (Caseinate; soy isolate)	29	2.6	2.6	1.24	300	0		104:1		
Newtrition Isotonic (liquid) (1,900)	56 (Maltodextrins)	14 (Caseinate; soy isolate)	30 (MCT; corn oil)	2.6	2.6	1.06	300	0		154:1		
Nutren 1.0[a] (liquid) (2,000)	51 (Maltodextrins; corn syrup; sucrose)	16 (Casein)	33 (MCT/LCT 24/76; corn oil, coconut oil)	2.17	3.2	1.0	300 (Unflavored); 380 (Vanilla, chocolate, strawberry)	0	Low	131:1	242/L	Oral or tube.
Nutren 1.5[a] (liquid) (2,000)	45 (Maltodextrins; corn syrup; sucrose)	16 (Casein)	39 (MCT/LCT 48/52; coconut oil; corn oil)	3.31	4.88	1.5	420 (Unflavored); 600 (Vanilla, chocolate, strawberry)	0	Low	131:1	363/L	Oral or tube.

Nutren 2.0 (liquid) (2,000)	39 (Maltodextrins; corn syrup; sucrose)	16 (Casein)	45 (MCT/LCT 73/27; coconut oil; corn oil)	4.35	6.41	2.0	800 (Vanilla)	0	Low	131:1	484/L	
Nutrex Besure[a] (powder) (1,887)	54.5 (Corn syrup solids; sucrose)	14 (Caseinate; soy isolate)	30 (Soy oil; mono- and diglycerides)	3.7	4.0	1.06	450	0	Low	153:1		
Nutrex Encare[a] (powder) (1,600)	55.6 (Corn syrup solids; sucrose)	14.4 (Egg white solids; caseinate)	30 (Soy oil; lecithin)	0.74	4.4	1.46	460	0	Low	146:1		
Nutrex Encare with Fiber[a] (powder) (1,200)	66 (Corn syrup solids; sucrose)	11 (Egg white solids; caseinate)	23 (Soy oil)	0.74	4.4	1.46	460 (Vanilla, chocolate strawberry)	0	4 g/serving	208:1		For oral feeding, full liquid diet; added fiber.
Nutrex Protamin[a] (powder) (1,180)	60.3 (Corn syrup solids, sucrose)	12.6 (Caseinate)	27.1 (Corn oil, lecithin)	0.74	4.36	1.3	450	0	Low	174:1		
Nutri-Aid[d] (powder) (2,075)	53.7 (Corn syrup solids; sucrose)	14.8 (Caseinate)	31.5 (Corn oil; mono- and diglycerides)	3.04	3.07	1.1	290/L (Vanilla, chocolate, strawberry)	0	Low	167:1		Oral or tube.
Osmolite HN[b] (liquid) (1,400)	53.3 (Hydrolyzed cornstarch)	16.7 (Caseinate; soy isolate)	30 (⅓ soy oil; ⅓ corn oil)	4.05	4.0	1.06	300	0	Low	125:1		Tube feeding.
Pediasure[f] (powder) (1,100)	11 (Hydrolyzed Cornstarch; sucrose)	3 (Caseinate; whey protein concentrate)	5 (50% safflower and 30% soy oil; 20% MCT)			1.00	325	0		20/100 kcal		
Portagen[b] (powder) (960)	45 (Corn syrup solids; sucrose; lactose)	14 (Caseinate)	41 (95% MCT; 5% corn oil)	2.0	3.2	0.68 (infants); 1.0 (adults)	320	0.3/quart	Low	153:1	15/dl	
Pre-Attain[e] (liquid) (800)	48 (Maltodextrins)	16 (Caseinate)	36 (Corn oil)	1.5	1.45	0.5	150	0	Low	134:1		
Precision HN[d] (powder) (1,850)	82.2 (Maltodextrins; sucrose)	16.7 (Lactalbumin; caseinate)	1.1 (Soy oil)	4.26	2.33	1.05	525	0	Low	153:1		
Precision Isotonic[d]	60 (Sucrose; glucose; oligosaccharides)	11.8 (Egg albumin)	1.3 (Soy oil)	1.97	2.46	0.96	300 (Vanilla, orange)	0	Low	239:1		
Precision LR[d] (powder) (1,710)	89.2 (Sucrose; maltodextrins)	9.5 (Egg albumin)	1.3 (Soy oil)	3.04	2.26	1.11	500–545 (Cherry, lemon, lime, orange, vanilla)	0	Low	183:1		Oral or tube.
Profiber[e] (liquid) (1,500)	48 (Hydrolyzed cornstarch)	16 (Caseinate)	36 (Corn oil)	3.2	3.2	1.00	300	0	12/L	134:1		
Renu[e]	50 (Maltodextrins; sucrose)	14 (Soy isolate; caseinate; l-methionine)	36 (Soy oil)	2.2	3.2	1.0	300	0	Low	154:1		Oral or tube.
Replete (liquid) (2,000)	45 (Maltodextrins; sucrose)	25 (Caseinate)	30 (Corn oil)	2.17	4.0	1.0	350	0		75:1		
Resource Instant[d] (crystals) (2,010)	54.5 (Maltodextrins; sucrose)	14 (Caseinate; soy isolate)	32 (Corn oil)	3.68	4.0	1.0	450 (Vanilla, chocolate)	0	Low	153:1		
Resource Plus[d] (liquid) (2,400)	53.31 (Maltodextrins; sucrose)	14.7 (Caseinate; soy isolate)	32 (Corn oil)	3.9	4.5	1.5	600 (Vanilla)	0	Low	146:1		
Sustacal[b] (liquid) (1,080)	55 (Sucrose; corn syrup solids)	24 (Skim milk; caseinate; soy isolate)	21 (Soy oil)	4.1	5.4	1.0	625 (Vanilla); 700 (Chocolate)	0	Low	79:1	364/quart	Oral feeding; tube feed with caution; also available as powder or pudding.

(continued)

Table G-3. (Continued)

Product (form) (kcal to meet vitamin RDA)	Composition (source)			Electrolytes (mEq/dl at usual dilution)		Caloric Density (kcal/ml at usual dilution)	Osmolality (mOsm/kg) (flavors)	Lactose	Residue	Nonprotein kcal:N ratio	Renal solute load (mOsm)	Notes
	Carbohydrate (% of kcal)	Protein (% of kcal)	Lipid (% of kcal)	Na	K							
Sustacal HC[b] (liquid) (1,800)	50 (Corn syrup solids; sucrose)	16 (Caseinate)	34 (Soy oil)	3.7	3.8	1.5	650 (Vanilla; eggnog)	0	Mix with milk	80:1		
Sustacal with fiber[b] (liquid) (1,500)	53 (Maltodextrins; sucrose; soy fiber)	17 (Caseinate; soy isolate)	30 (Soy oil)	3.16	3.58	1.06	450	0	6 g/1,000 kcal	120:1		Oral or tube.
Sustagen[b] (powder) (1,050)	68 (Corn syrup; sucrose lactose)	24 (Caseinate)	8 (Milk fat)	5.5	8.65	1.7	N/A			77:1		
Travasorb MCT[e] (powder) (2,000)	50 (Corn syrup solids)	20 (Lactalbumin; caseinate)	30 (80% MCT; 20% sunflower oil)	1.52	2.56	1.0	312	0	Low	100:1		
Travasorb MCT Liquid Diet[e] (liquid) (1,333)	50 (Maltodextrins)	20 (Lactalbumin; caseinate)	30 (Safflower oil)	2.28	2.56	1.5	420	0		100:1		
TwoCal HN[f] (liquid) (1,600)	43.2 (Hydrolyzed cornstarch; sucrose)	16.7 (Caseinate)	40.1 (Corn oil; MCT)	4.58	5.94	2.0	690	0	Low	125:1		Oral or tube; use 12F tube or higher if gravity-fed.
Blenderized formulas												
Carnacal[b]	48 (Corn syrup solids; green beans; peaches)	16 (Beef, nonfat dry milk; whey; soy isolate)	36 (Soy oil)			1.0	625					
Citrotein[d] (powder) (263 g dry weight)	73 (Maltodextrins; sucrose)	25 (Egg albumin)	2 (Soy oil; mono- and disaccharides)	3.1	1.8	0.66	480–515	0	Low	76:1		Protein supplement to clear liquid diet.
Compleat Regular[d] (liquid) (1,605)	48 (Maltodextrins; lactose; vegetable and fruit puree; orange juice)	16 (Beef, milk)	36 (Corn oil; beef; milk fat)	5.6	3.4	1.07	405	2.4	Moderate	131:1		Tube feeding.
Compleat Modified[d] (liquid) (1,605)	54 (Hydrolyzed cereal; fruit and vegetable puree)	16 (Beef; caseinate)	30 (Corn oil; beef)	2.9	3.6	1.07	300	0	Moderate	131:1		
Vitaneed[d] (liquid) (1,500)	48 (Fruit; vegetable; maltodextrins; soy fiber)	16 (Beef caseinates)	36 (Corn oil)	2.96	3.2	1.0	300	0	8 g/L	134:1		Tube feeding.

Disease-specific formulas

Product	Carbohydrate	Protein	Fat				mOsm (Flavor)		Na	Ratio		Comments
Amin-Aid[m] (powder)	74.8 (Maltodextrins; sucrose)	4.0 (Essential amino acids; histidine)	21.2 (Soy oil)	<1.5	<0.2	2.00	700 (Orange, lemon-lime, berry, strawberry)	0	Low	640:1		Indicated for renal disease; no added vitamins or electrolytes.
Glucerna[l] (liquid) (1,422)	33.3 (Glucose polymers; fructose; soy fiber)	16.7 (Caseinate)	50 (85% safflower oil; 15% soy oil)			1.0	375	0	3.4 g/8 oz.	150:1	36/dl	Indicated for diabetes mellitus.
HepaticAid II[l] (powder)	57.3 (Maltodextrins; sucrose)	15 (Amino acids; 46% BCAA)	27.7 (soy oil; mono- and di-glycerides; lecithin)	<1.5	<0.6	1.2	560	0	Low	340:1		Indicated for hepatic disease; no added vitamins or electrolytes.
Impact[d] (liquid) (1,500)	53 (Hydrolyzed cornstarch)	22 (Caseinate)	25 (Palm oil; sunflower oil; MCT)			1.0	375	0		71:1		Indicated for immune incompetence; added RNA, arginine, omega-3 fatty acids.
Pulmocare[l] (liquid) (1,420)	28.1 (Hydrolyzed cornstarch; sucrose)	16.7 (Caseinate)	55.2 (Corn oil)	5.7	4.88	1.5	490	0	Low	125:1		Indicated for ventilatory dependency; oral or tube; limit to 1.7 × kcal need or less.
Replena[l] (liquid) (960)	51 (Hydrolyzed cornstarch; sucrose)	6 (Caseinate)	43 (90% safflower oil; 10% soy oil)	3.0	2.9	2.0	615 (Vanilla)	0	Low	427:1		Indicated for non-dialyzed renal patients; fortified with carnitine and taurine, oral or tube.
Stresstein[d] (powder) (2,400)	57 (Maltodextrins)	23 (L-amino acids; 44% BCAA)	20 (MCT; soy oil)	2.9	2.87	1.2	910	0	Low	97:1		Indicated for severe metabolic stress.
Traum-Aid[l] (powder) (3,000)	66.4 (Maltodextrins)	22.4 (Amino acids; 50% BCAA)	11.2 (4.5 MCT; 6.7 soy oil)	2.3	3.0	1.0	760 (Grape; lemon cream; berry)	0	Low	102:1		Indicated for metabolic stress.
Traum-Aid HN[l]	71.9 (Maltodextrins; sucrose)	17.3 (Amino acids; 60% BCAA)	10.8 (Soy oil; MCT)	2.3	2.1	1.0	800 (Grape; lemon cream; berry)	0	Low			Indicated for catabolic states.
Traumacal[b] (liquid) (3,000)	38 (Corn syrup solids; sucrose)	22 (Caseinate)	40 (28 soy oil; 12 MCT)	5.2	3.6	1.5	490	0	Low	90:1		125 g BCAA/100 kcal.
Travasorb Hepatic[l] (powder) (2,100)	77.5 (Glucose oligosaccharides; sucrose)	22 (Amino acids; 50% BCAA; low AAA)	11.9 (70% MCT; 30% sunflower oil)	1.01	2.24	1.1	600 (Eggnog; custard; chocolate; apricot; strawberry)	0	Low	211:1		Indicated for hepatic disease.
Travasorb Renal[l] (powder) (2,100)	81.1 (Glucose oligosaccharides; sucrose)	6.9 (Amino acids; includes histidine)	12 (70% MCT; 30% sunflower oil)	0	0	1.4	590 (Apricot; strawberry)	0	No	340:1		Indicated for renal disease; no electrolytes; no fat-soluble vitamins.

Appendix H. Revised Daily Food Guide Food Groups

PROTEIN FOODS

Protein foods include both animal and vegetable foods. Animal protein foods supply protein, iron, riboflavin, niacin, vitamins B_6 and B_{12}, phosphorus, zinc, and iodine. Vegetable protein foods supply folacin, magnesium, and thiamine, in addition to the nutrients just mentioned for animal-protein foods.

Animal-Protein Foods

A serving is 2 oz. (60 g) unless otherwise noted.

Beef (ground, cube, roast, or chop)	
Eggs	2 medium
Fish (fillet or steak)	
Fish sticks	3 sticks
Frankfurters	2
Lamb (ground, cube, roast, or chop)	
Luncheon meat	3 slices
Organ meats: heart, kidney, liver, tongue	
Oysters	8–12 medium
Pork, ham (ground, roast, or chop)	
Poultry: chicken, duck, turkey	
Rabbit	
Sausage links	4 links
Shellfish: crab, lobster, scallops, shrimp	
Spareribs	6 medium ribs
Tuna fish	
Veal (ground, cube, roast, or chop)	

Adapted from "Eating Right for Your Baby," prepared by the California Department of Health Services.

Vegetable-Protein Foods

Beans are the best choice from vegetable-protein foods. A serving of beans contains more vitamins and minerals than a serving of nuts or seeds. A serving is 1 cup cooked unless otherwise stated.

Canned beans (garbanzo, kidney, lima, pork and beans)	
Dried beans and peas	
Nut butters (cashew butter, peanut butter, etc.)	$\frac{1}{4}$ cup (60 ml)
Nuts	$\frac{1}{2}$ cup (120 ml)
Sunflower seeds	$\frac{1}{2}$ cup (120 ml)
Tofu (soybean curd)	

MILK AND MILK PRODUCTS

Milk and milk products are the best food sources of calcium. In addition, these foods supply protein, phosphorus, vitamins A, D, E, B_6, and B_{12}, riboflavin, magnesium, and zinc. For some people, milk and milk products serve as primary sources of protein in the diet.

A serving is 8 oz. (1 cup or 240 cc) unless otherwise noted.

Cheese (except camembert, cream)	1 slice ($1\frac{1}{2}$ oz or 45 g)
Cheese spread	4 Tbsp. (60 ml)
Cocoa made with milk	$1\frac{1}{4}$ cups (10 oz. or 300 ml)
Cottage cheese	$1\frac{1}{3}$ cups (320 ml)
Custard (flan)	
Ice cream	$1\frac{1}{2}$ cups (360 ml)
Ice milk	$1\frac{1}{4}$ cups (10 oz. or 300 ml)

Milk
  Buttermilk
  Chocolate (not
    drink)
  Evaporated   ½ cup (4 oz. or 120
                        ml)
  Goat
  Low-fat
  Nonfat
  Nonfat (made
    from dry milk
    powder)
  Nonfat dry milk   ⅓ cup (80 ml)
    powder
  Whole
  Milkshake
  Pudding
  Soups made with   1½ cups (12 oz. or
    milk   360 ml)
  Yogurt (plain)

BREADS AND CEREALS

Breads and cereals supply thiamine, niacin, riboflavin, iron, phosphorus, and zinc. This food group is divided into two parts: whole-grain items and enriched products. The enriched breads, cereals, and pastas provide significantly lower amounts of magnesium, zinc, and fiber. For this reason, patients should be urged to choose whole-grain products.

Whole-Grain Items

Bread: cracked,   1 slice
  whole wheat, or
  rye
Cereal, hot: ½ cup cooked (120
  oatmeal (rolled   ml)
  oats), rolled
  wheat, cracked
  wheat, wheat
  and malted
  barley
Cereal, ready-to-   ¾ cup (180 ml)
  eat: puffed oats,
  shredded wheat,

wheat flakes,
  granola
Rice (brown)   ½ cup cooked (120
                        ml)
Wheat germ   1 Tbsp. (15 ml)

Enriched Items

Bagel   1 small
Bread (all except   1 slice
  those listed
  above)
Cereal, hot: cream   ½ cup cooked (120
  of wheat, cream   ml)
  of rice, farina,
  cornmeal, grits
Cereal, ready-to-   ¾ cup (180 ml)
  eat (all except
  those listed
  above)
Crackers   4
Macaroni, noodles,   ½ cup cooked (120
  spaghetti   ml)
Pancake, waffle   1 medium (5 inch
                        or 13 cm
                        diameter)
Rice (white)   ½ cup cooked
Roll, biscuit,   1
  muffin,
  dumpling
Tortilla   1 (6 inch or 15 cm
                        diameter)

VITAMIN C–RICH FRUITS AND VEGETABLES

Vitamin C–rich fruits and vegetables supply ascorbic acid. Fresh, frozen, or canned forms may be used although vitamin C content of canned products is lower.

A serving is ¾ cup (180 ml) unless otherwise noted.

Vegetables

Bok choy
Broccoli   1 stalk
Brussels sprouts   3–4

Cabbage
Cauliflower
Chili peppers   ¼ cup
   (green or red)
Greens: collard,
   kale, mustard,
   turnip
Peppers (green or   ½ medium
   red)
Tomatoes   2 medium
Watercress

Fruits

Cantaloupe   ½ medium
Grapefruit   ½ large
Guava   ½ small
Mango   1 medium
Orange   1 medium
Papaya   ½ small
Strawberries
Tangerine   2 large

Juices

Fruit juices and
   drinks with
   vitamin C added
Grapefruit   ½ cup (4 oz. or 120
                          ml)
Orange   ½ cup (4 oz. or 120
                          ml)
Pineapple   1½ cups (12 oz. or
                          360 ml)
Tomato   1½ cups (12 oz. or
                          360 ml)

DARK GREEN VEGETABLES

Dark green vegetables are an excellent source of folacin. In addition, these foods supply vitamins A, E, and B_6, riboflavin, iron, and magnesium. Cooking temperatures destroy folacin, so eat dark green vegetables raw whenever possible.

A serving is 1 cup (240 ml) raw or ¾ cup (180 ml) cooked.

Asparagus
Bok choy
Broccoli
Brussels sprouts
Cabbage
Chicory
Endive
Escarole
Greens: beet, collard, kale, mustard, turnip
Lettuce (dark leafy: red leaf, romaine)
Scallions
Spinach
Swiss chard
Watercress

OTHER FRUITS AND VEGETABLES

Other fruits and vegetables include yellow fruits and vegetables that supply significant amounts of vitamin A. Other fruits and vegetables also contribute varying amounts of B complex vitamins, vitamin E, magnesium, zinc, phosphorus, and also fiber. A serving is ½ cup (120 ml) unless otherwise noted.

Fruits

Apple   1 medium
Apricot   2 medium
Banana   1 small
Berries
Cherries
Dates   5
Figs   2 large
Fruit cocktail
Grapes
Kumquats   3
Nectarine   2 medium
Peach   1 medium
Pear   1 medium
Persimmon   1 small
Pineapple
Plums   2 medium

Prunes   4 medium
Pumpkin $\frac{1}{4}$ cup (60 ml)
Raisins
Watermelon

Vegetables

Artichoke   1 medium
Bamboo shoots
Beans (green, wax)
Bean sprouts
Beet
Burdock root
Carrot
Cauliflower
Celery
Corn
Cucumber

Eggplant
Hominy
Lettuce (head,
   Boston, bibb)
Mushrooms
Nori seaweed
Onion
Parsnip
Peas
Pea pods
Potato   1 medium
Radishes
Summer squash
Sweet potato   1 medium
Winter squash
Yam   1 medium
Zucchini

Appendix I. Age-Specific Lipid Values

Table I-1. Normal Value (mg/dl) for Blood Lipids in White Males

Age (years)	Total Cholesterol				Total Triglycerides				LDL Cholesterol				HDL Cholesterol			
		Percentiles				Percentiles				Percentiles				Percentiles		
	Mean	5	50	95	Mean	5	50	95	Mean	5	50	95	Mean	5	50	95
0–4	155	114	151	203	56	29	51	99	—	—	—	—	55.5	38	54	74
5–9	160	121	159	203	56	30	51	101	93	63	90	129	55.0	37	55	74
10–14	158	119	155	202	66	32	59	125	97	64	94	132	46.0	30	46	63
15–19	150	113	146	197	78	37	69	148	94	62	93	130	45.0	30	45	63
20–24	167	124	165	218	100	44	86	201	103	66	101	147	45.0	31	44	63
25–29	182	133	178	244	116	46	95	249	117	70	116	165	45.5	28	45	63
30–34	192	138	190	254	128	50	104	266	126	78	124	185	43.0	29	43	62
35–39	201	146	197	270	145	54	113	321	133	81	131	189	44.0	27	43	67
40–44	207	151	203	268	151	55	122	320	136	87	135	186	45.0	30	45	64
45–49	212	158	210	276	152	58	124	327	144	98	141	202	44.0	28	44	63
50–54	213	158	210	277	152	58	124	320	142	89	143	197	48.0	28	46	71
55–59	214	156	212	276	141	58	119	286	146	88	145	203	51.5	30	49	74
60–64	213	159	210	276	142	58	119	291	146	83	143	210	51.0	30	49	78
65–69	213	158	210	274	137	57	113	267	150	98	146	210	50.0	31	48	75
70+	207	151	205	270	130	58	111	258	143	88	142	186				

Adapted from U.S. Department of Health and Human Services, Public Health Service, National Institute of Health, Lipid Metabolism Branch, NHBLI; Lipid Research Clinic, Population Studies Data Book, vol. 1. Bethesda, Md.: NIH Publication No. 80–1527, 1980.

Table 1-2. Normal Value (mg/dl) for Blood Lipids in White Females (non-sex-hormone users)

Age (years)	Total Cholesterol				Total Triglycerides				LDL Cholesterol				HDL Cholesterol			
		Percentiles				Percentiles				Percentiles				Percentiles		
	Mean	5	50	95	Mean	5	50	95	Mean	5	50	95	Mean	5	50	95
0–4	156	112	156	200	64	34	59	112	—	—	—	—	53.0	36	52	73
5–9	164	126	163	205	60	32	55	105	100	68	98	140	52.0	37	52	70
10–14	160	124	158	201	75	37	70	131	97	68	94	136	52.0	35	51	73
15–19	157	120	154	200	72	39	66	124	95	60	93	135	52.0	—	50	—
20–24	164	122	160	216	72	36	64	131	98	—	98	—	56.0	37	55	81
25–29	171	128	168	222	75	37	65	145	106	70	103	151	55.0	38	55	75
30–34	175	130	172	231	79	39	69	151	109	67	108	150	55.0	34	52	82
35–39	184	140	182	242	86	40	73	176	119	76	116	172	57.0	33	55	87
40–44	194	147	191	252	98	45	82	191	125	77	120	174	58.0	33	56	86
45–49	203	152	199	265	105	46	87	214	130	80	127	187	60.0	37	59	89
50–54	218	162	215	285	115	52	97	233	146	90	141	215	59.0	36	58	86
55–59	231	173	228	300	125	55	106	262	152	95	148	213	62.0	36	60	91
60–64	231	172	228	297	127	56	105	239	156	100	151	234	60.5	34	60	89
65–69	233	171	229	303	131	60	112	243	162	97	156	223	60.0	33	60	91
70+	228	169	226	289	132	60	111	237	149	96	146	207				

Adapted from U.S. Department of Health and Human Services, Public Health Service, National Institutes of Health, Lipid Metabolism Branch, NHBLI; Lipid Research Clinic, *Population Studies Data Book*, vol. 1. Bethesda, Md.: NIH Publication No. 80–1527, 1980.

Appendix J. Exchange Lists for Protein-, Sodium-, and Potassium-Restricted Diets

Table J-1. *Average Nutrient Values Summarized for Quick Calculations*

Food List	Calories	Protein (g)	Sodium (mg)	Potassium (mg)
High-sodium meat	90	8.0	200	75
Low-sodium meat	60	8.0	30	100
Dairy	Varies	4.0	70	185
Regular bread, cereal, and starch	90	2.0	200	30
Low-sodium bread, cereal, and starch	65	2.0	5	30
Fruit:				
List 1	60	0.5	5	100
List 2	65	0.6	5	175
List 3	70	0.7	5	250
Vegetables:				
List 1	15	1.0	10	100
List 2	20	1.0	20	170
List 3	30	1.0	15	250
List 4	50	2.5	20	Varies

Tables J-1 through J-16 were compiled from *A Guide to Protein Controlled Diets for Dietitians*. Los Angeles: Los Angeles District of the California Dietetic Association, 1977; Department of Nutrition, *Manual of Clinical Dietetics*. Los Angeles: University of California, 1986; and Pemberton, C.M., Moxness, K.E., German, M.J., Nelson, J.K., and Gastineau, C.F., *Mayo Clinic Diet Manual*, 6th ed. Toronto: Decker, 1988.

Table J-2. *High-Sodium Meat List*[a]

Food Item	Measure	Weight (g)
Bacon, cured, cooked	5 slices	25
Beef, kidney, cooked	¼ c.	35
Cheese, natural		
Bleu	1 oz.	28
Cheddar	1 oz.	28
Edam	1 oz.	28
Gruyere	1 oz.	28
Monterey	1 oz.	28
Mozzarella	1 oz.	28
Provolone	1 oz.	28
Swiss	1 oz.	28
Parmesan, grated	3 Tbsp.	15
Cottage, creamed	2 oz. (¼ c.)	56
Cottage, low fat, 2%	2 oz. (¼ c.)	56
Corned beef, canned	1 oz.	28
Egg substitute, frozen (made from egg white, corn oil, and nonfat dry milk)	¼ c.	60
Pork, cured	1 oz.	28
Seafood		
Lobster, northern, fresh	¼ c.	36
Salmon, canned, drain	¼ c.	55
Sardines, 8/can, drain	1 oz. or 2 medium	28
Tuna, canned, drain	¼ c.	40

[a] Averages: calories, 90; protein, 8.0 g; sodium, 200 mg; potassium, 75 mg.

Table J-3. Low-Sodium Meat List (cooked without salt)[a]

Food Item	Measure	Weight (g)
Beef, lamb, pork, veal, game	1 oz.	28
Cheese		
Low-Na cheddar, Cellu	1 oz.	28
Low-Na colby, Cellu	1 oz.	28
Low-Na cottage	¼ c.	60
Poultry, without skin	1 oz.	28
Egg, chicken, raw	1 whole	50
Organ meats		
Beef heart, liver, tripe	1 oz.	28
Beef tongue	1 oz.	30
Calf liver	1 oz.	28
Chicken or turkey gizzard	¼ c.	36
Chicken liver	1 liver	25
Rabbit	1 oz.	28
Seafood		
Fresh or unsalted waterpacked (catfish, freshwater; cod; halibut; sole; flounder; perch, Atlantic; red snapper; salmon, fresh)	1 oz	28
Salmon, canned, low-Na	1 oz.	28
Tuna, canned, low-Na	¼ c.	40
Shellfish		
Clams	¼ c. or 4–5 small	57
Oysters	⅓ c. or 3–4 small	80
Shrimp	1 oz.	28

[a] Averages: calories, 60; protein, 8.0 g; sodium, 30 mg; potassium, 100 mg.

Table J-4. Dairy List[a]

Food Item	Measure	Weight (g)	kcal
Cream, half and half	½ c.	120	158
Cream, light whipping	¾ c.	180	524
Cream, heavy whipping	¾ c.	180	616
Ice cream, (10% fat) plain	¾ c.	100	202
Ice cream, (16% fat) rich	¾ c.	110	262
Ice milk, vanilla, hardened	¾ c.	100	138
Milk:			
Whole (3.3% fat)	½ c.	122	75
Low-fat (2% fat)	½ c.	122	60
Nonfat (skim)	½ c.	122	43
Evaporated, whole, canned	¼ c.	63	84
Chocolate, whole	½ c.	125	104
Chocolate, low-fat (2%)	½ c.	125	90
Special Milks			
Buttermilk, cultured	½ c.	122	50
Cocoa, hot, homemade with whole milk	½ c.	125	109
Dry, nonfat milk	2 Tbsp.	15	54
Dry, whole milk	2 Tbsp.	16	80
Goat's milk	½ c.	122	84
Low-fat milk, protein fortified	½ c.	123	68
Nonfat milk, protein fortified	½ c.	123	50
Low-sodium milk	½ c.	122	74
Yogurt, plain, low-fat	½ c.	133	72
Yogurt, fruited, low-fat	½ c.	113	116

[a] Averages: protein, 4.0 g; sodium, 70 mg; potassium, 185 mg.

Table J-5. Regular Bread, Cereal, and Starch List[a]

Food Item	Measure	Weight (g)
Breads and crackers		
Animal crackers, plain	10 crackers	26
Baking powder biscuit	average 1–2-in. diameter	28
Bread crumbs, dry	3 Tbsp.	19
Cracked-wheat bread	1 slice	25
Doughnut, cake type, plain	1 small	42
Doughnut, yeast raised	1 small	42
French, Italian, or Vienna bread	1 slice	20
Graham cracker, plain	2 squares	14
Hamburger or hot dog bun, enriched, plain	½ large	30
Kaiser roll	½ large	30
Melba toast	4 slices	15
Muffin, plain	1 small	30
Pancakes, homemade	1–4-in. diameter	27
Pancake from mix	1–4-in. diameter	27
Parkerhouse roll	2-in. roll	28
Rye bread, American	1 slice	25
Sugar wafers	5 wafers	48
Vanilla wafers	10 wafers	40
White bread, enriched	1 slice	25
Cooked cereals (cooked with salt as directed on package)		
Cornmeal, cooked	½ c.	120
Cream of Rice, cooked	½ c.	122
Farina (Cream of Wheat), cooked	½ c.	122
Hominy grits, cooked	½ c.	122
Malt-O-Meal, cooked	½ c.	120
Oatmeal, cooked	½ c.	120
Dry cereals		
Cheerios	½ c.	12
Cocoa Krispies	1 c.	28
Corn Chex	¾ c.	20
Cornflakes	1 c.	21
Frosted Flakes	¾ c.	28
Honeycomb	1 c.	28
Kix	1 c.	25
Product 19	¾ c.	21
Rice Chex	1 c.	25
Rice Krispies	¾ c.	21
Wheaties	½ c.	14
Starches (cooked with salt as directed on package)		
Macaroni, enriched, cooked	⅓ c.	47
Noodles, enriched, cooked	⅓ c.	53
Rice, white, cooked	½ c.	102
Rice, instant, cooked	½ c.	82
Spaghetti, enriched, cooked	⅓ c.	47

[a] Averages: calories, 90; protein, 2.0 g; sodium, 200 mg; potassium, 30 mg.

Table J-6. Low-Sodium Bread, Cereal, and Starch List[a]

Food Item	Measure	Weight (g)	Food Item	Measure	Weight (g)
Breads and crackers (low-protein breads are in the free list)			Malt-O-Meal, cooked	½ c.	120
			Oatmeal, cooked	½ c.	120
Low-Na crackers, Cellu	4 small	20	*Dry cereals*		
			Frosted Mini Wheats	3 biscuits	21
Low-Na melba toast, cellu	4 slices	20	Puffed Rice	1 c.	15
			Puffed Wheat	1 c.	15
Low-Na rice wafers, Cellu	4 wafers	20	Shredded Wheat, miniatures	⅓ c.	16
Low-Na white bread, average	1 slice	25	*Starches*		
Regular corn tortilla	1–6-in. diameter	30	All-purpose flour, unsifted	2 Tbsp.	17
Regular matzo cracker	1–6-in. diameter	20	Macaroni, enriched, cooked	⅓ c.	47
Venus Wheat wafers	4 small	30	Noodles, enriched, cooked	⅓ c.	53
Cooked cereals			Popcorn, plain, popped with oil, no salt	1 c.	6–12
Cornmeal, cooked	½ c.	120			
Cream of Rice, cooked	½ c.	122	Rice, white, cooked	½ c.	102
Farina (Cream of Wheat)	½ c.	122	Spaghetti, enriched, cooked	⅓ c.	47
Hominy grits, cooked	½ c.	122			

[a] Averages: calories, 65; protein, 2.0 g; sodium, 5 mg; potassium, 30 mg.

Table J-7. Vegetable List 1[a]

Food Item	Measure	Weight (g)
Asparagus, fresh, cooked	4 medium spears	60
Asparagus, canned, low Na	⅓ c.	79
Asparagus, frozen, cooked	3 medium spears	45
Bean snaps, wax, fresh, cooked	½ c.	65
Beans, frozen, French cut, cooked, drained	½ c.	65
Beans, green, low Na, canned, drained	½ c.	65
Cucumber, raw, pared	10 slices, ¼-in. thick	70
Cabbage, raw, shredded	½ c.	45
Cabbage, cooked, shredded	½ c.	72
Cabbage, red, raw, shredded	½ c.	45
Cabbage, Chinese, raw, cut 1-in. pieces	½ c.	37
Carrots, canned, low Na, drained	½ c.	77
Cauliflower, fresh, cooked	½ c.	68
Endive, raw, chopped	½ c.	25
Lettuce, all varieties, chopped	½ c.	27
Mustard greens, frozen, cooked	½ c.	75
Onion, raw, sliced	½ c.	58
Onion, cooked, sliced	½ c.	105
Onion, green, chopped, bulb and top	½ c.	50
Pepper, sweet green, cooked, 2¾ × 2½ in.	1 whole	73

[a] Averages: calories, 15; protein, 1.0 g; sodium, 10 mg; potassium, 100 mg.

Table J-8. Vegetable List 2[a]

Food Item	Measure	Weight (g)
Bamboo shoots, raw	¼ c.	33
Beets, fresh slices, cooked	½ c.	85
Beets, canned, low Na	½ c.	123
Carrots, fresh, sliced, cooked	½ c.	73
Cauliflower, raw	½ c.	50
Cauliflower, frozen, cooked	½ c.	90
Celery, raw, diced	½ c.	60
Celery, diced, cooked	½ c.	75
Eggplant, diced, cooked	½ c.	100
Mushrooms, raw, sliced	½ c. (3–4 small)	35
Mushrooms, canned, low Na	½ c.	100
Mustard greens, leaves, cooked, drained	½ c.	70
Okra, fresh, cooked, sliced	½ c.	80
Peppers, sweet green, raw 2¾ × 2½ in.	1 whole	90
Radishes, raw	10 medium	50
Rutabagas, sliced, cooked	½ c.	85
Squash, summer, cubes, cooked	½ c.	105
Squash, winter, boiled, mashed	⅓ c.	82
Turnips, cubed, cooked	½ c.	78

[a] Averages: calories, 20; protein, 1.0 g; sodium, 20 mg; potassium, 170 mg.

Table J-9. Vegetable List 3[a]

Food Item	Measure	Weight (g)
Beet greens, cooked	½ c.	73
Carrot, raw	7-in. long	81
Chard, fresh, cooked, leaves and stalks	1½ c.	73
Potato, pared, diced, or sliced	½ c.	78
Pumpkin, boiled	scant ½ c.	100
Squash, winter, baked	¼ c.	51
Tomato, cooked	⅓ c.	80
Tomato, raw, unpeeled	1 small	100
Tomato, canned, low Na	½ c.	120
Tomato catsup, low Na	2 Tbsp.	30
Tomato chili sauce, low Na	2 Tbsp.	30

[a] Averages: calories, 30; protein, 1.0 g; sodium, 15 mg; potassium, 250 mg.

Table J-10. Vegetable List 4[a]

Food Item	Measure	Weight (g)	Potassium (mg)
Artichoke, cooked	1 medium bud	250	301
Broccoli, fresh, cooked, stalk cut ½-in.	½ c.	78	207
Broccoli, frozen, chopped, cooked	½ c.	93	196
Brussels sprouts, fresh, cooked	3 sprouts	63	172
Collard greens, cooked leaves and stems	½ c.	73	170
Collard greens, frozen, chopped	½ c.	85	202
Corn, fresh, cut off cob	½ c.	83	136
Corn, frozen, on cob	½ ear	114	145
Corn, canned, low Na, whole kernel	½ c.	128	124
Peas, canned, low Na	⅓ c.	83	80
Peas, frozen, cooked	⅓ c.	53	72
Peas and carrots, frozen, cooked	½ c.	80	126
Potato, raw or baked	1–2¼-in. diameter	100	391
Spinach leaves, fresh, cooked	½ c.	90	292
Spinach, frozen, chopped, cooked	½ c.	102	341
Sweet potato, baked in skin	5 × 2 in.	146	342
Sweet potato, mashed	½ c.	127	310
Turnip greens, frozen, cooked	½ c.	82	123
Vegetable, mixed, frozen	½ c.	91	174
			205

[a] Averages: calories, 50; protein, 2.5 g; sodium, 20 mg.

Table J-11. Fruit List 1[a]

Food Item	Measure	Weight (g)
Sweetened		
Applesauce, canned	½ c.	128
Blueberries, frozen	¾ c.	172
Boysenberries, frozen	½ c.	72
Figs, canned	2 small	80
Grape juice, frozen (diluted 1:3)	1 c.	250
Grape drink, canned	1 c.	250
Orange/apricot juice drink, canned	½ c.	124
Pear halves, canned	2 small halves	96
Pear nectar, canned	1 c.	250
Pineapple chunks, canned	½ c.	128
Pineapple slices, canned	1 large or 2 small slices	105
Pineapple chunks, frozen	½ c.	122
Pineapple/grapefruit juice drink, canned	½ c.	125
Pineapple/orange juice drink, canned	½ c.	125
Raspberries, red, frozen	½ c.	125
Unsweetened (no sugar added)		
Apple, fresh	1 small, 2¼-in. diameter	115
Apple juice, canned	½ c.	124
Applesauce, canned	½ c.	122
Blackberries, fresh	½ c.	72
Blueberries, fresh	¾ c.	109
Blueberries, frozen	¾ c.	124
Boysenberries, fresh	½ c.	72
Boysenberries, canned	½ c.	122
Boysenberries, frozen	½ c.	63
Cherries, sweet, fresh	8 large	60
Cherries, sour, fresh	8 large	57

(continued)

Table J-11. (Continued)

Food Item	Measure	Weight (g)
Coconut, fresh	1 piece, 2 × 2 × ½ in.	45
Coconut, fresh, grated	½ c.	40
Cranberries, fresh	1 c.	95
Figs, fresh	1 medium (2-in. diameter).	50
Figs, canned	2 small	76
Loganberries, fresh	½ c.	72
Orange, fresh	½ small (2½-in. diameter)	66
Pear, Bartlett, fresh	½ large (2½-in. diameter)	90
Pear, D'Anjou, fresh	½ large (3-in. diameter)	110
Pear halves, canned	2 small	90
Persimmon, native, fresh	1 small	30
Pineapple, fresh, diced	½ c.	78
Pineapple chunks, canned	½ c.	123
Plums, Japanese, fresh	1 medium (2-in. diameter)	70
Prunes, dried	2 medium	15
Raspberries, red, fresh	½ c.	62
Strawberries, fresh	6 large	60
Tangerine, fresh	1 medium (2½-in. diameter)	116
Watermelon, fresh	½ c.	80

[a] Averages: calories, 60; protein, 0.5 g; sodium, 5 mg; potassium, 100 mg.

Table J-12. Fruit List 2[a]

Food Item	Measure	Weight (g)
Sweetened		
Apricot nectar, canned	½ c.	126
Blackberries, canned	½ c.	128
Cherries, sweet, canned	½ c.	140
Figs, canned	4 small	113
Fruit cocktail, canned	½ c.	128
Fruit salad, canned	½ c.	128
Grapefruit sections, canned	½ c.	127
Grapefruit juice, canned	½ c.	125
Grapes, canned, seedless	½ c.	128
Peach halves, canned	2 medium halves	162
Peach slices, frozen	½ c.	125
Peach nectar, canned	1 c.	248
Plums, purple, canned	3 large	140
Strawberries, frozen slices	½ c.	128
Unsweetened (no sugar added)		
Apricots, fresh	2 medium	76
Banana, fresh	3-in. piece	75
Blackberries, canned	½ c.	122
Blackberry juice, canned	½ c.	122
Cherries, sour, canned	½ c.	122
Cherries, sweet, canned	½ c.	135
Dates	4 medium	32
Figs, fresh	2 medium (2-in. diameter)	100
Figs, canned	4 small	107
Fruit cocktail, canned	½ c.	122

(continued)

Table J-12. (Continued)

Food Item	Measure	Weight (g)
Fruit salad, canned	½ c.	122
Grapefruit, fresh	½ medium (4-in. diameter)	268
Grapefruit sections, canned	½ c.	122
Grapefruit juice, fresh	½ c.	123
Grapefruit juice, canned	½ c.	124
Grapefruit juice, frozen (diluted 1 : 3)	½ c.	124
Grapes, seedless, fresh	16 or ½ c.	80
Grapes, seeded, fresh	16 or ½ c.	80
Grapes, seedless, canned	½ c.	122
Grape juice, canned	½ c.	126
Nectarine, fresh	½ medium (2½-in. diameter)	75
Orange sections, fresh	½ c.	82
Peach, fresh	1 medium (2½-in. diameter)	115
Peach halves, canned	2 medium halves	154
Pineapple juice, canned	½ c.	125
Pineapple juice, frozen (diluted 1 : 3)	½ c.	125
Plums, Damson, fresh	6 (1-in. diameter)	66
Plums, prune type, fresh	3 (1½-in. diameter)	90
Plums, purple, canned	3 medium	100
Pomegranate, fresh	½ (3½-in. diameter)	138
Prune juice, canned	⅓ c.	85
Raisins, dried	2 Tbsp.	18
Raspberries, red, canned	½ c.	122
Strawberries, canned	½ c.	121

[a] Averages: calories, 65; protein, 0.6 g; sodium, 5 mg; potassium, 175 mg.

Table J-13. Fruit List 3[a]

Food Item	Measure	Weight (g)
Sweetened		
Apricot halves, canned	4 medium halves	110
Apricots, frozen	½ c.	114
Melon balls, frozen (cantaloupe and honeydew)	½ c.	115
Orange juice, canned	½ c.	125
Rhubarb, cooked	½ c.	135
Tangerine juice, canned	½ c.	125
Unsweetened (no sugar added)		
Apple, fresh	1 large (3½-in. diameter)	230
Apple juice, canned	1 c.	248
Apricot halves, canned	4 medium halves	100
Banana, fresh	5-in. piece	100
Melons:		
Cantaloupe, fresh	⅙ (5-in. diameter)	177
Cantaloupe, fresh	12 melon balls	100
Honeydew, fresh	1/12 (6½-in. diameter)	198
Honeydew, fresh	12 melon balls	100
Orange juice, fresh	½ c.	124
Orange juice, canned	½ c.	124
Orange juice, frozen (diluted 1 : 3)	½ c.	124

[a] Averages: calories, 70; protein, 0.7 g; sodium, 5 mg; potassium, 250 mg.

Table J-14. "Protein-Free" List

Food Item	Measure	Weight (g)
Fats—unsalted		
Butter, unsalted	1 Tbsp.	14
Low-Na French dressing, Cellu	1 Tbsp.	14
Lard, regular	1 Tbsp.	14
Margarine, unsalted	1 Tbsp.	14
Vegetable oil	1 Tbsp.	14
Whipping cream, heavy unwhipped	1 Tbsp.	15
Low-protein products		
Arrowroot	1 Tbsp.	8
Cornstarch	¼ c.	32
Wheatstarch cookie, average	1 cookie	30
Low-protein bread, average	1 slice	30
Aproten low-protein products		
Semolino, hot cereal, cooked	½ c.	100
Annellini and Tagliatelle imitation pasta, cooked	½ c.	115
Rigatini imitation pasta, cooked	½ c.	65
Rusks	1 slice	12
Nondairy products		
Coffee-Mate	1 Tbsp.	2
Dessert topping, frozen	¼ c.	19
Dessert topping, powdered	¼ c. prepared	20
Dessert topping, pressurized	¼ c.	18
D'Zerta whipped topping	1 Tbsp.	15
Spices and seasonings		
All dry spices and herbs	Average serving	—
Diazest, Milani (low-Na beef flavoring)	4 drops	—
Garlic, fresh	1 clove	2
Tabasco sauce	½ tsp.	3
Vinegar, distilled	½ c.	120
Sweets		
Cranberry sauce	¼ c.	60
Danish dessert	½ c.	120
Gum drops	3 large	30
Hard candy	1 oz.	30
Honey	1 Tbsp.	20
Jam or preserves	1 Tbsp.	20
Jelly	1 Tbsp.	20
Jelly beans	10 beans	30
Sugar, granulated, white	1 Tbsp.	12
Sugar, powdered, white	1 Tbsp.	8

Table J-15. Miscellaneous List[a]

Food Item	Measure	Weight (g)	Energy (kcal)	Protein (g)	Sodium (mg)	Potassium (mg)
Alcoholic beverages						
Beer, average	8 oz.	240	101	0.7	17	60
Brandy, gin, vodka, rum, whisky (80 proof)	3 oz.	90	194	—	trace	3
Wine, sweet, dessert	4 oz.	120	164	trace	4	92
Wine, sherry	4 oz.	120	164	0.2	4	88
Wine, table, average	4 oz.	120	100	0.4	4	108
Beverages—carbonated						
Bubble Up	8 oz.	240	90	0	33	9
Coca Cola	8 oz.	240	110	0	30	2

(continued)

Table J-15. (Continued)

Food Item	Measure	Weight (g)	Energy (kcal)	Protein (g)	Sodium (mg)	Potassium (mg)
Gingerale	8 oz.	240	85	0	22	9
Hires Root Beer	8 oz.	240	100	0	41	3
Pepsi Cola	8 oz.	240	110	0	28	9
Royal Crown Cola	8 oz.	240	110	0	22	4
Tab, sugar free	8 oz	240	1	0	33	9
Beverages — coffee, tea, bouillon						
Coffee, regular instant	1 level tsp.	0.8	1	trace	1	26
Coffee, freeze dried instant	1 level tsp.	0.9	1	trace	1	29
Coffee, instant, prepared from 2 g powder	6 oz.	180	2	trace	2	65
Coffee, brewed, weak	6 oz.	180	(2)	(trace)	(1)	(112)
Postum	6 oz.	180	36	0.6	4	136
Tea	8 oz.	240	2	0.1	5	60–130
Bouillon, salted	1 cube	4	5	0.8	960	4
Bouillon, salted powder	1 level tsp.	2	2	0.4	480	2
Beverages — fruit drinks						
Awake (imitation orange juice)	4 oz.	124	51	trace	5	41
Cranberry juice cocktail	8 oz.	240	164	0.3	3	25
Grape Tang	8 oz.	240	120	0	110	2
Kool Aid, regular	8 oz.	240	100	0	1	1
Kool Aid, presweetened	8 oz.	240	90	0	1	1
Lemon Tang	8 oz.	240	100	0	30	2
Lemonade, frozen diluted	8 oz.	240	107	0.1	1	40
Limeade, frozen diluted	8 oz.	240	102	0.1	trace	32
Orange Tang	8 oz.	240	100	0	<20	42
Start Instant Breakfast drink	8 oz.	240	100	0	(47)	(47)
Tart Orange Tang	8 oz.	240	120	0	45	trace
Fats – salted						
Butter, salted	1 Tbsp.	15	108	0.1	123	3
Bacon, fried crisp	1 slice	8	43	1.9	77	18
Cream cheese	2 Tbsp.	28	99	2.1	84	34
French dressing	1 Tbsp.	14	66	0.1	219	13
Margarine, salted	1 Tbsp.	14	102	0.1	140	3
Mayonnaise, regular	1 Tbsp.	14	101	0.2	84	5
Mayonnaise, imitation	1 Tbsp.	14	40	0	95	—
Miracle Whip	1 Tbsp.	14	70	0	90	—
Peanut butter, regular	1 Tbsp.	16	94	4.0	97	100
Fats — unsalted						
Low-Na mayonnaise, Cellu	1 Tbsp.	14	100	0	6	26
Peanut Butter, Low-Na Cellu	1 Tbsp.	15	90	4.0	1	(87)
Sour cream	2 Tbsp.	24	52	0.8	34	12
Low-protein products						
Low-Protein baking mix, Paygel	¾ c.	100	410	0.3	55	10
Low-Protein Gelled Dessert, Prono	½ c.	—	55	0	5	77
Wheatstarch, Paygel	3 Tbsp.	25	92	0.1	16	3
Wheatstarch, Cellu	¼ c.	35	125	0.1	12	2
Wheatstarch cookie, Paygel	1 cookie	14	70	0.1	28	11
Nondairy products						
Coffee Rich liquid	¼ c.	60	96	0.2	24	24
Coffee whiteners, liquid (frozen) average	¼ c.	60	80	0.6	48	116
Coffee whiteners, powder, average	2 Tbsp.	12	66	0.6	24	96
Cremora, Borden	2 Tbsp.	12	66	0.6	1	10
Dessert Whip, liquid	¼ c.	60	164	0.6	40	20
Imitation sour cream	¼ c.	56	118	1.4	58	92

(continued)

Table J-15. (Continued)

Food Item	Measure	Weight (g)	Energy (kcal)	Protein (g)	Sodium (mg)	Potassium (mg)
Mocha Mix	¼ c.	60	75	0.2	43	28
Party Pride Whip, liquid	2 Tbsp.	30	99	0.6	13	1
Poly Rich liquid	¼ c.	60	88	0.2	12	40
Rich's Whip Topping, whipped	½ c.	23	63	0	13	trace
Spices, seasonings, and flavorings						
A-1 Sauce	1 Tbsp.	17	12	0.2	275	49
Catsup, regular	2 Tbsp.	30	32	0.6	312	108
Catsup, Low-Na, Featherweight	2 Tbsp.	30	12	1.0	9	224
Chili sauce, regular	2 Tbsp.	30	32	0.8	402	(112)
Chili sauce, Low-Na, Featherweight	2 Tbsp.	30	16	1.0	9	154
Green pepper, chopped	1 Tbsp.	10	2	0.1	2	20
Horseradish, prepared	1 tsp.	5	2	0.1	5	15
Lemon juice, fresh	1 Tbsp.	15	4	0.1	trace	21
Lime juice, fresh	1 Tbsp.	15	4	trace	trace	16
Mustard, regular	1 tsp.	5	4	0.2	63	7
Mustard, Low-Na, Featherweight	1 tsp.	5	4	0.2	1	24
Onion, fresh, chopped	1 Tbsp.	15	4	0.2	1	16
Vinegar, cider	½ c.	120	17	trace	1	120
Worcestershire sauce	1 tsp.	5	4	0.1	105	24
Sweets—chocolate						
Hershey's Chocolate products						
Chocolate Kisses	10 pieces	40	217	3.4	42	150
Chocolate bar, plain	1 oz.	28	152	2.2	30	105
Chocolate bar, almonds	1 oz.	28	142	2.4	10	75
Krackel bar	1 oz.	28	148	2.3	35	85
Mr. Goodbar	1 oz.	28	153	3.9	20	120
Chocolate syrup	1 oz.	28	69	0.7	15	55
Cocoa powder	1 Tbsp.	7	28	1.7	5	90
Chocolate Chips, semisweet	¼ c.	43	216	1.8	1	139
Bitter chocolate squares	1 square	28	142	(1.6)	1	232
Sweets—Other						
Canned cake, Low-Na, Cellu	½ slice	50	191	2.2	8	28
Fruit ice, lime	1 c.	—	247	0.8	trace	6
Gelatin, regular, flavored	½ c.	—	71	1.8	61	—
Gelatin, Low-Na, D'Zerta	½ c.	—	8	2.0	10	50
Honey cake, Holland, Low Na	½ slice	45	132	1.9	15	225
Log Cabin maple-flavored syrup	1 Tbsp.	20	35	0	13	1
Maple syrup, regular	1 Tbsp.	20	50	—	2	35
Marshmallows, white	4 large	30	92	0.4	12	1
Popsicles, Kool Pop	1 bar	36	26	trace	12	trace
Sherbet, orange	½ c.	96	135	1.1	44	99
Sugar, brown, packed	1 Tbsp.	14	52	0	4	47

ª Numbers in parentheses are approximate.

Note: The foods and beverages in the miscellaneous list do not fit into any other group. Averages are not given for this list because the figures vary too much. The items in the miscellaneous list cannot be used freely within the diet.

Table J-16. Low-Sodium Specialty Items

Food Item	Measure	Weight (g)	Energy (kcal)	Protein (g)	Sodium (mg)	Potassium (mg)
Chili con carne, Campbell	½ can	100	155	7.0	30	338
Chili con carne, Featherweight	½ can	120	150	8.5	18	—
Beef ravioli, Featherweight	½ can	120	115	4.0	68	166
Spaghetti with meat balls, Featherweight	½ can	120	110	4.0	28	—

(continued)

Table J-16. (Continued)

Food Item	Measure	Weight (g)	Energy (kcal)	Protein (g)	Sodium (mg)	Potassium (mg)
Beef stew, Featherweight	½ can	120	105	5.5	24	178
Chicken stew, Featherweight	½ can	100	80	4.5	16	95
Lamb stew, Featherweight	½ can	100	115	4.5	23	119
Spanish rice, Featherweight	½ can	100	70	1.5	14	203
Low-sodium soups						
Bouillon, Featherweight, unsalted, beef	1 cube	4	12	0	10	475
Bouillon, Featherweight, unsalted, chicken	1 cube	4	12	0	5	502
Chicken noodle, Featherweight	½ can	120	60	3.0	26	463
Chunky beef, Campbell	½ can	100	90	5.0	35	192
Chunky chicken, Campbell	½ can	100	75	5.0	30	93
Green pea soup, Campbell	½ can	100	65	3.0	20	62
Green pea soup, Featherweight	½ can	120	90	4.0	14	707
Mushroom cream, Campbell	½ can	100	65	trace	15	35
Mushroom cream, Featherweight	½ can	120	60	1.0	30	—
Tomato, Campbell	½ can	100	50	1.0	15	151
Tomato, Featherweight	½ can	120	60	2.0	14	798
Turkey noodle, Campbell	½ can	100	30	1.0	20	24
Vegetable, Campbell	½ can	100	40	1.0	15	84
Vegetable Beef, Campbell	½ can	100	40	2.0	25	72
Vegetable Beef, Featherweight	½ can	120	90	4.0	24	492
Beef soup base, Cellu	1 tsp.	5.3	20	0.5	6	360
Chicken soup base, Cellu	1 tsp.	5.3	25	0.2	1	193

Table J-17. High-Salt Items (400 mg sodium or 1 g salt each)

Food Item	Quantity
Meats and meat substitutes	
Hot dog	1 small
Lunchmeat, except braunschweiger, liverwurst, or salami	1 oz. or 1 slice
Bacon	4 slices
Pork sausage, ham, corned beef	1½ oz.
Tuna, regular, canned	1½ oz.
Salmon, regular, canned	3 oz.
Crab, regular, canned	1½ oz.
Cottage cheese	¾ c.
Cheese	2 oz.
Breads and cereals	
Pretzels, small	20
Pretzels, twisted medium	3
Pretzels, Dutch or soft	1
Vegetables	
Canned vegetables, regular, canned	2 servings
Sauerkraut, regular, canned, drained	⅓ c.
Potato chips	20 (or 1 oz.)
Soups, canned, diluted with equal volume of water	
Beef broth	⅔ c.
Vegetarian vegetable	⅔ c.
Tomato bisque, Manhattan-style clam chowder, tomato rice, tomato, cream of celery, cream of asparagus, chicken gumbo, golden vegetable noodle-O's	½ c.
Cream of mushroom	⅓ c.

(continued)

Table J-17. (Continued)

Food Item	Quantity
Seasonings	
Salt	$\frac{1}{4}$ tsp.
Soy sauce	1 tsp.
Worcestershire sauce	4 tsp.
Catsup	7 tsp.
Mustard, prepared	6 tsp.
Chili sauce	6 tsp.
Barbecue sauce	6 tsp.
Salad dressings	
Tartar sauce or mayonnaise	$4\frac{2}{3}$ Tbsp.
Thousand Island dressing	$\frac{1}{4}$ c.
French dressing	2 Tbsp.
Russian dressing	3 Tbsp.
Italian dressing	4 tsp.
Relishes	
Pickles, dill large	$\frac{1}{2}$
Olives	4 medium, 3 extra large, 2 giant
Pickle relish, sweet	$\frac{1}{4}$ c.

Appendix K. Appropriate Serving Sizes of Usual Foods for Infants and Children

Table K-1. Guidelines for Evaluation of Infant Diets

Age (months)	Mean Weight (kg)	Energy (kcal/kg BW/ 24 hr.)	Fluid (ml/kg BW/ 24 hr.)	Number of Feedings/ 24 hr.	Size of Formula Feeding[b] (oz.)	Solid Foods
0	3.3	115(95–145)	125–145	8+	2½–4	No
1	4.1	115(95–145)	125–145	7–8	3½–5	No
2	5.0	115(95–145)	125–145	6–7	4–6	No
3	5.7	115(95–145)	125–145	4–5	5–7	No
4	6.4	115(95–145)	125–145	4–5	6–8	No
5	7.0	115(95–145)	125–145	4–5	7–8	At 4–6 months or 6–7 kg, begin iron-fortified cereal (rice or mixed grains); teething biscuits.
6	7.5	115(95–145)	125–145	3–4	7–8	At 6–8 months, vegetables (strained/pureed): carrots, squash, beans, peas. At 7–10 months, use chopped foods.
7	8.0	105(80–135)	125–145	3–4	6–8	At 6½–9 months, fruits and juices: applesauce, pears, peaches, banana. At 7–10 months, use chopped foods.
8	8.5	105(80–135)	125–145	3–4	6–8	At 7–10 months, use strained meats, cheese, yogurt, cooked beans, egg yolk.
9	8.9	105(80–135)	125–145	3–4	6–8	At 10–12 months, use table foods: whole egg, orange juice.
10	9.2	105(80–135)	125–145	3–4	6–8	
11	9.6	105(80–135)	125–145	3	7–6	
12	9.9	105(80–135)	125–145	3	7–6	Whole milk.

[a] Mean weight for National Center for Health Statistics 50th percentile.
[b] Breast milk or infant formula during the first 12 months of life; whole cow's milk thereafter.

Table K-2. Guidelines for Evaluation of Diets in Childhood

		Milk or Meat and Meat Alternates					Fruits and Vegetables			Breads and Cereals				
Age (years)	kcal/kg/ day[a]	Equiv- alent	Egg	Meat, Poultry, Fish	Peanut Butter	Legumes	Citrus, Tomatoes	Green or Yellow	Other	Bread	Cold Cereal	Cooked Cereal, Pasta	Butter, Margarine	Desserts, Sweets
1	100	2 c.	1	2 Tbsp.	—	4 Tbsp.	$\frac{1}{4}$ c.	2 Tbsp.	2 Tbsp.	$\frac{1}{2}$ slice	$\frac{1}{2}$ c.	$\frac{1}{4}$ c.	1 Tbsp.	To meet caloric needs
2–3	90	2–3 c.	1	3 Tbsp.	1 Tbsp.	4 Tbsp.	$\frac{1}{2}$ c.	3 Tbsp. (3/week)	3 Tbsp.	1 slice	$\frac{3}{4}$ c.	$\frac{1}{3}$ c.	1 Tbsp.	To meet caloric needs
4–5	75	2–3 c.	1	4–6 Tbsp.	2 Tbsp.	$\frac{1}{2}$ c.	$\frac{1}{2}$ c.	$\frac{1}{4}$ c.	$\frac{1}{2}$ c.	$1\frac{1}{2}$ slices	$\frac{1}{2}$ c.	$\frac{1}{2}$ c.	1 Tbsp.	To meet caloric needs
6–9	60	3–4 c.	1	3–4 oz.	2–3 Tbsp.	$\frac{3}{4}$ c.	1 c.	$\frac{1}{4}$ c.	$\frac{1}{2}$ c.	1–2 slices	$\frac{1}{2}$ c.	$\frac{1}{2}$ c.	2 Tbsp.	To meet caloric needs
10–12	55	4 c.	1	4–5 oz.	3 Tbsp.	1 c.	1 c.	$\frac{1}{3}$ c.	$\frac{1}{2}$ c.	2 slices	$1\frac{1}{2}$ c.	$\frac{3}{4}$ c.	2 Tbsp.	To meet caloric needs

[a] Approximately 1,000 kcal + 100 kcal for each year of age.

Appendix L. Growth and Development Charts for Infants and Children

GIRLS: BIRTH TO 36 MONTHS
PHYSICAL GROWTH
NCHS PERCENTILES*

NAME _____ RECORD # _____

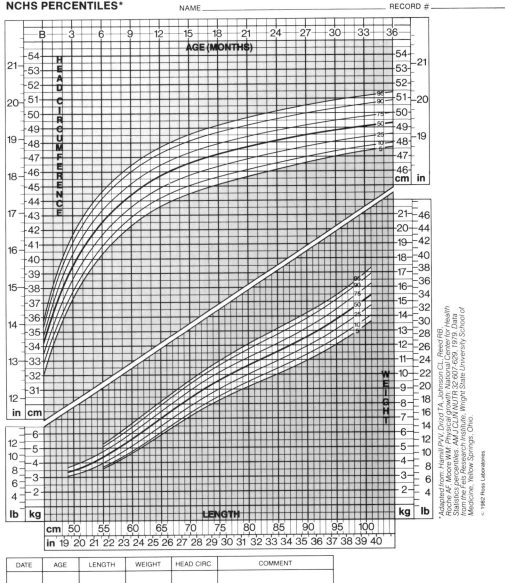

*Adapted from: Hamill PVV, Drizd TA, Johnson CL, Reed RB, Roche AF, Moore WM. Physical growth: National Center for Health Statistics percentiles. AM J CLIN NUTR 32:607-629, 1979. Data from the Fels Research Institute, Wright State University School of Medicine, Yellow Springs, Ohio.

© 1982 Ross Laboratories

DATE	AGE	LENGTH	WEIGHT	HEAD CIRC.	COMMENT

GIRLS: BIRTH TO 36 MONTHS
PHYSICAL GROWTH
NCHS PERCENTILES*

NAME _____   RECORD # _____

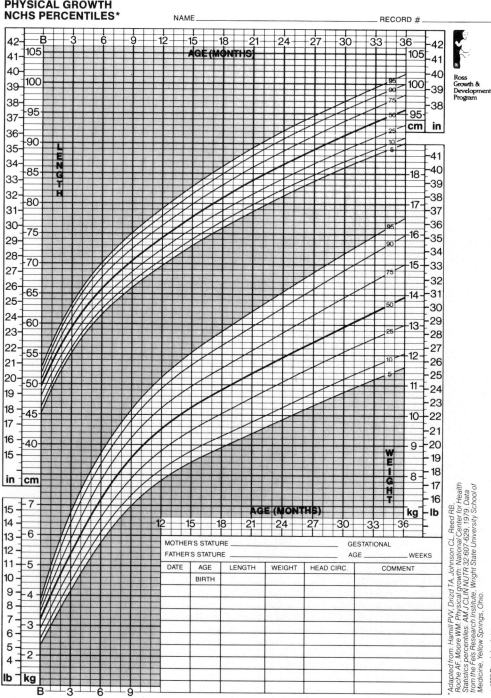

Ross
Growth &
Development
Program

*Adapted from: Hamill PVV, Drizd TA, Johnson CL, Reed RB, Roche AF, Moore WM. Physical growth: National Center for Health Statistics percentiles. AM J CLIN NUTR 32:607-629, 1979. Data from the Fels Research Institute, Wright State University School of Medicine, Yellow Springs, Ohio.

© 1982 Ross Laboratories

MOTHER'S STATURE _____   GESTATIONAL
FATHER'S STATURE _____   AGE _____ WEEKS

DATE	AGE	LENGTH	WEIGHT	HEAD CIRC.	COMMENT
	BIRTH				

BOYS: BIRTH TO 36 MONTHS
PHYSICAL GROWTH
NCHS PERCENTILES*

NAME _____ RECORD # _____

Ross
Growth &
Development
Program

MOTHER'S STATURE _____ GESTATIONAL
FATHER'S STATURE _____ AGE _____ WEEKS

DATE	AGE	LENGTH	WEIGHT	HEAD CIRC.	COMMENT
	BIRTH				

*Adapted from: Hamill PVV, Drizd TA, Johnson CL, Reed RB, Roche AF, Moore WM. Physical growth. National Center for Health Statistics percentiles. AM J CLIN NUTR 32:607–629, 1979. Data from the Fels Research Institute, Wright State University School of Medicine, Yellow Springs, Ohio.

© 1982 Ross Laboratories

BOYS: BIRTH TO 36 MONTHS
PHYSICAL GROWTH
NCHS PERCENTILES*

NAME_____ RECORD #_____

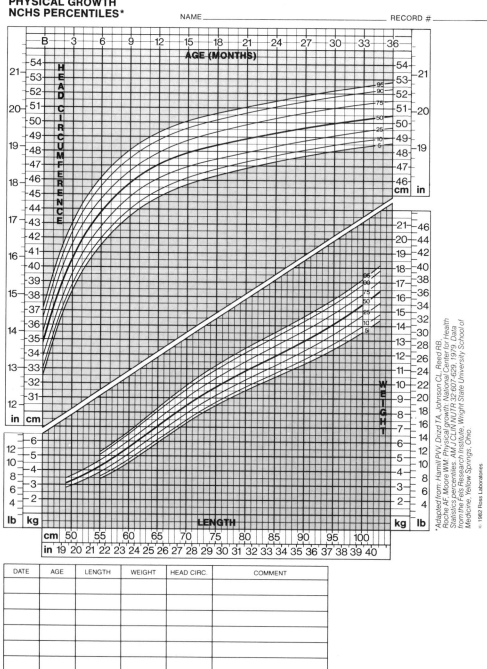

*Adapted from: Hamill PVV, Drizd TA, Johnson CL, Reed RB, Roche AF, Moore WM: Physical growth: National Center for Health Statistics percentiles. AM J CLIN NUTR 32:607-629, 1979. Data from the Fels Research Institute, Wright State University School of Medicine, Yellow Springs, Ohio.

© 1982 Ross Laboratories

DATE	AGE	LENGTH	WEIGHT	HEAD CIRC.	COMMENT

GIRLS: 2 TO 18 YEARS
PHYSICAL GROWTH
NCHS PERCENTILES*

NAME _____ RECORD # _____

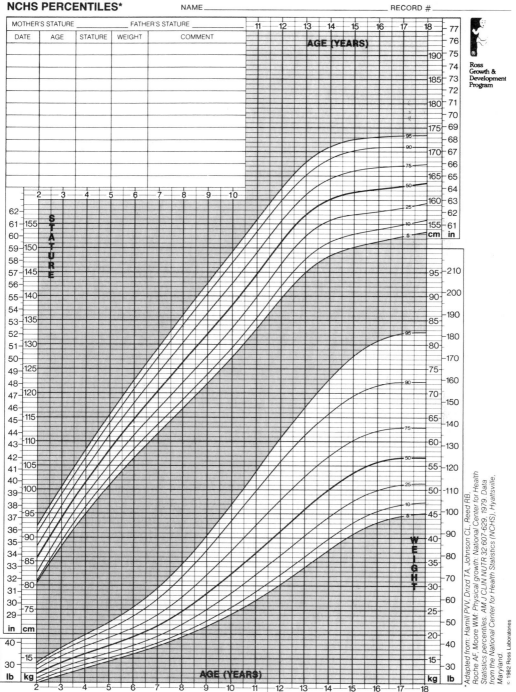

*Adapted from: Hamill PVV, Drizd TA, Johnson CL, Reed RB, Roche AF, Moore WM. Physical growth: National Center for Health Statistics percentiles. AM J CLIN NUTR 32:607-629, 1979. Data from the National Center for Health Statistics (NCHS), Hyattsville, Maryland.

© 1982 Ross Laboratories

Ross
Growth &
Development
Program

GIRLS: PREPUBESCENT
PHYSICAL GROWTH
NCHS PERCENTILES*

NAME _____   RECORD # _____

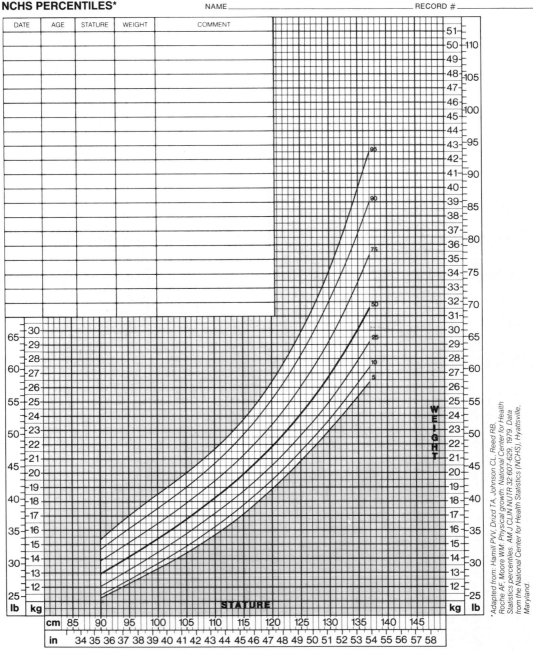

*Adapted from: Hamill PVV, Drizd TA, Johnson CL, Reed RB, Roche AF, Moore WM. Physical growth: National Center for Health Statistics percentiles. AM J CLIN NUTR 32:607-629, 1979. Data from the National Center for Health Statistics (NCHS), Hyattsville, Maryland.

© 1982 Ross Laboratories

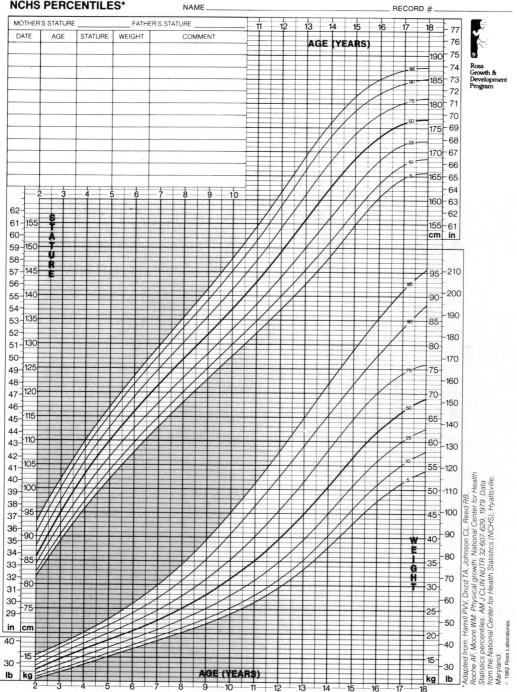

BOYS: 2 TO 18 YEARS
PHYSICAL GROWTH
NCHS PERCENTILES*

NAME_____ RECORD #_____

Ross
Growth &
Development
Program

*Adapted from: Hamill PVV, Drizd TA, Johnson CL, Reed RB,
Roche AF, Moore WM. Physical growth: National Center for Health
Statistics percentiles. AM J CLIN NUTR 32:607-629, 1979. Data
from the National Center for Health Statistics (NCHS), Hyattsville,
Maryland.*

© 1982 Ross Laboratories

BOYS: PREPUBESCENT
PHYSICAL GROWTH
NCHS PERCENTILES*

NAME _____ RECORD # _____

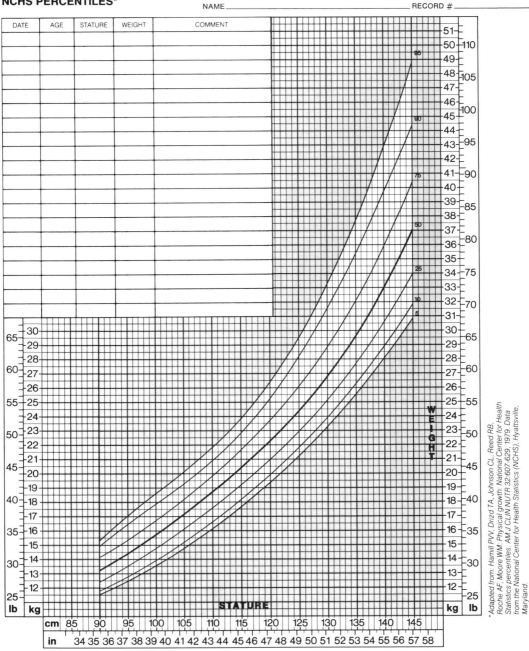

*Adapted from: Hamill PVV, Drizd TA, Johnson CL, Reed RB. Roche AF, Moore WM. Physical growth: National Center for Health Statistics percentiles. AM J CLIN NUTR 32:607-629, 1979. Data from the National Center for Health Statistics (NCHS), Hyattsville, Maryland.

© 1982 Ross Laboratories

Index

A

Abbreviations, in medical records, 753–759
Abdominal-to-gluteal circumference, 481
Abetalipoproteinemia, 255
Absence seizures, 719
Absorption. *See also* Malabsorption
  alcohol, 527
  drugs, 89
  nutrients and drugs, 101–104, 109
  small intestine and, 222–225
Absorptive cells, 219
Acanthocytosis, 255
Accelerated rejection, grafts, 167
Accumulation, degeneration and, 11
Acesulfame-K, diabetic diet, 439
Acetaldehyde, 716
  in ethanol metabolism, 527–529, 530
Acetate, 139
Acetylcholine, production of, 537
Achalasia, 199
Acid, buffering of, 30–31
Acid-base balance
  blood buffers, 30–31
  blood gas analysis, 33
  in diagnosis of diabetes, 419–420
  disturbances of, 29, 31–33
  in hepatic encephalopathy, 542–543
  hydrogen and, 30
  kidneys and, 31
  liver disease and, 539
  normal balance, 29
  peritoneal dialysis and, 310–311
  problems related to, 610
  respiratory system and, 31

Acidosis, 29–30, 240
  in chronic renal failure, 299, 301
  metabolic acidosis, 32–33, 38, 420
  respiratory acidosis, 31
Acinus, 228, 519
Acquired immune deficiency syndrome (AIDS), 161
  nutritional assessment, 258
  nutritional care, 258
  nutritional effects from drugs, 257, 258
  stages of, 256, 258
Acquired immunity, 150
Acrodermatitis enteropathica, 676–677
  characteristics of, 676–677
  diagnosis, 677
  nutritional care, 677
Acromegaly, 402
ACTH (adrenocorticotropic hormone), 354, 462, 559, 738
Active transport, 20, 89, 222
Activity energy expenditure, injury and, 560
Acupuncture, weight reduction and, 498
Acute degeneration, 11
Acute diarrhea, 239
Acute glomerulonephritis, 328–329
Acute inflammation, 10
Acute necrotizing ulcerative gingivitis, 193
Acute pancreatitis, 260
Acute-phase proteins, 158, 159, 558
Acute phase response, 153, 157–158
Acute rejection, grafts, 167
Acute renal failure
  categories of, 323
  causes of, 322–323
  clinical course, 324

fluid/electrolyte balance, control of, 327
  nutritional management, 324–326
  parenteral nutrition, 326–327
  pathogenesis, 323
  pathophysiology, 323–324
  patient monitoring, 326
Acute tubular necrosis, 10, 323
Adaptive thermogenesis, 478
Addison's disease
  hormonal aspects, 461–462
  treatment of, 462
Additives
  anticarcinogenic aspects, 575
  drug interactions, 94
  food hyperactivity and, 171–172
Adenoma, 572
Adenosylcobalamin-dependent methylmalonyl-CoA mutase, 674
Adenyl cyclase, 239–240
Adipomuscular ratio, 485
Adipose cells, 5, 471
  size and metabolism, 486
Adipose index, diagnosis of obesity, 481
Adipose tissue
  dieting and, 487
  functions of, 472–473
  lipase systems, 473
  regulation of food intake, 476
  in starvation, 556
  types of, 471–472
Adiposity, 12
Adipsin, 487
Administration routes, drugs, 88–89
Adrenal corticoids. *See* Corticosteroids; Glucocorticoids; specific hormones
Adrenergic fibers, 476, 536
Adrenergic inhibitors
  hypertension and, 360–361, 362

Adrenergic inhibitors *(continued)*
    types of, 360–361, 362
Adrenocortical dysfunction,
    461–462
    adrenocortical hyperfunction
        (Cushing's disease), 463
    adrenocortical insufficiency
        (Addison's disease),
        461–462
    hormonal treatment, 462
Adrenocorticotropic hormone
    (ACTH), 354
    rheumatoid arthritis, 738
    stress and, 559
    treatment with, 463
Adynamic ileus, 567
Aerobic exercise, hypertension
    and, 356
Aerophagia, 268
Afferent loop, 211
Aflatoxin B$_1$, 575
Age
    cancer and, 577
    drug effects and, 93
    hypertension and, 355
    immunologic deficiency and,
        162
    onset of obesity and, 485–486
    oral cavity changes, 196–197
Agenesis, 7
Agglutination, 154
Air swallowing, 268
Airways, anatomy of, 599–600
Alanine, 127
Albumin
    assessment in renal patients,
        318
    concentration of, 64
Albuminuria, 291
Alcohol
    absorption, 527
    categories of alcoholic
        beverages, 527
    diabetic diet and, 440
    dose-response relationship,
        526–527
    drug interactions and, 113,
        114–115
    excretion, 527
    fat metabolism and,
        374–375
    fetal alcohol syndrome,
        715–716

heart disease and, 393
hyperlipidemia and, 374–375
hypertension and, 355, 359
jejunoileal bypass and, 501
liver synthesis of, 521
metabolism of, 527–529
peptic ulcer disease and, 207–
    208
tolerance to, 529
Alcohol dehydrogenase, 527
Alcoholic cirrhosis, 532,
    545–546
    clinical manifestations of,
        545–546
    etiology of, 545
    nutritional care, 540–541,
        543–545, 546
Alcoholic liver disease, 531–532
    alcoholic cirrhosis, 532,
        545–546
    alcoholic hepatitis, 524, 525,
        532
    nutritional care, 532
    steatosis, 531–532
Alcoholism, 526. *See also*
        Alcoholic liver disease
    alcohol dementia, 732
    cancer and, 576
    cardiovascular disease and,
        393
    congeners in, 531
    food intake and, 530
    hepatocyte injury, mecha-
        nism of, 529–530
    intoxication, effects of, 531
    malabsorption in, 234
    nutrient metabolism and, 98,
        530–531
    nutritional deficiencies,
        530–531
    pancreatic, acute and
        chronic, 260
Aldehyde dehydrogenase, 528
Aldosterone
    Addison's disease and,
        461–462
    arterial blood pressure and,
        350
    Cushing's syndrome and, 462
    functions of, 27
Alimentary hypoglycemia, 212
Alimentary tract, components
    of, 186. *See also* Gastro-

intestinal disorders;
    Gastrointestinal tract
Alkaloids, 575, 583–584
Alkalosis, 29–30
    metabolic alkalosis, 33, 38
    respiratory alkalosis, 31
Alkaptonuria, 641
Alkylating agents, 584
Alleles, 618
Allergen, 164
Allergic rhinitis, 164
Allergy, 162. *See also* Food
        allergy; Hypersensitivity
Alloantigens, 167
Allogeneic, bone marrow
        transplant, 591
Allografts, 167
Alpha-2-globulin, 8
Alpha-agonists, regulation of
        food intake, 476–477
Alpha$_1$ antitrypsin deficiency,
        606
Alpha blockers, 361–362, 476,
        477
    food intake and, 476, 477
    hypertension and, 361–362
Alpha-linolenic acid, 351
Alpha-thalassemia, 697
Alstrom syndrome, 483
Aluminum toxicity, Alzheimer's
        disease, 732
Alveolar ducts, 599–600
Alveolar process, 188
Alveolar sacs, 599
Alveoli, 601
Alzheimer's disease, 731–732
    nutritional care, 732
    progression of, 731, 732
Amenorrhea, in anorexia
        nervosa, 507
Amino acid intake
    in acute renal failure, 326
    in hemodialysis, 306
    injury and, 561
    in jejunoileal bypass, 501
    parenteral feeding and, 135,
        140
    problems in PKU patient,
        638
    in respiratory failure, 610
    tube feeding and, 127
Amino acid metabolism
    cancer and, 579–580

liver disease and, 535, 537–538
liver and, 520–521
Amino acid metabolism disorders, 625–659
 branched-chain ketoaciduria, 644–650
 diagnosis/treatment summary, 660–662
 homocystinuria, 650–656
 isovaleric acidemia, 650
 nutritional care, amino acid administration methods, 625
 phenylketonuria, 625–640
 tyrosinemia, 640–644
 urea cycle disorders, 656–659
Amino acid profile, protein, 126
Amino acids. *See also* Branched-chain amino acids
 aromatic amino acids, 535, 538
 branched-chain type, 521
 cancer and, 580
 in chronic renal failure, 293
 deficiency in PKU patient, 638
 oxidation of, 603
4-aminobutyrate, production of, 537
Aminophylline, 181
5-aminosalicylic acid, 248
Ammonia
 in cirrhosis, 540
 liver disease and, 535–536, 537–538
 urea cycle disorders and, 656, 657, 658
Amniocentesis, 624
Amphetamines
 effects of, 713
 weight reduction and, 496
Amputations, diabetes and, 416
Amylase, serum, 259, 261
Amyloid, 12
Amyloidosis, 12
Amylopectin, 254
Amyotrophic lateral sclerosis, 730–731
 forms of, 730
 nutritional care, 731
 symptoms, 730
Amyotrophy, 417

Anabolism, 557, 558
Anamnestic response, 150
Anaphylactic responses, 164, 171
Anaphylactic shock, 164
Anaplasia, 574
Anasarca, 330
Anastamosis, 205
Anastamotic ulcer, 205
Android, 484
Anemia. *See also* specific types of anemia
 athletic performance and, 699
 chemotherapy and, 584
 chronic renal failure and, 303
 cirrhosis and, 539
 gastric surgery patients and, 213
 hematological assessment, 67–71
 hemodialysis, 307
 hemoglobinopathies
  sickle cell anemia, 696–697
  thalassemia, 697
 hemolytic anemia, 697–699
 laboratory tests for, 68
 megaloblastic anemias, 693–695
 microcytic anemias, 695–696
 normocytic anemias, 691–693
Anergy, 67, 161
Aneurysm, 722
Angina pectoris, 385–386
 cause of, 385
 dietary management, 385
 drug management, 385–386
 stable/unstable type, 385
Angioedema, 171
Angiography, liver function, 524
Angiopathy
 diabetes and, 416
 types of, 416
Angiotensin I, 350
Angiotensin II, 350
Angiotensinogen, 350
Anion gap, 32–33
Anion gap acidosis, 33
Anorectic drugs
 obesity treatment, 496, 497
 types of, 496, 497
Anorexia

cardiac cachexia and, 390–391
 definition of, 473
 drug-related, 97, 100
Anorexia nervosa, 484, 505–509
 clinical manifestations, 506–507
 diagnostic criteria for, 505, 506
 etiology of, 506
 high-risk groups, 505
 mortality in, 505, 507
 nutritional assessment, 508
 treatment of, 508–509
Anoxia, 10
Antacids, 200, 206
 nutrition-related side effects, 207
Antagonism, drug interaction, 94
Anterior interventricular artery, 343
Anthraquinone cathartics, 270
Antibiotics
 as chemotherapeutic agents, 584, 585
 in typhoid, 563
Antibodies. *See* Hypersensitivity; Immunoglobulins
Antibody-mediated immunity, 153
Anticholinergic drugs, 206
Anticonvulsant drugs, epilepsy, 721–722
Antidepressants, 111
Antidiuretic hormone, 26, 283–284, 349
Anti-GBM disease, 328
Antigen/antibody complex, 154–155
Antigenic determinant, 153
Antigens, 149, 150. *See also* Hypersensitivity
 histocompatibility antigens, 159–160
 immune response, 153–154
 intestinal absorption, 238–239
 markers, 160
Antihistamines, 181
Antihyperuricemia, gout, 673
Anti-inflammatory drugs

Anti-inflammatory drugs
 (*continued*)
 aspirin as, 352
 chronic ulcerative colitis, 248
 Crohn's disease, 247
 gout, 673
 rheumatoid arthritis, 738
Antimetabolites, 584
Antineoplastic enzyme, 584
Antiperistaltic drugs, small
 bowel syndrome, 251
Anuric, 290
Anus, 230
Aorta, 346
Aortic stenosis, 392
Aortic valves, 340
Aplasia, 7
Aplastic anemia, 692–693
Apoferritin, 227
Appetite
 definition of, 473
 drug effects, 97, 100, 101
APUDoma, 255
Arachidonic acid, 351, 352
Argentaffin cells, 202, 219
Arginine, 135
 urea cycle disorders, 658
Arnold-Chiara malformation,
 716
Aromatic amino acids, 535, 538
Arterial blood gases, 33
Arteries, types of, 347
Arteriovenous fistulas, 305
Arteriovenous malformation,
 722
Arthritis
 juvenile rheumatoid arthritis,
 738
 osteoarthritis, 737
 rheumatoid arthritis,
 737–738
Ascites
 in cirrhosis, 533–534,
 541–542
 in congestive heart failure,
 389
 in pancreatitis, 261
Ascorbic acid
 in acute renal failure, 326
 drug metabolism and, 108
 in spina bifida, 717
Asparaginase, 584
Aspartame, diabetic diet, 439

Aspartate, production of, 537
Aspiration, in tube feeding, 130
Aspirin
 anemia and, 693, 699
 anti-inflammatory effects,
 352
 rheumatoid arthritis, 738
Asterixis, 535
Asymmetric tonic neck reflex,
 food intake and, 706
Ataxia, 255
 branched-chain ketoaciduria,
 649
 cerebral palsy, 714
Atelectasis, 264, 601
Atheromas, 12, 382, 383, 384
Atherosclerosis, 12, 382–385
 cerebrovascular accident and,
 390
 etiology of, 382–383
 hypertension and, 358
 lesions in, 383
 pathogenesis of, 383–385
 renal transplantation and, 312
 risk factors, 383
Atherothrombotic brain infarct,
 390
Athetosis, 714
Athletic performance, anemia
 and, 699
Atonic constipation, 269
Atonic muscle tone, 705
Atonic seizures, 720
Atopy, 164
Atrial natriuretic factor, 284, 354
Atrophy, 7
Atypical PKU, 639
Auerbach's plexus, 186
Autoimmune diseases, 165–166
 classification of, 166
 diet, effects of, 166
 nutritional care, 166
 nutritionally significant
 diseases, 165
 theories of autoimmunity, 166
Autologous, bone marrow
 transplant, 591
Autonomic neuropathy, 417
Autoregulation, coronary blood
 flow, 344
Autosomal changes, 7
Autosomal recessive traits, 624
Autosomes, 619

Avoidance diets
 corn-free diet, 178–180
 egg-free diet, 178, 179
 milk-free diet, 176–177
 wheat-free diet, 177–178
Azotemia, 290, 291
Azothioprine, 312

B
Backward versus forward
 failure, heart, 388
Bacterial overgrowth
 causes of, 232
 iron and, 695–696
 lipid malabsorption and,
 232–233
Bacterial translocation, tube
 feeding, 131
Balloon tamponade, 541
Baroreceptors, 349
Basal energy expenditure,
 80–81
Basal granular cells, 219
Basal lamina, 4
Basal metabolic rate
 cancer and, 580
 estimation difficulty in
 hospitalized patients,
 559–560
Base. *See also* Acid-base balance
 base deficit, 420
 buffering of, 31
Basedow's disease, 463
Basement membrane, 4
Basic diabetes guidelines,
 diabetic diet, 441
Basic nutrition guidelines,
 diabetic diet, 441
Basophils, 151, 156
Bassen-Kornzweig syndrome,
 255
B cells, 151, 153, 156, 160. *See
 also* Lymphocytes
Bedsores, 140. *See also* Pressure
 sores
Behavioral problems, developmental disabilities, 712
Behavior modification, 494–
 495
 classical conditioning, 494
 observational learning, 494
 operant conditioning,
 494–495

weight reduction and, 495

Belching, 267

Belt test, obesity assessment, 482

Beniflex feeder, 702

Benign hyperphenylalaninemia, 639

Beta-2-thienylalanine, PKU testing, 630

Beta blockers
angina and, 385–386
hypertension and, 361–362

Beta granules, 404

Beta-thalassemia, 697

Beutler fluorescent test, galactosemia, 664

Bezoars, gastric surgery patients, 213

Bicarbonate, 32–33
bicarbonate ion imbalances, 38

Bile, 223, 521
drainage from liver, 518–519
production of, 227–228

Bile acid breath test, 235

Bile acids
bile-acid binding resin, 379
intraluminal binding of, 232
sequestrants and hyperlipidemia, 380, 381

Bile ducts, 518
biliary dyskinesia, 259

Bile ductules, 518

Bile salts, 224, 228
reduction in, 233

Biliary cirrhosis, 546–547
clinical manifestations, 546
nutritional care, 547

Biliary tract, 227–228
anatomy of, 227
lipid malabsorption and, 233
normal physiology, 227–228

Biliary tree, 518

Biliopancreatic bypass, obesity treatment, 499, 501

Bilirubin, 521–522
concentration tests, 522
unconjugated, 522

Billroth I reconstruction, 210

Billroth II reconstruction, 210

Binge eater, 484. *See also* Bulimia nervosa

Bioelectrical impedance, diagnosis of obesity, 482

Biological value, protein, 126

Biotransformations, drugs, 91

Bipolar disorders, 736

Bisacodyl, 270

Bite reflex, food intake and, 707

Bladder, 281

Blastoma, 573

Bleeding tendencies, cirrhosis and, 540

Blind loop, 211

Blindness, diabetes and, 417

Bloating, cancer patient, 588, 590

Blood-brain barrier, drugs and, 91

Blood buffers, acid-base balance, 30–31

Blood cells, 5. *See also* Erythropoiesis; Leukocytes; Lymphocytes
effects of burns on, 566

Blood flow. *See* Vascular system

Blood pressure, 346–354. *See also* Hypertension
cardiac output, 347–348
diastolic pressure, 348
measurement of, 348
peripheral vascular resistance, 347–348
regulation of
eicosanoids, 351–352
kidney, 350–351
kinins, 354
natriuretic factors, 352, 354
renin-angiotensin system, 349–350
sympathetic nervous system, 349
systolic pressure, 348

Blood testing
blood gas analysis, 33
commercial tests, 421
complete blood count, 64, 67
diabetic monitoring, 421–422
hematological assessment, 67–71
in renal disease, 287–288

Blood transfusions, normocytic anemias and, 693

Blood urea nitrogen, 71
renal disease, diagnosis, 288

renal patients, assessment, 319

Blood vessels, 345–346
structure of, 345–346
types of, 346

"Blue bloater," 606

B lymphocyte, 151

Body build, types of, 485

Body image, in anorexia nervosa, 507

Body-mass index, diagnosis of obesity, 481

Body weight
assessment of, 50–52
dry weight, 318

Body weight disorders. *See* Obesity; Underweight

Bolus feeding, 129

Bone, 5

Bone disease. *See also* Musculoskeletal disorders
chronic renal failure and, 302
gastric surgery patients and, 213–214
hemodialysis and, 307
renal transplant patients, 593

Bone marrow failure, normocytic anemias and, 692

Bone marrow transplantation, 591, 593–594
categories of, 591
complications
graft-versus-host disease, 593
opportunistic infections, 593
veno-occlusive disease, 592–593
nutritional care, 591, 593–594
total body irradiation, 591

Bottle caries syndrome, 193

Bowel habits, gastric surgery patients, 212–213, 215

Bowman's capsule, 281, 283

Brain
blood-brain barrier, 91
cerebral circulation, 344

Brain injury, 722–727
causes of, 722
coma, 723
metabolic effects, 722
nutritional assessment, 723

Brain injury *(continued)*
  nutritional care, 723–727
  prenatal causes of, 704
  treatment goals, 723
Branched-chain amino acids,
    521
  cancer patients, 578
  hepatic encephalopathy,
    543
  liver and, 520
  liver disease and, 535, 538
Branched-chain keto acid
    decarboxylase, 645
Branched-chain ketoaciduria,
    644–650
  diagnosis, 645–646
  forms of, 644, 649–650
  metabolic abnormalities, 645
  monitoring in, 646
  nutritional care, 647–650
    formula products, 646–647
  symptoms of, 644–645
Breads
  enriched, 787
  low-sodium, 795
  whole-grain, 787
Breast feeding
  allergic infant and, 172, 176
  diabetes and, 455, 457
  PKU and, 631, 636
Breath tests
  breath hydrogen test, 253
  diagnosis of malabsorption,
    235–236
  labeled carbon breath test,
    235
  for lactose intolerance, 253
Breck feeder, 702
Broca index, obesity assess-
    ment, 482
Bromsulphalein retention test,
    liver function, 522
Bronchi, 599, 601
Bronchiectasis, 264
Bronchiole-associated lymph-
    oid tissue, 150
Bronchioles, 599, 601
Bronchopulmonary dysplasia,
    611–612
  nutritional assessment, 612
  nutritional care, 612
  pathology of, 611
  phases of, 613

premature birth and, 611
  prevention of, 611
Bronchoscopy, 605
Brown adipose tissue, 472
Brunner's glands, 219
Bulbar palsy, 716
Bulbar poliomyelitis, 563
Bulimia nervosa, 509–510
  effects of, 509
  nutritional assessment, 509,
    510
  treatment of, 510
Bulk-forming laxatives,
    269–270
Bulking agents, obesity
    treatment, 496, 498
Burn injuries
  effects on blood cells, 566
  effects on skin, 565–566
  effects on vascular system,
    566
  full-thickness burn, 565
  management of, 567–568
    for fluid losses, 567
    formulas for nutritional
      requirements, 567–568
    skin grafts, 567
  metabolic effects, 566–567
  partial-thickness burn, 565
  percent determination, 565
  superficial burn, 564–565
Bursa of Fabricius, 151

C
Cachexia, 77
  cancer, 577, 585
Caffeine
  absorption of, 769
  drug sources of, 770
  excretion of, 769
  metabolism of, 769
  methylxanthines
    food sources of, 770
    pharmacologic uses, 769
  physiologic effects, 769
  related compounds, 769
  withdrawal symptoms, 769
Caffeine intake
  congestive heart failure and,
    389
  esophagus and, 197
  hypertension and, 356
  hyperthyroidism and, 463

lithium and, 736
  lower esophageal pressure,
    197
  MAO inhibitors and, 113
  myocardial infarction and,
    387
  peptic ulcer disease and, 207
Calcification of teeth, 191
Calcium
  absorption of, 227
  chronic renal failure and,
    301–302
  graft-versus-host disease
    and, 593
  hemodialysis and, 307–308
  hypermetabolic patient and,
    562
  hypertension and, 357, 359
  imbalances, 37
  in immobilized patient, 728
  intracellular degeneration
    related to, 13
  lactose intolerance and, 254
  in muscular dystrophy,
    733–734
  parenteral feeding, 139
  regulation of, 286
Calcium carbonate, 299
Calcium channel blockers, hy-
    pertension and, 361, 363
Caloric needs. *See* Energy needs
Caloric restriction, anticarcino-
    genic aspects, 575–576
Calorie count, 74
Calorie counting system,
    diabetic diet, 442
Calorie-nitrogen (C:N) ratio,
    126
Calorie-protein count, 74
Canals of Hering, 518
Cancer
  age and, 577
  cause of death in, 585
  dietary guidelines to reduce
    risk, 576
  effects on specific organs,
    580–581
  etiology and
    dietary factors, 575–576
    hormone-nutrient interac-
      tions, 576
    inflammation, chronic, 577
    radiation, 577

stress, 576
viruses, 577
gender and, 577
leukemia, 574, 590–594
metabolic effects, 577–580
  on amino acids, 580
  cachexia, 577, 585
  on carbohydrate metabolism, 579
  competition of tumors for nutrients, 578–579
  decreased food intake, 578
  on lipid metabolism, 579
  on protein metabolism, 579–580
nutritional care, 585–590
  benefits of, 585, 588
  nutritional assessment, 588
  oral feeding guidelines, 589
nutritional consequences
  of chemotherapy, 584, 586–587
  of immunotherapy, 585
  of radiation therapy, 582–583
  of surgery, 581–582
nutritional deprivation and, 580
pathogenesis of, 574–575, 577
Cancer enteropathy, 580
Candy, avoidance by diabetic, 438
Capillaries, 346
Capsular space, 282
Carbohydrate counting method, diabetic diet, 442
Carbohydrate intake
  in cirrhosis, 540–541
  in diabetic diet, 428, 429–430, 437, 441
  in failure to thrive, 719
  in hepatic encephalopathy, 543
  in hepatitis, 525
  low-carbohydrate diet, 492
  parenteral feeding and, 135–136, 140
  peritoneal dialysis and, 310
  in restricted-calorie diet, 489
  tube feeding and, 125

in underweight treatment, 505
Carbohydrate intolerance, 252–255
  glucose-galactose malabsorption, 254–255
  lactase deficiency, 252–254
  sucrase-isomaltase deficiency, 254
Carbohydrate metabolism
  cancer and, 579
  in diabetic, 406, 407
  liver and, 520
  liver disease and, 538
  process of, 406
Carbohydrate metabolism disorders, 659–671
  fructosuria, 666
  galactosemia, 663–666
  glycogen storage diseases, 668–670
  hereditary fructose-1, 6-bisphosphatase deficiency, 666–668
Carbohydrate-protein complexes, 11
Carbohydrates
  chronic renal failure and, 304
  digestion of, 222, 226
  drug effects, 100, 104
  intracellular degeneration related to, 11
  malabsorption of, 233–234
  types of, 125
Carbon dioxide, in respiration, 603
Carcinoid syndrome, 255–256
Carcinomas, 573. *See also* Cancer
Carcinosarcomas, 573
Cardiac beriberi, 393
Cardiac cachexia, 390–391
  causes of, 390–391
  clinical manifestations, 390
  treatment of, 391
Cardiac cycle, 341
Cardiac decompensation, 387
Cardiac edema, 389
Cardiac muscle, 4
Cardiac output, 347–348
Cardia glands, 203
Cardiomegaly, 393
Cardiomyopathies, 388

Cardiospasm, 199
Cardiovascular disease
  alcoholism and, 393
  atherosclerosis, 382–385
  cardiac cachexia, 390–391
  cerebrovascular accident, 390
  chronic renal failure and, 304
  congestive heart failure, 387–389
  coronary heart disease, 385–387
  diabetes and, 416
  hemodialysis patients, 306
  peripheral vascular atherosclerotic occlusive disease, 390
  rheumatic heart disease, 391–392
  transient ischemic attacks, 389–390
Cardiovascular system
  blood pressure, 346–354
  heart, 340–342
  hypertension, 354–363
  plasma lipid abnormalities
    hypercholesterolemia, 379
    hyperlipidemia, 363, 371–375, 379–382
    hyperlipoproteinemia, 375–379
  vascular system, 342–346
Cariogenic, 192
Carnitine, urea cycle disorders, 658
Carotenes. *See* Vitamin A
Carriers, sex-linked traits, 619
Cartilage, 5
Castor oil, 270
Catabolic hormones, insulin and, 405–406
Catabolic response, injury, 557
Catabolism, 557. *See also* Hypermetabolic illness; Hypermetabolic response
Catalase, 528, 698
Cataracts, galactosemia, 664
Catecholamines
  production of, 536
  regulation of food intake, 476
  stress effects, 558–559
Cathartics, constipation and, 269–270

Catheter insertion, parenteral feeding, 134–135
Cation exchange resins, 37
Celiac disease, 239, 244
Cell death, 10–11
Cell-mediated hypersensitivity, 166
Cell-mediated immunity, 49–50
assessment of, 66–67
Cell-mediated response, 151
Cell-mediated system, 166
Cells, differentiation, 3, 5
Cellular reproduction, normal, 571–572
Cementum, 188
Central adrenergic inhibitors, 360, 362
Central veins, liver, 518
Central venous alimentation, parenteral feeding, 134
Centroacinar cells, 228
Centromere, 617
Cephalic phase, 201
Cephalocaudally, 705
Cereal extract, 177
Cereals
enriched, 787
low-sodium breads, 795
whole-grain, 787
Cerebral arteries, 344
Cerebral edema, hepatitis and, 525
Cerebral palsy, 713–714
feeding problems, 714
forms of, 713–714
growth retardation, 714
medications in, 714
nutritional care, 714
Cerebrovascular accident, 390
atherosclerosis and, 382
renal transplantation and, 312
Cervical esophagostomy, 128
Cheilosis, 191
Chemical senses, 96
Chemical thermogenesis, 478
Chemoreceptor trigger zone, 584
Chemotherapy
cancer patients, 583–584, 586–587
classification of drugs, 583–584

log kill hypothesis, 584
mechanisms of action, 583
nutritional effects, 584, 586–587
resistance to drugs, 584
toxic effects, 584
Chenodeoxycholic acid, 227, 228, 259
Chewing
development of, 708
rotary chewing, 708, 709
Chief cells, 202
Children. *See also* Pediatric patient
daily requirements for nutrients, 626–627
elimination diet, 175, 176
guidelines for diet assessment, 806
weight/height assessment, 51
Chloride, 29
electrolytes, 29
imbalances, 37–38
minimum requirements, 749
parenteral feeding, 139
Cholecystectomy, 259
Cholecystitis, 258–259
Cholecystokinin-pancreozymin, 222, 223
Cholelithiasis, 258
Cholera, 240
Cholerrheic diarrhea, 249
Cholestatic hepatitis, 524
Cholesterol, 363–364. *See also* Lipid metabolism; Plasma lipid abnormalities; Plasma lipids
absorption of, 364
acceptable levels of, 375
dietary effects of, 371–372, 375
dietary sources of, 372
excretion of, 363–364
functions in body, 363
hypercholesterolemia, 379, 382
hypothyroidism and, 463
liver disease and, 539
organs in synthesis of, 364
Cholesterol ester transfer protein, 370
Cholesterol Lowering Atherosclerosis Study, 383

Cholestyramine, small bowel syndrome, 251
Cholic acid, 227
Chondroma, 572
Chordae tendinae, 341
Chorda tympani, 95
Chromatids, 617
Chromosomal abnormalities, 620–621
Chromosomal diseases, 7
Chromosomes, 616–619
Chronic active hepatitis, 524
Chronic bronchitis, characteristics, 606
Chronic degeneration, 11
Chronic glomerulonephritis, 329
Chronic granulomatous inflammation, 10
Chronic obstructive pulmonary disease, 605–608
characteristics of, 605–606
chronic bronchitis and, 606
cor pulmonale and, 606
emphysema and, 606
etiology of, 606
incidence of, 605
management of
drug therapy, 607
nutritional care, 607–608
nutritional assessment, 606–607
pathogenesis, 606
type A, 606
type B, 606
Chronic pancreatitis, 260–261
causes of, 260
clinical manifestations, 261
nutritional management, 261
pathogenesis, 260
Chronic rejection, grafts, 167
Chronic renal failure. *See also* Dialysis; Renal transplantation
conservative management, 291
dialysis, 305–311
diet planning, 293, 304–305
etiology, 289
malnutrition and, 312–313
manifestations of, 290, 291
metabolic changes
acidosis, 299, 301

amino acid abnormalities,
293
calcium balance abnormal-
ities, 301–302
carbohydrate metabolism
disorders, 304
energy needs and, 293–294
fluid balance abnormali-
ties, 296–298
iron balance abnormalities,
303
lipid-related abnormalities,
304
mental changes, 304
pediatric patient, 304
phosphorus balance ab-
normalities, 302–303
potassium balance
abnormalities, 298–299
protein abnormalities,
291–293
sodium balance abnormal-
ities, 294–296
vitamin needs and,
303–304
zinc deficiency, 303
pathophysiology, 289–290
progression of, 290
renal transplantation,
311–322
Chronic ulcerative colitis,
247–248
complications of, 248
symptoms of, 247–248
treatment of, 248
Chylomicrons, 224, 365, 367
Chyme, 203
Cigarette smoking
atherosclerosis and, 382, 384,
385
hypertension and, 356
peripheral vascular atherosclerotic occlusive
disease and, 390
pulmonary disease and, 606
Cimetidine
peptic ulcer disease, 206
small bowel syndrome, 251
Circle of Willis, 344
Circulatory system. *See*
Cardiovascular system;
Vascular system
Circumflex artery, 343

Cirrhosis, 533–547
causes of, 533
classification of, 533
clinical manifestations, 533
anemia, 539
ascites, 533–534
coagulatory problems,
540
hepatic encephalopathy,
535–537
malabsorption, 540
portal hypertension, 533–
534
renal failure, 540
varices, 534
end-stage cirrhosis, 545
metabolic changes in
acid-base balance, 539
amino acid metabolism,
535, 537–538
ammonia synthesis,
535–536, 537–538
carbohydrate metabolism,
538
fluid-electrolyte imbal-
ances, 539
lipid metabolism, 539
protein metabolism, 535,
537–538
protein synthesis, 535
urea synthesis, 535
vitamin metabolism, 539
nutritional care
feeding methods, 543–545
general care, 540–541, 547
treatment of
ascites, 541–542
control of gastrointestinal
bleeding, 541
edema, 542
hepatic encephalopathy,
542–543
types of
alcoholic cirrhosis, 532,
545–546
biliary cirrhosis, 546–547
postnecrotic cirrhosis, 546
Wilson's disease, 547
Classical conditioning, 494
Clear liquid diet, 119
Cleft lip/palate, 702–703
incidence of, 702
nutritional care, 702–703

prenatal development, 702
surgical repair, 703
Clinical observations
food intake, 74
nutritional assessment, 71
Clinical risk, calculation of, 81
Cloudy swelling, 11
Coagulopathy
in cirrhosis, 540
hepatitis, 525
treatment of, 525
Coarctation of the aorta, 354,
392
Cobalamin. *See* Vitamin B_{12}
Codeine, side effects, 241
Codominant, genes, 619
Codon, 618
Coenzymes, vitamin depen-
dency syndromes, 622,
674–676
Coffee. *See* Caffeine
Collagen, 5
Collateral circulation, 344
Colloid osmotic pressure, 21
Colon
anatomy of, 230
surgery of
colostomy, 273–274
ileostomy, 272–273
Colostomy, 273–274
nutritional management, 274
position of, 273–274
Coma
brain injury and, 723
causes of, 723
diabetes and, 412, 413, 414
Common bile duct, 227, 229
Compensated failure, heart, 388
Compensated metabolic
acidosis, diabetes and,
412
Complement, 154
Complement cascade, 154
Complete blood count, 64, 66,
67
Complex-partial seizures, 720
Compliance, lungs, 601–602
Composition disturbances,
correction of, 36–38
Computerized tomography (CT)
kidney, 289
liver function, 524
Concentration, drugs, 89

Concentration disturbances
  correction of, 35–36
  potassium, 29
  sodium, 27–28
Congeners, 531
Congenital conditions, 7
Congenital heart disease
  effects of, 392
  nutritional care, 392
  types of, 392
Congenital lactose intolerance,
  252
Congestive heart failure,
  387–389
  clinical manifestations, 389
  hypertension and, 358
  management of
    drug treatment, 389
    nutritional care, 389
    sodium-restricted diet,
    389
  pathogenesis of, 388
  salt/water retention in, 388
  types of, 388
Conjugase, 226
Conjugating agent, 92
Conjugations, drugs and, 92
Connective tissue, 5
Constipation, 268–270
  atonic constipation, 269
  causes of, 268
  developmental disabilities,
    713
  obstructive constipation,
    268–269
  spastic constipation, 269
  treatment of, 269–270
Contactants, in allergies, 170–
  171
Contaminated bowel syn-
  drome, 233
Continent ileostomy, 272
Contingency contracting, modification of eating
  behaviors, 495
Continuous ambulatory
  peritoneal dialysis, 308
Continuous arteriovenous
  hemofiltration, 327
Continuous cyclic peritoneal
  dialysis, 308
Contractures of the legs, 717
Conventional feeding, 119–123
  cultural influences, 123

increasing nutrient intake,
  121–122
modified diets, purposes of,
  119
types of diets, 119–121
vegetarian modification,
  122–123
Conventional therapy, insulin
  treatment, 425
Converting enzyme, 350
Converting enzyme inhibitors,
  361, 363
Copper
  in cirrhosis, 546, 547
  parenteral feeding and, 140
  in Wilson's disease, 676
Corn-free diet, 178–180
Coronary arteries, 343
Coronary bypass surgery,
  myocardial infarction,
  387
Coronary heart disease,
  385–387
  angina pectoris, 385–386
  hypertension and, 358
  myocardial infarction, 386–
    387
  risk factors, 363
Coronary occlusion, atherosclerosis, 382
Coronary Primary Prevention
  Trial, 375
Cor pulmonale, chronic
  obstructive pulmonary
  disease and, 606
Corticosteroids
  allergy treatment, 181
  hepatitis and, 525
Cortisol, insulin and, 405–406
Cortisone oral glucose tolerance test, in diagnosis of
  diabetes, 419
Counting systems, diabetic
  diet, 442–443
C peptide, 404
  chain assay, in diagnosis of
  diabetes, 419
Cranial nerves
  pairs of, 581–582
  types/functions, 755
Creatine phosphokinase, in
  muscular dystrophy, 734
Creatinine
  elimination of, 286

formation of, 56
renal disease, diagnosis, 288
Creatinine clearance test, 288
Creatinine-height index, 56, 59
Critical micellar concentration,
  223
Crohn's disease, 246–247
  causes of, 246
  clinical manifestations, 246
  diagnosis of, 246
  treatment of, 246–247
    drug treatment, 247
    nutritional care, 247
    surgical treatment, 247
Cromolyn sodium, 181
Crown, of tooth, 188
Crypts of Lieberkuhn, 219
Cultural factors
  diabetic diet, 444
  diet, 123
Cultured foods, lactose
  intolerance and, 253–
  254
Curling's ulcer, 567
Cushing's syndrome, 354, 402,
  483
  causes of, 462
  treatment of, 462
Cutaneous testing, food
  allergy, 174
Cyclamates, diabetic diet, 439
Cyclic adenosine monophosphate, 239
Cyclic parenteral nutrition, 143
Cycling, weight loss/gain,
  504
Cyclooxygenase, 352
Cyclophosphamide, 584, 590
Cyclosporin A, 312
Cystic duct, 227
Cystic fibrosis, 261, 263–265
  causes of, 261
  clinical manifestations, 261,
    264
  diagnosis, 265
  incidence of, 261
  life expectancy, 264
  nutritional assessment,
    264–265
  pathophysiology of, 261, 263
  treatment
    medications, 265
    nutritional care, 265
Cystic fibrosis transmembrane

conductance regulator, 261
Cystine, 135
    hemocystinurias, 655
Cytokines, 151, 156–158
    acute phase response, 157–158
    classes of, 157
    effects on metabolism, 157, 158
    types of, 157
Cytosine arabinoside, 584
Cytotoxic lymphocytes, 151
Cytotoxic responses, 164–165

D
Daily Food Guide, 76
Data collection methods, dietary assessment, 74–76
Dawn phenomenon, hypoglycemia, 413
Debridement, burns, 567
Decompensated metabolic acidosis, diabetes and, 412
Decubitus ulcers, 140. *See also* Pressure sores
Degeneration, 11–13
    degrees of, 11
    types of, 11–13
Deglutition, 191
Dehydration, 240. *See also* Fluid/electrolyte imbalances; Fluids; Water
    diabetes and, 411, 414
Delayed cutaneous hypersensitivity, 66
    renal patients assessment, 318
    skin tests, 162
Delayed-type sensitivity, 165
Deletion, chromosomes, 621
Delirium tremens, 530
Dementia, 731–732
    alcohol dementia, 732
    Alzheimer's disease, 731–732
    causes of, 731
    multi-infarct dementia, 732
Dental calculus, 192
Dental caries, 192–193
    bottle caries syndrome, 193
    causes of, 192
    fluoridation and, 192
    rampant caries, 192–193

Dental diseases, 191–194
    cerebral palsy and, 714
    dental caries, 192–193
    Down syndrome and, 715
    etiology of, 191–192
    gingivitis, 191, 193
    masticatory insufficiency, 194
    periodontal disease, 193–194
    stomatitis, 191, 193
Dental plaque, 192
Dentin, 188
Deoxycholic acid, 227
Depolarization wave, 536
Depression, treatment of, 736
Dercum's disease, 484
Detoxification, drugs, 91
Developmental disabilities
    behavioral problems, 712
    causes of, 704
    classification of, 7
    diet texture in, 710–711
    feeding skills, 705–710
    nutritional assessment, 711–712
    special problems
        constipation, 713
        drug-related, 713
        fluid intake, 713
        growth retardation, 713
        obesity, 713
        underweight, 713
    types of
        cerebral palsy, 713–714
        Down syndrome, 715
        failure to thrive, 718–719
        fetal alcohol syndrome, 715–716
        Prader-Willi syndrome, 716
        spina bifida, 716–718
Dextran, 192, 414
Dextrose in saline solutions, IV, 39
Dextrose in water solutions, IV, 38
Diabetes mellitus, 399–458
    brain injury and, 722
    clinical manifestations, 399–400, 411–412
    complications of
        angiopathies, 416
        coma, 412, 413, 414
        hypoglycemia, 412–413
        injection site problems, 414–415

        ketoacidosis, 413–414
        metabolic lesions, 415–416
        nephropathy, 416
        neuropathy, 416–417
        retinopathy, 417, 452
    diagnosis of, 417–420
    drug management of
        goals of management, 422
        insulin, 424–426
        sulfonylureas, 422–424
    etiology of, 402–403
    exercise and, 446–448
    incidence of, 400
    mental status and, 446
    metabolic changes in
        amino acid metabolism, 410–411
        carbohydrate metabolism, 406
        endogenous insulin, 403–406
        lipid metabolism, 406–410
        protein metabolism, 410
    monitoring in
        blood testing, 421–422
        urine testing, 420–421
    nutritional assessment, 420
    nutritional care
        ADA recommendations, 426–427
        basic diabetes guidelines, 441
        basic nutrition guidelines, 441
        counting systems, 442–443
        daily menu planning, 437–438
        determination of diet prescription, 427–429
        exchange system, 429–436, 441–442
        food choice plan, 443
        glycemic index, 443–444
        missed meal adjustments, 445
        practical considerations in, 444–445
        sample menus, 436
        special foods in diabetic diets, 438–440
        vitamin/mineral supplements, 440
    patient education, 448–449
    pediatric patient, 452

Diabetes mellitus (*continued*)
  pregnancy and, 452–457
    breast feeding, 455, 457
    gestational diabetes,
      454–455
    infants of diabetic mothers,
      453
    labor/delivery, 455
    pregestational diabetes,
      453–454
    self-management, 455
  risk factors in, 401–402
  self-management, 449–452,
    455
  surgical patient, 457–458
  tube feedings/TPN and,
    457–458
  types of
    gestational diabetes, 401,
      453
    insulin-dependent
      diabetes, 401
    malnutrition-related
      diabetes, 401
    non-insulin dependent
      diabetes, 401
    primary diabetes, 400–401
    secondary diabetes, 402
Diabetic renal disease
  clinical manifestations, 333
  nutritional care, 333
Diagnosis-related groups, 45
Dialysate, 305
Dialysis, 305–311. *See also*
    specific methods
  dialyzer, 305
  hemodialysis, 305–308
  home dialysis, 306
  parenteral nutrition and,
    326–327
  peritoneal dialysis, 308–311
Dialysis dementia, 302
Diaphragm, respiration and,
    600, 601
Diarrhea, 239–242
  causes of, 240
  classification
    acute diarrhea, 239
    intractable diarrhea, 239
    osmotic diarrhea, 239
    secretory diarrhea,
      239–240
  definition of, 239
  diagnosis of, 240

intestinal resection and, 250
jejunoileal bypass and, 499,
    500
lipid malabsorption and, 231,
    233
metabolic consequences, 240
pathogenesis, 239
treatment of, 241
Diastole, 341
Diastolic pressure, 348
Dietary assessment, 71–77
  data collection methods, 74–
    76
  evaluation of diet, 76–77
Dietary Standard for Canada, 77
Diet history, food allergy and,
    173
Diet-induced thermogenesis,
    477–478
Diets, hospital
  clear liquid diet, 119
  full liquid diet, 119
  house diet, 121
  lactoovovegetarian, 122
  lactovegetarian, 122
  medical liquid diet, 120
  modified diets, 121
  new vegetarians, 123
  ovovegetarian, 122
  partial vegetarians, 122
  pureed diet, 121
  qualitative diets, 121
  quantitative diets, 121
  soft diet, 120
  strained soft diet, 121
  surgical liquid diet, 120
  test diets, 121
  vegan, 122
Diets in obesity
  fad diets, 492–493
  fasting, 491
  formula diets, 491, 492
  packaged food programs, 492
  restricted-calorie diet,
    488–491
  very low calorie diet,
    491–492
Diet testing, food allergy,
    174–175
Differential blood cell count, 66
Differentiation, cells, 3, 5
Diffusion, 19–20
Digestion
  liver and, 521

process of, 220–221
small intestine, 222
Digestive system. *See* specific
    organs
Digitalis
  angina and, 385
  congestive heart failure and,
    389
  myocardial infarction and,
    386
Dihydropteridine reductase
    deficiency, 640
Dihydroxy acid, 227
3, 4-dihydroxyphenylalanine,
    production of, 536
Dihydroxyphenyl isatin, 269
Dilution syndrome, 23
Dimer, 156
Dinitrophenylhydrazine,
    branched-chain ketoaci-
    duria, 646
Dioctyl calcium sulfosuccinate,
    269
Dioctyl sodium sulfosuccinate,
    269
Dipeptidases, 225
Dipeptides, 127
Diploid, 617
Diplopia, 458
Direct smooth muscle vasodila-
    tors, 361, 362–363
Disaccharidases, 222
Disaccharides, 125
Discharge summary, 48
Disease
  causes of, 6
  diagnosis of, 6
  manifestations of, 6
Disorderly regeneration, 533
Distribution, drugs, 90
Disulfiram
  alcohol dependency treat-
    ment, 532
  reactions to drug, 110
Diuretics
  angina and, 385
  congestive heart failure and,
    389
  hypertension and, 360, 362,
    363
  nephrotic syndrome and,
    331, 332
  types of, 360, 362
Diverticular disease, 270–271

diet and, 270
management of, 270–271
symptoms of, 270
DNA, 616–618
Docosahexanoic acid, 351
Documentation
    problem-oriented medical
        record, 45–48
    source-oriented medical
        record, 48
Docycline, 104
Dominant trait, 619
Dopamine, 111
    foods containing, 122–113
    production of, 536
Dopamine-receptor blockers,
        side effects, 736
Down syndrome, 392, 715
    growth retardation, 715
    levels of dysfunction, 715
    nutritional care, 715
Drooling, infant, 707
Drug addiction, 736
    nutritional care, 736
Drugs
    affecting factors
        absorption, 89
        distribution, 90
        routes of administration,
            88–89
        size/frequency of dosage,
            87–88
    classification of, 94
    definition of, 87
    drug interactions, 94
    excretion, 91
    individual responses to,
        93–94
    malabsorption and,
        234–235
    mechanisms of action, 87
    metabolism of, 91
        biotransformations, 91
        influencing factors,
            92–93
        nonsynthetic reactions,
            91–92
        synthetic reactions, 92
    modification of drug effects,
        93
    most commonly used drugs,
        95
    naming of, 94
    obesity related to, 483–484

    properties of drug molecule,
        89
    side effects, 87
Drugs and nutrition
    alcohol–drug interactions,
        113, 114–115
    appetite effects, 97, 100, 101
    drug effects, on taste/odor,
        96–97, 99
    food–drug interactions, 108,
        111, 113
    food effects
        on drug absorption,
            101–104, 109
        on drug metabolism, 104,
            108
        nutrient absorption and,
            97–98
        nutrient metabolism and, 98,
            100–101
Drug treatments. *See* specific
        disorders
Duchenne muscular dystrophy,
        733
Duct cells, 229
Duct of Santorini, 229
Ductus arteriosus, 345
Ductus venosus, 345
Duct of Wirsung, 228–229
Dumping syndrome
    gastric surgery patients,
        212–213, 215
    nutritional management, 212
    organic reactive hypoglyce-
        mia, 461
Duodenal ulcer, 205, 206
    surgical procedures for, 210–
        211
Duodenum, 219, 222
    lipid malabsorption and, 233
Durand's syndrome, 252
D-xylose absorption test, 236
Dx, 46
Dyskinesia, cerebral palsy, 714
Dysphagia, 197–198
Dysphagia diet, 726
Dysplasia, 574
Dyspnea, 389, 412
Dystrophic calcifications, 13

E
Early dumping syndrome, 212
Eclampsia, 355
Ectoderm, 3

Ectomorphs, 484
Ectopic, 166
Ectopic hormones, 255
Eczema, 171
Edema, 11, 291
    areas for, 330
    cancer and, 580
    cerebral, 723
    cirrhosis and, 542
    nephrotic syndrome and,
        330, 331
Efflux, fluids, 239
Egg-free diet, 178, 179
Ehlers-Danlos syndrome, 392
Eicosanoids
    compounds related to, 351
    fish oil and, 374
    in regulation of blood
        pressure, 351–352
Eicosapentanoic acid, 351
Elastic arteries, 346
Elastin, 5
Electrocardiogram, 341–342
Electroencephalograph,
        diagnosis of epilepsy, 720
Electrolytes. *See also* Fluid/
        electrolyte imbalance
    absorption of, 226
    chloride, 29
    fluid/electrolyte imbalances,
        16, 24
    functions of, 24
    in oral rehydration solutions,
        241
    parenteral feeding, 141
    potassium, 28–29
    sodium, 24–28
Elimination diet, food allergy,
        175, 176
Embryonic development, 3–4
Emiocytosis, 404
Emphysema, characteristics of,
        606
Enamel, tooth, 188
Enamel pellicle, 191
Endocardium, 340
Endocrine disorders. *See also*
        Inborn errors of metabo-
        lism
    adrenocortical dysfunction,
        461–462
    diabetes mellitus, 399–458
    hypoglycemia, 458–461
    obesity in, 483

Endocrine disorders *(continued)*
   thyroid dysfunction, 462–
      463
Endocrine functions, of kidney,
   286–287
Endocrine glands, 4
Endocrine-secreting tumors, of
   gastrointestinal tract,
   255–256
Endocrine system
   components of, 399, 400
   effects of burns on, 566
   effects of injury on,
      558–559
Endoderm, 3
Endogenous pyrogens, 562
Endogenous transport system,
   lipoproteins, 368, 370
Endomorphs, 484
Endoscopic sclerotherapy, 541
Endothelial cells, 346
Endothelial-injury hypothesis,
   atherosclerosis and,
      384–385
Endothelium, 4
Endothermic thermogenesis,
   477
End-stage cirrhosis, 545
End-stage renal disease, 290
   nutritional care, pediatric pa-
      tient, 316–317
Energy, calculation in nutrients,
   473
Energy balance
   calculation of, 80–81
   food intake, controls in,
      474–477
   negative, 478
Energy expenditure
   control of, 478–479
   injury and, 559–560
   types of, 477–478
Energy needs
   in acute renal failure, 325
   in anorexia nervosa treat-
      ment, 509
   in bone marrow transplanta-
      tion, 591
   in branched-chain ketoaci-
      duria, 648
   in burn patient, 568
   in cancer patient, 588
   in cerebral palsy, 714

   in chronic renal failure,
      293–294
   in diabetic diet, 427–428
   in Down syndrome, 715
   excess energy intake,
      141–142
   in failure to thrive, 719
   height/weight chart, 748
   in hemodialysis, 306
   in hepatitis, 525
   in hypermetabolic illness,
      559–560
   in hyperthyroidism, 463
   in muscular dystrophy, 734
   in nephrotic syndrome, 332
   parenteral feeding and,
      140–141
   in peritoneal dialysis,
      309–310
   in PKU diet, 634–635, 636
   in pulmonary disease, 607
   in respiratory failure, 610
   restricted calories diet,
      488–489
   in spina bifida, 717
   in spinal cord injury, 728
   supplemental feeding and,
      39, 42
   tube feeding and, 125
   in underweight treatment,
      505
   in urea cycle disorders,
      656–657, 659
Energy stores, estimation of,
   52–56
Enteral administration, drugs,
   88
Enteral feeding. *See* Parenteral
   feeding
Enterochromaffin, 219
Enterocytes, 219
Enterogastric reflex, 203
Enterohepatic circulation, 224
Enterokinase, 222
Enterostomal therapists, 274
Enterotoxins, 239–240
Entoderm, 3
Environmental management, of
   eating behaviors, 495
Enzymes. *See also* Inborn errors
   of metabolism
   in alcohol metabolism,
      527–529

   control of dangerous
      oxidants, 698–699
   enzyme defects, 621–622,
      623
   intestinal tract, 222, 226
   liver damage and, 524
   metabolic pathway, 621, 622
   pancreatic, 220–221, 225,
      229
Eosinophils, 151–153
Epicardium, 340
Epiglottis, effects of surgery on,
   582
Epilepsy, 719–722
   diagnosis of, 720
   drug treatment of, 721–722
   incidence of, 719
   nutritional care, 721–722
   types of seizures in, 719–720
Epinephrine
   allergy treatment, 181
   food intake and, 476
   production of, 536
Epithelium, 4
Eructation, 267
Erythema, 67
Erythroblasts, 683
Erythrocytes, 5, 67, 687
Erythropoiesis, 683–691
   erythropoietic stimulating
      factor, 684
   hemoglobin, synthesis/deg-
      radation of, 685, 687
   nutrients involved in, 683,
      687–691
   red blood cells
      development of, 683–684
      maturation of, 684–687
Erythropoietin, 286, 303
   red blood cell maturation, 685
Eschar, 565
Escherichia coli, 240
Esophageal disease
   achalasia, 199
   in cirrhosis, 541
   dysphagia, 197–198
   esophageal ulcers, 205, 206
   esophagitis, 200
   lower esophageal incompe-
      tence, 200–201, 214
   odynophagia, 198
   stricture of esophagus,
      199–200

surgical procedures in, 129, 199, 201
Esophagitis, 200
Esophagomyotomy, 199
Esophagostomy, 129
Esophagus. *See also* Esophageal disease
  anatomy of, 197
  caffeine and, 197
  replacement of, 201
Essential fatty acids
  omega families of, 351, 352
  parenteral feeding and, 136, 141
  tube feeding and, 125
Essential hypertension, 355–357
  etiology of, 355–356
  protective minerals, 357
  sodium intake and, 356–357
Ethanol, metabolism of, 527–528. *See also* Alcohol
Exchange system, diabetic diet, 429–436, 441–442
Excretion
  alcohol, 527
  drugs, 91
  liver and, 521
  nitrogen, 66
  sodium, 27
  urine, 283–284
  water, 22–23
Exercise
  angina and, 385
  diabetes and, 446–448
  energy expenditures in, 494
  metabolic effects, 446
  obesity treatment, 493–494
  thermic effect of, 477
  weight loss and, 477
Exocrine glands, 4
Exogenous hypoglycemia, 459
Exogenous pyrogens, 562
Exogenous transport system, lipoproteins, 368
Exophthalmic goiter, 463
Extensor thrusting, food intake and, 706
External limiting membrane, 346
Extinction, in conditioning, 495
Extracellular fluid, 17, 26

Exudate, 8
Eye–hand coordination, infant, 707

F
Fab portion, 155
Facial nerves, 581
Facilitated diffusion, 20
Facilitated transport, 222
Factitious hypoglycemia, 459
Factor D, 487
Facultative excretion, 23
Facultative thermogenesis, 477
Fad diets, weight loss and, 492–493
Failure-to-thrive, 611, 718–719
  definitions of, 718
  diet history in, 718
  nutritional care, 718–719
  organic/inorganic, 718
False neurotransmitters, 537
Familial combined hyperlipidemia, 379
Familial dysbetalipoproteinemia, 378
Familial hypercholesterolemia, 379, 384
Familial hypertriglyceridemia, 378
Familial vitamin D–resistant rickets, 675–676
Fasting
  in diagnosis of hypoglycemia, 459
  weight loss and, 491
Fasting blood glucose
  in diagnosis of diabetes, 417
  in diagnosis of hypoglycemia, 459
Fasting hypoglycemia, 459
Fasting lipid profile, in diagnosis of diabetes, 420
Fasting plasma glucose, in diagnosis of diabetes, 417
Fat, body. *See* Adipose tissue; Obesity
Fat, dietary. *See* Lipid intake
Fat cells, size and metabolism, 486–487
Fat intake, cancer and, 576
Fat requirements. *See* Lipid intake
Fat-restricted diets, types of, 237

Fat substitutes
  Olestra, 491
  Simplesse, 491
Fatty acids. *See also* Lipid metabolism
  adipose tissue, 472–473
  red blood cell formation and, 691
  response to injury, 559
  saturation, effects of, 372–373
  synthesis/storage of, 408
  utilization of, 409
Fatty liver, 531–532
Fatty metamorphosis, 12
Fatty streaks, atherosclerosis and, 383, 384, 385
Fava beans, hemolytic anemia and, 699
Fc portion, 155
Fecal fat assay, 235
Fecal nitrogen, 235
Feeding problems. *See* Food intake
Feeding skills
  assessment of, 709
  learning of, 708
  self-feeding skills, 708–709
Fenfluramine, weight reduction and, 496
Ferric chloride, PKU testing, 630
Ferritin, 688
Fetal alcohol syndrome, 715–716
  features of, 715
Fetor hepaticus, 535
Fetus, circulation in, 344–345
Fever
  causes of, 562
  hypothalamus and, 562
  metabolic effects, 562–563
Fiber, 265–267
  classification of, 266
  dietary versus crude, 266
Fiber intake
  anticarcinogenic aspects, 576
  constipation and, 269
  in Crohn's disease, 247
  in diabetic diet, 437, 441
  diet modifications for, 167
  diverticular disease and, 270–271
  hemorrhoids and, 274

Fiber intake *(continued)*
  hypocholesterolemic effects, 374
  in periodontal disease, 194
  physiological effects, 266–267
  in spinal cord injured, 728
Fibric acid derivatives, hyperlipidemia, 381
Fibroblasts, 4, 10
Fibroma, 572
Filtration, 21
Fish oil, beneficial effects, 373–374
Fistulas
  intestinal, 243–244
  surgically created, 305
Fixed ratio formulas, tube feeding, 127
Flaccid muscle tone, 705
Flare, 67
Flatulence, 267
Flavonoids, 575
Flavor, 95
Flow sheets, 48
Fluid/electrolyte imbalances
  in acute renal failure, control of, 327
  cancer and, 581
  clinical manifestations of, 24
  correction of
    composition disturbances, 36–38
    concentration disturbances, 35–36
    energy supply, 39, 42
    intravenous fluids, 38–39, 40–41
    volume disturbances, 34–35
  jejunoileal bypass and, 501
  liver disease and, 539
  prevention of, 33–34
  types of, 16
Fluid intake
  in acute renal failure, 324
  burns and, 566, 567
  in chronic renal failure, 296–298
  in cirrhosis, 542
  in congenital heart disease, 392
  in developmental disabilities, 713

  in dialysis, 307, 310
  in glomerulonephritis, 329
  in renal transplantation, 311
  in tube feeding, 131
Fluid restriction, cerebral edema, 723
Fluid retention, congestive heart failure, 388
Fluids
  abnormal losses of, 34, 36
  hemodialysis and, 307
  hydration status, evaluation of, 71
  peritoneal dialysis and, 310
  shifts in, 22
  transfer of, 19–22
Fluoridation, dental caries and, 192
5-fluorouracil, 584
Flush reactions, 110
  nicotinic acid and, 380, 382
Focal tissue reactions, 7
Folate
  alcoholism and, 531
  folate dependency, 674
  urea cycle disorders and, 658
Folic acid
  anemias and, 693, 694
  causes of deficiency, 689, 692
  digestion/absorption of, 226
  hemoglobin synthesis and, 689–690
Food, cancer-causing, 575–576
Food allergy, 167–181
  clinical manifestations, 171–172
  diagnosis of, 172–175
    cutaneous testing, 174
    diet history, 173
    diet testing, 174–175
    elimination diet, 175, 176
    food diary, 173–174
  food allergens, 167, 170
  prevention of, 172
  treatment of, 175–181
    avoidance diets, 175–180
    drug therapy, 181
    food restrictions, 180–181
Food choice plan, diabetic diet, 443
Food diary, food allergy, 173–174
Food–drug interactions, 108, 111, 113

  alcohol–drug interactions, 113, 114–115
  effects, 101–108
    on absorption, 101–104, 109
    on metabolism, 104, 108
  monoamine oxidase inhibitors and, 111–113
  types of, 110
Food frequency lists, 74, 78–79
Food intake
  activity level and, 479
  alcoholism and, 530
  anatomy/physiology of, 704–705
  brain injured patient and, 726
  cancer patients and, 577–578
  control of, 474–477
    adipose tissue, 476
    central controls, 474–475
    gastrointestinal tract, 476
    hormones, 476
    liver, 476
    sensory factors, 477
  increasing, methods of, 121–123
  problems of developmentally disabled, 705–709
  problems in PKU patient, 637
  problems in psychiatric patients, 735
  reflexes in, 705–708
  thermogenic response, 479
Food poisoning, 240
Food records, 74
Foramen ovale, 345
Force fluids, 296
Foregut tumors, 255
Formula diets, weight-loss and, 491, 492
Formula feeding products, listing of, 772–785
Frank-Starling law, 347
Free radicals, 611
French tube measure, 130
Fructose-1-phosphate aldolase, 666, 667
Fructose, in diabetic diet, 439–440
Fructose loading test, in diagnosis of hypoglycemia, 459
Fructose metabolism, metabolic pathways, 667

Fructose metabolism disorders,
461, 666–668
  fructosuria, 666–668
    essential fructosuria, 666
  hereditary fructose-1,
    6-bisphosphatase defi-
    ciency, 666–668
  hereditary fructose intoler-
    ance, 666–668
    biochemical abnormalities,
      666
    clinical manifestations,
      666–668
    diagnosis, 668
    nutritional care, 668
  nutritional care, 668–669
Fructose-restricted diet, 668–669
Fructose tolerance test, 668
Fruits
  sodium content, 777–779
  sources of Vitamin A, 788
  sources of Vitamin C, 788
Full diet, 121
Full liquid diet, 119
Full-thickness burn, 565
Fulminant hepatitis, 524
  complications, 525
Functional abnormalities, 6
Functional renal failure,
  322–323
Function tests, nutritional
  assessment, 71
Fungal infections, parenteral
  feeding and, 141
Furazolidone, 111

G
GABA (gamma-aminobutyric
  acid), 537, 538
Gag reflex, food intake and, 707
Galactokinase deficiency, 663
Galactose-1-phosphate uridyl
  transferase, 664–665
Galactose, metabolic pathways,
  663
Galactosemia, 663–666
  biochemical abnormalities,
    663–664
  clinical manifestations,
    664–665
  diagnosis, 664
  forms of, 663–664
  monitoring in, 666
  nutritional care, 665–666

Gallbladder, 227
  diseases of
    cholecystectomy and, 259
    cholecystitis, 258–259
    gallstones, 258
  lipid malabsorption and, 232
Gallstones, 260
  formation of, 258
  intestinal resection and, 249
  pancreatitis and, 260
Gametes, 618
Gamma-aminobutyric acid, 538
  production of, 537
Gammopathies, 160
Gangrene, 10
Garren-Edwards Gastric
  Bubble, 499
Gas, intestinal, 267–268
Gastrectomy, 208
Gastric bypass, nutritional care,
  501–502
Gastric emptying, drugs and, 89
Gastric juice, secretion of,
  201–203
Gastric phase, 202
Gastric pits, 202
Gastric resections, 210–211
  conditions associated with,
    248–249
  obesity treatment, 501–502
  post-operative adaptations,
    250
  short bowel syndrome and,
    248–252
Gastric ulcer, 205. *See also*
  Peptic ulcer disease
Gastrocarcinogenic, 575
Gastroesophageal reflex, 200
  drug treatment, 200
  nutritional care, 200
Gastrointestinal allergy, 171
Gastrointestinal bleeding
  in cirrhosis, 541–542
  control of, 541
Gastrointestinal disorders
  abetalipoproteinemia, 255
  abnormal antigen absorption,
    238–239
  AIDS patients, 256–258
  carbohydrate intolerance,
    252–255
  diabetes and, 417
  diarrhea, 239–242
  endocrine-secreting tumors

  of gastrointestinal tract,
    255–256
  gluten-induced enteropathy,
    244–245
  inflammatory bowel disease,
    245–248
    chronic ulcerative colitis,
      247–248
    Crohn's disease, 246–247
  intestinal fistulas, 243–244
  intestinal lymphangiectasia,
    242–243
  malabsorption syndromes,
    230–238
  protein-losing enteropathies,
    242
  short bowel syndrome,
    248–252
  tropical sprue, 245
Gastrointestinal tract. *See also*
  specific organs
  alcoholism and, 530
  biliary tract, 227–228
  cancer of, 580
  large intestine, 230
  pancreas, 228–230
  regulation of food intake, 476
  small intestine, 219, 222–227
  splanchnic circulation, 344
Gastroparesis diabeticorum, 417
Gastrostomy, 129
G cells, 203
Gender
  cancer and, 577
  drug effects and, 93
  sex-linked traits, 619
Genetic counseling, 624
Generic name, drugs, 94
Genes, 618
Genetic factors
  in anemia, 693
  in branched-chain ketoaci-
    duria, 644
  in cirrhosis, 545, 547
  in diabetes, 402–403
  in fructose intolerance, 666
  in homocystinurias, 651, 652
  in obesity, 483
  in phenylketonuria, 630
  in pulmonary disease, 606
  in Refsum's disease, 671
  in tyrosine metabolism
    disorders, 640
  in xanthinuria, 674

Genetic regulation, immune response, 159–160
Genetic resistance, to chemo-therapy, 584
Genetics
chromosomal abnormalities, 620–621
genotype, 618–619
mutations, 619, 620
phenotype, 619
sex-linked traits, 619
transmission of genetic code, 616–618
Genotype, 618–619
Gestational diabetes, 401, 453
Gingiva, 188
Gingivitis, 191, 193
Glasgow Coma Scale, 723, 724
Glial cells, 5
Globin, 687
Globulins. *See* Immunoglobulins
Glomerular filtration rate, 283
Glomerulonephritis
acute glomerulonephritis, 328–329
chronic glomerulonephritis, 329
etiology of, 327–328
immune reactions in, 327–328
nephrotic syndrome, 329–332
nutritional care, 329
pathology in, 328
Glomerulus, 281
Glossitis, 191
Glossopharyngeal nerves, 582
Glucagon
insulin and, 405–406
production of, 403
regulation of food intake, 477
stress effects, 558, 559
Glucagon kit, 445
Glucocorticoids
Addison's disease and, 461–462
Cushing's syndrome and, 462
regulation of thermogenesis, 478
treatment with, 462
Glucomylase, 254

Gluconeogenesis, 520
primary organs in, 555
Glucose-6-phosphate dehydro-genase deficiency, 699
Glucose
cancer and, 579
diabetes and, 401–402
dieting and, 487
effects of exercise on, 446
fasting blood glucose, 417, 459
glucogenesis, 406
injury and, 559
metabolism/utilization of, 406
monitoring
blood tests, 421–422
urine·tests, 420–421
starvation and, 555
Glucose-galactose malabsorp-tion, 254–255
Glucose polymers, 125
Glucose tolerance test, 455
in diagnosis of diabetes, 418–419
in diagnosis of hypoglyce-mia, 459
Glucuronic acid, 92
Glutamate, 538
production of, 537
Glutamic oxaloacetic transami-nase, 144
Glutamic pyruvic transaminase, 144
Glutamine, function of, 127, 538
Glutamyloxalotransaminase assay, liver function, 524
Glutathione insulin transhy-drogenase, 404
Glutathione peroxidase, 698–699
Gluten, 244
Gluten-free diet, 245
Gluten-induced enteropathy, 244–245, 276
clinical manifestations, 244
diagnosis, 245
pathogenesis, 244
treatment, 245
Gluten intolerance, 244
Gluten-sensitivity, diabetes and, 417
Glycemic index, diabetic diet, 443–444

Glycine, 227
isovaleric acidemia, 650
production of, 537
Glycogen, 11
metabolic pathways, 672
metabolism of, 406
Glycogenesis, 520
Glycogenolysis, 520
Glycogen storage diseases, 668–670
biochemical abnormalities, 669–670
diagnosis of, 670–671
nutritional care, 670–671
Glycoproteins, diabetes and, 415
Glycosuria, 411
Glycosylated hemoglobin, in diagnosis of diabetes, 418
Goblet cells, 219
Gout, 673–674
biochemical abnormalities, 673
clinical features of, 673
nutritional care, 674
treatment of, 673–674
Graft, 305
Graft rejection, 167
forms of, 167
Graft-versus-host disease, 167
bone marrow transplanta-tion, 593
Graham, 177, 245
Grand-mal seizures, 719
Granulation tissue, 14
Granulocytes, 151
Granuloma, 574
Graves' disease, 463
Gravity drip method, tube feeding, 130
Griseofulvin, 104
Gross body deformities, 7
Gross organ deformities, 7
Growth charts, 51, 810–814
Growth disturbances, response to injury, 7
Growth hormone
insulin and, 405–406
regulation of food intake, 477
regulation of thermogenesis, 479
Growth hormones, stress effects, 559

Growth inhibitors, in muscular dystrophy, 734
Growth retardation
in cerebral palsy, 714
in chronic renal failure, 304, 318
in congenital heart disease, 392
in developmental disabilities, 713
in Down syndrome, 715
hemodialysis and, 308
Guillain-Barré syndrome, 730
Gull's disease, 463
Gut-associated lymphoid tissue, 150
Guthrie bacterial inhibition assay
branched-chain ketoaciduria, 646
PKU testing, 630
Gynecoid, 484

H
Hageman factor, 354
Half-life, drugs, 91
Haploid, 618
Haptens, 154
Harris-Benedict equation, 607
Hashimoto's thyroiditis, 463
Haustra coli, 230
Hay fever, 164
H chains, 155
Head/neck cancer
effects of radiation, 583
effects of surgery on, 581–582
malnutrition and, 581
nutritional care, 590
Healing, 13–15
affecting factors, 15
processes in, 13–14
Heart, 340–342
anatomy of, 240–241
cardiac cycle, 341
coronary circulation, 343–344
electrocardiogram, 341–342
Heartburn, 200
Heart disease, 387–389. *See also* Cardiovascular disease
Heavy chain disease, 160

Height
assessment in handicapped children, 712
calculation of, 50
height of age, 318
height-weight ratios in diagnosis of obesity, 480–482
Helper/inducer cells, 151
Hematocrit, 67, 692
Hematological assessment, 67–71
Hematoma, types of, 722
Heme, 687
Hemiparesis, 713
Hemizygous, 619
Hemochromatosis, 402
Hemodialysis, 305–308
attachment to machine, 305
complications of, 307–308
nutritional care, 306–307
Hemoglobin
erythropoiesis and, 685
hemoglobin variants, 696
synthesis/degradation of, 685, 687
Hemoglobin A, glucose monitoring, 421–422
Hemoglobinopathies
sickle cell anemia, 696–697
thalassemia, 697
Hemolytic anemia, 697–699
causes of, 697–699
fava beans and, 699
Hemolytic jaundice, 526
Hemopoietic stem cells, 151
Hemorrhoids, 274–275
hemorrhoidectomy, 275
Hemosiderin, 688
Hemothorax, parenteral feeding and, 141
Henderson–Hasselbalch equation, 30
Hepatic-Aid, 542, 545, 547
Hepatic artery, 518
Hepatic cords, 518
Hepatic decompensation, 535
Hepatic duct, 227
Hepatic encephalopathy, 535–537
acute type, 535–536
chronic type, 536
etiology of, 536

grading of, 542
precipitating factors, 542
protein metabolism and, 537–538
treatment of, 542–543
Hepatic failure
nutritional assessment, 548–549
nutritional care, 547–548
Hepatic fructokinase, 666
Hepatitis, 524–525
alcoholic, 524, 525, 532
clinical manifestations, 524–525
complications of, 525
treatment, nutritional care, 525
types of, 524
Hepatitis A, 524
Hepatitis B, 524
Hepatitis C, 524
Hepatocarcinogen, 575
Hepatocellular jaundice, 526
Hepatocytes, 12, 227, 518
destruction of, 533
Hepatolenticular degeneration, 676
Hepatoma, 532
Hepatorenal syndrome, 533, 535
Hepatostatic theory, food intake, 476
Hereditary disorders. *See* Genetic factors; Inborn errors of metabolism
Hereditary fructose-1, 6-bis-phosphatase deficiency, 666–668
Hereditary fructose intolerance, 666–668
biochemical abnormalities, 666
clinical manifestations, 666–668
diagnosis, 668
nutritional care, 668
Hereditary tyrosinemia, 640
Hereditary xanthinuria, 674
Heterozygous, 619
Hiatal hernia, 200
High-density lipoproteins, 365, 367
metabolism of, 370–371

High-fructose corn sweetener, in diabetic diet, 440
High-output failure
  heart, 388
  renal failure, 323
Hilus hepatis, 518
Hindgut tumors, 255
Histamine, 8, 164
  in humoral response, 156
Histamine H_2-receptor antagonist, ulcer treatment, 206
Histidine, 293
Histocompatibility antigens, 159–160
Histocompatibility marker HLA-8, 244
Histocompatibility testing, 311
HLA (human leukocyte antigen) histocompatibility marker, 244
  HLA identity, 311
HMG-CoA reductase, 364
  inhibitor in hyperlipidemia, 380, 381
Hodgkin's disease, 573
Holzel's syndrome, 252
Homeostasis
  kidney and, 283
  potassium and, 28–29
  sodium and, 26–27
Homocystinuria, 650–656
  biochemical abnormalities in, 651–652
  clinical manifestations, 651–652
  diagnosis of, 652
  forms of, 651, 652
  incidence of, 650
  monitoring in, 652
  nutritional care, 653, 655
  formula products, 655–656
Homogentisic acid oxidase, 641
Homografts, 167
Homologous pairs, 618
Homozygous, 619
Hora somni feeding, 428
Hormone-producing tumors
  carcinoid syndrome, 255–256
  diarrhea and, 240
  foregut tumors, 255
  hindgut tumors, 255
  midgut tumors, 255
Hormones. *See also* specific hormones

cancers and, 576, 581
  as chemotherapeutic agents, 584
  primary effects of, 399
  regulation of food intake, 476
Hormone-sensitive lipase, 408, 473
Host defense mechanisms, iron and, 695
House diet, 121
Human chorionic gonadotropin, weight reduction and, 498
Human growth hormone, weight reduction and, 498
Human immunodeficiency virus (HIV), AIDS, 256–258
Human leukocyte antigen histocompatibility marker, 244
  HLA identity, 311
Humoral autoimmunity, 166
Humoral response, immune system, 154–156
Hunger, definition of, 473
Huntington's chorea, 732
Hurler's syndrome, 392
Hyaline, 12
Hyaline membrane disease, 611
Hydration status, nutritional assessment, 71. *See also* Fluid intake; Fluids
Hydrogen
  acid-base balance, 30
  imbalances, 38
Hydrogen breath test, 235
Hydrogen ion, kidney and, 286
Hydrogen ions, 410
Hydrolyzed proteins, 126
Hydropic degeneration, 11
Hydrostatic pressure, 21
Hydrothorax, 389
5-hydroxyindoleacetic acid, 256
Hyperactive gag reflex, food intake and, 707
Hyperactivity
  in anorexia nervosa, 507
  food additives and, 171–172
  in psychiatric patients, 735
Hyperacute rejection, grafts, 167

Hypercalcemia, correction of, 37. *See also* Calcium
Hypercellular obesity, 485
Hyperchloremia, correction of, 37
Hyperchloremic acidosis, 33
Hypercholesterolemia, 379
  atherosclerosis and, 382
Hyperglycemia
  diabetes and, 399–400, 411, 426–427
  injury and, 558, 559
  parenteral feeding and, 141
Hyperkalemia, 29, 298, 359. *See also* Potassium
  in chronic renal failure, 298–299
  correction of, 36
Hyperlipidemia, 363, 371–375, 379–382
  dietary effects, 371–375
  drug management, 379–382
  familial combined type, 379
  nephrotic syndrome, 330–331
  treatment of, 375
Hyperlipoproteinemia, 375–379
  causes of, 375, 377
  classification of, 377–379
  dietary management, 377
Hypermagnesemia, correction of, 37. *See also* Magnesium
Hypermetabolic illness
  nutritional requirements
    energy needs, 559–560
    protein-energy ratio, 561
    protein needs, 561
    vitamins, 561–562
Hypermetabolic response
  to brain injury, 722
  to burn injury, 566–567
  to cancer, 577–580
  to injury, 557–559
  to starvation, 554–557
Hypernatremia, 28. *See also* Sodium
  correction of, 36
Hyperosmolar nonketotic coma, parenteral feeding and, 141
Hyperostosis frontalis interna, 483

Hyperphenylalaninemias. *See also* Phenylketonuria
differential diagnosis, 639–640
Hyperplasia, 7, 574
Hyperplastic obesity, 485
Hyperpnea, 412
Hypersensitivity, 151, 153, 163–165
  anaphylactic responses, 164
  cytotoxic responses, 164–165
  delayed-type sensitivity, 165
  immune complex disease, 165
  modes of contact, 170–171, 172
Hypertension, 354–363
  atherosclerosis and, 382
  essential hypertension, 355–357
  hemodialysis and, 307
  management of
    drug treatments, 360–361, 362–363
    nutritional management, 358, 362
    stepped-care approach, 362
  secondary hypertension, 355–356
  symptoms of, 358
  untreated, consequences of, 357–358
Hyperthermia, 562
Hyperthyroidism, 463
Hypertonic muscle tone, 705
Hypertonic saline, IV, 39
Hypertonic solution, 21
Hypertrophic obesity, 485
Hypertrophy, 7
Hypertyrosinemia, 640
Hypervolemia, 23
  correction of, 35
Hypnosis, obesity and, 503
Hypoactive gag reflex, food intake and, 707
Hypoalbuminemia, 291
Hypocalcemia
  correction of, 37
  in nephrotic syndrome, 331
Hypochloremia, correction of, 37
Hypoglossal nerves, 582
Hypoglycemia, 157, 458–461
  branched-chain ketoaciduria and, 649

classification of, 458–459
definition of, 458
diagnosis of, 459
in ex-alcoholics, 532
fasting hypoglycemia, 459–460
functional type, 461
liver disease and, 538–539
management of, 413, 414
mental status in, 412, 458
nutritional care, 459, 461
oral hypoglycemic drugs, 424–426
parenteral feeding and, 141
reactive hypoglycemia, 461
symptoms of, 458
tumor-related, 460
Hypoglycemic reactions, 110
Hypogonadism, 483
Hypokalemia, 29, 108, 240, 359, 363. *See also* Potassium
  correction of, 36
Hypomagnesemia, correction of, 37
Hyponatremia, 28, 240, 294. *See also* Sodium
  correction of, 35–36
Hypophosphatemia. *See* Phosphate
Hypoplasia, 7
Hypoproteinemia, 242, 291
  liver disease and, 535
  nephrotic syndrome and, 330
Hypothalamus
  body temperature regulation, 562
  fever and, 563
  hypothalamic obesity, 483
Hypothyroidism, 463
Hypotonic muscle tone, 705
Hypotonic saline, IV, 39
Hypotonic solution, 21
Hypovolemia, 23, 558
  correction of, 34–35

I

Iatrogenic deficiency, of immunity, 162–163
Iatrogenic disease, 240
Ideal weight tables, diagnosis of obesity, 480
Idiopathic disease, 240

Idiosyncrasy, response to drug, 93
Ileostomy, 272–273
  ileostomy bag, 272
  nutritional management, 272–273
  post-operative problems, 273
Ileum, 219, 222, 230
  lipid malabsorption and, 233
Immediate rejection, grafts, 167
Immune complex disease, 165
Immune complex glomerulonephritis, 327
Immune response. *See also* Hypersensitivity
  antigens, 153–154
  categories of, 153
  cell-mediated response, 154, 158
  humoral response, 154–156
  regulation of, 156–160
    cytokines, 156–158
    genetic regulation, 159–160
    local immunity, 160
    nutritional regulation, 158–159
Immune response genes, 160
Immune system
  components of
    central and peripheral systems, 150
    fixed tissues/organs of, 153
    mobile cells, 151, 153
  function of, 149
Immune system disorders
  autoimmune disease, 165–166
  categories of, 160
  food allergy, 167–181
  graft rejection, 167
  hypersensitivity, 163–165
  immunologic deficiency, 161–163
  immunoproliferative disease, 160
  tests of immunocompetency, 163
Immunity
  obesity and, 487
  types of, 149–150
Immunoblasts, 156
Immunocompetency tests, types of, 163

Immunogens, 149, 153. *See also*
    Antigens
Immunoglobulins, 154–156
    actions of, 154
    immunoglobulin A, 156
    immunoglobulin G, 155–156
    immunoglobulin M, 156
    immunoglobulin D, 156
    immunoglobulin E, 156
Immunologic deficiency, 161–
        163
    age-related disease, 162
    iatrogenic deficiency,
        162–163
    malnutrition and, 161, 162
    stress-related, 161–162
    viral disease and, 161
Immunoproliferative disease,
        160
    nutritional care, 160–161
    types of, 160
Immunosuppressive agents,
        renal transplantation,
        312, 313
Immunotherapy
    bone marrow transplanta-
        tion, 593
    cancer treatment, 585
    side effects, 585
Inborn errors of metabolism.
        See also individual
        disorders
    amino acid metabolism
        disorders, 625–659
    carbohydrate metabolism
        disorders, 659–671
    clinical manifestations, 623
    diagnosis, 623–624
    lipid transport disorders,
        671–673
    management of
        metabolic intervention, 624
        nutritional care, 624–625
    mineral metabolism dis-
        orders, 676–677
    nutritional care, 617
    pathophysiology, 621–623
    purine and pyrimidine
        metabolism disorders,
        672–674
    vitamin dependency dis-
        orders, 674–676
Incomplete dominance, 619

Incomplete penetrance, genes,
        619
Increased intracranial pressure,
        brain injury, 723
Indomethacin, rheumatoid
        arthritis, 738
Induration, 66–67
Infants. *See also* Pediatric patient
    allergies in, 172, 176–177
    bronchopulmonary dyspla-
        sia, 611–613
    cleft lip/palate, 702–703
        reflexes and food intake,
        705–708
    daily requirements for
        nutrients, 626–627
    of diabetic mothers, 453
    diarrhea in, 241
    growth charts, 807–814
    guidelines for diet assess-
        ment, 805
    respiratory distress syn-
        drome, 611
Infarct, 10
Infections. *See also* Sepsis
    agents and, 562
    branched-chain ketoaciduria
        and, 649
    cancer and, 576
    fever and, 562–563
    renal transplantation and, 312
Infectious disease
    infectious hepatitis, 524
    poliomyelitis, 563
    tuberculosis, 563
    typhoid fever, 563
Infiltration, degeneration, 11
Inflammation, 7–10. *See also*
        Sepsis
    cancer and, 577
    cellular response to, 8
    drugs and, 91
    duration of, 10
    influencing factors, 8, 10
    systemic manifestations, 8
    vascular response to, 8
Inflammatory bowel disease,
        239, 245–248
    chronic ulcerative colitis,
        247–248
    Crohn's disease, 246–247
    nutritional assessment, 248
    nutritional care, 248

Inflammatory response, 153
Influx, fluids, 239
Infusion pumps, insulin
        treatment, 425–426
Ingestants, in allergies, 170
Inhalants, in allergies, 170
Inhalation, drugs, 88
Initiators, cancer cells, 574–575
Injectants, in allergies, 171
Injury
    cellular responses to, 7–13
    metabolic effects, 557–559
        catabolic response, 557
        development of malnutri-
            tion, 559
        endocrine alterations,
            558–559
        increased metabolic rate,
            558
Insensible losses, 22
Insulin, 424–426. *See also*
        Insulin treatment
    amino acid metabolism and,
        410–411
    antihypertensives and, 363
    carbohydrate metabolism
        and, 406–407
    catabolic hormones and,
        405–406
    diabetic renal disease, 333
    lipid metabolism and,
        408–410
    normal actions of, 405
    pancreatic production, 403–
        404
    protein metabolism and,
        410–411
    regulation of food intake, 476
    regulation of thermogenesis,
        478–479
    response to injury, 558
Insulin-dependent diabetes, 401
Insulin-producing islet cell
        tumors, 460
Insulin shock, 412
Insulin treatment, 424–426
    conventional therapy, 425
    infusion pumps, 425–426
    intensive therapy, 425–426
    meal planning and, 426
    pregnant diabetic patients,
        454, 455, 456
    properties of, 424, 425

sources of insulin, 424
types of insulins, 424–425
Intact nephron hypothesis, 289
Intact proteins, 127
Intensive therapy, insulin treatment, 425–426
Intercellular material, 5
Intercostal muscles, 601
Interferon, 157
Interleukin 1, 157
fever and, 562
Interleukin-1 *a*, 157
Interleukin-2, 157
Interleukin-2 *b*, 157
cancer treatment, 585
Interleukin 6, 157
Intermediate branched-chain ketoaciduria, 644, 649
Intermediate-density lipoproteins, 365, 367
Intermittent branched-chain ketoaciduria, 644, 649
Intermittent claudication, 416
Intermittent feeding, 129–130
Intermittent peritoneal dialysis, 308
Internal elastic lamina, 346
Interstitial fluid, 17
Intestinal fistulas, 243–244
Intestinal gas, 267–268
components of, 267–268
management of, 268
Intestinal lymphangiectasia, 242–243
Intestinal phase, 202
Intestinal stasis syndrome, 233
Intestinal tract. *See* Gastrointestinal disorders; Gastrointestinal tract
Intracellular fluid, 17
Intracellular triglyceride lipases, 408
Intractable diarrhea, 239
Intradermal administration, drugs, 88–89
Intradialytic parenteral nutrition, 326–327
Intragastric balloon therapy, obesity treatment, 499–500
Intragastric tube feeding, 128, 129

Intramuscular administration, drugs, 88–89
Intrarenal failure, 323
Intrathecal administration, drugs, 88–89
Intravascular fluid, 17
Intravenous administration, drugs, 88–89
Intravenous feeding, energy supply and, 39, 42. *See also* Parenteral feeding
Intravenous fluids, types of, 38–39, 40–41
Intravenous pyelogram, kidney, 288
Intravenous tolbutamide response test, in diagnosis of hypoglycemia, 459
Intravenous tolerance test, in diagnosis of hypoglycemia, 459
Intrinsic factor, 226, 689, 694
Intussusception, 255–256
Inversion, chromosomes, 621
Ionized drugs, 89
Iron
absorption of, 227
in anemia, 695–696
bacterial proliferation and, 695–696
chronic renal failure and, 303
hemodialysis and, 307
hemoglobin synthesis and, 688–689
host defense mechanisms and, 695
parenteral feeding and, 139–140
pregnancy needs, 695
regulation of, 688
respiration and, 605
in sickle cell anemia, 697
solubility aspects, 689
supplements at mealtime, 695
Irritable bowel syndrome, 269
Ischemia, 10
Ischemic atrophy, 10
Islets of Langerhans, 403
Isoniazid, tuberculosis, 563
Isotonic dehydration, 28
Isotonic solution, 21
Isotopic renogram, kidney, 288

Isovaleric acidemia, 650
clinical manifestations, 650
diagnosis of, 650
metabolic abnormalities, 650
monitoring in, 650
nutritional care, 650
Isovaleryl-CoA dehydrogenase, 650

J
Jacksonian seizures, 720
Jaundice
causes of, 526
in hepatitis, 524
nutritional care, 526
types of, 526
Jaw
food intake and, 704, 708
jaw bone, 188
jaw surgery, 194
jaw wiring in obesity treatment, 502
J chain, 156
Jejunal ulcers, 205, 206
Jejunocolic bypass, obesity treatment, 499, 500
Jejunoileal bypass, obesity treatment, 499–500
Jejunostomy, 129
Jejunum, 219, 222
lipid malabsorption and, 231
Joule, definition of, 473
Juices, sources of Vitamin C, 788
Juvenile rheumatoid arthritis, 738
classification of, 738
incidence of, 738
nutritional assessment, 738
nutritional care, 738–739
Juxtaglomerular apparatus, 282

K
Kallikreins, 256, 354
Karyotype, 574
Kayser-Fleischer rings, 676
Kerckring's folds, 219
Ketoacidosis, 409, 412, 413–414
classification for severity, 413
pregnancy and, 455
Ketoaciduria. *See* Branched-chain ketoaciduria
Ketone bodies
commercial tests for, 421

Ketone bodies *(continued)*
diabetes and, 409, 412
formation of, 409
hypoglycemic drugs,
422–426
insulin, 424–426
sulfonylureas, 422–424
Ketonemia, 412
Ketonuria, 412
Ketosis, in epileptic patient, 722
Kidney disease. *See also* Renal
disease; Renal failure
anemia and, 692–693
diabetes and, 416
Kidneys
acid-base balance, 31
anatomy of, 281–283
fructose intolerance and, 667
functions of, 283–287
gluconeogenesis, 555
hypertension and, 358
in regulation of blood pressure, 350–351
Kidney stones, intestinal
resection and, 249
Kilocalories, definition of, 473
Kinetic resistance, to chemotherapy, 584
Kininases, 354
Kinins, 8
in regulation of blood
pressure, 354
Korsakoff's psychosis, 531
Kupffer cells, 518, 521
Kussmaul respiration, 299, 412
Kwashiorkor, 48
Kwashiorkor-like syndrome, 80

L
Labeled carbon breath test, 235
Labile cells, 5
Laboratory abnormalities, 6
Laboratory values, listing of
normal values, 760–766
Labor/delivery, diabetes and,
455
Lactase deficiency, 252–254
Lactase enzyme, 253
Lactic dehydrogenase, 144
Lactobezoars, 213
Lactoovovegetarian, 122

Lactose, in galactosemia, 664,
665
Lactose intolerance, 252–254
diagnosis of, 253
forms of, 252
nutritional care, 253–254
Lactose-restricted diet, 253
Lactose tolerance test, 253
Lactosuria, 252
Lactulose, 542
Laennec's cirrhosis, 532
Lamellar bodies, 600
Lamina propria, 219–220
Laminar air flow room, 593
Laminar flow, 601
Lanugo, 507
Large intestine, 230
anatomy of, 230
colon surgery
colostomy, 273–274
ileostomy, 272–273
diseases of
constipation, 268–270
diverticular disease,
270–271
intestinal gas, 267–268
normal physiology, 230
rectal surgery, 274–275
Late dumping syndrome, 212
Laurence-Moon-Biedl syn-
drome, 483
Laxatives, constipation and,
269–270
LCAT (Lecithin-cholesterol
acyl-transferase), 370
L chains, 155
L-DOPA, Parkinson's disease,
729
Lecithin cholesterol acyl-transferase, 370
Left ventricular heart failure,
388
Leucine
branched-chain ketoaciduria,
648, 644–650
leucine sensitivity, 461
Leucine sensitivity test, in diagnosis of hypoglycemia,
459
Leukemia, 574, 590–594
cause of, 591
characteristics of, 592
classification of, 590–591,
592

nutritional care, 593–594
treatment
bone marrow transplanta-
tion, 591, 593–594
goal of, 591
Leukemias, 160
Leukocytes, 5, 151
Leukopenia, 584
Leukotrienes, 351, 352
Levodopa, 108
Light chain disease, 160
Linoleate supplement, in multiple sclerosis, 732
Linoleic acid, 125, 351
Lipase, 259, 261
adipose tissue and, 473
Lipectomy, obesity treatment,
498–499
Lipemia, 408
diabetes and, 411–412
Lipid-infiltration hypothesis,
atherosclerosis and, 384
Lipid intake
in cirrhosis, 540
in diabetic diet, 408–410,
428, 430
in hepatic encephalopathy,
543
in hepatitis, 525
parenteral feeding and,
136–138, 141
in pulmonary disease, 607
in respiratory failure, 610
in restricted calorie diet, 489
types of lipids, 125–126
in underweight treatment,
505
Lipid metabolism, 406,
408–409
cancer and, 579
fatty acid synthesis/storage,
408
liver and, 364, 369
liver disease and, 539
Lipids. *See also* Plasma lipid
abnormalities; Plasma
lipids
chronic renal failure and, 304
digestion of, 222, 224–225
drug effects, 98, 100, 103, 104
drug metabolism and, 104,
108
intracellular degeneration
related to, 11–12

ketoacidosis, 409–410
ketone body formation, 409
malabsorption of, 231–233
Lipid-soluble drugs, 89, 90
Lipid storage disease, 484
Lipid transport disorders, 671–673
Refsum's disease, 671–672
Lipiduria, nephrotic syndrome, 331
Lipoatrophy, diabetes and, 414
Lipolysis, 223, 408
Lipomas, 484
diabetes and, 414
Lipoprotein lipase, 408, 473
Lipoproteins, 364–371
apoproteins, 364–365
classification of
chylomicrons, 365–367
high-density lipoproteins, 365, 367
intermediate-density lipoproteins, 365, 367
low-density lipoproteins, 365, 367, 370, 372, 373
very-low density lipoproteins, 365, 367, 368, 373
metabolism of, 368–371
endogenous transport system, 368, 370
exogenous transport system, 368
HDL metabolism, 370–371
structure of, 364
Liposarcomas, 484
Liposuction, obesity treatment, 498
Lipoxygenase, 352
Lip. *See* Cleft lip and palate
Liquid diets, types of, 119–120
Liquid nutritional supplements, 122
Lithium, side effects, 736
Lithocholic acid, 227–228
Liver
anatomy/physiology of, 518–519
cancer of, 581
ethanol metabolism, 528–529
fatty metamorphosis, 12
fructose intolerance and, 667
functions of
alcohol metabolism, 521

carbohydrate metabolism, 520
circulatory function, 522
digestive function, 521
excretion function, 521–522
lipid synthesis, 521
lymph production, 522
mineral storage, 521
protein metabolism, 520–521
vitamin synthesis, 521
gluconeogenesis, 555
glycogen storage disease, 669–670
lipid malabsorption and, 232
lipids synthesis, 364, 369
regenerative capacity of, 533
regulation of food intake, 476
Liver disease
alcoholic liver disease, 531–532
cirrhosis, 533–547
diagnosis of, 522–524
hepatic failure, nutritional care, 547–548
hepatitis, 524–525
jaundice, 526
jejunoileal bypass and, 499–500
nutritional assessment, 548–549
Liver lobule, 519
Liver transplant
indications for, 549
pre-transplant diet, 549
survival rates, 549
Lobules, lungs, 600
Local immunity, 160
Locus, genes, 618
Logarithmic dose–response curve, 87, 88
Logic dose, drugs, 94
Log kill hypothesis, chemotherapy, 584
Lomotil, side effects, 241
Long-chain triglycerides, 125–126, 223
Loop diuretics, 360, 362
Low-density lipoproteins, 365, 367, 370, 372, 373
Lower body obesity, 484
Lower esophageal incompetence, 200–201, 214

Lower esophageal sphincter, 197
disorders of, 199–200
factors affecting pressure, 197, 200, 201
Low-fat diet
in acute pancreatitis, 260
in gallbladder disease, 259
in hypertension, 359, 362
in multiple sclerosis, 732–733
Low-microbial diet, 593–594
Lundh test meal, 259
Lungs
anatomy of, 600
elasticity of, 601–602
functions of, 603
Lymphadenitis, 8
Lymphatics
intestinal lymphangiectasia, 242
lipid malabsorption and, 233
Lymph nodes, 153
Lymphoblasts, 156
Lymphocytes, 8
in the peripheral circulation, 162
types of, 151
Lymphocytic leukemia, 590
Lymphokines, 157
Lymphomas, 160
Lymph production, liver and, 522

M

Macroangiopathy, 416
Macromolecules, digestion of, 238
Macronodular liver, 533
Macrophages, 8, 151
"Magic 36" test, obesity assessment, 482
Magnesium
alcoholism and, 530
hypertension and, 357, 359
imbalances, 37
parenteral feeding and, 139
respiration and, 605
Major histocompatibility complex, 159
Malabsorption, 275–276
in cirrhosis, 540
drug effects, 98, 102
flatulence and, 269

Malabsorption *(continued)*
  in gastric surgery patients, 213
  primary/secondary, 98
Malabsorption syndromes,
    230–238
  carbohydrate malabsorption,
    233–234
  causes of, 230–231, 232
  diagnosis of, 235–236
  drug-induced, 234–235
  lipid malabsorption, 231–233
  protein malabsorption, 234
  symptoms of, 235
  treatment, 236–238
    medium-chain triglyceride
      oil, 237–238
    nutritional care, 236–237
  Vitamin B_{12} malabsorption,
    234
Malignant tumors, 572. *See also*
    Cancer
Mallory-Weiss syndrome, 205
Malnutrition, 45
  alcoholism and, 530, 545
  biochemical indices, 548
  chronic renal failure and,
    312–313
  Crohn's disease and, 246
  degrees of, 55, 56
  diabetes and, 401
  in hospitalized patients, 48,
    162
  immunologic deficiency and,
    161, 162, 163
  oral cavity abnormalities
    and, 191
  protein-calorie malnutrition,
    77, 80
  respiratory failure and, 602,
    605, 607
  in surgical patient, 564
Malonyl-CoA, 409
Mandible, 188
  food intake and, 704, 708
Mania, treatment of, 736
Manifestations
  of disease, 6
  pathognomonic, 6
Mannitol, diabetic diet, 440
MAO inhibitors. *See* Mono-
    amine oxidase (MAO)
    inhibitors
Maple syrup urine disease. *See*

Branched-chain ketoaci-
    duria
Marasmic kwashiorkor, 80
Marasmus, 48, 77, 80
Marfan's syndrome, 392
Markers, antigens, 160
Mast cells, 156
Mastication, 187–188
Masticatory insufficiency, 194
Matrix, 5
Maxilla, 188, 704
Maxillomandibular fixation, 194
Mazindol, weight reduction
    and, 496
Meal frequency, weight loss
    and, 490
Mean corpuscular hemoglobin,
    67
Mean corpuscular hemoglobin
    concentration, 69
Mean corpuscular volume, 67
Meat
  high-sodium meats, 792
  low-sodium meats, 793
  protein foods, 786
Mechanical ventilation
  problems related to, 610
  in respiratory failure, 610
Meconium ileus, 261, 265
Mediastinum, 600
Mediators, 156
Medical liquid diet, 120
Medical records, abbreviations
    used, 753–759
Medicare Prospective Payment
    System, 45
Medium-chain triglyceride oil,
    237–238
Medium-chain triglycerides,
    125–126, 224–225
Megaloblastic anemias,
    693–695
  cause of, 693–694
  nutritional care, 695–696
  pernicious anemia, 694
  symptoms of, 694
Megaloblastic cells, 694
Meiosis, 618
Meissner's plexus, 186
Melanin, in PKU, 629
Membrane, 4
Memory cell, 151
Mental disorders

drug addiction, 736
  mood disorders, 736
  psychosis, 734–735
  schizophrenia, 735–736
Mental retardation
  Down syndrome, 715
  galactosemia, 664, 665, 666
  in PKU, 629
Mental status
  chronic renal failure, 304
  diabetes and, 446
  hemodialysis and, 307
  hepatic encephalopathy and,
    535
  hypoglycemia and, 412, 458
Mercaptans, 535
6-mercaptopurine, 584
Mesangial cells, 282
Mesenchymal cells, 5, 683
Mesoderm, 4
Mesomorphs, 484
Mesothelium, 4
Metabolic acidosis, 420
  correction of, 38
  diabetes and, 412
Metabolic affectors, obesity
    treatment, 498
Metabolic alkalosis, correction
    of, 38
Metabolic disorders. *See* Inborn
    errors of metabolism
Metabolic pathway, enzymes,
    621, 622
Metabolic rate increases,
    cardiac cachexia and,
    391
Metabolic wastes, kidney and,
    286
Metaplasia, 574
Metastases, 572, 574
Metastatic calcification, 13
Methionine, homocystinuria,
    651–652, 653
Methotrexate, 584
Methyl-cellulose, 270
Methyl-cobalamin-dependent
    homocysteine-N^5-meth-
    yltetrahydrofolate
    methyltransferase, 674
3-methylhistidine, 66
Methylmalonic acidemia, 674
Methylxanthines
  food sources of, 770

myocardial infarction and, 387

pharmacologic uses, 769

Micelles, 223–224

Microalbuminemia, 333

Microangiopathy, 416

Microcirculation, 346

Microcytic anemia, 695–696, 699

  causes of, 695, 696

  heavy metal intoxication and, 696

  iron deficiency in, 695–696

  protein deficiency in, 696

Microencephaly, in PKU, 629

Micronodular liver, 533

Microsomal ethanol oxidizing system, 528

Microvilli, 219

Midarm circumference method, 55, 56

  renal patient assessment, 318

Midarm fat area method, 55–56

Midarm muscle area method, 56

Midgut tumors, 255

Milk-free diet, 176–177

  lactose intolerance, 252–254

  milk-substitutes, 177, 253, 265

Milk products

  sodium content, 793

  tetracycline and, 103

  types of, 786–787

Mineral metabolism disorders, 676–677

  acrodermatitis enteropathica, 676–677

  Wilson's disease, 676

Minerals. *See also* specific minerals

  alcoholism and, 530–531

  in diabetic diet, 440

  digestion/absorption of, 226–227

  drug effects, 100–101

  drug metabolism and, 105–107, 108

  liver synthesis of, 521

  parenteral feeding and, 139–140

  safe/adequate daily intake, 749

  tube feeding, 127

Minimal residue diet, 267

Mirror test, obesity assessment, 482

Missense mutations, 620

Mitogenic response, 162

Mitogens, 162

Mitosis, 571

Mitral valve, 340

Mixed-function oxidizing system, 92

Modified diets, 121

Modular formulas, 127, 545

Molecular weight, 20

Monoamine oxidase, 111, 113

Monoamine oxidase (MAO) inhibitors

  avoidance of amphetamines and, 496

  categories of, 111

  food reactions, 111–113

Monoclonal, 160

Monocycline, 104

Monocytes, 8, 151, 155

Monokines, 157

Monomer, 156

Mononeuropathy, 417

Mononuclear cells, 151

Mononuclear/phagocyte system, 153

Monosaccharides, 125

Monounsaturated fatty acids, 373

Mood disorders, 736

  drug treatment, 736

  types of, 736

Morbid obesity, 479

Morgagni-Stewart-Morel syndrome, 483

Moro's reflex, food intake and, 706

Mucin degenerations, 11

Mucopolysaccharides, diabetes and, 416

Mucosa, 186

Mucositis, 583

Mucous chief cells, 202

Mucous colitis, 269

Mucous neck, 202

Multi-infarct dementia, 732

Multiple electrolytic solutions, IV, 39

Multiple endocrine neoplasia-type I, 206

Multiple sclerosis, 732–733

  clinical course, 732

  nutritional care, 732–733

  symptoms of, 732

Muscles

  contraction of, 704

  muscle layer, 186

  muscle tissue, 4

  nervous system and, 705

  tone of, 704–705

Muscular dystrophy, 733–734

  death and, 733

  management of, 734

  nutritional assessment, 734

  nutritional care, 734

  pathogenesis, 733–734

  progression of, 733

Muscularis mucosa, 186

Musculoskeletal disorders

  classification of, 737

  juvenile rheumatoid arthritis, 738

  osteoarthritis, 737

  rheumatoid arthritis, 737–738

Mutagens

  atherosclerosis and, 385

  in food, 575

Mutations, 619, 620

  cancer cells, 574–575

  missense mutations, 620

  modes of inheritance and, 619

  no-sense mutations, 620

  point mutations, 620

  silent mutations, 620

Myasthenia gravis, 733

Mycobacterium tuberculosis, 563, 695

Myelin, 5

Myelocytic leukemia, 590–591

Myenteric plexus, 186

Myocardial infarction, 386–387

  atherosclerosis and, 382

  clinical course, 386

  clinical manifestations, 386

  diagnosis of, 386

  management of, 386–387

    coronary bypass surgery, 387

    drug treatment, 386–387

    nutritional care, 386, 398

    sodium restriction, 387

Myocardium, 340

Myxedema, 463
Myxomas, 11

N

Nasoduodenal tube feeding, 128
Nasojejunal tube feeding, 128
National Cholesterol Education
    Program, 375, 377
Natriuretic factors, in regula-
    tion of blood pressure,
    352, 354
Natural immunity, 149–150
Natural killer (NK) cells, 151
Nausea, 203, 204
    disease related, 204
    drug related, 97, 100
Necrobiosis, 10
Necrosis, modes of action,
    10–11
Needle biopsies, lung, 605
Needle catheter jejunostomy,
    129
Negative inotropic effect, 347
Neomycin, 542
Neonatal hepatitis, 524
Neonatal tyrosinemia, 640
Neoplasia, 7, 574
Neoplasms
    classification of, 572–574
        by embryonic origin,
            573–574
        by histologic type, 573
        by tissue of origin, 572–573
    growth stages, 574
    proliferative cells and,
        571–572
    staging of, 574
Nephron, 281
Nephropathy, diabetes and, 416
Nephrotic syndrome, 291
    clinical manifestations, 329–
        331
    treatment
        diuretics, 331, 332
        nutritional care, 331–332
Nervous system
    diabetes and, 416–417
    muscles and, 705
    neurotransmitters and, 536
Nervous tissue, 4
Neurilemma, 14
Neurogenic bladder, 717

Neurogenic bowel, 717
Neurological disorders
    brain injury, 722–727
    dementia, 731–732
    epilepsy, 719–722
    nutritional effects of drugs,
        720–721
    Parkinson's disease, 729–730
    spinal cord injury, 727–729
Neuromuscular disorders. *See
    also* Developmental
    disabilities
    amyotrophic lateral sclerosis,
        730–731
    Guillain-Barré syndrome, 730
    Huntington's chorea, 732
    multiple sclerosis, 732–733
    muscular dystrophy,
        733–734
    myasthenia gravis, 733
Neuromuscular junction, 536
Neuron, 4
Neuropathy
    classification of, 417
    diabetes and, 416–417
Neurotransmitters
    false neurotransmitters, 537
    hepatic encephalopathy and,
        537
    nerve impulses and, 536
    types of, 536–537
Neutrophils, 8, 151, 155
New vegetarians, 123
Niacin
    alcoholism and, 531
    drug metabolism and, 108
Nicotinic acid, hyperlipidemia
    and, 380, 382
Night-eater syndrome, 484
Nitrogen
    calculation of nitrogen
        balance, 66, 81
    cancer and, 579–580
    chronic renal failure abnor-
        malities, 291–292
    parenteral feeding and, 138
Nitrogen-energy ratio
    injury and, 561
    parenteral feeding and, 138
    pulmonary disease and, 608
Nitrogen mustard, 584
Nitrogen retention, 291
Nitroglycerin, angina and, 385

Nitroprusside, homocystinuria,
    652
Nitrosamines, 575
Nocturia, 290, 296
Non-anion gap acidosis, 33
Noncongenital condition, 7
Non-insulin dependent
    diabetes, 401
Nonpancreatic tumors,
    hypoglycemia and, 460
Nonshivering thermogenesis,
    472, 478
Nonsynthetic reactions, drugs,
    91–92
Nonvolatile acids, 30
Norepinephrine
    food intake and, 476
    hepatic coma and, 538
    production of, 536
Normochloremic acidosis, 33
Normocytic anemias, 691–693
    aplastic anemia, 692–693
    treatment of, 693
No-sense mutations, 620
Nothing by mouth, 211, 247,
    260, 564
Null cells, 151
Nursing bottle syndrome, 193
Nutrient absorption, drug
    effects, 97–98
Nutrient intake. *See* Food intake
Nutrient metabolism, drug
    effects, 98, 100–101
Nutritional assessment, 72–73
    cell-mediated immune
        function, 66–67
    clinical observations, 71
    conditions related to nutri-
        tional risk, 49, 77
    dietary assessment, 71–77
    energy stores, estimation of,
        52–56
    evaluation requirements,
        80–81
    function tests, 71
    hematological assessment,
        67–71
    hydration status, 71
    nitrogen balance, 66
    problem-identification, 77,
        80–82
    somatic protein, estimation
        of, 56, 59

visceral protein, estimation of, 59, 64–66

vitamin assays, 70, 71

weight in relation to height, 50–52

Nutritional care, documentation, 45–48. *See also* specific disorders

Nutritional support. *See also* specific methods

conventional feeding, 119–123

parenteral feeding, 132–144

planning for, 118

transitional feeding, 144

tube feeding, 123–132

Nutrition history, 74

O

Oat bran, 374

Obesity, 12, 479–504

acupuncture treatment, 498

age of onset classification, 485–486

behavior modification and, 494–495

definition of, 479

developmental disabilities and, 713

diabetes and, 403, 427–428

diagnosis of

bioelectrical impedance, 482

height-weight ratios, 480–482

ideal weight tables, 480

research methods, 479–480

self-assessment methods, 482

triceps skinfold, 480, 485

dietary treatment

fad diets, 492–493

fasting, 491

formula diets, 491, 492

packaged food programs, 492

restricted-calorie diet, 488–491

very low calorie diet, 491–492

drug treatment, 496–498

anorectic drugs, 496, 497

bulking agents, 496, 498

metabolic affectors, 498

etiological classification, 482–484

drug-related factors, 483–484

endocrine disorders, 483

environmental factors, 484

genetic factors, 483

hypothalamic obesity, 483

nutritional factors, 483

psychological factors, 484, 503

exercise and, 493–494

exogenous and endogenous, 482

fat distribution classification

generalized fat accumulation, 484–485

localized fat accumulation, 484

hyperlipidemia and, 374

hypertension and, 356, 358

hypnosis and, 503

immune factors in, 487

immunological deficiency and, 163

metabolic alterations and, 486–487

in muscular dystrophy, 734

nutritional assessment in, 504

in Prader-Willi syndrome, 716

prevention of, 504

psychotherapy and, 502–503

recommended treatment for, 503, 504

respiratory failure and, 606

risks related to, 486

self-help groups, 496

spina bifida, 716

surgical treatment, 498–502

biliopancreatic bypass, 499, 501

complications of, 499–500, 502

gastric restrictive surgery, 501–502

intragastric balloon therapy, 499–500

jaw wiring, 502

jejunocolic bypass, 499, 500

jejunoileal bypass, 499–500

lipectomy, 498–499

liposuction, 498

nutritional care and, 500–501

treatment considerations, 487–488

treatment goals, 487

weight loss/gain cycles, 504

Obesity hypoventilation syndrome, 486

Obligatory thermogenesis, 477

Obligatory water excretion, 22

Obligatory water loss, 284

Observational learning, 494

Obstructive constipation, 268–269

Obstructive jaundice, 526

Obstructive nephropathy, 323

Obturator, in cleft lip/palate, 703

Ochronosis, 641

Octopamine, 537

Oddi's sphincter, 227

Odynophagia, 198

Olestra, 491

Olfaction

anatomy of, 95–96

drug effects, 96–97, 99

types of odors, 95

Oligopeptidases, 225

Oliguric, 290

Omega-3 fatty acids, 351, 362

coronary heart disease and, 373–374

Oncogenic viruses, 577

Operant conditioning, 494–495

Operator gene, 618

Operon, 618

Opportunistic infections, 161, 258

bone marrow transplantation, 593

Opsonization, 154

Optimum body weight, 51

Oral cavity

components of, 187

salivary glands, 189–190

swallowing, 190, 191, 197

teeth, 187–189

Oral cavity abnormalities

age and, 196–197

dental disease, etiology of, 191–192

Oral cavity abnormalities
   (continued)
   dental diseases, 191–194
      dental caries, 192–193
      gingivitis, 191, 193
      masticatory insufficiency,
         194
      periodontal disease,
         193–194
      stomatitis, 191, 193
   jaw surgery, 194
   malnutrition and, 191, 194
   swallowing abnormalities,
      195
Oral glucose tolerance test
   in diagnosis of diabetes, 418–
      419, 455
   in diagnosis of hypoglyce-
      mia, 459
Oral hypoglycemic agents,
      sulfonylureas, 424–426
Oral rehydration solutions, 241
Organization, tissue repair, 13
Orogastric tube, 129
Orthomolecular psychiatry,
      psychiatric patients, 735
Orthopnea, 389
Osmolarity, 20–21
   kidney and, 283
   measurement of, 768
   parenteral feeding, 140, 142
   serum, 71
   serum osmolarity formula,
      768
   tube feeding, 123
Osmosis, 19, 20–21
Osmotic diarrhea, 239
Osmotic injury, 10–11
Osmotic pressure, 20
Osteitis fibrosa cystica, 302
Osteoarthritis, 737
Osteodystrophy, forms of, 302
Osteomalacia, 302
   gastric surgery patients, 214
Osteopenia, 302
Osteoporosis
   gastric surgery patients, 214
   renal transplant patients, 593
Osteoradionecrosis, 583
Osteosclerosis, 302
Overfeeding, 478
   obesity in, 483, 504
Overhydration, 23

Overweight. *See* Obesity
Ovovegetarian, 122
Ovum, 618
Oxidations, drugs and, 92
Oxidative deamination, liver,
      520
Oxygen
   damaging oxidants, 699
   free radicals, 611
   in respiration, 603
   toxicity, 611
Oxygen therapy, in pulmonary
      disease, 607

P
Pacemaker cells, 341
Packaged food programs,
      weight loss and, 492
Packed cell volume, 67
Palate. *See also* Cleft lip/palate
   prenatal development of, 703
Palmar grasp, food intake and,
      707–708
Palm-chin reflex, food intake
      and, 708
Pancreas, 228–230
   anatomy of, 229–230
   diseases of
      acute pancreatitis, 260
      chronic pancreatitis,
         260–261
      cystic fibrosis, 261,
         263–265
      diagnosis, 259
   insulin production, 403–404
   lipid malabsorption and, 231
   pancreatic enzymes, 220–
      221, 225, 229
Pancreatic cholera, 255
Pancreatic enzyme extracts,
      cystic fibrosis, 265
Pancreatic insufficiency, 231,
      264
Pancreatic lipase, 223
Paneth cells, 219
Papillary muscle, 341
Paralytic ileus, 131
Paraparesis, 714
Parathyroid hormone, 286
Paregoric, side effects, 241
Parenchymal cells, 13
Parenchymal renal failure, 323
Parenchymal tissue, 12

Parenteral administration,
      drugs, 88–89
Parenteral feeding, 132–144
   in bone marrow transplanta-
      tion, 593
   in bronchopulmonary
      dysplasia, 611
   catheter insertion, 134–135
   central venous alimentation,
      134
   commercially available
      products, 135
   complexity of, 133–134
   complications of, 141–142
   composition of solutions,
      135–140
   cyclic parenteral nutrition,
      143
   in diabetic patients, 457–458
   energy needs, 140–141
   in hepatic encephalopathy,
      543–544
   in hepatic failure, 547
   indications for, 133
   intradialytic parenteral
      nutrition, 326–327
   compared to IV feeding, 133
   osmolarity, 140, 142
   in Parkinson's disease, 730
   patient monitoring, 143–144
   peripheral venous alimenta-
      tion, 142–143
   in respiratory failure,
      609–610
Pargyline, 111
Parietal cells, 202
Parietal cell vagotomy, 210
Parkinson's disease, 729–730
   clinical manifestations, 729
   feeding problems, 729
   L-DOPA, 729
   nutritional care, 730
Partial gastrectomy, 208
Partial-thickness burn, 565
Partial vegetarians, 122
Passive diffusion, 222
Passive transfer, 89
Pathogenicity, 8
Pathology, 3
   cellular responses to injury
      degeneration, 11–13
      developmental disorders, 7
      growth disturbances, 7

inflammation, 7–10
necrosis, 10–11
disease, 6–7
healing, 13–15
Patient education, diabetes
and, 448–449
Patient profile, 46
Pedal edema, 330
Pediatric patient. *See also*
Children; Infants; De-
velopmental disabilities
cancer, 576
chronic renal failure, 304
congenital heart disease, 392
diabetes, 452
end-stage renal disease,
nutritional care, 316–
317
hemodialysis, 308
Pellagrous psychosis, 531
Pendular movements, 222
Penicillamine, 87
Wilson's disease, 547
Penicillin, 91
sensitivity to, 180
Penicillium, 180
Peptic cells, 202
Peptic ulcer disease
clinical manifestations,
206
conservative management,
206–208
drug treatment, 206–207
pathogenesis, 206
sites for ulcers, 205
surgical treatment, 208–211
postoperative nutrition,
211
post-surgical complica-
tions, 212–214
types of procedures,
208–211
Peptidases, 222
Percutaneous endoscopic
gastrostomy, 129
Perimololysis, in anorexia
nervosa, 507
Periodontal disease, 193–194
etiology of, 193–194
prevention of, 194
Periodontal ligament, 188
Periodontium, 189
Periorbital edema, 330

Peripheral neuronal inhibitors,
360, 362
Peripheral neuropathy, 531
Peripheral vascular atherosclerotic occlusive
disease, 390
Peripheral vascular resistance,
347–348
Peripheral venous alimentation, parenteral feeding,
142–143
Peristalsis
small intestine, 222
stomach, 203
Peristaltic pump, tube feeding,
130
Peritoneal dialysis, 308–311
indications for, 308
nutritional care, 309–310
protocols for, 308–309
Peritoneum, 308
Permanent cells, 6
Pernicious anemia, 694
Persistent flexor reflex, food
intake and, 705–706
Persistent vegetative state, 723
Petit mal seizures, 719
pH. *See* Acid-base balance
Pharmacologic dose, drugs, 94
Pharmacology
classification of drugs, 94
drug action, mechanisms of,
87
drug effects, influencing
factors, 87–91
drug metabolism, 91–93
drug safety/effectiveness, 93
individual responses to,
93–94
Pharmacy, 87
Phenistix, 630
Phenolphthalein, 270
Phenotype, 619
Phenylacetate, urea cycle
disorders, 657–658
Phenylalanine
in PKU, 628–629, 637–638,
639
in tyrosine metabolism
disorders, 640, 641, 644
Phenylethanolamine, 537
Phenylketonuria (PKU),
625–640

clinical manifestations,
629–630
diagnosis of, 630, 639–640
feeding problems, 637
forms of, 639–640
genetic factors, 630
incidence of, 630
maternal phenylketonuria,
638–639
metabolic abnormalities,
628–629
nutritional care, 630–637
age adjustments, 636–637
in breast feeding, 631, 636
duration of diet, 638
extra energy sources, 636
follow-up procedures,
637–638
formula products, 632–
633, 634–635
low-phenylalanine diet,
631–636
Pheochromocytoma, 354, 402
Phosphate
acute renal failure and, 326
parenteral feeding and, 139
regulation of, 286
respiration and, 605
Phosphate binders, 302
Phospholipase, 352
Phosphorus
chronic renal failure abnormalities, 302–303
food sources of, 303
hemodialysis, 307
peritoneal dialysis, 310
Physical condition, drug effects
and, 93
Physiologic cell death, 10
Phytanic acid, 671–672
Phytanic acid storage disease.
See Refsum's disease
Phytobezoars, 213
Pickwickian syndrome, 486
Pinch test, obesity assessment,
482
"Pink puffer," 606
Pinocytosis, 89, 222
Placental barrier, drugs and, 91
Plaque, atherosclerosis and, 383
Plasma cell dyscrasias, 160
Plasma cells, 8, 151, 154
Plasma lipid abnormalities

Plasma lipid abnormalities
    (*continued*)
  dietary management,
      373–375, 377–378
  hypercholesterolemia, 379,
      382
  hyperlipidemia, 363,
      371–375, 379–382
  hyperlipoproteinemia,
      375–379
Plasma lipids
  age-specific values
    females, 791
    males, 790
  effects of diet
    alcohol, 374–375
    caloric intake, 374
    cholesterol, 371–372,
        375
    fatty acid saturation,
        372–373
    fiber intake, 374
    omega-3 fatty acids,
        373–374
Plasma protein binding, drugs
    and, 90
Platelet aggregation, 374
Platelet-derived growth factor,
    383
Platelets, 151
Pleiotropic, genes, 619
Pleural cavity, 600
Pleural effusion, 389
Plicae circularis, 219
Plummer-Vinson syndrome,
    200
Pluripotential cells, 5
Pneumocystis carinii, 161
Pneumocytes, 600
Pneumothorax, parenteral
    feeding and, 141
Podocytes, 282
Point mutations, 620
Point system, diabetic diet, 443
Poliomyelitis, 563
Polyclonal, 160
Polycyclic hydrocarbons, 575
Polydactyly, 483
Polydipsia, 411
Polyneuropathy, 417
Polyol sweeteners, diabetic
    diet, 439, 440
Polyphagia, 411
Polyphoretic phosphate,

    regulation of food in-
        take, 477
Polysaccharides, 125
Polyunsaturated fats, 372
Polyunsaturated fatty acids,
    158–159, 162
Polyuria, 290, 296, 411
Pompe's disease, 392
Ponderal index, diagnosis of
    obesity, 481
Pores of Kohn, 600
Portacaval shunts, 536
Porta hepatis, 518
Portal hypertension, in
    cirrhosis, 533–534
Portal lobule, 519
Portal system, 344
Portal tracts, 519
Portal vein, 344, 518
Portasystemic shunts, 536, 538
Positive reinforcement,
    modification of eating
    behaviors, 495
Postcholecystectomy syn-
    drome, 259
Postnecrotic cirrhosis, 546
Postpartum renal failure, 326
Postrenal failure, 323
Postvagotomy diarrhea, 213
Potassium
  acute renal failure and,
      325–326
  causes of altered levels, 29
  chronic renal failure and,
      298–299
  in cirrhosis, 541
  concentration disturbances,
      29
  congestive heart failure and,
      389
  content and distribution in
      body, 28
  electrolytes, 28–29
  food sources of, 299, 300–301
  function of, 28
  glomerulonephritis and, 329
  hemodialysis and, 307
  homeostasis, 28–29
  hypertension and, 357, 359
  imbalances, 36–37
  jejunoileal bypass and,
      500–501
  kidney and, 285–286
  minimum requirements, 749

  nephrotic syndrome and, 332
  normal requirements, 28
  parenteral feeding and, 139
  peritoneal dialysis and, 310
  for prevention of deficit, 34
  removal from body, 37
  renal transplantation and, 311
  signs of deficiency, 359
Potassium-restricted diet, 299
Potassium-sparing agents, in
    hypertension, 360–362,
    363
Prader-Willi syndrome, 483,
    716
Precipitation, 154
Precursor to toxic levels, 621,
    624
Prednisone
  Crohn's disease, 247
  in muscular dystrophy, 734
  in renal transplant, 312
Preeclampsia, 355
Preformed insulin, 423
Pregestational diabetes, 453–
    454
Pregnancy
  amniocentesis, 624
  diabetes and, 452–457
  hypertension in, 355
  iron needs in, 695
  maternal PKU, 638–639
  postpartum renal failure, 326
  premature labor, drugs in, 455
Premature infants, bronchopul-
    monary dysplasia,
    611–613
Premature labor, drugs in, 455
Preoptic area, hypothalamus,
    562
Prepared foods, avoidance by
    diabetic, 438
Prerenal failure, 322
Pressure overload, 388
Pressure sores, 717
  affecting factors, 724
  prevention of, 724
  staging of, 724
Prick tests, 174
Primary aldosteronism, 354
Primary diabetes, 400–401
Primary familial xanthomatosis,
    483
Primary lactose intolerance,
    252, 253

Primary malabsorption, 98
Primary protein-losing gas-
    troenteropathy, 242
Problem-oriented medical
    record, 45–48
Probucol, hyperlipidemia, 381
Procarbazine, 111
Prodromal period, hepatitis, 524
Prognostic nutritional index, 81
Progress notes, 47–48
Proinsulin, 403–404
Prolapse, rectum, 274
Promoters, cancer cells,
    574–575
Pronated grasp, 709
Proprietary, drugs, 94
Prospective payment system, 45
Prostacyclins, 351, 352
Prostaglandin, 352
    functions of, 351
    regulation of food intake, 477
    ulcer treatment, 207
Prostanoid synthetases, 352
Protein
    chronic renal failure and,
        291–293
    digestion of, 222, 225–226
    drug effects, 98, 103
    drug metabolism and, 104
    fever, effects of, 563
    forms of, 126–127
    genetic abnormalities of, 623
    intracellular degeneration
        related to, 12–13
    malabsorption of, 234
    oxidation of, 603
    quality, measures of, 126
    red blood cell formation and,
        691
    renal solute load in, 22–23
    response to injury, 558
    starvation and, 556–557
Protein catabolic rate, renal pa-
    tients assessment, 319,
    321
Protein intake
    acute renal failure, 325, 326
    animal sources of protein, 786
    in bone marrow transplanta-
        tion, 591
    in burn patient, 568
    in chronic renal failure,
        292–293
    in cirrhosis, 540

in diabetic diet, 428
in diabetic renal disease, 333
in glomerulonephritis, 329
hemodialysis and, 306
in hepatic encephalopathy,
    543
hepatitis, 525
in hypermetabolic illness,
    561
in hyperthyroidism, 463
in isovaleric acidemia, 650
in jejunoileal bypass, 501
needs under stress, 141
in nephrotic syndrome, 331–
    332
in Parkinson's disease, 730
peritoneal dialysis and, 309,
    310
protein-free foods, 800
in pulmonary disease, 608
renal patients assessment,
    319, 321
in renal transplantation,
    311–312
in respiratory failure, 610
in restricted calorie diet, 489
in spinal cord injury, 728
tube feeding and, 126–127
in underweight treatment,
    505
in urea cycle disorders, 658,
    659
vegetable sources of protein,
    786
Protein-losing enteropathies,
    242
    diseases related to, 242
Protein metabolism
    cancer and, 579–580
    liver and, 520–521
    liver disease and, 535,
        537–538
    in muscular dystrophy, 733
Protein-restricted diets, chronic
    renal failure, 292–293
Protein-sparing therapy, 39, 42
Proteinuria, 291
    nephrotic syndrome,
        329–330
Prothrombin time, liver
    function, 522, 524
Proximal gastric vagotomy, 210
Prudent diet, 121
Psoriasis, 674

Psychiatric patient. *See* Mental
    disorders
Psychological factors, obesity,
    484, 503. *See also*
    Mental status
Psychosis, 734–735
    feeding problems in, 735
    nutritional care, 735
    outpatient care, 735
    vitamin mega-doses in, 735
Psychotherapy, obesity and,
    502–503
Psyllium, 270
Pulmonary arteries, 340
Pulmonary disease
    bronchopulmonary dyspla-
        sia, 611–612
    chronic obstructive pulmo-
        nary disease, 605–608
    diagnosis of, 603–605
    malnutrition and, 605
    respiratory failure, 608–610
Pulmonary veins, 340
Pulmonic valves, 340
Pulp, of tooth, 188
Pump, in tube feeding, 130
Pureed diet, 121
Purine, gout, 673, 675
Purine and pyrimidine metabo-
    lism disorders, 672–674
    gout, 673–674
    hereditary xanthinuria, 674
P wave, in ECG, 342
Pyloric glands, 203
Pyridoxine, 108
    hemoglobin synthesis and,
        690
    urea cycle disorders, 658
Pyridoxine dependency, 675
Pyridoxine-dependent anemia,
    696
Pyrogens, 8
    types of, 562
Pyrosis, 200

Q
QRS complex, in ECG, 342
Qualitative diets, 121
Quantitative diets, 121
Quinacrine hydrochloride, 90

R
Radiation, cancer and, 577
Radical neck dissection, 582

Radiculopathy, 417
Radioallergosorbent test, 174
Raffinose, 268
Rampant caries, 192–193
Ranitidine, 206, 541
Recall antigen skin testing, 66
Recessive trait, 619
Recommended Dietary
    Allowances, 76, 77,
    746–747
Rectum, 230
    hemorrhoids, 274–275
    prolapse, 274
Red blood cells, 67, 151
    development of, 683–684
    maturation of, 684–687
Reference data, 55
Reflexes
    in food intake, 705–708
    normal infant compared to
        developmentally
        disabled, 705–708, 710
Refsum's disease
    characteristics of, 671–672
    metabolic abnormalities, 671,
        673
    nutritional care, 672
Regeneration, healing, 13–14
Regional enteritis. *See* Crohn's
    disease
Regulator gene, 618
Regurgitation, 203
Rehydration, diarrhea, 241
Reinforcers, in behavior
    modification, 494–495
Relaxation methods, hyperten-
    sion and, 356
Remission, cancer, 591
Renal arteriography, kidney,
    288
Renal biopsy, kidney, 289
Renal corpuscle, 281
Renal disease. *See also* specific
    diseases
    diabetic renal disease,
        332–333
    diagnosis
        diagnostic tests, 287–288
        direct examination,
            288–289
        renal function tests, 288
    end-stage, 290
    glomerulonephritis, 327–329

nephrotic syndrome,
    329–332
Renal failure, 290, 533. *See also*
    Acute renal failure;
    Chronic renal failure
    in cirrhosis, 540
    functional renal failure,
        322–323
    in hepatitis, 524, 525
    nutritional care, 314–315
Renal function tests, 288
Renal insufficiency, 290
Renal solute load, 22–23
    tube feeding and, 124
Renal transplantation, 290,
    311–322
    death, causes of, 312
    donor and, 311
    immunosuppressive agents,
        312, 313
    nutritional assessment, 312
    special procedures,
        318–322
    nutritional care, presurgical,
        311–312
    preparation for transplant,
        311–312
Renin, 286, 350
Renin-angiotensin system, in
    regulation of blood
    pressure, 349–350
Residue, tube feeding, 124
Resin cholestyramine, 232
Respiration, mechanisms in,
    601–602
Respiratory acidosis, 31, 610
Respiratory alkalosis, 31
Respiratory failure, 608–610
    causes of, 608
    malnutrition and, 602, 605,
        607
    mechanical ventilation, 611
    nutritional assessment,
        608–609
    nutritional care, 609–610
    patient monitoring, 610–611
    symptoms of, 608
Respiratory quotient, 142
Respiratory system
    acid-base balance, 31
    airways, 599–600
    energy needs, 602
    lungs, 600

respiration, 601–602
ventilation, 602–603
Resting energy expenditure,
    injury and, 560
Resting metabolic expenditure,
    477
Restricted-calorie diet, weight
    loss and, 488–491
Reticular fibers, 5
Reticulocytes, 685
Reticuloendothelial cells, 153
Retinitis pigmentosa, Refsum's
    disease, 671
Retinol-binding protein, 561
Retinopathy, diabetes and, 417,
    452
Retroviruses, 161
Reverse transcriptase, 161
Rheumatic heart disease, 391–
    392
Rheumatoid arthritis, 737–738
    drug treatment, 738
    nutritional care, 738
    symptoms of, 737
Rheumatoid factor, 737
Rickets
    familial Vitamin D–resistant
        type, 675–676
    Vitamin D–dependent type,
        675
Right ventricular heart failure,
    388
Root, of tooth, 188
Rooting reflex, food intake and,
    706
Rotary chewing, 708, 709
Roughage. *See* Fiber; Fiber in-
    take
Rule of nines, burn injuries, 565
Ruler test, obesity assessment,
    482
Rx, 46

S
Saccharin, diabetic diet,
    438–439
Sulfasalazine, 247
Salicylates, sensitivity to, 171,
    180, 181
Saline cathartics, 270
Saline solution, IV, 39
Saliva
    affecting factors, 190

artificial, 195
functions of, 189–190
Salivary glands, 189–190
abnormalities of
loss of taste, 196
xerostomia, 195–196
stimulation of, 195–196
Salmonella, 695
Salmonella typhosa, 563
Salt. *See also* Sodium
salt-sensitivity in hypertension, 357
salt substitutes, 296
salt-wasters, 294, 305
Sarcolemma, 14
Sarcomas, 573
Saturated fats, hypertension and, 359, 362
Scalene muscles, 601
Scarring, 13
Schilling test, 236
Schizophrenia, 735–736
genetic factors, 736
medication side-effects, 736
symptoms of, 736
Schwann cells, 5
Scintiscan, liver function, 524
Scleroderma, 166, 200
Scoliosis, 717
in muscular dystrophy, 733, 734
Scratch test, 174
Seasonal affective disorder, 736
Secondary diabetes, 402
Secondary hypertension, 355–356
etiology of, 355–356, 357
Secondary lactose intolerance, 252, 253
Secondary malabsorption, 98
Secretin, 222
Secretin-pancreozymin test, 259
Secretion, 284
Secretory diarrhea, 239–240
Secretory IgA, 156
Secretory piece, 156
Segmentation, small intestine, 222
Selective necrosis, 10
Selective vagotomy, 208, 210
Self-blood glucose monitoring, 421

Self-feeding, development of, 708–709
Self-help groups, obesity treatment, 496
Self-management, diabetes and, 449–452, 455
Semipermeable membranes, 20
Sengstaken-Blackemore tube, 541
Sensible losses, 22
Sensory factors, regulation of food intake, 477
Sepsis
definition of, 554, 562
infection producing agents, 562–563
metabolic effects, 562–563
symptoms of, 562
Serosal layer, 186
Serotonin, 536, 538, 578
Serous saliva, 189
Serum osmolarity, 71
formula for, 768
Sex chromosomes, 619
Sex-linked traits, 619
Shaping, in conditioning, 495
Shock organs, 164
Short bowel syndrome, 248–252
etiology, 248–249
nutritional assessment, 252
pathophysiology, 249–250
treatment
drug treatment, 251
nutritional management, 250–251
Shunt, 305
liver, 536
SIADH (syndrome of inappropriate ADH secretion), 722
Sickle cell anemia, 696–697
incidence of, 697
nutritional care, 697
Sideroblastic anemia, 696
Sideroblasts, 696
Signs, definition of, 6
Silent mutations, 620
Simple-partial seizures, 720
Simplesse, 491
Sinoatrial node, 341
Sinusoids, 518
Sitophobia, 195

Skeletal muscles, 4
Skin, effects of burns, 565–566
Skinfold measurements, 53–59
diagnosis of obesity, 480, 485
renal patients assessment, 318
Skin grafts, burn injuries, 567
Skin-window test, 174
Slow continuous ultrafiltration, 327
Small intestine, 219, 222–227
disorders of
abetalipoproteinemia, 255
carbohydrate intolerance, 252–255
endocrine-secreting tumors of gastrointestinal tract, 255–256
fistula, 243
gluten-induced enteropathy, 244–245
inflammatory bowel disease, 245–248
short bowel syndrome, 248–252
tropical sprue, 245
food receptors, 476
functions of, 222–227
normal structure, 219, 222
protective mechanisms, 227
Smooth muscles, 4
Snacks, diabetic diet, 428
SOAP, 46, 47
Sodium, 16
absorption of, 226–227
acute renal failure and, 325
chronic renal failure and, 294–296
concentration disturbances, 27–28
content and distribution in body, 24–26
electrolytes, 24–28
excretion, 27
in glomerulonephritis, 329
in hemodialysis, 307
homeostasis, 26–27
hypertension and, 356–357
minimum requirements, 749
in nephrotic syndrome, 332
normal requirements, 26
parenteral feeding and, 139
peritoneal dialysis and, 310
for prevention of deficit, 34

Sodium (continued)
  regulation of, 284–285
  in renal transplantation, 311
  respiration and, 605
Sodium benzoate, urea cycle
      disorders, 657–658
Sodium bicarbonate, 87, 104,
      299
Sodium in foods
  dairy products, 793
  fruits, 777–779
  high-sodium items, 803–804
  high-sodium meats, 792
  low-sodium bread/cereals/
      starches, 795
  low-sodium meats, 793
  low-sodium specialty items,
      802–803
  vegetables, 795–797
Sodium-restricted diet
  adrenocorticotropic hormone
      therapy, 432
  in cardiac cachexia, 391
  chronic renal failure,
      294–297
  in cirrhosis, 542
  in congestive heart failure,
      389
  in hypertension, 359
  in myocardial infarction, 387
  procedure/methods in, 297
  in rheumatic heart disease,
      392
  types of, 359
Soft diet, 120
Solubility, drugs, 89
Solute diuresis, 296
Solution, 20
Solvent, 20
Somatic proteins, 49
  estimation of, 56, 59
Somatostatin, 403
Somatotype, types of, 484
Somogyi effect, 413
Sonography, kidney, 288
Sorbitol
  accumulation in diabetes, 414
  in diabetic diet, 440
Source-oriented medical
      record, 48
Spastic colon, 269
Spastic constipation, 269
Spastic diplegia, 714

Spasticity, cerebral palsy, 713,
      714
Specialized transport, 89
Specific gravity, 768
Sperm, 618
Sphygmomanometer, 348
Spina bifida, 716–718
  associated problems,
      716–717
  etiology of, 717
  nutritional assessment,
      717–718
Spinal cord injury, 727–729
  causes of, 727
  effects and location of injury,
      727
  malnutrition and, 727–728
  nutritional assessment, 729
  nutritional care, 728–729
Spleen, 153
Spontaneous hypoglycemia,
      459
Sports anemia, 699
Sprue, tropical, 245, 693. See
      also Gluten-induced
      enteropathy
Stable, cells, 6
Stachyose, 268
Staging, cancer, 574
Stagnant loop syndrome, 233
Staphylococcus aureus, 240
Starvation. See also Malnutrition
  in cancer patients, 577, 578,
      581
  metabolic effects, 554–557
    early starvation, 555–556
    prolonged starvation,
      556–557
Status epilepticus, 720
Steatorrhea, 231
Stein-Leventhal syndrome, 483
Stem cells, 151
Step-One diet, 375
Stepped-care approach,
      hypertension, 362
Step-Two diet, 375
Sterile diet, 593
Sternocleidomastoid muscles,
      601
Steroids. See also Corticosteroids
  effects of, 713
  renal transplant patient, 593
Stimulant cathartics, 270

Stimulus control, modification
      of eating behaviors, 495
Stoma, 128
Stomach
  components of, 202
  digestion, 203
  functions of, 201
  peptic ulcer disease, 205–215
  secretion of gastric juice,
      201–203
  storage/motility, 203
Stomatitis, 191, 193
Strained soft diet, 121
Streptococcus mutans, 192
Stress
  cancer and, 576
  constipation and, 269
  immunologic deficiency and,
      161–162
  metabolic effects, 558
  obesity and, 484
Striated muscles, 4
Stricture of esophagus,
      199–200
Stroke
  atherosclerosis and, 382
  hypertension and, 358
  prediction of, 481
Structural abnormalities, 6
Structured lipids, 126
Subacute inflammation, 10
Subchondral bones, 673
Subcutaneous administration,
      drugs, 88–89
Subcutaneous fat obesity, 485
Subendothelium, 346
Submucosa, 186
Sucking reflex, food intake
      and, 706–707
Sucralfate, ulcer treatment,
      207
Sucrase-isomaltase deficiency,
      254
Sucrose-free diet, 254
Sucrose-restricted diet, 254
Sugar alcohol sweeteners, dia-
      betic diet, 440
Sugar intake, diabetes and,
      403, 437–438
Sulcus, 188
Sulfasalazine, 248
Sulfobromophthalein, liver
      function, 522

Sulfonamide compounds, 360, 362
Sulfonylureas, 422–424
    advantages/disadvantages of, 423
    extrapancreatic effects, 423
    types of, 423
Summation, drug interaction, 94
Superficial burn, 564–565
Superoxide dismutase, 698
Superoxide radical, 698
Suppressor cells, 151
Supraglottic laryngectomy, 582
Surface mucous cells, 203
Surfactant, lungs, 600, 602
Surgical liquid diet, 120
Surgical patient, 563–564
    cancer patients, nutritional effects, 581–582
    diabetes and, 457–458
    postoperative nutrition, 564
    preoperative nutrition, 564
Swallowing
    abnormalities of, 194–195
    brain injured patient, 725–726
    development of, 708
    dysphagia, 197–198
    Parkinson's disease and, 729
    process of, 190, 191, 197
Sweaty feet syndrome. *See* Isovaleric acidemia
Sympathetic nervous system
    parts of, 349
    in regulation of blood pressure, 349
Sympathoadrenal system, regulation of thermogenesis, 478
Symptoms, 6
Synapses, 536
Synergism, drug interaction, 94
Syngeic, bone marrow transplant, 591
Synovium, 737
Synthetic reactions, drugs, 92
Synthetic tripeptide test, 259
Systemic effects, drugs, 88
Systemic lupus erythematosus, 165
    incidence of, 738
Systole, 341

Systolic versus diastolic failure, heart, 388
Systolic pressure, 348

T
Tachycardia, 343
Target organs, 399
Taste
    anatomy of, 95–96
    cancer therapy and, 583, 584
    drug effects, 96–97, 99
    loss of, 196
    types of tastes, 95
Taurine, 227
T cells, 151, 153, 156
    blast formation, test of, 162
Teeth, 187–189
    in anorexia nervosa, 507
    dental disease, 191–194
    edentulous patient, 194
    formation of, 191
    parts of, 188
    supporting structures, 188–189
Temperature of food, myocardial infarction and, 386, 387
Teniae coli, 230
Teratomas, 573
Test diets, 121
Tetracycline, food interactions, 103–104
Tetrad, 618
Tetrachloroethylene, 104
Tetraparesis, 714
T_4 cells, 151, 161
Thalassemia, 697
T helper cells, 154
Thenar eminence, 708
Theophylline, 181
Thermic effects
    of exercise, 477
    of feeding, 477–478
Thermogenesis
    control of, 478–479
    types of, 477–478
Thiamine
    alcoholism and, 531
    branched-chain ketoaciduria, 644, 649, 650
    thiamine-responsive beriberi, 393
Thiazides, 360, 362

Thickening agents, use of, 726
Third spaces, 17
3-in-1 formulas, 138
Threshold dose, 87–88
Thrombocytopenia, 584
Thromboxanes, 351, 352
Thymus, 153
Thyrocalcitonin, 462, 581
Thyroid dysfunction, 462–463
    hyperthyroidism, 463
    hypothyroidism, 463
Thyroid gland, cancer of, 581
Thyroid hormone, 462
    regulation of thermogenesis, 479
    weight reduction and, 498
Thyrotoxicosis, 463
Thyroxine, 462
Tissue
    physiologic changes, 5–6
    regenerative capacity of, 13
    types of, 4–5
Tissue wasting, in nephrotic syndrome, 331
T lymphocytes, 151, 161
TNM system, cancer staging, 574
Tolerance, response to drug, 93–94
Tongue
    eating and, 708
    taste perception, 95
    tongue thrust, 708
Tonic-clonic seizures, 719
Tonic labyrinthine reflex, food intake and, 706
Topical administration, drugs, 88
Total allergic load, 172
Total available glucose counting method, diabetic diet, 443
Total body weight, 52
Total daily energy expenditure, 81
Total gastrectomy, 208
Total iron-binding capacity, 65
Total lymphocyte count, 66
    renal patients assessment, 318
Total nutrient admixtures, 138
Total parenteral feeding. *See* Parenteral feeding
Toxicity, response to drug, 93

Toxic megacolon, 248
Toxicogenic diarrhea, 239
Trace elements, parenteral
feeding, 140, 141
Trachea, 599
Trade-off hypothesis, 290, 302
Transamination, liver, 520
Transcellular fluid, 17
Transcobalamin, 226
Transferase deficiency
characteristics of, 664
galactosemia, 664, 665
homocystinuria, 653
Transferrin, 65
assessment of renal patient,
318
Transient ischemic attacks
cardiovascular disease and,
389–390
hypertension and, 358
Transient PKU, 639
Transitional feeding, 144
Translocation, chromosomes,
621
Transposition of the great
arteries, 392
Transudate, 8
Trauma. *See* Injury, metabolic
effects
Travasorb Hepatic, 542, 545,
547
Traveler's diarrhea, 240
Trench mouth, 193
Triceps skinfold method, 53–54
diagnosis of obesity, 480, 485
renal patients assessment, 318
Trichobezoars, 213
Trichorrhexis nodosa, 656
Tricuspid valve, 340
Trigeminal nerves, 581
Triglycerides. *See also* Lipid
metabolism; Lipids
in adipose tissue, 472
digestion of, 223–225
liver and, 521
long-chain, 125–129, 223
medium-chain, 125–126, 224
oxidation of, 603
peritoneal dialysis and, 310
synthesis from glucose, 603
synthesis/storage of, 408
Triglyceride storage diseases,
483

Trihydroxy bile acid, 227
Triiodothyronine, 462
Tripeptidases, 225
Tripeptides, 127
Trismus, 583
Tropical sprue, 245, 693
Truncal vagotomy, 208, 210
Tryptophan, 536, 537, 538, 578
Tube feeding, 123–132
administration, routes of,
128–129
in brain injured patient, 725
in burn patient, 568
in cancer patient, 590
carbohydrates, 125
in cerebral palsy, 714
contraindications for, 131
in diabetic patient, 457–458
energy needs, 125
evaluation of, 127–128
in hepatic encephalopathy,
545
in hepatic failure, 547
indications for, 123, 124
lipids, 125–126
methods of, 129–130
minerals, 127
nutrition-related problems
in, 132
osmolarity, 123
in Parkinson's disease, 730
patient monitoring, 131–132
protein, 126–127
rate/frequency of, 130–131
renal solute load, 124
residue, 124
in respiratory failure, 609
types of, 127
types of tubes, 130
viscosity, 124
vitamins, 127
Tuberculosis, 563
Tumors. *See also* Cancer;
Neoplasms
competition for nutrients,
578–579
hormone-producing tumors,
255–256
hypoglycemia and, 460
tumor necrosis factor, 157
Tunica adventitia, 345
Tunica intima, 345
Tunica media, 345

Turner's syndrome, 196
T wave, in ECG, 342
Twenty-four-hour recall, 74, 75
2-in-1 formulas, 138
Type A, chronic obstructive
pulmonary disease, 606
Type B, chronic obstructive
pulmonary disease, 606
Typhoid fever, 563
Tyramine
as false neurotransmitters,
537
foods containing, 112–113
MAO inhibitors and, 111
Tyramine reactions, 110
Tyrosine
in hepatic failure, 538
in PKU, 629
production of, 536
Tyrosine metabolism disorders
diagnosis of, 641, 644
forms of, 640–641
nutritional care, 644
formula products, 642–
643, 644
Tyrosinemia, 640–644
Tyrosinosis, 640

U
Ulcers. *See also* Peptic ulcer
disease
types of, 205
Ultrafiltration, in hemodialysis,
306
Ultraviolet light, cancer and, 576
Undernutrition, 67
Underweight
in anorexia nervosa, 505–509
in bulimia nervosa, 509–510
causes of, 505
definition of, 504
in developmental disabilities,
713
effects of, 505
treatment of, 505
Unipolar disorders, 736
Unsaturated fatty acids, 351,
353
Upper body obesity, 484
Upper esophageal sphincter,
197
Urea, 286

liver disease and, 535
synthesis and liver, 520
Urea cycle disorders, 656–659
diagnosis, 656
metabolic abnormalities, 656
monitoring in, 658
treatment of, 656–658
Urea generation rate, renal
patients assessment, 321
Urea nitrogen, renal patients
assessment, 288,
320–321
Uremia, 291
Uremic syndrome, 290
Uremic toxins, chronic renal
failure, 292–293
Ureters, 281
Urethra, 281
Uric acid, 286
bronchopulmonary dyspla-
sia, 611
gout, 674–674
renal disease, diagnosis, 288
Urinary system, components
of, 281
Urinary tract infection, 717
Urine, excretion of, 283–284
Urine amylase, 259
Urine testing
commercial tests, 420
diabetic monitoring, 420–421
renal disease diagnosis, 287
Urticaria, 164, 171

V
Vagotomy, 208–210
Vagus nerves, 582
Van den Bergh's test, liver
function, 522
Variable expressivity, genes, 619
Varices
in cirrhosis, 534, 541
complications from, 534
Vasa vasorum, 346
Vascular system, 342–346. *See
also* Blood pressure
blood vessels, 345–346
cerebral circulation, 344
coronary circulation,
343–344
divisions of, 342
fetal circulation, 344–345

splanchnic circulation, 344
Vasoactive amines, in food, 111
Vasoactive intestinal peptide,
255
Vasodilators
hypertension and, 361,
362–363
types of, 361, 362–363
Vasomotor center, 349
Vasopressin, 26, 541
Vegan, 122
Vegetables
intestinal gas and, 268
protein foods, 786
sodium content, 795–797
sources of Vitamin A, 789
sources of Vitamin C,
787–788
Vegetarianism, 122–123
categories of, 122, 123
recommended nutrients,
122–123
Veins, 346
Veno-occlusive disease, bone
marrow transplantation,
592–593
Ventilation, mechanisms in,
602–603
Ventricular septal defect, 392
Venules, 346
Verner-Morrison syndrome, 255
Very low calorie diet, weight
loss and, 491–492
Very-low density lipoproteins,
365, 367, 368, 373, 408
Vibrio cholerae, 240
Villi, 219
Vinblastine, 584
Vincent's gingivitis, 193
Vincristine, 583
Viruses
cancer and, 577
immunologic deficiency and,
161
Visceral fat obesity, 485
Visceral proteins, 49
estimation of, 59, 64–66
Viscosity, tube feeding, 124
Vitamin A
anticarcinogenic aspects, 575,
576
in cirrhosis, 541
deficiencies, 162

hemoglobin synthesis and,
690
hypermetabolic patient and,
561
intoxication, 303
liver and, 521
respiration and, 605
toxicity, 561, 690
Vitamin assays, nutritional
assessment, 70, 71
Vitamin B complex
in cirrhosis, 541
in underweight treatment,
505
Vitamin B_6
hemoglobin synthesis and,
690
urea cycle disorders, 658
Vitamin B_6 dependency, 675
Vitamin B_6 dependent anemia,
696
Vitamin B_{12}
in anemias, 693, 694
causes of deficiency, 689, 692
digestion/absorption of, 226
hemoglobin synthesis and,
689–690
malabsorption of, 234
Vitamin B_{12} dependency, 674–
675
Vitamin C. *See also* Ascorbic acid
anticarcinogenic aspects, 575
bronchopulmonary dyspla-
sia, 611
respiration and, 605
vegetable/fruit/juice
sources, 787–788
Vitamin dependency disorders,
622, 674–676
familial vitamin D–resistant
rickets, 675–676
folate dependency, 674
pyridoxine dependency, 675
Vitamin B_{12} dependency,
674–675
Vitamin D–dependent
rickets, 675
Vitamin D
in acute renal failure, 326
anticonvulsants and,
721–722
calcium metabolism and, 286
in chronic renal failure, 302

Vitamin D *(continued)*
  liver and, 521
  in osteomalacia, 214
  peritoneal dialysis, 310
Vitamin D–dependent rickets, 675
Vitamin E
  bronchopulmonary dysplasia, 611
  drug metabolism and, 108
  hemoglobin synthesis and, 690–691
  in hemolytic anemia, 697–698
  liver and, 521
Vitamin K
  in coagulopathy, 525
  drug metabolism and, 108
  liver and, 521
  parenteral feeding and, 138
  tube feeding and, 127
Vitamins
  absorption of, 226
  in acute renal failure, 326
  in cirrhosis, 541
  in diabetic diet, 440
  drug effects, 100–101
  drug metabolism and, 105–107, 108
  in homocystinuria, 653
  in hemodialysis, 307
  in hepatitis, 525
  in hypermetabolic illness, 561–562
  in jaundice, 526
  liver disease and, 531, 539
  liver synthesis of, 521
  mega-doses, psychiatric patients, 735
  needs in chronic renal failure, 303–304
  parenteral feeding and, 138–139, 141
  peritoneal dialysis and, 310

safe/adequate daily intake, 749
  in sickle cell anemia, 697
  tube feeding and, 127
  in underweight treatment, 505
Volatile acids, 30
Volume disturbances, 16, 23
  correction of, 34–35
Volume overload, heart, 388
Vomiting, 203–205
  in anorexia nervosa, 507
  disease related, 204
  drugs related to, 97, 100
  metabolic effects, 204, 205
  nutritional care in, 205

W
Warfarin sodium, 108
Wasting syndrome, chronic renal failure, 293
Water. *See also* Fluid intake; Fluids
  absorption of, 226
  content and distribution in body, 17
  excretion, 22–23
  fluid shifts, 22
  fluid transfer, 19–22
  intracellular degeneration related to, 11
  normal requirements, 17–19
  sources for intake, 19
  water deficit, 23
  water excess, 23
Water intoxication, 23
WDHA syndrome, 255
Weber-Christian disease, 484
Weight
  drug effects and, 93
  optimum body weight, 51
  total body weight, 52
  weight age, 718

Weight loss. *See also* Obesity
  in cancer patients, 578–579
  exercise and, 477
  in gastric surgery patients, 213
  hypertension and, 358
  pulmonary disease and, 606
  weight loss measures, 489
Weight tables, diagnosis of obesity, 480
Wernicke-Korsakoff syndrome, 531
Wernicke's encephalopathy, 531
Wheal, 67
Wheal-and-flare reaction, 164, 174
Wheat-free diet, 177–178
White adipose tissue, 471–472
White blood cells, 8
Wilm's tumor, 573
Wilson's disease, 547, 676
  cause of, 547
  characteristics of, 676
  diagnosis of, 676
  drug treatment, 547
  nutritional care, 547, 676
Withdrawal, alcohol, 530, 532

X
Xerostomia, 195–196
X-linked traits, 619

Z
Zinc
  in acrodermatitis enteropathica, 677
  chronic renal failure and, 303
  deficiencies, 140
  parenteral feeding and, 140
  in sickle cell anemia, 697
Zollinger-Ellison syndrome, 206, 233, 240, 255
Zymogen granules, 229
Zymogenic cells, 202